SPINAL CORD INJURIES
Management and Rehabilitation

ABOUT THE AUTHORS

Sue Ann Sisto is a Distinguished Professor of Physical Therapy and Research Director of the Rehabilitation Sciences Division at the School of Health Science and Technology, Stony Brook University (Stony Brook, N.Y.). Before joining the University, she was the Director of the Human Performance and Movement Analysis Laboratory at Kessler Medical Rehabilitation Research and Education Center (West Orange, N.J.). She was an employee of the Kessler Institute and Kessler Research Center for 28 years.

Dr. Sisto graduated cum laude from St. Louis University in 1979 with a Bachelor of Science in physical therapy and graduated magna cum laude from New York University (NYU) in 1985 with a Master's degree in physical therapy and pathokinesiology. After she was a recipient of the Mary E. Switzer Fellowship from the National Institute on Disability and Rehabilitation Research (NIDRR), the full-time NIDRR doctoral clinical traineeship from NYU, and a Doctoral Research Award from the Foundation for Physical Therapy of the American Physical Therapy Association (APTA), she graduated magna cum laude from NYU in 1997 with a PhD in physical therapy and pathokinesiology. She has been the principal investigator for more than $1.5 million in grants, including most recently a postdoctoral training grant on Neuromusculoskeletal Rehabilitation funded by the NIDRR and another grant funded by the Christopher and Dana Reeve Foundation and Centers for Disease Control and Prevention for the NeuroRecovery Network to study locomotor training in spinal cord injury (SCI).

Dr. Sisto's university appointments have included Associate Professor of Physical Medicine and Rehabilitation at the University of Medicine and Dentistry of New Jersey (UMDNJ)–New Jersey Medical School (Newark, N.J.); Clinical Assistant Professor of Physical Therapy, School of Health Related Professions, UMDNJ; Assistant Professor of Clinical Physical Therapy at Columbia University (New York, N.Y.); and Associate Research Professor of Biomedical Engineering at the New Jersey Institute of Technology (Newark, N.J.).

Her research interests include the integration of biomechanics and motor control to evaluate bipedal and wheelchair locomotion with three-dimensional videography, kinetic, electromyography (EMG), and metabolic and autonomic measurement tools. These interests extend to mathematical modeling of human movement, mechanical and cardiopulmonary efficiency of the wheelchair users and others with disabilities, EMG signal assessment of spasticity and its influence during human movement, the effect of locomotor training on recovery of walking in SCI, the effect of wheelchair propulsion biomechanics on pain and disease in paraplegia and tetraplegia, the kinematics and kinetics of patients with knee conditions, and interventions to improve gait and balance in SCI and other disability groups, including the effect of orthotics on foot pressure maps, the impact of rehabilitation interventions on cortical and neuromuscular excitability, and the relationship of these quantitative gait measures to functional and global outcomes.

Dr. Sisto is on the Executive Board of the Gait and Clinical Movement Analysis Society, the Board of Governors of the American Congress of Rehabilitation Medicine, the Rehabilitation and Recovery Advisory Board of the National Stroke Association, and the New Jersey APTA Research Committee. She is on several editorial boards, including those of the *Journal of Spinal Cord Medicine,* the *Journal of Head Trauma Rehabilitation,* and the *Journal of Neuroengineering and Rehabilitation,* and is on the Assistive Technology Panel of the *Journal of Disability and Rehabilitation.* She is also a member of the APTA, the American College of Sports Medicine (ACSM), American Congress of Rehabilitation Medicine American Spinal Injury Association, American Society of Biomechanics, and the American Paraplegia Society (APS).

Erica Druin received her bachelor of science in biology from Carnegie Mellon University (Pittsburgh, Pa.) and her Master's degree in physical therapy from Hahnemann University (Philadelphia, Pa.). She has worked with individuals with SCIs for more than 18 years.

Ms. Druin has published numerous articles on SCI and has presented extensively on topics related to SCI both nationally and internationally, including a course in Singapore at the invitation of the Health Ministry Development Program. Ms. Druin has served as Program Director for Adventist Rehabilitation Hospital of Maryland, Director of Rehabilitation Services at Kessler Adventist Rehabilitation Hospital in Maryland, and Clinical Specialist for SCI at Kessler Institute for Rehabilitation in New Jersey, one of the model SCI centers in the United States.

Ms. Druin has also lectured on the treatment of patients with SCI at the UMDNJ, Howard University (Washington, D.C.), and George Washington University (Washington, D.C.) where she also serves as a member of the Physical Therapy Program Advisory Board.

Martha Macht Sliwinski graduated magna cum laude with her bachelor's degree in physical therapy from Temple University (Philadelphia, Pa.) in 1979. She began her professional career in rehabilitation at the Kessler Institute, where she continues to practice on a part-time basis. Motivated by a passion to understand pathophysiological movement, she pursued both her Master's degree and doctorate at New York University in physical therapy and pathokinesiology and graduated magna cum laude.

Early in her career, Dr. Sliwinski became interested in the clinical education process and has been an APTA trainer for the Clinical Instructor Credentialing Program for more than 10 years. In addition, she has been trained to conduct the Advanced Clinical Instructor Credentialing Program. She joined academia as an adjunct in 1984, moving to the faculty at Hunter College (New York, N.Y.) in 1993 and to Columbia University (New York, N.Y.) in 2004.

Dr. Sliwinski's research interests focus on SCI, and she is currently collaborating with the SCI team at Mount Sinai Medical Center (New York, N.Y.). Her professional expertise includes patient evaluation and rehabilitation of neurological dysfunction specifically related to SCIs and traumatic brain injury. Facilitating students' growth into compassionate physical therapists is her most rewarding endeavor.

SPINAL CORD INJURIES
Management and Rehabilitation

Sue Ann Sisto, PT, MA, PhD
Distinguished Professor and Research Director
Division of Rehabilitation Science
Stony Brook University
Stony Brook, New York

Research Scientist III, Human Performance and Movement Analysis Laboratory
Kessler Medical Rehabilitation Research and Education Center
West Orange, New Jersey

Associate Professor of Physical Medicine and Rehabilitation
Clinical Assistant Professor, School of Health Related Professions
University of Medicine and Dentistry of New Jersey–New Jersey Medical School
Newark, New Jersey

Erica Druin, MPT
Clinical Specialist
Adventist Rehabilitation Hospital of Maryland
Rockville, Maryland

Martha Macht Sliwinski, PT, MA, PhD
Assistant Professor of Clinical Physical Therapy
Columbia University
New York, New York

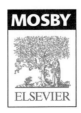

MOSBY

ELSEVIER

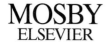

11830 Westline Industrial Drive
St. Louis, Missouri 63146

SPINAL CORD INJURIES: MANAGEMENT AND REHABILITATION   ISBN: 978-0-323-00699-6
Copyright © 2009 by Mosby, Inc., an affiliate of Elsevier Inc.

Library of Congress Control Number: 2007939682

Vice President and Publisher: Linda Duncan
Senior Editor: Kathy Falk
Senior Developmental Editor: Christie M. Hart
Publishing Services Manager: Patricia Tannian
Project Manager: Claire Kramer
Design Direction: Kimberly Denando

Printed in the United States of America

Last digit is the print number: 9 8 7 6 5 4 3 2 1

I dedicate this book to Kessler Institute for Rehabilitation and Kessler Medical Rehabilitation Research and Education Center, the two places where I have worked with and experienced people with spinal cord injury who will always inspire me. These organizations have given me the opportunity to develop an expertise in the treatment of patients with spinal cord injury and to examine the research questions related to mobility problems that they experience. Throughout my career at Kessler, I have been privileged to collaborate with outstanding colleagues, many of whom have contributed to this volume. In my practice and research at these premier rehabilitation and research centers, I am grateful to have formed relationships with talented faculty and scientists from other institutions, many of whom also have contributed to this book.

I thank my undergraduate institution, St. Louis University, and graduate institution, New York University, Department of Physical Therapy, for enabling me to first receive the education to become a physical therapist, and then in graduate school, for enabling me to conduct research in a rigorous manner and leading me to become an independent researcher, and I thank, most especially, Arthur Nelson and Wen Ling for my experiences at NYU. Through my foundation in the research process, I became more and more curious about the evidence supporting therapeutic interventions in spinal cord injury, which led me to push forward to complete this book. *Spinal Cord Injuries: Management and Rehabilitation* will fill a need for clinicians who treat patients with spinal cord injury, for faculty and students who strive for greater depth of understanding of spinal cord injury rehabilitation, and for researchers who need benchmarks for scientific pursuits.

I thank my co-editors, Erica and Martha, who have stayed the course in the completion of this project. Most of all, I thank my family for their patience and support during this long endeavor. I hope that they will enjoy the journey of reading about rehabilitation of individuals with spinal cord injury as much as I have compiling it. My parents have inspired me to pursue my education rigorously. My husband, Michael, and daughters, Jackie and Gabby, keep me on track throughout all my endeavors but also ground me in leading a balanced life.

Sue Ann Sisto, PT, MA, PhD

In loving memory of my mother, Marilyn, whose creativity and enthusiasm will always serve as an inspiration to me.

In honor of my friend and former patient Christopher Reeve, who fought tirelessly to better the lives of those with spinal cord injury.

To my family, whose love and support mean everything to me.

To the many therapists and countless patients with whom I have had the opportunity to work over the years; you have taught me so much.

To Sue Ann, Martha, and Sue for their hard work and dedication to this project.

To Roger, Mattix, and Melanie, who make my life complete . . . I am truly blessed.

Erica Druin, MPT

My life has been touched by so many remarkable patients who have taught me to be the best that I can be. This book is dedicated to those patients whom I have met along the journey and who inspired me to push beyond what I believed possible. And to my parents, Jean and Paul, thank you for believing in me throughout the years.

To my children Brian, Mark, and Lauren, may you be the best that you can be.

For Rick, we love you and miss you.

Martha Macht Sliwinski, PT, MA, PhD

CONTRIBUTORS

Paula M. Ackerman, OTR/L, MS
SCI Post-Acute Rehabilitation Manager
Shepherd Center
Atlanta, Georgia

Joan P. Alverzo, RN, CRRN, PhD
Chief Clinical Officer
Kessler Institute for Rehabilitation
West Orange, New Jersey

John R. Bach, MD
Professor, Physical Medicine and Rehabilitation
Vice Chairman, Department of Physical Medicine and Rehabilitation
Professor of Neurosciences
Department of Neurosciences
University of Medicine and Dentistry of New Jersey–New Jersey Medical School
Newark, New Jersey

Director of Research and Associate Medical Director
Department of Physical Medicine and Rehabilitation
Co-director, Jerry Lewis Muscular Dystrophy Association Clinic
Medical Director of the Center for Ventilator Management Alternatives
University Hospital
Newark, New Jersey

Andrea Behrman, PT, PhD
Associate Professor
Department of Physical Therapy
University of Florida
Gainesville, Florida

Research Investigator
Brain Rehabilitation Research Center
Malcom Randall VA Medical Center
Gainesville, Florida

Barbara Benevento, MD
Director
Ventilator Program
Kessler Institute for Rehabilitation
West Orange, New Jersey

Assistant Clinical Professor
Physical Medicine and Rehabilitation
University of Medicine and Dentistry of New Jersey–New Jersey Medical School
Newark, New Jersey

Gina Bertocci, PE, PhD
Associate Professor
Endowed Chair, Biomechanics
Mechanical Engineering
University of Louisville
Louisville, Kentucky

Mark Bowden, PT, MS
Brain Rehabilitation Research Center
North Florida/South Georgia Veterans Affairs Health System
Gainesville, Florida

Amy Boyles, BA
Human Engineering Research Laboratories
VA Pittsburgh Healthcare Systems
Pittsburgh, Pennsylvania

Sarah Broton, OTR/L
SCI Program
Shepherd Center
Atlanta, Georgia

Terrence Carolan, PT, ATP, MS
Clinic Manager
Kessler Institute for Rehabilitation
West Orange, New Jersey

Pratiksha P. Chesney, PT, DPT
Clinical Practitioner
Verona, New Jersey

Scott Chesney
Professional Speaker and Life Coach
Scott Chesney, LLC
Verona, New Jersey

Rory A. Cooper, PhD
Distinguished Professor and FISA Foundation–Paralyzed Veterans of America Chair
Department of Rehabilitation Science and Technology
University of Pittsburgh
Pittsburgh, Pennsylvania

Director
Human Engineering Research Laboratories
VA Rehabilitation Research and Development Center of Excellence
VA Pittsburgh Healthcare System
Pittsburgh, Pennsylvania

Rosemarie Cooper, ATP, MPT
Assistant Professor
Department of Rehabilitation Science and Technology
University of Pittsburgh
Pittsburgh, Pennsylvania

Kim Davis, MSPT
Clinical Research Scientist
Crawford Research Institute
Shepherd Center
Atlanta, Georgia

Sandra Shultz DeLeon, CRRN, CCM, MS, BSN
Spinal Cord Coordinator
SCI Services
Kessler Institute for Rehabilitation
West Orange, New Jersey

Erica Druin, MPT
Clinical Specialist
Adventist Rehabilitation Hospital of Maryland
Rockville, Maryland

Pouran D. Faghri, MD, FACSM, MS
Professor
Department of Allied Health Sciences
College of Agriculture and Natural Resources
University of Connecticut
Storrs, Connecticut

Martin Forchheimer, MPP
Senior Research Associate
University of Michigan Model Spinal Cord Injury Care System
Department of Physical Medicine and Rehabilitation
Ann Arbor, Michigan

Barbara Garrett, PT
Senior Physical Therapist
Kessler Institute for Rehabilitation
West Orange, New Jersey

Susan V. Garstang, MD
Assistant Professor
Department of Physical Medicine and Rehabilitation
University of Medicine and Dentistry of New Jersey–New Jersey Medical School
Newark, New Jersey

David R. Gater, Jr., MD, PhD
Chief, Spinal Cord Injury and Disorders
Hunter Holmes McGuire VA Medical Center
Richmond, Virginia

Professor
Physical Medicine and Rehabilitation
Virginia Commonwealth University
Richmond, Virginia

Amanda Gillot, OTR/L, MS
SCI Program
Shepherd Center
Atlanta, Georgia

Susan Harkema, PhD
Associate Professor and Rehabilitation Director
Owsley B. Frazier Chair in Neurological Rehabilitation
Kentucky Spinal Cord Injury Research Center
Rehabilitation Research Director
Department of Neurological Surgery
University of Louisville
Frazier Rehabilitation Institute
Louisville, Kentucky

Julie Hartrich, OTR/L
SCI Program
Shepherd Center
Atlanta, Georgia

Polly Hopkins, OTR/L
SCI Program
Shepherd Center
Atlanta, Georgia

Katharine Hunter-Zaworski, PE, PhD
Director
National Center for Accessible Transportation
Oregon State University
Corvallis, Oregon

Claire Z. Kalpakjian, PhD, MS
Research Assistant Professor
Department of Physical Medicine and Rehabilitation
University of Michigan Model Spinal Cord Injury Care System
Ann Arbor, Michigan

Annmarie Kelleher, OTR/L, MS
Human Engineering Research Laboratories
VA Pittsburgh Healthcare Systems
Pittsburgh, Pennsylvania

Bryan Kemp, PhD
Director, RRTC on Aging with a Disability
Ranchos Los Amigos Medical Center
Downey, California

Clinical Professor of Medicine
University of California Irvine School of Medicine Program in Geriatrics
Irvine, California

Sue Kida, PT, MHA
Vice President, Administration
Kessler Institute for Rehabilitation
Chester, New Jersey

Steven Kirshblum, MD
Medical Director
Director, Spinal Cord Injury Program
Co-director, Northern New Jersey Spinal Cord Injury Model System
Kessler Institute for Rehabilitation
West Orange, New Jersey

Professor
Physical Medicine and Rehabilitation
University of Medicine and Dentistry of New Jersey–New Jersey Medical School
Newark, New Jersey

Alicia Koontz, RET, ATP, PhD
Research Health Scientist
Human Engineering Research Laboratories
VA Pittsburgh HealthCare System
Pittsburgh, Pennsylvania

David Kreutz, PT, ATP
Seating and Mobility Clinic
Shepherd Center
Atlanta, Georgia

Chris Maurer, ATP, MPT
Seating and Mobility Clinic
Clinical Research Scientist
Shepherd Center
Atlanta, Georgia

Sean McCarthy, OTR/L, ATP, MS
Kessler Institute for Rehabilitation
West Orange, New Jersey

Mary Jane (M.J.) Mulcahey, OTR, PhD
Director of Rehabilitation Services and Clinical Research
Shriners Hospitals for Children–Philadelphia
Philadelphia, Pennsylvania

Cynthia Nead, Senior COTA
Kessler Institute for Rehabilitation
West Orange, New Jersey

Richard Nead, CDRS
Driver's Training Program
Kessler Institute for Rehabilitation
West Orange, New Jersey

Phil Parette, EdD
Kara Peters Endowed Chair
Editor, *Assistive Technology Outcomes and Benefits*
SEAT Center
Illinois State University
Normal, Illinois

Kim Ratner, PT, BS
Assistant Vice President of Rehabilitation Services
Kessler Institute for Rehabilitation
West Orange, New Jersey

Ian Rice, OTR/L, MS
Human Engineering Research Laboratories
VA Pittsburgh Healthcare Systems
Pittsburgh, Pennsylvania

Jay H. Rosenberg, CRRN, BSN
Nurse Manager
Spinal Cord Injury Unit
Kessler Institute for Rehabilitation
West Orange, New Jersey

Marcia J. Scherer, PhD
President
Institute for Matching Person and Technology
Webster, New York

Professor of Orthopaedics and Rehabilitation
University of Rochester Medical Center
Research Associate
International Center for Hearing and Speech Research at
the University of Rochester and National Technical Institute
for the Deaf/Rochester Institute of Technology
Rochester, New York

Hania Shatzer, CCC-SLP
Livingston, New Jersey

Mary Shea, OTR, ATP, MA
Clinical Manager
Wheelchair Clinic
Kessler Institute for Rehabilitation
West Orange, New Jersey

Sue Ann Sisto, PT, MA, PhD
Distinguished Professor and Research Director
Division of Rehabilitation Science
Stony Brook University
Stony Brook, New York

Research Scientist III, Human Performance and Movement Analysis
Laboratory
Kessler Medical Rehabilitation Research
and Education Center
West Orange, New Jersey

Associate Professor of Physical Medicine and Rehabilitation
Clinical Assistant Professor, School of Health Related Professions
University of Medicine and Dentistry of New Jersey–New Jersey
Medical School
Newark, New Jersey

Sarah Everhart Skeels, MPH
Teaching Associate in Community Health
Brown University Health, Wellness, and Empowerment Educator
Brown University
Providence, Rhode Island

Martha Macht Sliwinski, PT, MA, PhD
Assistant Professor of Clinical Physical Therapy
Columbia University
New York, New York

Carolyn A. Sorensen, RN, CRRN, MSN
Clinical Specialist/Educator
Adventist Rehabilitation Hospital of Maryland
Rockville, Maryland

Stephen H. Sprigle, PT, PhD
Director
Center for Assistive Technology and Environmental Access
Associate Professor
Applied Physiology and Industrial Design
Georgia Institute of Technology
Atlanta, Georgia

Gabriella Stiefbold, OTR, ATP
Clinical Manager
Inpatient Occupational Therapy
Kessler Institute for Rehabilitation
West Orange, New Jersey

Denise G. Tate, PhD
Chair for Research
Professor in the Division of Rehabilitation Psychology
and Neuropsychology
Associate Chair for Research
Department of Physical Medicine and Rehabilitation
University of Michigan Model Spinal Cord Injury Care System
Ann Arbor, Michigan

Lilli Thompson, PT
Director
Physical Therapy Department
Ranchos Los Amigos Medical Center
Downey, California

Loran C. Vocaturo, ABPP (Rp), EdD
Director
Department of Psychology and Neuropsychology
Kessler Institute for Rehabilitation
West Orange, New Jersey

FOREWORD

There has been heightened interest in spinal cord injury, particularly over the last two decades. This is reflected in the number of research reports, the number of scientists studying spinal cord injury, the number of clinical trials being conducted, and the amount of money available for supporting basic and clinical research. This focus has been a more thorough understanding of the nature of the problems facing individuals with spinal cord injury and, to some extent, a better understanding of some of the mechanisms that underlie the changes observed in daily functions, such as sleep patterns, bladder and bowel function, cardiovascular control, sexual function, and motor functions related to hand control and to posture and locomotion. This has resulted in some elevation in the level of optimism regarding the potential development of interventions that can significantly improve some of these lost or impaired functions and in some cases has actually produced more effective rehabilitative interventions, resulting in the recovery of higher levels of ambulatory functions caused by the use of activity-dependent approaches to regain the ability to stand and to step.

There have been a number of other incremental improvements and interventions that may have some effect in minimizing the magnitude of the secondary injury that occurs after a spinal trauma. Although these improved interventions are significant, everyone generally recognizes that they are incremental. During these last two decades, though, a fundamental change has occurred in the attitude toward the rehabilitative strategies. There is a growing optimism regarding what the future holds. Unlike in the past when rehabilitation was totally focused on adaptive mechanisms that would improve motor function above the lesion, now there is more concentration and greater realization of the potential to improve motor function below the lesion, particularly in those individuals who are considered to have "incomplete" but severe injures. There are numerous examples reported in the literature of remarkable levels of recovery of weight-bearing ambulatory capability as a result of locomotor training in individuals who have had a severe spinal cord injury for many years.

Although *Spinal Cord Injuries: Management and Rehabilitation* reflects some of these particular changes in rehabilitative strategies, it actually accomplishes much more. In fact one of the most important features of this book is that it is excitingly comprehensive. This is important because individuals with spinal cord injuries must seek advice and clinical care from a variety of experts, each of whom can be critical to survival, particularly those related to cardiovascular function, pulmonary function, bladder and bowel function, sexual function, and depression. A major problem is that in many cases the whole individual is not treated. Often there is inadequate consideration or knowledge of how one specific function or dysfunction affects other systems. The point here is that this book provides a resource for those individuals directly interacting with individuals with the injuries and the intermittent complications associated with the injury. It provides a foundation for the more resourceful rehabilitation team to gain a better understanding of the complications of the whole individual. It provides a resource for a better understanding of those problems most frequently encountered by individuals with a spinal cord injury. The authors have engineered a text that helps us move toward "one stop" clinical care. It identifies what can be done, how to do it, and what expectation the individual can have regarding the outcome. Because we are able to more successfully merge our technical capability and our knowledge about the biology of therapy, in the near future it appears that continued and even more significant therapeutic advances are likely to occur.

V. Reggie Edgerton, PhD
Departments of Physiological
Science and Neurobiology
Brain Research Institute
UCLA
Los Angeles, California

PREFACE

The genesis for *Spinal Cord Injuries: Management and Rehabilitation* sprang from our day-to-day experience with patients and clients whose determination to live fully motivated us to bring together outstanding clinicians, academicians, and researchers to compile this evidence-based book. The comprehensive model found in this book differs from the medical model and the more restricted scope of rehabilitation-oriented books currently available in the marketplace.

Spinal cord injury (SCI) remains a serious condition, but during the past 25 years the dedication of comprehensive, interdisciplinary neurorehabilitation care models has improved outcomes and encouraged hopeful prognoses for all injury levels. Today's emphasis includes pharmaceuticals to decrease injury and promote neuroplasticity; neurosurgical techniques to enhance spinal stability to prevent further injury and allow for early rehabilitation; respiratory and integumentary management; therapeutic strategies to enhance movement; wheelchair or ambulatory mobility techniques; and fitness and sports activities to improve quality of life. These strategies are further enhanced by new technologies for orthotics, neuromuscular electrical stimulation, wheelchair seating, assistive devices, and modes of safe transportation to gain greater access within the environment. Specialized rehabilitation teams can focus on the importance of patient-centered goals that enable many individuals to approach their recovery and rehabilitation after an SCI in a manner that results in optimal lifestyles.

THE AUDIENCE

Conceived as a textbook to aid students and clinicians working with people with SCI, as well as SCI academicians and researchers, this book aims for the broad audience of physical and occupational therapists, nurses, physicians, rehabilitation professionals, educators, psychologists, case managers—in a word, everyone on the interdisciplinary rehabilitation team. In addition, care has been taken to make the volume a useful resource for patients and clients with SCI and their families.

THE BOOK

In accordance with our premise that the patient and client are of utmost importance in the discussion of SCI, the introductory chapter focuses on the lives and accomplishments of those with the condition. This introduction is essential to embed the reader in the real lives of individuals with SCI. The client quotations that open each chapter and the Client's Perspective boxes in many chapters continue a dialogue of honest assessment that promotes understanding along with helpful hints for the practical application of skills.

This book is organized to reflect the general order and importance of specific steps in the care of individuals with SCI, beginning with the medical perspective, nursing care,

and respiratory management of people with SCI. The book progresses to the psychological adjustment of sustaining an SCI and then provides a thorough presentation of evaluation procedures and therapeutic interventions that improve opportunities for daily life. Detailed interventions and instructional activities are reviewed for movement and position changes, daily living, transfer skills, wheelchair skills, and ambulation. Matching and using assistive technologies for home, work, and school, as well as the importance of home modifications, wheelchair transportation and safety, and community access, are reviewed in preparation for home and community living. Specialty chapters focus on the management of the upper limb in tetraplegia, seating and positioning for individuals at all injury levels, functional electrical stimulation, exercise and fitness, sports and recreation, aging with an SCI, and quality of life issues in individuals with SCI.

Individuals affected by an SCI set the stage for each chapter with their opening quotations relative to the content in that chapter. Chapters are also supplemented with boxes and tables to highlight salient content, Clinical Notes that emphasize important clinical treatment, and Case Studies that promote an individualized perspective toward each patient-client. People First language has been adopted throughout the book to highlight the individuality of each person over his condition. For clarity, we have designated people with SCI as "he" and clinicians as "she." Content from Case Studies is reinforced with review questions designed to promote critical thinking with suggested answers printed at the end of each chapter. The more than 500 illustrations in the book provide visual understanding of anatomy, physiology, interventions, and care modalities.

THE DVD

In addition to the carefully illustrated text, a DVD with video components accompanies the book. Although a picture may equal a thousand words, in clinical care, a movie shows even more. We have included the DVD to capture key therapeutic interventions that can aid the student, clinician, faculty member, and researcher in understanding, practicing, teaching, and studying highly specific movements. The video has been organized to reinforce interventions and includes therapeutic mobility activities such as basic and advanced position changes, transfers to multiple surfaces including floor and car transfers, ambulation training for complete and incomplete injuries, high-level wheelchair activities, and high-technology electronic aids for daily living.

NOTE TO READERS

Readers should review each Case Study in the context of the chapter as it is presented before accessing the discussion of solutions at the end of the chapter.

We welcome your comments. As you read this book, please let us know what you found the most helpful and what your suggestions are for future editions. Our goal is to provide in-depth coverage of content in a readable and understandable format. You may contact us through Sue Ann Sisto, PT, MA, PhD, at sue.sisto@stonybrook.edu.

SUMMARY

In our daily care of individuals with SCI, we are constantly encouraged and enlightened by our patients, clients, and their families and clinical, academic, and research colleagues. It has been a privilege to coordinate compilation of this book.

Sue Ann Sisto

ACKNOWLEDGMENTS

Spinal Cord Injuries: Management and Rehabilitation is the first comprehensive research-based book on this topic that combines the academic, clinical, and research perspectives of physical and occupational therapists, nurses, physicians, psychologists, engineers, rehabilitation and case management specialists, and educators. In doing so, it mirrors the interdisciplinary rehabilitation team collaboration that makes model spinal cord injury (SCI) centers effective.

Among the many contributors to this project, our patients, clients, and colleagues have been steadfast in their support and gracious gifts of time and energy to ensure its successful completion. We especially thank Ian James Brown, Scott Chesney, Pratiksha Chesney, Jerri Fortunato, Trevor Dyson-Hudson, Karen Hwang, Alicia Kemp, Nick LaBassi, Leigh Ann Martinez, Ronald Moore, Christopher Reeve, Wayne Sipes, Sarah Everhart Skeels, and Janine Valenti.

The team at Kessler Institute for Rehabilitation and Kessler Medical Rehabilitation Research and Eduction Center (KMRREC) also supported our work through daily, weekly, and ongoing input. Guidance from KMRREC's Chief Operating Officer Mitch Rosenthal and Medical Director and Director of Spinal Cord Injury Services Steven Kirshblum was invaluable. We also thank Barbara Benevento, Joan Alverzo, Jay Rosenberg, Sandy Shultz DeLeon, Barabara Garrett, Hania Shatzer, Loran Vocaturo, Kim Ratner, Gabriella Stiefbold, Terry Carolan, Sean McCarthy, Cindy Nead, Mary Shea, Sue Kida, and Richard Nead for their contributions of expertise and wise counsel.

In addition, our colleagues around the country working at other model SCI centers and academic institutions have shared their breadth of knowledge and varied perspectives. We thank Paula Ackerman and her co-contributors Sarah Broton, Amanda Gillot, Julie Hartrich, and Polly Hopkins, Shepherd Center, Atlanta; John Bach, University Hospital, Department of Physical Medicine and Rehabilitation, University of Medicine and Dentistry of New Jersey–New Jersey Medical School, Newark; Andrea Behrman, University of Florida, Gainesville; Gina Bertocci, Mechanical Engineering Department, University of Louisville; Mark Bowden, North Florida/South Georgia Veterans Affairs Health System, Gainesville, Fla.; Rory A. Cooper and co-contributors Ian Rice, Rosemarie Cooper, Annmarie Kelleher, and Amy Boyles, Human Engineering Research Laboratories, University of Pittsburgh and VA Rehabilitation Research and Development Center of Excellence; Pouran Faghri, University of Connecticut; Susan Garstang, University of Medicine and Dentistry of New Jersey–New Jersey Medical School, Department of Physical Medicine and Rehabilitation; David Gater, Hunter Holmes McGuire VA Medical Center, Richmond, Va.; Susan Harkema, University of Louisville and Frazier Rehabilitation Institute; Claire Kalpakjian and co-contributors Denise Tate and Martin Forchheimer, University of Michigan Model Spinal Cord Injury Care System; Bryan Kemp and co-contributor Lilli Thompson, Ranchos Los Amigos Medical Center; Alicia Koontz, Human Engineering Research Laboratories, University of Pittsburgh; Mary Jane (M.J.) Mulcahey, Shriners Hospitals for Children, Philadelphia; Phil Parette, SEAT Center, Illinois State University; Carolyn Sorensen, Adventist Rehabilitation Hospital of Maryland; Stephen Sprigle and his co-contributors David Kreutz, Kim Davis, and Chris Maurer, Georgia Institute of Technology and Shepherd Center; Marcia Scherer, Institute for Matching Person and Technology; Katharine Hunter-Zaworski, National Center for Accessible Transportation.

Columbia University Physical Therapy students Bradley Epstein and Nicole Benedetti provided invaluable assistance during videography for the DVD. Mahlon Stewart did the DVD voice-overs.

Our many colleagues and friends who have shared input and advice throughout the project include William DeTurk, Irene Marchesano-DeMasi, and Kim Ratner We deeply appreciate Kessler Institute and Kessler Medical Rehabilitation Research and Education Center for allowing us to use their facilities and patients for capturing the photographic media. We also thank Sue Bredensteiner, our developmental editor, for her "Goliath" effort in helping us complete this book; photographer Patrick Watson; videographer Joan Banks; and Elsevier editors Kathy Falk and Christie Hart. They have worked together to tremendously encourage and significantly support our efforts.

CONTENTS

AN INTRODUCTION: PROFILES IN TENACITY, RESILIENCE, COURAGE, AND HOPE

The individuals who contributed to this Introduction are spinal-cord injured. They have shared their feelings and backgrounds with us to add the richness of personal experience to this book.

In an instant, the world as we knew it turned upside down. Instead of jumping up from the TV and walking into the kitchen to get a soda, we were dependent and relearning every physical skill we thought we knew. Whether caused by an accident, a violent act, or disease, spinal cord injury (SCI) is a life-changing event. We are among the 500,000 individuals worldwide who are paralyzed. We survive by choosing to accept our situations and understanding the duality of pain and pleasure that SCI carries. Every hour of every day, another man or woman is paralyzed by SCI.

Sometimes our experiences generate pain, frustration, depression, and anger. But without a doubt, our experiences result in huge changes in our daily lives. How we act and react to these changes is a choice. Because no two SCIs are exactly alike, our lives are unique. They also are full of challenges. Learning to create fulfilling and rewarding futures is one of our main priorities after completing in-patient rehabilitation. Our progress is tempered by an understanding that after such a monumental disruption, time is needed to adjust.

Realizing the importance that time adds to developing perspective to any traumatic experience is a beginning step. With SCI, there is no specific time frame for getting over it. Some of us take a few years and others, a lifetime. What matters is that we keep plugging away at defining and redefining what life means to us and then leading it because having an SCI does not diminish our choice to lead a quality life filled with hopes, dreams, love, fulfillment, and reward. We are, after all, still ourselves.

Although life will change, some years will be better than others, and living with SCI will improve as long as we want it to. We can choose to be angry and never leave the house, or we can choose to get involved in our community, in other people, and in the many wonderful things life has to offer. Maybe the answer lies in making both choices: accepting the anger and then looking beyond it.

Scott Chesney and Sarah Everhart Skeels

◆ ◆ ◆ ◆ ◆ ◆ ◆ ◆ ◆ ◆ ◆ ◆ ◆ ◆ ◆

In an Instant . . .

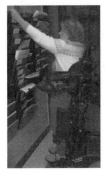

Janine (C6-7 SCI)
At 2:00 in the afternoon in November of 2001, a drowsy driver crossed the highway median and broad-sided my SUV, causing it to flip. I am the mother of three children who were 3, 6, and 7 at the time of the accident. I also was a full-time Spanish teacher, a Sunday school teacher, active in my church and community, volunteering with the poor and the mentally retarded, and an avid exerciser. I loved to ski!

During my 4-month in-patient rehabilitation at Kessler, I requested an extra hour of physical therapy each day, and it helped to speed my recovery. I couldn't wait to get my strength back and be independent enough to get home to my husband and children. I was determined to have a normal life again.

Despite my hard work, initially I was heartbroken. But my marriage and faith in God got stronger. And with extreme support from my family and friends, I am once again high on life! I am absorbed with family, friends, lots of volunteer work, and travel. I even snorkel with my husband on trips to the Caribbean.

I use a wheelchair that can stand, and it enables me to do almost everything independently. My accessible van has a lift so I can scoot right in and drive to the store as necessary. I can stop at the bookstore, do the weekly grocery shopping, pick up a prescription at the pharmacy, and be back home before 9:00 AM. I cook, clean, and do the laundry just like always. I chose not to go back to work because keeping the house in order, preparing delicious meals, juggling our schedule, and keeping family life running smoothly fills all my time now.

Attitude is EVERYTHING when recovering from such a trauma. If you focus on your blessings and nurture them, you will shine beyond your expectations, and your grateful heart will attract others to you like a magnet. You become a blessing to those around you.

And to the able-bodied, I say: Smile, even on your worst days, because you have no idea how good you really do feel.

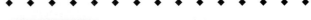

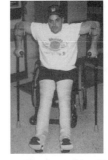

Nick (T10 Para SCI)
At the time of my injury, I was an active, determined-to-succeed, happy 26-year-old. My career goal was to be a carpenter, particularly a home builder in the influential area of Bergen County, New Jersey.

I'd been skydiving for many years and loved the thrill of jumping and flying through the air. But on November 16, 1996, I was involved in a midair collision.

The main thing I learned in rehab was that you are basically starting over—just like you've been born again. Every aspect of life changes, and you need to learn how to adjust to your injury at the same time that you adapt to how other people are responding to you.

Just like many other people who have life-changing accidents or injuries, my initial reactions were depression and a sense of loss. Trying to maintain friends was probably the hardest part of my recovery because I constantly needed to emphasize that I was not different. I was so lucky to have a tremendous family support group; without them I wouldn't have made it.

Early on, I promised myself that I would not once say the phrase "I used to . . ." I always looked for things that I could do. I built on each small step, each progression. And even before I left the in-patient unit, I was driven to walk either on my own or with the assistance of long leg braces.

Did SCI make me change my goals? No. My SCI did not change my goals. It just made me more determined, which helps me find new ways to achieve them. And that relates to how I encourage others. It is so important to get to know your body. After SCI, things work differently, and the faster you know what is happening to you in certain situations, the faster you will be able to get on with your life. You can't give in to negativity. You have to work extra hard to make sure you remain the same person you were. NEVER SAY NEVER!

To people without SCI, I say: Allow us to grow and adjust. Don't baby us. Don't make us feel less than we were before.

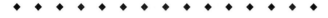

Sarah (T4 SCI)

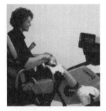

I was hit by a car while out on a training ride on my bicycle in 1990. I sustained a complete T4 level SCI, as well as losing significant use of my right arm. Since then, I have earned a master's degree, participated in two cross-country handcycle rides, and become an adaptive snow sports instructor and avid sailor. I run holistic therapy and recreation programs for children, adolescents, and adults with neurological disabilities focusing on health promotion, disease prevention, and disability.

I was 23 years old at the time of my injury, and as far as I was concerned, on top of the world. I had just been accepted into my school of choice for a master's degree in PT, was competing very successfully as an amateur triathlete, and had a wonderful relationship with a great guy. I was planning to spend the summer backpacking around Europe with my best friend and felt as though life was falling into place, just as planned. In one fell swoop, it all came to an abrupt halt. It was a great lesson in life planning.

Waking up in the ICU, one of my first thoughts was that I felt like Humpty Dumpty. Little did I know how accurate I was, when it came to putting me back together again. I spent the next 4 months in rehab, moved back in with my parents, and continued as an outpatient for the next 2 years because of additional surgery on my right arm and shoulder to increase function.

Along the way I learned that my most powerful assets were my family and friends. When I think about the support I have received from these amazingly wonderful people, it moves me to tears. I think they are the major reasons for my adjustment to disability. My support system was so strong that I chose to go back to the D.C. area, where many of my friends lived, when I moved out of my parents' home. I knew that if anything went wrong, any one of my friends would be there for me, and this gave me a huge boost of confidence. I remember feeling both completely excited and scared to death about living alone. I didn't know how successful I was going to be, but I knew I had to start doing it or I'd never know.

As my confidence grew, I continued to take on new challenges, many of them athletic. I swam laps at the pool and rode my handcycle on a regular basis. I joined a group that was biking across the country, some of them using handcycles. I took internships in interesting places and roamed cities feeling quite confident and able. My disability became a part of me, but I was becoming MORE than it, I was becoming MYSELF.

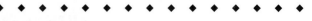

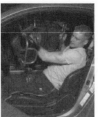

Ian (T2 ASIA C SCI)

In 2002, I was injured in a line-of-duty vehicle accident: someone called 911, threw a blanket over me, and moved on. I was 24 years old and a combat rescue officer and pilot in the United States Air Force. I planned to go to medical school.

Initially, there were a few curves. My girlfriend of 3 years left me while I was in a coma. We had lived together and were stationed in the Boston area. So I moved back with my parents in New Jersey. And I finished graduate school at Harvard while waiting for medical retirement from the Air Force.

During rehabilitation, the most important lessons I learned were the details and consequences of my spinal injury. My body was going through an adjustment period as it relearned new pathways to adapt to former functions and tasks. My interest in medicine was a real plus to understanding the renewal process. I also recognized that wheelchair skills, including floor to wheelchair transfers, skin checks, and ascending and descending stairs, were key ingredients to successful mobility.

I have not changed my life goals and I am not required to . . . I only need to adapt to the new situation. My spinal injury is merely a matter of logistics. I will still complete medical school and work in SCI research.

I have found that it is most important to look at adversity with the excitement of figuring out new ways to conquer prior tasks: in the gym; at school; at work; and with friends, family, and loved ones. Frustration and anger only waste time and energy, and in the end, we still have to face our challenges. So I go at them headstrong, eager, and determined.

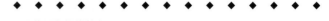

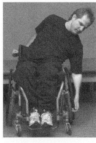

Trevor (C6-7 ASIA A SCI)

I was 27 years old and had just finished my third year in medical school. It's a very intensive clinical year and had increased my interest in surgery, orthopedics, trauma, and rehab. I played rugby on the med school team as a weekend outlet; it was a sport I'd played all my life. But that day in 1992, I was tackled the wrong way and got firsthand experience in trauma and rehab.

It never occurred to me to give up, and I was fortunate not to have a period of withdrawal and depression. I'd been raised to always look ahead and go forward. And while it obviously was the worse thing I'd ever faced, it was also the best because of the outpouring of concern and care from the hospital, friends, and other med students. I felt I had to show them all it would be OK.

Learning how to balance again when the rest of your body is dead weight is so hard. Just the sitting forward to sitting back and fear about moving your arms is huge. I had to reframe my mental ability to make my body work.

Before I began wheelchair skills, I fantasized about doing wheelchair marathons. The first day in a manual chair, I couldn't push it and I couldn't stop it from rolling. It was devastating. I had to build up my strength, and 6 months out I had regained enough physical strength to control the chair, start transfers, and move forward in functional skills.

In July of 1994, 1 year after my injury, I began my fourth year of med school. It wasn't a hard transition, but my quad hand function was now impaired so surgery wasn't an option. I did a radiology and nuclear medicine rotation, followed with a 1-month elective in rehab medicine with Allan Brown, who also was spinal-cord injured. Allan drove a Saab and was very active. His motivation really encouraged me. Later that year during a pediatric rotation, my chair started to bottom out, and I developed severe pressure ulcers that resulted in more down time for surgery and healing. I've been fanatical about good skin care and air cushions ever since.

Being a patient really opens your eyes. And other patients respond differently as well because they know you've walked in their shoes. I've found that I can do most things, so I advise my patients to keep pushing themselves. My work in a research lab focuses on medical complications in folks with SCI and allows me to share what I've learned as I help others.

Along the way I've had tendon transfer surgery to help regain finger function, and the results have been wonderful. Being able to drive my car with hand controls and the sunroof open gives me a great sense of independence and satisfaction.

◆ ◆ ◆ ◆ ◆ ◆ ◆ ◆ ◆ ◆ ◆ ◆ ◆ ◆ ◆

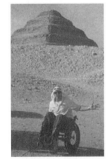

Scott (T8 SCI)

The morning I woke up with a numb big toe, I began to be more aware of my body. During the 48 hours when numbness in my left toe spread to the entire lower half of my body from my navel down both legs to all my toes, I recall a feeling of overwhelming uncertainty, but also a sense of peace, which I didn't understand at the time. It was as if my body was leaving and returning at the same time. Never before had I given my body that much attention. Today, after spending half my life in a wheelchair, I can honestly say that I know my body. I take care of it. And more than ever, I love it . . . the whole package.

When I sustained spinal cord injury in 1985, it was the result of a rare arterial-venous malformation (AVM), which can best be described as a stroke in the spinal cord. I did not lose my personality and self-discipline. Those characteristics may have faded temporarily with all the confusion and fear, but soon I was the same person I had been before.

Lying in my hospital beds—and there were several—I always had a big smile on my face and was in a good mood. Family and friends visited constantly and brought me food, cards, letters, and gifts. I was the center of attention. And that love helped me to survive and endure.

I have made wonderful friends of the doctors, nurses, therapists, and fellow patients whom I have met over the years. Each has played a vital role in helping me become the man I am today. And the most precious jewel in the world, my wife, Pratiksha, is my best friend.

We always need to remember that gifts can be found in everything in this world. Some of life's greatest challenges and obstacles open up doors that allow us to move forward in life. Sometimes it may feel as if the world is ending, but looking back those experiences teach us about ourselves and others. I know the 3 years I spent at the Miami Project to Cure Paralysis were filled with growth-oriented experiences.

The first 15 years of my life were about physical movement; the last 22 have been about the emotional and spiritual. I remember being an able-bodied athlete and pushing my body to the point where I could not move. I liked the exhilaration when I put my body to the test, and it responded with great strength and conviction. There was knowledge and certainty that I could achieve something if I worked hard enough and believed in myself. Now the power of belief has become my driving force allowing me to achieve my goals and for that I am eternally grateful.

CHAPTER ONE

Understanding Spinal Cord Injury and Advances in Recovery

Steven Kirshblum, MD, and Barbara Benevento, MD

In a moment, your life is completely changed. Yes, life will go on; yes, you can still be functional; but nothing will ever be the same again. Understanding that fact will be the most difficult lesson you will ever learn. Nothing is easy anymore, the simple tasks you used to do seem like they are impossible now. In rehab, you will learn about your bladder, bowels, skin, and nutrition. You will learn how to be functional in a wheelchair, maybe even how to be independent. But at the end of the day, it all comes down to one question—do you want to go on living? As you ponder that question, think about family, friends, a hug from your son or daughter, a kiss from your lover, sunsets, your favorite food. Whatever you need to think about to choose life—just do it. You'll have all the time in the world to learn about SCI once you've chosen life.

Tara (T12 SCI)

The multidisciplinary spinal cord injury (SCI) rehabilitation team includes physicians who specialize in SCI medicine. This specialty depends on a thorough knowledge of spinal cord neuroanatomy and spine anatomy that endows an understanding of the neurological sequelae associated with SCI and spinal cord disease. SCI physicians are responsible for managing medical and rehabilitation care. They must know how to prognosticate the degree to which a patient is likely to recover from complete and incomplete injuries and are responsible for prescribing medications or procedures to manage problems related to SCI that may affect body systems, such as pain, bowel and bladder symptoms, spinal stability, spasticity, and autonomic dysreflexia.

The physician coordinates patient care with the rehabilitation team through discharge to the home or to an alternate living environment. This involves working closely with physical, occupational, speech, and respiratory therapists; nurses; psychologists; urologists; wheelchair seating and orthotic specialists; social service representatives; and case managers. Social service and case management representatives provide the skilled investigation of reimbursement for care and equipment during the patient's transition into the home, community, and workplace environments. This chapter supplies the foundation of knowledge about SCI from a historical and epidemiological aspect. In addition, it presents the anatomy of the spinal cord and defines how to diagnose complete and incomplete injuries. Algorithms for predicting outcomes on the basis of patient presentation early after injury are provided. Finally, an overview of pharmaceutical and surgical clinical trials to promote recovery are discussed.

HISTORY AND EPIDEMIOLOGY

The earliest reference to SCI was approximately 5000 years ago by an unknown Egyptian physician in the so-called Edwin Smith Papyrus as "an ailment not to be treated."[1] Only during the past half century have individuals with SCI been given hope for survival. Before World War II, life expectancy for a person with SCI was rarely greater than 2 years; most succumbed to septic infections, renal failure, and pressure ulcers. With the advent of antibiotics and improved therapeutic techniques, remarkable progress has been made toward effectively preventing and managing the numerous medical complications of SCI. Improved acute-care management and early provision of comprehensive rehabilitation

services have helped individuals with SCI maximize their self-care and mobility skills, which usually permits them to reintegrate into their communities. As the annual incidence of SCI has remained unchanged in the United States, with decreased mortality each year after injury, there has been a gradual increase in the prevalence and the importance of this condition as a health issue for society has occurred.

Traumatic SCI has an incidence of approximately 11,000 patients per year in the United States with a prevalence of 250,000,[2] thus affecting a small but significant portion of the population over the years. Although the overall incidence has remained constant in the last few decades, the epidemiology has changed (Box 1-1). Motor vehicle crashes (MVC) are still the primary cause of SCI, followed by falls and violence-related causes.[2] The proportion of injuries related to sports has decreased over time, whereas the proportion of injuries from falls has increased. Acts of violence caused 13% of SCI before 1980, and peaked between 1990 and 1999 at 25% before declining to 14% since 2000. The mean age at traumatic SCI has increased to 37.6 years, although the majority of injuries still occur in 16- to 30-year-olds.[2-4] The percentage of people older than 60 years has increased from 5% before 1980 to 11% among injuries since 2000. The etiology of the injury differs in the various age groups, with violence and sports-related injuries more common in the younger individuals and falls higher in the older population.

Males are predominately affected, with African Americans and Hispanics disproportionally affected relative to their percentages in the general population.[2-4] There is a greater incidence of injuries in the warmer months and on weekend days. There has been a recent trend toward an increased number of incomplete lesions, possibly as a result of changes in etiology (i.e., falls are more likely to cause an incomplete injury and violence a complete injury), improved treatment at the site of injury by emergency medical technicians, and subsequent immediate medical care. At the time of injury, more than 50% of people with SCI are at least high school graduates and employed. The majority are single at the time of injury, with fewer than one third being married (30%).[4] Approximately one half of all traumatic SCIs are cervical lesions, and one third are thoracic. The most common neurological level of injury (NLI) is C5, followed by C4 and then C6 in the cervical region, and T12 is the most common level of paraplegia[3,4] (Box 1-2).

BOX 1-1 | **Epidemiology of Traumatic Spinal Cord Injury**

Incidence: 11,000/year
Prevalence: 250,000
Average age: 37.6 years
Sex: 80% male
Ethnicity: Disproportionally African Americans and Hispanics
Etiology: Motor vehicle crashes (MVCs) (48%), falls (23%), violence (14%), sports (9%), other (6%)

Adapted from Spinal cord injury: facts and figures at a glance, *J Spinal Cord Med* 28:379-380, 2005.

BOX 1-2 | **Percentage of Injuries by ASIA Classification**

Incomplete tetraplegia (34.5%)
Complete paraplegia (23.1%)
Complete tetraplegia (18.4%)
Incomplete paraplegia (17.5%)

Adapted from Spinal cord injury: facts and figures at a glance, *J Spinal Cord Med* 28:379-380, 2005.

ANATOMY

To understand SCI and its treatment, it is imperative to understand the basic anatomy of the vertebral column, the spinal cord, coverings, the spinal cord and associated nerves, its vascular supply, the spinal tracts with the spinal cord, and the autonomic nervous system.

Vertebral Column

The vertebral column (Figure 1-1) is composed of seven cervical, twelve thoracic, five lumbar, five sacral, and four coccygeal vertebrae. Each vertebrae consists of a body and an arch. The arch or lamina is connected to the vertebral body by the pedicle. Spinous processes project posteriorly from the lamina and the transverse processes project laterally (Figure 1-2). Each vertebra articulates with the vertebrae superiorly and inferiorly by the superior and inferior articular process. The spinal cord is then protected within the vertebral foramen, which is formed by the vertebral body and arch.

The intervertebral discs separate each vertebra and constitute 20% to 33% of the vertebral column. The disc is composed of the nucleus pulposus, which is the central aspect and composed of fine fibrous strands in a mucoprotein gel of mucopolysaccharides. The water content is 70% to 90% and decreases with age. In the lumbar spine the nucleus lies more posterior than in the cervical spine. The annulus fibrosis forms the outer boundary of the disc, and it is composed of fibrous tissue in concentric laminated bands, which is arranged in a helix. The fibers in each adjacent band run in opposite directions. The peripheral bands attach to the vertebral body and are called Sharpey's fibers, which form a much stronger attachment than those fibers attached centrally.

The ligaments function to stabilize the vertebral column (Figure 1-3). The anterior longitudinal ligament (ALL) connects the anterior aspect of the vertebral bodies, and the posterior longitudinal ligament (PLL) attaches the posterior aspect of the vertebral bodies. These ligaments act to limit flexion and extension, respectively. Both the ALL and PLL are thicker in the thoracic region. Unlike the ALL, the PLL is connected to the intervertebral disc. The ligamenta flava extend from the anterior inferior border of the laminae above to the posterosuperior borders of the laminae below, thereby connecting the borders of adjacent lamina from the second cervical vertebrae to the first sacral vertebrae.

The interspinous ligaments connect adjacent spines. They are narrow and longer in the thoracic region and wider and thicker in the lumbar region and only somewhat developed in the cervical region. The supraspinous ligament originates in the ligamentum nuchae and is attached to the tip of the spinous processes down to the sacrum. These are thicker and broader in the lumbar region than in the thoracic region. Intertransverse ligaments pass between the transverse processes in the thoracic region and connect with the deep muscles in the back. The capsular ligaments attach the adjacent articular processes. These are more taut in the thoracic and lumbar regions.

Coverings of the Spinal Cord

The coverings (i.e., meninges) of the spinal cord include the dura mater, arachnoid membrane, and pia mater (Figure 1-4). The spinal dura is located between the meningeal layer of the dura and the vertebra and is single layered, unlike the cranial dura. The venous plexuses are located in this space and are used clinically for the administration of epidural anesthesia. Caudally, the spinal dura ends at the level of the second sacral vertebra, where the dura becomes a thin extension (i.e., the coccygeal ligament or filum terminale externum) and serves to anchor the spinal dura to the base of the vertebral canal. The arachnoid membrane loosely invests the spinal cord and is connected to the dura by connective tissue trabeculae. The arachnoid extends from the foramen magnum and surrounds the cauda equina (i.e., nerve roots of the spinal nerves caudal to the second lumbar vertebra). The subarachnoid space contains cerebrospinal fluid (CSF). The spinal pia is a vascular membrane that projects into the ventral fissure of the spinal cord. At intervals, dentate ligaments (i.e., ligaments of pial tissue) extend from the lateral surfaces of the spinal cord, serving to anchor the spinal cord to the arachnoid and through it to the dura. The pia mater extends from the cranial pia mater to the filum terminale that anchors the spinal cord to the dura at the level of the second sacral vertebra.

Spinal Cord

The spinal cord is a cylindrical structure that extends from the medulla oblongata rostrally and ends at the lower border of the first lumbar vertebra (Figure 1-5). At the caudal end, the spinal cord is conical and is known as the conus medullaris. A filament extending from the conus medullaris is called the filum terminale. This filament is enclosed in pia and consists of glial cells, ependymal cells, and astrocytes. The coccygeal ligament is an extension of spinal dura. This ligament surrounds the filum terminale internum of the spinal cord and attaches to the coccyx to anchor the spinal cord.

The spinal cord initially occupies the entire length of the vertebral canal. After the third month of life, however, the spinal cord lengthens at a slower rate than the vertebral column. By adulthood, the spinal cord occupies only the upper two thirds of the vertebral column, with its caudal end located at the level of

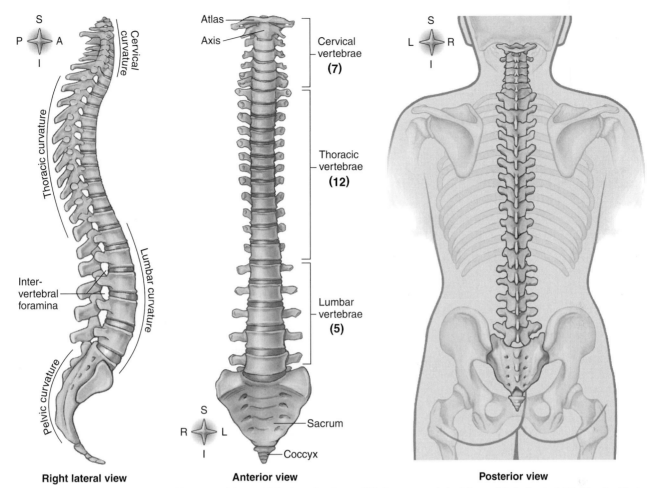

FIGURE 1-1 The vertebral column (three views) (From Thibodeau GA, Patton KT: *Anatomy and physiology*, ed 5, St. Louis, 2003, Elsevier Mosby, Figure 8-13, p. 233.)

the first lumbar vertebra. For this reason, it is necessary for the lumbar and sacral nerve roots to descend some distance within the vertebral canal to exit from their respective intervertebral foramina. The filum terminale is surrounded by lumbosacral nerve roots that resemble a horse's tail, and it is called the cauda equina (see Figure 1-5).

The lumbar cistern extends from the caudal end of the spinal cord at the L2 vertebra to the second sacral vertebra. The subarachnoid space is widest at this site and contains the filum terminale internum and nerve roots of the cauda equina. Because of the large size of the subarachnoid space and relative absence of neural structures, this space is most suitable for the withdrawal of CSF by lumbar puncture (LP). The LP is usually preformed between the third and fourth lumbar vertebra (L3 to L4).

Spinal Nerves

Thirty-one pairs of spinal nerves emerge from the spinal cord and at each level of the spinal cord and exit through the intervertebral foramina. The 31 segments include 8 cervical, 12 thoracic, 5 lumbar, 5 sacral, and 1 coccygeal pairs of spinal nerves. In the thoracic level and below the spinal cord, nerves exit through the intervertebral foramina just caudal to the vertebra of the same name. In the cervical region, however, these nerves exit through the intervertebral foramina just rostral to the vertebra of the

same name. This is because there are eight cervical nerve roots and only seven cervical vertebrae; the eighth cervical spinal nerve exits through the intervertebral foramen just rostral to the first thoracic vertebra.

Each spinal nerve consists of a dorsal root, which contains afferent fibers, and a ventral root, which contains efferent fibers. The dorsal root is absent in the first cervical and coccygeal nerves. The dorsal and ventral roots enter the intervertebral foramen, but because of the length difference between the spinal cord and the vertebral column, cervical and upper thoracic roots run at right angles to the spinal cord, whereas lower thoracic and more caudal roots are increasingly oblique. Within the intervertebral foramen is the dorsal root ganglion.

The dorsal and ventral roots then join to form the common spinal nerve trunk (see Figures 1-4, *B* and 1-5). Usually the following four branches (i.e., rami) arise from the common spinal nerve trunk: (1) the dorsal ramus, which innervates the muscles and skin of the back; (2) the ventral ramus, which innervates the ventrolateral part of the body wall and all limbs; (3) the meningeal branch, formed by several small branches arising from the common nerve trunk and the ramus communicantes, which re-enters the intervertebral foramen and innervates the meninges, blood vessels, and vertebral column; and (4) the ramus communicans, which consists of the white and gray portions. The white ramus

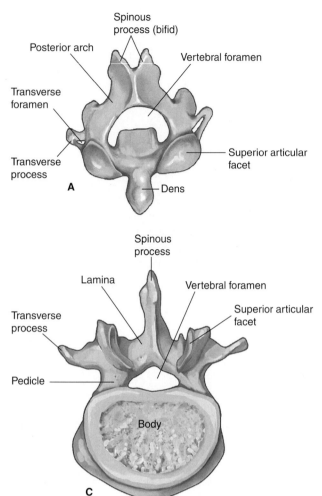

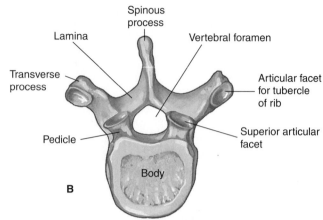

FIGURE 1-2 The spinous and transverse processes seen in the vertebrae. **A,** Axis (second cervical vertebra), slightly posterior and superior view. **B,** Thoracic vertebra, superior view. **C,** Lumbar vertebra, superior view. (From Thibodeau GA, Patton KT: *Anatomy and physiology*, ed 5, St. Louis, 2003, Elsevier Mosby, Figure 8-14, p, 234.)

communicans carries myelinated preganglionic fibers from the spinal cord to the sympathetic ganglion, whereas the gray ramus communicans contains the unmyelinated postganglionic fibers.[5]

The spinal cord has two enlargements; cervical and lumbar (see Figure 1-5). The cervical enlargement includes the C5 through T1 nerve roots to form the brachial plexus, which innervates the upper limbs. The lumbar plexus, comprising nerve roots L1 to L4, and the lumbosacral plexus, consisting of nerve roots from L4 to S2, emerge from the lumbar enlargement. The lumbar plexus innervates the lower limbs. The sacral spinal nerves emerge from the conus medullaris and contain parasympathetic and somatic motor fibers innervating the muscles of the bladder wall and external sphincter, respectively.

Vascular Supply

The spinal cord receives its blood supply from one anterior and two posterior spinal arteries and anterior and posterior radicular arteries. The anterior spinal artery arises in the upper cervical region and is formed by the union of two small branches of the vertebral arteries. The anterior spinal artery supplies the anterior two thirds of the spinal cord, including the gray matter and

anterior and anterolateral white matter. It travels in the ventral median fissure for the entire length of the spinal cord. The anterior spinal artery varies in diameter according to its proximity to a major radicular artery. It usually is narrowest in the T4 to T8 region of the spinal cord. There are two posterior spinal arteries, which originate as a small branch of either the vertebral artery or the posterior inferior cerebellar artery. The posterior spinal arteries supply the posterior one third of the spinal cord, consisting of posterolateral and posterior white matter of the spinal cord.

The blood supply from the anterior and posterior arteries is sufficient for the upper cervical segments. Segmental arteries that arise from the aorta supply the anterior and posterior spinal arteries in the thoracic and lumbar regions. The radicular arteries supply the remaining segments of the spinal cord. These arteries arise from the vertebral, cervical, intercostal, lumbar, and sacral arteries. They have anterior and posterior divisions that supply the vertebrae, meninges, and spinal arteries. The posterior arteries are joined by communicating vessels except in the area of the conus medullaris. The major radicular artery that supplies the lumbosacral enlargement of the spinal cord is known as the artery of Adamkiewicz. It arises from the left intercostal or lumbar artery at the level of T6 to L3 and provides the main blood supply to the lower two thirds of the spinal cord. There are fewer radicular arteries supplying the midthoracic region of the spinal cord; they are smaller in diameter and therefore create a watershed zone of the spinal cord at this level. In clinical situations where there is low blood flow to the spinal cord, this level of the cord is most affected at the T4 to T6 level.

Spinal Tracts

The internal structure of the spinal cord is such that a transverse section of the spinal cord reveals a butterfly-shaped central gray matter surrounded by white matter (see Figure 1-5). The gray matter of the spinal cord contains cell bodies and primarily neurons, dendrites, and myelinated and unmyelinated axons, which are either exiting from the gray matter to the white matter or projecting from the white matter to innervate neurons located in the gray matter. Autonomic neurons are located laterally and exit by the ventral root and innervate smooth muscle. Lower motor neurons are located ventrally, exit by the ventral roots, and innervate striated muscle. The white matter consists of ascending and descending bundles of myelinated and unmyelinated axons (i.e., tracts or fasciculi). The ascending pathways relay sensory information **to** the brain (Figure 1-6), whereas the descending pathways relay motor information **from** the brain (Figure 1-7).

Ascending Pathways

Sensory tracts or ascending pathways are composed of bundles of axons that are continuations of the peripheral sensory nerves whose cell bodies are located in the dorsal root ganglion and ascend toward the brainstem (Figure 1-6). The lateral spinothalamic tract transmits pain and temperature sensation. Receptors for pain and temperature travel from the dermis and epidermis of the skin toward the spinal cord and synapse in the dorsal horn of the gray matter. The fibers cross over within one or two vertebral segments and then travel in the lateral spinothalamic tract and ascend to the ventral posterolateral nucleus of the thalamus. The fibers then ascend in the internal capsule to reach the postcentral gyrus, which is the primary somatic sensory area of the brain.

The nerve fibers of the receptors in the dermis of the skin for pressure and light touch enter the cord in the same fashion; however, on entering, the axons pass into the ipsilateral dorsal white column and bifurcate. One branch immediately enters the dorsal horn gray matter, synapses, and crosses over within one or two segments, and the other branch remains ipsilateral and ascends in the dorsal column for as many as 10 spinal segments. The ipsilateral branch ultimately enters the dorsal horn, synapses, and crosses over to join the other branch in the ventral white column. This bundle of fibers forms the ventral spinothalamic tract. These axons travel in the same pathway as the lateral tract to reach the post central gyrus, which interprets these sensations.

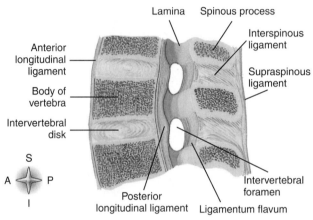

FIGURE 1-3 Vertebrae and their ligaments. Sagittal section of two lumbar vertebrae and their ligaments. (From Thibodeau GA, Patton KT: *Anatomy and physiology*, ed 5, St. Louis, 2003, Elsevier Mosby, Figure 9-11, p, 266.)

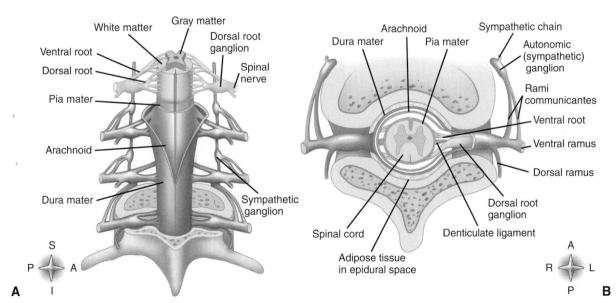

FIGURE 1-4   A, The meninges, the inner coverings of the spinal cord, are composed of three distinct layers. The dura mater extends to cover the spinal nerve roots and nerves and sheaths the arachnoid membrane and the pia mater. **B,** Rami arising from the common spinal nerve trunk (dorsal, ventral, and communicantes). (From Thibodeau GA, Patton KT: *Anatomy and physiology*, ed 5, St. Louis, 2003, Elsevier Mosby, Figure 13-3, p. 377.)

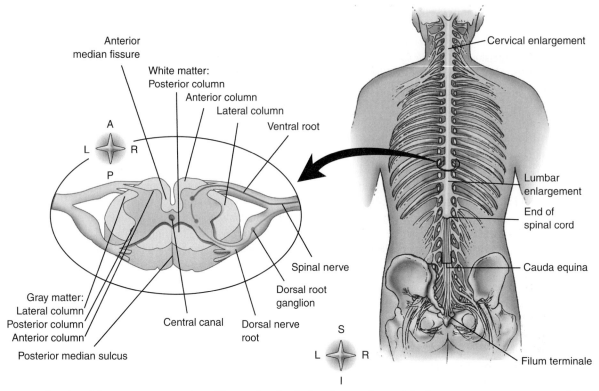

FIGURE 1-5   Spinal cord. *Inset,* A transverse section of the spinal cord in the broader view. (From Thibodeau GA, Patton KT: *Anatomy and physiology,* ed 5, St. Louis, 2003, Elsevier Mosby, Figure 13-6, p. 381.)

The posterior columns transmit three different sensations: proprioception (conscious awareness of movement), fine touch, and vibration sense. The receptors for proprioception are located in muscles, tendons, and joints, whereas those for fine touch and vibration are located in the dermis. Their nerve fibers reach the dorsal root ganglion in the same manner as the above tracts. Once the axons enter the spinal cord they immediately pass into the ipsilateral dorsal white columns and ascend to the medulla. Axons that enter the cord at the sacral and lumbar levels are situated in the medial part of the dorsal column, called the fasciculus gracilis, and convey information from the lower part of the body. Those axons that enter at the thoracic and cervical levels are situated in the lateral part of the column, termed the fasciculus cuneatus, and convey information from the upper part of the body. Both axons of each fasciculus synapse in the medulla and form a bundle termed the medial lemniscus. These axons also ascend by the same pathway as the above tract to reach the postcentral gyrus.

The cerebellum is the control center for the coordination of voluntary muscle activity, equilibrium, and muscle tone. The spinocerebellar pathways supply information regarding the condition of the muscles, the amount of tone, and the position of the body by unconscious proprioceptive fibers, whose receptors are found in joints, tendons, and muscles. This enables an individual to walk and perform other complex acts subconsciously without having to think about which joints are flexed and extended.

Descending Pathways

The lateral corticospinal tract is the main tract for voluntary muscle activity. Its origin is the precentral gyrus of the frontal lobe of the brain, where large pyramidal-shaped cell bodies are located

(Figure 1-7). Their axons exit the cortex and descend through the internal capsule to the medulla oblongata. At this point approximately 80% to 90% of the axons cross at the pyramidal decussation to the contralateral side of the medulla and descend in the lateral white columns of the spinal cord in the lateral corticospinal tract. At each level of the spinal cord the axons from the lateral tract peel off and enter the gray matter of the ventral horn and synapse with secondary neurons. The 10% to 20% of uncrossed axons that continue down on the same side of the cord travel in the ventral corticospinal tract. The axons of the ventral tract then cross over at the corresponding level of muscles that it innervates. Both tracts travel from the precentral gyrus to the ventral horn as a single uninterrupted neuron and are termed upper motor neurons (UMN), whereas the secondary neurons that they synapse on are termed lower motor neurons (LMN). Injury to the UMN versus the LMN presents with different effects on the muscles they innervate.

Autonomic Nervous System

The autonomic nervous system regulates involuntary functions such as blood pressure, heart rate, respiration, digestion, glandular secretion, reproduction, and body temperature. The autonomic nervous system is divided into three divisions: sympathetic, parasympathetic, and enteric. Preganglionic neurons of the sympathetic nervous system originate in the intermediolateral cell column from the first thoracic to second lumbar (T1 to L2) area. Generally, the axons of these preganglionic neurons exit the spinal cord through the ventral roots and enter the main trunk of the spinal nerve. The axons of the sympathetic preganglionic neurons exit through the white ramus and reach one of the sympathetic ganglia to ultimately innervate its target organ.

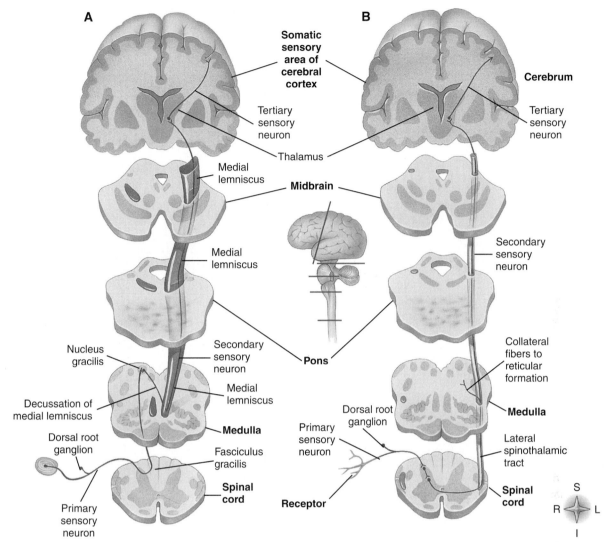

FIGURE 1-6   Examples of somatic sensory ascending pathways. **A,** A pathway of the medial lemniscal system that conducts information about discriminating touch and kinesthesia. **B,** A spinothalamic pathway that conducts information about pain and temperature. (From Thibodeau GA, Patton KT: *Anatomy and physiology,* ed 5, St. Louis, 2003, Elsevier Mosby, Figure 13-22, p. 399.)

The sympathetic division of the autonomic nervous system is activated in stressful situations, resulting in increases in heart rate, blood pressure, blood flow in the skeletal muscles, blood sugar, and pupillary dilatation. All of these responses prepare the individual for fight or flight. For example, an increase in blood flow in the skeletal muscles will help in running away from the site of danger (i.e., flight), an increase in heart rate and blood pressure will help in better perfusion of various body organs, an increase in blood sugar will provide energy, and pupillary dilatation will provide for better vision under these circumstances.[5]

For the parasympathetic nervous system, the preganglionic neurons arise from the brainstem, which includes the midbrain, pons and medulla oblongata, and the sacral region (S2 to S4) of the spinal cord, therefore often referred to as the craniosacral division. From the spinal cord, the axons exit through the ventral roots, travel through pelvic nerves, and synapse on postganglionic neurons that are located close to or within the organs being innervated. The postganglionic parasympathetic nerve fibers are very short compared with the sympathetic postganglionic nerve fibers.

Activation of the parasympathetic division of the autonomic nervous system results in conservation and restoration of body energy. For example, decreases in heart rate by the parasympathetic system will also decrease the demand for energy while the increased activity of the gastrointestinal (GI) system will promote restoration of body energy. The effects of parasympathetic activation are localized and last for a short time.

The enteric nervous system consists of neurons in the wall of the gut (i.e., intrinsic innervation), which regulates GI motility and secretion. The GI system is also controlled by sympathetic and parasympathetic innervation (i.e., extrinsic innervation). The extrinsic system can override the intrinsic system under certain conditions.

CLINICAL ASSESSMENT OF SPINAL CORD INJURY

The most accurate way to assess SCI is to perform a standardized physical examination based on the *International Standards for Neurological Classification of Spinal Cord Injury*,[6,7] previously referred to as the American Spinal Injury Association (ASIA) guidelines.

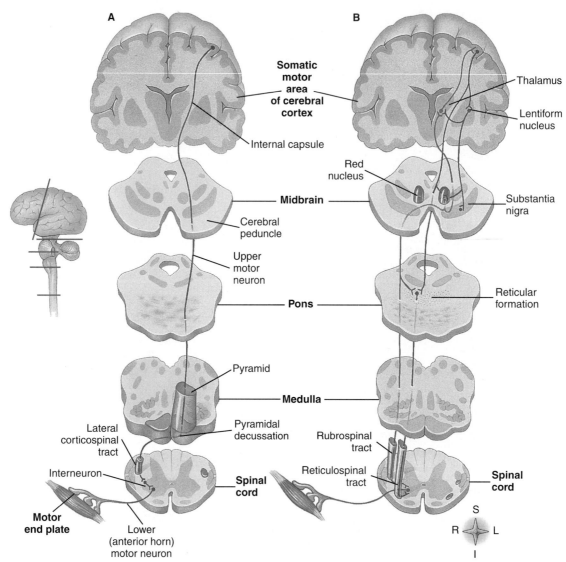

FIGURE 1-7 Examples of somatic motor descending pathways. **A,** A pyramidal pathway, through the lateral corticospinal tract. **B,** Extrapyramidal pathways, through the rubrospinal and reticulospinal tracts. (From Thibodeau GA, Patton KT: *Anatomy and physiology*, ed 5, St. Louis, 2003, Elsevier Mosby, Figure 13-22, p. 401.)

This allows the examiner to determine the motor, sensory, and neurological level of injury (NLI) and the degree of completeness of the injury and to determine the ASIA Impairment Scale (AIS).

The neurologic examination of a person with SCI has two main components: the sensory and motor, with certain required and optional elements. The required elements include determination of the sensory, motor, and neurological levels, generation of sensory and motor scores, and determination of the completeness of the injury. Also required is a rectal examination that tests for voluntary anal contraction and anal sensation. This information should be recorded on the standardized neurological flow sheet (see Figure 1-8), which can be included in the medical records. The optional elements involve aspects of the neurological examination that may better describe the patient's clinical condition but that are not used for numerical scoring and include testing of additional muscles, proprioception, and reflexes. To learn how to use the international standards, an instructional manual and video tapes are available through the ASIA office in Atlanta,

Georgia. These standards provide basic definitions of the most common terms used by clinicians in the assessment of SCI and describe the neurological examination.

The international standards are the most valid and reliable classification to assess SCI and are used by the Model System Spinal Cord Injury database. This database, which is maintained by specially designated SCI model system centers in the United States, tracks information regarding the injury, functional, and behavioral status from the time of injury through follow-up over the years. Key terms frequently used in the treatment of SCI are defined in Box 1-3.

Twenty-eight key dermatomes are used for the sensory examination (i.e., C2 to S4-5), each separately tested for pinprick with a safety pin and light touch with a cotton-tipped applicator (Figure 1-8). A numerical scale is used, with 0 representing absent sensation, 1 representing impaired sensation, which is defined as partial or altered sensation including hyperesthesia, and 2 representing normal sensation, with the face being the normal reference point (Figure 1-8).

BOX 1-3 | Key Terms Important to the Assessment of Spinal Cord Injury

Key muscle groups: Ten muscle groups that are tested as part of the standardized spinal cord examination.

Root Level	Muscle Group
C5	Elbow flexors
C6	Wrist flexors
C7	Elbow extensors
C8	Long finger flexors
T1	Small finger abductors
L2	Hip flexors
L3	Knee flexors
L4	Ankle dorsiflexors
L5	Long toe extensor
S1	Ankle plantar flexors

Motor level: The most caudal key muscle group that is graded 3/5 or greater with the segments cephalad graded normal (5/5) strength.

Motor index score: Calculated by adding the muscle scores of each key muscle group; a total score of 100 is possible.

Sensory level: The most caudal dermatome to have normal sensation for both pinprick and light touch on both sides.

Sensory index score: Calculated by adding the scores for each dermatome; a total score of 112 is possible for each pinprick and light touch.

Neurological level of injury: The most caudal level at which both motor and sensory modalities are intact.

Complete injury: The absence of sensory and motor function in the lowest sacral segments.

Incomplete injury: Preservation of motor or sensory function below the neurological level of injury that includes the lowest sacral segments.

Sacral sparing: Presence of motor function (voluntary external anal sphincter contraction) or sensory function (light touch, pinprick at S4/5 dermatome, or anal sensation on rectal examination) in the lowest sacral segments.

Zone of partial preservation: All segments below the neurological level of injury with preservation of motor or sensory findings; used only in complete SCI.

For the pinprick examination the patient must be able to distinguish between the pin (i.e., sharp) and dull edge of the safety pin (dull). The inability to distinguish between the two yields a score of 0. A score of 1 for impaired response to the pinprick testing is given when the patient can distinguish between sharp and dull, but the pin is not felt as sharp as on the face. The normal score of 2 is only given if the pin is felt as sharp as when tested on the face.

For light touch, a cotton-tipped swab is used, with a normal score of 2 being the same touch sensation as on the face and an impaired score of 1 indicating less sensation than on the face. The sensory level is defined as the most caudal dermatome to have normal sensation for both pinprick and light touch on both sides of the body. Sensory index scoring is calculated by adding the scores for pinprick and light touch separately, for each dermatome, for a total score possible of 112 (56 on each side).

To test deep anal sensation, a rectal digital examination is performed. The patient is asked to report any sensory awareness, touch or pressure, with firm pressure of the examiner's digit on the rectal wall. Deep anal sensation is recorded as either present or absent. The optional elements of the sensory examination include proprioception (i.e., joint position and vibration), temperature, and deep pressure sensations.

If accurate sensory testing in any dermatome cannot be performed, "not tested" (NT) should be recorded, or an alternate location within the dermatome can be tested with notation that an alternate site was used. If NT has been documented, then a sensory score cannot be calculated.

The required elements of the motor examination consist of testing 10 key muscles on each side of the body, five in the upper limb and five in the lower limb (see Box 1-3). Muscles should be examined in a rostral to caudal sequence, starting with the elbow flexors (i.e., C5 innervated muscles), and finishing with ankle plantarflexors (Sl). All muscles are tested with the patient in the supine position and graded on a numerical scale from 0 to 5 (see Figure 1-8). Although most muscles are innervated by more than one nerve root segment, the muscles tested have been chosen because of their consistency for being innervated primarily by the segment indicated and for their ease of testing in the supine position. If a particular muscle has a grade of 3/5, it is considered to have full innervation by at least one of its innervating segments, in SCI the more cephalad segment. A muscle graded 5 (i.e., normal) is considered to be fully innervated by both its spinal root segments. A muscle with strength greater than 3 has antigravity strength and is considered useful for functional activities.[8] A number of optional muscles (e.g., diaphragm, deltoids, abdominal muscles, and hip adductors) may also be tested, which may be helpful in determining involvement of certain regions of the spinal cord, but are not used to obtain a motor score.

In addition to the key muscles, the external anal sphincter should be tested by digital examination to sense for voluntary contraction. Care must be taken not to confuse a reflex contraction of the anal sphincter with voluntary contraction.

The motor level is defined as the most caudal key muscle group that is graded 3 or greater with the segments cephalad to it graded normal in strength.[6] Motor scores for each muscle are entered on a standard form and the motor index score is calculated. The maximum total motor score is 50 on each side, for a total of 100. Often the patient's clinical condition may prevent the completion of an accurate examination, such as when a patient is comatose from an associated traumatic brain injury, has injury to the brachial or lumbosacral plexi, or has a limb immobilized because of a fracture. When the patient is not fully testable for any reason, the examiner should record NT for not tested instead of a numerical score.

The NLI is the most caudal level at which both motor and sensory modalities are intact on both sides of the body. For example, if the motor level is C7 and the sensory level is C8, the overall NLI is C7. The motor or sensory level may be different from side to side, and therefore it is recommended to record each separately if it presents a clearer picture of the patient's status (i.e., right C6 motor, C7 sensory, left C7 motor, C6 sensory). The motor level and upper limb motor score better reflect the degree of function and the severity of impairment and disability, relative to the NLI, after motor complete tetraplegia.[9]

CLASSIFICATION OF SPINAL CORD INJURY

In 1969, Frankel et al[10] introduced a five-grade system of classifying traumatic SCI, with a division into complete and incomplete injuries. This scale was adapted by ASIA in 1982. A complete injury was defined as the patient having no preservation of motor or sensory function more than three levels below the NLI. The three levels distal to the NLI were termed the zone of partial preservation (ZPP). In an incomplete injury, there was preservation of motor or sensory function below the ZPP. The amount of preserved sensory or motor function determined the specific Frankel classification. Changes were subsequently made to the Frankel classification and the 1982 ASIA Guidelines.[7] The Frankel classification was replaced in 1992 by the ASIA Impairment Scale (AIS),[11] which was revised in 1996[12] and 2000[6] and reprinted in 2006 with corrections to the 2000 edition.

Tetraplegia, the preferred term instead of quadriplegia, is defined as loss of motor or sensory function in the cervical segments of the spinal cord. It does not include brachial plexus lesions or injury to the peripheral nerves outside the neural canal. Paraplegia is defined as an impairment of motor or sensory function in the thoracic, lumbar, or sacral segments of the cord. With paraplegia, neurological function in the upper limbs is spared, but depending on the level of injury, the trunk, legs, and pelvic organs may be involved. Paraplegia can refer to cauda equina and conus medullaris injuries but not to lumbosacral plexus lesions or injuries to peripheral nerves outside the

neural canal. Use of the terms quadriparesis, tetraparesis, and paraparesis are discouraged because they describe incomplete lesions imprecisely.

A complete injury is defined as the absence of sensory or motor function in the lowest sacral segments (i.e., no sacral sparing). An incomplete injury is defined as preservation of motor function or sensation below the NLI that includes the lowest sacral segments (i.e., sacral sparing). Sacral sparing is tested by light touch and pinprick at the anal mucocutaneous junction (S4 to S5 dermatome), on both sides, and testing voluntary anal contraction and deep anal sensation as part of the rectal examination. If any of these are present, indicating sacral sparing, the individual has a neurologically incomplete injury. According to this definition, a patient with cervical SCI can have sensory and motor function in the trunk or even in the legs, but unless sacral sparing is present, the injury must be classified as complete with a large ZPP (Clinical Note: Classification of Spinal Cord Injury). The ZPP is now defined as the segments below the NLI with preservation of sensory or motor findings and is used only in patients with a complete (ASIA A) SCI.[6] The ASIA Impairment Scale, which describes five categories of SCI, is listed in Box 1-4.

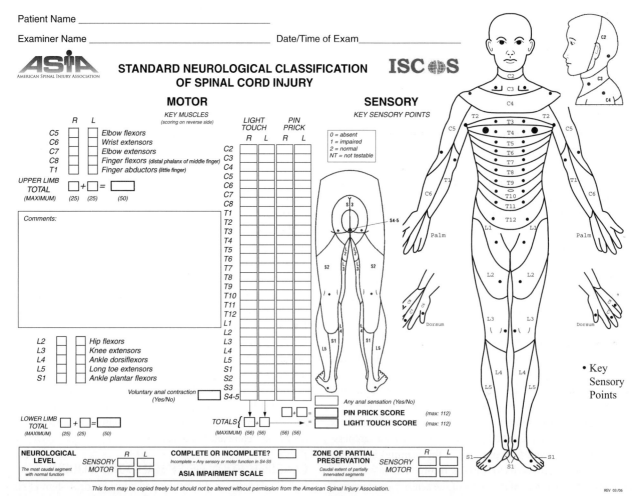

FIGURE 1-8   American Spinal Injury Association (ASIA) Standard Neurological Classification of Spinal Cord Injury. (Courtesy American Spinal Injury Association, Atlanta, GA, 2006.)

MUSCLE GRADING

0 total paralysis

1 palpable or visible contraction

2 active movement, full range of motion, gravity eliminated

3 active movement, full range of motion, against gravity

4 active movement, full range of motion, against gravity and provides some resistance

5 active movement, full range of motion, against gravity and provides normal resistance

5* muscle able to exert, in examiner's judgement, sufficient resistance to be considered normal if identifiable inhibiting factors were not present

NT not testable. Patient unable to reliably exert effort or muscle unavailable for testing due to factors such as immobilization, pain on effort or contracture.

ASIA IMPAIRMENT SCALE

☐ **A = Complete**: No motor or sensory function is preserved in the sacral segments S4-S5.

☐ **B = Incomplete**: Sensory but not motor function is preserved below the neurological level and includes the sacral segments S4-S5.

☐ **C = Incomplete**: Motor function is preserved below the neurological level, and more than half of key muscles below the neurological level have a muscle grade less than 3.

☐ **D = Incomplete**: Motor function is preserved below the neurological level, and at least half of key muscles below the neurological level have a muscle grade of 3 or more.

☐ **E = Normal**: Motor and sensory function are normal.

CLINICAL SYNDROMES (OPTIONAL)

☐ Central Cord
☐ Brown-Sequard
☐ Anterior Cord
☐ Conus Medullaris
☐ Cauda Equina

STEPS IN CLASSIFICATION

The following order is recommended in determining the classification of individuals with SCI.

1. Determine sensory levels for right and left sides.

2. Determine motor levels for right and left sides.
   Note: in regions where there is no myotome to test, the motor level is presumed to be the same as the sensory level.

3. Determine the single neurological level.
   This is the lowest segment where motor and sensory function is normal on both sides, and is the most cephalad of the sensory and motor levels determined in steps 1 and 2.

4. Determine whether the injury is Complete or Incomplete (sacral sparing).
   *If voluntary anal contraction = **No** AND all S4-5 sensory scores = **0** AND any anal sensation = **No**, then injury is COMPLETE. Otherwise injury is incomplete.*

5. Determine ASIA Impairment Scale (AIS) Grade:

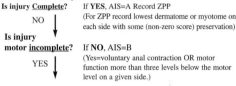

Is injury **Complete**?   If YES, AIS=A Record ZPP
   NO   (For ZPP record lowest dermatome or myotome on each side with some (non-zero score) preservation)

Is injury
motor **incomplete**?   If **NO**, AIS=B
   YES   (Yes=voluntary anal contraction OR motor function more than three levels below the motor level on a given side.)

Are at least half of the key muscles below the (single) neurological level graded 3 or better?

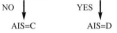

NO   YES

AIS=C   AIS=D

If sensation and motor function is normal in all segments, AIS=E
Note: AIS E is used in follow up testing when an individual with a documented SCI has recovered normal function. If at initial testing no deficits are found, the individual is neurologically intact; the ASIA Impairment Scale does not apply.

FIGURE 1-8, cont'd   American Spinal Injury Association (ASIA) Standard Neurological Classification of Spinal Cord Injury. (Courtesy American Spinal Injury Association, Atlanta, GA, 2006.)

INCOMPLETE SPINAL CORD INJURY

Different clinical syndromes of SCI are frequently referred to by clinicians and in the literature, including central cord, Brown-Sequard, anterior cord, conus medullaris, and cauda equina syndromes. In general, these syndromes do not accurately describe the extent of the neurological deficit (Table 1-1).

Central Cord Syndrome

The most common of the incomplete syndromes is central cord syndrome (CCS). CCS is characterized by motor weakness in the upper limbs greater than the lower limbs, in association with sacral sparing. In addition to the motor weakness, other features include bladder dysfunction and varying sensory loss below the level of the lesion. In his original description, Schneider and others[14] noted that the etiologic factor was hyperextension with simultaneous compression of the cord by anterior osteophytes and posterior impingement caused by buckling of the ligamentum flavum. Although CCS most frequently occurs in older adults with cervical spondylosis with hyperextension injuries, the syndrome may occur in individuals of any age and is associated with other etiologies, predisposing factors, and injury mechanisms. The pathology of central cord syndrome is commonly believed to result from an injury that primarily affects the center of the spinal cord. Depending on the degree and severity of the lesion, there may be paralysis of both the upper and lower limbs, with relatively more involvement of the upper limbs. This is due to the proposed lamination of the fibers in the corticospinal tract, with the cervical fibers most centrally located in relation to the thoracic, lumbar, and sacral fibers.[13,14] Others have not, however, found this lamination to exist in humans.[15,16] Quencer et al,[17] in a study that used magnetic resonance imaging (MRI) and pathological observations, found that CCS is predominantly a white matter peripheral injury and that intramedullary hemorrhage is not a common feature. Central cord syndrome generally has a favorable prognosis.[18-21] The typical pattern of recovery usually occurs earliest and to the greatest extent in the lower limbs, followed by bladder function, upper limb (proximal), and intrinsic hand function. Although there is a reported generally good outcome for persons with CCS, the prognosis for functional recovery should consider the patient's age, with a less optimistic prognosis in older relative to younger patients.[20] Specifically, younger people (less than 50 years of age) are more successful in becoming independent in ambulation than are older adults (97% versus 41%). Similar differences are seen between the younger and older patients in independent bladder function (83% versus 29%), independent bowel function (63% versus 24%), and dressing (77% versus 12%).[20] All patients, regardless of age, whose injuries initially are classified as ASIA D within 72 hours, are usually able to regain ambulatory function.[21]

Classification of Spinal Cord Injury

The following steps should be followed to classify a patient's SCI:
- Perform sensory examination in 28 dermatomes bilaterally for pinprick and light touch including S4-S5 dermatome and test for anal sensation
- Determine sensory level (right and left) and total sensory score
- Perform motor examination in the 10 key muscle groups including anal contraction
- Determine motor level (right and left) and motor index score
- Determine NLI
- Classify injury as complete or incomplete
- Categorize according to the ASIA Impairment Scale (see Box 1-4)
- Determine zone of partial preservation if ASIA A

BOX 1-4 | ASIA Impairment Scale

A = Complete: No motor or sensory function is preserved in the sacral segments S4-S5.
B = Incomplete: Sensory but not motor function is preserved below the neurological level and includes the sacral segments S4-S5.
C = Incomplete: Motor function is preserved below the neurological level, and more than half of key muscles below the neurological level have a muscle grade less than 3.
D = Incomplete: Motor function is preserved below the neurological level, and at least half of key muscles below the neurological level have a muscle grade of 3 or more.
E = Normal: Motor and sensory function are normal.

American Spinal Injury Association (ASIA) Standard Neurological Classification of Spinal Cord Injury. (Courtesy American Spinal Injury Association, Atlanta, GA, 2006.)

TABLE 1-1 | Incomplete Clinical Syndromes

Syndrome Recovery	Main Symptoms	Prognosis
Central cord	Greater weakness in the upper limbs than in the lower limbs Occurs almost exclusively in the cervical region Frequently seen in older adults and those with cervical stenosis	Favorable prognosis for walking and activities of daily living on the basis of age (<50 years old greater improvement than >50 years) Recovery occurs earliest in legs, followed by bladder, then proximal upper extremity muscles, and intrinsics last
Brown-Sequard	Greater ipsilateral proprioceptive and motor loss and contralateral loss of sensitivity to pain and temperature	Best prognosis for ambulation Recovery starts in ipsilateral proximal extensors then the distal flexors
Anterior cord	Variable loss of motor function and pain and temperature, while preserving proprioception	Poor prognosis for recovery of lower limb function and ambulation
Cauda equina	Injury to the lumbosacral nerve roots resulting in an areflexic bladder, bowel, and lower limbs	A lower motor neuron injury Regrowth is possible, but better prognosis for proximal muscles
Conus medullaris	Injury of the sacral cord and lumbar nerve roots Sacral segments may show preserved reflexes (e.g., bulbocavernosus with high conus lesions) Results in areflexic bladder, bowel, and lower limbs with a low lesion	As above Depends on the level of injury to the conus

Data from Kirshblum S, O'Connor K: Levels of injury and outcome in traumatic spinal cord injury, *Phys Med Rehabil Clin North Am* 11:1-27, 2000.

Brown-Sequard Syndrome

Brown-Sequard syndrome (BSS) consists of asymmetric paresis with hypalgesia more marked on the less paretic side. It accounts for 2% to 4% of all traumatic SCIs.[22-24] In the classical presentation, BSS consists of the following:
- Ipsilateral loss of all sensory modalities **at** the level of the lesion
- Ipsilateral flaccid paralysis **at** the level of the lesion
- Ipsilateral loss of position sense and vibration **below** the lesion
- Contralateral loss of pain and temperature **below** the lesion
- Ipsilateral motor loss **below** the level of the lesion

Neuroanatomically, this is explained by the crossing of the spinothalamic tracts, which carry pain and temperature fibers, in the spinal cord, as opposed to the corticospinal (i.e., motor tract fibers) and dorsal columns (i.e., light touch), which cross for the most part in the brainstem.

Only a limited number of patients have the pure form of BSS; Brown-Sequard plus syndrome (BSPS) is much more common.[25] BSPS refers to a relative ipsilateral hemiplegia with a relative contralateral hemianalgesia. Although BSS has traditionally been associated with knife injuries, stab wounds are rarely the cause of BSPS. A variety of etiologies, including those that result in closed spinal injuries with or without vertebral fractures may be the cause.

Despite the variation in presentation, considerable consistency is found in the prognosis of BSS. Recovery takes place in the ipsilateral proximal extensors and then the distal flexors.[26,27] Motor recovery of any limb having a pain and temperature sensory deficit occurs before the opposite limb and these patients may expect voluntary motion, strength, and functional gait recovery by 6 months.

Overall, patients with BSS have the best prognosis for functional outcome. Many patients ambulate independently at discharge from rehabilitation (75%) and nearly 70% perform functional skills and activities of daily living independently.[25] The most important predictor of function is whether the upper or lower limb is the predominant site of weakness: when the upper limb is weaker than the lower limb, patients are more likely to ambulate at discharge. Recovery of bowel and bladder function is also favorable, with continent bladder and bowel function achieved in 89% and 82%, respectively.[25]

TABLE 1-2 | **Comparison of Epiconus, Conus Medullaris, and Cauda Equina Lesions**

Symptom	Epiconus	Conus Medullaris	Cauda Equina
Pain	Uncommon	Uncommon	Very common and may be severe
Bowel and bladder reflexes	Present	Absent	Absent
Anal and BC reflex	Present	Absent*	Absent
Muscle tone	Increased	†	Decreased
MSRs	Increased‡	†	Decreased
Symmetry of weakness	Yes	Yes	No
Sensation	In dermatomal distribution	Absent in saddle distribution and may be dissociated	In root distribution
Recovery prognosis	Limited	Limited	Possible

Data from Kirshblum S, Donovan WH: Neurological assessment and classification of traumatic spinal cord injury. In Kirshblum S, Campagnolo DI, DeLisa JA, editors: *Spinal cord medicine,* pp. 82-95, Philadelphia, 2002, Lippincott Williams & Wilkins.
*Unless a high conus lesion.
†Depends on whether nerve roots are affected. If so, then is decreased.
‡Ankle plantarflexors and hamstrings, not knee jerks.
BC, Bulbocavernosus; *MSR,* muscle stretch reflexes.

Anterior Cord Syndrome

Anterior cord syndrome involves a lesion affecting the anterior two thirds of the spinal cord while preserving the posterior columns. This may occur with retropulsed disc or bone fragments,[28] direct injury to the anterior spinal cord, or with lesions of the anterior spinal artery, which provides the blood supply to the anterior spinal cord.[29] Lesions of the anterior spinal artery may result from diseases of the aorta, cardiac or aortic surgery, embolism, polyarteritis nodosa, or after an angioplasty. There is a variable loss of motor and pinprick sensation with a relative preservation of light touch, proprioception, and deep pressure sensation. Usually patients with an anterior cord syndrome have only a 10% to 20% chance of muscle recovery, and even in those with some recovery there is poor muscle power and coordination.[30]

Conus Medullaris and Cauda Equina Injuries

The conus medullaris, which is the terminal segment of the adult spinal cord, lies at the inferior aspect of the L1 vertebrae. The segment above the conus medullaris is termed the epiconus, consisting of spinal cord segments L4 to S1. Nerve roots then travel from the conus medullaris caudal as the cauda equina.

Lesions of the epiconus will affect the lower lumbar roots supplying muscles of the lower part of the leg and foot, with sparing of sacral segments. The bulbocavernosus reflex and micturition reflexes are preserved, representing a UMN lesion. Spasticity will most likely develop in sacral innervated segments including the toe flexors, ankle plantar flexors, and hamstring muscles. Recovery is similar to other UMN SCIs.

The conus medullaris consists of neural segments S2 and below. Injuries to the conus will present with LMN deficits of the anal sphincter and bladder as a result of damage to the anterior horn cells of S2 to S4. Bladder and rectal reflexes are diminished or absent, depending on the exact level of the lesion. Motor strength in the legs and feet may remain intact if the nerve roots (L3 to S2) are not affected. The lumbar nerve roots may be spared partially or totally in the conus medullaris; this is referred to as root escape. If the roots are affected as they travel with the sacral cord in the spinal column, this will result in LMN damage with diminished reflexes. In low conus lesions,

the S1 segment is not involved and therefore the ankle jerks are normal, a finding accounting for most instances of failure to make the diagnosis. Because of the small size of the conus medullaris, lesions are more likely to be bilateral compared with those of the cauda equina. With conus medullaris lesions, recovery is limited.

Injuries below the L1 vertebral level do not cause injury to the spinal cord but rather to the cauda equina or nerve roots supplying the lumbar and sacral segments of the skin and muscle groups. This usually produces motor weakness and atrophy of the lower limbs (L2 to S2) with bowel and bladder involvement (S2 to S4) and areflexia of the ankle and plantar reflexes. Often the patient may have spared sensation in the perineum or lower limbs but complete paralysis. In cauda injuries there is loss of anal and bulbocavernosus reflexes and impotence.

There is consensus that cauda equina injuries have a much better prognosis for recovery than other SCI syndromes. This is most likely because the nerve roots are more resilient to injury and because many of the biochemical processes that occur in the spinal cord and produce secondary damage occur to a much lesser extent in the nerve roots. Progressive recovery may occur over a course of weeks and months.

Separation of cauda equina and conus lesions in clinical practice is difficult because the clinical features of these lesions overlap. Isolated conus lesions are rare because the roots forming the cauda equina are wrapped around the conus. The conus may be affected by a fracture of L1, whereas a fracture of L2 or lower can impinge on the cauda equina. Sacral fractures and fractures of the pelvic ring also frequently damage the cauda equina. Bullet wounds can penetrate the bony structures to traumatize the cauda equina and conus. Differences between these lesions are outlined in Table 1-2.

PROGNOSIS FOR RECOVERY AND PREDICTION OF OUTCOME

The physical examination is the most important component in determining future neurological improvement after injury. After classification of the patient's injury is made, prognostication early after the injury can be determined. There are a number of clinical methods to assist in prognosticating neurological recovery after

BOX 1-5 | **Prognostic Indicators of Complete Tetraplegia**

- From 1 week to 1 year after injury, 30% to 80% of patients will regain one motor level
- Initial strength of the muscle is a significant predictor of its rate of recovery and its prognosis for achieving antigravity strength
- The faster an initially 0/5 muscle starts to recover some strength, the greater the prognosis for recovery
- Most upper limb recovery occurs during the first 6 months, with the greatest rate of change during the first 3 months
- Most patients with some initial strength plateau earlier but at a higher level than patients who are initially 0/5
- Motor recovery can continue with lesser gains seen in the second year, especially for patients with initial 0/5 strength

SCI, including the neurological examination and the use of radiological and electrodiagnostic tests.[31,32]

The most important determinant of recovery is whether the person has a neurological complete or incomplete injury as determined by the neurological examination. Other key determinants on examination include the initial level of injury, the initial strength of the muscles, and the age of the individual. Box 1-5 lists some generalizations regarding prognostication based on an early examination.

Individuals with a motor complete injury will usually regain one motor level of recovery by 1 year after injury. Recovery of strength is greater and earlier in those patients with some initial motor strength immediately caudal to the level of injury. The greater the initial strength of the muscle, the faster the muscle will recover to strength of greater or equal to 3/5. Those with an initially incomplete injury have a better prognosis for future ambulation if there is motor sparing as opposed to sensory sparing only. For individuals with an initially sensory incomplete lesion, sparing of pinprick sensation may be a better predictor of functional ambulation at 1 year relative to those with light touch alone spared. Approximately 70% of individuals with a diagnosis of an incomplete cervical injury may regain the ability to ambulate at 1 year, with approximately 46% regaining the ability for community ambulation.

Recovery from injuries below the cervical spine, resulting in paraplegia, has not been studied to the degree of tetraplegia, but some of the generalizations regarding prediction of recovery is the same. In thoracic level and high lumbar level injuries (NLI above L2), the clinician can usually only test for sensory modality change to document an improvement in NLI because there are no corresponding key muscle groups between T1 and L2. The prognosis for regaining functional ambulation in people with complete paraplegia is 5%; however, the lower the level of injury, the greater the potential functional capability. Individuals with incomplete paraplegia have the best prognosis for ambulation. Eighty percent of individuals with incomplete paraplegia regain hip flexors and knee extensors at 1 year.

For the purposes of prognostication, MRI is the most superior of all radiological tests. A number of studies have related MRI findings to the neurological status and recovery after SCI and found that the degree and type of MRI change correlates with the severity and prognosis of the injury. A hemorrhage displayed on the initial MRI correlates with the poorest prognosis, followed by contusion, and edema. A normal study (no MRI abnormality) correlates with the best prognosis. If a hemorrhage is initially seen, this usually suggests a complete injury. If a hemorrhage is present in patients with an incomplete injury, those patients usually have less chance of recovery relative to patients with other MRI findings. If no hemorrhage is seen on the initial MRI, those patients will most likely have an incomplete lesion and have a significantly better prognosis for motor recovery in the upper and lower limbs as well as improvement in the ASIA Impairment Scale classification. The degree and extent of cord edema on MRI has an inversely proportional effect as a prognostic indicator for initial impairment level and future recovery. If the edema involves multiple levels, there is a poorer prognosis and a greater chance of having a complete lesion. In general, MRI can be used to augment the physical examination in prognosticating recovery of patients with a cervical SCI; however, by itself it is not as accurate a predictor as the physical examination.

There are a number of electrophysiological tests that have been used in the acute period after SCI to assess the level and severity of the SCI and to prognosticate neurological and functional outcomes. Techniques include nerve conduction studies, late responses (H-reflex and F-wave), somatosensory evoked potentials, motor evoked potentials, and sympathetic skin responses, all of which can supplement clinical and neuroradiological examinations.[32] These tests, however, are most useful in differentiating lesions of the central and peripheral nervous system and in uncooperative or unconscious patients because they do not require the cooperation of the patient. They are not recommended as a routine part of the acute workup of a newly injured individual to offer prognosis for neurological or functional outcome.

PHARMACOLOGICAL AND SURGICAL INTERVENTIONS TO ENHANCE RECOVERY AND REGENERATION

After the initial injury, numerous changes occur within the spinal cord that hinder return of function.

Table 1-3 lists areas of research in each of the categories of treatment after SCI. The text summarizes recently completed trials, trials currently in progress, or human clinical trials planned for the near future.

Over the last few decades there have been a number of pharmacological strategies in the initial treatment of SCI to enhance recovery. Methylprednisolone (MP) was initially studied in the National Acute Spinal Cord Injury Study (NASCIS) I, which randomized patients into high- versus low-dose regimens.[33] No statistical difference in neurological or functional outcome was found between the two regimens at 6 months or 1 year; however, the high dose used was below the theoretical therapeutic threshold. The NASCIS II study randomized patients with acute SCI into placebo, high MP, and naloxone treatment groups.[34] Patients with penetrating wounds and cauda equina injuries were excluded. This study found that MP given within 8 hours after the injury (30 mg/kg bolus and 5.4 mg/kg/hour for 23 hours) improved neurological recovery at 6 weeks, 6 months, and 1 year, although functional recovery was not clearly studied. Patients treated after 8 hours demonstrated

TABLE 1-3 | Overview of Spinal Cord Injury Research

Category of Treatment	Areas of Research
Protection	Previously studied: Methylprednisolone, naloxone, calcium channel blockers, GM-1
	Present and future studies: Minocycline, erythropoietin, riluzole, sulfonylureas, hyperdynamic therapy, and CSF drainage
Stimulating axonal growth	Electrical stimulation (oscillating field stimulator [OFS], IN-1 (Nogo-blocking antibody), MAG (myelin-associated glycoprotein), OMgp (oligodendrocyte myelin glycoprotein), Rho inhibitors (e.g., BA-210 [Cethrin]), activated macrophages, chondroitin sulfate proteoglycans (CSPGs), inosine, heparan sulfate proteoglycans (HSPGs), keratan sulfate proteoglycans (KSPGs), nerve growth factors, estrogen and serotonin selective reuptake inhibitors
Bridging	Peripheral nerve grafts, Schwann cells, olfactory ensheathing glial cells, nanotubes
Enhancing axonal transmission	Schwann cells, olfactory ensheathing glial cells, 4-aminopyridine, HP-184, neuroprogenitor cell transplants (stem cells)
Rehabilitation	Electrical stimulation, weight supported ambulation

no beneficial effect. Although the initial report of NASCIS II indicated no beneficial effects of naloxone, a subsequent report found that patients with incomplete lesions treated with naloxone within 8 hours had significantly greater recovery than patients treated with placebo.[35] One of the keys to NASCIS II was the evidence that medication may improve neural recovery, thus indicating that secondary injury (i.e., injury occurring after the initial trauma to the cord) occurs. Mechanisms of action for MP include improving blood flow to the spinal cord, preventing lipid peroxidation, being a free radical scavenger, and having anti-inflammatory function.

NASCIS III randomized patients into 24- or 48-hour treatment with MP or tirilazad mesylate.[36] Tirilazad is a potent steroid with no glucocorticoid effect, thus offering the positive effects of MP (e.g., lipid peroxidation and antioxidant activity) without the side effects. This study concluded that patients treated within 3 hours of the injury should receive 24 hours of steroids and those treated between 3 to 8 hours after injury should receive 48 hours of treatment. This newer protocol using 48 hours of treatment has not been universally accepted, and there are a number of recent reports that question the current routine use of steroids.[37-39]

GM-1 ganglioside (Sygen) is present in high concentrations in the central nervous system (CNS) and forms the major component of cell membranes. It is thought that GM-1 ganglioside can augment neurite outgrowth and decrease CNS tissue damage, prevent glutamate-induced neuronal excitotoxicity, and stimulate and preserve protein kinases. An initial small study treating patients within 48 hours of injury for an average of 26 days found greater mean recovery at 1 year including some improved recovery in muscles with no strength at entry of the study.[40] A subsequent large multicenter study reported a trend toward improvement in neurological recovery in ASIA B individuals at 26 weeks after being treated for 8 weeks and a significant effect in individuals who received GM-1 ganglioside but who did not have surgery relative to those who did have surgery and did not receive GM-1 ganglioside. No significant effect was noted at the principal end point of 26 weeks in the total group of patients studied.[41]

A medication trial was performed for subjects with chronic incomplete spinal cord injury with fampridine-SR, a long-acting formulation of 4-aminopyridine (4-AP). 4-AP is a potassium (K^+) channel blocker that blocks fast internodal axonal K^+, which blocks conduction of the nerve action potentials.

Preliminary work in SCI (Phase II studies) showed trends toward improvement in pain and spasticity.[42-44] Phase III multicenter trials were completed but did not show significant results, although there were improvements in multiple sclerosis trials and further study is currently underway.

A Phase II trial was also performed with HP-184. This medication is a potassium (K^+) and sodium (Na^+) channel blocker that in a Phase I trial in 48 subjects with chronic incomplete SCI resulted in increased motor index scores.[45] The Phase II trial recruited 240 subjects with chronic incomplete SCI (ASIA C, D) with injury levels C4-T10. Outcome measures include motor index score and gait improvement. Results have not been published to date.

The study with ProCord (activated macrophages) (Proneuron Biotechnologies, Ness-Ziona, Israel) was an international multicenter trial for individuals with an acute neurologically complete SCI (ASIA A). The basis of this study was to impose an appropriate inflammatory response encouraging a self-operating chain of reactions needed for spinal cord regeneration and regrowth. Macrophages isolated from the patient's own blood were activated through Proneuron's proprietary process and then injected directly into the patient's injured spinal cord by day 14 after injury. In a Phase I trial in Israel initiated in 2000, five of 16 subjects showed an AIS improvement from ASIA A to incomplete status, with three subjects to ASIA C and two to ASIA B by 1 year.[46] The Phase II trial, however, was halted because of financial restraints after approximately two thirds of the subjects were recruited. Results should be forthcoming.

A Phase 1 clinical trial was performed on 10 subjects with oscillating field electrical stimulation (OFS) for individuals with a neurologically complete SCI. Their levels of injury were between C5 and T10, with no evidence of cord transection demonstrated on MRI. Implantation of the OFS was within 18 days of the injury and the subjects underwent evaluation every 2 weeks after implantation; the unit was removed at 15 weeks. At 1 year, their degree of pain as measured by the visual analog scale pain score was decreased, with improvement noted in light touch and pinprick sensation and some muscle strength improvement as well.[47] The use of OFS treatment in patients with acute SCI was found to be safe and perhaps efficacious, and the Food and Drug Administration has given permission for enrollment of 10 additional acutely injured patients. Further results and clinical trials in this area are expected.

A recently initiated trial is using BA-210 (Cethrin), a Rho pathway antagonist that may promote neuroregeneration and neuroprotection in the CNS. This is applied to the surface of the dura mater of the spinal cord together with a fibrin sealant normally used to repair small dural tears, within 7 days of injury. The study is being performed in a number of centers in the United States and Canada for individuals with a neurologically complete SCI. Minocycline, a semisynthetic tetracycline antibiotic, showed good improvement in hind limb function and strength in animal model studies, and human trials have begun.[48]

A number of surgical procedures using either fetal stem cells (Huang in China) or adult olfactory cell transplants (Lima in Portugal) are being performed. Although Huang has reported some results,[49] this was not a prospective research project and many questions remain regarding these results. Additional results are pending from these surgical approaches.[50]

There has been great excitement within the field of SCI medicine regarding research that has moved from the laboratory to human clinical trials. Despite the excitement with respect to cure and the optimism regarding the development of therapies, at present no pharmacological, surgical, or rehabilitative therapy exists that can cure all of the impairments caused by the injury. Most likely a combination of the above mentioned treatments will be required to address the complex issues of SCI. Further study is required to not only find treatments to enhance neurological and functional recovery but also to decrease medical complications and optimize the quality of lives of persons with SCI.

SUMMARY

While the overall incidence of traumatic spinal cord injury has remained relatively stable, there has been a change in the epidemiology of SCI. Although MVCs remain the primary cause of SCI, falls rank second, primarily among older adults, and injury related to violence, most often seen in young men, is third. There also is a recent trend toward an increased number of incomplete lesions, possibly the result of changes in etiology and improved treatment at the site of injury by emergency medical technicians and subsequent immediate care.

Understanding the neurological anatomy of the spinal cord is essential to comprehension of the mechanisms of SCI. In addition, knowledge of the autonomic nervous system anatomy and function is critical to appreciation of the impairments of the multiple body systems that it controls.

Classification of an SCI enables the determination of impairment and helps prognosticate outcomes and plan for the patient's ongoing needs. The ASIA examination is the standard neurological examination for SCI and is used to determine the neurological level of injury, the motor impairment scale, the sensory impairments, and the zone of partial preservation. There are several types of incomplete injuries and classification of these types also aids in determining outcomes. Clinical mastery of methods for prognosis of functional recovery is important to give the patient a realistic picture of his future. In the acute stages after injury, however, patients and their families may focus completely on this information and every attempt must be made to avoid depleting all hope of recovery.

Finally, some completed and new clinical trials concentrating on spinal cord injury cure and recovery are reviewed. Research is constantly changing as new technologies in the basic and clinical sciences emerge. Thus, the field of rehabilitation must continue to build and maintain the physical capacity of individuals with SCI so that when a cure becomes available their body systems will be in optimal condition.

REFERENCES

1. Guttman L: *Spinal cord injuries: comprehensive management and research*, Oxford, 1973, Blackwell Scientific Publications.
2. Spinal cord injury: facts and figures at a glance, *J Spinal Cord Med* 28:379-380, 2005.
3. Go BK, DeVivo MJ, Richards JS: The epidemiology of spinal cord injury. In Stover SL, DeLisa JA, Whiteneck GG, editors: *Spinal cord injury: clinical outcomes from the model systems*, Gaithersburg, MD, 1995, Aspen Publishers.
4. DeVivo MJ: Epidemiology of traumatic spinal cord injury. In Kirshblum S, Campagnolo DI, DeLisa JA, editors: *Spinal cord medicine*, Philadelphia, 2002, Lippincott Williams & Wilkins.
5. Sapru HN: Spinal cord: anatomy, physiology and pathophysiology. In Kirshblum S, Campagnolo DI, DeLisa JA, editors: *Spinal cord medicine*, Philadelphia, 2002, Lippincott Williams & Wilkins.
6. American Spinal Injury Association and International Spinal Cord Society: *International standards for neurological classification of spinal cord injury*, ed 6, Chicago, IL, 2006, ASIA and ISCS.
7. Kirshblum S, Donovan W: Neurological assessment and classification of traumatic spinal cord injury. In Kirshblum S, Campagnolo DI, DeLisa JA, editors: *Spinal cord medicine*, Philadelphia, 2002, Lippincott Williams & Wilkins.
8. Welch RD, Lobley SJ, O'Sullivan SB, et al: Functional independence in quadraplegia: critical levels, *Arch Phys Med Rehabil* 67:235-240, 1986.
9. Marino RJ, Rider-Foster D, Maissel G, et al: Superiority of motor level over single neurological level in categorizing tetraplegia, *Paraplegia* 33:510-513, 1995.
10. Frankel HL, Hancock DO, Hyslop G, et al: The value of postural reduction in initial management of closed injuries of the spine with paraplegia and tetraplegia, I, *Paraplegia* 7:179-192, 1969.
11. American Spinal Injury Association: *International standards for neurological and functional classification of spinal cord injury patients* [revised)] Chicago, IL, 1992, ASIA.
12. American Spinal Injury Association: *International standards for neurological and functional classification of spinal cord injury patients*, Chicago, IL, 1996, ASIA.
13. Schneider RC, Cherry GR, Patek H: The syndrome of acute central cervical spinal cord injury; with special reference to mechanisms involved in hyperextension injuries of cervical spine, *J Neurosurg* 11:546-577, 1954.
14. Foerster O: Symptomatologie der erkrankungen des Ruclenmarks und seiner surzeln. *Handbook Neurol* 5:1-403, 1936.
15. Nathan PW, Smith MC: Long descending tracts in man, I: review of present knowledge, *Brain* 78:248-303, 1955.
16. Hopkins A, Rudge P: Hyperpathia in the central cervical cord syndrome, *J Neurol Neurosurg Psychiatry* 36:637-642, 1973.
17. Quencer RM, Bunge RP, Egnor M, et al: Acute traumatic central cord syndrome: MRI pathological correlations, *Neuroradiology* 34:85-94, 1992.
18. Roth EJ, Lawler MH, Yarkony GM: Traumatic central cord syndrome: clinical features and functional outcomes, *Arch Phys Med Rehabil* 71:18-23, 1990.

19. Merriam WF, Taylor TK, Ruff SJ, et al: A reappraisal of acute traumatic central cord syndrome, *J Bone Joint Surg Br* 68:708-13, 1986.

20. Penrod LE, Hegde SK, Ditunno JF: Age effect on prognosis for functional recovery in acute, traumatic central cord syndrome, *Arch Phys Med Rehabil* 71:963-8, 1990.

21. Burns SP, Golding DG, Rolle WA Jr, et al: Recovery of ambulation in motor- incomplete tetraplegia, *Arch Phys Med Rehabil* 78: 1169-1172, 1997.

22. Brown-Sequard CE: Lectures on the physiology and pathology of the central nervous system and the treatment of organic nervous affections, *Lancet* 2:593-595, 659-662, 755-757, 821-823, 1868.

23. Bohlman HH: Acute fractures and dislocations of the cervical spine: an analysis of three hundred hospitalized patients and review of the literature, *J Bone Joint Surg Am* 61:1119-1142, 1979.

24. Bosch A, Stauffer ES, Nickel VL: Incomplete traumatic quadraplegia: a ten-year review, *JAMA* 216:473-478, 1971.

25. Roth EJ, Park T, Pang T, et al: Traumatic cervical Brown-Sequard and Brown-Sequard-plus syndromes: the spectrum of presentations and outcomes, *Paraplegia* 29:582-589, 1991.

26. Little JW, Halar E: Temporal course of motor recovery after Brown-Sequard spinal cord injuries, *Paraplegia* 23:39-46, 1985.

27. Graziani V, Tessler A, Ditunno JF: Incomplete tetraplegia: sequence of lower extremity motor recovery, *J Neurotrauma* 12:121, 1995.

28. Bauer RD, Errico TJ: Cervical spine injuries. In Errico TJ, Bauer RD, Waugh T, editors: *Spinal trauma*, Philadelphia, 1991, JB Lippincott.

29. Cheshire WP, Santos CC, Massey EW, et al: Spinal cord infarction: etiology and outcome, *Neurology* 47:321-330, 1996.

30. Bohlman HH, Ducker TB: Spine and spinal cord injuries. In Rothman RH, Simeone FA, editors: *The spine*, ed 3, Philadelphia, 1992, WB Saunders.

31. Kirshblum SC, O'Connor KC: Levels of spinal cord injury and predictors of neurologic recovery, *Phys Med Rehabil Clin North Am* 11:1-27, 2000.

32. Ditunno JF, Flanders AE, Kirshblum S, et al: Predicting outcomes in traumatic spinal cord injury. In Kirshblum S, Campagnolo DI, DeLisa JA, editors: *Spinal cord medicine*, Philadelphia, 2002, Lippincott Williams & Wilkins.

33. Bracken MB, Collins WF, Freeman DF et al: Efficacy of methylprednisolone in acute spinal cord injury, *JAMA* 251:45-52, 1984.

34. Bracken MB, Shephard MJ, Collins WF et al: A randomized, controlled trial of methylprednisolone or naloxone in the treatment of acute spinal-cord injury: results of the Second National Acute Spinal Cord Injury Study, *N Engl J Med* 322:1405-1141, 1990.

35. Bracken MB, Holford TR: Effect of timing of methylprednisolone or nalaxone administration on recovery of segmental and long-tract neurological function in NASCIS 2, *J Neurosurg* 79:500-507, 1993.

36. Bracken MB, Shephard MJ, Holford TR, et al: Administration of methylprednisolone for 24 or 48 hours or tirilizad mesylate for 48 hours in the treatment of acute spinal cord injury: results of the Third National Acute Spinal Cord Injury Randomized Controlled Trial, National Acute Spinal Cord Injury Study, *JAMA* 277:1597-1604, 1997.

37. Nesathurai S: Steroids and spinal cord injury: revisiting the NASCIS 2 and 3 trials, *J Trauma* 45:1088-1093, 1998.

38. Short DJ, El Masry WS, Jones FW: High dose methylprednisolone in the management of acute spinal cord injury—a systematic review from a clinical perspective, *Spinal Cord* 38:278-286, 2000.

39. Hurlbert RJ: The role of steroids in acute spinal cord injury: an evidenced-based analysis [review], *Spine* 26(24 Suppl):S39-S46, 2001.

40. Geisler FH, Dorsey FC, Coleman WP: Recovery of motor function after spinal-cord injury: a randomized, placebo-controlled trial with GM-1 ganglioside, *N Engl J Med* 324:1829-1838, 1991.

41. Fehlings MG, Bracken MB: Summary statement: the Sygen (GM-1 ganglioside) clinical trial in acute spinal cord injury, *Spine* 26(24 Suppl):S99-S100, 2001.

42. Segal JL, Brunnemann SR. 4-Aminopyridine alters gait characteristics and enhances locomotion in spinal cord injured humans, *J Spinal Cord Med* 21:200-204, 1998.

43. Davis FA, Stefoski D, Rush J: Orally administered 4-aminopyridine improves clinical signs in multiple sclerosis, *Ann Neurol* 27: 186-192, 1990.

44. Segal JL, Brunnemann SR: 4-Aminopyridine improves pulmonary function in quadriplegic humans with longstanding spinal cord injury, *Pharmacotherapy* 17:415-423, 1997.

45. Gorman P, Mody V, Jariwala N, et al: Safety and tolerability of HP 184, an oral sodium and potassium channel blocker, in chronic incomplete SCI: a phase II study, *J Spinal Cord Med* 27:165, 2004.

46. Baptiste DC, Fehlings MG: Pharmacological approaches to repair the injured spinal cord, *J Neurotrauma* 23:318-334, 2006.

47. Shapiro S, Borgens R, Pascuzzi R et al: Oscillating field stimulation for complete spinal cord injury in humans: a phase 1 trial, *J Neurosurg Spine* 2:3-10, 2005.

48. Festoff BW, Ameenuddin S, Arnold PM: Minocycline neuroprotects, reduces microgliosis, and inhibits caspase protease expression early after spinal cord injury, *J Neurochem* 97:1314-1326, 2006.

49. Huang H, Chen L, Wang H, et al: Influence of patients age on functional recovery after transplantation of olfactory ensheathing cells into injured spinal cord injury, *Chin Med J (Engl)* 116:1488-1491, 2003.

50. Lima C, Protas-Vital J, Escada P et al: Olfactory mucosa autografts in human spinal cord injury: a pilot clinical trial, *J Spinal Cord Med* 29:191-203, 2006.

CHAPTER TWO

Medical Management and Complications of Spinal Cord Injury

Steven Kirshblum, MD

Due to my spinal cord injury I suffered severe spasticity, for which I was treated with many different medications to try and control the spasms. After months of trial and error, my doctor introduced the idea of the Baclofen Pump. I had it implanted and to great success I now live virtually spasm free allowing me to perform daily activities such as transfers, driving a van, and working.

John (C6 SCI)

The primary goals for management of a person who has had an acute spinal cord injury (SCI) include saving the individual's life, minimizing the neurological damage, stabilizing the spine, and preventing secondary medical complications. When the injury occurs, emergency medical personnel initially secure spinal immobilization by placing the patient supine on a spinal board with straps, immobilizing the entire spine from the skull to the sacrum. Spinal traction should not be applied until the specific diagnosis of spinal injury is firmly established, that is, after completion of proper imaging studies of the entire spine at the hospital. If spinal stability and decompression of the nervous tissue cannot be obtained by nonsurgical means, surgery may be indicated.

SCI results in the dysfunction of multiple organ systems and, therefore, places the individual with SCI at high risk for medical complications, particularly during the acute phase after injury. If the early medical complications of SCI can be prevented, the rehabilitation course is facilitated, institutional lengths of stay are shortened, functional gains are greater, human suffering is reduced, and the total cost of medical care is decreased. Secondary medical complications after SCI may develop even in the finest institutions, but the incidence of these complications appears to be inversely related to the quality of care and the expertise available. Premorbid clinical conditions may place the patient with acute SCI at higher risk for development of complications, which are more likely to occur in older individuals than in the young. Similarly, injuries sustained to body parts other than the spine make treatment more difficult and the development of secondary medical complications more likely. Frequently associated injuries include traumatic brain injury, contusion of the lungs and abdominal organs, rupture of major blood vessels, and fractures of the long bones of the extremities. Most patients with SCI require eventual admission to a short-term inpatient rehabilitation service. This should occur as soon as the spine has been stabilized and the medical condition does not require the continued monitoring and interventions of the intensive care unit.

It is important to review the primary differences in SCI diagnoses discussed in Chapter 1 before considering the various complications that may arise with treatment. Tetraplegia is defined as loss of motor or sensory function in the cervical segments of the spinal cord, impairing upper and lower limbs, the trunk, and function of the abdominal and pelvic organs. Individuals with lesions above C5 also will have compromised respiratory function. Paraplegia is defined as an impairment of motor or sensory function in the thoracic, lumbar, or sacral segments of the cord. With paraplegia, neurological function in the upper limbs is spared, but depending on the level of injury, the trunk, legs, and pelvic organs may be involved. In addition, a complete neurological injury is defined as the absence of sensory or motor function in the lowest sacral segments (i.e., no sacral sparing). An incomplete injury is defined as preservation of motor function or sensation below the neurological level of injury that includes the lowest sacral segments (i.e., sacral sparing). It is helpful to understand the motor capabilities and sensations mediated by each spinal cord level (Table 2-1).

This chapter focuses on spinal orthotics and medical complications that occur in the subacute and rehabilitation phases after SCI.

MANAGEMENT OF SPINAL STABILITY: SPINAL ORTHOSES

Spinal orthoses are commonly used after SCI to limit spinal movement, protect the spine during healing, and to provide mechanical unloading.[1-3] Numerous designs of spinal orthoses are available, providing different degrees of support to different segments of the spine. Few spinal orthoses provide complete immobilization of the spine, but in general, the longer and better fitting the orthosis, the greater its effectiveness. When an orthosis is used to protect the spine during healing of a fracture or postoperatively after a surgical fusion, it generally is worn for 10 to 12 weeks. To ensure that a patient's spinal stability is not compromised, there may be limitations placed on his ability to participate in certain functional activities (i.e., certain types of transfers or weight shifts, prone or high-level position changes, advanced wheelchair skills) while in an orthosis. It is important that these precautions are clearly communicated between the physician and treating therapists.

Two main biomechanical principles are used in the design of spinal orthoses. The orthosis must either provide counteractive horizontal forces through use of the three-point pressure system or create a longitudinal traction-distraction force. Different orthoses restrict spinal motions in different ways and to different degrees. Some primarily limit flexion and extension, whereas others restrict lateral flexion or rotation. Other designs provide unloading of the spinal segments through longitudinal traction. The success of spinal bracing depends on the goal of bracing and the ability of the chosen brace to serve that purpose.

Different nondescriptive eponyms are frequently used for orthotic devices. To reduce confusion, a descriptive nomenclature for orthotic devices was developed in which orthoses are named according to the body segments involved and the planes of movement restricted. Consequently, spinal orthoses include cervical orthoses (CO), head cervical orthoses (HCO), cervical thoracic orthoses (CTO), thoracolumbosacral orthoses (TLSO), lumbosacral orthoses (LSO), sacral orthoses, and cervical thoracolumbosacral orthoses (CTLSO).

TABLE 2-1	**Functional Abilities Associated with Complete Spinal Cord Injury at Various Levels**	
Level of Lesion	Motor Capability*	Intact Sensation
Brainstem	Facial, pharyngeal, laryngeal movements	Neck and head (cranial nerves from face; C2: posterior head, upper neck; C3: lower neck)
Above C4	Facial, pharyngeal, laryngeal movements	Neck and head (cranial nerves from face; C2: posterior head, upper neck; C3: lower neck)
C4	Scapular elevation, adduction	
C5	Deltoids, elbow flexion (C5, C6)	Lateral upper arm
C6	Pectoralis major, radial wrist extensors, serratus anterior	Lateral forearm and lateral hand
C7	Triceps (C7, C8), latissimus dorsi	Middle finger
C8	Flexor digitorum muscles	Medial hand
T1	Finger abduction	Medial forearm
T1 to T6	Erector spinae above the injury	T2: medial upper arm; T3 to T6: torso
T7 to T12	Abdominal muscles above the injury	T7 to T12: torso (T10: level of umbilicus)
L1	Psoas	Anterior upper thigh
L2	Iliacus	Mid thigh, below L1
L3	Quadriceps (L3, L4)	Anterior knee
L4	Tibialis anterior	Medial leg
L5	Extensor hallucis longus	Lateral leg, dorsum of foot
S1	Peroneus longus and brevis, triceps surae, hamstrings, gluteus maximus	Posterior calf and lateral foot
S2	—	Posterior thigh
S3	—	Ring surrounding S4 to S5
S4 to S5	Voluntary and contraction	Ring surrounding anus

From Lundy-Ekman L: *Neuroscience: fundamentals for rehabilitation*, Philadelphia. 2002, WB Saunders, Table 12-5, p 285.
*Each additional level adds functions to the capabilities of the higher levels. Muscles listed may be only partially innervated at the level indicated. Thus the quadriceps usually has some voluntary activity if the L3 level is intact; however, the action is weak unless the L4 level also is intact.

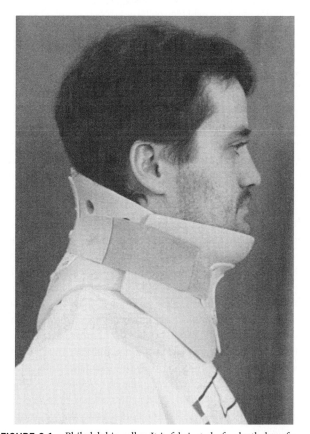

FIGURE 2-1 Philadelphia collar. It is fabricated of polyethylene foam with rigid anterior and posterior plastic strips and can be easily applied with Velcro closures. (From Umphred DA: *Neurological rehabilitation,* ed 4, St. Louis, 2001, Mosby, Figure 16-4, p 482.)

Cervical Orthoses

The simplest COs are soft cervical collars made of cloth or foam rubber. These are usually comfortable to wear and restrict neck motion primarily through sensory feedback rather than by mechanical restriction.[4] They have little indication for use in traumatic SCI. Other COs includes a more rigid collar, but this also does not offer enough immobilization for a traumatic injury. Prefabricated HCOs, made of various plastic materials in different designs to provide greater support and restriction, include the Philadelphia (Figure 2-1), Aspen, and Miami collars, and other collars with a similar design.[5] These collars are useful for some spinal immobilization but do not stabilize the spine. A good rule to remember is that any brace that can be taken off by the patient cannot offer stability for a traumatic spinal injury. HCOs are usually indicated for stable midcervical bony or ligamentous injuries or postoperatively when rigid control is no longer needed.

Poster cervical appliances are examples of CTOs, which usually consist of chin and occipital pieces that are connected by two to four adjustable metal uprights to sternal and back plates. Such devices provide greater restriction of neck motion than collars do. The sternal occipital mandibular immobilizer (SOMI) is lightweight and usually more comfortable because there are no posterior rods, making it easier to use in a patient who is bedridden. In addition, a headband that encircles the forehead can be used if the chin piece needs to be removed (e.g., during eating). The SOMI can be applied and easily fitted and provides substantial restriction of motion in the mid to low cervical region. Another type of CTO is a Yale orthosis, which is similar to an extended Philadelphia collar, thus increasing the restriction of motion.

Maximum immobilization of the cervical spine is obtained by application of head-cervical-thoracic orthoses, including the rigid

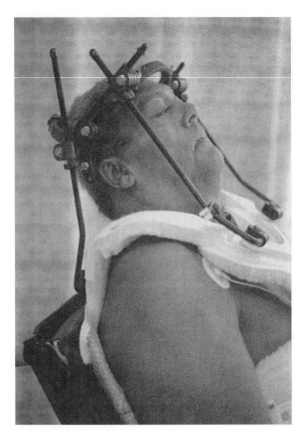

FIGURE 2-2   Halo vest. The basic components include the halo ring, distraction rods, and jacket. (From Umphred DA: *Neurological rehabilitation,* ed 4, St. Louis, 2001, Mosby, Figure 16-5, p 483.)

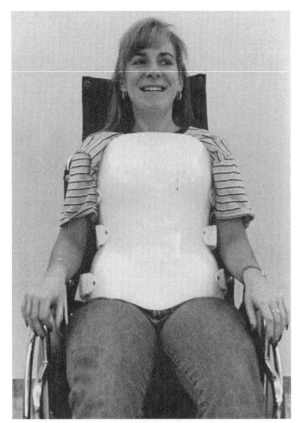

FIGURE 2-3   Custom thoracolumbosacral orthosis. This molded plastic body orthosis has a soft lining on the interior. It controls flexion, extension, and rotary movements until healing can occur. (From Umphred DA: *Neurological rehabilitation,* ed 4, St. Louis, 2001, Mosby, Figure 16-8, p 484.)

halo (Figure 2-2) and the semirigid Minerva orthosis. During the acute phase of cervical SCI, a halo orthosis is frequently applied for external support after a period of cervical traction or after surgical spinal fusion. Although the halo orthosis provides the maximum restriction of flexion and extension of the potentially unstable cervical spine, it does not guarantee maintenance of alignment and ultimate fusion. The halo consists of a halo ring, a vest, and upright posters. The ring is made of lightweight magnetic resonance imaging (MRI)–compatible metal and should be large enough to provide 1-cm clearance around the head.

The ring is placed approximately 1 cm above the ears and is tilted so that it is slightly higher anteriorly than posteriorly, placing the neck in slight extension. Four pins attach the ring to the head, two anterolaterally on the forehead and two posteriorly. To prevent infection, the pin sites should be cleaned twice daily with normal saline solution. The halo vest is made of prefabricated plastic material and lined with sheepskin or a soft fabric. The vest should fit the body well to prevent pressure ulcers and loss of spinal reduction. When the halo orthosis has been securely applied, the patient can usually get out of bed and participate in physical activities, either ambulatory or in a wheelchair. Most rehabilitation exercises do not seem to cause any greater motion to the spine than does daily motion and activity[6,7]; however, shoulder shrugging and overhead activities should be avoided because this can push on the straps of the vest and increase the load on the cervical spine.

The Minerva orthosis is a custom-molded total contact appliance made of plastic materials that are shaped over a positive body cast. It encloses the upper part of the trunk, the neck, and the back of the head and may have a band around the forehead. It provides excellent restriction of lateral and rotational neck motions and limits flexion and extension. This brace may be the only true noninvasive orthosis that offers the support of the halo for injuries below C2. The halo, however, is still better at controlling the occiput to C2 levels.[8]

Thoracolumbosacral Orthoses

Immobilization of the thoracic spine by simple orthotic means is difficult. In general, a custom thoracolumbosacral orthosis (TLSO) is necessary to limit motion in the upper half of the thoracic spine (Figure 2-3). A well-constructed TLSO can provide adequate protection for the lower thoracic spine. In the upper thoracic spine, an intact rib cage provides relative stability and minimizes displacement of a fracture. This is fortunate because this part of the spine is difficult to immobilize by simple orthoses. Effective immobilization of the lumbar spine, especially its lower part and the lumbosacral junction, is difficult to achieve by orthotic means, although frequently attempted. To achieve maximum external immobilization for the lowest spine regions, a molded rigid pelvic girdle, or a hip spica, may be required. The orthosis must then extend upward to the thoracolumbar region. In general, a hip spica is not well tolerated and its efficacy has been disputed.

Flexible LSO or TLSO corsets made of different fabrics with adjustable sets of braces or straps are relatively ineffective in mechanically restricting motion but are usually comfortable and effective in reducing pain for various painful back disorders when spinal stability is not in question. When greater restriction of spinal motion is needed, a variety of prefabricated, adjustable, and more rigid orthoses are available. These include the Knight-spinal LSO, Knight-Taylor TLSO, and hyperextension orthoses such as the Jewett and CASH (cruciform anterior spinal hyperextension) braces. These effectively reduce gross motion and provide trunk support but are inadequate for treatment of unstable spinal fractures. The Jewett TLSO is occasionally used after surgical stabilization of fractures at the thoracolumbar junction. This prefabricated, adjustable orthosis uses a three-point pressure system where pressure is applied anteriorly on the sternum above and on the pelvis or pubic bone below by means of pads attached to a firm metal frame (Figure 2-4). Posteriorly, pressure is applied over the lower thoracic and upper lumbar spine by a pad that is attached to the anterior metal frame by adjustable straps. The Jewett and CASH TLSOs provide no abdominal muscle support and limit only flexion. They are lightweight but may be uncomfortable because the corrective forces are spread over a relatively small area.

The most rigid design is a custom-molded total contact TLSO, sometimes referred to as a body jacket. It is prescribed for maximum restriction of flexion, extension, and rotation. The orthosis is usually bivalved, and Velcro straps attach the anterior and posterior halves. The jacket is molded to firmly fit the pelvis below and may extend anteriorly to the manubrium of the sternum and posteriorly to the midportion of the scapula. A cervical extension may be attached to provide restriction of motion of the upper thoracic and cervical spine. A rigid, total contact TLSO is particularly indicated for unstable fractures of the spine when surgical stabilization is not indicated or when the adequacy of the surgical stabilization is in question. Because of the total contact, this orthosis tends to be warm and somewhat uncomfortable.

MEDICAL COMPLICATIONS
Cardiovascular Complications

Direct cardiovascular (CV) complications after SCI are due to the interruption of communication between receptor organs and brainstem centers as well as interruption of the autonomic nervous system (ANS). CV complications after SCI include orthostasis, cardiac arrhythmia, thermoregulatory disorders, autonomic dysreflexia (AD), and thrombophlebitic disorders including deep venous thrombosis (DVT) and pulmonary embolism (PE).

The CV derangements typically seen in acute SCI are hypotension and bradycardia, which are due to loss of sympathetic tone. The classic triad of neurogenic shock includes hypotension, bradycardia, and hypothermia (Clinical Note: Classic Triad for Neurogenic Shock). The initial loss of sympathetic tone produces hypotension because of a decrease in systemic vascular resistance and dilation of the venous vessels, thereby reducing preload to the heart. Hypotension during acute SCI may also be the result of hypovolemia caused by severe hemorrhage or inadequate administration of fluids. Initially, hypotension is treated with fluids and vasopressor drugs as needed.[9] Careful monitoring is important to prevent pulmonary edema.

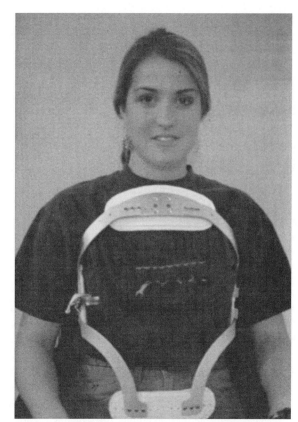

FIGURE 2-4 Jewett hyperextension brace. A single three-point force system is provided by sternal pad, suprapubic pad, and thoracolumbar pad. Forward flexion is restricted in the thoracolumbar area. (From Umphred DA: *Neurological rehabilitation*, ed 4, St. Louis, 2001, Mosby, Figure 16-9, p 485.)

CLINICAL NOTE **Classic Triad for Neurogenic Shock**

- Hypotension
- Bradycardia
- Hypothermia

Orthostatic Hypotension

Orthostatic hypotension is a fall in blood pressure that results from a change in body position toward the upright. Symptoms include lightheadedness, dizziness, syncope, numbness about the face, and pallor (Clinical Note: Symptoms of Orthostatic Hypotension). Orthostasis is more likely to occur in persons with a complete injury above the T6 level. The mechanism of orthostatic hypotension includes interruption of the CV sensory input to the brainstem and preganglionic sympathetics in the spinal cord. When the patient is moved toward an upright position, there is a decrease in blood pressure that is sensed by the aortic and carotid baroreceptors. This would usually cause an increase in sympathetic outflow resulting in tachycardia and vasoconstriction. In SCI, however, the efferent pathway is interrupted and therefore there is no increase in sympathetic outflow (i.e., epinephrine and norepinephrine). This results in an only minimal increase in heart rate that is not sufficient to counterbalance the decrease in blood pressure. Venous pooling also occurs, which limits venous return to the heart and thus limits cardiac output. The symptoms of orthostasis depend on cerebral blood flow rather than on absolute blood pressure.[10] This syndrome lessens with time as a result of the development of spinal postural reflexes that cause vasoconstriction and improved autoregulation of cerebrovascular circulation in response to low perfusion pressures.[11]

CLINICAL NOTE   **Symptoms of Orthostatic Hypotension**

- Lightheadedness
- Dizziness
- Syncope
- Numbness about the face
- Pallor

The treatment of orthostatic hypotension involves the use of abdominal binders, compression stockings, or lower limb Ace wraps while gradually bringing the patient toward an upright position (Clinical Note: Treatment of Orthostatic Hypotension). Various therapeutic treatment techniques to address orthostatic hypotension are discussed in Chapter 6. In addition, the patient should be adequately hydrated. Pharmacological interventions include the use of salt tablets, midodrine, and fludrocortisone (i.e., a salt-retaining steroid) in a progressive manner.[9] Patients receiving these medications should be monitored carefully because these drugs should not be used for a longer period of time than absolutely necessary because they can potentially increase the blood pressure response during an episode of AD.

CLINICAL NOTE   **Treatment of Orthostatic Hypotension**

- Abdominal binders
- Compression stockings or lower limb Ace wraps
- Gradually bring patient to an upright position
- Ensure adequate hydration
- Pharmacological interventions

Cardiac Arrhythmias

Cardiac arrhythmias are most commonly seen in the early weeks after injury and they occur in patients with lesions above the T5 level. This is due to inadequate supraspinal control of the sympathetic nervous system and unopposed vagal tone. Sympathetic innervation to the heart is from T1 through T4, and parasympathetic control to the heart is by the vagus nerve that originates in the brainstem. Bradycardia is the most common arrhythmia and it may be worsened by activities that stimulate the vagus nerve, such as tracheal suctioning, turning and placing the patient in the prone position, defecation, and even belching. This usually resolves within a few weeks after injury, as spinal shock resolves, but patients should be monitored for possible severe bradycardia when the previously mentioned activities are performed. Especially at risk are older adults, those with high level tetraplegia, and those with complete neurological injuries. Bradycardia resulting from unopposed vagal influence on the heart acutely after SCI usually does not require treatment unless the heart rate falls below 44 beats per minute or if the patient is symptomatic. Anticholinergic agents, such as atropine, may be needed intermittently. When bradycardia is profound or sustained, a cardiac pacemaker may be required, at least temporarily, to regulate the heart rate.[12]

Thermoregulation

Body temperature (i.e., thermoregulation) is normally regulated by the hypothalamus. When core temperature requires an adjustment, the hypothalamus can use shivering and vasoconstriction, generating increased heat and decreasing heat loss, to increase core temperature. Likewise, sweating and vasodilation decrease temperature by increasing heat loss. SCI decreases the ability of the hypothalamus to direct the periphery. Patients with lesions above T5 are at times poikilothermic, adapting to the temperature of the local environment.[13] For example, an individual with a high-level SCI who is in a hot room or outdoors in the heat may have a high core temperature, which can be confused with a fever caused by an infectious source. It is therefore vital that patients be instructed in strategies to protect themselves from both hypothermia and hyperthermia.

Autonomic Dysreflexia

AD, also known as autonomic hyperreflexia, is a syndrome of massive imbalanced reflex sympathetic discharge occurring in patients with SCI above the splanchnic outflow (T6 level). AD is a medical emergency that requires quick recognition and treatment. The incidence is reported from 48% to 85% of susceptible individuals,[14,15] and it is caused by a noxious stimulus below the level of injury that the patient is unaware of because of lack of sensation. These noxious stimuli most often arise from the urinary bladder, with overdistention being the predominant cause. This can also occur from a blocked indwelling Foley catheter or a missed intermittent catheterization. Any noxious stimulus, however, may precipitate the syndrome, including an impacted rectum, pressure ulcer, ingrown toenail, tight clothing, or fracture. These stimuli incite a reflex release of sympathetic activity. Descending inhibitory tracts to the sympathetic surge is interrupted and therefore cannot control the sympathetic output. The result is regional vasoconstriction that increases peripheral vascular resistance with a marked rise in arterial blood pressure. A reflex bradycardia may be seen in response to this arterial blood pressure rise, from vagal stimulation, but is not enough to lower the blood pressure significantly (see Figure 3-1). Hypertension is particularly important in older adult patients who may have a baseline hypertensive nature.

The symptoms of AD include headache, sweating above the level of the lesion, and piloerection from sympathetic stimulation of hair follicles (Clinical Note: Signs and Symptoms of Autonomic Dysreflexia). Flushing may occur above the level of lesion and eye symptoms are variable. Typically, the patient also complains of nasal congestion and anxiety. Potential complications of AD include retinal hemorrhage, subarachnoid or intracerebral hemorrhage, myocardial infarction, seizure, and potentially death. AD is rarely detected before 1 month after injury and is present in most patients by 6 months after injury, with 92% of patients exhibiting their the first episode of AD by 1 year after injury.[14]

CLINICAL NOTE — Signs and Symptoms of Autonomic Dysreflexia

- Hypertension: Increase of systolic blood pressure >15 mm Hg to 20 mm Hg above baseline
- Headache: Pounding and severe, usually bilateral, in back of head or behind the eyes
- Sweating: Above level of lesion
- Flushing of the skin: Above level of lesion
- Piloerection (i.e., goosebumps): Sympathetic stimulation of hair follicles below the level of injury
- Eye symptoms: Lid retraction, mydriasis, conjunctival injection
- Nasal congestion
- Anxiety
- Temperature elevation
- Cardiac changes: Classically bradycardia, but may have tachycardia, arrhythmias, and chest pain
- Blurry vision
- Skin rash

Treatment of AD involves recognition of its symptoms along with prompt removal of the precipitating stimuli. The Consortium of Spinal Cord Medicine has outlined recommendations[16] that are summarized in Clinical Note: Treatment Recommendations for Autonomic Dysreflexia. If the patient is in bed, the head of the bed should be raised. If seated, the patient should be brought to the fully erect position and his clothes loosened. Effective treatment may include drainage of the bladder, disimpaction of fecal material from the rectum, or resection of an ingrown toenail. Nasal decongestants with sympathomimetic properties, such as pseudo-ephedrine, may cause or worsen AD. Therefore, in general, nasal congestion in patients with SCI who are susceptible to AD should not be treated with these products. Pharmacologic intervention for AD includes the use of various vasodilators such as nitroglycerin paste or oral blood pressure medications with a rapid onset of action. Occasionally intravenous medications are required and the reader is referred elsewhere for greater details.[9,16] Early education of the patient and his caregivers is of utmost importance.

CLINICAL NOTE — Treatment Recommendations for Autonomic Dysreflexia

- Recognize the symptoms and check the blood pressure
- Sit the patient up and loosen any clothing or constrictive devices
- Survey the patient for causes, beginning with the urinary system
- Check for catheter kinks if indwelling or external catheter
- Flush the catheter
- If on intermittent catheterization, catheterize by using lidocaine jelly before catheterization if immediately available
- *Monitor blood pressure frequently
- *Consider pharmacological intervention if the systolic blood pressure remains elevated above 150 mm Hg
- Check rectum for fecal impaction if suspected, after lidocaine jelly is placed
- If source is not found, the patient should be seen by a specialist in SCI medicine

Deep Vein Thrombosis

Deep vein thrombosis (DVT) is the most common of the CV complications after the acute period after SCI. Its incidence varies between 8% and 100% depending on the diagnostic tests used.[17,18]

Recent data indicate that the incidence of DVT may be decreasing,[18,19] perhaps as a result of effective prophylaxis. The risk factors associated with the development of a DVT in SCI include Virchow's triad of stasis, intimal injury, and hypercoagulability. Further risk factors include lower limb fracture, older age, obesity, history of previous thrombosis, diabetes, and arterial vascular disease.[20] DVT is more common in patients with tetraplegia and in patients with neurologically complete injuries. The onset is typically within 2 weeks, with the incidence decreasing after 8 weeks. PE occurs in 1% to 7% of patients with SCI and is one of the leading causes of death in patients in the acute phase.[19] Most cases develop from the deep veins of the lower limbs. PE is not influenced by the degree or level of SCI.

Prophylaxis of DVT is critical after SCI. Clinical monitoring is important, but not as effective in the SCI population because of an absence of some of the usual signs and symptoms, such as tenderness to palpation. There is poor correlation between the extent of thrombosis and leg circumference; however, a 1-cm difference between the two lower limbs at the calf or thigh should raise suspicion. The Consortium in Spinal Cord Injury has published clinical recommendations regarding the prophylaxis and treatment of DVT in SCI.[21] A method of mechanical prophylaxis (i.e., pneumatic compression devices) and anticoagulant prophylaxis is recommended. Mechanical prophylaxis is usually recommended for 24-hour use while the patient is in bed. Anticoagulant prophylaxis, with either low-molecular-weight or unfractionated heparin, should be initiated within 72 hours after injury provided that there is no active bleeding, evidence of head injury, or a coagulopathy. The length of time for DVT prophylaxis depends on the level and extent of the SCI and on the coexistent medical issues that are present.[21] Vena cava filter placement is indicated in patients who have failed anticoagulant prophylaxis or who have a contraindication to anticoagulation, but it is not a substitute for pharmacological thromboprophylaxis. With a documented clot, mobilization and exercise of the lower limbs are usually withheld for 48 to 72 hours after appropriate medical therapy has been implemented.

Respiratory Complications

The incidence of respiratory complications after SCI is high,[22] including aspiration, atelectasis, and pneumonia. In general, the older the patient, the higher the neurological level, and the more complete the neurological lesion, the more likely these conditions are to develop. Preexisting respiratory conditions (e.g., history of cigarette smoking, chronic obstructive pulmonary disease, bronchial asthma, intrinsic lung disease, and marked obesity) make the patient with SCI more vulnerable for development of respiratory complications.

Respiratory insufficiency during acute SCI may occur for several reasons. Paralysis of some or all of the respiratory muscles develop with high-level SCI. Patients with injuries at or above C3 are usually initially unable to breathe on their own and require mechanical ventilation. Injuries below C3 may also require mechanical ventilation for a period of time. These patients may be unable to clear their secretions because there is a loss of the ability to cough as a result of varying levels of abdominal muscle paralysis. Injuries to the chest, such as rib fractures, hemopneumothorax, and lung contusions, are commonly associated with thoracic SCI and may result in temporary respiratory insufficiency.

Good respiratory care during acute SCI is important to prevent any potential respiratory complications. A prophylactic respiratory therapy program should be started as soon as possible after SCI (Clinical Note: Components of a Prophylactic Respiratory Therapy Program). Breathing treatments with saline solution or bronchodilators should be provided for individuals with high-level SCI. Active chest physical therapy (PT) including percussion, postural drainage as tolerated, and assistive coughing techniques are important aspects of respiratory care. Placing the patient regularly in the Trendelenburg and reverse Trendelenburg positions should encourage postural drainage, as well as side-lying positions if possible. Because the cough is weak in persons with high-level SCI, assistive coughing is provided by various manual techniques (e.g., quad cough) or by use of a mechanical insufflation-exsufflation machine (see Figure 4-31). Caution should be used with the quad coughing technique in a patient with a newly inserted inferior vena cava filter. Individuals with SCI prefer mechanical insufflation-exsufflation compared with suctioning for management of their secretions.[23] As soon as possible, an active exercise program should begin to increase the strength of the diaphragm and other innervated accessory respiratory muscles. The diaphragm may decondition rapidly during mechanical ventilation and may not be able to sustain adequate pulmonary function immediately after its discontinuation.

CLINICAL NOTE Components of a Prophylactic Respiratory Therapy Program

- Breathing treatments with saline solution or bronchodilators (for patients with high-level SCI)
- Active chest PT including percussion and postural drainage as tolerated (placing the patient regularly in the Trendelenburg and reverse Trendelenburg positions as well as side-lying position if possible)
- Assistive coughing techniques (manual or mechanical)
- Active exercise program to increase the strength of the diaphragm and other innervated accessory respiratory muscles

Mechanical ventilation should be provided either by intubation or by tracheotomy and is usually indicated when the vital capacity decreases to 1 liter or less, when arterial blood gasses become increasingly abnormal, when atelectasis occurs frequently or persists, and when chest radiographs show consolidation (Clinical Note: Indications for Mechanical Ventilation). Tidal volumes for patients with SCI on mechanical ventilation are generally kept higher than normally provided for nonparalyzed people on ventilators, or at least 10 to 15 ml per kilogram of body weight. Weaning off the ventilator can begin when the patient's respiratory status has been stabilized and is best accomplished by progressively increasing time off the ventilator rather than by reducing intermittent mandatory tidal volume.[24] When atelectasis and pneumonia occur, antibiotics should promptly be administered. Vaccinations for influenza and *Pneumococcus* are recommended in these patients. A detailed review of respiratory considerations, equipment, and treatment strategies can be found in Chapter 4.

CLINICAL NOTE Indications for Mechanical Ventilation

- Vital capacity decreases to 1 L or less
- Increasingly abnormal arterial blood gas values
- Frequent or persistent atelectasis
- Consolidation seen on chest radiographs

Genitourinary Complications
Bladder Management

Although no longer among the leading causes of death for individuals with SCI, bladder dysfunction remains a major care management problem. During the immediate postinjury period, an indwelling catheter is recommended. During this period of spinal shock, urinary retention is the rule because the bladder is areflexic. An indwelling catheter provides adequate bladder drainage and allows constant measurement of urine output when the patient with SCI may be hemodynamically unstable. Retention of urine or the presence of foreign bodies in the bladder, including the catheter, may lead to frequent urinary tract infections (UTIs). Intermittent catheterization is recommended as early as possible provided that the patient is medically stable, can tolerate fluid restriction, is not orthostatic and that the nurse staffing is adequate and well trained.

The goals of management of the neurogenic bladder are to achieve an acceptable method of bladder drainage, preventing complications including infection, stone formation, hydronephrosis, and bladder-associated AD. After some time post injury, usually 1 month, the bladder may contract reflexively with loss of voluntary control, generally with frequent spontaneous voiding at abnormally low bladder volumes (i.e., hyperreflexic or upper motor neuron [UMN] neurogenic bladder). However, if the injury involves the conus medullaris or cauda equina, the bladder and sphincter may be denervated and a condition of urinary retention with overflow incontinence results (i.e., areflexic or lower motor neuron [LMN] neurogenic bladder).

There are a number of options for bladder management in the chronic stage after SCI (see Chapter 3). This includes the use of a condom catheter in males with a hyperreflexic bladder (i.e., reflex voiding), the use of indwelling catheters, and intermittent catheterization. Using a condom catheter with an external collecting system is an option for men who have a hyperreflexic bladder; voiding occurs when the bladder contracts. Suprapubic tapping to trigger the reflex bladder contraction can augment this type of voiding. Unfortunately, reflex voiding in SCI is often associated with detrusor-sphincter dyssynergia (DSD) and elevated voiding pressures, thereby placing the person at risk for vesicoureteral reflux and hydronephrosis. Means to relax the sphincter mechanism to reduce DSD include medications, botulinum toxin injections, and surgical procedures (e.g., sphincterotomies). Reflex voiding is a poor option for women because there is no consistently acceptable external collection device available to act as a receptacle.

Bladder drainage by an indwelling Foley or suprapubic catheter is an option for women and for men unable to perform self-intermittent catheterization or tolerate condom devices, either because of skin breakdown from the condom catheter or inability to obtain a secure fit. Use of indwelling catheters is associated with a higher rate of short- and long-term complications, including UTIs, stone formation, and cancer.

Intermittent catheterization (IC) four to six times per day has physiological advantages over an indwelling catheter. An IC program allows for bladder filling and periodic emptying and has been shown to be associated with fewer complications than long-term indwelling catheters. Patients are advised to limit their fluid intake to approximately 2 liters per day, with the desired volumes per catheterization not to exceed 500 ml. Frequently, the use of anticholinergic medications is needed to relax the smooth muscle of the bladder to prevent incontinence between catheterizations. These medications are often associated with side effects of constipation and dry mouth. IC is not a good option for every patient with SCI. A person with high-level (C1 to C6) tetraplegia may be unable to perform this procedure independently because of the lack of hand and finger motion and therefore may require another method of management. The use of the HouseHold device available from Flexlife in Texas may improve the capability for individuals with higher-level injuries to perform this procedure.[25] If a person with SCI can perform his own IC, then it can be performed with a clean technique; however, if another person performs the catheterization, then sterile technique should be used.[26]

To improve bladder capacity and to permit more successful IC in either men or women who cannot become more continent with medications, surgical procedures may be appropriate. Augmentation cystoplasty involves incising the hyperreflexic bladder and using a portion of the patient's intestine to create a low-pressure, high-capacity reservoir. The patient may then catheterize the bladder as previously mentioned. For certain clinical conditions, such as intractable skin breakdown or difficulty performing the IC, the augmentation cystoplasty may be combined with a bladder neck closure and the creation of a continent stoma in the abdominal wall. There are a number of surgical techniques available to enhance bladder management.[26]

UTIs are an extremely common complication in SCI. Symptoms of a UTI in individuals with SCI include fever, spontaneous voiding between catheterizations, increased spasticity, hematuria, AD, nausea, malaise, and vague abdominal discomfort (Clinical Note: Symptoms of a Urinary Tract Infection in Individuals with Spinal Cord Injury). The urine may become increasingly malodorous and cloudy. Bacterial colonization can lead to epididymitis, orchitis, and prostatism in men. Although the treatment of an obvious UTI with antibiotics is not in question, there is considerable disagreement as to what constitutes a UTI. Individuals with neurogenic bladder dysfunction often have significant bacteriuria, especially when the bladder management involves some type of indwelling catheter. Frequent treatment with antibiotics for asymptomatic UTIs may lead to highly resistant pathogens.

CLINICAL NOTE **Symptoms of a Urinary Tract Infection in Individuals with Spinal Cord Injury**

- Fever
- Spontaneous voiding between catheterizations
- Increased spasticity
- Hematuria
- Autonomic dysreflexia
- Nausea
- Malaise
- Vague abdominal discomfort
- Increasingly malodorous and cloudy urine

Renal failure was formerly the most common cause of death in persons with SCI but currently is not as prevalent. Improved surveillance and effective treatment of UTIs are the primary reasons for this decline. Preventing urinary tract morbidity depends on a lifetime of proper evaluation and management. Evaluation should be by both anatomical (e.g., ultrasonography, intravenous pyelography, excretory cystography, and renal scintigraphy) and physiological (e.g., urodynamic) testing.[26]

Urinary tract calculi (i.e., stones) are common in people with SCI and may be present in the bladder, ureters, or kidneys. Presence of bacteria, sediment, and catheters are major reasons for the development of urinary tract stones. Urinary tract stones should be suspected in the presence of blood in the urine, recurrent UTIs, or unexplained AD. The treatment is removal of the stones, but the method of removal depends on the location and size of the stone.

Sexuality

Sexuality is an integration of physical, emotional, intellectual, and social aspects of an individual's personality that expresses maleness or femaleness.[27] SCI can have a significant impact on an individual's body image and self-esteem, which has an effect on sexuality. These issues as well as the physical aspects of sexuality need to be addressed. Unfortunately, individuals with SCI report that they receive little information regarding sexuality after their injury.

The impact of SCI on sexuality physiologically is dependent on the severity of injury (e.g., complete versus incomplete) and the level of injury (e.g., UMN versus LMN).[28] Women after a complete UMN injury can have reflex vaginal lubrication with tactile stimulation, but not psychogenic lubrication. Those with incomplete UMN lesions may have both psychogenic and reflex vaginal lubrication.[29] An estimated 25% of women with a complete LMN lesion that affects the sacral segments have the capacity for psychogenic lubrication, with almost no capacity for reflex lubrication. Women with incomplete LMN lesions have a greater chance of both psychogenic and reflex lubrication.[30] Women with SCI can achieve orgasms.[31-33]

Men with complete UMN lesions (above the T11 level) similarly are usually able to have reflex erections but are unable to have psychogenic erections. The reflex erections may, however, be poorly sustained so that they are not successful at having intercourse. Only a small percent of these individuals can achieve ejaculation,[34,35] although some individuals have retrograde ejaculation (i.e., into the bladder), in which case the ejaculation may go undetected. Men with LMN lesions have less ability to achieve erections, usually by psychogenic rather than reflex pathways, but they do have a higher chance of achieving ejaculation. Those with incomplete injuries have a greater chance of erection and ejaculation.

A number of options to assist men with SCI in achieving erections are available.[36] Implants are effective but carry a risk of infection and erosion of the penis. Intracavernous injections with papaverine and prostaglandins may be used but should be used with caution. Individuals who cannot achieve an erection can use a vacuum pump with a constriction ring, whereas those who can achieve an erection can use only the constriction ring to occlude venous outflow to sustain the erection. Negative pressure produced by the pump causes engorgement of the penis, with the erection maintained by the application of a constriction ring placed at the base of the penis. This device should not be used for greater than 30 minutes because the lack of blood flow may cause necrosis of the penis. Phosphodiesterase medications are an effective and well-tolerated treatment for erectile dysfunction in SCI[37-39]; however, there are a number of side effects of which the patient should be aware. Of greatest importance is the contraindication of this medication to be given with nitrates. Patients with AD, who may use nitrates for treatment, should be cautioned about this serious interaction.

For males and females, the desire and opportunity for sexual activity decreases after injury.[40-42] Partner availability, and the additional time required for sexual activity, may influence the levels of sexual satisfaction. Continued research about the influence of both physiological and psychological factors in sexual functioning is important to identify treatment interventions to maximize sexual satisfaction for those with SCI.

GASTROINTESTINAL DISTURBANCES

Gastrointestinal (GI) disorders are common after an acute SCI. Virtually all patients have paralytic ileus, gastric atony, and distention during the early phases of spinal shock, but this condition rarely lasts beyond 5 days. Oral feeding should not begin until after bowel sounds are present. Management during this time can include nasogastric decompression and alternative means for nutrition, including total peripheral nutrition. Peptic ulcer, esophagitis, and GI hemorrhage may occur. Prophylactic treatment is effective with administration of a histamine 2 receptor antagonist and adequate nutritional support. Pancreatitis has its highest incidence in the first month after injury and may be related to steroid use. This should be considered if adynamic ileus does not resolve, or if it recurs after resolving.

Abdominal complaints in people with SCI are difficult to diagnose because of their limited ability to localize pain. There should be a high index of suspicion, and the necessary diagnostic tests ordered, if the patient has worsening vague abdominal complaints without apparent cause.

Cholecystitis or cholelithiasis is the most common cause of emergency abdominal surgery in persons with SCI.[43] The incidence is greater in those over age 40 years and with injury levels above T10. Gallstones may remain asymptomatic, cause cholecystitis, or migrate into the common bile duct, causing cholangitis or pancreatitis. Treatment for this includes continued observation, surgical removal, or medical dissolution.

Superior mesenteric artery (SMA) syndrome is seen mostly in patients with tetraplegia who have abdominal distention, discomfort, and recurrent emesis after eating.[44] It is caused by obstruction in the distal part of the duodenum as it passes behind the SMA and in front of the spine and aorta. It often occurs in patients who are immobilized and who have lost a significant amount of weight and retroperitoneal fat. Symptoms are worse when the person is in the supine position, especially if he is wearing a body jacket. An upper GI series reveal an abrupt cessation of barium in the third part of the duodenum. Treatment includes sitting the patient upright or positioning him in the left side-lying position after meals, nourishment to restore weight, and applying a lumbosacral corset to push the abdominal contents upward. Surgery is rarely indicated.

Bowel Management

The most frequent GI problem after SCI is altered bowel elimination. It has been reported that 27% of individuals with chronic SCI have complaints relating to bowel elimination, hemorrhoids, abdominal distention, and AD caused by rectal impaction.[45] Factors contributing to such symptoms include altered colonic compliance, impaired transit time, and poor dietary intake. The key to preventing such problems is the use of an effective bowel program, which allows the patient to have control over the time and frequency of his bowel elimination. The combination of oral medications (e.g., stool softeners, bulk formers, and oral stimulants), suppositories, and digital stimulation is usually effective for elimination of stool.[46] A bowel program should begin as soon as bowel sounds return and the patient is receiving feedings. An ineffective bowel evacuation program may adversely affect most aspects of the patient's life and the pursuit of physical, psychological, social, vocational, and sexual goals. The Consortium of Spinal Cord Medicine has published recommendations regarding bowel care.[47]

The goals of an effective bowel program are to minimize or eliminate the occurrence of unplanned bowel movements, to evacuate stool at a regular and predictable time within 1 hour from start to finish, and to minimize GI symptoms.[47] Key components of a bowel program are listed in the Clinical Note: Key Components of a Bowel Program. There are differences in bowel programs for reflexic (UMN lesions) and areflexic bowels (LMN lesions). Reflex bowel programs rely on digital stimulation and initially suppository insertion to assist in evacuation of the stool, whereas areflexic bowel programs require gentle Valsalva maneuvers with manual disimpaction to assist in evacuation. The goal for stool consistency in a reflexic bowel is a soft, formed stool, whereas in an areflexic bowel it is firm formed stool that can be retained between bowel sessions so that there is no incontinence from a lax external sphincter.[47] For individuals with a reflexic bowel program, bowel care should be scheduled at the same time of day to develop a predictable response, foods should be ingested approximately 30 minutes before the gastrocolic reflex is stimulated and should be performed at least every 2 days to avoid long-term colonic distention. Those with an areflexic bowel may need to perform disimpaction up to two times per day. See Chapter 3 for nursing management of the bowels in SCI.

CLINICAL NOTE **Key Components of a Bowel Program**

- Timing and frequency of medications
- Proper diet and fluid management
- Activity level
- Attendant care provisions
- Life schedules

Neurological Complications
Spasticity
Spasticity is a velocity-dependent increase in resistance of muscle tone. It is usually direction dependent with some initial free motion and associated pathological reflexes. Spasticity

TABLE 2-2	Positive and Negative Symptoms of Spasticity in the Upper Motor Neuron Syndrome
Positive Symptoms (Abnormal Behaviors)	Negative Symptoms (Performance Deficits)
Hyperreflexia	Weakness
Clonus	Incoordination
Spasms	Fatigue
Postural abnormalities	Pain

may be characterized by positive (i.e., abnormal behaviors) and negative (i.e., performance deficits) UMN symptoms (Table 2-2). Positive UMN symptoms are more likely to respond to antispasticity treatment than are negative symptoms. Relief of spasticity, therefore, does not necessarily enhance performance. The pathophysiology of spasticity at this time is not completely known.[48] The loss of descending inhibitory pathways is thought to be a main mechanism; however, formation of new synapses by motor neurons that have lost supraspinal input also may be involved.[49]

Spasticity is one of the most common and potentially disabling complications affecting patients with SCI. Approximately 70% of patients have spasticity 1 year after injury,[50] although not all patients require treatment. Spasticity is often less severe in patients with either complete injuries or with functional voluntary movements and more severe in patients with minimal sparing of voluntary movement.[51] In some patients, the increased tone may offer benefits, such as providing stability in the sitting or standing position and helping maintain muscle bulk by preventing atrophy. It also may increase venous return, thus decreasing orthostasis, and improve a patient's cough, helping to better clear secretions. Spasticity may also allow a patient to improve his functional skills. Examples include inducing flexor spasms of the lower limbs to assist in lower body dressing or inducing a Babinski response to more easily place a bed pan. In many other patients, however, spasticity interferes with numerous aspects of their lives, including medical, physical, social, vocational, and recreational activities. Complications of spasticity include direct functional impairment, consisting of diminished mobility and activites of daily living (e.g., grooming, hygiene, and self-care skills) and interference with sleep, cosmesis, self-esteem, mood, and sexual function. Spasticity also can be a source of inactivity, contractures, and pain. Treatment should therefore be guided by the patient's ability to function.

Although there are a number of ways to quantify the degree of spasticity, the severity of spasms may vary from moment to moment and may be difficult to accurately measure. The most frequently used scales include the Ashworth,[52] the Modified Ashworth,[53] and the Spasm Frequency scales[54] (Box 2-1). Other techniques used in research include the pendulum test[55] and electrophysiological methods.[56]

The basic principle underlying the management of spasticity is to use the most conservative tactics to minimize the adverse effects of spasticity without compromising function. Classic treatment for spasticity is based on a stepwise approach in which a stretching and therapy program is attempted before pharmacological intervention. Thus treatment begins with rehabilitation modalities then progresses to pharmacological interventions,

BOX 2-1	Three Standard Spasticity Scales

Ashworth Scale Grade	Description
1	No increased tone
2	Slight increase in tone, giving a catch when the affected parts are moved in flexion or extension
3	More marked increased in tone but affected part is easily flexed
4	Considerable increase in tone, passive movement is difficult
5	Affected part is rigid in extension

Modified Ashworth Scale Grade	Description
0	No increased muscle tone
1	Slight increase in muscle tone, manifested by a catch and release, or by minimal resistance at end ROM when affected part is moved in flexion or extension
1+	Slight increase in muscle tone, manifested by a catch, followed by minimal resistance throughout the remainder (<50%) of ROM
2	More marked increase in muscle tone through most of ROM, but affected part is easily moved
3	Considerable increase in muscle tone, passive movement difficult
4	Affected part is rigid in flexion or extension

Spasm Frequency Score Grade	Description
0	No spasms
1	Mild spasm induced by stimulation
2	Infrequent full spasm occurring less than once per hour
3	Spasms occurring more than once per hour
4	Ten or more spasms per hour, or continuous contraction

Data from Ashworth B: Preliminary trial of carisoprodol in multiple sclerosis, *Practioner* 192:540-542, 1964; Bohannon RW, Smith MB: Interrator reliability on modified Ashworth scale of muscle spasticity, *Phys Ther* 67:206-207, 1987; Penn RD, Savoy SM, Corcos DC et al: Intrathecal baclofen for severe spinal spasticity, *N Engl J Med* 320:1517-1521, 1989.
ROM, Range of motion.

injection techniques, intrathecal baclofen, and surgery.[56] It is generally understood that no one intervention will effectively reduce spasticity in all patients. When a neurologically stable patient demonstrates an increased amount of spasticity, a thorough evaluation for precipitating factors should be completed before medications are increased. The clinician should first try to find out if there are any underlying causes for the spasticity including pressure ulcers, GI or genitourinary complications, DVT, or the presence of heterotopic ossification. Stress and emotional or physical factors may also have an impact on the degree of spasticity present. Similarly, drugs that are being taken for other comorbid disorders may adversely affect spasticity. For example, some antidepressants, including trazodone and selective serotonin reuptake inhibitors, have been reported to increase spasticity[57] by interfering with the pharmacological actions of antispasticity medications.

Therapeutic Treatment Techniques

Proper bed positioning early after SCI may reduce long-term spasticity. Daily range of motion (ROM) and stretching (i.e., once to twice daily) diminishes tone and has a carryover effect. Modalities such as cold and topical anesthesia may decrease tendon reflex excitability, reduce clonus, and increase ROM, thus facilitating improved motor function.[58,59] A cold pack should be used for approximately 20 minutes for maximal effect. Its duration of effectiveness, however, is less than 1 hour. Electrical stimulation,[60,61] transcutaneous electrical nerve (TENS) stimulation,[62] and biofeedback have been shown to modulate spasticity,[63] but their usefulness is believed to be limited.[64] Because prolonged stretch to the ankle plantarflexor muscles decreases tone, the use of standing (e.g., on a tilt table or standing frame) will decrease spasticity.[65] Serial casting and splinting techniques can improve more severe ROM limitations that develop as a result of spasticity or contracture, and positioning the limb in a tonic stretch can decrease reflex tone.[66] A tone-reducing plastic molded ankle foot orthosis or a tone-reducing foot plate can maintain the ankle or foot in a rigid position, thereby diminishing the input that causes the mass extensor response when the ankle is stretched such as that which occurs from the wheelchair footrest. Maintaining proper sitting posture also is extremely important. Postural considerations for seating are discussed in detail in Chapter 11.

Pharmacological Interventions

Many medications are available to treat spasticity, and no single medication may have a beneficial effect in all patients. Almost all medications have potentially serious side effects, and this should be carefully considered before any drug is begun. The most common medications are discussed here, but for additional information the reader is referred to other sources.[48,56]

Oral Medications. Baclofen (Lioresal), an analog of gamma aminobutyric acid (GABA), is involved in presynaptic inhibition, increasing inhibitory influences on the stretch reflex. The believed mechanism of action is by binding to the GABA-B receptor, inhibiting calcium influx into presynaptic terminals and suppressing release of excitatory neurotransmitters. Baclofen may interfere with attention and memory in patients, which is especially of concern in persons with concomitant brain injury. The initiating dosage is 5 to 12 mg two or three times a day. This can be increased every 2 to 3 days, up to a dosage of 80 mg/day,[67] but many SCI practitioners use higher dosages of baclofen, up to 200 mg/day, with good effect.[68,69] Sudden withdrawal from this medication should be avoided because of possible precipitation of seizures and hallucinations.

Benzodiazepines, including diazepam (Valium) and clonazepam (Klonopin), also increase inhibitory mechanisms but in a manner slightly different than baclofen. Benzodiazepines decrease reflexes and painful spasms but have little effect on non-velocity-dependent muscle responses. These drugs are generally well tolerated except for their sedative effect. Evidence of abuse and addiction is rare, but true physiological addiction may occur with this medication.

Dantrolene sodium (Dantrium) is the only medication that works directly on the muscle tissue, rather than at the spinal cord level, to weaken muscles that are overexcited. Dantrolene prevents calcium release from the sarcoplasmic reticulum to the active myosin fibers, decreasing the force produced by excitation-contraction coupling.[70] Because it is less likely to cause lethargy or cognitive disturbances than baclofen or diazepam, dantrolene is preferred for cerebral forms of spasticity but may be a useful adjunct in the treatment of SCI spasticity. It is not, however, devoid of central nervous system side effects. In addition, liver function test monitoring is indicated during titration and long-term treatment.

Clonidine (Catapres) is a centrally acting alpha-2 adrenergic agonist that has been shown to be effective for spasticity in patients SCI.[71] The transdermal system (Catapres-TTS) that releases clonidine at a fixed rate over a 1-week period has been shown to be effective for treatment of spasticity with minimal adverse effects noted. Tizanidine (Zanaflex), a newer centrally acting alpha-2 agonist, has been studied in patients with multiple sclerosis and SCI,[72] and has been shown to offer similar efficacy to that provided by baclofen and diazepam. It may, however, be better tolerated because it causes less weakness than baclofen and less sedation than diazepam. Unlike clonidine, tizanidine does not induce a consistent change in blood pressure.[73]

Other medications occasionally used in treating SCI-related spasticity include cyproheptadine, a potent antihistaminic antiserotonergic medication with mild anticholinergic activity,[74-76] and gabapentin.[77,78]

Injection Techniques. Injection techniques to address spasticity include peripheral blocks (e.g., nerve blocks and motor point blocks) and botulinum toxin injections. Peripheral nerve blocks may help facilitate management of contractures and prevent recurrences after surgical correction. They can help reduce hip adductor spasticity (i.e., scissoring), relieve painful spasms, and block spastic ankle plantarflexor muscles. The blocks may be used to facilitate nursing care, hygiene, positioning, healing, or prevention of pressure ulcers and to improve gait. Therapeutic nerve blocks can be performed with alcohol or phenol. They are used to relieve spasticity that interferes with function or is a source of morbidity such as pain, contractures, or skin breakdown. An example is an obturator nerve block for the reduction of adductor muscle hyperactivity. Alcohol and phenol denature protein have a duration of 3 months but cause painful paresthesias in roughly 10% of patients. If paresthesias occur, they may be treated with oral steroids, medications used for neuropathic pain, TENS, or a repeat block.

Upper limb motor point blocks can help functional activities. They may allow for additional movement by blocking an antagonist muscle, for example, helping to open the hand for hygiene care. The effects of motor point blocks are not permanent. However, concurrent therapy may produce longer-lasting results by permitting the development of good habits and strengthening of other muscle groups. Injections are most useful when the agonists appear to have sufficient strength for functional purposes when freed from hyperactive antagonists.

Botulinum toxin is a potent neurotoxin produced by the anaerobic bacteria *Clostridium botulinum*. Injected into a muscle at its end plate zone region, botulinum toxin reduces the release of acetylcholine from presynaptic motor axons and thereby weakens the muscle without affecting the synthesis of acetylcholine. Because of the complex mechanism of action involved, this chemical denervation develops over the course of a few days, peaks at 2 to 6 weeks, and lasts for several months (approximately 3 months). Although the effect of botulinum toxin is irreversible, the clinical response slowly subsides, probably from collateral sprouting at the nerve terminals. The effectiveness of the botulinum toxin does not last as long as phenol or alcohol does. If the botulinum toxin is effective, the injections can be repeated. Although botulinum toxin is not recommended for generalized spasticity, isolated muscle groups can be injected to improve nursing care, hygiene, patient comfort, and functional activity.[79,80] A small percentage of patients may have antibodies develop after numerous injections, thereby making the injections no longer functional. Currently two toxins are available in the United States: type A (Botox) and type B (MyoBloc).

The overall benefits of botulinum toxin include a procedure that is not as painful relative to alcohol or phenol in individuals with sensation (although pediatric patients may still require anesthesia), effects that are local and dose dependent, and pain associated with tone is reduced. Drawbacks to its use include cost to use ratio (i.e., spasticity lasts a relatively short period of time), the possibility of antibody formation, and the time it takes for results to occur. The definitive indications for neurolytic agents versus botulinum toxin have not been fully delineated. They should, however, be based on the severity and prognosis of the patient and the goals of treatment.

Intrathecal Baclofen. Intrathecal baclofen is an option that combines pharmacological intervention with a surgical technique. Intrathecal baclofen is indicated for patients who do not respond to, or have intolerable side effects from, oral medication and in whom other techniques have been attempted and failed.[81-83] Advantages of the intrathecal delivery of a drug lie in its bypassing the blood-brain barrier and allowing smaller doses to deliver a greater effect with less systemic toxicity. Doses necessary for a therapeutic effect are approximately 1% of the oral dose; therefore, systemic side effects are minimized. This technique should be considered before definitive surgical intervention. The use of intrathecal baclofen decreases pain and improves sleep and results in improved activities of daily living (ADLs) and bowel and bladder programs.

Before insertion of the baclofen pump, a screening trial is performed in which the patient is observed after the trial dosage and monitored with the Modified Ashworth Score (MAS), the degree and frequency of spasms, and the duration of drug effectiveness. Patients who have a decreased average score of 1 to 2 on the MAS and a beneficial drug effect lasting greater than 4 hours will benefit from pump insertion.

The pump is approximately four inches in circumference, situated subcutaneously in the abdomen, and connected to a catheter that is threaded into the subarachnoid space (Figure 2-5). The pump reservoir is accessed by a percutaneous puncture into the access port. The pump can be refilled with baclofen that will last up to 3 months at a time. Communication with the computer chip is achieved by telemetry from an external computer. The dosage and flow rate can be individualized by use of this mechanism. The battery within the pump is usually replaced within 5 years after implantation. Aside from the potential for accidental overdose and surgical complications, device-related complications reported have included pump failure, battery depletion, catheter kinks, dislodgment, disconnection, and migration.

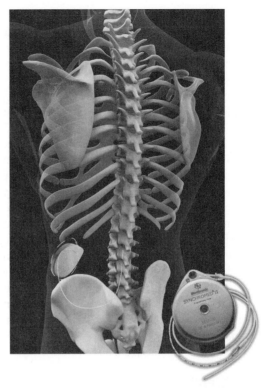

FIGURE 2-5   Intrathecal baclofen pump. The intrathecal baclofen pump is situated subcutaneously in the abdomen and connected to a catheter that is threaded into the subarachnoid space. The pump reservoir is accessed by a percutaneous puncture into an access port. (Courtesy © Medtronic, Inc., Minneapolis, MN.)

Surgical Procedures

A variety of neurosurgical procedures to control spasticity may be performed as a last resort. Nerves may be surgically cut rather than chemically disrupted to create a more permanent disturbance of nerve function.[84] The most common of these procedures is obturator neurectomy along with adductor release. Selective posterior (i.e., dorsal) rhizotomy has been useful in patients with cerebral palsy; however, is not as frequently used in patients with SCI. Microsurgical dorsal root entry zone lesions (DREZ-tomy) relieve both pain and spasticity by destroying the laterally placed small nociceptive fibers without producing loss of large fiber sensation. Although they are invasive procedures, DREZ-otomy and selective dorsal rhizotomy are replacing the more destructive neuroectomy and rhizotomy. With the advent of more effective and less destructive therapies, fewer patients may require procedures of these sorts.

Posttraumatic Cystic Myelopathy (Syringomyelia)

A syrinx is a fluid-filled cavity within the spinal cord. It is the most common cause of progressive myelopathy in persons with SCI and is particularly devastating because it may cause weakness or sensory loss after a patient has stabilized after the injury. The incidence of this condition, frequently referred to as posttraumatic syringomyelia (PTS), had been reported to occur in just over 3% of people with SCI, but since the introduction of MRI, a higher incidence of 12% to 22% has been reported.[85,86] This condition may develop in any person with SCI regardless of level of injury, neurological severity, or initial management. A syrinx may develop at any time, as early as 2 months or as late as decades after SCI. PTS should be included in the differential diagnosis of neck and shoulder pain in the patient with chronic SCI. Early diagnosis can minimize the potentially devastating effects of PTS.

The most common presenting symptom of PTS is pain, usually described as a dull ache that is generally increased by straining (Clinical Note: Symptoms of Posttraumatic Cystic Myelopathy [Syringomyelia]). Other symptoms of PTS include hyperhidrosis (i.e., excessive sweating) above or below the level of the lesion, an increase or decrease in muscle tone and spasticity, hypertension, neuropathic joints, change of bladder evacuation, orthostasis, and Horner's syndrome. With progression of a high cervical syrinx, the clinician may see symptoms of diaphragmatic paralysis and cranial nerve involvement including sensory loss in the trigeminal nerve distribution. Symptoms may be worse in the sitting position because of the gravitational forces on the lower part of the cyst. The earliest sign of a syrinx may be the loss of deep tendon reflexes. Other common signs include an ascending sensory level, with light touch sensation less affected than pinprick because of the usual central location of the syrinx. Motor weakness occurs but rarely in isolation from other symptoms.

CLINICAL NOTE | **Symptoms of Posttraumatic Cystic Myelopathy (Syringomyelia)**

- Pain, usually described as a dull ache and usually increased by straining
- Hyperhidrosis above or below the level of the lesion
- An increase or decrease in tone and spasticity
- Hypertension
- Neuropathic joints
- Change of bladder evacuation
- Orthostasis
- Horner's syndrome
- Diaphragmatic paralysis and cranial nerve involvement with progression of a high cervical syrinx
- Loss of deep tendon reflexes
- Ascending sensory level, with light touch sensation less affected than pinprick because of the central location of the syrinx
- Motor weakness that rarely occurs in isolation from other symptoms
- Symptoms may be worse in the sitting position because of the gravitational forces on the lower part of the cyst

---

A syrinx is best visualized with a gadolinium-enhanced MRI study. The presence of a spinal cord cyst on MRI does not, however, constitute a clinically significant syrinx and may not always be the cause of symptoms. On routine MRI scanning, cysts at the level of trauma have been reported in half of patients who were either asymptomatic or tolerating symptoms, none of whom had ascending myelopathy. Electrophysiological studies may be of some value in diagnosing and monitoring of the syrinx.[87]

The natural progression of PTS is variable. The neurological status may remain unchanged or slowly progress. Nonprogressive asymptomatic PTS may be treated conservatively by pain control and avoiding straining. Surgical treatment is only recommended for progressive neurological deterioration or severe pain.

Surgical treatment involves drainage of the cavity and placement of a shunt to the subarachnoid space or peritoneal cavity. Relief of pain postoperatively and improvement of motor weakness is usually found, but sensory recovery is not usually as favorable.

Skeletal Complications
Osteoporosis

After SCI, there is marked calcium resorption and associated hypercalciuria, resulting in osteoporosis of the bones of the paralyzed limbs. Bone loss in the lower limbs after complete lesions is rapid, with approximately 22% of the bone depleted 3 months after injury.[88] An additional 5% is lost between the third and fourth months, and at 14 months post injury approximately one third of the bone has been lost. This bone loss increases the risk of lower limb fractures. It also appears to follow a selective pattern, with the most significant loss occurring from distal to proximal in the lower limb and at the hips with the lumbar spine relatively preserved, probably as a result of weight bearing during sitting.[89]

A number of interventions have been studied to minimize osteoporosis. Functional electrical stimulation (FES) may reduce the rate of bone loss but has not been found to reduce osteoporosis after it has developed in people with chronic SCI.[89,90] In addition, there is conflicting evidence in its efficacy and clinical role in acute SCI.[91] Standing and ambulation may decrease hypercalciuria, but such activities have not been shown to prevent or reduce osteoporosis, although early performance of such activities may be helpful. Pharmacological agents, including calcitonin and recombinant human growth hormone, have been studied but none of these have yet been shown to be effective in reducing osteoporosis in people with SCI. The use of bisphosphonates may be effective,[92] and further study is in progress in both acute and chronic SCI.

Fractures

The incidence of lower limb fractures in individuals with chronic SCI has been reported to be between 1.5% and 6%.[93,94] The most common site of fracture after SCI is the femur. Fractures are more common in persons with paraplegia and in those with neurologically complete injuries. The most commonly reported cause is a fall during transfers, but fractures may also occur during ROM exercises or without any known cause. The diagnosis of these fractures may be difficult, especially in the absence of pain. The presenting symptoms may be a low-grade fever, malaise, and a swollen limb. A plain radiograph gives a more definitive diagnosis.

Lower limb fractures in ambulatory individuals with SCI are treated similarly to those occurring in able-bodied people, with the goal of maintaining normal leg length and alignment (Clinical Note: Goals for Treating Fractures in Individuals with Spinal Cord Injury). In those with SCI who are not able to ambulate, normal femoral length and angular alignment is not the primary goal and some degree of shortening and angulation is acceptable, but rotational deformity is not. Most fractures in individuals with SCI are treated without surgery, using soft, well-padded splints and frequent skin inspections. Splints made of hard materials must be liberally padded. The majority of these fractures heal well, often with rapid union and exuberant callus formation, often within 3 to 4 weeks. Weight-bearing activities, such as tilt table, standing, and stand pivot transfers, however, should be postponed for a longer period. The patient does not need to remain in bed and should be permitted to be mobile in his wheelchair. Good functional positioning is maintained with the legs flexed at the hips and knees and the feet flat on the footrests.

CLINICAL NOTE   **Goals for Treating Fractures in Individuals with Spinal Cord Injury**

- Restore prefracture functional capability
- Minimize interference with the individual's daily routine
- Minimize the risk of complications
- Allow for proper bone healing with satisfactory alignment

Some methods commonly used for fracture management in able-bodied patients, including surgery, casting, and external fixation, are not usually indicated for the person with SCI because of their possible complications. Circumferential plaster casts and skeletal traction may cause problems in the anesthetic limbs. Open reduction is only occasionally necessary.[94] Surgical interventions may be indicated when nonsurgical methods do not control rotational deformity of proximal femur fractures, severe muscle spasm is present, splints are too bulky and interfere with function, vascular supply is compromised, or leg shortening and angulation results in unacceptable function or cosmesis.

Upper limb fractures should be treated in the same fashion as those occurring in able-bodied individuals. The clinician must, however, consider the impact of the fracture on functional activities, such as the ability to perform transfers, pressure relief, wheelchair propulsion, and activities of daily living (ADL).

Heterotopic Ossification

Heterotopic ossification (HO), the formation of mature lamellar bone in the soft tissue, occurs in up to 53% of individuals with SCI.[95] Approximately 20% of HO results in limitations of joint ROM, interfering with ADLs, and in 3% to 5% of patients severe restrictions or ankylosis of the joint develop. Mature HO is pathologically similar to fracture callus and forms in the connective tissue between the muscle planes but not within the muscle itself. Heterotopic ossification occurs below the level of the spinal cord lesion unless there are other causative factors, such as a concomitant head injury or burns. The incidence of HO is higher in those with a neurologically complete injury, spasticity, and pressure ulcers. Most HO occurs 1 to 4 months after SCI, although HO has been reported to develop several years after injury. The most common location of HO is the anterior aspect of the hip, followed by the medial aspect of the knee. The shoulders and elbows may occasionally be affected in persons with high-level tetraplegia and in those with concomitant brain injury.

The cause of HO is poorly understood. A yet-unknown factor may induce a metaplasia of multipotential connective tissue (i.e., mesenchymal cells) to chondroblasts and osteoblasts. The presence of a fracture, DVT, or pressure ulcer may increase the risk of HO formation. The early clinical features of HO include swelling, warmth, and fever. After the initial phase the swelling becomes more firm and localized. Occasionally, the early inflammatory phase is not clinically detected and the HO occurs with a decreased ROM of the joint. Alkaline phosphatase levels become elevated early, but this is not specific. Additional laboratory tests that can be helpful include C-reactive protein, creatine phosphokinase, and erythrocyte sedimentation rate.[96,97] Plain radiographs also are helpful for detection of HO but do not reveal the process during the earliest phase. A specific method for early detection includes a triple-phase bone scan, which returns to normal in 6 to 18 months.

HO may cause pressure ulcers resulting from bony pressure or a change in sitting posture secondary to the extra bone. After the acute inflammatory phase of HO is over (i.e., a few days), it is important to initiate joint ROM with gentle stretching to prevent additional joint mobility loss. Administration of disodium etidronate is effective in limiting the extent of the ossification. Aggressive stretching should be avoided. Treatment is usually continued for 6 months, with the dosage used dependent on the degree of laboratory test abnormalities.[97,98] Nonsteroidal anti-inflammatory medications can be used as well to decrease the extra bone growth and for pain management associated with HO formation and progression. When HO severely limits ROM and impairs function, wedge resection surgery is indicated after the heterotopic bone is mature to prevent recurrence. Normal radiograph and alkaline phosphatase levels are not reliable markers for bone maturity; the best method to ascertain HO bone maturity is through serial bone scans.

Integumentary Complications

Pressure Ulcers

Pressure ulcers are an extremely common and costly sequela after SCI.[99] In the acute stage after SCI, more than one third of patients have pressure ulcers. Pressure ulcers may delay the onset of rehabilitation therapies, lengthen the total hospitalization, and make the ultimate adjustment to disability more difficult. In the long term, these ulcers impair an individual's quality of life because of activity restriction and the increased need for medical and nursing care, often by hospitalization or surgery.

Pressure ulcers are caused by pressure and shear forces. Ischemia develops when vascular structures are compressed between bony prominences and external surfaces. Individuals with SCI often have many major secondary factors that predispose them to the development of pressure ulcers, including paralysis, loss of sensation, incontinence of urine and stool, infections, obesity, spasticity, joint contracture, edema, anemia, and poor nutrition. Pressure ulcers are most commonly located at the sacrum, ischial tuberosities, heels, and trochanters (see Figure 6-10). The sacrum, followed by the heels, are the most common sites of ulceration during acute SCI because of prolonged supine positioning.[100] Ischial tuberosity ulcers occur when the person is sitting without adequate pressure relief. Other sites of pressure ulcers include trochanteric ulcers about the hip, usually from side lying; the scapulae, often when wearing a halo vest; and the occiput. All bony prominences must be considered as potential sources of pressure ulceration, especially in those areas that are insensate.

Several classification systems for pressure ulcers exist, each describing the pressure ulcers on the basis of depth and extent of tissue damage, with higher numbers indicating deeper ulcers.

The staging system of pressure ulcers most commonly used is based on the National pressure Ulcer advisory Panel Consensus Development Conference (Box 2-2), which incorporates several of the most commonly used staging systems.[101]

Initial prevention of pressure ulcers after SCI involves the use of specialty mattresses and beds, vigilance in weight shifting, and securing adequate nutrition. To prevent pressure ulcer development when in bed, the patient should be turned and the skin inspected every 2 hours. Ankle positioning orthoses are recommended because they provide support and cushioning to the malleoli and a relief for the heel while also preventing plantar flexion contractures.

The best method for preventing pressure ulcers is proper education about the importance of maintaining a life-long rigorous prevention program of avoiding prolonged pressure to susceptible areas. No mattress or cushion alone can prevent ulcers. Frequent and regular repositioning of the patient and careful skin inspection is necessary. Clothing should be inspected for appropriate fit. Attention to appropriate bowel and bladder management to avoid incontinence and skin maceration and nutritional instruction to minimize the metabolic effects of the early catabolic state are important at all stages after SCI.

When the rehabilitation phase begins, emphasis is placed on mobility. As more time is spent out of bed, the risk for development of ischial pressure ulcers related to sitting increases. Prescribing an appropriate wheelchair is vital because a poorly fitting wheelchair increases risk of ulcer development. Cushion selection also is important to provide equal pressure distribution in the ischial region. Options for cushions and recommendations for generating appropriate wheelchair prescriptions are discussed in Chapter 11. As soon as sitting is initiated, the patient should be instructed in weight-shifting techniques to relieve pressure. If the individual cannot independently perform the pressure-relieving maneuver, a caregiver should be trained and the patient should take responsibility for directing her in it. Specific maneuvers include tilting the wheelchair backward, leaning forward or to the side, and performing a pushup. Some patients with high-level tetraplegia may benefit from a power tilt-in-space or reclining wheelchair to allow for independence in weight shifts. These techniques are discussed in more detail in Chapter 7.

After an ulcer has developed, the treatment depends primarily on the depth and degree of tissue involvement. Stage I ulcers, which appear as erythematous areas over a bony prominence, require no specific skin care, although more vigilant positioning or a change in equipment should be addressed after this warning sign. With proper nutrition and pressure relief, these ulcers usually heal well. When the ulcer has penetrated the skin, however, more aggressive topical therapy is required. Most important is proper wound debridement of devitalized tissue to create a healthy, clean base. Some form of dressing should then be applied. There are many products that promote wound healing including gels, pastes, enzymes, bio-occlusive dressings, and growth factors. Whatever product is used, it does not take the place of regular inspection, pressure relief, and debridement of necrotic material (see Chapter 3).

After the ulcer has reached sufficient depth to expose muscle or bone, treatment most commonly involves surgery. At this stage, if the deep ulcer involves the ischial tuberosities, limiting or prohibiting wheelchair use may be necessary. Before surgical reconstruction is undertaken, the situation producing the ulcer should be addressed and, if possible, rectified. For example, a wheelchair should be replaced if it cannot accommodate the presence of a pelvic obliquity and thus results in uneven ischial weight bearing; pressure mapping can be performed to see whether there is proper weight distribution from the individual's cushion.

The most common surgical procedure is a myocutaneous rotational flap using local tissue. After surgery, the patient is positioned to remove all pressure from the repaired segment. Most commonly the patient is placed on a specialized bed for 3 to 4 weeks. ROM to the involved joints (e.g., hip or knee) is avoided and spasticity should be controlled as aggressively as possible. When the sutures and drains are removed, the individual gradually resumes activity that allows contact between the flap and external surfaces, with increases as tolerated over a 1- to 2-week time course as dictated by the physician.

Pain

Pain is a common, yet poorly defined, occurrence in patients with SCI. There is no accepted classification system for pain after SCI, and as such it is difficult to accurately document its prevalence. The prevalence of severe pain in SCI seems to be lowest in patients with tetraplegia (10% to 15%), followed by thoracic-level lesions (25%), and highest in those with cauda equina lesions.[102-106] The perception of pain severity may be influenced by external factors, including depression and adjustment disorders.

Although there are numerous ways to categorize pain in SCI, the recent Bryce-Ragnarsson Classification can be helpful in describing the type and location of pain (see Figure 3-7).[107] It specifically differentiates pain as nociceptive or neuropathic pain (i.e., pain related to injury to the nerve roots, spinal cord, or cauda equina) and whether the pain is above, at, or below the level of injury. The understanding of the type and etiology of the pain can then help determine the best approach for management. For discussion later, SCI pain has been differentiated between nociceptive and neuropathic pain.

TABLE 2-3 | Goals and Treatment for Upper Limb Nociceptive Pain

Goal	Treatment
Decrease pain	Rest
	Pharmacological intervention and injections
Address secondary disability	Use of compensatory techniques and equipment
Prevent recurrence	Balance of strength and flexibility in the upper limb musculature
	Instruct in proper posture
	Limit overhead activities
	Avoid unnecessary upper limb weight bearing

Nociceptive Pain

Nociceptive pain occurs in those body parts that are innervated in the patient with SCI (i.e., above the level of the injury). Upper limb musculoskeletal problems are often encountered in patients with SCI yet are underappreciated.[108-110] The most common causes are impingement syndrome of the shoulder, overuse injuries, degenerative joint diseases, bursitis, capsulitis, myofascial pain syndrome, and cervical radiculopathy. Overuse syndromes may become major contributing factors to chronic disability in this population, with the shoulder the most common joint involved because upper limbs become weight-bearing structures for mobility during wheelchair activities, transfers, and ADLs instead of for their designed use in prehensile activities. Patient age and the length of time since injury are correlated to a greater incidence of upper limb musculoskeletal problems, with patients with paraplegia having a slightly higher prevalence of musculoskeletal pain, although it is usually less disabling.

The diagnosis of upper limb pain is similar in patients with SCI to that of the able-bodied population. Treatment goals are to decrease pain, address secondary disability, and prevent recurrence (Table 2-3). Rest, if possible, and pharmacological intervention and injections are used to address pain as needed. Secondary disability as caused by the musculoskeletal problems may be addressed by using compensatory techniques and equipment. Prevention of recurrence is important and may be achieved by obtaining a balance of strength and flexibility of the upper limb musculature surrounding the shoulder.[111] In addition, proper posture should be emphasized, overhead activities limited, and unnecessary upper limb weight bearing avoided.

Carpal tunnel syndrome is reported in up to two thirds of patients with SCI.[112,113] Its incidence increases in relationship to time after injury. This may be secondary to the repetitive weight bearing and extension forces placed on the wrist during activities. Pressures within the carpal tunnel are greatly increased during functional activities. Treatment includes rest if possible, splinting, and injections into the carpal tunnel. Functional activities must be modified including transfers, pressure relief techniques, and wheelchair propulsion to decrease excessive flexion-extension of the wrist. Padded gloves can be used for wheelchair propulsion. Surgical release is indicated as in the able-bodied population. Ulnar neuropathy at the elbow has also been reported in up 20% of patients, with the highest incidence in wheelchair athletes.[114]

Neuropathic Pain

Neuropathic pain, also referred to as neurogenic pain, has been categorized as radicular, segmental, and central pain. Almost half of patients with this type of pain report that it interferes with daily activities.[115,116] Radicular pain is caused by injury to one or more nerve roots at the level of the injury. It is usually limited to specific dermatomal distributions and can be described as burning, aching, tingling, or tightness.

Central pain is perhaps the most common, least understood, and most difficult to treat. It can be described as cutting, burning, piercing, radiating, or nagging pain, usually in the saddle distribution and lower limbs. This type of pain usually begins within 6 months of injury.

Because patients with high-level injuries (above T6) cannot perceive pain from their visceral organs (e.g., abdomen, bladder), they may have visceral-type pain, which is characterized by deep, diffuse pain in abdominal and pelvic areas. Visceral pain and the possibility of other SCI-specific disorders that can cause pain including PTS, HO, DVT, fracture, and spasticity, which have been discussed previously, should be considered for patients who have pain after their injury without an inciting event.

Treatment of neuropathic pain is extremely difficult because few medications have been developed specifically to target this type of pain. Neither has the use of modalities including TENS, functional electrical stimulation, and dorsal column stimulation proved effective.[116-118] Establishing an accurate diagnosis is an important first step. Relieving stress-related activities is important because these intensify most pain disorders and may be helped by psychological counseling or psychiatric intervention. In addition, no one pharmacological protocol can be used in the treatment of all patients. Usually the approach is to try one agent until pain relief is achieved, a maximum dose is obtained, or side effects prohibit increasing the dose, before trying another agent. The most common medications used in the management of neuropathic pain include antidepressants, anticonvulsant agents, narcotics, and intrathecal medications.[107,108] Antidepressants used include tricyclic agents (e.g., nortriptyline, amitriptyline, doxepin) and serotonergic reuptake inhibitors such as fluoxetine, sertraline, and paroxetine. Anticonvulsant agents frequently used include carbamazepine, gabapentin, and phenytoin. If these options have proved ineffective, narcotic agents can be used, but cautiously, because of their side effects. These include effects on the bowel program (e.g., constipation), fatigue, tolerance, dependence, and potential abuse. The use of intrathecal baclofen, morphine, and clonidine are newer approaches to decrease this type of pain.

Surgical intervention is only considered if all else has failed and the neuropathic pain interferes with daily activities. Few individuals have significant improvement from surgery, unless a syrinx is the cause of the pain. The most common surgical techniques include dorsal root rhizotomy, cordotomy, and lumbar sympathectomy.

SUMMARY

Understanding the potential medical complications that may arise in the acute and chronic stages after SCI is extremely important. When a clinician recognizes potential complications and treats them appropriately, morbidity and mortality are diminished. Prevention and treatment of medical issues, along with proper rehabilitation allow individuals with SCI to maximize their functional capability and return to a community setting.

It is important to understand the implications of spinal stability during rehabilitation and how spinal orthotics enable rehabilitation activities while providing support and protection to the spine. In addition, management of individuals with SCI including the possibility of numerous complications affecting body systems (e.g., cardiovascular, respiratory, genitourinary, GI) must be addressed while planning rehabilitation activities because symptoms and medical treatments can affect a patient's tolerance. Patients also will be concerned with sexual function and the more education and treatment that can be provided, the more they will be able to focus on the recovery process. Other complications relate to the musculoskeletal system such as osteoporosis, fractures, and heterotopic ossification. These conditions as well as integumentary conditions such as pressure ulcers can place significant restrictions on physical activities that are desirable during rehabilitation and home/community living. Although the presence of nociceptive pain can be aided by pharmacological and medical management to allow participation in the rehabilitation process, solutions to neuropathic pain are often more complex. Understanding the scope and impact of the medical complications in SCI can better help the clinician effectively accelerate rehabilitation.

REFERENCES

1. Kirshblum S, O'Connor K, Benevento B et al: Spinal orthotics. In DeLisa JA, Gans BM, Bockeneck WL, editors: *Rehabilitation medicine: principles and practice*, ed 3, Philadelphia, 1998, Lippincott-Raven.

2. Goldberg B, Hsu JD: *Atlas of orthoses and assistive devices*, ed 3, St. Louis, 1998, Mosby.

3. Kirshblum S, Ho C, Druin E et al: Rehabilitation after spinal cord injury. In Kirshblum S, Campagnolo DI, DeLisa JA, editors: *Spinal cord medicine*, Philadelphia, 2002, Lippincott Williams & Wilkins.

4. Johnson RM, Owen JR, Hart DL et al: Cervical orthoses: a guide to their selection and use, *Clin Orthop Rel Res* 154:34-45, 1981.

5. Askins V, Eismont FJ: Efficacy of five cervical orthoses in restricting cervical motion: a comparison study, *Spine* 22:1193-1198, 1997.

6. Lind B, Sihlbom H, Nordwall A: Forces and motions across the neck in patients treated with halo-vest, *Spine* 13:162-167, 1988.

7. Koch RA, Nickel VL: : The halo vest: an evaluation of motion and forces across the neck, *Spine* 3:103-107, 1978.

8. Sharpe KP, Rao S, Ziogas A: Evaluation of the effectiveness of the Minerva cervicothoracic orthosis, *Spine* 20:1475-1479, 1995.

9. Campagnolo DI, Heary RF: Acute medical and surgical management of spinal cord injury. In Kirshblum S, Campagnolo DI, DeLisa JA, editors: *Spinal cord medicine*, Philadelphia, 2002, Lippincott Williams & Wilkins.

10. Gonzalez F, Chang JY, Banovac K et al: Autoregulation of cerebral blood flow in patients with orthostatic hypotension after spinal cord injury, *Paraplegia* 29:1-7, 1991.

11. Corbett JL, Frankel HL, Harris PJ: Cardiovascular reflex responses to cutaneous and visceral stimuli in spinal man, *J Physiol* 215: 395-409, 1971.

12. Gilgoff IS, Ward SLD, Hohn AR: Cardiac pacemaker in high spinal cord injury, *Arch Phys Med Rehabil* 72:601-603, 1991.

13. Schmidt KD, Chan CW: Thermoregulation and fever in normal persons and in those with spinal cord injuries, *Mayo Clin Proc* 67: 469-475, 1992.

14. Lindan R, Joiner E, Freehafer AA et al: Incidence and clinical features of autonomic dysreflexia in patients with spinal cord injury, *Paraplegia* 18:285-292, 1980.

15. Erickson RP: Autonomic hyperreflexia: pathophysiology and medical management, *Arch Phys Med Rehabil* 61:431-440, 1980.

16. Consortium for Spinal Cord Medicine: *Acute management of autonomic dysreflexia: adults with spinal cord injury presenting to healthcare facilities*, ed 2, Washington, DC, 2001, Paralyzed Veterans of America.

17. Green D, Hull RD, Mammen EF et al: Deep vein thrombosis in spinal cord injury summary and recommendations, *Chest* 102(6 Suppl):633S-635S, 1992.

18. Green D, Sullivan S, Simpson J, et al: Evolving risk for thromboembolism in spinal cord injury (SPIRATE Study), *Am J Phys Med Rehabil* 84:420-422, 2005.

19. Ragnarsson KT, Hall KM, Wilmot CB, et al: Management of pulmonary, cardiovascular and metabolic conditions after spinal cord injury, In Stover SL, DeLisa JA, Whiteneck GG, editors: *Spinal cord injury: clinical outcomes from the model systems*, Gaithersburg, MD, 1995, Aspen Publishers.

20. Green D, Hartwick D, Chen D, et al: Spinal cord injury risk assessment for thromboembolism (SPIRATE Study), *Am J Phys Med Rehabil* 82:950-956, 2003.

21. Consortium for Spinal Cord Medicine: *Prevention of thromboembolism in spinal cord injury: clinical practice guidelines*, Washington, DC, 1997, Paralyzed Veterans of America.

22. Jackson AB, Groomes TE: Incidence of respiratory complications following spinal cord injury, *Arch Phys Med Rehabil* 75:270-275, 1994.

23. Garstang SV, Kirshblum SC, Wood KE: Patient preference for inexsufflation for secretion management in spinal cord injury, *J Spinal Cord Med* 23:80-85, 2000.

24. Peterson P, Kirshblum SC: Respiratory management in spinal cord injury. In Kirshblum S, Campagnolo DI, DeLisa JA, editors: *Spinal cord medicine*, Philadelphia, 2002, Lippincott Williams & Wilkins.

25. Adler US, Kirshblum SC: A new assistive device for intermittent self-catheterization in men with tetraplegia, *J Spinal Cord Med* 26:155-158, 2003.

26. Linsenmeyer TA: Neurogenic bladder following spinal cord injury. In Kirshblum S, Campagnolo DI, DeLisa JA, editors: *Spinal cord medicine*, Philadelphia, 2002, Lippincott Williams & Wilkins.

27. Ducharme S, Gill K, Biener-Bergman S: Sexual functioning: medical and psychological aspects. In DeLisa JA, editor: *Rehabilitation medicine: principles and practice*, ed 2, , Philadelphia, 1993, JB Lippincott.

28. Linsenmeyer TA: Sexual function and fertility following spinal cord injury. In Kirshblum S, Campagnolo DI, DeLisa JA, editors: *Spinal cord medicine*, Philadelphia, 2002, Lippincott Williams & Wilkins.

29. Sipski ML, Alexander CJ: Sexuality and disability. In DeLisa JA, Gans BM, Bockeneck WL, editors: *Rehabilitation medicine: principles and practice*, ed 3, Philadelphia, 1998, Lippincott-Raven.

30. Sipski ML: Spinal cord injury: what is the effect on sexual response? *J Am Paraplegia Soc* 14:40-43, 1991.

31. Komisaruk BR, Gerdes CA, Whipple B: 'Complete' spinal cord injury does not block perceptual responses to genital self-simulation in women, *Arch Neurol* 54:1513-1520, 1997.

32. Sipski ML, Alexander CJ, Rosen RC: Orgasm in women with spinal cord injury: a lab-based assessment, *Arch Phys Med Rehabil* 76:1097-1102, 1995.

33. Talbot HS: The sexual function in paraplegia, *J Urol* 73:91-100, 1955.

34. Bors E, Comarr AE: Neurological disturbances of sexual function with special reference to 529 patients with spinal cord injury, *Urol Surg* 10:222, 1960.

35. Rivas DA, Chancellor MB: Management of erectile dysfunction. In Sipski ML, Alexander CJ, editors: *Sexual function in people with disability and chronic illness,* Gaithersburg, MD, 1997, Aspen Publishers.

36. Linsenmeyer TA: Evaluation and treatment of erectile dysfunction following spinal cord injury: a review, *J Am Paraplegia Soc* 14:43-51, 1991.

37. Solar JM, Previnaire JG, Dennys P et al: Phosphodiesterase inhibitors in the treatment of erectile dysfunction in spinal cord injured men, *Spinal Cord* 15:165-173, 2007.

38. Giuliano F, Hutling C, El Masry WS et al: Randomized trial of sildenafil for the treatment of erectile dysfunction in spinal cord injury: Sildenafil Study Group, *Ann Neurol* 46:15-21, 1999.

39. Goldstein I, Lue T, Padma-Nathan H et al: Oral sildenafil in the treatment of erectile dysfunction: Sildenafil Study Group, *N Engl J Med* 338:1397-1404, 1998.

40. Sipski ML, Alexander CJ: Sexual activities, response and satisfaction in women pre and post-spinal cord injury, *Arch Phys Med Rehabil* 74:1025-1029, 1993.

41. Alexander CJ, Sipski ML, Findley TW: Sexual activities, desire and satisfaction in males pre and post-spinal cord injury, *Arch Sex Behav* 22:217-228, 1993.

42. Black K, Sipski ML, Strauss SS: Sexual satisfaction and sexual drive in spinal cord injured women, *J Spin Cord Med* 21:240-244, 1998.

43. Neumayer LA, Bull DA, Mohr JD et al: The acutely affected abdomen in paraplegic spinal cord injury patients, *Ann Surg* 212:561-566, 1990.

44. Gore RM, Mintzer RA, Calenoff L: Gastrointestinal complications of spinal cord injury, *Spine* 6:538-544, 1981.

45. Stone JM, Nino-Murcia M, Wolfe VA et al: Chronic gastrointestinal problems in spinal cord injury patients: a prospective analysis, *Am J Gastroenterol* 85:1114-1119, 1990.

46. Stiens SA, Bergman SB, Goetz LL: *Neurogenic bowel dysfunction after spinal cord injury: clinical correlation and rehabilitative management Arch Phys Med Rehabil* 78(3 Suppl):S86-S102, 1997.

47. Consortium for Spinal Cord Medicine: *Neurogenic bowel management in adults with spinal cord injury,* Washington, DC, 1998, Paralyzed Veterans of America.

48. Preibe MM, Goetz LL, Wuermser LA: Spasticity following spinal cord injury. In Kirshblum S, Campagnolo DI, DeLisa JA, editors: *Spinal cord medicine,* Philadelphia, 2002, Lippincott Williams & Wilkins.

49. Young RR: The physiology of spasticity and its response to therapy, *Ann N Y Acad Sci* 531:146-149, 1988.

50. Maynard FM, Karuns PS, Waring WP: Epidemiology of spasticity following traumatic spinal cord injury, *Arch Phys Med Rehabil* 71:566-569, 1990.

51. Little JW, Mickelsen P, Umlauf R, et al: Lower extremity manifestations of spasticity in chronic spinal cord injury, *Am J Phys Med Rehabil* 68:32-36, 1989.

52. Ashworth B: Preliminary trial of carisoprodol in multiple sclerosis, *Practioner* 192:540-542, 1964.

53. Bohannon RW, Smith MB: Interrator reliability on modified Ashworth scale of muscle spasticity, *Phys Ther* 67:206-207, 1987.

54. Penn RD, Savoy SM, Corcos DC, et al: Intrathecal baclofen for severe spinal spasticity, *N Engl J Med* 320:1517-1521, 1989.

55. Wartenberg R: Pendulousness of the legs as a diagnostic test, *Neurology* 1:18-24, 1951.

56. Kirshblum S: Treatment alternatives for spinal cord related spasticity, *J Spinal Cord Med* 22:199-217, 1999.

57. Stolp-Smith KA, Wainberg MC: Antidepressant exacerbation of spasticity, *Arch Phys Med Rehabil* 80:339-342, 1999.

58. Lightfoot E, Varrier M, Ashby P: Neurophysiological effects of prolonged cooling of the calf in patients with complete spinal transection, *Phys Ther* 55:251-258, 1975.

59. Price R, Lehmann JF, Boswell-Bessette S et al: Influence of cryotherapy on spasticity at the human ankle, *Arch Phys Med Rehabil* 74:300-304, 1993.

60. Stefanovska A, Rebersek S, Bajd T et al: Effects of electrical stimulation on spasticity, *Crit Rev Phys Med Rehabil* 3:59-99, 1991.

61. Robinson CJ, Kett NA, Bolam JM: Spasticity in spinal cord injured patients: short term effects of electrical stimulation, *Arch Phys Med Rehabil* 69:598-604, 1988.

62. Bajd T, Gregoric M, Vodornik L et al: Electrical stimulation in treating spasticity resulting from spinal cord trauma, *Arch Phys Med Rehabil* 66:515-517, 1985.

63. Basmajian JV: Biofeedback in rehabilitation; a review of principles and practice, *Arch Phys Med Rehabil* 62:469-475, 1981.

64. Wolf SL, Binder-MacLeod SA: Electromyographic biofeedback applications to the hemiplegic patient: changes in lower extremity neuromuscular and functional status, *Phys Ther* 63:1404-1413, 1983.

65. Bohannon RW: Tilt table standing for reducing spasticity after spinal cord injury, *Arch Phys Med Rehabil* 74:1121-1122, 1993.

66. Collins K, Oswald P, Burger G et al: Customized adjustable orthoses: their use in spasticity, *Arch Phys Med Rehabil* 66:397-398, 1985.

67. Physicians' *desk reference,* ed 51, Woodcliff Lake, NJ, 1997, Medical Economics.

68. Kirkland LR: Baclofen dosage: a suggestion, *Arch Phys Med Rehabil* 65:214, 1984.

69. Bianchine JR: Drugs for Parkinson's disease, spasticity, and acute muscle spasms. In Goodman LS, Gilman A, Gilman AG, editors: *Goodman and Gilman's the pharmacological basis of therapeutics,* ed 7, New York, 1985, Macmillan.

70. Herman R, Mayer N, Mecomber SA: Clinical pharmaco-physiology of dantrolene sodium, *Am J Phys Med Rehabil* 51:296-311, 1972.

71. Weingarden SI, Belen JG: Clonidine transdermal system for treatment of spasticity in spinal cord injury, *Arch Phys Med Rehabil* 73:876-877, 1992.

72. Wallace JD: Summary of combined clinical analysis of controlled clinical trials with tizanidine, *Neurology* 44(11 Suppl 9):S60-S69, 1994.

73. United Kingdom Tizanidine Trial Group: A double blind, placebo-controlled trial of tizanidine in the treatment of spasticity caused by multiple sclerosis, *Neurology* 1994; 44(11 Suppl 9):S70-S78, 1994.

74. Nance P: A comparison of clonidine, cyproheptadine, and baclofen in spastic spinal cord injured patients, *J Am Paralegia Soc* 17:150-156, 1994.

75. Norman KE, Pepin A, Barbeau H: Effects of drugs on walking after spinal cord injury, *Spinal Cord* 36:699-715, 1998.

76. Wainberg M, Barbeau H, Gauthier S: The effects of cyproheptadine on locomotion and on spasticity in patients with spinal cord injuries, *J Neurol Neurosurg Psychiatry* 53:754-763, 1990.

77. Cutter N, Scott D, Johnson J et al: Gabapentin effect on spasticity in multiple sclerosis: a placebo-controlled randomized study, *Arch Phys Med Rehabil* 81:164-169, 2000.

78. Mueller ME, Gruenthal M, Olson WL et al: Gabapentin for relief of upper motor neuron symptoms in multiple sclerosis, *Arch Phys Med Rehabil* 78:521-524, 1997.

79. Snow BJ, Tsui JK, Bhatt MH, et al: Treatment of spasticity with botulinum toxin: a double blind study, *Ann Neurol* 28:512-515, 1990.

80. Brin MF: Dosing, administration, and a treatment algorithm for use of botulinum toxin A for adult-onset spasticity. *Spasticity Study Group, Muscle Nerve* Suppl 6 S208-S220, 1997.

81. Abel NA, Smith RA: Intrathecal baclofen for treatment of intractable spinal spasticity, *Arch Phys Med Rehabil* 75:54-58, 1994.

82. Coffey JR, Cahill D, Steers W, et al: Intrathecal baclofen for intractable spasticity of spinal origin: results of a long-term multicenter study, *J Neurosurg* 78:226-232, 1993.

83. Ivanhoe CB, Tilton AH, Francisco GE: Intrathecal baclofen therapy for spastic hypertonia, *Phys Med Rehabil Clin North Am* 12:923-938, 2001.

84. Burchiel KJ, Hsu FPK: *Pain and spasticity after spinal cord injury: mechanisms and treatment, Spine* 26(24 Suppl):S146-S160, 2001.

85. Biyani A, El Masry WS: Post-traumatic syringomyelia: a review of the literature, *Paraplegia* 32:723-731, 1994.

86. Schurch B, Wichmann W, Rossier AB: Post-traumatic syringomyelia (cystic myelopathy): a prospective study of 449 patients with spinal cord injury, *J Neurol Neurosurg Psychiatry* 60:61-67, 1996.

87. Little JW, Stiens SA: Electrodiagnosis in spinal cord injury, *Phys Med Rehabil Clin North Am* 5:571-593, 1994.

88. Garland DE, Marie E, Adkins RH, et al: Bone mineral density about the knee in SCI patients with pathological fractures, *Contemp Orthop* 26:375-379, 1993.

89. Saltzstein RJ, Hardin S, Hartings J: Osteoporosis in SCI: using an index of mobility and its relationship to bone density, *J Am Paraplegia Soc* 15:232-234, 1992.

90. BeDell KK, Scremin AM, Perell KL et al: Effects of functional electrical stimulation-induced lower extremity cycling on bone density of spinal cord-injured patients, *Am J Phys Med Rehabil* 75:29-34, 1996.

91. Clark JM, Jelbart M, Rischbieth H et al: Physiological effects of lower extremity functional electrical stimulation in early spinal cord injury: lack of efficacy to prevent bone loss, *Spinal Cord,* 45:78-85, 2007.

92. Nance PW, Schryvers O, Leslie W, et al: Intravenous pamidronate attenuates bone density loss after acute spinal cord injury, *Arch Phys Med Rehabil* 80:243-251, 1999.

93. Ragnarsson KT, Sell GH: Lower extremity fractures after SCI: a retrospective study, *Arch Phys Med Rehabil* 62:418-423, 1981.

94. Freehafer AA: Limb fractures in patients with spinal cord injury, *Arch Phys Med Rehabil* 76:823-827, 1995.

95. van Kuijk AA, Geurts AC, van Kuppevelt HJ: Neurogenic heterotopic ossification in spinal cord injury, *Spinal Cord* 40:313-326, 2002.

96. Estores IM, Harrington A, Banovac K: C-reactive protein and erythrocyte sedimentation rate in patients with heterotopic ossification after spinal cord injury, *J Spinal Cord Med* 27:434-437, 2004.

97. Sherman AL, Williams J, Patrick L et al: The value of serum creatine kinase in early diagnosis of heterotopic ossification, *J Spinal Cord Med* 26:227-231, 2003.

98. Banovac K, Sherman AL, Estores IM, et al: Prevention and treatment of heterotopic ossification after spinal cord injury, *J Spinal Cord Med* 27:376-382, 2004.

99. Consortium for Spinal Cord Medicine: *Pressure ulcer prevention and treatment following spinal cord injury: a clinical practice guideline for health care professionals,* Washington, DC, 2000, Paralyzed Veterans of America.

100. Yarkony GM, Heineman AW: Pressure ulcers. In Stover SL, DeLisa JA, Whiteneck GG, editors: *Spinal cord injury: clinical outcomes from the model systems,* Gaithersburg, MD, 1995, Aspen Publishers.

101. Nutritional Pressure Ulcer Advisory Panel: *Pressure ulcer definition and stages:* www.npuap.org. Washington, DC, 2007.

102. Jensen TS, Hoffman AJ, Cardenas DD: Chronic pain in individuals with spinal cord injury: a survey and longitudinal study, *Spinal Cord* 43:704-712, 2005.

103. Bockeneck WL, Stuart PJB: Pain in patients with spinal cord injury. In Kirshblum S, Campagnolo DI, DeLisa JA, editors: *Spinal cord medicine,* Philadelphia, 2002, Lippincott Williams & Wilkins.

104. Elliot T, Harkins SW: Psychosocial concomitant of persistent pain among persons with spinal cord injuries, *J Neurorehabil* 1:7-16, 1991.

105. Woolsey RM: Pain in spinal cord disorders. In Young RE, Woolsey RM, editors: *Diagnosis and management of disorders of the spinal cord,* Philadelphia, 1995, WB Saunders.

106. Mariano AJ: Chronic pain in spinal cord injury [review], *Clin J Pain* 8:119-122, 1992.

107. Bryce TN, Ragnarsson KT: Pain after spinal cord injury, *Phys Med Rehabil Clin North Am* 11:157-168, 2000.

108. Ragnarsson KT: Management of pain in persons with spinal cord injury, *J Spinal Cord Med* 20:186-199, 1997.

109. Subbarao JV, Klopfstein J, Turpin R: Prevalence and impact of wrist and shoulder pain in patients with spinal cord injury, *J Spinal Cord Med* 18:9-13, 1995.

110. Sie IH, Waters RL, Adkins RH, et al: Upper extremity pain in the postrehabilitation spinal cord injury patient, *Arch Phys Med Rehabil* 73:44-48, 1992.

111. Kirshblum S, Druin E, Planten K: Musculoskeletal conditions in chronic SCI, *Top Spinal Cord Injury Rehabil* 2:23-35, 1997.

112. Gellman H, Chandler DR, Petrasek J et al: Carpal tunnel syndrome in paraplegic patients, *J Bone Joint Surg Am* 70:517-519, 1988.

113. Davidoff G, Werner R, Waring W: Compressive mononeuropathies of the upper extremity in chronic paraplegia, *Paraplegia* 29:17-24, 1991.

114. Boninger ML, Robertson RN, Wolff M et al: Upper extremity nerve entrapment in elite wheelchair racers, *Am J Phys Med Rehabil* 75:170-176, 1996.

115. Beric A, Demitrijevic M, Lindblom U: Central dysesthesia syndrome in spinal cord injury patients, *Pain* 34:109-116, 1988.

116. Anke AG, Stenehjem AE, Stanghelle JK: Pain and life quality within 2 years of spinal cord injury, *Paraplegia* 33:555-559, 1995.

117. Edgar RE, Best LG, Quail PA et al: Computer assisted DREZ microcoagulation: post traumatic spinal deafferentation pain, *J Spinal Disord* 6:48-56, 1993.

118. Richardson DE, Akil H: Pain reduction by electrical stimulation in man, I acute administration in periaqueductal and periventricular sites, *J Neurosurg* 47:178-183, 1977.

CHAPTER THREE

Nursing Care and Education for Patients with Spinal Cord Injury

Joan P. Alverzo, RN, CRRN, PhD, Jay H. Rosenberg, CRRN, BSN, Carolyn A. Sorensen, RN, CRRN, MSN, and Sandra Shultz DeLeon, CRRN, CCM, MS, BSN

My main goal when I entered rehab was to get out of there and back to school right away. To do that I needed to learn all there was about my injury. My family also needed to learn all aspects of my care. We learned everything from wound care to transfers. As we became more educated, our confidence increased and I began to realize that I really could complete college and lead a productive life.

Jason (C6 SCI)

The practice of rehabilitation nursing, which was formally organized in 1964, is defined as "the diagnosis and treatment of human responses of individuals and groups to actual or potential health problems stemming from altered functional ability and altered lifestyle."[1] One of the central principles of rehabilitation nursing is the prevention of complications and any further disability in patients who have sustained a disability from an illness or injury. Spinal cord nursing is a highly specialized subset of rehabilitation nursing, integrating its fundamental principles together with elements of critical care nursing, urological nursing, and community nursing to provide a holistic approach and plan of care to support patients in their recovery.

Spinal cord nursing can be conceptualized in many different ways on the basis of a range of nursing theories, conceptual frameworks, and models of care. In a global sense, it encompasses a range of nursing roles, from assuming total responsibility for all physiological needs of the patient with a catastrophic spinal cord injury (SCI) to educating the patient and family on self-care management in preparation for community re-entry.[2]

Dorothy Orem's self-care model that defines nursing care agency as legitimized by the gap between a patient's needs and his ability to provide for his own self-care supplies a good framework for this specialty.[3] Spinal cord nursing is dynamic, requiring a shift in role of the rehabilitation nurse from wholly compensatory (a total substitution of nursing for a patient's own self-care needs) to supportive or educational on the basis of assessment and cues of the patient's readiness to participate in direct care.

Rehabilitation nurses who treat spinal cord injuries develop very special relationships with their patients. The multisystem alterations that threaten survival after an SCI necessitate nursing care and interventions of the highest caliber. Although the needs of the patient with SCI are greatest early in their recovery, for many patients the need for continuing nursing care and support may be life long. The initial injury is often catastrophic, and the nurse who is frequently closest to the patient during the early hours and days after injury must demonstrate tremendous strength to sustain the patient and family when they are facing such significant loss.[4]

The ability to engender trust in the patient and family is central to their ability to both survive and recover from such loss. The recovery from SCI is ever changing, with new research and technology supporting the survival of patients who may not have survived less than a decade ago. The complexity of care that is required for patients who are ventilator dependent or who survive repeated life-threatening complications is tremendous.[5]

Patients who are very fragile need to be carefully moved along the trajectory from injury to recovery. Subtle cues and symptoms need to be understood in the context of this fragility, and the assessment and response of the rehabilitation nurse is ever more important to avert catastrophe. Critical thinking must be used to determine what is important and to alert the physiatrist and other team members of important changes in a patient's condition.

In general, the path of recovery for the patient with SCI is from some level of dependence toward self-care. Given the extent of the loss of function, adaptation cannot begin until a sense of reality has begun to be assimilated by the patient. During the early days and weeks after injury, nurses take over for many of the functional deficits of the multisystem failure and often patient or family participation in care may be delayed. The length of time a patient remains in each stage of recovery varies according to the individual patient, his history of adaptation, the family involvement, and the nature of the injury and loss.

Recognizing cues for readiness by the patient or family to become more involved is critical for the rehabilitation nurse to shift his/her role from wholly compensatory to supportive/educative. There are many cues for readiness for learning (see Clinical Note: Indicators of Readiness to Participate in Care). A nurse's relationship with the patient is intimate, based on their close involvement with all bodily functions. This creates an opportunity for trust and bonding that may set the stage for involving the patient or family in care activities. Key to success is providing just the right amount of information at the right moments to entice further investment of the patient in his recovery. In addition, the interdisciplinary team may provide critical information and feedback about the readiness of the patient and family to become more involved in care.

The impact of interdisciplinary collaboration in the management and rehabilitation of patients who have sustained an SCI cannot be overstated.[6] The unique role of nursing on the team is a multisystem view of the patient, incorporating both physiological and psychological aspects of recovery. Aside from providing context regarding how a patient or family may be progressing toward self-care, nursing has a principal role throughout the rehabilitation stay in early recognition of symptoms that may be potentially life threatening. This "rescuing" role of nurses is critical to the patient with an SCI because of the dynamic nature of potential multisystem failure.[7] In addition, nursing provides a balance to the perspective of the patient's ability to participate in self-care or direct care by giving feedback of progress on the nursing unit,

CLINICAL NOTE **Indicators of Readiness to Participate in Care**

- The patient asks questions about nursing care as it proceeds and inquires regarding what is to be expected in the near future around care activities.
- The patient watches or closely observes care as it is unfolding, cooperating and anticipating activities.
- The patient interacts with other patients with SCIs, participating in some dialog about the process of recovery.
- The patient demonstrates some anticipation of care activities and daily schedules or reminds the nurse of what is due to occur.

a more realistic setting that mimics the home environment more closely than the therapy gym.

Spinal cord nursing requires a range of nursing skills from traditional critical care skills such as managing patients on ventilators or responding to sudden fluctuations in cardiovascular homeostasis to establishing programs of self-care for the individual patient that can be assimilated into the home environment on discharge. Knowledgeable patients and families have a tremendous advantage both in successfully managing the transition into community living and in averting potentially life-threatening complications by reporting signs and symptoms early to the primary care physiatrist or physician. This chapter focuses on the short-term management of patients with SCI after their injury and the transition to patient- and family-managed care through patient and family education.

ALTERED AUTONOMIC FUNCTION

Autonomic dysfunction is associated with injuries above the level of T6. This is largely because the major sympathetic outflow for the body stems from vasculature between T1 and T7. During the period of spinal shock that follows an acute injury, there may be a loss of sensory function, motor function, and autonomic reflexes for a period of a few days to as long as 6 weeks. After the period of spinal shock, function may return along with autonomic reflexes; however, although a complete lesion above the sacral level may allow some reflexive function, more serious disruption of the autonomic system occurs with higher-level injuries.[8,9] Lesions above T6 cause a loss of descending spinal cord control and result in dysfunctions of the autonomic nervous system that affect the following functions:

- Thermoregulation
- Bradycardia
- Hypotension
- Autonomic dysreflexia (AD)

Thermoregulation

The body's ability to maintain its core temperature by balancing heat production and heat loss is important to homeostasis[10]; however, disrupted thermoregulation is one of the cardiovascular sequelae of an SCI. Hyperthermia, defined as an increase in body temperature, occurs in the patient with SCI as a result of an absence of normal temperature control that should begin in the hypothalamus and that is normally regulated through perspiration and vasodilation. Individuals with lesions above T6 are at

risk for heat stroke when exposed to high ambient temperature. Signs and symptoms of heat stroke include rapid pulse, high core temperature, and dry and flushed skin.

A condition called partial poikilothermia results when a patient's body temperature changes with the environment because perspiration has not occurred. This reaction is more pronounced during an infection (e.g., when fever is present) or when the room is too hot. Management of hyperthermia includes maintaining the proper ambient temperature and ensuring that the patient is well hydrated. If the hyperthermia is extreme, a cool bath immersion may be required to lower the patient's core body temperature.

Hypothermia, defined as a decrease in body temperature, is countered in the healthy person by shivering to increase body temperature. In the patient with SCI, the mechanism of shivering does not occur below the level of the injury, and therefore the body does not have the ability to raise its temperature. Patient care to prevent hypothermia includes maintaining the proper ambient temperature as well as the use of lap blankets and other garments to warm the body. Irritability, lethargy, clumsiness, slowed respiration and heartbeat, and mental confusion may be signs of hypothermia.

Bradycardia

Bradycardia is defined as a pulse rate that is slower than normal. This phenomenon is seen during the first 2 to 3 weeks after an SCI, and it often resolves after about 6 weeks or with the resolution of spinal shock. In patients with an SCI, parasympathetic function is largely intact, which results in the cardiovascular system impact of slowing of the heart rate. The injury and spinal shock interfere with the sympathetic function that should increase the heart rate. As a result, there is no counterbalance for bradycardia. If the bradycardia is nonsymptomatic, intervention may not be necessary. When a patient is going to have vagal stimulation such as during tracheal suctioning, however, care should be taken to limit the activity or length of time or to pretreat with administration of intravenous atropine. In rare cases, if the problem does not resolve, a pacemaker may be necessary.

Hypotension

Orthostatic hypotension is defined as an extreme decrease in blood pressure that results from a postural change as from lying down to an upright position.[11] Orthostatic hypotension in the patient with an SCI is caused, in part, by the loss of sympathetic responses such as vasoconstriction and tachycardia. In general, when a person moves from lying to sitting or standing, vasoconstriction and tachycardia compensate for the demand for increased blood supply, and the blood pressure is maintained. In patients with SCI, there is a pooling of blood in the venous system in dependent areas such as the legs and a resultant drop in blood pressure. Symptoms of orthostatic hypotension include lightheadedness, nausea, dizziness, and syncope.

The immediate management of orthostatic hypotension includes tilting the patient back until the symptoms resolve. If syncope occurs, the patient should be brought to a supine or close to supine position and the patients' legs may also need to be elevated. Prevention of orthostatic hypotension is central to proper care. Interventions include any of the following: pressure gradient stockings, abdominal binders, medications, and adequate hydration. The resolution of spinal shock after several weeks will tend to resolve issues of orthostatic hypotension. In addition, the repeated postural challenges each time the patient is moved to an upright position will help the body to adapt to the drop in pressure by developing compensatory spinal postural strategies.

Autonomic Dysreflexia

AD is defined as a syndrome of massively uncontrolled sympathetic nervous system discharge that is unique to patients who have sustained an SCI (Figure 3-1). It is characterized by a sudden and exaggerated reflex and with an increase in blood pressure. The mechanism of this syndrome begins with patient exposure to noxious stimuli such as pain or pressure below the level of injury. A signal is sent through a sympathetic pathway, which triggers an exaggerated reflex (e.g., vasoconstriction and a subsequent increase in blood pressure). Baroreceptors in the aorta sense this increase in blood pressure and send a signal to the brainstem, which in normal physiologic conditions responds by transmitting a signal for vasodilatation and a slowing of the heart rate. These signals are interrupted by the spinal cord lesion and, as a result, no compensatory action occurs. The blood pressure remains elevated and the cycle continues until noxious stimuli are removed.

AD occurs in patients with injuries at T6 or above, but rarely occurs during the acute phase after SCI. In general, the onset of AD begins after the resolution of spinal shock. Prevalence estimates vary from 66% to 85% of patients with lesions at or above T6.[12] Symptoms of AD include the following (see Box 2-4):

- Hypertension (systolic pressure possibly as high as 300 mm Hg)
- Headache: severe or pounding
- Perspiration: above the level of injury
- Flushing: above the level of injury
- Piloerection: below the level of injury
- Vision: blurred; dilated pupils
- Nasal congestion
- Anxiety
- Bradycardia

Because AD is typically seen only in patients with SCI, clinicians who do not regularly work with these individuals may fail to recognize symptoms, delaying critical treatment. There are many causes of AD (Box 3-1). Determining the cause is essential so the reflex can be stopped by removing the stimuli at the source.

Treatment of AD involves a number of interventions (Box 3-2). The administration of nitroglycerin as a topical paste is typically the first step, followed by having the patient bite and swallow nifedipine to reduce the blood pressure. Xylocaine 2% jelly is used if the nurse is checking for fecal impaction or changing or inserting a urinary catheter. In addition, note that problems with temperature regulation may follow an incidence of AD because the dysreflexia can result in the patient sweating with heat loss and then being unable to compensate with resultant shivering. Interventions to correct the hypothermia may be required.

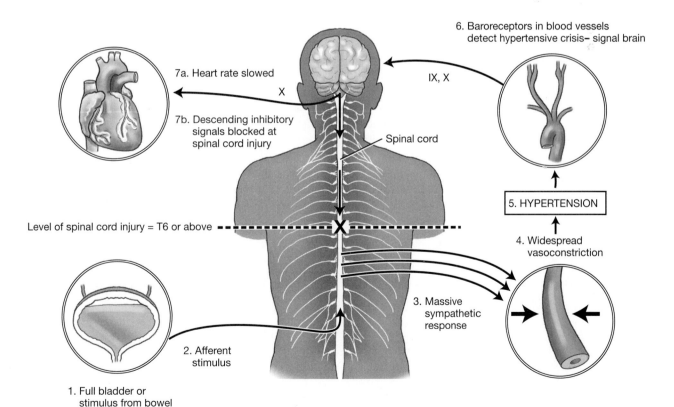

FIGURE 3-1 How AD occurs in a person with SCI. The afferent stimulus, in this case a distended bladder, triggers a peripheral sympathetic response, which results in vasoconstriction and hypertension. Descending inhibitory signals, which would normally counteract the rise in blood pressure, are blocked at the level of the SCI. The roman numerals *(IX, X)* refer to cranial nerves. (From Blackmer J: Rehabilitation medicine, 1: Autonomic dysreflexia, *CMAJ* 169:931-935, 2003, © 2003 Canadian Medical Association or its licensors.)

BOX 3-1 | Potential Causes of Autonomic Dysreflexia

1. Most common causes
   - Tight clothing
   - Body positioning
   - Bladder distention, including an obstructed catheter
   - Bowel distention or impaction
   - Pain
   - Intercourse
2. Less frequent causes
   - Ingrown toenail
   - Menstruation

3. Medical conditions
   - Deep vein thrombosis
   - Pulmonary embolus
   - Invasive procedures
   - Acute abdomen
   - Heterotopic ossification
   - Labor and delivery
   - Pressure sores
   - Fractures

BOX 3-2 | Clinical Practice Guidelines for Acute Management of Autonomic Dysreflexia: Summary of Treatment Recommendations

NOTE: Pregnant women should be referred to an appropriate consultant.

1. Check patient's blood pressure.
2. If blood pressure is not elevated, refer to a consultant, if necessary.
3. If blood pressure is elevated and patient is supine, immediately sit the person up.
4. Loosen any clothing or constrictive devices.
5. Monitor the blood pressure and pulse frequently.
6. Quickly survey patient for instigating causes, beginning with urinary system.
7. If an indwelling urinary catheter is not in place, catheterize patient.
8. Before inserting catheter, instill 2% lidocaine jelly (if readily available) into the urethra and wait several minutes.
9. If patient has an indwelling urinary catheter, check the system along its entire length for kinks, folds, constrictions, or obstructions and for correct placement of the indwelling catheter. If problem is found, correct immediately.
10. If the catheter appears to be blocked, gently irrigate the bladder with a small amount of fluid, such as normal saline solution at body temperature. Avoid manually compressing or tapping on the bladder.
11. If the catheter is draining and the blood pressure remains elevated, proceed to step 16.
12. If catheter is not draining and blood pressure remains elevated, remove and replace catheter.
13. Before replacing the catheter, instill 2% lidocaine jelly (if readily available) into the urethra and wait several minutes.
14. If catheter cannot be replaced, consider attempting to pass a coude catheter or consult a urologist.
15. Monitor patient's blood pressure during bladder drainage.
16. If acute symptoms of autonomic dysreflexia persist, including a sustained elevated blood pressure, suspect fecal impaction.
17. If elevated blood pressure is at or above 150 mm Hg systolic, consider pharmacological management to reduce the systolic blood pressure without causing hypotension before checking for fecal impaction. If blood pressure remains elevated but is less than 150 mm Hg systolic, proceed to step 20.
18. Use an antihypertensive agent with rapid onset and short duration while the causes of autonomic dysreflexia are being investigated.
19. Monitor the patient for symptomatic hypotension.
20. If fecal impaction is suspected, check the rectum for stool, using the following procedure: With a gloved hand, instill a topical anesthetic agent such as 2% lidocaine jelly generously into the rectum. Wait approximately 5 minutes for sensation in the area to decrease. Then, with a gloved hand, inset a lubricated finger into the rectum and check for the presence of stool. If present, gently remove, if possible. If autonomic dysreflexia becomes worse, stop the manual evacuation. Instill additional topical anesthetic and recheck the rectum for the presence of stool after approximately 20 minutes.
21. Monitor patient's symptoms and blood pressure for at least 2 hours after resolution of the autonomic dysreflexia episode to make sure that it does not recur.
22. If there is poor response to treatment as specified above or if cause of dysreflexia has not been identified, strongly consider admitting the patient to the hospital to be monitored, to maintain pharmacological control of blood pressure, and to investigate other causes of the dysreflexia.
23. Document the episode in patient's medical record. This record should include presenting signs and symptoms and their course, treatment instituted, recordings of blood pressure and pulse, and response to treatment. The effectiveness of the treatment may be evaluated according to the level of outcome criteria reached:
    - Cause of autonomic dysreflexia episode has been identified.
    - Blood pressure has been restored to normal limits (usually 90 to 110 mm Hg systolic for a tetraplegic person in sitting position).
    - Pulse rate has been restored to normal limits.
    - Patient is comfortable, with no signs or symptoms of autonomic dysreflexia, increased intracranial pressure, or heart failure.
24. Once patient with SCI has been stabilized, review the precipitating cause with patient, members of the patient's family, significant others, and caregivers. This process entails adjusting the treatment plan to ensure that future episodes are recognized and treated to prevent a medical crisis or, ideally, are avoided altogether. The process also entails discussion of autonomic dysreflexia in the SCI education program so that individuals with SCI will be able to recognize early onset and obtain help as quickly as possible. It is recommended that an individual with SCI be given a written description of treatment for autonomic dysreflexia at the time of discharge that can be referred to in an emergency. Alert cards that individuals with SCI can carry to alert health care providers of possible episodes of autonomic dysreflexia are also helpful.

Data from Acute management of autonomic dysreflexia: adults with spinal cord injury presenting to health-care facilities, Consortium for Spinal Cord, *J Spinal Cord Med* 20:284-308, 1997; Acute management of autonomic dysreflexia: individuals with spinal cord injury presenting to health-care facilities, Consortium for Spinal Cord Medicine, *J Spinal Cord Med* 25(1 Suppl):S67-S88, 2002; Sabharwal S: Cardiovascular dysfunction in spinal cord disorders. In Lin VW, editor: *Spinal cord medicine: Principles and practice*, New York, 2003, Demos.

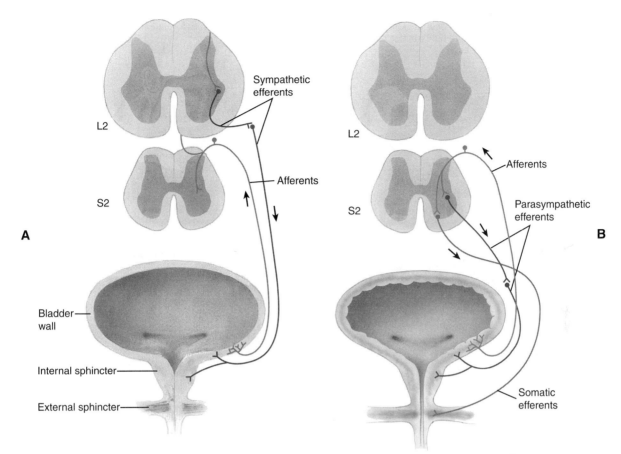

FIGURE 3-2 Reflexive control of the bladder. **A,** Bladder is filling. Afferents convey information regarding stretch of the bladder wall to the spinal cord. Signals in sympathetic efferents maintain relaxation of the bladder wall and constriction of the internal sphincter. **B,** When the bladder is full, reflexive voiding is initiated by signals in the parasympathetic efferents, producing contraction of the bladder wall and relaxation of the internal sphincter. Somatic efferent activity produces relaxation of the external sphincter.(From Lundy-Ekman L: *Neuroscience: fundamentals for rehabilitation*, ed 2, p 278, Philadelphia, 2002, WB Saunders.)

Preventive measures for AD are critical and reduce the chance that noxious stimuli will occur. Ensuring that clothing is loose, the bladder is nondistended, the bowel program is effective, linen under the patient is smooth, and podiatric care is regularly performed (to prevent ingrown toe nails) all help limit the possibility that AD will develop. The patient and family must be taught to recognize the symptoms of AD and to either take action or instruct care providers to take action. In addition, patient and family education needs to focus on reducing the risk of AD by using the prevention strategies discussed above.

A number of complications can result if AD goes untreated. The patient may have retinal hemorrhages. A more serious complication may be a subarachnoid or intracranial hemorrhage, potentially resulting in a cerebrovascular accident. Myocardial infarction is also a potential complication and, in some cases, AD may be fatal.

ALTERED BLADDER FUNCTION

One of the biggest challenges for many patients with SCI is the establishment of a bladder program that achieves continence or urine containment and that supports community reintegration for the patient. Designing a bladder program that will be effective depends on the proper diagnosis of the type of bladder dysfunction combined with creative strategies that will allow the patient to have maximum control.[13] A basic understanding of normal micturition is necessary to understand the impact of upper and lower motor neuron alterations. Strategies for managing bladder function are based on the type of bladder dysfunction and on patient characteristics and preferences.

Normal Micturition

Bladder function is based on the principles of both the storage of urine and the emptying of urine from the bladder. In the healthy adult, bladder tone and pelvic floor muscle tone are intact and the bladder will store urine up to a quantity of 200 to 300 ml before a signal is emitted from the stretch receptors located on the wall of the bladder.[14] This sensory signal is transmitted to the spinal cord at the level of S2 to S4. The spinal cord relays several signals: first a signal goes up the cord to the brain signaling bladder fullness (Figure 3-2, *A*); second, a reflexive signal stimulates the sympathetic and parasympathetic branches to initiate bladder emptying (Figure 3-2, *B*).

The autonomic innervation for bladder emptying involves coordinated actions that result in complete emptying of the bladder. The parasympathetic innervation (S2 to S4) results in bladder contraction and some bladder neck relaxation. The sympathetic

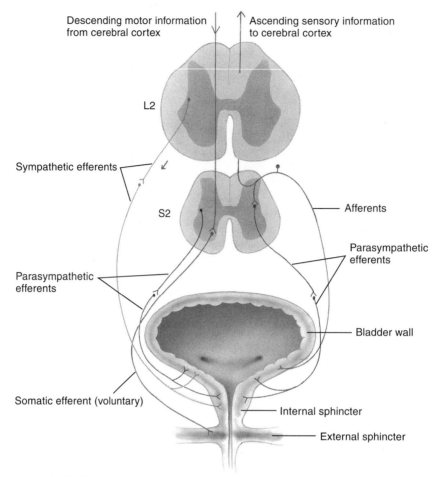

FIGURE 3-3 Neural control of the bladder. Descending activating neurons and efferents are indicated on the left side of the illustration. Ascending sensory neurons, afferents, and a reflexive connection between an afferent and parasympathetic efferent are shown on the right side. (From Lundy-Ekman L: *Neuroscience: fundamentals for rehabilitation*, ed 2, p. 279, Philadelphia, 2002, WB Saunders.)

innervation T12 to L2 allows the bladder to fill and maintains contraction of the sphincter. The somatic innervation originates at S2 to S4 and results in voluntary inhibition through neural control of the external sphincter (Figure 3-3). These activities combine to initiate micturition by reflex with complete emptying of the bladder contents at one time. The conscious component of bladder emptying is a relay from the brain by an upper motor neuron to the lower spinal cord, with a relay by a lower motor neuron to the external sphincter to "delay the urge" to void, accomplished by sphincter contraction. If the signal from the brain is interrupted, bladder emptying will go forward by reflexive voiding.[15]

Neurogenic Bladder

The term neurogenic bladder is broadly defined and describes general rather than specific bladder alterations after SCI. Two alterations that fall under the category of neurogenic bladder are discussed here. First, patients with lower motor neuron alterations from T12 and below have a flaccid bladder that is often unable to store urine and that is categorized as an autonomous neurogenic bladder (Figure 3-4, *A*).[14] The lower segments of the spinal cord form the cauda equina, meaning "horse tail." It is actually composed of many lower motor neurons that exit the

cord akin to a horse's tail. Injuries in this region often result in damage to multiple lower motor neurons, affecting bladder function, lower segments of the gastrointestinal tract, and genitalia, including sphincters. Patients with this dysfunction tend to have a bladder and sphincters that have very little or no ability to store urine.

A second alteration common in upper motor neuron defects is categorized as failure to empty, or reflex neurogenic bladder.[16] Patients with upper motor neuron alterations from T12 to L1 and above generally have a reflexive bladder, which may, in some cases, be hyperreflexive or hypertonic (Figure 3-4, *B*). The brain does not receive the signal of a full bladder because of the nature of the spinal cord damage, and, more important, the motor neuron impulse that provides conscious control of voiding by signaling to "delay the urge" is not transmitted. Here too, just as with other reflexes in patients who have sustained upper motor neuron injuries, the bladder reflex is often exaggerated, resulting in hyperreflexia. Patients with this dysfunction may have intermittent spontaneous bladder emptying but may often additionally have residual urine after voiding as a result of detrusor sphincter dyssynergia.[14] The ability to initiate voiding may be problematic for some patients because of lack of coordination between bladder contraction and sphincter relaxation.[13]

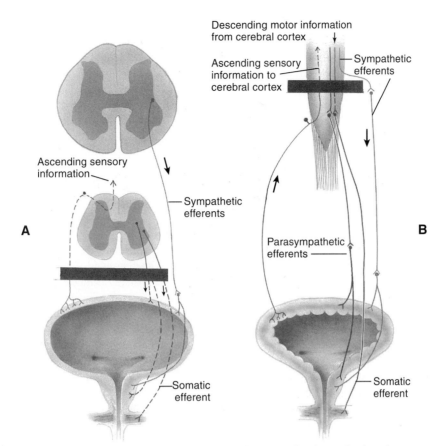

FIGURE 3-4 Bladder dysfunction after spinal region injury. Dotted lines indicate neural pathways that have been interrupted and do not convey information. **A,** Flaccid bladder resulting from a complete lesion of the cauda equina. All neural connections with the bladder are severed, except the sympathetic efferents. A complete lesion of spinal cord levels S2 to S4 would also produce a flaccid bladder, owing to interruption of the reflexive bladder emptying circuit. **B,** Hypertonic bladder caused by a complete lesion above the S2 level. Communications between the brain and the sacral level parasympathetic neurons controlling the bladder are interrupted, preventing voluntary control. The reflexive connections between the bladder and spinal cord are intact, so reflexive emptying of the bladder can occur. (From Lundy-Ekman L: *Neuroscience: fundamentals for rehabilitation,* ed 2, p 284, Philadelphia, 2002, WB Saunders.)

Assessment

Proper diagnosis of urinary alteration is central to any bladder program. This assessment begins with the American Spinal Injury Association (ASIA) classification to determine the level and extent of the spinal cord damage (see Figure 6-11).[17] In many cases, the patient arrives at the rehabilitation hospital in spinal shock and with an indwelling catheter. As previously discussed, spinal shock is "a temporary condition of flaccid paralysis and loss of all reflex activity below the level of the lesion" (see Chapter 2).[14]

When the patient is admitted for short-term rehabilitation, laboratory tests include an analysis of the urine and a culture and sensitivity to determine whether there is any active infection. The indwelling catheter, if present, is generally changed on admission and every 10 to 14 days thereafter. Urine is evaluated for color, particulate matter, and clarity. In addition, assessment includes the appearance of the urinary meatus and, in men who are uncircumcised, the appearance of the foreskin to rule out any swelling, redness, or signs of irritation or excoriation.

For patients who do not have an indwelling catheter on admission, the clinician must track bladder patterns, including urine volume and frequency and ask the patient to describe when he has voided. Assessing for the postvoiding residual volume (PVR)

within 15 minutes of voiding is generally done several times after admission by bladder ultrasonography and the volume is recorded. In the case of a PVR that is greater than 20% of the voided volume, emptying of the bladder is recommended by intermittent catheterization.[13] Bladder tracking of volumes, frequency, and PVR may continue for several days or weeks, depending on the nature of the bladder dysfunction.

Urinary incontinence may be an issue for patients with either an upper or a lower motor neuron deficit. Male patients may be using condom catheters to contain urine. If a condom catheter is in use, the nurse must assess the shaft of the penis and urinary meatus for any signs of irritation or infection; the fit of the condom catheter, including any indication of overcompression; and the free flow of urine into the leg bag or bedside bag with a secure attachment to prevent backflow. Male or female patients may be using adult briefs, and assessment must include a careful evaluation of the skin for any signs of irritation or breakdown.[16]

Assessing urinary dysfunction requires the nurse to also assess the patient for hydration and nutritional status. Underhydration can have a significant impact on urinary function and the ability of the patient to be successful in a bladder program.[14] Because of the multisystem failures associated with SCI, normal autoregulation such as temperature regulation and electrolyte balance may be flawed. Thirst mechanisms may also be affected, and if the patient is on an alternate fluid consistency, ingesting sufficient amounts of liquids may be a challenge. Indicators of dehydration include poor skin turgor, appearance of oral mucous membranes, orthostatic hypotension, dark color of the urine, and low urine volume. Ensuring adequate hydration is critical both to the homeostasis of the patient and to a successful bladder program.

The importance of nutrition for patients with an SCI cannot be overstated. After the initial injury, the nutritional demands of the patient with SCI are greatly increased. A balanced diet enhanced with nutritional supplements is important on many levels. Nutritional assessment begins with the patient's height and weight and includes a diet history, blood work to determine protein levels (blood albumin), and tracking of food intake. The dietitian, physiatrist, and nurse must collaborate to ensure that nutritional needs continue to be met and monitored. Malnutrition is associated with increased urinary incontinence and often goes hand in hand with proper hydration.[18]

Assessment of urinary function must include an assessment of the patient's awareness of his bladder function, including symptoms such as pain, urgency, or fullness. The patient may or may not be aware of the current bladder management devices or techniques that are being used. It is important to involve the patient in understanding the rationale for the bladder device or techniques and to elicit his feedback both of the physiological symptoms he may experience and the psychological impact of the overall experience.

Interventions

Some general nursing principles are central to a successful bladder program regardless of the devices or techniques used (Clinical Note: Nursing Principles Central to a Successful Bladder Program). Bladder control is a very personal and intimate issue for most patients, so providing privacy and discretion both in conversations and teaching as well as in any hands-on interventions is critical to the patient's self-esteem. Wherever possible, normalcy should be maintained. This may include use of the bathroom toilet versus a commode, good positioning to promote complete emptying, and, in the case of adult briefs, ensuring that the briefs are changed promptly after bladder emptying to reduce skin irritation, odor, and wet clothing. Assessing for changes in bladder function and any signs of complication such as infection must be continuous. Bladder programs are dynamic and very often the program needs to be re-evaluated and modified in accordance with the patient's feedback to promote patient control of the program and to accommodate changing needs. Components of a successful bladder program may include indwelling catheters, suprapubic catheters, intermittent catheterization, condom catheters, adult briefs, bladder tapping, Crede method, and medication.

CLINICAL NOTE **Nursing Principles Central to a Successful Bladder Program**

- Provide privacy and discretion.
- Normalcy should be maintained whenever possible.
- Assessment for changes in bladder function and signs of complications is continuous.
- Bladder programs are dynamic and may need to be re-evaluated and modified.

Indwelling Catheter

An indwelling catheter is often used early in the recovery phase for both upper and lower motor neuron deficits (Figure 3-5). It provides complete urine containment and complete bladder emptying. In patients with upper motor neuron injuries, an indwelling catheter may cause spasms, and any defect in drainage may be a causative factor in AD.[14] In patients with lower motor neuron injuries, an indwelling catheter may be the only urine containment device that is effective. Condom catheters are not an option for female patients, making an indwelling catheter the only option for urine containment.

Regardless of the type of neurogenic bladder, an indwelling catheter presents its own problems, which include risk of infection, formation of bladder stones, and aesthetics related to the catheter placement, including clothing management.[16] Care of the patient with an indwelling catheter must include the following:

- Regular change schedule using sterile technique
- Minimal interruptions in the system that can lead to contamination
- Assurance of free flow of urine
- Secure placement of the catheter to support good anatomical positioning, particularly in males
- Continuous monitoring for infection and obstruction

Suprapubic Catheter

Some patients with an SCI may require a suprapubic catheter placed through the urinary meatus as an alternative to an indwelling catheter. This catheter is surgically implanted through the abdominal wall directly into the bladder. The drainage system is the same as with an indwelling catheter. Infection is a critical issue with a suprapubic catheter, however, because any breach in the system could introduce bacteria directly into the bladder.

Intermittent Catheterization

Many patients with SCI use intermittent catheterization (IC) as either a short- or long-term strategy. One primary reason for using an IC strategy may be the presence of a PVR that exceeds a reasonable volume.[16] This may be a time-limited need early in the establishment of a bladder program or may become a lifetime strategy. A second reason for using an IC strategy may be the inability to initiate voiding. In the case of upper motor neuron lesions, hyperreflexia may result in either the presence of PVR requiring intermittent catheterization or in an inability to initiate voiding. IC is not an option for patients with complete lower motor neuron deficits because their bladders cannot store urine.

Initially, IC may be performed by the nurse. If IC is to be part of the long-term bladder program, on the basis of the level of the patient's injury, the goal is to teach the patient to perform IC himself or to supervise an assistant. When the IC is being performed by a nurse in a hospital setting, sterile technique is required. Self-catheterization or catheterization by a family member or friend in the home environment can be done as a clean technique. Although there is some risk of infection as with any invasive technique, the risk is substantially lower for IC than for an indwelling catheter.

For a female, the urinary meatus may be challenging to locate, and a mirror should be used for good visualization. Initially, this procedure may be upsetting and offensive to the patient or

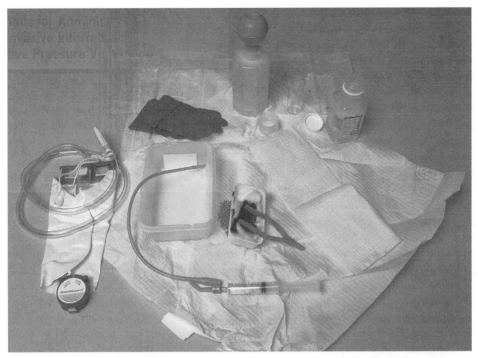

FIGURE 3-5 Preparation for insertion of an indwelling catheter and attachment to a bedside drainage bag.

family care person. After the initial objections are addressed with a rationale and the IC has been performed several times, the patient and family generally adjust reasonably well to the idea. A long-term strategy with a family member performing the IC may be very burdensome and should be carefully discussed before a final decision is reached.

Condom Catheter

A condom catheter is an option as a bladder containment strategy for men who have problems with urinary incontinence. In the case of upper motor neuron deficits, there may be episodes of urinary incontinence that can be managed with this technique. In the case of lower motor neuron deficits, the condom catheter may be part of the long-term strategy to contain urine.[19]

Nursing challenges when managing patients with condom catheters fall into three categories. First is the proper fit and application of the catheter, which depends on use of the correct-sized catheter, and the application technique, which may be an issue of trial and error until an acceptable and successful method is achieved. Options include self-adhering catheters, straps, or adhesive spray or liquid. The goal is to achieve a reasonable seal while ensuring a minimal amount of pressure on the shaft of the penis. Patient preference is a key to choice of products, and a period of trial and error is to be expected.

Second is maintenance of skin integrity and cleanliness of the penis. Removing any crystal or urine residue buildup is critical to the prevention of skin breakdown and infection. In the case of a man who is uncircumcised, the foreskin must be fully extended except during hygiene. Any retraction of the foreskin can result in swelling of the penis and associated complications (see discussion of AD).

Ensuring free flow of urine to prevent backflow and possible displacement of the condom catheter represents the third challenge. The catheter must be secured in a way that promotes gravity drainage to either a leg bag or a bedside drainage bag. In addition, the bags must be frequently emptied both for comfort and to avert urine leakage. For the patients going to the therapy gym, endorsing the use of the condom catheter is important so that as the patient changes position the placement of the tubing and bag can be adjusted to ensure free flow.

Adult Briefs

Adult briefs are often seen as a last resort method of urine containment. They may be used alone or in conjunction with other devices or techniques. The quality of adult briefs has substantially improved and new products have an increasingly better ability to contain large quantities of urine and protect the skin surface from direct urine contact.

In patients with upper motor neuron lesions, some degree of urinary incontinence may be a continuing issue. For patients with lower motor neuron lesions, urine containment is the central issue, requiring that adult briefs be used alone or as a backup in conjunction with other urine containment devices such as a condom catheter. Adult briefs present an aesthetic challenge and the need to avert adverse skin condition problems. It is most important is to make sure the briefs are changed regularly and that the patient is washed with soap and water at each changing. Skin barriers may be used to prevent any skin breakdown. In addition, odor control products may be used to address the buildup of unpleasant urine odor. It is also important to monitor female patients for signs and symptoms of urinary tract infections and vaginitis.

Patients may respond in one of two ways to using adult briefs. For some, the fear of having wet clothing or having an accident may result in their reliance on this device both short and long term. For others, the idea of wearing an adult brief is so offensive that other containment strategies must be considered. In either case, the discretion, privacy, and sensitivity by nurses and other staff members to the potential embarrassment of urinary incontinence and to the use of an adult brief are critical to the patient's self-esteem.

Bladder Tapping

The technique of bladder tapping is used in patients with upper motor neuron lesions who have difficulty initiating a urine stream. This technique involves placing two fingers over the apex of the bladder and using two fingers of the opposite hand to tap on top in sequences of ten interrupted with pauses of 5 to 20 seconds. It is designed to stimulate the bladder reflex and to result in voiding. In general, it is done while the patient is sitting on the toilet. Patients with upper extremity movement can use this technique themselves to initiate voiding. There are few negative effects from this technique, aside from it not always being successful for every patient.

Crede Method

The Crede method is used in patients with upper motor neuron lesions to initiate voiding. Caution must be exercised, however, in using this technique because it can cause damage if too much force is applied.[13] The flat part of the hand is placed over the apex of the full bladder and the bladder is massaged from top to bottom with a smooth, firm stroke. This technique, which is similar to bladder tapping, is designed to initiate voiding and has few adverse effects. The patient can perform this technique himself as long as he has sufficient upper body movement and strength. Again, the technique may not be effective in every patient.

Medications

Medications can be adjunctive to a bladder program, especially in patients with upper motor neuron deficits (see Chapter 2). In addition to medications to manage urinary track infections, there are a number of medications that can be used alone or in combination to increase sphincter tone, decrease sphincter tone, increase bladder contraction, or diminish bladder contraction (Table 3-1).

Outcomes

The Functional Independence Measure (FIM) instrument, which includes an assessment of bladder function, is the industry standard and used by the U.S. Center for Medicare and Medicaid Services (see Figure 6-13). Assessing bladder function on admission to short-term rehabilitation and discharge provides some insight into patient outcomes. This measure is very limited in the SCI population because of the inherent functional limitations of the patient with an SCI on the basis of the level of injury and, therefore, inability to improve in functional areas defined by the instrument.

An individual patient's potential for achieving a successful bladder program may or may not be based on the achievement of bladder continence. Other critical outcome measures include the ability of the patient to self-manage the bladder program or

to supervise by directing others in the management of the bladder program. Episodes of incontinence may be unavoidable, but the patient's sense of control in managing the episodes of incontinence may be the more important indicator.

A number of factors may confound a successful bladder program and affect patient outcome. Infection is a continuous threat for most patients with SCI, and every effort to minimize the risk must be used. Infections in patients with SCI are not as easily defined as in other populations and effort must be made not to overtreat with antibiotics.[13] In addition, bladder stones are a particular problem for patients with indwelling catheters. Regular screening and removal of bladder stones is critical to a successful bladder program for patients with indwelling catheters.

Regulation of medication is a continuing challenge, and patients with SCI may be taking medication for other symptoms such as an antihistamine for a cold without realizing its impact on sphincter tone and the potential not to be able to initiate voiding. Skin integrity must be considered in the design of the bladder program and every effort made to minimize the risk of skin breakdown from incontinence.

Finally, sexuality is a continuing challenge based on the integration of the genitourinary system.[20] Establishing bladder programs specifically designed to facilitate sexual intimacy are critical to the patient's sense of control and self-esteem. Emptying the bladder before sexual encounters combined with using a shower as the place where the sexual encounter takes place minimizes the potential embarrassment of urinary incontinence during the activity.

THE CLIENT'S PERSPECTIVE Bladder and Bowel Care

I learned how to manage my bladder and bowel care so that I could return to work and be out and about in the community.
Helpful Hints:
- Be prepared with plenty of urological supplies
- Check ahead to make sure the bathroom is accessible to ensure comfort and security
- Have an extra change of clothes available in anticipation of the unexpected
- Drink more fluids when you know you will not have meetings or conference calls, and less when you know you will
- Have patience when it comes to bladder and bowel routine; the meeting or function will be there when we get back and most important, we will be in the moment without worry
- Drink when you need to—not drinking liquids can lead to urinary tract infections or dehydration
- Prepare for any possible scenario so that you are not caught by surprise—it is the difference between being inconvenienced or embarrassed

Sarah Everhart Skeels and Scott Chesney

ALTERED BOWEL FUNCTION

Alterations in bowel function are a central concern in patients who have sustained an SCI because of issues of control and the potential for fear and embarrassment if control is not achieved. The term neurogenic bowel refers to general bowel dysfunction after SCI. Designing a bowel program that is successful both in

TABLE 3-1 | Medications to Treat Voiding Disorders

Drug Class	Action	Adverse Effects	Nursing Considerations
Drugs That Inhibit Contractility and Promote Urine Storage			
Anticholinergics (propantheline bromide, hyoscyamine, methantheline bromide, dicyclomine hydrochloride, tincture of belladonna, atropine sulfate, glycopyrrolate)	Reduces spasm or smooth muscle contraction by blocking or inhibiting the effects of acetylcholine at the muscarinic receptor	Dizziness, drowsiness, blurred vision, dry mouth, increased HR; contraindicated in many disease states—check before administration	Give 30-60 min before meals and at bedtime; monitor vital signs and urine output; use gum or sugarless candies to relieve dry mouth
Antispasmodics/direct smooth muscle relaxants (oxybutynin chloride, flavoxate hydrochloride, B&O suppositories)	Inhibits muscarinic action of acetylcholine on smooth muscle; direct antispasmodic effect on detrusor smooth muscle	Same as for anticholinergics	Same as for anticholinergics
Beta-adrenergics (terbutaline)	Increases bladder capacity through beta-stimulatory effect on bladder body	Palpitations, insomnia, hypertension	Monitor pulse and blood pressure
Tricyclic antidepressants (imipramine, doxepin)	Anesthetic-like action at nerve terminals; produces strong inhibitory effect on bladder smooth muscle	Weakness, fatigue, sedation, postural hypotension, rash, parkinsonian effect, fine tremors, abdominal distress, nausea and vomiting, headache, lethargy, irritability	Older adults require close observation; inform patient of possible side effects
Drugs That Increase Bladder Outlet Resistance			
Alpha-adrenergics (ephedrine sulfate, imipramine, phenylpropanolamine hydrochloride, pseudoephedrine)	Exaggerates alpharesponse in the bladder neck and urethra to increase bladder outlet resistance	Tachycardia, precordial pain, cardiac arrhythmias, vertigo, headache	Used to treat stress urinary incontinence, postprostatectomy incontinence; monitor vital signs
Beta-adrenergic blocks (propranolol)	Blocks beta-adrenergic receptors in the urethra, thereby increasing urethral pressure	Bradycardia, lightheadedness	Used when alpha-adrenergics are contraindicated
Estrogens	Increases periurethral blood flow; strengthens periurethral tissues	Headaches, nausea, edema, hypertension, weight changes, breast tenderness	Assess for vaginal bleeding, GU or abdominal pain; monitor blood pressure and weight
Drugs That Stimulate Detrusor Contractility and Promote Bladder Emptying			
Cholinergics (bethanechol chloride, neostigmine methylsulfate, myotonachol, carbachol)	Stimulates muscarinic cholinergic receptors in the bladder to increase bladder tone and sensations to bladder filling	Increased GI motility; vasodilation; decreased HR	Used for postoperative and nonobstructive urinary retention; do not give bethanechol IM or IV; give oral bethanechol on empty stomach; monitor vital signs; contraindicated in many disease states—check before administering
Drugs That Decrease Bladder Outlet Resistance			
Alpha-adrenergic blockers (phenoxybenzamine hydrochloride, phentolamine, reserpine, prazosin, terazosin, doxazosin)	Blocks alpha-adrenergic receptors of the bladder neck, posterior urethra, and external sphincter	Postural hypotension	Have patient change positions slowly; give with food or milk; avoid use with alcohol; avoid cold products containing sympathomimetics
External Sphincter or Striated Muscle Relaxants (baclofen, diazepam, dantrolene sodium)	Relaxes the external sphincter by inhibiting postsynaptic reflexes of striated muscles	Weakness; sedation	Often used in patients with multiple sclerosis or high-cord lesions; implement safety precautions

B&O, Belladonna and opium; *HR,* heart rate; *GU,* genitourinary; *IM,* intramuscular *IV,* intravenous. From Karlowicz K, editor: *Urological nursing principles and practice,* p 391, Philadelphia, 1995, WB Saunders.

avoiding accidents and achievable by the patient or family is the goal regardless of the level of injury. Unlike bladder continence, bowel continence is achievable for most patients with SCI as long as the patient and family are highly motivated and disciplined.[21]

Normal Bowel Function

Bowel elimination is the removal of waste products from the body and is a function of the GI tract. The human GI tract is unique because of the enteric nervous system that lies within the walls of the gut extending from the esophagus to the anus. The neural circuitry present in this system supports a reflexive pathway, which can function without central nervous system input and allows for continuing physiological function, including the transportation of nutrients and enzymes as well as bowel motility.

There are a number of triggers that promote bowel evacuation. First, the rectum has stretch receptors that send a signal to the cord when the rectal cavity is full. Similarly to bladder function, the signal goes to the cord and splits with a signal traveling to the brain, where a decision can be made and sent along an upper motor neuron to delay the urge. If the brain does not reply to the signal, reflexive bowel evacuation will occur. Other triggers may also initiate a bowel movement, including the gastrocolic reflex that initiates peristalsis when food or fluid is ingested into the stomach. Ultimately, in the normal bowel reflexive evacuation involves a lower motor neuron from the cord transmitting signals to the cord of rectal distention and parasympathetic enervation results in increased GI activity and defecation. The sympathetic enervation results in a decrease in GI activity.

Upper Motor Neuron Reflexive Bowel

An upper motor neuron lesion interferes with conscious control of bowel evacuation, which results in reflexive bowel emptying (Figure 3-6, *A*). Reflexive bowel emptying will occur whenever a reflex is triggered, and the amount of feces will depend on the fullness of the rectum and lower bowel at the time the reflex is triggered, along with the consistency of the stool. Reflexive bowel evacuation may be triggered by food or fluid entering the stomach, movement of additional feces into the rectal cavity, or the insertion of a suppository or other artificial stimulant.[21]

Typically, upper motor reflexive bowel is present in injuries at T12 to L1 and above. Upper motor neuron injuries may have associated hyperreflexia that can result in more frequent bowel emptying, a more exaggerated reflex as a result of a trigger, or contraction of the rectal sphincter that can, at times, interfere with bowel emptying. Continence is dependent on triggering reflexes and complete bowel evacuation, generally once a day. Parasympathetic innervation creates sphincter tone and reduces the chance of fecal incontinence.

Lower Motor Neuron Areflexive Bowel

A lower motor neuron lesion interferes with reflexive bowel evacuation. The lack of nerve innervation and bowel reflexes that involve a lower motor neuron results in a loss of motor tone and a flaccidity of the rectal sphincter (Figure 3-6, *B*). Ultimately, this affects a patient in two ways. First, peristalsis and movement of the bolus of stool into the lower intestines

and rectal cavity may be slowed with reabsorption of water. This leads to a risk of constipation and hard stool that can cause an impaction and AD. Second, the rectal sphincter may fail to contain stool and, depending on the amount of stool and its consistency, bowel incontinence can result. Lower motor neuron lesions occur in injuries below T12 to L1. Continence is dependent on keeping the rectal cavity empty and triggering bowel evacuation on demand with complete bowel evacuation.

Assessment

Assessment of bowel function begins with the ASIA classification to determine whether the SCI lesion is complete or incomplete as well as its level (see Figure 6-11). When the patient first arrives in the rehabilitation setting it is important to establish how long it has been since his last bowel movement and to assess the abdomen for distention, cramping, pain, and bowel sounds. An abdominal x-ray may be used to determine the presence and extent of a bowel impaction and, in some facilities, is routinely done as part of the admission assessment to rule out impaction. The presence of diarrhea is a potential indicator of any of the following: impaction, infection, dietary alteration, disease process, or medication side effect. Determining the patient's normal evacuation pattern, including the timing and triggers for defecation, is important in developing a bowel program for that individual. Continuing assessment of bowel function should include the frequency of evacuation, time of day, amount, consistency, and any skin problems that may be associated with incontinence.

Interventions

Care for altered bowel function begins with the establishment of a "clean" bowel, indicating that any impaction or residual stool has been removed and bowel motility is active given the underlying SCI. Initially, establishing a clean bowel is dependent on a combination of any of the following: suppositories, bulk-forming supplements, laxatives, and enemas.[21] One of the challenges is to introduce these interventions with some caution to avoid triggering diarrhea, which can present its own set of management challenges.

Treatment of diarrhea must be based on the underlying cause of the condition. If an impaction is present, it must be removed. In addition, reviewing and modifying medications may be necessary if there is a strong suspicion that medication(s) are contributing to the condition. A stool culture may be necessary to rule out infection and antibiotics may be indicated to treat the condition. Overall, it is necessary to increase hydration, ensure proper nutrition, and assess and treat electrolyte imbalances.

Constipation can be quite challenging from a treatment perspective. Once the bowel is clean, consideration is given to reducing the risk of continued or repeated constipation. Diet may need to be modified to increase both fluid and fiber intake, which support effective bowel evacuations. Again medication(s) are evaluated with a particular focus on narcotic analgesics that can have a substantial effect on slowing peristalsis (Box 3-3).[22] The longer stool remains in the large intestine or rectum, the more water will be reabsorbed, with resultant hard and often impacted stool. For

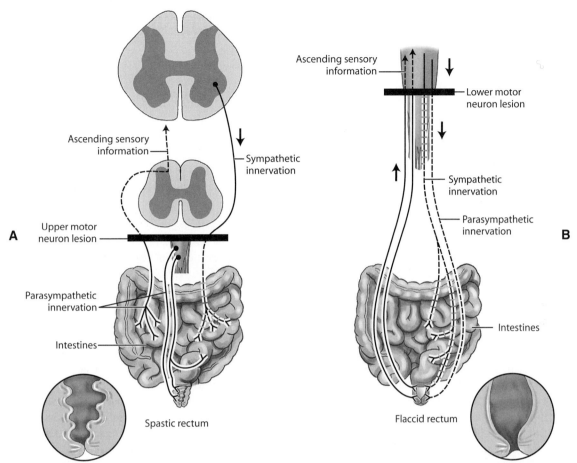

FIGURE 3-6 Bowel dysfunction after SCI. The dotted lines indicate a break in the neural circuitry. **A,** Upper motor neuron reflexive bowel function is typically associated with lesions at the T12 to L1 and above. Such lesions interrupt the pathways from the vagus, mesenteric, and hypogastric nerves and interfere with voluntary control of defecation and the anal sphincter. The innervation of the parasympathetic system, however, is intact and results in rectal and sphincter tone. Sacral nerve (S2 to S4) segments also remain intact, allowing some patients to develop a stimulus response bowel control. In addition, hyperreflexia associated with such injuries can cause a spastic bowel and anal response. **B,** Lower motor neuron areflexive bowel function occurs when lesions are at or below the T12 to L1 level. Lesions at this level interfere with reflexive bowel evacuation because parasympathetic innervation is interrupted and result in a loss of rectal or sphincter tone that causes flaccidity of the rectal sphincter, which then provides little anal resistance, resulting in fecal incontinence.

this reason, the goal must be bowel evacuation every day or, at the very least, every other day.

Bowel Program

The establishment of a bowel program ensures that the bowel is evacuated daily and it depends on timing it for success (Clinical Note: Guidelines for Bowel Program). Research indicates that

> **CLINICAL NOTE** **Guidelines for Bowel Program**
>
> • Perform the bowel program at the same time each day.
> • Follow a diet high in fiber.
> • Drink at least eight glasses of water per day.
> • Drink a hot liquid 30 minutes before initiating the bowel program.
> • Perform the bowel program in an upright position.
> • Consider premorbid bowel schedule.

From Umphred D, editor: *Neurological rehabilitation*, ed 4, p. 509, St. Louis, 2001, Mosby.

bowel programs administered in the morning are most successful.[23] Bowel programs are also more effective when they follow a meal or ingestion of a hot liquid such as coffee or tea. A hot liquid trigger initiates the gastrocolic reflex and begins peristalsis, supporting the full evacuation of stool from the rectum and lower large intestine. Typically, administering a bowel program takes 1 to 1.5 hours.

The use of gravity and position to maximize the bowel evacuation is important. Evacuation is best accomplished in the bathroom on the commode with the proper support for sitting up comfortably. Initially, checking for an impaction or the presence of stool in the rectal cavity and possible removal of stool may be indicated. Inserting a suppository is often the first step in the bowel program, making sure placement is against the wall of the rectum. If the rectum is full of stool, the suppository may not be effective. After 5 to 15 minutes, the patient may have an urge to push by using Valsalva's maneuver. Changing position by leaning forward may also assist in facilitating a bowel movement.

BOX 3-3 | **Medications That May Cause Constipation**

Anticholinergic Medications
- Antihistamines
- Antispasmodics
- Tricyclic antidepressants
- Antipsychotics

Cardiovascular Medications
- Calcium-channel blockers
- Beta-adrenergic antagonists
- Diuretics
- Antiarrhythmics

Central Nervous System Depressants
- Anticonvulsants
- Antiparkinsonian drugs

Narcotic Analgesics
- Opiates
- Barbiturates

Antineoplastics
- Vinca alkaloids

Cation-Containing Medications
- Antacids
- Sucralfate
- Calcium, iron, barium

Others
- Bile acid–binding agents (e.g., cholestyramine)
- Nonsteroidal anti-inflammatory drugs (e.g., ibuprofen, naproxen)
- Oral hypoglycemics
- Chronic laxative use (bisacodyl and anthraquinones)
- Parasympatholytics
- Acetylsalicylic acid

From Doughty D: *Urinary and fecal incontinence management*, ed 2, St. Louis, 2000, Mosby.

In the presence of a clean bowel, good hydration, and proper dietary intake, a bowel program with a suppository trigger as the only intervention can be effective for some patients. This is more common in patients with upper motor neuron lesions. For patients with a lower motor neuron defect, digital removal of stool from the rectal cavity may be required before suppository insertion and it may also be necessary to administer a small enema to facilitate bowel evacuation.[21] In addition, bulk-forming supplements and laxatives may be necessary to establish complete and regular bowel evacuation.

A bowel program that can be self-administered by the patient is most desirable whenever feasible. Given the amount of time involved, the intimacy of activity and potential impact on self-esteem, reliance on a helper such as a family member or significant other can be very difficult. After the administration of the bowel program, patients often prefer to schedule their daily shower. The bowel program that is established should take into consideration the degree of independence that can be achieved and the patient should participate in all decision making. A bowel program is only as effective as the degree to which the patient and, in some cases, the family is compliant and disciplined.

Outcomes

One of the principal measures of bowel function in rehabilitation is the FIM score on admission, on discharge, and sometimes on 90-day follow-up. The measure of function is a combination of the number of accidents and the amount of assistance required. Often the FIM measure on admission does not fully reflect a correct level of function because the patient may not have had a bowel movement for many days before his admission to rehabilitation because of constipation or an impaction. Once a bowel program is established, the number of accidents is an important indicator of its effectiveness and of the patient's outcome.

Ultimate measurements of goal achievement in a bowel program are twofold: (1) achievement of a bowel movement as a result of a bowel program in a short period of time and (2) minimizing or eliminating the occurrence of bowel accidents. The potential to achieve bowel continence is often critical to patient self-esteem, regardless of whether it is achieved as a self-managed program or one directed by the patient and administered by a care provider. It is an important factor in the achievement of social reintegration and participation in community activities. An effective bowel program is necessary to support a patient returning to work. Finally, an effective bowel program supports a return to sexuality and intimacy.[20]

SEXUALITY

Sexuality is a natural part of the human experience. After an SCI, patients vary a great deal regarding when they first inquire about how their sexual ability has been affected. For some patients, particularly younger men, questions may be asked very shortly after their injury. Older patients, and more often female patients, may not ask any questions for many months. Although patients can pose their questions to any member of the interdisciplinary team, nurses may be among the first to whom questions about sexuality are addressed. The response to these questions is important in setting the stage for future sexual education and counseling. Nurses who work with patients with an SCI must have basic knowledge about sexuality to provide correct information and the right environment for future dialog.

Sexuality is a complex phenomenon and the physiological processes that support sexual functions are only one component of sexuality. Psychological components, including emotions and psychosexual stimuli, are integral parts as well. Each patient has his own sexual history before the injury and unique relationships that may support his sexuality as he moves forward. From the onset, nurses and other team members must be tolerant and not impose their own morality or sexual boundaries on the patient or family member.[24] Sexual education and counseling generally addresses three basic areas: alterations in sexual function associated with SCI, factors that enhance and diminish sexuality, and compensatory strategies and devices.

Normal sexual function is also complex, requiring the integration of a number of neural pathways, autonomic innervations, sufficient vascular supply, and psychosexual components. Sexual excitement can be the result of physical stimulation, psychosexual stimulation, or a combination of both. In the male, it is important to note that physical stimulation alone produces a weak erection, whereas psychosexual stimulation produces an erection that is more sustained.[20] To understand the impact of SCI on sexuality, the starting point is to understand the level and extent of the injury. For patients with upper motor neuron lesions, physical stimulation that triggers a reflex erection in the male and vaginal secretion in the female as well as psychosexual stimulation may be used. Although the patient cannot feel the physical stimulation, it can contribute to the overall experience for both partners. Psychosexual stimulation is an important component for patients with upper motor neuron injury and can result in creating and sustaining an erection in the male and providing the central pleasure for the patient with SCI. In addition, psychosexual stimulation is closely associated in orgasm both for males and females. Although ejaculation for the male with an upper motor neuron injury is often not possible,[25] "new understanding of the physiology of sexual function and improved treatment can enable most cord-injured men to achieve erections suitable for sexual satisfaction."[26]

For patients with lower motor neuron injury, psychosexual stimulation is the key component of sexuality after SCI for both men and women. Because reflexes are not present, physical stimulation is generally not successful in producing an erection in the male. It is important to note here, however, that a patient with complete lower motor neuron lesions may have psychogenic erections in spite of the absence of reflex erections.[27] Men may be able to ejaculate in some cases. For the female patient, psychogenic stimulation and arousal are also possible. In patients with SCI regardless injury level, research indicates that approximately half experience orgasm.[28]

Numerous factors may affect sexuality for the SCI patient (Box 3-4). To begin with, variables that affect sexuality in the general population may have the same impact on patients with SCI. These include physiological factors such as chronic diseases, medications, and vascular supply, as well as psychological factors such as mood and self-concept.[29] For the patient with SCI, there are a number of additional factors that are unique. The first of these is the patient's bladder program. For the patient who uses an indwelling catheter, the options are either to remove the catheter or to secure it to minimize its interference with sexual intimacy. Securing the catheter for a man can be accomplished by folding the catheter back along the shaft of the penis and covering it with a condom.[20] For a woman, the catheter should be secured so that it has minimal interference, such as securing the catheter to the side and back along the body. Patients who perform IC should time their sexual intimacy immediately after the IC to minimize the risk of bladder distention or contractions that can trigger AD and to minimize the risk of incontinence.

The second factor for the patient with SCI is the patient's bowel program. Timing sexual intimacy after a bowel program will help to mitigate bowel incontinence during the sexual activity for patients with lower motor neuron lesions and will decrease the risk of bowel distention and potential AD for those with upper motor neuron injury. These considerations do interfere with sexual spontaneity and both patient and partner will determine how important this is to them. Because timing related to bladder program is also critical, patients may find having a sexual encounter in the shower a good alternative that adds to the comfort of the couple in addressing concerns with incontinence.

Another factor applies to patients at risk for AD. Sexual intimacy can be a trigger for AD. The patient with SCI should be very knowledgeable regarding the causes and symptoms of AD and should immediately stop sexual stimulation if symptoms occur.[30] In addition, the interventions that the patient uses for AD may need to be activated, such as the application of nitroglycerin paste as prescribed.

The psychological impact of SCI that may alter body image causes social isolation, or depression is the fourth factor.[31] Supportive counseling is an important part of the treatment plan. Addressing psychological issues in a counseling forum is the starting point for developing strategies that may assist in overriding their interference in a patient's sexual life. For patients who are in a relationship, couple counseling may be the most effective intervention and can assist in helping achieve satisfying sexual intimacy for both partners.

BOX 3-4 | Factors Affecting Sexuality Among Patients with Spinal Cord Injury

1. All factors that affect sexuality in the able-bodied population also affect sexuality in the SCI population.
2. Bowel and bladder programs or regimens must be taken into account as follows:
   - Minimizing equipment/catheter interference
   - Minimizing the risk of incontinence during the activity
   - Minimizing the risk of bladder distention during the activity
   - Bowel programs or regimens should be administered in advance of a sexual encounter to minimize the risk of either abdominal distention or incontinence during the sexual encounter.
3. Patient with a risk of AD must take steps before a sexual encounter and be knowledgeable to take necessary steps if symptoms occur during the activity.
4. Additional psychological factors including body image, mood, and adjustment affect both interest in sexual activity and success and satisfaction related to the encounter.
5. Positioning must be modified, and often advance planning may be necessary to support a good sexual experience both for the patient and the partner.
6. Alternative methods of stimulation may be necessary to support satisfaction both for the patient and the partner.

Finally, positioning and stimulation are factors that enhance satisfaction in sexual intimacy. Based on the patient's level of injury, the partners must be flexible in finding a sexual position that is satisfying for both. Sometimes having the patient with SCI sit upright may provide the opportunity for more participation. Very often, the individual with SCI may need to be in the dependent position. Because of the impairment in normal sensory function, it is important to focus on areas where the patient has sensation. The areas for each patient may be somewhat different but can include the breasts, ears, eyes, neck, lower abdomen, groin, and inner thigh.[32] Creative strategies may include incorporating stimulation to these areas along with psychosexual stimulation such as visualization.

Compensatory strategies for the patient with SCI include alternative strategies, pharmacological agents, and devices to enhance performance. Alternative strategies include sexual activities that vary from traditional male-female intercourse. For many patients, masturbation may be an alternative by either the patient or the partner. Cunnilingus and fellatio may be other options that provide satisfaction to patient, partner, or both. Techniques used for erectile dysfunction (ED) in the general population such as the "stuffing technique" can be effective.[33] Vacuum entrapment systems or pumps may be used for ED, but caution should be exercised because damage to the shaft of the penis can occur if they are used incorrectly.

Pharmacological agents to manage impotence are increasingly common. The main category of medications enhances male erection. Sildenafil citrate (Viagra) relaxes smooth muscles, leading to an erection. Male patients with SCI reported a 75% improvement with sildenafil[34] and a cost-utility analysis in 2005 that compared various treatment options for ED in SCI concluded that sildenafil is a cost-effective treatment in this population.[35] Caution must be exercised to use the drug properly, and patients with AD may not be candidates. Testosterone injections, patches, and gels may enhance libido in men with low levels[36] but have no impact if levels are already normal. Recent research by Schoop et al,[37] however, has documented the prevalence of low testosterone levels among men with SCI. The medicated urethral system (MUSE, VIVUS, Mountain View, Calif.) has been on the market since 1997 and has been demonstrated to be effective in patients with an SCI.[38,39] It may be used in combination with a venous constrictor band to prevent system absorption and enhance the erection.

Devices to enhance sexual function include penile implants and penile prostheses as well as artificial penises and vibrators. Penile devices may be hydraulic inflatable, noninflatable semirigid, or malleable.[20] These devices do enhance erection but do not enhance orgasm or the achievement of orgasm. The decision to have a penile implant should be delayed until all other options have been explored. Artificial penises are devices that can be strapped onto the groin and can simulate a natural erection. Vibrators can enhance sexual function for some patients, but caution should be exercised because the patient can become dependent on intense stimulation. They should be used with water-soluble lubricant.

ALTERED SENSATION: PAIN

Pain is a significant problem for patients who have sustained an SCI. Patients with SCI have nociceptive pain as the result of intact peripheral receptors in areas of the body that remain innervated, including musculoskeletal pain that is often chronic, particularly

in shoulders and hands bearing the brunt of body movement in, between, and out of the wheelchair. Table 2-3 discusses goals and treatment for nociceptive pain.

Neuropathic pain includes pain related to injury of nerve roots, the spinal cord, or the cauda equina.[40] Despite the common occurrence of neuropathic pain in patients with SCI, the actual causative factors are poorly understood (see Chapter 2). Neuropathic pain generally presents within the first 6 months after an SCI. It results from nerve injury, whether from surgery, disease, or trauma, and is characterized by constant aching sensations that may be interrupted by burst of burning and shock-like pain in the affected area.[41] Research shows reports of chronic pain from individuals with SCI as high as 4 in 5; additionally one third report severe chronic pain that interferes with daily life. No classification of pain in SCI has been universally accepted; however, the Bryce and Ragnarsson Classification offers an algorithm tree that helps explain differences in patient physiologic response (Figure 3-7).[40,42] This classification identifies 15 types of pain, which indicates the complexity of altered sensation after SCI.

Recent research by Werhagen et al[43] concludes that neuropathic pain related to SCI occurs more often in patients injured at older ages regardless of sex (pain is at the level of injury up to 39 years of age; pain below the level of injury at ages 40 and above) and indicates the importance of neuroanalgetic intervention. Because long-standing pain after SCI is one of its most challenging medical problems and may affect social reintegration and the challenge of a patient's return to work, clinicians need to be aware of current treatments, including cognitive-behavioral therapy.

Factors Associated with Pain

As shown in the Bryce and Ragnarsson Classification, pain is associated with a number of factors including location in regard to the level of injury, etiology, and intensity.[40,42] Both nociceptive and neuropathic pain would appear to be influenced by environmental and psychological factors (Clinical Note: Contributing Factors Associated with Pain). A more complete understanding of the neurobiology of pain based on continuing research will be necessary to elucidate its mechanisms.

CLINICAL NOTE — **Contributing Factors Associated with Pain**

- Prolonged sitting
- Fatigue
- Muscle spasms
- Presence of infection
- Negative mood
- Limited sense of control
- Cold weather
- Sudden movements

Clinicians must instruct patients that prolonged sitting and fatigue often contribute to pain in individuals with SCI. The presence of neck pain in particular is often associated with an upright position and with the presence of orthostatic hypotension. In addition, patients who have muscle spasms are at a greater risk for pain. Psychological factors include negative mood, depression,

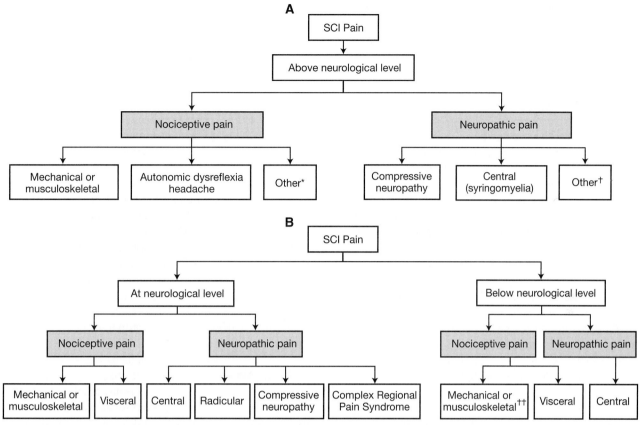

FIGURE 3-7 **A,** Four common subtypes of above-level SCI pain. Other nociceptive *(asterisk)* and neuropathic *(dagger)* subtypes include all other types of pain that are not necessarily more common to persons with SCI. **B,** Nine subtypes of at-level and below-level SCI pain. SCI below-level mechanical or musculoskeletal pain *(double dagger)* is found only in people who have incomplete lesions or who have partially innervated dermatomes at the level of the pain. (Adapted from Bryce TN, Ragnarsson KT: Pain after spinal cord injury, *Phys Med Rehabil Clin North Am* 11:157-168, 2000.)

and a limited sense of control of life—all recognized responses to SCI.[44] Cold or changing weather, sudden movements, and infection may contribute to pain as well.

Assessment

Pain assessment in the patient with SCI presents many of the same challenges as in other populations. Pain is, first and foremost, a subjective experience.[45] Health care providers and family members must guard against judging whether the reported pain is valid or exaggerated. Establishing the characteristics of a patient's pain should include the location, description, factors that worsen the pain, factors that improve the pain, and any associated symptoms such as nausea or changes in sensation such as numbness. The McGill pain scale is generally a reliable assessment tool (see Figure 6-12).[45] In addition, rating pain on a scale from 1 to 10 both before and after interventions to reduce the pain is a central part of a complete pain assessment.

Bryce and Ragnarsson[40] emphasize the importance of a multistep approach in evaluating pain in patients with SCI:
- Determine the neurological level and completeness of injury
- Localize pain to one of three regions of injury: above level, at level, below level
- Categorize pain as nociceptive or neuropathic
- Subdivide pain into specific subtype (see Figure 3-7)
- Establish an evidence-based treatment plan

Objective observations associated with pain are also important. These may include facial grimacing, altered muscle tone or spasticity, diaphoresis, and changes in vital signs. The patient's posture and any change in the activity level, including a drop in functional independence, may also be indicators of pain. Autonomic responses to pain can be very challenging to manage, and for patients with injuries above T6, AD may be a serious risk.

Assessment of pain must include an understanding of the patient's history and baseline data about both the history of pain and the patient's pain tolerance. Differentiating acute from chronic pain is as important as understanding the differences in nociceptive and neuropathic pain. The potential contributing factors in acute and chronic pain may vary and it must be recognized that, although chronic pain may be managed by a number of therapies, a permanent cure may not result.[46]

Interventions

Foremost, the removal of potential or immediate causes of pain must be undertaken. A change in a patient's position may include weight shifting or transferring a patient from a sitting position to supine. Ensuring proper positioning and support of the head and neck and limbs can enhance comfort and reduce spasticity that may be a causative factor of pain. Ensuring the proper position and function of catheters, intravenous lines, or other tubes is important to alleviating pain.

Analgesic management of pain is a common approach to all types of chronic pain in the patient with SCI. The selection of medication is dependent on the patient's history, the severity of the pain, and the presence or absence of associated factors such as spasticity. The prompt administration of ordered medication is critical because pain that goes untreated tends to worsen quickly, making effective treatment more challenging. Medications may be administered in response to a complaint of pain or may be prophylactic to prevent pain exacerbations (see Chapter 2).

Other interventions for pain may be helpful, either alone or in combination. Massage and the use of heat or cold therapies or a combination of these strategies can be very helpful in some patients.[47] The use of injections to treat spasticity associated with pain with blocks or botulinum toxin has shown positive results.[48,49] Psychological support can also be an effective adjunct to a pain program. It may be as limited as supportive counseling or as involved as a pain management program using relaxation, hypnotic, and cognitive-behavioral techniques tailored for the patient through a learning protocol that enables him to perform the techniques and help manage his pain over the long term.[42,50] Although the treatment plan "may include physical measures, pharmacological treatments, behavioral interventions, surgery, or an eclectic combination program" and provide some relief, "complete relief often is not possible."[40]

Outcomes

Pain management in patients with SCI is important to numerous areas of outcomes. The frequency and severity of pain and the effectiveness of pain relief can be evaluated as continuous indicators of trend data across time. Patient reports of pain remain a good interval indicator of both episodes of pain and effectiveness of intervention strategies. Tracking daily reports of pain graphically provides important feedback on the overall plan for pain relief. For instance, evaluating the effectiveness of slow-acting opioids or changes in reported pain as a result of the introduction of antidepressants are important steps in the effort to control chronic pain.

In addition, a patient's ability to assume functional independence related to activities of daily living and social reintegration is closely related to successful pain management. For patients who are unable to perform their own self-care, the ability and initiative in directing care providers in performing self-care activities is a valid indicator of their sense of well-being and interest in maintaining a good routine and social reintegration. Overall, the best indicators of an effective pain management program are the patient's self-report of pain and his sense of well-being and optimism.[45]

ALTERED SKIN INTEGRITY

Maintaining skin integrity is essential for patients who have sustained SCI, both immediately after the injury and for the rest of their lives. Altered skin integrity is defined as any break in the normal skin surface or the destruction of a skin surface. The central challenge is to avoid the development of a pressure ulcer, which is defined as a lesion caused by unrelieved pressure most often over a bony prominence resulting in damage to the underlying tissue (Figure 3-8). Many factors are associated with skin integrity, including pressure, shearing, friction, immobility, nutrition, and moisture (Box 3-5).

In the able-bodied person, sensory perception gives continual feedback that results in position change, sometimes very subtle and sometimes very dramatic. The sensory feedback may include pain, a sensation of moisture, pressure, heat, or burning. The lack of sensory feedback coupled with impaired motor function place the patient with SCI at a very high risk for skin breakdown.

The prevalence of impaired skin integrity in the patient with an SCI ranges from 3% to 30%, depending on sources.[51] If we assume that, on average, 17% have skin breakdown, a total of more than 38,000 persons with SCI will have a pressure ulcer in their lifetimes.[52] Pressure ulcers, which are the leading cause of unplanned rehospitalization in individuals with SCI, may prove fatal.[53] A simple case of skin breakdown can cost up to $30,000 to treat successfully and to heal.[53] In the case of a more complex full-thickness ulcer, the cost increases substantially to as much as $70,000. The estimated national cost of pressure ulcers is more than $1.3 billion, with some estimates as high as $3.6 billion.[51,54] Pressure ulcers account for as much as 25% of the cost of caring for a patient with SCI.[55] It is important to note that prevention costs only a tenth of treatment.

Pathophysiology

The skin consists of three layers: epidermis, dermis, and subcutaneous tissue. An area of pressure over a bony prominence is distributed in a cone-like fashion (see Figure 3-8). At the skin level, there may be a very small opening, but the area widens quickly lower from the skin surface. The greater amount of damage is usually seen at the muscle layer rather than at the skin layer.

The immobility associated with SCI often leads to unmitigated pressure at certain areas of the body, particularly over bony prominences. The pressure causes capillary closure and the cessation of blood flow to the area, resulting in ischemia and tissue death. Patients with SCI have a slower blood reflow rate to the pressure area once the pressure has been relieved, delaying the supply of oxygen and nutrients to the area. This delay contributes even more to the process of skin breakdown. The location of pressure ulcers can be predicted, with approximately 37% of ulcers occurring over the sacrum, 16% on the heels, and 9% over ischial tuberosities.

Prevention of Pressure Ulcers

Prevention of pressure ulcers necessitates a multipronged approach.[56] In a rehabilitation setting, the patient and family must learn to take responsibility for themselves rather than relying on the health care team for all of their care needs. From the beginning, it is important to stress that a pressure ulcer after SCI is *not* inevitable. Knowledge and vigilance are the keys to preventing pressure ulcers.

Patients with a new spinal cord injury should be turned at least every 2 hours from side to side at an oblique angle to avoid direct pressure on the trochanteric processes. A central concern is to avoid pressure on the sacrum because it is the area most susceptible to breakdown. This time interval for turning may lengthen as time goes on and skin tolerance to prolonged pressure increases. If medically appropriate, the patient may be positioned prone as well.

Stage I

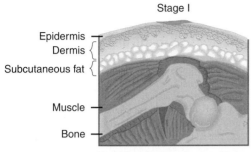

Epidermis
Dermis
Subcutaneous fat
Muscle
Bone

Non-blanching erythema of intact skin;
the heralding lesion of skin ulceration

Stage II

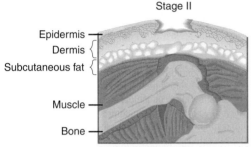

Epidermis
Dermis
Subcutaneous fat
Muscle
Bone

Partial-thickness skin loss involving
epidermis and/or dermis. The ulcer is
superficial and presents clinically as an
abrasion, blister, or shallow crater.

Stage III

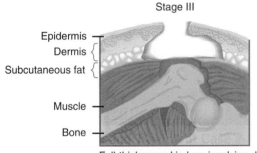

Epidermis
Dermis
Subcutaneous fat
Muscle
Bone

Full-thickness skin loss involving damage
or necrosis of subcutaneous tissue, which
may extend down to, but not through, the
underlying fascia. The ulcer presents
clinically as a deep crater with or without
undermining of adjacent tissue.

Stage IV

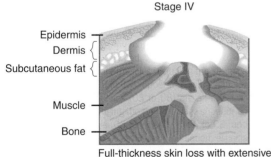

Epidermis
Dermis
Subcutaneous fat
Muscle
Bone

Full-thickness skin loss with extensive
destruction, tissue necrosis, or damage
to muscle, bone, or supporting structures
(e.g., tendon, joint capsule, etc.)

FIGURE 3-8 Stages of pressure ulcers. (From Black JM, Hawks JH: *Medical-surgical nursing: clinical management for positive outcomes,* ed 7, p 1404, St. Louis, 2005, Mosby.)

Pillows and foam wedges are also used to enhance pressure relief. Sometimes patients use up to seven or eight pillows at various anatomic locations. Specialty suspension boots designed to avoid pressure on the heels, such as Multi Podus (Restorative Care of America, Inc., St. Petersburg, Fla.), Posey Heel (Posey Company, Arcadia, Calif.), and Heelift Supension boots (DM Systems Inc., Evanston, Ill.), may be used to suspend the heel in space while supporting the rest of the lower leg with soft padding. Heel protectors such as booties or heel pads are ineffective in dissipating pressure on heels in this population.

To avoid friction-related injury, a draw sheet should be used to reposition the patient in bed. This allows the caregivers to move the patient around the bed easily and safely. Keeping the head of the bed as flat as possible is good practice because the risk of shearing to the patient's body during movement increases as the head is elevated. Checking the bed linen for wrinkles and smoothing them out is important because wrinkles often cause pressure that can result in skin breakdown. Friction and bumping are major concerns during transfers from surface to surface. Use of a mechanical lift is advised if a patient is dependent for transferring for both patient and caregiver safety. When an individual can transfer by himself, proper use of a transfer board decreases friction and the chance of skin breakdown.

Pressure ulcers may also be a result of problems related to wheelchair seating (see Chapter 11). The areas of the body most susceptible to pressure ulcers while seated are the bony prominences over the ischial tuberosities, the sacrum, and the coccyx. Proper seating includes making sure that the chair is the correct size, type, and configuration for the individual. Once a patient is transferred from bed to wheelchair, visual inspection should be done to determine whether the patient's buttocks is well back in the chair and his weight centered. If the pelvis is tilted posteriorly, shearing or pressure can occur at the sacral and coccygeal areas.

The Consortium for Spinal Cord Medicine (2000) recommends a 30-second weight shift every 30 minutes or a 1-minute weight shift every 60 minutes.[57] Recent studies recommend more frequent and longer weight shifts, but to date these have not been incorporated in Consortium guidelines. Several sources indicate that weight shifts should be done for 30 seconds at a time every 15 minutes.[58,59] In addition, research done in 2003 showed that 30 seconds was not enough time to achieve complete revascularization of the area and concluded "alternative pressure relief measures (e.g., leaning forward, side to side, and tilt back) would be more sustainable and efficient because the extended duration required (range 42 seconds to 3 minutes 30 seconds) was not practical or desired for most patients when using a traditional lifting up technique."[60]

In reality, most patient's arms get too tired to sustain a long-duration weight shift using the traditional press-up lifting technique that is typically thought to be the most effective although most difficult to perform (see Chapter 7).[59] For this reason the following options may be more feasible:

- Anterior weight shift: The patient leans forward at the waist until pressure is removed from the ischial tuberosities.
- Posterior weight shift: The patient leans back in the chair until pressure shifts from ischial tuberosities to the sacral area; this is performed in a power wheelchair by hitting a lever that tilts the chair back.

BOX 3-5 | Factors Associated with Skin Integrity

- **Pressure:** Defined as an uninterrupted mechanical loading of tissue that occurs most often over a bony prominence where skin and the underlying tissue are compressed
- **Shearing:** Occurs when the skin remains stationary while the underlying tissue shifts. This typically occurs as a patient slides down in bed when the head of the bed is elevated more than 30 degrees
- **Friction:** The movement of skin against a surface; most commonly occurs during surface-to-surface transfers or during bed repositioning
- **Immobility:** Significant contributory factor to impaired skin integrity. Lack of mobility increases the likelihood that there will be prolonged skin pressure. Among all the factors associated with impairment to skin integrity, immobility is considered to have the greatest impact.

- **Nutrition:** Critical to maintaining healthy tissue. Low serum albumin levels can lead to interstitial edema that decreases the cell's ability to carry oxygen and nutrients.
- **Moisture:** Often associated with bladder or bowel incontinence, has a profound impact on skin integrity. Moisture in general can cause the skin to become macerated, increasing the susceptibility to breakdown. The contents of urine and stool can be very caustic to the skin and may lead to rashes or other skin alterations that can progress very quickly.

- Lateral weight shift: The patient leans to one side, which off-loads pressure from one ischial tuberosity at a time.

Patients must be encouraged to advocate for their own care particularly when working to prevent pressure ulcers. They are instructed to ask care providers or family members to assist with weight shifts, repositioning in bed, and help with skin inspection as needed. Such patient education needs to begin as soon as a patient demonstrates ability to participate in his own care. In short-term rehabilitation, this training starts on the day of admission and may include both the patient and family members.

From the beginning, the health care team must encourage a patient's family and friends to provide weight shifting, turning in bed, and use of preventive devices to help the patient avoid skin breakdown. This model of self-care is different from the one used in many acute-care settings because the health care team focuses on empowering others to provide safe patient care rather than providing all of the primary care for the entire length of rehabilitation stay. Before discharge, a home care team may need training about how to prevent pressure ulcers.

Proper nutrition is also important in the prevention of pressure ulcers. Research has shown that low serum albumin levels are associated with increased risk of pressure ulcer development.[58] In addition, the Agency for Health Care Policy and Research recommends eating at least 1 g of protein per kilogram of body weight daily for prevention of skin breakdown.[51] The importance of dietary protein and oral liquid supplements between meals in patients who have pressure ulcers has been documented.[51,61,62] Because the presence of a pressure ulcer is a catabolic process that includes inflammation and sometimes infection, loss of body protein and calories further increases the need for sufficient protein and calorie intake.[57]

Assessment

Assessing the risk for skin breakdown is essential to ensure that an effective program of preventing pressure ulcers is established. A number of scales can be used, but the most common ones are the Braden scale and the Norton scale.[63,64] There has been little research to indicate the effectiveness of these scales in the SCI population because these patients typically fall into a high-risk category as a result of their injuries. A specific tool for assessment,

the Pressure Ulcer Risk Assessment Scale for Persons with Paralysis, was developed in 1998 but needs further testing in the SCI population for validation.[52]

Skin inspection is critical to the nursing plan for all patients with an SCI. Initially, the inspections are done by the nurse. As soon as feasible, the patient should be instructed to perform his own skin check by using a hand-held mirror. Skin checks should be performed after any period of sitting in a wheelchair, toilet, or commode, or lying in bed. Any area of redness that does not dissipate after 30 minutes is considered at high risk for skin breakdown. An immediate plan to reduce pressure must be implemented so that the condition does not worsen.

Prevention strategies for maintaining skin integrity among patients with SCI are essential and must be interdisciplinary. An evaluation of risk factors along with skin assessment and use of devices to support good skin integrity are essential to a coordinated plan of care. Table 3-2 highlights cross-disciplinary steps to prevent skin breakdown and indicates the broad scope of responsibilities that contribute to a comprehensive skin care program.

Interventions

Important basic principles for treatment of pressure ulcers in patients with SCI include the following:

- Begin treatment as soon as skin breakdown is detected
- Relieve pressure and avoid any friction or shearing
- Keep the wound bed clean, moist, and free from infection
- Remove (i.e., by debridement) any devitalized tissue from the ulcer[65]

Wound assessment is critical when the wound is first discovered and at regular intervals along the course of treatment and recovery. Wound assessment should include a number of key observations in addition to the pressure ulcer stage. The location of the wound along with its size and depth in centimeters should be part of each wound assessment and reassessment. Staging of the wound can occur only when there is no necrotic tissue or eschar that would prevent full visibility (see Figures 3-8 and 6-11). The color of the tissue along with the presence of any odor or exudates is important to report. The inspection should also include any observation of undermining or tunneling and the presence of any necrotic tissue. Finally, the observation of granulation tissue should be noted.

TABLE 3-2 | Skin Breakdown Prevention and Pressure Relief

Prevention Strategy	Nursing	Physical Therapy	Occupational Therapy	Patient, Family, and Caregivers
Begin an interdisciplinary pressure relief program from day 1 of onset of SCI	Conduct comprehensive, systematic, and consistent assessment of pressure ulcer risk factors in individuals with SCI: Assess and document on admission and reassess on a routine basis. Use clinical judgment and a risk assessment tool. Assess demographic, physical/medical, and psychological factors associated with pressure ulcer prevention			Learn about the importance of comprehensive, systematic, and consistent assessment of pressure ulcer risk factors
Avoid prolonged immobilization	Implement bed turning every 2 hours	Ensure proper positioning for optimal skin protection for therapy interventions	Provide wheelchair seating and adaptive equipment for ADLs	Learn about pressure relief guidelines and individualized risk factors
Areas of daily skin inspections: ischii, sacrum, coccyx, trochanters, heels, malleoli, anterior knee, shoulder, side of head, elbow, occiput, rim of ear, dorsal thoracic spine	Inspect; educate and train patient and family related to the patient's bed position, mobility status, and medical confounding factors	Educate and train patient and family about areas of inspection and use of adaptive equipment and functional activities related to inspection		Learn about methods of daily skin inspection dependent on mobility status and level of injury
Evaluate support surface	Select appropriate bed surface and monitor medical issues that may change these needs	Identify hazards of support surfaces during interventions. Provide appropriate bridging for skin relief. Monitor wheelchair seating and support surfaces for optimal protection	Identify hazards of support surfaces for ADLs and optimize protection and prevention. Evaluate optimal seating support and monitor needs for altering these surfaces	Learn about moisture, surface shear, surface friction, and medical issues that may affect support surfaces and potential risks for skin vulnerability
Wheelchair pressure relief program	Perform and educate about weight shift in upright every 15 to 30 minutes, allowing adequate oxygen replenishment to muscles	Train and educate about weight shift techniques individualized to level of injury, strength, cognitive status (power relief or manual)	Train and educate about maintenance of equipment and weight shift options (power relief or manual)	Learn about and teach caregivers the individualized skin relief schedule and methods
Mobility program training for prevention of deconditioning	Encourage patient in self direction of care. Educate about the importance of mobility to decrease the incidence of pressure ulcer development	Educate and provide individual guidelines for mobility and exercise programs for the prevention of pressure ulcer development	Educate about the importance of mobility to decrease the incidence of pressure ulcer development	Practice self-direction of care. Learn about the importance of mobility in relation to decreased incidence of pressure ulcer development
Individualized patient education program	Consider the learning styles of patients and family. Assess understanding by questions. Clarify and give explanations considering psychosocial issues			Ask lots of questions

Wound cleansing can be accomplished by irrigating the wound with normal saline solution. The amount of pressure used is important so that the wound is sufficiently cleansed but there is no damage to any granulation tissue. The most appropriate pressure is between 3 and 15 pounds per inch, which can be accomplished with a 35-ml syringe barrel with a 19-gauge needle or angiocatheter attached.[66]

A number of wound dressings are available on the market and the decision regarding the appropriate dressing depends first on the wound assessment (Table 3-3).

Wet-to-dry dressings and enzymatic agents may be used to debride a wound with necrotic tissue. Alginates and foams can be used to contain heavy exudates from a wound. Protective films and barriers may be used on stage I and II pressure ulcer wounds to prevent friction. Antimicrobial dressing products are designed to reduce the bacterial load in a wound.

The type of bed an individual with SCI uses is an important consideration, both in the prevention and treatment of skin breakdown. Specialty beds are available for use during the acute-care stay immediately after the injury, during short-term rehabilitation, and after discharge into the community. Beds with pressure reduction surfaces are available that use air suspension to redistribute body weight away from bony prominences. The patient will spend 6 to 8 hours a night on the surface, and the

choice of a mattress or overlay should take into account his height, weight, and skin care needs. Two common specialty beds used in the SCI population are low-air-loss beds and high-air-loss beds. Low-air-loss beds allow for air movement around the skin and a pressure-relieving surface (Figure 3-9, *A*). It may be used for prevention of pressure ulcers and an adjunctive therapy for people with low-grade skin breakdown. High-air-loss beds or beds with bead fluidization allow the patient to rest on a supporting surface while underneath a sea of ceramic microbeads are pumped with air (Figure 3-9, *B*). This results in a surface where pressure on the skin is greatly relieved. Such pressure-reduction beds with controlled air pressure encourage wound healing.[57]

Surgery may be used to close a stage III or IV pressure ulcer wound. The advantages of surgery include a reduced healing time, intervention to help prevent infection, lower cost, and a decrease in the amount of care required. Patients may undergo direct closure, skin grafting, or a procedure called flap surgery. Flap surgery involves the removal of necrotic tissue followed by bringing the intact muscle and skin together with a sutured skin closure. This surgery provides the patient with a well-padded, well-vascularized new area of intact skin and muscle in place of the pressure ulcer.

After skin surgery to treat a pressure ulcer, patients often spend 4 to 8 weeks lying supine on a high-air-loss bed while the incision heals and strengthens. Over time, the patient will be allowed to participate in a gradual sitting program, beginning with 15 minutes daily and progressing to full sitting capacity. Patient education is critical to achieving good outcome after skin surgery for a pressure ulcer. Patients will need to carefully evaluate their own skin after each sitting trial and adjust the length of sitting time on the basis of how their skin has reacted to that particular trial.

Wound healing can be delayed as a result of factors that interfere both in natural wound healing and in wound healing after surgery. Obesity and nonadherence to pressure relief or sitting trials interfere with good wound healing. In addition, smoking affects wound healing, in part because of vasoconstriction, as do incontinence and infection.

TABLE 3-3	Types of Wound Dressings and Their Indications for Use
Type of Dressing	Indications for Use
Wet to dry dressings and enzymatic agents	Debridement of a wound with necrotic tissue
Alginates and foams	Containment of heavy exudates
Protective films and barriers	Prevent friction at grade 1 and 2 wounds
Antimicrobial dressing products	Reduce bacterial load in a wound

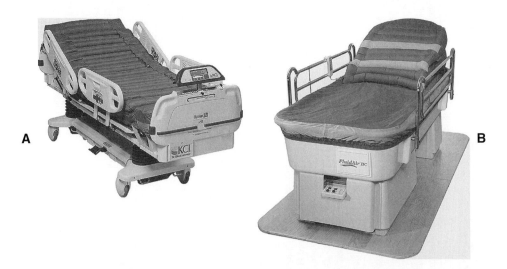

FIGURE 3-9 Pressure reduction surfaces. **A,** Kinair Medsurg beds provide controlled air suspension to redistribute body weight away from bony prominences. **B,** FluidAir Elite beds use air flow and bead fluidization. Both these beds are covered with GORE-TEX fabric, which resists tearing. This fabric is also waterproof and acts as a barrier against bacteria. (From Black JM, Hawks JH: *Medical-surgical nursing: clinical management for positive outcomes*, ed 7, p. 1405, St. Louis, 2005, Mosby. Courtesy of Kinetic Concepts, Inc., San Antonio, TX.)

In some patients who have skin surgery for pressure ulcers, a temporary colostomy may be performed to divert stool away from the fragile surgical site. This decreases the risk of wound infection and ensures that the skin will be free from maceration as a result of the contact of feces. Some patients opt to keep the colostomy after wound healing has been achieved because it may be a more convenient way to manage their bowel program and will permanently eliminate the risk of bowel incontinence on future skin integrity.

Pressure ulcers may be associated with a number of complications. Infection is a principal concern in the patient with an SCI because it can lead very quickly to sepsis and may be life threatening.[67] Prompt recognition of the presence of infection is critical, and long-term courses of antibiotic therapy may be necessary. Other complications associated with pressure ulcers include AD, contractures, osteomyelitis, and heterotopic ossification.

Outcomes

The best outcome for patients with SCI is to maintain skin integrity and to have no incidences of pressure ulcers over their lifetime. Establishing this as a central goal is important early in the patient's recovery. Achievement of this goal depends on the effectiveness of patient and family education combined with the intrinsic motivation of the patient and family to do everything possible to support good skin integrity. Establishment of a collaborative plan between the team, the patient, and the patient's family will increase the likelihood of success.

Once a pressure ulcer has occurred, the likelihood of recurrence is higher because the skin is only approximately 80% as strong as it was originally.[66] One study indicated that patients who had a pressure ulcer in the first month after injury were significantly more likely to have recurrent skin breakdown in the future.[52] Additional research indicates a recurrence rate of approximately 35%, regardless of whether the pressure ulcer healed naturally or as a result of surgery.[55] Patient and family may also be discouraged after the initial pressure ulcer, anticipating a recurrence.[59]

ALTERED MOBILITY

Altered mobility in patients with SCI is associated both with specific challenges to nursing care and successful patient outcome. Over the course of the 24-hour day, the delivery of nursing care includes a number of patient transfers to different surfaces or equipment and assistance with patient mobility in association with activities of daily living (ADLs). Impaired patient mobility makes achievement of patient care physically demanding for the caregiver and increases the opportunity of medical complications for the patient. The five complications that challenge mobility and require special knowledge and nursing interventions include the following:

- Spasticity
- Heterotopic ossification (HO)
- Deep vein thrombosis (DVT)
- Osteoporosis
- Respiratory complications

Spasticity

Spasticity affects almost everything many patients with SCI do, particularly those who have upper motor neuron lesions. Research indicates that 67% of patients who sustain an SCI have some spasticity.[68] The assessment of spasticity must include the following: triggers, location and muscle groups, associated pain, associated autonomic reflexes, severity, and response to interventions.

> ### THE CLIENT'S PERSPECTIVE   Spasticity
>
> A spasm is an involuntary muscle movement, similar to when your eye twitches and you are unable to control it. On many occasions, when I sleep, my legs and abdomen shake and will jar my upper body to the point where no matter how tired I am, physically or mentally, I still cannot sleep. How's that for lack of control!
>
> It took a year to understand how spasticity was going to affect my life, but it can be managed with medication, stretching, and exercise. When people have extreme difficulty with spasticity, the baclofen pump may offer relief.
>
> *Scott Chesney*

Position and posture can act as triggers of spasticity. Mobility includes how a patient transfers from one surface to another and must take into account position and posture that may either trigger spasticity or limit functional range. ADLs must be administered with consideration of position and posture and the timing of the activity to minimize the trigger of spasticity during the activity. Position and posture during sleep may trigger spasticity and thus affect sleep patterns; every effort must be made to minimize triggers that can interfere with a patient's ability to get a full night of sleep. Spasticity can be a central source of neuropathic pain, so efforts to minimize triggers of spasticity or intervene to reduce spasticity or manage pain are very important. In addition, the overall problem of spasticity can negatively affect patient mood.

Nursing interventions to manage spasticity must be carefully selected on the basis of individual patient characteristics. Positioning and stretching can be opportunities to avoid spasticity and decrease the presence of spasms with a general focus on good body alignment and slow movement. A number of modalities can be used to treat spasticity, including transcutaneous electrical nerve stimulation and biofeedback.[68] Therapeutic exercise as an adjunct to therapy may be useful and an individualized program designed by the physical therapist can be applied by nurses during care activities. The proper management of orthoses is important, ensuring correct application, positioning, and slow movement to minimize spasms.

Pain management is essential both before activities where pain or spasm are anticipated and to manage acute episodes of pain related to spasm so that fear does not interfere with physical activities. Medications to manage spasms may be an important part of the plan and may focus on spasticity related to bladder or bowel functions or spasticity associated with movement. Peripheral nerve blocks and motor point blocks can also be an important adjunct to the reduction of spasticity.[69]

Heterotopic Ossification

HO can have a significant impact on mobility and comfort and on the performance of functional activities. Depending on which joints are involved, movement limitations can significantly impair self-care and may necessitate special strategies or equipment to enhance self-care.[8] The medical management of HO can include surgery, serial casting, and medications. Nursing care should focus on supporting the medical strategies being used to treat the HO, developing functional alternatives to promote self-care in spite of the HO, and management of pain.

Deep Vein Thrombosis

Impaired mobility results in additional medical problems including the risk for DVT. DVT and pulmonary embolism can be life threatening, and prevention of these complications is critical to the plan of care. The loss of mobility and weight bearing place the patient with an SCI at particular risk for DVT and prevention of any clot formation is the first step in prevention.[70] Nurses must consider the signs and symptoms of DVT when assessing a patient with SCI as well as its potential differential diagnosis with the onset of new symptoms. Collaborative care with the physician achieves effective prophylaxis and prevents DVT.

Prescription of pharmaceutical agents to reduce the formation of clots is central to the medical management of the patient. Nursing care is designed to support the careful management of medications such as low-molecular-weight heparin and warfarin (Coumadin). This requires that nurses are knowledgeable about blood tests that monitor therapeutic levels or potentially dangerous levels of these drugs. Careful adherence to dose and scheduled administration times is essential to ensure therapeutic levels and avoid risks associated with overdose.

Osteoporosis

Osteoporosis is a long-term concern in patients who have sustained SCI. Decreased mobility combined with a loss of weight bearing in the lower and the upper extremity are contributory factors. Prevention is the best approach to this complication from the outset.[71] The establishment of mobility training and exercise based on the individual's injury and abilities is critical both immediately after the injury and in a longer-term basis. Adaptive equipment must be prescribed to encourage as much functional challenge as reasonable and promote muscle tone through physical activity. Medication to support good bone formation and decrease the risk of osteoporosis may be indicated. In addition, patient education should motivate patients to adopt an active lifestyle and exercise customized to their functional abilities.

Respiratory Complications

The risk of respiratory compromise associated with SCI is a serious concern because of decreased mobility and the level of injury with its potential impact on respiratory enervation. Decreased movement combined with postural changes and other factors results in a decrease in tidal volume and a risk for atelectasis. The combination of a decreased tidal volume combined with an increase in respiratory secretions significantly elevates the risk of complications such as pneumonia. Nursing goals for the patient with SCI include the following:

- Promotion of deep breathing and an increased tidal volume
- Promotion of pulmonary toileting
- Removal of respiratory secretions

A number of interventions target both an increase in tidal volume and a reduction in respiratory secretions. Deep breathing both at rest and during activity is one of the first steps to decrease atelectasis and mobilize secretions. Cueing the patient to perform several deep breaths in association with particular activities or according to a clock schedule sets the stage for patient and family education to initiate deep breathing on their own. Adding a deep cough at the end of several deep breaths changes pressures in the chest cavity and promotes pulmonary toileting.[72]

Ensuring adequate hydration is critical to good pulmonary care, liquefying secretions, and preventing mucus plugs. Assessing the lungs regularly for lung sounds and the presence or absence of rales, rhonchi, and wheezes is essential. Medications combined with treatments to manage pulmonary conditions may be an integral part of the care plan and should be preceded and followed by respiratory assessment to determine their effectiveness. In addition, the use of a CoughAssist mechanical insufflation-exsufflation (J.H. Emerson Co., Cambridge, Mass.), quad cough, or an intrapulmonary percussive ventilator device may be indicated to support good tidal volume and improved pulmonary toileting (see Chapter 4).

PATIENT AND FAMILY EDUCATION

Whether the patient is a 14-year-old boy with a T12 (ASIA A) SCI who is preparing for discharge to home and return to school, a 46-year-old father of three who sustained a C1 (ASIA A) SCI and will be returning home on a ventilator with limited nursing care, or a 25-year-old newlywed with a C6 (ASIA C) SCI who is heading home after rehabilitation to her new husband and home, patient and family fears can be addressed and alleviated through effective educational tools and rehabilitation programs.

Developing an educational program for patients with SCI is also a proactive method for working with decreased inpatient lengths of stay and preventing rehospitalization.[73] In fact, patient and family education should be an integral part of the mission and vision for any hospital specializing in SCI. Patient education should have a clear purpose and aim at helping fulfill each patient's individual needs and goals.

A formal series of classes covering all aspects of SCI designed to provide the patient and family with a knowledge base that will assist the patient in returning to a productive and healthy lifestyle is an excellent way to present vital information to patients with SCI. The series should be composed of different components that complement each other (Box 3-6).

BOX 3-6 | Components of a Spinal Cord Injury Education Program

- SCI manual
- Audio and video tapes
- Education lectures for both patients and their families
- Practical hands-on instruction provided by the nursing and therapy staff
- Peer support and resource groups

Spinal Cord Injury Education Manual

A rehabilitation education program for individuals who have experienced SCI has a very steep learning curve because the patient must relearn how to navigate most ADLs and come to terms with psychological aspects of the situation and attendant perceptions on the parts of loved ones and the community at large. In the same way that a textbook reinforces classroom skills in other learning environments, this manual is an important reinforcement tool of the information provided in the various education lectures and of therapies and procedures on the nursing unit. It gives patients and family members a document to review or to jot notes in for later discussion and reminders and becomes a handy reference guide after a patient's discharge that will increase everyone's sense of security when facing new care tasks on their own.

A good SCI education manual reinforces the complete range of subjects covered during the class series (Box 3-7). It should be written by the interdisciplinary treatment team and given to patients on admission to the SCI unit. In addition, it should be written in layman's terms and at a level so that even those patients with a limited educational background can comprehend the information. If possible, the manual should be available in both audio and printed form and in more than one language.

Patient and Family Education Programs

For those inpatients who are newly diagnosed with SCI, this series of educational lectures should provide an overview of all aspects of living with an SCI, starting with the anatomy of the spinal column, definition of a spinal cord injury, explanation of medical complications associated with SCIs and ways of preventing them, coverage of bowel and bladder management, discussion of sexuality, and explanation of discharge planning. Content should review how SCI affects physical function and the latest spinal cord injury research. These classes enhance the discussions that the patient and family may have with the physician and the therapists. They also help with the transition from the rehabilitation facility to home. In addition, the classes can also benefit patients with chronic injuries and their families by providing access to refresher courses.

Because of decreased inpatient lengths of stay, it is recommended that these classes be held several times per week to ensure that patients complete all classes before discharge. The importance of attending all lectures should be reinforced with the patient by each member of the treatment team. In addition, the class time should be a set part of the patient's schedule and all members of the treatment team are encouraged to reinforce the information provided during classes. For example, during the skin care lecture, types of weight shifts and skin checks are reviewed with patients. The patient's therapist can reinforce weight shifts during the following therapy session similar to the information addressed in class. Nurses can also reinforce weight shifts and review skin inspection with the patient while preparing for bed.

The formal class program also reviews the continuing education that nurses provide to patients and their families about bladder and bowel management, respiratory care, skin care, and medication during daily and evening care in the residential unit. When the therapy part of the day is over, visiting family members must be encouraged to participate in the care of their loved one (Figure 3-10). This participation can include something as simple as setting up a meal and utensils for the loved one or observing the bowel training program with plans to practice and demonstrate the procedures on the next bowel night. Teaching how to switch from the leg to the overnight bag is something health care professionals may take for granted but actual hands-on care can be new and frightening for the layman.

Family members should be encouraged to attend therapy sessions with patients for training. They will learn patient care skills that include the following:

- Techniques to move a patient in a wheelchair up and down a curb, ramp, or stairs
- How to perform upper and lower extremity passive range of motion exercises with the patient
- Practice of functional transfers including transfers to the bed, tub, toilet, car, and floor
- Equipment needs for home modifications
- How to provide assistance required during ambulation

The ideal educational facility will have an accessible on-site apartment for patients to use with their families. This allows the patient and family members a chance to perform practical applications of all the skills they have been taught during rehabilitation classes during on overnight stay in the accessible

---

BOX 3-7 | Contents of a Spinal Cord Injury Education Manual

I. The basics	XI. Emotional adjustment
• Anatomy	XII. Range of motion exercises
• Complete versus incomplete injuries	XIV. Moving around and position changes
• Functional expectations	XV. Transfers
II. Complications	XVI. Discharge planning
III. Bowel program	XVI. Items and issues
IV. Bladder program	• Assistive devices for ambulation
V. Skin care	• Upper and lower extremity bracing
VI. Nutrition	• Home modifications
VII. Sex after SCI	XVII. Wheelchair management and maintenance
VIII. Medications	XVIII. Adaptive driving
IX. Recreation	
X. Getting back to work	

Adapted courtesy of Kessler Institute for Rehabilitation in West Orange, New Jersey.

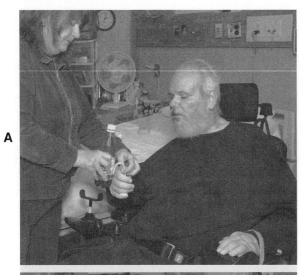

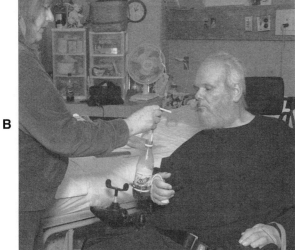

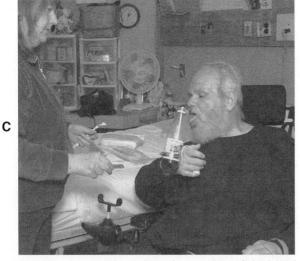

FIGURE 3-10 A patient directs his wife to attach a soft drink bottle onto his hand brace adapter (**A**) and add a straw (**B**) so that he can drink independently (**C**).

apartment. It provides privacy for families and an interim step before discharge.

Table 3-4 lists various topics that should be covered during patient and family education lectures and training.[74] It is important to remember that the educational program will vary depending on the patient's level of injury and personal needs. Different members of the SCI team will teach the family education series sessions. In addition, a peer educator is encouraged to present in a consumer capacity.

Family members must be informed about these scheduled programs in advance to optimize attendance. The schedule can be displayed in patients' rooms and on dining tables and can be inserted in the SCI education manual. To further promote attendance, patients and family members can be reminded by flyers, volunteers, and general announcements made on the public address system.

Support Groups

Support groups help patients and their family members discuss and adjust to the life changes imposed by SCI. Inpatient support groups need not be topic specific and can be facilitated by a psychologist and a nurse who works in the SCI unit. The sessions allow patients to verbalize feelings and discuss constructive ways to handle difficult situations. Outpatient peer resource groups are composed of former patients with SCIs who meet regularly with inpatients to offer practical advice to the newly injured patient and their family members. Family support groups should also be held, where the discussions are driven by family needs.[75]

The more the patient and family members know before discharge, the more successful will be their transition to home and into the community. The ideal situation is when the patient and all family members are independent and knowledgeable in all aspects of care on discharge from short-term rehabilitation. This process, however, is most successful when the patient and family are psychologically ready to learn. Furthermore, they need to be open to constantly modifying their lives so that life can work for them all in the easiest, most effective manner. Unfortunately, time for adjustment to the huge changes in lifestyle imposed by SCI is a luxury with shortened lengths of stay in rehabilitation facilities. Patients are discharged to home in a matter of weeks rather than months. Therefore it is imperative that education be initiated as early as possible, even if the patient and family may not be ready to fully accept the information presented. All members of the treatment team must reinforce education to expedite a safe discharge that will enable the highest possible level of functional independence for the patient.

TABLE 3-4 | Education Topics Concerning Spinal Cord Injuries

Issue	Patient Education	Family Training
Neurological level of injury	Understand basic anatomy of spinal cord, neurological level of injury, functional levels to address needs and direct care	Understand basic anatomy of the spinal cord and neurological level of injury for better understanding of patient needs
Breathing	Direct tracheotomy and ventilator care	Perform tracheotomy care and know how to use and troubleshoot the ventilator
Removing secretions	Direct use of CoughAssist mechanical insufflation-exsufflation device and direct or perform assistive cough techniques	Use CoughAssist device and perform assistive cough techniques as directed by the patient
Respiratory infections	Know signs and symptoms and avoid respiratory infections	Know signs and symptoms of respiratory infections and decrease risks of transmitting them
Skin management	Know causes of skin breakdown and how to prevent it. Perform or direct skin inspection. Know various types of weight shifts, proper positioning in the wheelchair, types of cushions and their care, and seasonal precautions. Identify and troubleshoot problem areas	Know causes of and techniques to prevent skin breakdown Perform skin inspection Troubleshoot skin problems Know seasonal precautions, types and care of various cushions, and proper positioning in the wheelchair
Bowel management	Know what a neurogenic bowel means. Know potential complications that may arise and how to avoid and troubleshoot them (e.g., constipation, AD). Understand need for and techniques used for bowel management. Direct or perform bowel program	Manage and care of a neurogenic bowel
Bladder management	Know what a neurogenic bladder is and the different ways to empty the bladder (i.e., Foley, suprapubic, or condom catheter, ICX). Direct or perform bladder management. Know medical complications of a neurogenic bladder and how to recognize and manage them (i.e., urinary tract infection, kidney infection, epididymitis, AD)	Know meaning of a neurogenic bladder. Care for the selected option of bladder management. Know signs and symptoms of complications (e.g., urinary tract infections) and how to troubleshoot and manage them
Sexuality	Understand how body responds sexually after SCI. Know what methods, techniques, and devices are available to enhance sexual function	Know how partner's body responds sexually after SCI. Know what methods, techniques, and devices are available to enhance pleasure
Medications	Know what, why, and the potential side effects of prescribed medications	Know what medications the patient takes, why medications are taken, and the possible side effects of the medications
Transfers	Know what various transfer techniques are and how to perform or direct transfers	Know what various transfers are and how to assist during transfers
Mobility	Know that various types of wheelchairs are available. Understand what to look for in selecting one. Know how to perform or direct the care and maintenance of the wheelchair. Understand vendor follow-up for wheelchairs. Know how to perform or direct breakdown of the wheelchair for transport. Know how to direct or perform advanced wheelchair skills	Know what types of wheelchairs are available and how to select one. Understand the care, maintenance, and vendor follow-up with wheelchairs. Know how to break down wheelchair and assist during advanced wheelchair skills.
Accessibility issues and adaptive equipment	Know about home modifications, travel, the Americans with Disabilities Act, and high- and low-tech adaptive equipment options	Know about home modifications, travel, the Americans with Disabilities Act, and high- and low-tech adaptive equipment options
Vocation	Understand what agencies and government programs are available for job retraining and employment. Know how to access them	Understand what agencies and government programs are available for job retraining and how to assist in accessing them
Insurance	Know your insurance company's name, numbers and codes, contact information, and case manager. Understand what your insurance covers and how to access it (i.e., are you assigned a vendor or are you free to choose?)	Understand the importance of knowing the insurance coverage and how to use it
Preparation for discharge	Understand how to direct your family to prepare a home emergency folder containing history of current medical needs (a form should be created with the following: name, address, phone number, insurance company's name and number/codes, case manager's name and phone number, ambulance, police, power company, name and phone number of equipment vendor, respiratory vendor, pharmacy, and medical supplier). Place this folder in one location and inform each caregiver	Understand the need to complete a home emergency folder. Contact the local police and fire departments to visit the home to inspect for safety, plan emergency exit routes, and place patient on their emergency response list

Continued

TABLE 3-4 | Education Topics Concerning Spinal Cord Injuries—cont'd

Issue	Patient Education	Family Training
Identify equipment vendors	Understand what supplies and equipment are needed and where to obtain them. Give consideration to the following: is the price competitive? do they deliver? is it mail order? does the insurance case manager establish and contact the vendors or do I? is there 24-hour on-call respiratory care? do they supply a backup ventilator in the home? what is their service policy? identify ways to locate vendors (e.g., insurance case manager, rehabilitation case manager, telephone directory, other patients)	Understand what equipment and supplies are needed and how to identify the suppliers
Continued medical care at home	Understand the need to locate accessible medical care or a facility to provide home visits	Understand the need to identify and contact a physician for continued medical care
Nursing or attendant care	Know how to locate nursing or attendant care. Understand how to hire, train, and fire a caregiver. Direct needs in an assertive, not passive or aggressive, manner	Understand how to locate nursing or attendant care using rehabilitation case manager or insurance case manager. Contact agencies for training before discharge
Loss of power or heat	Understand the need to contact local power and heating companies and be placed on emergency list in the event of power failure	Understand the need to contact local power and heating companies and be placed on emergency list in the event of power failure
Community resources	Know what government agency resources are available to assist with nursing or attendant care, transportation, home modifications, van or car purchase or modifications	Understand what government agency resources are available to assist with nursing or attendant care, transportation, home modifications, van or car purchase or modifications

CLINICAL CASE STUDY Critical Nursing Care

Patient History

Stephen Mills is a 20-year-old man with a C7 tetraplegia ASIA A diagnosis. He is a college student in his junior year and was injured in a motor vehicle accident (MVA) in which he was traveling as an unrestrained rear passenger when the vehicle hit a tree. Stephen is 3 weeks post injury and medically stable. He received acute care at a hospital near his college where his injury was stabilized surgically with a posterior fusion and wiring and reinforced with a sternal-occipital-mandibular immobilizer (SOMI) orthotic collar. Currently all collar restrictions have been removed and he does not have any positional precautions because he is orthopedically stable.

Stephen was admitted to inpatient rehabilitation near his home 3 days ago and he is scheduled to receive rehabilitation services for a total of 5 weeks. He is in resolving stages of spinal shock and occasionally complains of lightheadedness when suddenly placed upright in his wheelchair and is unable to tolerate extreme ambient temperatures. Stephen also complains of feeling flushed when his bladder is full.

Patient's Self-Assessment

Stephen hopes to return to his college 100 miles away from home and graduate with a degree in biology and ultimately attend medical school. His parents live in a split-level single-family home with his younger brother (age 17 years) and sister (age 12 years). His father is a certified public accountant and his mother works for a health insurance company. He consents to evaluation for treatment.

Clinical Assessment
Patient Appearance
- Height 6 feet 0 inches, weight 185 lb, body mass index 25.1

Cognitive Assessment
- Alert, oriented X 3

Cardiopulmonary Assessment
- BP 118/70, HR at rest 68, RR 12, cough flows are ineffective (<360 L/min), vital capacity is reduced (between 1.5 and 2.5 L), and breathing pattern incorporates accessory muscles and upper chest wall only. There is marked decrease in the anterior and lateral chest wall with a slight decrease in the posterior wall expansion

Musculoskeletal and Neuromuscular Assessment
- Motor assessment reveals ASIA A motor and sensory C7
- Deep tendon reflexes 3+ below the level of lesion

Integumentary and Sensory Assessment
- Skin is intact throughout; sensory level is intact to C7

Range of Motion Assessment
- Passive and active motion is within normal limits

ADL Assessment
- Currently dependent

Equipment
- No equipment has been ordered

Evaluation of Clinical Assessment
Stephen Mills is a 20-year-old male with a C7 tetraplegia diagnosis resulting from an MVA 3 weeks ago. ASIA classification: C7 A. All orthopedic restrictions have been removed and patient is now clear for training in all ADLs and instrumental activities of daily living (IADLs). Patient and family education regarding ADL and IADL activities and prevention of cardiopulmonary and integumentary complications will be concurrent with all functional training.

Patient's Care Needs
1. Inability to perform skin care management for adequate pressure relief
2. Inability to perform self-care for bowel and bladder needs
3. Inability to perform ADLs: dressing and grooming
4. Instruction and training in pulmonary hygiene

Diagnosis and Prognosis
Diagnosis is C7 tetraplegia, ASIA A with a prognosis of full independence in skin care, bowel and bladder management, and maintaining good pulmonary hygiene.

Preferred Practice Patterns*
Impaired Muscle Performance (4C), Joint Mobility, Motor Function, Muscle Performance, and Range of Motion Associated With Fracture (4G), Primary Prevention/Risk Reduction for Cardiovascular/Pulmonary Disorders (6A), Prevention/Risk Reduction for Integumentary Disorders (7A)

Team Goals
1. Patient to perform skin care management for prevention independently
2. Patient to perform self-care bowel and bladder management independently
3. Patient to perform dressing and grooming independently
4. Team to educate the patient regarding complications and prevention of medical problems after an SCI with impaired sensation and AD

Patient Goals
"To be able to take care of myself without relying on my parents."

Care Plan
Treatment Plan and Rationale
• Nursing education training for skin care
• Nursing education for bowel and bladder care
• Nursing education for complications and prevention of medical problems after a C7 SCI

Interventions
• Group, individual, and family education training

Documentation and Team Communication
• Nurse education documentation sheet is completed and signed by both nursing staff and the patient weekly

Follow-Up Assessment
• Weekly nurse education team meetings

Critical Thinking Exercises
Consider factors that will influence patient education and nursing care decisions unique to Stephen when answering the following questions:
1. Based on the level of Stephen's injury, what patient education should be provided regarding four autonomic dysfunctions?
2. What type of bladder dysfunction would be expected with Stephen's level of injury? How would this be managed?
3. What patient education should Stephen receive regarding prevention of pressure ulcers?

Guide to physical therapist practice, rev. ed. 2, Alexandria, VA, 2003, American Physical Therapy Association.

SUMMARY
Patients with SCI require highly specialized nursing care immediately after their injuries and often for the rest of their lives. The integration of all of the therapeutic interventions into a synthesized plan of care is critical to ensure that all components work together toward the goal of wellness. The role of the nurse is to begin by nurturing the patient and family and to slowly develop their knowledge and skills to move the patient from total dependence toward modified independence, depending on his level of injury. A holistic approach is necessary because the multiple modalities and complexities of the patient injury and response can affect one another. Ultimately, the practice of spinal cord nursing within the interdisciplinary team ensures coordinated, collaborative care for the patient.

REFERENCES

1. American Nurses Association and Association of Rehabilitation Nurses: *Rehabilitation nursing: scope of practice; process and outcome criteria for selected diagnoses*, p. 4, Kansas City, MO, 1998, American Nurses Association.
2. Ter-Matt ML: Diversity in nursing practice roles and settings. In Nelson A, Zejdlik CP, Love L, editors: *Nursing practice related to spinal cord injury and disorders: a core curriculum*, Jackson Heights, NY, 2001, Eastern Paralyzed Veterans Association.
3. Orem D: *Nursing concepts of practice*, ed 5, St. Louis, 1995, Mosby.
4. Nelson A: Rehabilitation. In Nelson A, Zejdlik CP, Love L, editors: *Nursing practice related to spinal cord injury and disorders: a core curriculum*, Jackson Heights, NY, 2001, Eastern Paralyzed Veterans Association.
5. Davis AE: Acute care management of patients with spinal cord injuries, *Crit Care Curr* 9:1-4, 1991.
6. Dunn M, Sommer N, Gambina H: A practical guide to team functioning in spinal cord injury rehabilitation. In Zejdlik CP, editor: *Management of spinal cord injury*, ed 2, pp 229-239, Boston, 1992, Jones & Barlett.
7. Benner P, Tanner CA, Chesla CA: *Expertise in nursing practice: caring, clinical judgement, and ethics*, New York, 1996, Springer.
8. Zejdlik CP: *Management of spinal cord injury*, ed 2, Boston, 1992, Jones & Bartlett.
9. Lundy-Ekman L: *Neuroscience: fundamentals for rehabilitation*, ed 2, Philadelphia, 2002, WB Saunders.
10. Colachis S: Hypothermia associated with autonomic dysreflexia after traumatic spinal cord injury, *Am J Phys Med Rehabil* 81:232-235, 2002.
11. Campagnolo DI, Merli GJ: Autonomic and cardiovascular complications of spinal cord injury. In Kirshblum S, Campagnolo DI, DeLisa JA, editors: *Spinal cord medicine*, Philadelphia, 2002, Lippincott Williams & Wilkins.
12. Schmitt JK, Midha M, McKenzie ND et al: Autonomic dysreflexia. In Eltorai IM, Schmitt JK, editors: *Emergencies in chronic spinal cord injury patients*, ed 3, Jackson Heights, NY, 2001, Eastern Paralyzed Veterans Association.
13. Linsenmeyer TA, Stone JM: Neurogenic bladder and bowel dysfunction. In DeLisa JA, Gans BM, editors: *Rehabilitation medicine principles and practice*, pp 733-762, Philadelphia, 1993, JB Lippincott.
14. Pires M: Bladder elimination and continence. In Hoeman S, editor: *Rehabilitation nursing: process, application, and outcomes*, ed 3, St. Louis, 2002, Mosby.
15. Gray MI: Physiology of voiding. In Doughty DB, editor: *Urinary and fecal incontinence: nursing management*, ed 2, pp 1-27, St. Louis, 2000, Mosby.
16. Alverzo JP, Jacalan CL: Nonpharmacologic treatment of voiding dysfunctions: a nursing perspective, *Neurorehabilitation* 4:237-244, 1994.
17. American Spinal Injury Association: *International standards for neurological and functional classification of spinal cord injury worksheet*, Atlanta, GA, 2006, The Association.
18. Jeter KF, Faller N, Norton C: *Nursing for continence*, Philadelphia, 1990, WB Saunders.
19. Giroux J: Bladder elimination and continence. In Nelson A, Zejdlik CP, Love L, editors: *Nursing practice related to spinal cord injury and disorders: a core curriculum*, Jackson Heights, NY, 2001, Eastern Paralyzed Veterans Association.
20. Greco S: Sexuality education and counseling. In Hoeman S, editor: *Rehabilitation nursing: Process, application, and outcomes*, ed 3, St. Louis, 2002, Mosby.
21. Gender AR: Bowel elimination and regulation. In Hoeman S, editor: *Rehabilition nursing: Process, application, and outcomes*, ed 3, St. Louis, 2002, Mosby.
22. Doughty D: *Urinary and fecal incontinence management*, ed 2, St. Louis, 2000, Mosby.
23. Venn MR, Taft L, Carpentier IB et al: The influence of timing and suppository use on efficiency and effectiveness of bowel training after a stroke, *Rehabil Nurs* 17:116-121, 1992.
24. Annon JS: The PLISST model: a proposed conceptual scheme for behavioral treatment of sexual problems, *J Sex Ed Ther* 2:1-15, 1976.
25. Horn LJ, Zasler ND: *Medical rehabilitation of traumatic brain injury*, Philadelphia, 1996, Hanley & Belfus.
26. Brown DJ, Hill ST, Baker HW: Male fertility and sexual function after spinal cord injury, *Prog Brain Res* 152:427-439, 2006.
27. Yarkony GM, Chen D: Sexuality in patients with spinal cord injury, *Phys Med Rehabil State Art Rev Sex Disabil* 9:325-344, 1995.
28. Tepper MS: Attitudes, beliefs, and cognitive processes that impede or facilitate sexual pleasure in people with spinal cord injury, unpublished dissertation, Philadelphia, 1999, University of Pennsylvania.
29. Burnette AL: Oral pharmacology for erectile dysfunction: current perspectives, *Neurology* 54:392-399, 1999.
30. Consortium for Spinal Cord Medicine: *Acute management of autonomic dysreflexia: adults with spinal cord injury presenting to healthcare facilities*, Washington, DC, 1997, Paralyzed Veterans of America.
31. Hirsch IH, Seager SW, Seldor J et al: Electroejaculatory stimulation of a quadriplegic man resulting in pregnancy, *Arch Phys Med Rehabil* 71:54-57, 1990.
32. Woods NF: *Human sexuality in health and illness*, ed 3, St. Louis, 1984, Mosby.
33. Griffith ER, Trieschmann RB: Sexual dysfunctions in the physically ill and disabled. In Nadelson CC, Marcotte DB, editors: *Treatment interventions in human sexuality*, pp 241-277, New York, 1983, Plenum Press.
34. Monga M, Bernie J, Rajesekaran M: Male infertility and erectile dysfunction in spinal cord injury: a review, *Arch Phys Med Rehabil* 80:299-312, 1999.
35. Mittmann N, Craven BC, Gordon M, et al: Erectile dysfunction in spinal cord injury: a cost-utility analysis, *J Rehabil Med* 37:358-364, 2005.
36. Jockenhovel F: Testosterone therapy—what, when and to whom? *Aging Male* 7:319-324, 2004.
37. Schopp LH, Clark M, Mazurek MO et al: Testosterone levels among men with spinal cord injury admitted to inpatient rehabilitation, *Am J Phys Med Rehabil* 85:678-684, 2006.
38. Padma-Nathan H, Hellstom WJ, Kaiser FE et al: Treatment of men with erectile dysfunction with transurethral alprostadil: Medicated Urethral System for Erection (MUSE) Study Group, *N Engl J Med* 336:1-7, 1997.
39. Raina R, Agarwal A, Ausmundson S et al: Long-term efficacy and compliance of MUSE for erectile dysfunction following radical prostatectomy: SHIM (IIEF) analysis, *Int J Impot Res* 17:86-90, 2005.
40. Bryce TN, Ragnarsson KT: Pain after spinal cord injury, *Phys Med Rehabil Clin North Am* 11:157-168, 2000.
41. Nelsen-Marsh JD, Banasik JL: Pain. In Copstead LEC, Banasik JL, editors: *Pathophysiology*, ed 3, St. Louis, 2005, Elsevier Saunders.
42. Bryce TN, Ragnarsson KT: Pain management in persons with spinal cord disorders. In Lin VW, editor: *Spinal cord medicine: principles and practice*, New York, 2003, Demos.
43. Werhagen L, Budh CN, Hultling C et al: Neuropathic pain after traumatic spinal cord injury—relations to gender, spinal level, completeness, and age at the time of injury, *Spinal Cord* 42:665-673, 2004.
44. Wall P, Melzack R, editors: *Textbook of pain*, ed 4, pp 1-12, Philadelphia, 1999, WB Saunders.

45. Melzack R, Katz J: The McGill pain questionnaire: appraisal and current status. In Melzack R, Katz J, editors: *Handbook of pain assessment*, New York, 1992, Guilford Press.

46. Balazy T: Clinical management of chronic pain in spinal cord injury, *Clin J Pain* 8:102-110, 1992.

47. Mariano A: Chronic pain and spinal cord injury, *Clin J Pain* 8:87-92, 1992.

48. Brin MF: Dosing, administration, and a treatment algorithm for use of botulinum toxin A for adult-onset spasticity: Spasticity Study Group, *Muscle Nerve Suppl* 6:S208-S220, 1997.

49. Burchiel KJ, Hsu FP: Pain and spasticity after spinal cord injury: mechanisms and treatment, *Spine* 26(24 Suppl):S146-S160, 2001.

50. NIH Technology Assessment Panel on Integration of Behavioral and Relaxation Approaches into the Treatment of Chronic Pain and Insomnia: Integration of behavioral and relaxation approaches into the treatment of chronic pain and insomnia, *JAMA* 276:313–318, 1996.

51. U.S. Department of Health and Human Services, Public Health Service: *Treatment of pressure ulcers: clinical practice guideline no. 15*, Rockville, MD, 1994, Agency for Health Care Policy and Research.

52. Salzberg CA, Byrne DW, Cayten CG et al: Predicting and preventing pressure ulcers in adults with paralysis, *Adv Wound Care* 11:237-246, 1998.

53. Chen Y, DeVivo MJ, Jackson AB: Pressure ulcer prevalence in people with spinal cord injury: Age-period-duration effects, *Arch Phys Med Rehabil* 86:1208-1213, 2005.

54. Langemo DK, Melland H, Hanson D, et al: The lived experience of having a pressure ulcer: A qualitative analysis, *Adv Skin Wound Care* 13:225-235, 2000.

55. Niazi ZB, Salzberg CA, Byrne DW, et al: Recurrence of initial pressure ulcer in persons with spinal cord injuries, *Adv Wound Care* 10:38-42, 1997.

56. Arnold MC: Pressure ulcer prevention and management: the current evidence for care, *AACN Clin Issues* 14:411-428, 2003.

57. Consortium for Spinal Cord Medicine: *Pressure ulcer prevention and treatment following spinal cord injury: a clinical practice guideline for health-care professionals*, Washington, DC, 2000, Paralyzed Veterans of America.

58. LaMantia JG: Skin integrity. In Hoeman S, editor: *Rehabilitation nursing: Process and applications*, ed 2, St. Louis, 1996, Mosby.

59. O'Connor KC, Salcido R: Pressure ulcers and spinal cord injury. In Kirshblum S, Campagnolo DI, DeLisa JA, editors: *Spinal cord medicine*, Philadelphia, 2002, Lippincott Williams & Wilkins.

60. Coggrave MJ, Rose LS: A specialist seating assessment clinic: changing pressure relief practice, *Spinal Cord* 41:692-695, 2003.

61. Breslow RA, Hallfrisch J, Guy DG et al: The importance of dietary protein in healing pressure ulcers, *J Am Geriatr Soc* 41:357-362, 1993.

62. Raffoul W, Far MS, Cayeux MC et al: Nutritional status and food intake in nine patients with chronic low-limb ulcers and pressure ulcers: importance of oral supplements, *Nutrition* 22:82-88, 2006.

63. Bergstrom N, Braden BJ: The Braden Scale for predicting pressure sore risk, *Nurs Res* 36:205-210, 1987.

64. Bergstrom N, Demuth PJ, Braden BJ: A clinical trial of the Braden Scale for predicting pressure sore risk, *Nurs Clin North Am* 22: 417-428, 1987.

65. Black JM, Hawks JH: *Medical-surgical nursing: clinical management for positive outcomes*, ed 7, St. Louis, 2005, Mosby.

66. Thomason SS: Skin. In Nelson A, Zejdlik CP, Love L, editors: *Nursing practice related to spinal cord injury and disorders: a core curriculum*, Jackson Heights, NY, 2001, Eastern Paralyzed Veterans Association.

67. Eltorai IM, Wisbnow RM: Decubitus ulcer emergencies in patients with SCI. In Eltorai IM, Schmitt JK, editors: *Emergencies in chronic spinal cord injury patients*, ed 3, Jackson Heights, NY, 2001, Eastern Paralyzed Veterans Association.

68. Maynard F, Karunas R, Maring W: Epidemiology of spasticity following traumatic spinal cord injury, *Arch Phys Med Rehabil* 71: 566-569, 1990.

69. Savoy SM, Gianino JM: Intrathecal baclofen infusion: an innovative approach for controlling spasticity, *Rehabil Nurs* 18:105-113, 1993.

70. Herzog JA: Deep vein thrombosis in the rehabilitation client, *Rehabil Nurs* 17:196-198, 1992.

71. Saltztein RJ, Hardin S, Hartings J: Osteoporosis in SCI: using an index of mobility and its relationship to bone density, *J Am Paraplegia Soc* 15:232-234, 1992.

72. Wirtz KM, La Favor KM, Ang R: Managing chronic spinal cord injury: issues in critical care, *Crit Care Nurse* 16:24-35, 1996.

73. Lindsey LL, Kurilla LL, DeVivo MJ: Providing SCI education during changing times, *SCI Nurs* 19:11-14, 2002.

74. Iacono J, Campbell A: *Patient and family education: the compliance guide to the JCAHO standards*, Marblehead, MA, 1997, Opus Communications.

75. Sheija A, Manigandan C: Efficacy of support groups for spouses of patients with spinal cord injury and its impact on their quality of life, *Int J Rehabil Res* 28:379-383, 2005.

SOLUTIONS TO CHAPTER 3 CLINICAL CASE STUDY

Critical Nursing Care

1. Autonomic dysfunction is associated with injuries above the level of T6. It causes a loss of descending spinal cord control that affects thermoregulation, bradycardia, hypotension, and AD.

   Thermoregulation is impaired, resulting in the potential for hyperthermia, which increases the patient's danger for heat stroke because of his body's inability to dissipate heat through sweat. Attention to the control of ambient room temperature is recommended. Room temperature must also be monitored to prevent hypothermia because the patient is unable to shiver to raise the body temperature below the level of the lesion.

   Bradycardia, a slowing of the heart rate, is typically seen during the period of spinal shock. Bradycardia usually resolves within 6 months after injury, but if it persists a pacemaker may be recommended.

   Hypotension is displayed as a decrease in blood pressure typically after a postural change from lying to an upright position. This is partially a result of loss of vasoconstriction and tachycardia from sympathetic involvement with this level of injury. Complaints of lightheadedness, nausea, dizziness, and at times fainting accompany orthostatic hypotension. To manage these symptoms, tilt the patient back, or if syncope occurs, bring the patient to supine, and elevate his legs. Prevention of orthostatic hypotension is important. Therefore, pressure gradient stockings, abdominal binders, medication, and adequate hydration are recommended and their use should be monitored. Each time the patient is moved to an upright position, it helps the body to adapt to the drop in pressure and develop compensatory spinal postural strategies. The resolution of spinal shock several weeks after injury will also help to resolve issues of orthostatic hypotension.

   Autonomic dysreflexia, a syndrome of massively uncontrolled sympathetic nervous system discharge, is characterized by a dangerous increase in blood pressure that begins with exposure to noxious stimuli such as pain or pressure below the level of injury. The first step in treatment is to determine the cause so that the reflex can be stopped by removing the source of the stimuli. Administration of nitroglycerin as a topical paste followed by having the patient bite and swallow nifedipine to reduce the blood pressure can be effective. Symptoms include hypertension, headache, perspiration (above the level of injury), flushing (above level of injury), piloerection (below level of injury), blurred vision, dilated pupils, nasal congestion, or anxiety. It is important to be aware of potential triggers, including bowel impaction, bladder distension, or other noxious stimulation such as an ingrown toenail.

2. Stephen will have a reflexive bladder, which may become hyperreflexive. Male patients may use condom catheters to contain urine; the flow of urine into the leg bag must be free without kinks. The penis and urinary meatus must be checked regularly for any signs of irritation or infection. Sufficient hydration and nutritional status must be monitored. Attention to changes in bladder function including any signs of infection must be continuous. Bladder programs are dynamic, and very often the program may need to be re-evaluated and modified in accordance with the patient's feedback to promote patient control of the program and to accommodate changing needs.

3. Maintaining skin integrity is essential for any patient who has sustained an SCI AISA A. Because Stephen is 20 years old, it is important that he establish effective skin care management immediately after his injury and maintain it as a standard practice for the rest of his life. Clinicians should stress the idea that a pressure ulcer after an SCI is not inevitable. Knowledge and vigilance are the keys to preventing pressure ulcers. A contract between the patient and his health care providers is often an effective care tool that enlists patient understanding and participation while emphasizing the patient's roles and responsibilities.

   Initially, in the acute stages of care, Stephen should be turned at least every 2 hours from side to side at an oblique angle by the nursing staff. He must be encouraged to advocate for his own care and request assistance with weight shifting when he is unable to accomplish movement on his own. During the rehabilitation process a routine of weight shift frequency and duration should be established by using a team approach (see Chapter 7). The most effective and efficient weight shift techniques will be determined by the care team for both bed positions and upright seating. It is hoped that Stephen will be able to perform these techniques independently because of his youth, injury level, and intact triceps muscles.

CHAPTER FOUR

Respiratory Treatment and Equipment

Barbara Garrett, PT, Hania Shatzer, CCC-SLP, and John R. Bach, MD

Getting off the vent meant freedom for me. I could go wherever I wanted to go without a machine trailing after me.
When I was weaning during the day, I hated going back on at night.
Dennis (C5 SCI)

The evaluation and treatment of respiratory function is a primary concern in the therapeutic program of all patients with a spinal cord injury (SCI). According to the SCI database, respiratory complications are second only to cardiac complications as the most common cause of death during the first year after injury and the leading cause of death beyond that first year.[1] Depending on the patient's neurological level of SCI, the impaired or absent innervation of respiratory musculature can cause significant pulmonary dysfunction, including limited inspiratory and expiratory capacity (Table 4-1). Resultant hypomobility of the thorax contributes to secretion pooling and limited ability to take deep inspirations. In addition, autonomic nervous system changes can impair the respiratory drive or cough reflex.

To address the respiratory dysfunction of a patient with an SCI, the clinician must first have an understanding of normal pulmonary anatomy and physiology. This chapter focuses on anatomy, physiology and pathophysiology, respiratory evaluation and complications, and treatment interventions for the patient with pulmonary dysfunction as a result of SCI. In addition, special considerations for patients with high tetraplegia including the use of ventilators and other respiratory equipment are discussed.

RESPIRATORY ANATOMY

The anatomy of the respiratory system includes the skeletal structures, muscles of respiration, and other structures within the upper and lower airways.

Skeletal Structures

The skeletal structures involved in respiration include the thoracic and cervical cage and spine, sternum, clavicle, and ribs (Figure 4-1). Although these structures have mobility between them, they also serve as places for the attachment of the muscles of respiration. During normal inspiration, the upper ribs elevate in what is known as a bucket handle motion, rotating on a fixed spine which brings the sternum forward. Simultaneously, the lower ribs elevate and rotate in a lateral and superior direction, simulating a bucket handle motion (Figure 4-2).

The increase in chest wall dimensions (anteroposterior and superoinferior) caused by these movements leads to the decrease in intrathoracic pressure necessary for ventilation[2] and are discussed in detail later. There must be adequate respiratory muscle strength and joint mobility at the intervertebral joints, costovertebral joints, costosternal joints, and sternoclavicular joints for these skeletal movements to occur (Figure 4-3).

In addition, adequate soft tissue mobility of the structures within the thoracic cavity, including the muscles, fascia, nerves, and blood vessels, is necessary to allow the appropriate range of motion (ROM) of the thorax for breathing. In other words, adequate ROM of the involved joints and soft tissues of the thorax allow for normal expansion and easier inspiration. The clinician should recognize that impaired innervation of the respiratory musculature after SCI, as well as the resulting decreased flexibility of joints and soft tissue, greatly diminish the respiratory capacity of the patient.

Muscles of Respiration

The diaphragm is the primary muscle of respiration, providing 60% to 70% of vital capacity and tidal volume.[3] It is a large, dome-shaped muscle separating the rib cage and the abdomen (Figure 4-3). Each half of the diaphragm is innervated by the phrenic nerve (C3 to C5). Its origin and insertion are on the inferior surface of the lower ribs. Its concentric contraction results in an inferior movement of the muscle and an upward and outward movement of the lower ribs in three dimensions. The resultant decrease in intrathoracic pressure results in the drawing of air into the lungs (Figure 4-4, *A* and *B*). The diaphragm is also used eccentrically for elongated phonation or expiration. It will be important to teach patients about this function when they are learning to operate a sip n' puff power wheelchairs for mobility or to use environmental control units (see Chapters 11 and 13). The diaphragm maximally contracts when it is on a slight stretch in a dome-shaped position.

After an SCI, the abdominal muscles are often weakened or no longer innervated, which allows the abdominal cavity to protrude anteriorly when the patient is in an upright position. This leaves the diaphragm in a flattened, weakened position. A patient without abdominal strength will often report easier breathing and will have larger vital capacity in the supine position because of the improved position of the diaphragm. Patients with such a condition should consistently use an abdominal binder when upright to restore alignment of the abdominal wall and to keep the diaphragm in a position that will have the greatest possible mechanical advantage (Figure 4-5).

The abdominal muscles (rectus abdominis, internal and external obliques, and transversus abdominis), innervated from T5 to T12, provide visceral support under the diaphragm and stability to the rib cage and are the primary muscles needed for forceful exhalation or cough. When they contract, these muscles

TABLE 4-1 | Neuromuscular Effects on Respiration in Spinal Cord Injury

Level of Injury	Weakened or Missing Muscle Innervation	Limited Planes of Respiration	Physical Indications
Paraplegia (T1-T5)	Abdominal Intercostal Erector spinae	Slight decrease in anterior expansion Slight decrease in lateral expansion	Decreased chest expansion Decreased VC Decreased ability to build up intrathoracic pressure Decreased cough effectiveness Possible paradoxical breathing pattern
Tetraplegia (C5-C8)	Above muscles and Pectoralis Serratus anterior Scalenes	Marked decrease in anterior and lateral expansion Slight decrease in posterior expansion	Marked decrease in chest expansion Marked decrease in VC Marked decrease in FEV Marked decrease in cough effectiveness Paradoxical breathing in acute phase or longer
Tetraplegia (C4)	Above muscles and Diaphragm	Marked decrease in anterior and lateral expansion Slight decrease in posterior expansion	Marked limitations in all three planes of ventilation Slight decrease in TV Possible need for mechanical ventilation
Tetraplegia (C1-C3)	Above muscles and sternocleidomastoid Trapezius	All planes severely limited Superior expansion limited	Marked decrease in TV Possible need for full-time mechanical ventilation

FEV, Forced expiratory volume; *TV,* tidal volume; *VC,* vital capacity.
Adapted from Frownfelter D, Dean E: *Principles and practice of cardiopulmonary physical therapy,* ed 3, Chicago, 1996, Mosby, pp. 690-691.

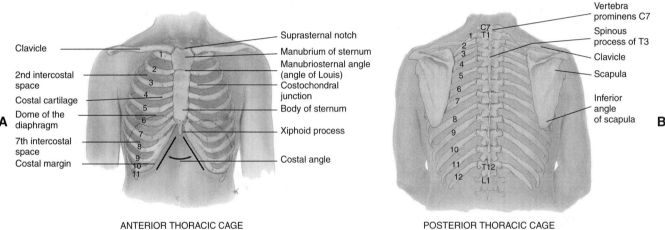

ANTERIOR THORACIC CAGE   POSTERIOR THORACIC CAGE

FIGURE 4-1 **A,** Anterior, and **B,** posterior views of the thoracic cage. (From Jarvis C: *Physical examination & health assessment,* ed 4, Philadelphia, 2004, WB Saunders.)

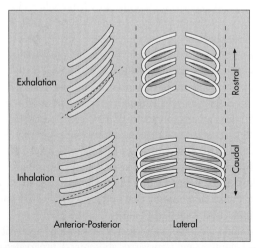

FIGURE 4-2 Mechanics of breathing. Chest wall dimension changes during breathing. The left column illustrates the pump-handle movement of the ribs; the right column illustrates the ribs' bucket-handle movement. (Modified from Leff AR, Schumacker PT: *Respiratory physiology: basics and applications,* Philadelphia, 1993, WB Saunders.)

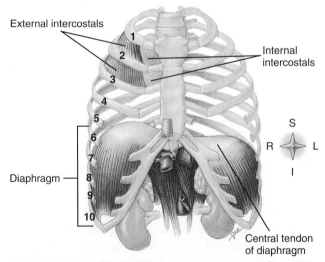

FIGURE 4-3 Muscles of the thorax. Anterior view. Note the relationship of the internal and external intercostal muscles and placement of the diaphragm. (From Thibodeau GA, Patton KT: *Anatomy & physiology,* ed 5, St. Louis, 2003, Mosby.)

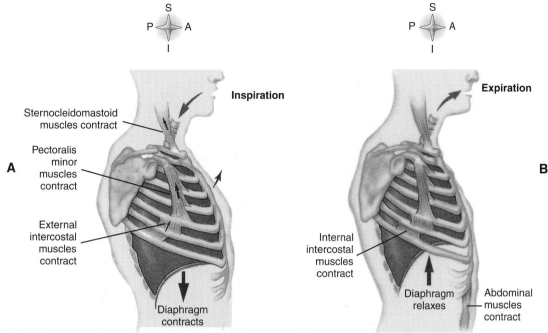

FIGURE 4-4 **A,** Mechanism of inspiration. Note the role of the diaphragm and the chest-elevation muscles (pectoralis minor and external intercostals) in increasing thoracic volume, which decreases pressure in the lungs and thus draws air inward. **B,** Mechanism of expiration. Note that relaxation of the diaphragm plus contraction of chest-depressing muscles (internal intercostals) reduces thoracic volume, which increases pressure in the lungs and thus pushes air outward. (From Thibodeau GA, Patton KT: *Anatomy & physiology*, ed 5, St. Louis, 2003, Mosby.)

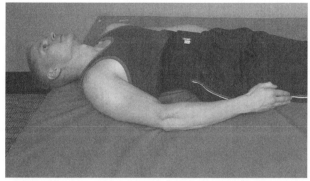

FIGURE 4-5 Abdominal binder supports weak abdominal muscles to aid in respiration. The upper border of the binder fits snugly under the lower border of the ribs at the level of the diaphragm. Care should be taken to ensure minimal wrinkles in the binder or pressure areas that can lead to skin breakdown. An undershirt can be worn under the abdominal binder if skin irritation occurs or is expected.

displace the relaxed diaphragm into the thoracic cavity, thereby forcing air quickly out of the lungs. They also pull the lower ribs downward and inward to decrease thorax dimensions during forced exhalation. Indirectly, they assist inhalation when high ventilatory demand or rapid breathing is needed but the passive recoil of the lungs and thorax is not fast enough.[2,4] A patient with an SCI who has poor or absent strength of the abdominals needs to rely on an assisted cough technique or other respiratory equipment to remove secretions or foreign objects from the airway.

The internal and external intercostal muscles are innervated by the adjacent intercostal nerves (T1 to T11) and are primarily responsible for stabilizing the rib cage during inspiration to prevent paradoxical inward movement of the chest but can also assist with controlled exhalation for speech or with forceful exhalation during cough. The internal and external intercostals run at right angles to each other between the ribs, and both muscle groups provide general rib cage stability. The external intercostals run inferiorly and anteriorly, causing rib elevation during inspiration while the internal intercostals run inferiorly and posteriorly and are considered expiratory in function.[4]

The accessory muscles of respiration include the sternocleidomastoid innervated by cranial nerves C2 to C4 and the accessory nerve (XI), the scalenus (C3 to C8), the trapezius (C1 to C4 and XI), the pectoralis muscles (C5 to T1), the serratus anterior muscles (C5 to C7), and the erector spinae muscles (C1 to L5) (Figure 4-6). When diaphragm function is impaired, the sternocleidomastoids along with the scalenes and the trapezius muscles become important to respiration by providing superior and anterior expansion of the thoracic cage. The pectorals become active when the arms are fixed, acting to elevate the sternum and ribs and assisting the intercostal muscles with rib cage stability. In addition, when the arms are fixed, contraction of the serratus anterior muscles results in a posterior expansion of the chest cavity. The deep back erector spinae muscles provide spinal stability required for adequate rib cage mobility. With deep inspiration, these muscles also extend the vertebral column to further elevate the ribs. Also of importance are the bulbar muscles of the pharynx and larynx innervated by the lower cranial nerves. In addition to producing speech, they serve to maintain the upper airway during inspiration, prevent aspiration while swallowing, allow glottic

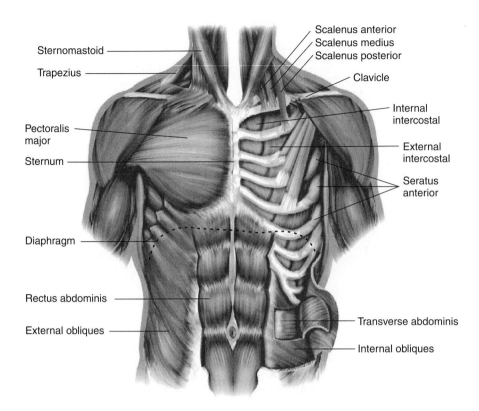

FIGURE 4-6 Muscles of respiration, including the accessory muscles. (From Wilkins RL, Stoller CL: *Eagan's fundamentals of respiratory care,* ed 8, St. Louis, 2003, Mosby.)

closure with cough, and act as a pump for air during glossopharyngeal breathing.[5]

Upper and Lower Airway

The upper airway or upper respiratory tract includes the nasal cavity, mouth, pharynx, and larynx (Figure 4-7). The primary function of these structures is to cleanse, heat, and humidify the inhaled air. They also prevent foreign materials from entering the lower airway. In addition, the vocal cords located within the larynx provide for phonation.

The lower airway, or lower respiratory tract, is composed of the tracheobronchial tree and lung parenchyma and starts with the trachea (windpipe) which is 11 to 13 cm in length with walls fortified by 16 to 20 horseshoe-shaped cartilaginous rings. It is lined by tracheobronchial epithelial cells containing cilia that beat in a cephalad direction (mucociliary elevator). These comprise the self-cleaning mechanism of the normal lung and provide a continuous blanket of mucus to trap secretions and foreign particles.

The trachea has a bifurcation called the carina at the level of T5. It splits into the right and left mainstem bronchi with the left at an approximate 50-degree angle and the right at an approximate 25-degree angle, which leads to aspirated materials usually ending up in the right lung with its more vertical position. The mainstem bronchi divide into lobar bronchi, three on the right and two on the left, which further divide into segmental bronchi

with ten on the right and eight on the left. Segmental bronchi then are divided into subsegmental bronchi, then bronchioles, terminal bronchioles, respiratory bronchioles, alveolar ducts, and finally alveoli. This continued division sets up a complex design engineered to distribute air rapidly and uniformly.[6,7] Respiratory zones consist of the lung parenchyma beyond the terminal bronchioles where molecular gas exchange between the blood and alveolar air occurs by diffusion. The alveoli have a thin lining and are covered by pulmonary capillaries to facilitate gas exchange. The central airway region is above the seventh division and the peripheral airway region is at the seventh division and below.

Lungs

The lungs are located in the thoracic cavity, with their apices reaching above the clavicles and bases extending to the region of the lower ribs. Covered by visceral pleura, each lung is attached to the heart and trachea by its root and the pulmonary ligament. The right lung is larger and has upper, middle and lower lobes, the upper and middle separated by the horizontal fissure and the middle and lower separated by the oblique fissure. The left lung is smaller, secondary to the heart, occupying space on the left side of the thoracic cage, and the oblique fissure divides the upper and lingula from the lower lobe (Figure 4-8). Bronchopulmonary segments lie within the lobes of the lungs, ten on the right and eight on the left, and will be

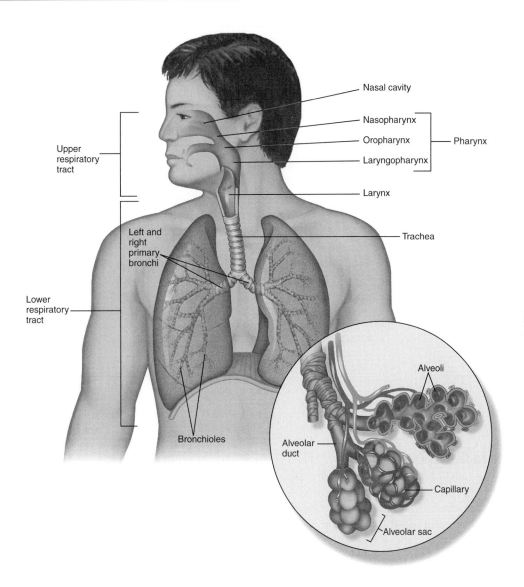

FIGURE 4-7 Structure of respiratory system includes the upper and lower respiratory tract. Note the inset shows the alveolar sacs where the interchange of oxygen and carbon dioxide takes place through the walls of the grapelike alveoli. (From Thibodeau GA, Patton KT: *Anatomy & physiology,* ed 5, St. Louis, 2003, Mosby.)

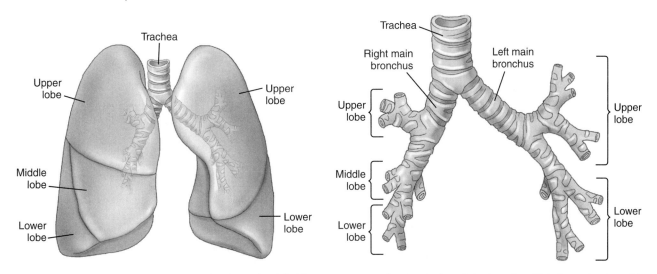

FIGURE 4-8 The bronchial tree and lobes of the lung. (Modified from Epstein O, Perkin GD, Cookson J, De Bono DP: *Clinical examination,* ed 3, St. Louis, 2003, Mosby.)

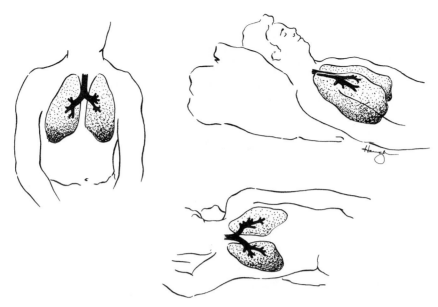

FIGURE 4-9 The effect of positioning on the perfusion of the lung. Note that gravity-dependent segments have the greatest amount of perfusion *(darker regions)*. (From Frownfelter D, Dean E: *Cardiovascular and pulmonary physical therapy: evidence and practice,* ed 4, St. Louis, 2006, Mosby.)

important to postural drainage positions described in the treatment section.

PHYSIOLOGY OF RESPIRATION

Respiration is a physical and chemical exchange process that moves oxygen to the body's tissue and removes oxidation byproducts (carbon dioxide and water). Normal respiration requires basic processes, which may be impaired in patients with SCI because of muscle weakness, trauma, and premorbid conditions. These processes include ventilation, which is simply the movement of air in and out of the lungs and alveolar-capillary diffusion, which is the process of gas exchange between the alveoli of the lungs and the pulmonary capillaries. Perfusion refers to the blood flow available for gas exchange.

Gravity tends to pull blood into the dependent areas of the lung. The ventilation-perfusion ratio is used in matching alveolar ventilation (of gas) to simultaneous capillary blood flow. It is affected by patient position in that the dependent or inferior areas of the lung are more perfused as a result of gravity. For example, in the right side-lying position, the right lung is better perfused than the left (Figure 4-9). An adequate oxygen transport system also is vital to the respiratory system, which allows oxygen to combine with hemoglobin to form oxyhemoglobin to be carried in the bloodstream.

These processes are mediated by the respiratory centers within the brainstem, which receive information from the central and peripheral chemoreceptors and mechanoreceptors to optimize the levels of oxygen and carbon dioxide in the body. The peripheral chemoreceptors specifically respond to the decrease in oxygen in the blood by increasing the ventilation rate and cardiac output.[7] Clinicians often need to be aware of blood carbon dioxide and oxygen partial pressures to understand the patient's respiratory status. Pulse oximetry measures the percent saturation of the hemoglobin (oxygen saturation or SpO_2) with a finger or ear probe and can be used to monitor blood oxygen saturation status during treatment sessions (Figure 4-10).

Pulmonary pathologic conditions can be defined in terms of either ventilatory or oxygenation impairment. Ventilatory impairment is usually due to respiratory muscle insufficiency (e.g., SCI) and leads to increased carbon dioxide in the blood (hypercapnia). Oxygenation impairment is related to conditions of the lungs and airways as seen in chronic obstructive pulmonary disease.[2]

MECHANICS OF VENTILATION

The mechanics of ventilation in the pulmonary system include compliance, airway resistance, and elasticity. Compliance is the ease with which the lungs expand during inspiration (i.e., the change in volume per change in pressure) and can be affected by various lung diseases and by increased rigidity of the thorax. Therefore, the greater the pressure needed to change the lung volume, the less compliant the lung and the more the work of breathing is increased. Both decreased chest compliance and laryngeal muscle dysfunction limit maximum insufflation capacity (MIC) and, therefore, the ability to clear airway secretions by coughing for patients with reduced vital capacity (VC).

Airway resistance is the pressure difference required for one unit flow change. Decreases in airway diameter increase the airway resistance. Increased secretions in the airways that add to the work of breathing can cause a reduction in the airway diameter. Elasticity is a property of the lung and chest wall tissue, which allows these tissues to return to their resting state after deformation by an external force. Thus, in ventilation, elasticity allows the passive process of relaxed exhalation. If the lungs and thoracic cage lose their elasticity, quiet exhalation and also cough are negatively affected.[2]

A function vital to the pulmonary system is a strong, productive cough. A normal cough requires the forceful expulsion of air from the lungs to clear secretions or other irritants from the airway. This can occur as a reflex or as a voluntary action. There are four stages of an effective cough (Figure 4-11). The first stage requires a sufficient inspiration or insufflation, which is defined as blowing of air into the lungs. A sufficient inspiratory volume corresponds to at least 60% of a patient's predicted vital capacity. The second stage corresponds to the closing of the glottis (vocal folds), which allows intrathoracic pressure to increase (stage three) by active contraction of the abdominal and intercostal muscles. The fourth stage corresponds to the opening of the glottis after an inspiratory pause of several seconds and the forceful exhalation of air, assisted by further contraction of the abdominal and intercostal muscles.[7] The explosive rush of air generates peak cough flow (PCF) of 6 to 20 liters per second (360 to 1200 L/min) in individuals with normal pulmonary function. If a patient's PCF is less than 160 L/min, the cough is ineffective.[8]

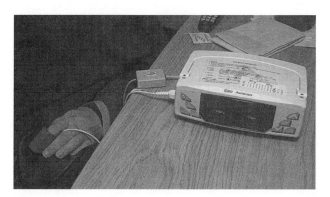

FIGURE 4-10 Pulse oximeter on finger tip with monitor to measure oxygen saturation (SpO$_2$).

EVALUATION
Pulmonary Function

Pulmonary function tests give clinicians information about the mechanical function of the lungs. Lung volumes that can be tested and analyzed include total lung capacity (TLC), VC, residual volume, inspiratory capacity, functional residual capacity, inspiratory reserve volume, and expiratory reserve volume (Figure 4-12). These volumes estimate unassisted inspiratory and expiratory muscle function. TLC is the volume of air in the lungs at the end of maximal inspiration (Box 4-1). VC represents the patient's maximum breathing ability and is commonly monitored, especially for patients with high cervical injuries to help determine their potential to be weaned from ventilatory support.

Maximal insufflation capacity (MIC) is another parameter used by clinicians working with patients with SCI. MIC is the maximum volume of air that a patient can hold with a closed glottis, and the difference between the MIC and VC strongly correlates with glottic function. This will be important to glossopharyngeal breathing (i.e., air stacking).

Normal values for pulmonary function including values for lung volumes, ventilation, mechanical breathing, gas exchange, alveolar gas, and arterial blood are listed in Table 4-2. Patients with SCI may have lower values depending on the level of injury. Pulmonary functions do not have a single normal value because these are based on an interaction between body surface area, age, height, weight, sex, and race. The normal values listed in Table 4-2 provide a frame of reference based on a young male with a body surface area of 1.7m^2. There are no universally accepted criteria for determining abnormalities.[9]

Although a subset of standard pulmonary function tests are typically performed on patients with SCI, it should be remembered that the lungs of these patients are normal unless an overriding disease process such as chronic obstructive pulmonary disease (COPD) or tumor exist. Therefore, the

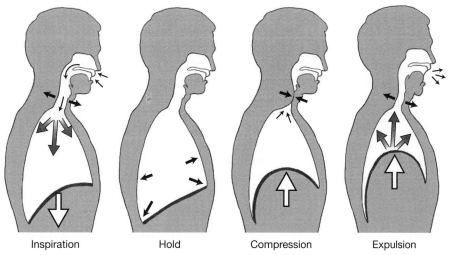

| Inspiration | Hold | Compression | Expulsion |

FIGURE 4-11 Schematic representation of a cough. Inspiration entails achieving an adequate inspiratory volume; hold involves an inspiratory pause to ensure optimal peripheral distribution or gas; compression depicts glottic closure and increasing intrathoracic pressure; expulsion depicts the opening of the glottis and rapid outward movement of gas. (Redrawn from Shapiro BA, Kacmarek RM, Cane RD et al: *Clinical application of respiratory care*, ed 4, St. Louis, 1991, Mosby.)

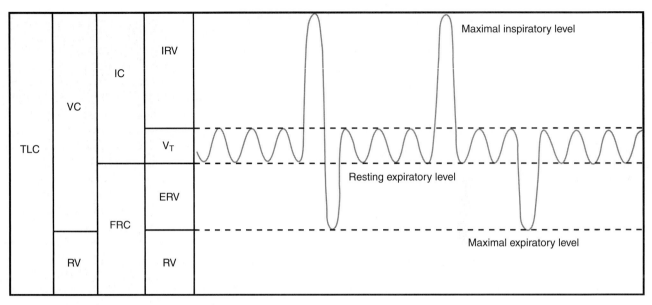

FIGURE 4-12 Pulmonary function test components. *TLC,* Total lung capacity; *VC,* vital capacity; *RV,* residual volume; *IC,* inspiratory capacity; *FRC,* functional residual capacity; *IRV,* inspiratory reserve volume; *V*$_T$, tidal volume; *ERV,* expiratory volume. (From Black JM, Hawks JH: *Medical-surgical nursing: clinical management for positive outcomes,* ed 7, St. Louis, 2005, Elsevier Saunders.)

BOX 4-1 | Lung Capacities

- Total lung capacity (TLC) = TV + IRV + ERV + RV
- Vital capacity (VC) = IRV + ERV + TV
- Inspiratory capacity (IC) = TV + IRV
- Functional residual capacity (FRC) = RV + ERV

TV, Tidal volume; *IRV,* inspiratory reserve volume; *ERV,* expiratory reserve volume; *RV,* residual volume

---

primary limitation to lung function in SCI is chest wall muscle paralysis.

Peak Cough Flow

It also is important to measure PCF. PCF measures the volume of air that can be forcefully expired in liters per minute and may be critical in determining the risk of pneumonia or other respiratory restrictions or obstructions. Simply coughing through a peak flow meter provides a spontaneous PCF value. Measuring an assisted PCF with a peak flow meter (Figure 4-13, *A* and *B*) best estimates the risk of serious pulmonary complications. An assisted PCF is obtained by having the patient build deep inspiration by using glossopharyngeal breathing (i.e., air stacking) followed by a manually applied abdominal thrust timed to glottic opening.

Pulmonary Capacity

The clinician with knowledge of normal pulmonary anatomy and physiology can determine the degree of respiratory impairment on the basis of evaluation of spirometry (VC in sitting, VC in supine, MIC), cough flows, and SpO$_2$ measurements. These objective parameters, along with capnography to assess blood carbon dioxide levels when available, provide an excellent estimate

of pulmonary capacity and risk of complications irrespective of the level of SCI. It is important to perform pulmonary function measurements both in sitting and supine positions because of the pattern of inspiratory muscle weakness (e.g., diaphragm versus accessory muscle involvement) varies in relation to body position.

Although a patient with a VC of 500 ml (10% of predicted normal) may maintain normal alveolar ventilation, he can only inflate or expand about 10% of his lungs and chest wall. Joint mobilization and ROM are the cornerstones of rehabilitation of patients with severe muscle weakness or paralysis and can be used to enhance the potential for maximal ventilation. Just as limb articulations can become hypomobile when not regularly mobilized, so too can intercostal articulations and soft tissue of the chest wall as a result of SCI.

Glossopharyngeal breathing (i.e., air stacking) to maximal insufflations, especially in patients with SCI who have intact laryngeal muscle function, can, however, provide the mobilization that can maintain compliance and elasticity. This is a learned technique that is accomplished by using a manual resuscitator (bag-valve mask) or volume-cycled ventilator to deliver increased volumes of air that are stacked into the lungs and held by the glottis (discussed in detail later). The greater the ability to stack air in the lungs, the greater the MIC and the greater the lung and chest wall can expand, which increases the ROM and pulmonary compliance that can be achieved.[10]

RESPIRATORY COMPLICATIONS AFTER SPINAL CORD INJURY

Respiratory complications after SCI are the result of weakened or no longer innervated respiratory muscles, as well as retained secretions, concomitant blunt chest trauma, and autonomic system

TABLE 4-2 | Pulmonary Function Test

Abbreviations	Definition	Normal Values*
Lung Volumes (BTPS)		
VC	Vital capacity: volume of air that is measured during a slow, maximal expiration after a maximal inspiration; normal range varies with age, sex, and body size	4.8 L
IC	Inspiratory capacity: largest volume of air that can be inhaled from resting expiratory volume	3.6 L
ERV	Expiratory reserve volume: largest volume of air exhaled from resting end-expiratory level	1.2 L
FRC	Functional residual capacity: volume of air remaining in lungs at resting end-expiratory level	2.4 L
IRV	Inspiratory reserve volume: volume of air that can be inhaled from a tidal volume level	—
RV	Residual volume: volume of air remaining in lungs at the end of maximal expiration	1.2 L (20% of TLC)
TLC	Total lung capacity: volume of air contained in the lungs after maximal inspiration	6 L
Ventilation (BTPS)		
V_T	Tidal volume: olume of air inhaled or exhaled during each respiratory cycle; normal range is 400-700 ml	500 ml
F	Frequency	12/min
Mechanics of Breathing		
FVC	Forced vital capacity: maximal volume of air that can be forcefully expired after a maximal inspiration to total lung capacity	4.8 L
FEV_1	Forced expiratory volume	—
$FEF_{25\%-75\%}$	Forced expiratory flow$_{25\%-75\%}$: average flow during the middle half of an FVC maneuver	
PEFR	Peak expiratory flow rate: maximal flow rate attained during an FVC maneuver	600 L/min
MVV	Maximal voluntary ventilation: largest volume that can be breathed during a 10- to 15-second interval with voluntary effort	170 L/min
MIP	Maximal inspiratory pressure: greatest negative pressure that can be generated during inspiration against an occluded airway	—
MEP	Maximal expiratory pressure: highest positive pressure that can be generated during a forceful expiratory effort against an occluded airway	—
Gas Exchange		
VCO_2	Carbon dioxide production	200 m/min
VO_2	Oxygen consumption	250 m/min
RQ	Respiratory quotient	0.8 (VCO_2/VO_2)
Alveolar Gas		
P_AO_2	Partial pressure of alveolar oxygen	109 torr
$P_{Ac}O_2$	Partial pressure of alveolar carbon dioxide	40 torr
Arterial Blood		
Pao_2	Partial pressure of arterial blood	99 torr
Sao_2	Oxygen saturation of arterial blood	>94%
Spo_2	Oxygen saturation as measured by pulse oximetry	>94%
PH	Hydrogen ion content	7.4
Airway Secretion Parameters		
MIC	Maximum insufflation capacity	—
PF (unassisted cough)	Unassisted cough peak flow	>360 L/min
PF (assisted cough)	Assisted cough peak flow	>360 L/min

Data from Black JM, Hawks JH: *Medical-surgical nursing: clinical management for positive outcomes,* ed 7, St. Louis, 2005, Elsevier Saunders; Oakes DF: *Clinical practitioners guide to respiratory care,* Old Town, ME, 1996, Health Educator Publications, Inc.; Wagner J: *Pulmonary function testing: a practical approach,* Baltimore, MD, 1992, Williams & Wilkins; American Medical Association: *AMA manual of style: a guide for authors and editors,* ed 9, Baltimore, 1998, Williams & Wilkins.
*Values are for a young male with a 1.7 m² body surface area.
BTPS, Body temperature pressure standard.

dysfunction. Patients lacking innervation of their abdominals and intercostals will have poor inspiratory ability and virtually no expiratory ability. With an impaired cough mechanism, secretion management becomes problematic. With decreased VC and tidal volume, the patient may be prone to atelectasis, pneumonia, and ventilatory failure.

Patients with an impaired cough must rely on mechanical means to remove secretions, including assisted cough techniques, suctioning, or noninvasive mechanical insufflation-exsufflation (MI-E) (all described in detail later). Even a patient with paraplegia who has a high to mid thoracic injury will have difficulty with secretion removal because he may have only partial abdominal

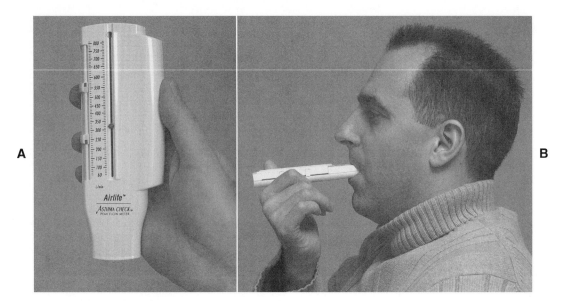

FIGURE 4-13 Peak flow meter. **A,** Calibrations on peak flow meter measure forced expiratory volume. **B,** After exhaling completely, client takes a deep breath, seals lips tightly around mouthpiece, and blows out as hard and fast as he can.

and intercostal innervation. A patient with paraplegia with a low thoracic injury may have a fairly productive cough because his abdominals and intercostals may be almost fully innervated.

Secretion retention must be avoided because it can lead to inflammation of the pulmonary mucosa, pneumonia, or atelectasis, which is the partial or complete collapse or airless condition of the lung. One of the most common causes of the production of excessive secretions is the presence of a tracheostomy tube and the most common treatment for the removal of excessive secretions uses a suctioning device. Although suctioning does remove secretions, long-term suctioning can damage the mucociliary elevator because of the mechanical irritation. MI-E can be successful in reducing secretions without the mechanical damage to the normal ciliary function and mucus composition, providing lung clearance at a cellular level (i.e., mucociliary elevator), which is necessary for airway secretion elimination. In addition, other factors that may inhibit this self-cleaning mechanism must be addressed, such as dehydration, infection, trauma, and smoking.

An individual who is ventilator dependent is at risk for development of atelectasis because of airway secretion retention, restricted chest wall and body movement, and the maintenance of the recumbent position. Atelectasis results in reduced chest wall movement and breath sounds and can involve the alveoli and blood vessels, leading to diminished blood flow and decreased gaseous exchange to the affected area. Untreated, atelectasis can lead to acidosis, hypoventilation, and ultimately respiratory failure.

Sleep apnea, the periodic cessation of breathing during sleep, is another complication that may affect patients with SCI. Sleep apnea is more common in males, in patients who are obese, and in those with tetraplegia. The use of antispasmodics and antianxiety medication adds to the problem because of the corresponding central depression of the breathing centers.[2,7]

Thorough respiratory care after SCI is important to prevent any potential respiratory complication. Prophylactic respiratory therapy should be initiated as soon as possible, which includes breathing treatments with saline solution or bronchodilators.

TREATMENT

Respiratory care for patients with SCI depends on whether the injury is acute or chronic (i.e., post injury 6 months to 1 year). After the patient's respiratory evaluation and armed with the results from appropriate tests and measurement parameters, the therapist can generate a problem list and a plan of care with interventions to achieve optimal outcomes (Table 4-3).

Respiratory care treatment techniques include postural drainage, percussion and vibration, assisted cough, deep breathing exercises, and stretching strategies. Percussion and vibration are more often needed for patients with concomitant lung disease such as COPD rather than for those primarily with chest muscle weakness resulting from SCI. The focus for patients with SCI is on cough production. Although there is little research evidence to support postural drainage and vibration as methods to increase peak cough flow, some patients with SCI may require them and so they will be reviewed. During each treatment session, if a cough is productive or secretions are removed by mechanical means, the clinician should document this, including a description of the secretions.

Postural Drainage

Frequent position changes and turning help patients with SCI keep their lungs free of secretions. When a patient is immobilized or recovering from an infection, passive positioning techniques using gravity or postural drainage may be necessary to mobilize secretions from the lungs. The goal of treatment is to centralize secretions from the regions beyond the segmental bronchi of the lungs to a larger airway where the mucociliary elevator and cough, suctioning, mechanical or insufflation-exsufflation (MI-E) can remove them. Indications and contraindications for postural

TABLE 4-3 | Respiratory Treatment Plan for a Patient with Spinal Cord Injury

Problem	Intervention	Functional Outcome
Ineffective secretion management	Patient and caregiver education on postural drainage, percussion and vibration, assisted cough, and use of suction or mechanical insufflation-exsufflation	Patient is independent with instruction of airway clearance techniques or applicable self-assisted cough resulting in an increase assisted peak cough flow with the SpO_2 >94%
Decreased strength of respiratory muscles	Therapeutic exercise of respiratory muscles including diaphragm, abdominal, intercostal, and accessory muscles	Patient improves strength of innervated respiratory muscles for a more effective cough, increased VC and more efficient breathing pattern and is independent (with caregiver as needed) in the home exercise program
Decreased ROM of thorax and upper limbs	Patient and family education on appropriate stretching and positioning to maintain/increase trunk and upper limb ROM and glossopharyngeal breathing (i.e., air stacking)	Patient maintains or increases ROM and flexibility of lungs and chest wall and increases maximal insufflation capacity with home exercises, assisted by a trained caregiver
Poor postural alignment in wheelchair	Patient and family education on proper positioning in wheelchair; refer for wheelchair evaluation and prescription of optimal equipment	Patient achieves optimal posture in sitting to maximize breathing capabilities and decrease dyspnea
Ventilator education needed	Patient and family training in use of ventilator and other equipment	Patient and family independent with ventilator use, including maintenance and alarm trouble shooting

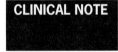 **CLINICAL NOTE** Indications and Contraindications for Postural Drainage

Indications
- Prophylaxis to prevent secretion accumulation
- Secretion mobilization for patients on bed rest, with invasive airway tubes, during respiratory tract infections

Contraindications
- Unstable cardiovascular system
- Untreated tension pneumothorax
- Pulmonary embolism
- Large pleural effusion
- Unstable spinal injury
- Recent neurosurgery with a contraindication for increased intracranial pressure
- Orthopedic conditions or fractures that limit position
- Acute hemoptysis

drainage are listed in the Clinical Note: Indications and Contraindications for Postural Drainage.

Classical or modified postural drainage positions may be used to allow maximal drainage for each lung segment (Figure 4-14). During the positioning procedure, the patient should be monitored for any adverse effects. Each position should be maintained for at least 5 to 10 minutes if tolerated. It may be beneficial to use techniques such as percussion and vibration and secretion removal with assisted cough, suctioning, or MI-E while the patient is in these positions with the secretions centralized. The clinician should assess the patient after postural drainage and any other respiratory treatment with auscultation, taking vital signs (including pulse oximetry), and monitoring the patient's response for signs of respiratory discomfort or distress.

If a patient is unable to be positioned into any of these positions, modifications may be considered, including the elimination of certain components of the position. For example, keeping a patient horizontal instead of placing him in Trendelenburg position with head down will decrease the risk of increased intracranial pressure. For patients unable to be positioned prone, modified

positions can be used. These include supine, side lying, side lying three fourths supine, side lying three fourths prone on the right or left side to drain each lung segment and lobe.[2]

Percussion and Vibration

Percussion and vibration are external manipulations of the thorax to dislodge and remove pulmonary secretions. Indications and contraindications should be considered before these treatments are applied (Clinical Note: Indications and Contraindications for Percussion and Vibration).

CLINICAL NOTE Indications and Contraindications for Percussion and Vibration

Indications
- Prophylaxis to prevent secretion accumulation
- Secretion mobilization for patients on bed rest, with invasive airway tubes, or with respiratory tract infections

Contraindications
- Unstable cardiovascular system
- Untreated tension pneumothorax
- Pulmonary embolism
- Large pleural effusion
- Unstable spinal surgery
- Recent neurosurgery with a contraindication for increased intracranial pressure
- Orthopedic conditions or fractures that limit position
- Acute hemoptysis
- Subcutaneous emphysema
- Recent spinal anesthesia
- Recent skin graft or flap to the thorax
- Other skin conditions, including burns, open wounds, or infection
- Advanced osteoporosis
- Metastatic bone cancer
- Fractured ribs
- Conditions prone to hemorrhage
- Acute onset of chest wall pain resulting from the techniques

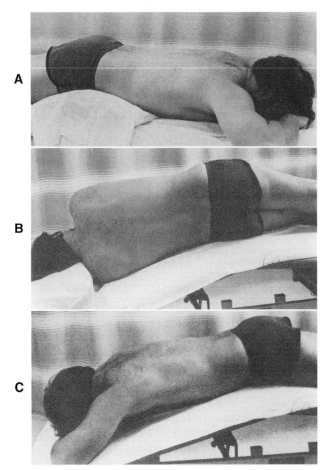

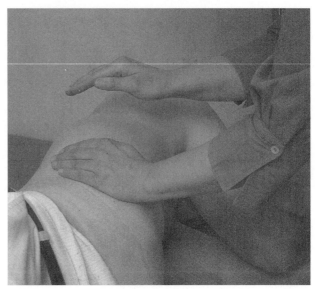

FIGURE 4-15   Chest percussion. Therapist uses cupped hands to promote lung drainage while patient is in side-lying position.

FIGURE 4-14   Postural drainage positions can be useful for maximal drainage of specific lung segments. **A,** Modification of position recommended for bronchial drainage of the superior segments of both lower lobes. **B,** Modification of position recommended for bronchial drainage of the right lateral basal segment. **C,** Modification of position recommended for bronchial drainage of both posterior basal segments. (From Irwin S, Tecklin JS: *Cardiopulmonary physical therapy: a guide to practice*, ed 4, St. Louis, 2004, Mosby.)

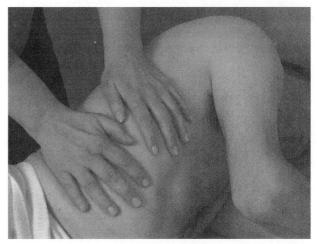

FIGURE 4-16   Therapist demonstrates the vibration technique to promote lung drainage by positioning her hands on one side of the patient's chest.

Percussion uses the rhythmic striking of the thorax with cupped hands (Figure 4-15) or placement of a hand-held mechanical percussor over the segment of lung to be drained. When manual percussion is performed, a sheet or gown should be used at all times as a protective barrier between the therapist's hands and the patient's chest wall. The therapist then cups his hands by adducting the fingers and thumb and rhythmically applies a striking force while moving over the congested area. The sound produced should be a "pop" and not a slap. The clinician should avoid the floating ribs (ribs 11 and 12) and take care to continuously monitor the patient's comfort to the intensity and duration of the percussion.

Vibration involves the application of a fine, tremulus, vibratory action to the ribs and soft tissue of the thorax during the expiratory phase of the respiratory cycle. A larger lung volume before the vibration can be achieved by taking a deep breath or by air stacking. Vibration can be applied to the lateral, anterior, or posterior aspect of the chest wall and should follow the

normal rib movement during exhalation (Figure 4-16). The clinician applies her hands on the segment to receive vibration either side by side or one hand on top of the other with the fingers following the angle of the ribs. The vibrating force should be applied with arms stiffened in a co-contraction.

Assisted Cough Techniques

Traditional methods of rehabilitation for an inadequate cough include the assisted cough technique.[11] This technique was described by Braun et al in 1984, who reported a significant improvement in cough coupled with an increased ROM.[12] Although the mucociliary elevator is the primary method for clearance of secretions, the cough is equally important for secretion clearance if, for example, a patient with SCI develops an upper respiratory infection in which excessive secretions are accumulated. Box 4-2 lists various assisted cough techniques that may be used in patients with

BOX 4-2 | Assisted Cough Techniques

- Heimlich type, quad cough, abdominal thrust
- Costophrenic assist
- Anterior chest compression
- Counterrotation assist
- Paraplegia long-sit self-assist
- Tetraplegia long-sit self-assist
- Short-sit self-assist
- Prone-on-elbows self-assist
- Self-assist in quadruped

CLINICAL NOTE | Indications and Contraindications for Assisted Cough

Indications
- Assist the patient with limited respiratory muscle capacity to remove secretions and foreign substances in the airway
- Secretion mobilization for patients on bed rest, with invasive airway tubes, or with respiratory tract infections

Contraindications
- Unstable cardiovascular system
- Untreated tension pneumothorax
- Pulmonary embolism
- Large pleural effusion
- Unstable spinal surgery
- Recent neurosurgery with contraindications for increased intracranial pressure
- Orthopedic conditions or fractures that limit position
- Acute hemoptysis
- Subcutaneous emphysema
- Recent spinal anesthesia
- Recent skin graft or flap to the thorax
- Other skin conditions, including burns, open wounds, or infection
- Advanced osteoporosis
- Metastatic bone cancer
- Fractured ribs
- Conditions prone to hemorrhage
- Acute onset of chest pain resulting from the technique
- Recent abdominal surgery or injury
- Aortic aneurysm
- Patient at risk for tussive syncope (syncope caused by decreased cardiac output with increased intrathoracic pressure)

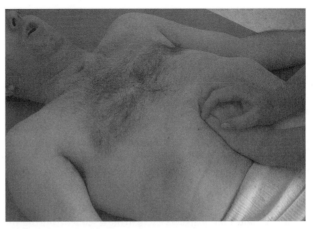

FIGURE 4-17 Therapist performs Heimlich-assisted cough technique with patient in supine position.

the highest measure, but not to average the measurements. The patient should be tested for both unassisted and assisted peak cough flows (see Table 4-2 for normative values). As mentioned earlier, cough assist techniques also can be used when the patient is in postural drainage positions, enabling secretions to be removed while centralized.

Clinicians need to understand the mechanisms of a normal cough (see Figure 4-11) to best assist a patient with productive coughing. In patients with an impaired cough reflex, which is mediated by the vagal nerve (cranial nerve X), or those who are unable to follow directions, a cough reflex can be stimulated with a sterile water mist inhaled or dropped into the trachea directly through the tracheostomy tube. In addition, a tracheal tickle can be applied by pressing a fingertip firmly on the trachea in the area above the sternal notch and using a circular motion. When the therapist is attempting to elicit a cough reflex, care should be taken to stand to the side of the patient to avoid contact with expelled sputum.

A number of assisted cough techniques require the patient to take a maximal inspiration, which can be augmented by maximum deep glossopharyngeal breathing (i.e., air stacking). These include the Heimlich, costophrenic, and short-sitting self-assist techniques.

Heimlich-Assisted Cough

The Heimlich-assisted cough technique is also called the quad cough or abdominal thrust assist. It is so named because of the similarity of hand placement to the Heimlich technique used to expel foreign objects in the airway (Figure 4-17). The therapist places the heel of one hand just proximal to the patient's navel while making sure to be distal to the lower ribs and xiphoid process of the sternum. The therapist instructs the patient to take a deep breath or air stack with hold for several seconds. Then as the therapist instructs the patient to cough, she simultaneously applies an anterior and superior force to increase the expiratory effort of the patient. This type of assisted cough also can be applied when the patient is sitting in a wheelchair or when in postural drainage positions, including supine or side lying (with one hand on the posterior thorax for stability).

limited respiratory muscle capacity to remove secretions and foreign substances in the airway. Refer to the Clinical Note: Indications and Contraindications for Assisted Cough.

The velocity of the air during a cough creates a turbulent flow in the trachea and large bronchi. When this turbulence is created, secretions are entrapped in this air flow and are moved toward the larynx. Peak cough flow can be measured with a PCF meter (see Figure 4-13, *A*). Patients should start with the meter set to 0, sit upright if possible or always measure in a consistent posture, close lips around meter with tongue under mouthpiece, and blow as hard and as fast as possible until all possible air is expired. This test should be administered three times to record

Costophrenic-Assisted Cough

The costophrenic assist is frequently used with patients who cannot tolerate the abdominal thrust applied during the Heimlich-type assist or with patients who can benefit from manual facilitation of the deep inspiration. The clinician places the palmar surface of her hands along the costophrenic angles of the rib cage with fingers laterally spread in the direction of the ribs (Figure 4-18). To assist with the inhalation phase, the clinician waits for the completion of an exhalation and then applies a quick stretch down and inward while instructing the patient to "take a deep breath." This quick stretch can facilitate an improved contraction of the diaphragm and intercostal muscles. After the patient completes the inspiration phase, the clinician instructs him to "hold the air in" and then instructs the patient to cough. During the cough phase, the clinician quickly applies a lateral and inferior manual force to enhance the force of the patient's exhaled air flow. This assisted cough technique is most easily accomplished with the patient in a side-lying position.

Anterior chest compression is a modification of the costophrenic assist, which facilitates the upper chest rather than the lower. The therapist places one hand or the entire forearm across the upper chest wall and the other across the lower chest wall (Figure 4-19). As the patient coughs, the lower hand or forearm still compresses to assist exhalation while the upper hand stabilizes and compresses the upper chest as well.[2]

Counterrotation-Assisted Cough

The counterrotation assist compresses the thorax in three planes for a maximal exhalation.[13] It is performed in side-lying patients when there are no contraindications for spinal rotation. With the patient in the left side-lying position with 45 degrees of hip flexion, the therapist kneels behind the patient diagonally facing his shoulder (Figure 4-20, *A*). The therapist's left hand should be on the patient's right scapula and the right hand on the patient's right anterior superior iliac spine. The patient is instructed to take a deep breath in while the therapist pushes the upper thorax superiorly and anteriorly with the left hand and pulls the pelvis inferiorly and posteriorly with the right hand. The patient is instructed to hold his breath while the therapist switches hand placement. The left hand slides forward over the pectoral region and the right hand slides posteriorly into the gluteal region (Figure 4-20, *B*). The patient is now told to cough while the therapist pulls the upper chest inferiorly and posteriorly with the left hand and simultaneously pushes the gluteal area superiorly and anteriorly with the right hand.[2,13] This maneuver is intended to function in the same manner as innervated intercostal muscles.

Self-Assisted Techniques

Other techniques described by Massery[13] require more participation from the patient, in particular his manual assist during exhalation. It is beneficial for individuals with adequate strength to learn self-assist techniques to clear secretions and foreign substances from the airways when no one is available to provide cough assistance.

The first technique is the tetraplegia long-sit self-assist. This is performed with the patient in long-sitting position or with

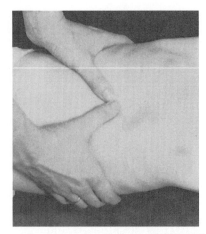

FIGURE 4-18 Therapist performs costophrenic-assisted cough technique with patient in supine position. (From Frownfelter D, Dean E: *Cardiovascular and pulmonary physical therapy: evidence and practice,* ed 4, St. Louis, 2006, Mosby.)

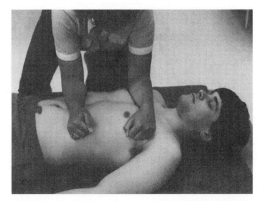

FIGURE 4-19 Therapist performs assistive cough technique with patient in supine position; variation of the anterior chest compression assist. (From Frownfelter D, Dean E: *Cardiovascular and pulmonary physical therapy: evidence and practice,* ed 4, St. Louis, 2006, Mosby.)

legs externally rotated and flexed (Figure 4-21). The patient is instructed to take in a deep breath with cues to extend the trunk and retract the scapulae to enhance inspiration. He then is instructed to cough as he throws his trunk and arms forward to enhance forced exhalation.

The tetraplegia long-sit self-assist requires less balance because the patient is supported on extended and externally rotated upper limbs. Again, the patient is asked to take a deep inhalation with cervical extension and scapular retraction. Then the patient is instructed to cough while bringing head forward to assist with upper chest compression.

The short-sitting self-assist is performed with the patient sitting in the wheelchair or on the side of a bed or mat. The patient is instructed to take a deep breath during extension of the upper body as much as his balance will allow (Figure 4-22, *A*). He is then instructed to cough and flex his trunk forward while his interlocked forearms or hands, in the Heimlich position, press inward and upward on his abdomen to assist with the forced exhalation (Figure 4-22, *B*). Even a patient with limited upper limb strength

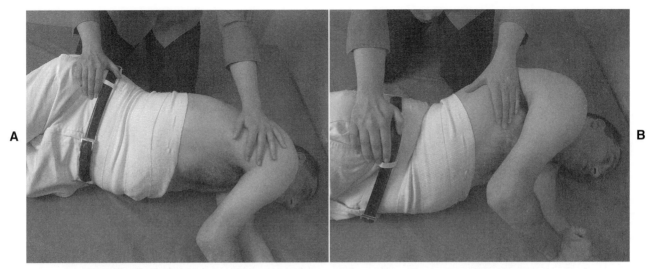

FIGURE 4-20 Massery[13] counterrotation assisted cough technique. **A,** Therapist demonstrates the starting position for hand placement with the upper hand on right scapula and lower hand on anterior pelvis. **B,** Therapist demonstrates the ending for hand placement with upper hand on anterior shoulder and pectoral region and lower hand on the gluteal region. Patient remains in left side-lying position.

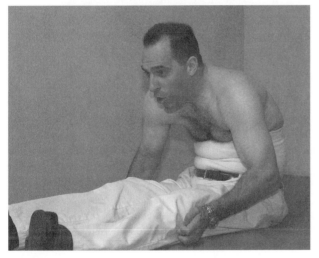

FIGURE 4-21 Client with tetraplegia demonstrates long-sitting self-assist cough technique while wearing an abdominal binder.

and balance can throw his trunk forward to attempt to clear his airway in an emergency situation.

The patient can also try a self-assist maneuver in the prone position on elbows if this position is not contraindicated. This position inhibits diaphragmatic excursion and the patient must use accessory muscles by extending his neck to enhance the deep inhalation. Then the head and neck are flexed as the patient coughs.

The self-assist technique in the quadruped position is the most advanced assisted cough technique and requires more balance and motor control from the patient. On hands and knees, he is instructed to rock forward extending his head and trunk as he inhales. Then he rocks back, bringing his hips posterior and inferior and flexing his trunk as he coughs.[2,13]

Deep Breathing Exercises

Appropriate goals for individuals with SCI that affect the respiratory muscles include maximizing the inspiratory and expiratory capacity. By focusing on increasing the MIC (i.e., air stacking),

the clinician can decrease the risk of atelectasis and prevent the accumulation of bronchial secretions. When expiratory capacity is improved, a more productive cough will result. The clinician first evaluates the patient to see which respiratory muscles are innervated and require strengthening (see Chapter 6). During a normal inspiration, the clinician first should see a rise of the abdomen because of the descending diaphragm, the flaring of the lower ribs also from diaphragmatic contraction, and then the rising of the upper chest as air fills the lungs.[2] After analyzing which components of normal inspiration are missing or affected, the clinician can determine what muscles need to be strengthened. The goal may be to strengthen the diaphragm, intercostals, or accessory muscles for a deeper inhalation or to focus on the abdominals and intercostals for a more forceful exhalation needed for a productive cough. To facilitate such strengthening, the following breathing exercises can be incorporated into a respiratory treatment program.

The clinician begins by observing the patient's natural breathing pattern. After SCI, a patient may use accessory muscles to augment inspiration in the presence of a weak or partially innervated diaphragm. To strengthen the diaphragm—the primary muscle of inspiration—the clinician positions the patient for a maximal contraction. Placing the patient supine with a pillow and a posterior pelvic tilt with arms resting at his side in shoulder adduction and internal rotation will slacken the accessory muscles and therefore enhance diaphragmatic contraction. The patient can be given verbal cues to "take a deep breath from your belly" and also can be told to relax his shoulders to discourage accessory muscle use. To further inhibit the accessory muscles, the clinician can provide firm manual pressure to the shoulders in an inferior direction. Manual cues to the diaphragm can be incorporated (Figure 4-23), providing a quick stretch just before inspiration, as in the costophrenic-assisted cough technique. As the patient gains greater control and strength of his diaphragm, the clinician can encourage the patient to work on diaphragmatic exercises in other positions and with functional activities and exercises.[2] The patient can use toys that require breathing efforts (such as blowing bubbles or a pinwheel) or an incentive spirometer to enhance sustained inspiratory effort.[14]

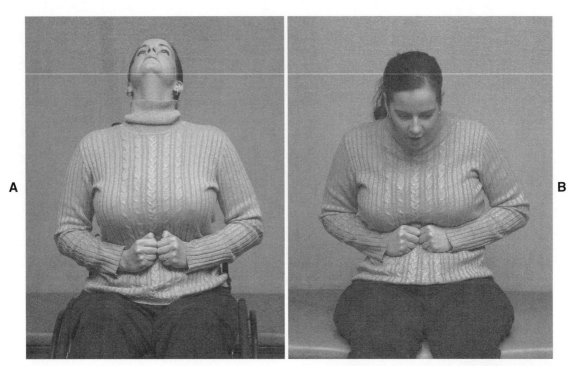

FIGURE 4-22 **A,** Client performs Heimlich-assisted cough in short-sitting position starting in extension, and **B,** in flexion.

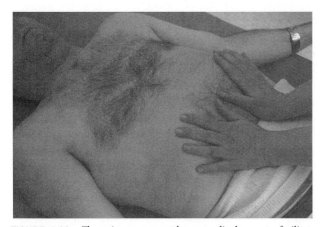

FIGURE 4-23 Therapist uses manual cues to diaphragm to facilitate diaphragmatic breathing.

To offer resistance to the diaphragm, the clinician can add weights to the abdomen when the patient is in the supine position. If weights are placed on the abdomen, the patient must be closely observed to ensure correct performance of the exercise. A common problem with this exercise occurs when, rather than working to raise the weights and strengthen the diaphragm, the weights inhibit the diaphragm and encourage accessory muscle breathing. An inspiratory muscle trainer can also be used (see Figure 6-8).

The clinician may also focus on strengthening the abdominal muscles to augment expiratory effort for a more productive cough. Patients with paraplegia or incomplete tetraplegia with partial innervation of the abdominal muscles may benefit from a program of exercises with emphasis on strengthening both the upper and lower abdominal muscles.

Additional goals include clinical facilitation of the accessory muscles to enhance inspiration. This is especially important for patients with high tetraplegia who have little or no active diaphragmatic contraction. The patient may be instructed to "take a deep breath" while raising his shoulders and contracting the innervated muscles in his neck and pectoral region (Figure 4-24). The accessory muscles can further be encouraged to stretch by not using a pillow under the patient's head and placing the patient's arms in shoulder abduction and external rotation with the trunk in an anterior pelvic tilt. The clinician may want to imitate the desired motion and use a mirror for patient feedback.

Patients also can be taught to use eye movements to facilitate inspiration, by learning to look up each time they inspire. Another strategy is to inhibit the diaphragm while a patient is learning to use his accessory muscles. As the patient exhales, the clinician applies manual pressure to the abdomen in the Heimlich position so that on the next inhalation the patient cannot use the diaphragm as efficiently. Prone on elbows is a diaphragm-inhibiting position mentioned earlier that allows the patient to better use his accessory muscles.[2]

Glossopharyngeal Breathing

It is very tiring to breathe only with the accessory muscles. If the diaphragm does not strengthen sufficiently to support normal spontaneous alveolar ventilation without the undue burden of exhausting accessory breathing, the patient should be taught glossopharyngeal breathing. Glossopharyngeal breathing (GPB), also called frog breathing or air stacking, is a method of breathing taught to patients who have extreme weakness or paralysis of the respiratory muscles as in high tetraplegia. With this technique, the muscles of the tongue, soft palate, pharynx, and larynx work in concert to create a pumping action that forces gulps of air into the trachea and lungs (Figure 4-25). Patients trap air in a pocket of negative pressure within their mouths, which allows them to maximize that space, pulling in more air, and then they close their lips and force the air back and down the throat with stroking maneuvers of the tongue, pharynx, and larynx.[2]

More than 60% of patients with high-level SCI who are unable to breathe without the ventilator (some with immeasurable VC) can achieve autonomous breathing for hours and even all day by using this technique.

Patients require practice to use GPB for successful breathing. GPB was developed in the 1950s when patients with poliomyelitis discovered that they could have freedom from body ventilators by using a technique of gulping air to achieve adequate inspiration. It is rarely very effective in the presence of a tracheostomy tube. At some medical centers, physicians remove the tracheostomy tubes (i.e., decannulate) of patients with high tetraplegia to permit glossopharyngeal breathing, thereby eliminating any fear of ventilator failure or accidental disconnection.[2,5,7,15]

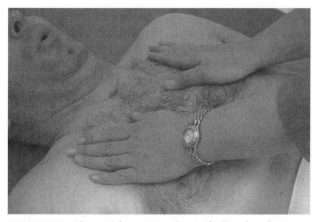

FIGURE 4-24 Therapist demonstrates how to facilitate breathing using manual contacts of the pectoral muscles for individuals with high tetraplegia.

Stretching Techniques

Muscle and joint stretching, as well as applying soft tissue manipulation, may be performed by the therapist to maximize the thoracic mobility and inspiratory abilities of a patient with SCI. Little evidence supports the use of stretching techniques to improve VC or MIC; however, in chronic SCI or after thoracic surgery, the chest wall may become restricted. Just as joint articulations can become hypomobile if they are not regularly stretched, the lungs and the chest wall can also suffer such restrictions. Long-term positioning in a flexed posture and increased tone can shorten the respiratory muscles and connective tissues. Thoracic incisions and trauma can create scar tissue that further decreases thoracic joint flexibility. The clinician, after evaluating the ROM of the various joints of the upper body and the soft tissue flexibility can design a program of stretching to maximize thoracic expansion. Muscle stretching, especially when focused on the pectoral muscles and other flexors of the shoulder and trunk, can improve the patient's ability to extend his neck and trunk for improved inspiration.

Mobilization and stretching techniques for the joints of the thoracic cage and shoulder may be indicated as well.[16] For example, a static stretch such as a supine stretch with the upper limbs at 90 degrees abduction and external rotation (as tolerated) will increase or maintain shoulder flexibility. Positioning in bed should also be addressed so that the patient avoids continually lying with excessive cervical and shoulder flexion. The clinician should also focus on cervical, thoracic, and lumbar flexibility in the treatment program of patients without spinal rotation or flexion-extension precautions.

Mobilization of the joints of the rib cage will allow for greater range of motion of the thorax and subsequently increased expansion of the lungs. Contraindications for this type of manual therapy include recent rib fractures, clavicular fractures, unstable spinal fractures, pelvic fractures, and osteoporosis. The rib cage can be passively stretched in the side-lying position over a pillow or rolled towel. Upper limb ROM and breathing exercises can be incorporated for even greater expansion. For example, in the side-lying position, the upper limb can be fully abducted with

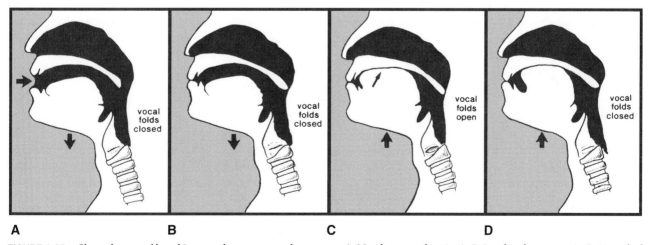

A **B** **C** **D**

FIGURE 4-25 Glossopharyngeal breathing uses the tongue muscles as pump. **A,** Mouth open to draw in air. **B,** Jaw closed to entrap air. **C,** Air pushed back with tongue into trachea. **D,** Vocal folds closed to prevent passive air leaks. Entire maneuver is then repeated. (From Frownfelter D, Dean E: *Cardiovascular and pulmonary physical therapy: evidence and practice,* ed 4, St. Louis, 2006, Mosby)

inspiration and adducted with controlled exhalation. This will emphasize expansion throughout the rib cage on the same side being stretched. In addition, this technique also will emphasize the separation of the ribs from the pelvis.

External rotation of the upper limb also can be used in the side-lying position with inhalation. This will emphasize active upper anterior chest and passive lateral chest expansion. Side sitting can be substituted if a side-lying position cannot be tolerated. In the supine position, the patient can lie on a rolled towel or thoracic roll horizontally or vertically to expand the rib cage. The upper limb is abducted with inspiration, which will emphasize lateral expansion, and the scapulae can be adducted with inhalation. This scapular adduction can emphasize lateral and anterior expansion primarily in the upper chest. If the upper limb is flexed with inspiration and returned to neutral with exhalation, the middle and upper chest will expand anteriorly.

Shoulder abduction or flexion and scapular adduction also can be used in a sitting or standing position. The patient inhales, lifts his head, and brings the upper limbs up and back, which emphasizes trunk extension. The patient exhales as the body is moved into a flexed position. These movements can be performed actively or passively. This emphasizes full anterior chest expansion bilaterally. Rotation can be added, thus emphasizing the intercostals and abdominal obliques and maximizing upper chest expansion on the side of rotation during inhalation.

Each of the individual ribs can be mobilized through manual manipulation of the soft tissue between the ribs to improve the ROM, which naturally occurs with inspiration. The patient can be positioned in the side-lying, supine, sitting, or prone position depending on the patient's tolerance and medical clearance. The clinician should start inferiorly and move superiorly in an area of limited rib motion. The patient is instructed to inhale and hold his breath. The soft tissue above and below the rib is then mobilized to facilitate further elevation of the rib with inspiration.

SPECIAL CONSIDERATIONS FOR THE PATIENT WITH HIGH-LEVEL TETRAPLEGIA

Special considerations must be made for patients with high tetraplegia (C3 and above) and those with lower spinal cord injuries with severe respiratory dysfunction. The majority of these patients will require mechanical ventilation of some form, more commonly with an artificial airway or noninvasive ventilation. Both forms of ventilation are discussed as well as airway secretion removal and weaning from the ventilator and concerns about communication and dysphagia.

Ventilatory Equipment

Ventilatory failure can occur in patients at the time of the SCI or insidiously as with late-onset ventilatory failure. The long-term inability to take a deep breath (chronic hypoventilation) results in permanent pulmonary restriction. When a patient with hypoventilation has an upper respiratory infection or conditions that weaken partially innervated respiratory muscles, there is a high risk for pneumonia and respiratory failure.[17]

The majority of patients with severe respiratory dysfunction are left with an artificial airway. This is a tube, either endotracheal (Figure 4-26) or tracheostomy, inserted in the trachea to bypass

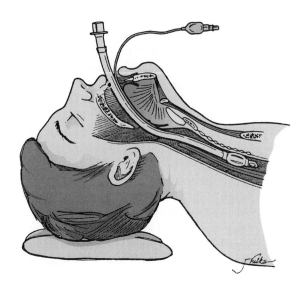

FIGURE 4-26 Oral endotracheal tube in position. The inflated cuff at the tip of the tube isolates the lower trachea and airways from the pharynx. (From Barnes TA: *Core textbook of respiratory care,* ed 2, St. Louis, 1994, Mosby.)

the upper airway.[6] An artificial airway relieves upper airway obstruction, facilitates clinical procedures to remove mucus from the airway, and provides a means of supplemental oxygen delivery that supports mechanical ventilation. Unfortunately, tracheostomy tubes can also cause an increase in secretions, as previously mentioned, and lead to ventilator dependence. The hazards of an artificial airway include pulmonary infection through contamination of the lower airway (often within 24 hours of placement), disruption of the normal mucociliary elevator, and interference with the cough mechanism.[7] These factors must be weighed by the physician, respiratory therapist, and rehabilitation team to optimize timing of extubation and ventilatory weaning (which are discussed later).

A tracheostomy tube is preferred over an endotracheal tube when noninvasive methods of ventilatory support and secretion removal cannot be used in the acute-care setting and it is evident that the patient will require mechanical ventilation for a prolonged period, as may be the case with a dual diagnosis of SCI and traumatic brain injury. Clinicians need to be knowledgeable regarding the usage and care of the particular tracheostomy tubes used by their patients as well as possible auxiliary attachments. After surgical placement of a tracheostomy site, a tracheostomy tube fits through the stoma (Figure 4-27, *A*). An obturator is placed within the tracheostomy tube's outer cannula to help guide the tube placement by gently separating the tissue of the trachea (Figure 4-27, *B*). Most tracheostomy tubes also have an inner cannula (often disposable) that acts as a lining to facilitate cleaning of the tube.[7,18]

The tracheostomy tube often has a tracheostomy cuff attached to the outer cannula, which can be filled with air through the cuff inflation line with a 10-ml syringe. The cuff inflation line has a pilot balloon, which fills when air is inserted into the tracheostomy cuff. The cuff is inflated with approximately 5 to 7 ml of air to prevent air leakage during insufflation by the mechanical ventilator and to prevent aspiration of food and liquid into the lower airway. Sometimes this can result in dysphagia (i.e., difficulty

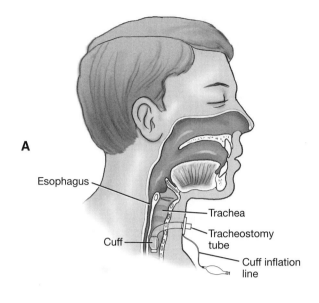

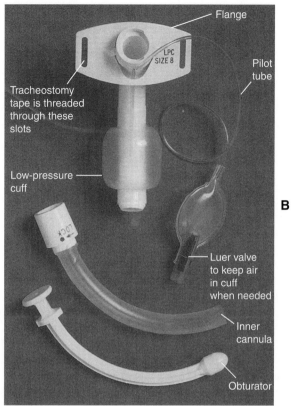

FIGURE 4-27 Tracheostomy tube. **A,** Tube inserted placed directly through the anterior neck into the tracheal stoma. **B,** Parts of a tracheostomy tube. (**B** from Black JM, Hawks JH: *Medical-surgical nursing: clinical management for positive outcomes,* ed 7, St. Louis, 2005, Elsevier Saunders. Courtesy Shirley Inc., Irvine, CA.)

swallowing) and changes in the structure of the trachea itself. The physician, speech-language pathologist, and rehabilitation team must carefully monitor dysphagia when making treatment decisions (discussed later).

The cuff may be inflated with the minimal leak technique, which means a minimal leak should be present at insufflation phase of the ventilator when tracheal diameter is at a maximum. An air pressure manometer can indicate air pressure in the cuff to prevent overinflation, which could hasten tracheal tissue ischemia. The clinical team should consult regularly about inserting and removing air from the tracheostomy cuff.

A tracheostomy tube also may be fenestrated with holes in the outer cannula. When the inner cannula is removed, this fenestration allows air from the lungs to exit through the vocal cords and upper airway to allow speech. Some fenestrated tubes also have a fenestrated inner cannula to allow vocalization during mechanical ventilation. Another method that enables vocalization is to deflate the cuff balloon as tolerated to allow air to escape over the vocal cords.[7,18,19]

Phonation valves, such as the Passy-Muir valve, allow patients with tracheostomy tubes to speak continuously (Figure 4-28). These one-way valves are especially effective when patients are not able to move enough air past a capped tube to speak adequately. The one-way valve opens during inspiration to allow air to go through the tube and into the lungs. It closes during expiration, thereby forcing air up through the vocal cords for speech. Capping the expiratory valve of the ventilator tubing can accomplish

the same outcome with no expense. It is, however, vital that the tracheostomy cuff be completely deflated when the phonation valves are used or the air will be trapped in the lungs and prevent exhalation.[2,20,21] Other attachments may include the Thermovent (Smiths Medical, Carlsbad, Calif.), a device with a filter that attaches to the tracheostomy tube in line with the ventilator and that can be used to provide warm, humidified, oxygenated air for patients breathing through the tracheostomy because their upper airway has been bypassed.

Although tracheostomy care is usually part of nursing care, physical and occupational therapists need to be adept at these procedures in the event adjustment or cleaning must occur during their treatment sessions. Gauze surrounding the stoma may become wet or soiled and need to be replaced with use of gloves and a clean technique. The tracheostomy ties and tracheostomy tube neck plate may need to be cleaned and dried as well. The inner cannula is often disposable and may need replacement if secretions build up on the inner lumen and begin to occlude the opening. To lock and unlock the inner cannula, the clinician may need to use a twist mechanism or a pincer-type clip that secures it to the outer cannula.[18,22]

If the tracheostomy tube becomes dislodged (i.e., inadvertent decannulation), the clinician can cover the stoma (with a sterile gauze, if possible) and use a valve-mask resuscitator (Ambu bag), with an oronasal (i.e., anesthesia) mask. If airway obstruction occurs and prevents ventilation, the clinician should check for a kink in the tubing, cuff slippage over the end of the

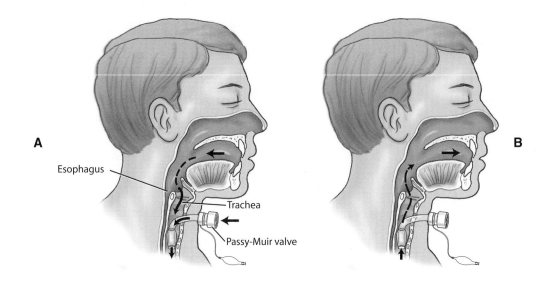

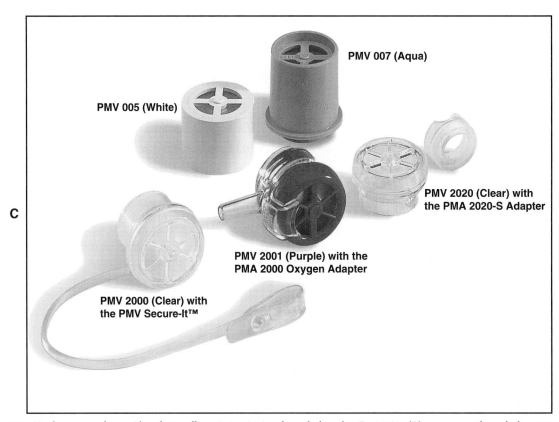

FIGURE 4-28   Tracheostomy adaptor. The adaptor allows **A,** inspiration through the valve. Expiration **(B)** must occur through the upper airway to allow speech. **C,** Family of Passy-Muir tracheostomy and ventilator speaking valves. (Courtesy Passy-Muir, Irvine, CA.)

tracheostomy tube, or mucus plug in the tracheostomy tube lumen. It is possible that the tracheostomy tube has slipped and become lodged against the wall of the trachea or carina. The clinician must try to manipulate the tube, deflate the cuff, or try suction. If not successful, the tube must be removed and reinserted by a physician or respiratory therapist.[7]

An Ambu bag can be attached to the tracheostomy tube to provide manual ventilation in case of ventilator failure or for patient resuscitation. It is squeezed fully with two hands at the rate of 12 squeezes per minute and oxygen can be added to the tubing

if the SpO_2 is low or the patient is still in respiratory distress. If distress is caused by airway mucus accumulation, the tube can be suctioned or MI-E used to clear the secretions.

When combined with mechanical ventilation, the ventilator tubing attaches with an adapter to the tracheostomy tube and may be further secured with rubber bands or Velcro ties to the tracheostomy tube neck plate to prevent disconnection. The tracheostomy tube also may be capped with a tracheal button or cap (Figure 4-29) when a patient is not using excessive mechanical ventilation to breathe. A tracheostomy button also may be used as a step between

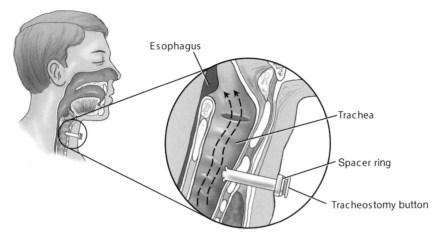

Esophagus

Trachea

Spacer ring

Tracheostomy button

FIGURE 4-29 Tracheostomy button. The button may be used as a step between mechanical ventilation and spontaneous breathing through the upper airway while maintaining a direct route to the lower airway if assistance is needed for removal of secretions or the tracheostomy must be reinserted.

mechanical ventilation and spontaneous breathing or invasive ventilation through the upper airway while keeping the skin open to allow for replacement of the tracheostomy tube as necessary. Noninvasive ventilation may be facilitated by the upper airway with a fenestrated tracheostomy or a downsized one with the cuff deflated.[7]

Airway Secretion Removal

Postural drainage, percussion and vibration, and the assisted cough techniques described previously can be used to centralize secretions to the tracheostomy tube where they can be expelled by suctioning or insufflation-exsufflation. Suctioning is the removal of excessive secretions by inserting a catheter through a tube and applying negative pressure. The clinician should be aware of the major complications of airway suctioning: hypoxemia, cardiac arrhythmia, lung collapse, and infections.

To avoid these complications, the clinician can take precautions such as preoxygenation before suctioning, limiting suctioning to 10 seconds each time, and using the correct size of catheter. For an adult patient, a catheter is used with an outer diameter no greater than half the inner diameter of the tracheostomy tube. Suction pressure (checked by occluding the

tube) should not exceed 7 to 15 mm Hg by portable suction machine or 100 to 120 mm Hg by wall suction. The clinician must be careful to keep the gloved hand on the catheter sterile; the other gloved hand that handles the tubing and adjusts dials must be kept clean (Clinical Note: Steps for Using Suction Catheter with Tracheostomy).

The suction catheter is inserted until gentle resistance is met at the carina (Figure 4-30, *A*) and is then withdrawn a few centimeters before suction is applied (Figure 4-30, *B*). Suction is applied intermittently while the catheter is rotated between the thumb and forefinger. The catheter should not be in the airway longer than 10 seconds and the total time between suctioning and re-establishing ventilation and oxygenation should not exceed 20 seconds. It may be necessary to replace the ventilator or use the Ambu bag for 5 breaths before repeating the suctioning process. The catheter may be rinsed with saline solution between each suction attempt to clear out the secretions. It is more difficult to suction the left mainstem bronchus because of the anatomical arrangement of the bronchus,[2] which may cause increased risk of pneumonias in the left lung. Use of a directed catheter[2] or MI-E may address this problem.[8]

CLINICAL NOTE **Steps for Using Suction Catheter with Tracheostomy**

1. Check equipment and make sure it is present and sterile; maintain a sterile field
2. Check monitors
3. Wash hands
5. Hyperoxygenate with 100% oxygen for three to five breaths with manual resuscitation bag
6. Place the patient's neck in extension
7. Put on sterile gloves and goggles
8. Lubricate the catheter with sterile saline solution or water-soluble gel
9. Place the catheter (without suction) upward and backward in short increments; continue until an obstruction (the carina) is reached
10. When the carina is stimulated, the patient will generally cough unless his reflexes are obtruded
11. Pull the catheter back slightly from the carina and then apply suction with no more than 120 mm Hg pressure (wall suction) as the catheter is withdrawn in a rotating motion
12. Suctioning time should be within 10 to 15 seconds total (a good guideline is for the therapist to hold her breath during suctioning because the patient is not breathing; this helps develop sensitivity for what the patient is experiencing)
13. Allow the patient to rest for several seconds and preoxygenate him again
14. Check the patient's breath sounds and repeat the procedure if necessary
15. Suction the pharynx
16. Observe the patient and monitor for any arrhythmias
17. Use pulse oximetry to monitor desaturation
18. Discard used equipment; remove gloves and goggles
19. Wash hands

Adapted from Frownfelter D, Dean E: *Cardiovascular and pulmonary physical therapy: evidence and practice*, ed 4, St. Louis, 2006, Elsevier Mosby, p. 781.

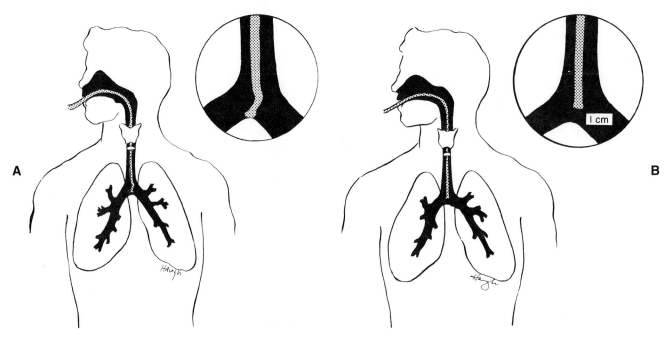

FIGURE 4-30 Placement of a suction catheter. **A,** The catheter will stimulate coughing when it contacts the carina (in patients with cough reflex). **B,** The catheter is withdrawn 1 cm after it reaches the carina, before suction is applied. (From Frownfelter D, Dean E: *Cardiovascular and pulmonary physical therapy: evidence and practice,* ed 4, St. Louis, 2006, Mosby.)

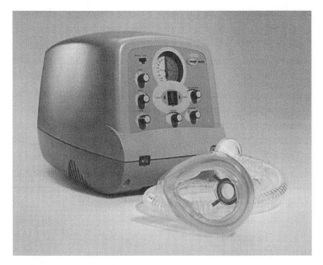

FIGURE 4-31 The CoughAssist Mechanical Insufflation-Exsufflation (MI-E) device is a noninvasive device that effectively clears bronchopulmonary secretions and reduces the risk of respiratory complications. It uses a gradual application of positive pressure to the airway and then rapidly shifts to negative pressure. The rapid shift in pressure produces a high expiratory flow from the lungs that simulates a cough. (Courtesy of JH Emerson Co., Cambridge, MA.)

An alternate method of airway secretion removal is MI-E, using the CoughAssist (Figure 4-31). This mechanical device delivers a maximal insufflation, usually at pressures of 35 to 60 cm H_2O, immediately followed by a decrease in pressure to create a forced exsufflation at pressures usually between −35 and −60 cm H_2O. The clinician applies insufflation for a count of three or less and then exsufflation for a count of three to four. The procedure can be applied four to five times with pauses to prevent hyperventilation.

CLINICAL NOTE Precautions and Contraindications for Mechanical Insufflation-Exsufflation (MI-E)

Precautions
- Patients with acute SCI who are susceptible to bradycardia
- Patients who have had airway or chest trauma, pneumothorax, or disease where deep insufflation could be harmful
- Patients with cardiac compromise (cardiac output is decreased with this technique)

Contraindications
- Bullous emphysema
- Susceptibility to pneumothorax
- Recent history of barotrauma

CoughAssist applied by endotracheal or tracheostomy tube can be more effective than tracheal suctioning and can eliminate the need for emergency bronchoscopy by clearing mucus plugs from distal airways where routine suctioning cannot. The efficacy of CoughAssist has been demonstrated clinically and in animal models, and because it is noninvasive, there is less chance of lower airway contamination compared with traditional suctioning, and it is more comfortable for patients.[23-26] CoughAssist is not without risk, however, and therefore certain precautions and contraindications must be considered (Clinical Note: Precautions and Contraindications for Mechanical Insufflation-Exsufflation [MI-E]).

Mechanical Ventilation

Clinicians need to be familiar with the two types of mechanical ventilation: invasive ventilation by an artificial airway (e.g., tracheostomy) that is attached to ventilator tubing and noninvasive ventilation by nasal or full-face masks attached to a bi-level positive airway pressure (BiPAP) device that provides bilevel positive airway pressure.[2,27] Mechanical ventilation provides preset volume and positive pressure breaths to patients as opposed to normal human physiology in which diaphragmatic contractions create negative pressure that pulls air into the lungs. Indeed, such differences in air flow and pressure in the thoracic cavity can cause adverse consequences.[2,6] When positive pressure ventilation pushes air into the lungs, areas of higher pressure are created in the thoracic cavity. This is important because the thoracic cavity becomes an area of higher pressure, which may create adverse cardiovascular and hemodynamic events. Monitoring of heart rate and blood pressure is critical when patients are placed on a mechanical ventilator.[2]

Invasive Mechanical Ventilation

Invasive mechanical ventilation with a positive pressure ventilator is delivered to the patient in a cyclic manner. During acute care, mechanical ventilation most commonly uses endotracheal and tracheostomy tubes. One type of positive pressure ventilation is pressure cycled and requires an operator to set the desired positive pressure (usually about 20 cm H_2O) to be delivered during the patient's inspiration. Sometimes, pressures may be set on the basis of the blood gas values and breathing patterns of the patient. It should be remembered that during positive pressure ventilation the tidal volume is always varying, so the pressures are going to be set to achieve a target volume. The ventilator delivers pressure until the set pressure has been obtained or the high pressure limit has been reached. Consequently, this type of ventilator delivers less air when the airway is obstructed (e.g., by mucus). In this case, suctioning or CoughAssist insufflation-exsufflation is warranted to clear the secretions. Ventilators used by a majority of patients with SCI are volume cycled so that a set volume of air (tidal volume) is delivered with each inspiration irrespective of the pressures generated in the lungs and tracheobronchial tree within the alarm limit (Figure 4-32). The ventilator only delivers air during inspiration and a positive end-expiratory pressure (PEEP) valve can be added to increase functional residual capacity.[27]

Ventilator Modes

When choosing the best ventilator options, the clinical team must carefully consider the patient's needs, including trigger (pressure, volume, or flow), flow rate, frequency, and spontaneous breathing.[2] Each new generation of ventilators provides increasing options to improve patient care, but five modes remain typical (Box 4-3).

1. Synchronized intermittent mandatory ventilation (SIMV), in which breaths delivered by the ventilator are synchronized to the patient's spontaneous breaths.[2] During SIMV, the patient is still breathing on his own, but the tidal volume between each machine breath is at his own tidal volume. The SIMV mode is often used in ventilator-weaning protocols.
2. Pressure and volume control ventilation, in which the ventilator delivers a set pressure or set volume of air at the set rate, and any breathing efforts by the patient are not supplemented.
3. In assist control (AC) ventilation the ventilator is preset to deliver pressure or volume, the number of breaths per minute, and flow rate even in the absence of triggered breaths by the

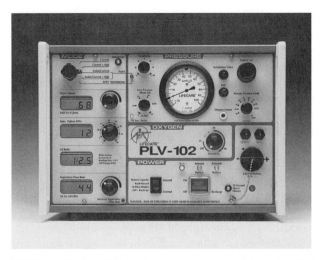

FIGURE 4-32 The PVL-102 is a light-weight ventilator well suited for portable applications in subacute, nursing home, or home settings. (Courtesy Respironics, Murrysville, PA.)

BOX 4-3 | Types of Ventilator Modes

- Synchronized intermittent mandatory ventilation (SIMV)
- Pressure and volume control ventilation modes
- Assist control (AC) ventilation mode
- Sigh mode
- Sensitivity control

---

user. The patient can breathe without help, but the tidal volume will always be at the volume set by the ventilator. Although the patient can trigger the ventilator to deliver another breath, no spontaneous breathing occurs.[2]

4. In sigh mode the ventilator delivers a sigh breath at approximately 150% of the set tidal volume every so many breaths (usually 100) to help prevent atelectasis and maintain compliance. The PLV-102 ventilator allows the sigh to be preset at 150% tidal volume; however, some ventilators allow the clinician to set the sigh volume.
5. Sensitivity control, in which the inspiratory effort needed by the patient to trigger the ventilator is determined, can then be adjusted according to patient ability.[27]

The respiratory therapist and ventilator manual should be consulted for a more thorough understanding of a particular unit.

Ventilator Alarms and Safety

The ventilator alarm system gives the clinician information about the status of both the patient and the ventilator (Box 4-4). When an alarm sounds, it may be necessary to use the Ambu bag to ventilate the patient until the problem is corrected, particularly if the clinician is uncertain whether the patient is receiving sufficient volumes of air.

The low-pressure alarm alerts the clinician when there is a partial or full disconnection in the ventilator circuit preventing the full preset volume of air to be delivered to the patient. If there is a full disconnection, no volume is being delivered. The disconnection source must be identified and reconnections made to restore proper volume delivery. The high-pressure alarm sounds when airway pressure exceeds the alarm setting. This alarm may be set off by the patient attempting to speak or cough or by obstructions caused by secretions, water, or kinks in the tubing.

Ventilators also can have a power source alarm that indicates the power source is low or has changed from alternating current (AC) to external battery or from the external to the internal battery.[27] Not all ventilators have internal alarms; these can only be switched from AC to an external battery. The clinician always should check the status of the battery when the patient arrives for therapy and ventilators should be plugged in to save the external and internal batteries.

Other alarms include an internal failure alarm that indicates a mechanical problem within the ventilator; the ventilator should be replaced and not be used until fixed. The oxygen system alarm will sound if the oxygen flow or source pressure is too low or oxygen flow is sensed during exhalation, indicating either a defective flow sensor or another internal problem. An alarm also may sound if its parameters have been set out of range, indicating that the parameters are set at a level the ventilator cannot perform such as tidal volumes that are set too high.

BOX 4-4 | Types of Ventilator Alarms

- Low pressure
- High pressure
- Power source
- Internal failure
- Oxygen settings
- Settings out of range
- Expiratory volume alarm (prevents the use of noninvasive ventilation because the alarm never turns off)

Each clinical institution will have policies to control ventilator use. Sometimes only the respiratory therapist can adjust the settings on the ventilator under orders from the physician. Safety policies at other facilities may direct the patient to travel with a log book of the current settings; only be transported by ventilator-certified staff and family members; or always travel with an Ambu bag, portable suction unit, or CoughAssist machine, and other supplies as needed for pulmonary care and hygiene.

Noninvasive Mechanical Ventilation

Noninvasive mechanical ventilation is another method of delivering positive pressure; it can be administered either through nasal masks, mouthpieces, oronasal interfaces, or full-face masks (Figure 4-33). These methods for delivering noninvasive ventilation, when removed, have the advantage of not interfering with speech or eating. This method of ventilation also avoids the complications associated with indwelling tubes.

BiPAP is a noninvasive form of mechanical ventilation delivered through nasal or full-face masks with inspiration and exhalation pressures above atmospheric levels that has gained broad clinical support.[2]

Continuous positive airway pressure (CPAP) ventilation delivers a continuous flow of air into the airways by nasal masks, mouthpieces, oronasal interfaces, or full-face masks. It keeps the airway open but does not directly assist inspiratory muscle activity.[7] The patient breaths spontaneously while supported by a constant preset level of pressure.[2]

Intermittent positive pressure ventilation (IPPV) is another type of noninvasive ventilation. It can also permit glossopharyngeal breathing (i.e., air stacking) for intermittent maximal insufflation to maintain pulmonary compliance and prevent atelectasis. The initial use of IPPV requires a significant time commitment, and difficulties may include insufflation leakage.

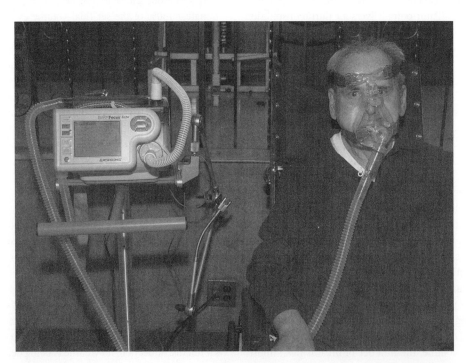

FIGURE 4-33 Patient uses nasal mask for intermittent positive pressure ventilation (IPPV) administration.

BOX 4-5	Methods for Administering Noninvasive Intermittent Positive Pressure Ventilation

- Nasal mask: commonly used at night to allow for relaxation of the mouth and less feeling of claustrophobia
- Mouthpiece: most commonly used during the day so that the patient is not attached to the ventilator and for the ability to use IPPV when desired
- Oronasal interface for patients with little or no bulbar-innervated muscle function who have excessive insufflation leakage with mouthpiece, lip seal, or nasal ventilation

When nasal interfaces are not chosen carefully, the nasal bridge pressure rises and a variety of nasal interfaces are not typically supplied as alternatives to permit options for nightly use. Aerophagia, or the swallowing of air, can also present difficulties when IPPV is administered.

Although IPPV is a less common means of ventilation in patients with SCI, it is an alternative to tracheostomy tubes for a patient with high-level tetraplegia. Patients must be alert and cooperative and avoid the use of sedatives, narcotics, and supplemental oxygen. Mouthpiece IPPV is the preferred method for daytime ventilatory assistance, and nasal IPPV, often with a nasal CPAP mask, is generally preferred for nighttime support. Mouthpiece ventilation can also be used overnight with a lip seal (e.g., an Oracle or an orthodontic bite plate)[28,29] (Box 4-5).

Noninvasive ventilation can also be accomplished with negative pressure body ventilation with either a tank (i.e., iron lung) or a chest shell style ventilator. The intermittent negative pressure created around the trunk with these devices expands the chest and abdomen to facilitate inspiration.[23,24] An intermittent abdominal pressure ventilator consists of an elastic, inflatable bladder incorporated within an abdominal corset. The sac is intermittently inflated, which pushes the diaphragm upward, causing a forced exsufflation. During bladder deflation, the abdominal contents and diaphragm fall to resting position and inspiration occurs passively. Because the method depends on gravity, it can only be used in the sitting position.[30] Therefore, only the IPPV method can be used during the night to allow the patient to sleep in the supine position.

Weaning from Mechanical Ventilation

Partial or complete weaning from mechanical ventilation can be considered as a goal for patients with SCI. An initial vital capacity of greater than 1 L at time of injury is a favorable prognosticator of success for patients with high-level injuries. Conventionally, weaning is attempted by interspersing increasing periods of ventilator-free breathing with oxygen supplementation with ventilator use, often in SIMV mode. Progressive ventilator-free breathing (PVFB) is another option. In a study comparing success of SIMV versus PVFB weaning, it was reported that SIMV was successful in only 35% of the weaning attempts; on the other hand, PVFB weaning resulted in success in 68% of attempts.[31]

After a patient is weaned from the ventilator, the clinician can consider decannulation. A typical weaning protocol from mechanical ventilation for patients with SCI includes specific patient criteria, close monitoring, and a graduated schedule (Box 4-6). Another approach involves making the lungs healthy (Spo_2 >94% in ambient air), decannulation, and then letting the patient wean himself by taking fewer and fewer IPPVs by a mouthpiece or nasal interface as tolerated.[32] Levels of hypercapnia must be taken into consideration during the weaning process.

Communication

The speech-language pathologist is often called on to assist tracheostomized or ventilator-dependent individuals with communication impairments. During an assessment, the speech-language pathologist will consider many factors, including size and type of tracheostomy tube, mode of mechanical ventilation, oral motor abilities, upper airway patency, cognitive status, and level of patient participation. She will then determine whether a verbal or nonverbal communication option is best suited for the individual on the basis of the findings of her assessment. Steps in the evaluation of patients who are ventilator dependent are summarized in Table 4-4.

An evaluation begins with a complete review of the medical history, including type and level of injury, surgical procedures, and ventilator or tracheostomy tube parameters. The speech-language pathologist then conducts a thorough interview with the patient and family to determine the patient's communication needs. An oral peripheral examination is completed to assess oral motor function. Other areas addressed during the evaluation are cognition and phonation. The speech-language pathologist assesses voicing capabilities and voice quality, taking note whether the voice is adequate, hoarse, breathy, or effortful, which can indicate vocal cord dysfunction. Nonverbal communication options for the individual with a high-level SCI are limited to facial expressions, eye blinks, lip reading, and head movements for yes or no responses. These nonverbal options are effective for communication of basic needs, but they are not practical for social communication.

Verbal communication for many individuals who have a tracheostomy tube can be attained if they have at least partially intact vocal cord function. Patients with SCI who have undergone emergency intubation or spinal cord stabilization surgeries may have damage to the recurrent laryngeal nerve or the vocal cords. Unilateral vocal cord paresis or paralysis can cause dysphonia but may still allow for verbal communication. The type and size of the tracheostomy tube can also affect verbal communication of patients with tracheostomies. A tracheostomy tube in which the inner and outer cannulas of the tube are fenestrated generally enables phonation because expired air can exit through the fenestrations and pass over the vocal cords and exit the upper airway. Another tracheostomy tube option is to slightly deflate the tracheostomy cuff again, allowing some air to enter the upper airway so vocalization can be produced. If a large tracheostomy tube occupies more space in the trachea, leaving less space for air to flow around the tube into the upper airway, verbal communication will again be blocked, but the type or size of the tracheostomy tube can be adjusted.

When tracheostomy tube adjustments are unsuccessful in producing speech, a phonation or speaking valve is an option

BOX 4-6 | Guidelines for Weaning a Patient from Mechanical Ventilation

Criteria to begin or increase the weaning process:
- Patient's level of injury is such that part- or full-time weaning is possible allowing for approximately 10 to 15 ml/kg vital capacity
- Patient agrees to and understands the procedure

Monitor each change closely and increase under the following conditions:
- Patient agrees to change the weaning time
- Oximetry during the change of weaning time is >94% in ambient air

Schedule for weaning periods:
- Start at 2 to 5 minutes three times a day and increase slowly as tolerated: 10 minutes three times a day (tid), 20 minutes tid, 30 minutes tid, 1 hour tid, 2 hours tid, 3 hours tid, 4 hours twice a day (bid), 5 hours bid, 12 hours a day (qd), 14 hours qd, 16 hours qd, 18 hours qd, 20 hours qd, 22 hours qd, 24 hours qd
- On the basis of the judgment of the physician or respiratory therapist, the patient may skip weaning steps progressing through the weaning schedule

Procedures for weaning:
- Weaning procedures should start in the bed, with the patient lying supine
- Weaning should be done with the cuff deflated and the patient talking through the trachea tube, as tolerated, with a fenestrated tube
- Titrate oxygen to saturation >94%
- Cuff should be inflated if the patient is nauseated or has reflux

- Once the patient can tolerate weaning for >30 minutes, weaning may be started in the wheelchair and then to therapy under supervision
- Weaning can occur in the shower after the patient is able to wean for >1 hour, under supervision
- Weaning may be discontinued or reduced in time if patient has persistent atelectasis

Documented parameters for all weaning:
- Vital capacity
- Respiratory rate
- Heart rate
- Oxygen saturation
- Negative inspiratory force
- Minute ventilation

Relative criteria to discontinue weaning:
- Respiratory rate increased to >30 respirations per minute
- Heart rate increased by 20 from baseline or is >130/minute or <50/minute
- Blood pressure change of plus or minus 30 points from baseline or systolic pressure <70 mm Hg or diastolic pressure >100 mm Hg
- Saturation <95% in room air
- Vital capacity decreasing
- Marked increase in spasms, diaphoresis, or change in mental status
- Marked increase of complaint of shortness of breath or fatigue
- Patient request

Adapted from Peterson WP, Kirshblum S: Pulmonary management of spinal cord injury. In Kirshblum S, Campagnolo DI, DeLisa JA, editors: *Spinal cord medicine*, Philadelphia, 2002, Lippincott Williams & Wilkins, p. 149.

TABLE 4-4 | Evaluation of Communication in Ventilator-Dependent Patients with Tracheostomy

Overview	History	Patient Information
Background Information		
	Medical diagnosis—level of injury	C3 tetraplegia
	Date of onset	2 months ago
	Surgical procedures	A-P cervical fusion
	Tracheostomy type, size, cuff status	Shiley No. 6 nonfenestrated with cuff deflated
	Ventilator settings	AC rate 12, PEEP 5
	Age	45 years
	Physical status	Tetraplegia
	Respiratory status and pulmonary toilet status	CoughAssist MI-E device as needed
Speech and Language Skills		
	Current means of communication and efficiency	Mouthing words with fair intelligibility
	Verbal expression	WFL
	Auditory comprehension	WFL
	Phonation (through leak speech or finger occlusion)	Good quality with finger occlusion
	Articulation	Good
	Speech intelligibility	Good with finger occlusion
Cognition		
	Orientation	×3
	Memory	WFL
	Attention	WFL
	Problem solving	WFL
	Thought organization	WFL
Oral Peripheral Examination		
	Labial strength/ROM	WFL
	Lingual strength/ROM	WFL
	Velar competence	WFL

The patient information used in this table is for an individual with a high-level spinal cord injury (level C3) who is ventilator dependent. A communication assessment revealed that the patient is a good candidate for trial of speaking valve.

AC, Assist control; *A-P,* anterior-posterior; *MI-E,* mechanical insufflation-exsufflation; *PEEP,* positive end-expiratory pressure; *×3,* times three; *WFL,* within functional limit.

that may help to extend speech. A speaking valve is a one-way valve placed on the hub of the tracheostomy tube or in the ventilator tubing (see Figure 4-28). The valve allows inspired air to enter the tracheostomy tube, but the expiratory flow is directed into the upper airway to produce speech. Patients must meet candidacy criteria before trial of a speaking valve; contraindications for the use of a speaking valve also must be considered (Clinical Note: Indications and Contraindications for Using a Speaking Valve).

CLINICAL NOTE **Indications and Contraindications for Using a Speaking Valve**

Indications
• Awake and alert
• Intact vocal cords
• Ability to tolerate complete cuff deflation
• Ability to remove or have help removing speaking valve if it becomes clogged
• Patent upper airway with ability to exhale
• Enough pulmonary compliance to exhale around the tracheostomy tube and out through the mouth and nose

Contraindications
• Tracheal or laryngeal stenosis
• Inability to tolerate cuff deflation
• Airway obstruction
• Chronic obstructive pulmonary disease
• Severe cognitive impairment
• Severe anxiety
• Anarthria (inability to speak)
• Laryngectomy
• Copious secretions

It is important to completely deflate the tracheostomy cuff when a speaking valve is used and to closely monitor the patient with tetraplegia because he cannot remove the valve independently. Consideration about the use of a speaking valve with patients who have thick or copious secretions is also important because, if expelled secretions become lodged in the speaking valve, the patient will not be able to exhale. To accommodate the speaking valve, it is recommended that the speech-language pathologist collaborate with the respiratory therapist, who can make the necessary adjustments to the ventilator settings such as increasing tidal volumes and resetting alarm limits. The patient must be monitored for signs of difficulty with breathing or speaking, oxygen desaturation, airway pressure changes, or discomfort.

A phonation valve is favored by ventilator-dependent patients because it is easy to use and permits speech during inspiration and expiration, allowing speech to be continuous and more pleasing to the listener. Other benefits of the speaking valve include improved olfaction and taste, a possible decrease in secretions, and an improved swallowing function.[20] Elimination of the need for finger occlusion decreases risk of infection and allows normalization of air flow and the automatic PEEP

feature in that the speaking valve traps a small amount of air in the lungs, which can have positive implications for patients with tracheostomies. The speech-language pathologist and respiratory therapist suggest parameters for use of the speaking valve or adjustments to the tracheostomy tube to the physician, who makes the final decision and writes orders for how the changes will be implemented.

Dysphagia

Dysphagia impairs the mechanics of swallowing. It may result if the processes of chewing and swallowing are interrupted by a high-level spinal cord or cranial nerve injury or by the presence of a tracheostomy tube, especially one with an inflated cuff. The primary concern is to prevent food or liquid from entering the patient's airway and lungs (i.e., aspiration). Such an occurrence could gravely compromise the patient's already susceptible pulmonary status. During the pharyngeal phase of swallowing, the food or liquid passes from the mouth into the pharynx. It then descends over the elevated larynx as the airway closes and passes on into the esophagus. Any dysfunction in this process, such as incomplete glottic closure, can cause possible aspiration of some food consistencies. Trauma and injury at the cervical spine level, including anterior cervical spinal surgery, can cause damage to the laryngeal structures and to the recurrent laryngeal nerve, resulting in pooling of food and possible aspiration.

The presence of the tracheostomy tube alters pressure within the pharynx and esophagus and can cause dysfunction in the pressure-driven process of swallowing. The tracheostomy tube can also reduce sensation and the natural operation of the valve mechanism of the vocal cords, leaving the airway unprotected and at risk for aspiration. In addition, a poorly fitting tube or overinflated cuff can contribute to the development of tracheomalacia, stenosis, or tracheoesophageal fistulas, all of which can be associated with dysphagia. For this reason, an ideal dysphagia evaluation is completed with the tracheostomy cuff deflated, if tolerated. Generally, cuff deflation can be tolerated if the ventilator volume is increased to compensate. Also, head position in a halo vest with cervical extension may to a certain degree cause reduced coordination of the upper esophageal sphincter and impaired movement of the food within the pharynx. A structural impingement caused by the cervical spine and spinal surgery hardware might also negatively affect the pharyngeal swallow evaluation.

A comprehensive dysphagia evaluation by the speech-language pathologist will include a review of the patient's medical history, clarification of the subjective complaint, inspection of the anatomy and structures, review of ventilator and tracheostomy tube status, and preliminary swallowing assessment. The patient may have a methylene blue dye test. The dye is introduced into the patient's saliva, food, or liquid. Immediate or delayed coloring of secretions found with suctioning or MI-E is an indication of aspiration. In addition, a videofluoroscopic swallowing study may be completed, allowing the speech-language pathologist and radiologist to directly observe and assess swallowing function. This procedure also permits the exploration of therapeutic techniques, postural changes, and the effect of altered food consistencies. The

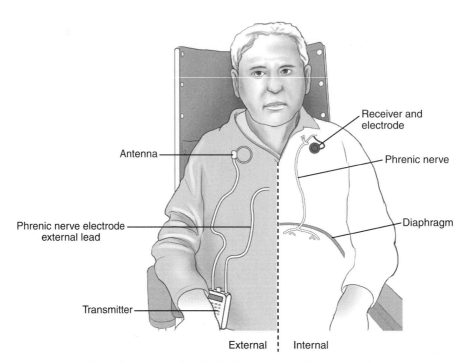

FIGURE 4-34 Phrenic pacemakers can be implanted to stimulate the diaphragm and provide respiratory function by allowing inhaled air to be drawn into the lungs by the musculature rather than forced into the chest under positive pressure ventilation.

flexible endoscopic evaluation of swallowing with an otolaryngologist also may be ordered to directly visualize the pharynx and larynx before and after the swallow.

Treatment for dysphagia may be prescribed for individuals for whom oral intake is not safe. A therapeutic program focuses on remediation of the deficit areas as identified on evaluation. Alternate methods of providing food are considered such as a percutaneous gastrostomy tube or nasogastric tube if oral intake is prohibited or limited to a degree that nutritional needs are not being met.

Early interventions by the speech therapist may include modifying the food consistency to that which is tolerated. For example, pureed food tends to remain cohesive and may not be aspirated as readily. If tolerated, a one-way phonation valve could be used to restore appropriate pressure levels within the pharynx and esophagus. Oromotor exercises can be used to improve movement and function within the oral cavity. Various techniques are encouraged to facilitate improved laryngeal elevation and vocal cord closure, such as the Mendelsohn maneuver, supraglottic swallow, base of tongue exercises, and vocal cord adduction exercises. Thermal stimulation using the application of cold to the faucial arches to stimulate the swallow reflex can facilitate the processes of swallowing.[21] Also, a method of transcutaneous neuromuscular electrical stimulation of the muscles of swallowing with an FDA-approved system, VitalStim Therapy, has shown to be effective in the treatment of dysphagia when used by certified health care professionals.[33]

Phrenic Nerve Pacing

Another invasive method of achieving artificial ventilation is phrenic nerve pacing (PNP).[34] The procedure is predominantly applied to ventilator-dependent people with tetraplegia and it

has several clinical advantages over a ventilator.[35] Some authors have found it to be only suboptimally effective for the majority of patients for which it is indicated.[36,37] The individual may be liberated from being connected to a mechanical ventilator through a tracheostomy tube.

This procedure once required a thoracotomy until the more recent use of laparoscopy.[34] PNP is achieved by surgically placing intramuscular electrodes on the right and left phrenic nerves to allow the transmission of a radiowave signal from antennas placed on the skin above the implanted receivers. The signal is converted to electrical impulses that are carried to the electrodes in contact with the phrenic nerves, which then stimulate diaphragmatic contraction (Figure 4-34). PNP may be indicated in the case of high tetraplegia with no measurable vital capacity.

Patients on PNP must be monitored closely for backup care in the event of failure of the electrical transmitter. Other problems include operative risks, atelectasis resulting from the inability to take a deep breath, infection, and trauma to the phrenic nerves. There is some risk of phrenic nerve injury because manipulation of the phrenic nerve is required for electrode placement.[38] Diaphragmatic pacing is an evolving technique that requires more research and involves direct diaphragm muscle stimulation with implanted electrodes. Patients who have had irreparable damage to the phrenic nerve may not be candidates for this technique.[35]

One report indicated success with intercostals to phrenic nerve transfer as an effective means of reactivating the diaphragm of patients with high cervical SCIs.[39] A later study evaluated the long-term effect of continuous pacing of 12 patients with tetraplegia.[40] Half the patients continued pacing and lived at home, three stopped after approximately 2 years, one converted from full-time to part-time pacing, and two were deceased but paced for 10 years and 1 year, respectively, before their deaths. Elefteriades et al[40] point out that evaluation of candidates for pacing involves a careful review of medical conditions and that social support and motivation are essential for successful long-term results.

RESPIRATORY CARE CERTIFICATION

Clinicians who treat patients with spinal cord injuries who are ventilator dependent or in need of assisted pulmonary hygiene must be competent in the areas of pulmonary assessment and treatment and in the management of respiratory equipment. It may be beneficial to have a formal education process that ensures the entire clinical staff can assess and treat these patients safely, especially in the therapy area, which may not be located near the nursing wing. In many successful institutions, all clinicians treating patients with SCI must undergo a respiratory certification process that includes demonstration of appropriate use of respiratory equipment and ventilator troubleshooting and maintenance. Examples of the recommended knowledge base for respiratory care certification are listed in Box 4-7.

BOX 4-7 | Knowledge Base for Respiratory Care Certification

Pulmonary Anatomy and Physiology
- Muscles of respiration—primary and accessory

Tracheostomy and Accessories
- Size of tracheostomy tube
- Thermovent
- Speaking valve
- Tracheostomy button/cap
- Supplemental oxygen options

Ventilator Settings
- Mode
- Tidal volume/pressure setting
- Rate
- PEEP
- Inspiratory/expiratory ratio
- Inspiratory time
- Percent of oxygen delivered
- Peak flow
- Sensitivity

Ventilator Alarms
- High pressure
- Low pressure
- Low minute ventilation
- Power source
- Oxygen alarm
- Expiratory volume

Power Sources
- Internal battery
- External battery
- AC source

Humidifier
- Proper temperature
- Use of heat moisture exchanger
- Set and reset humidifier

Supplemental Oxygen
- Parameters for use
- Ventilator dependent (in-line oxygen)
- Tracheostomy attachment
- Speaking valve attachment

Oxygen Tank
- Settings/reading gauges
- Life of tank: large versus small
- Changing tank with or without ventilator
- Storage of tank

Pulse Oximeter
- Parameter review, including alarm settings
- Probe placement
- Interpretation of readings

CoughAssist Mechanical Insufflation-Exsufflation Device
- Circuit setup
- Pressure settings and parameters
- Time settings
- Contraindications
- Technique review

Use of Ambu Bag
- Indications
- Technique
- Rate
- Verbal instructions
- Addition of supplemental oxygen
- Tracheostomy versus mouthpiece versus nasal mask

Respiratory Treatment Techniques
- Secretion centralization/removal
- Assisted cough by caregiver
- Patient self-assisted cough
- Postural drainage
- Percussion and vibration
- Facilitation of diaphragm and accessory muscles
- Breathing awareness with activities
- Stretching/mobilization of structures affecting respiration (neck, trunk, shoulder)
- Respiratory facilitation devices (inspiratory and expiratory muscle trainers)

AC, Alternating current; *PEEP,* positive end-expiratory pressure.

CLINICAL CASE STUDY Respiratory Care and Treatment Case 1

Patient History

Gary Fisher is a 41-year-old man who had both C4 and C5 cervical fractures when he fell 20 feet from a scaffold at a construction site 10 days ago. He also had multiple rib fractures with an open wound over the posterior thorax from T8 to T11. His cervical spine fracture was stabilized with a surgical anterior fusion and wiring. He is currently in a sternal occipital mandibular immobilizer (SOMI) collar. Gary has a C4 tetraplegia with American Spinal Injury Association (ASIA) B diagnosis and is in spinal shock. He is on a ventilator with a tracheostomy.

Gary Fisher is a construction supervisor with a history of smoking (one pack of cigarettes per day for 25 years). He is married and has a daughter age 6 years. His wife works as a dental hygienist. They live in a split-level single family home with four steps at the front door entrance; access to the family room from the garage is at ground level with no steps. There is a bathroom adjacent to the family room.

Patient's Self-Assessment

Gary is in acute care and has not processed the extent of his injuries sustained from his fall.

Clinical Assessment
Patient Appearance

- Height 5 feet 11 inches, weight 190 pounds, body mass index 26.5
- Posture: Gary is positioned with the head of his bed at 30 degrees

Cognitive Assessment

- Alert, oriented ×3
- Gary is not able to speak because of the ventilator; he communicates with one eye blink for "yes" and two eye blinks for "no."

Cardiopulmonary Assessment

- Blood pressure 108/62 mm Hg, heart rate at rest 60 beats/min, SpO_2 is 95 to 97, respiration is controlled by the ventilator at 12 respirations per minute
- Weaning from the ventilator will be assessed with alternate breathing strategies and instruction on pulmonary complications for optimal pulmonary hygiene.

Musculoskeletal and Neuromuscular Assessment

- Upper limb and lower limb key muscle grades are 0/5 except for 3+/5 for shoulder elevation bilaterally
- Deep tendon reflexes are 0 due to state of spinal shock

Integumentary and Sensory Assessment

- Skin is intact throughout, except for the healing wound 7 × 3 cm to the right of spinous processes T8 through T11.
- Sensation is absent below C4 to all modalities except deep anal sensation, which is intact.

Range of Motion Assessment

- Passive ROM is within functional limits (WFL) in both upper and lower limbs.

Mobility and Activities of Daily Living Assessment

- Dependent in all mobility
- Dependent in all self-care activities

Equipment

- Multipodus boots are in position on lower limbs bilaterally and the upper limbs are supported with pillows at the elbows. Gary is currently on a Clinitron bed and uses a reclining wheelchair, abdominal binder, compressive stockings, and resting hand splints.

Evaluation of Clinical Assessment

Gary Fisher is a 41-year-old male with a C4 tetraplegia, ASIA B diagnosis who remains in spinal shock. He is 10 days post injury and is currently ventilator dependent with a tracheostomy. He also has multiple rib fractures with an open wound lateral T8 to T11 spinous processes. His cervical spine fracture was stabilized with anterior surgical fusion and wiring. He is currently in a SOMI collar. He will remain in acute care until medically stable and then be transferred to an acute rehabilitation setting.

Patient's Care Needs

1. Evaluation for prescription of pulmonary assessment for pulmonary hygiene
2. Evaluation of speech dysphagia and method of vocalization with tracheostomy accessories
3. Evaluation for tolerance to upright relative to orthostatic hypotension in wheelchair, upright sitting on mat or on tilt table
4. Evaluation for wheelchair for optimal postural alignment and appropriate method of power mobility and weight shift
5. Instruction for pulmonary and skin prophylaxis and bowel and bladder management and maintenance of ROM to patient and caregiver
6. Evaluation for assistive technology and electronic aids for daily living (EADLs)
7. Evaluation for home assistive technology and optimal pressure relief bed

Diagnosis and Prognosis

Diagnosis is C4 tetraplegia, ASIA B. Prognosis for Gary is to be independent in power wheelchair mobility; a personal assistant will be required for all activities of daily living. It is likely that he will be weaned from the ventilator during the day with supplemental support of the ventilator at night.

Preferred Practice Pattern*

Impaired Muscle Performance (4C), Joint Mobility, Motor Function, Muscle Performance, and Range of Motion Associated With Fracture (4G), Impairments Nonprogressive Spinal Cord Disorders (5H) Impaired Ventilation and Respiration/Gas Exchange Associated with Ventilatory Pump Dysfunction or Failure (6E), Impaired Integumentary Integrity Associated with superficial skin involvement (7A)

Team Goals

1. Team to develop goals for tracheostomy management for pulmonary hygiene
2. Team to organize speech evaluation for assessment of speech capabilities with tracheostomy tube and complete a dysphagia evaluation
3. Team to explore ventilatory weaning for daytime
4. Team to help Gary improve orthostatic tolerance to upright postures
5. Team to schedule appointments for Gary to attend wheelchair seating clinic and assistive technology clinic to enable independence in wheelchair mobility and manipulation of environmental devices

CLINICAL CASE STUDY Respiratory Care and Treatment Case 1—cont'd

6. Team to establish education plan for pulmonary hygiene, skin care, ROM, and bowel and bladder maintenance for patient and caregiver
7. Team to consider psychological consultation to monitor adjustment to SCI

Patient Goals
"To walk and go home."

Care Plan
Treatment Plan and Rationale
- Complete a pulmonary assessment specific for PCF (peak cough flow), vital capacity, and oxygen saturation during functional wheelchair tasks
- Initiate a ventilator weaning protocol
- Initiate a patient and caregiver education plan for pulmonary hygiene, skin care, bowel and bladder management, and ROM maintenance
- Wean tolerance to upright postures in wheelchair, upright sitting, or on standing tilt table
- Schedule a wheelchair seating evaluation considering ventilator and assistive technology device needs on the wheelchair for EADLs
- Schedule a home evaluation to determine assistive technology needs to enhance independence in management of home environment, accessibility, and needs for additional home modifications and a specialized pressure relief bed

Interventions
- Evaluate and manage secretions (including suctioning requirements) that result from tracheostomy tube placement
- Instruct patient in positioning for postural drainage
- Practice ventilator weaning according to the weaning protocol
- Provide fluids during therapy on the basis of dysphagia evaluation and enable speech with adjustments to tracheostomy accessories
- Instruct patient in ROM management and skin relief techniques when in bed and in wheelchair
- Instruct patient in how to teach position changes to caregivers to prevent pressure ulcers, protect joints from pain and contracture, and use ideal seating and positioning in the wheelchair and the bed
- Monitor blood pressure and oxygen saturation during upright activities to address orthostatic hypotension
- Practice wheelchair mobility with sip n' puff or chin control
- Instruct patient and family to manage respiratory care, including education about suctioning and managing ventilator alarms
- Instruct patient and family on goals of daytime weaning off ventilator and nighttime ventilator use
- Instruct patient to manage his care including weight shifts, home exercise program, passive ROM, exercises, transfers, assisted cough, wheelchair management, wheelchair on stairs and curbs, transfers, bed mobility, use of mechanical lift

Documentation and Team Communication
- Team will document daytime weaning time and tolerance off ventilator
- Team will discuss and document short- and long-term goals and communicate these to the patient and family, including educational plan, functional mobility, home modifications, assistive technology, and durable medical equipment
- Team will discuss speech vocalization and dysphagia goals
- Team will document wheelchair prescription and communicate assistive technology goals for ventilator and EADLs on wheelchair and at home
- Team will discuss patient's understanding of prevention of respiratory and skin and bowel and bladder management and ability to instruct others in these prevention methods
- Team will communicate and document patient's adjustment to SCI

Follow-Up Assessment
- Reassessment of team goals every 2 weeks
- Reassessment for consultations with other services

Critical Thinking Exercises
Consider factors that will influence Gary's respiratory treatment and patient and family education regarding his continuing care, potential complications, and interventions when answering the following questions:
1. Identify which of Gary's muscles are intact for inspiration and expiration. Which of Gary's muscles are not innervated for inspiration and expiration?
2. What potential respiratory health and care complications could Gary face?
3. List three treatment interventions necessary to prevent a decrease in respiratory vital capacity.
4. Which cough stage(s) is/are impaired by Gary's injury?
5. List possible contraindications for percussion and vibration in Gary's history.
6. If the ventilator high pressure alarm sounds while you are performing passive ROM on Gary, what should you check?

*Guide to physical therapist practice, rev. ed. 2, Alexandria, VA, 2003, American Physical Therapy Association.

CLINICAL CASE STUDY Respiratory Care and Treatment Case 2

Patient History

Samantha Evans is a 62-year-old woman with a C8 tetraplegia, ASIA A diagnosis resulting from a motor vehicle accident. She had multi-level fractures: C7, T1, T2, and T3. Surgery including a decompression laminectomy and spinal fusion (C6 to T4) was performed 2 weeks ago and is being followed with halo traction. She has had no secondary complications. She is medically stable and preparations are in the process for discharge from an acute hospital setting to an acute rehabilitation unit in the next 2 days. She is emerging from spinal shock.

Samantha is an elementary school teacher and is married. Her husband is a retired CEO of a large bank, age 68 years. They live in a townhouse in an older adult community. Their master bedroom and bath are on the first floor. Both their married children live close by (within 10 miles) and they have four grandchildren.

Patient's Self-Assessment

Samantha does not want to retire until age 68 years but is currently uncertain about her future employment plans. She enjoys her work and delights in playing with and educating her grandchildren. She is an avid golfer.

Clinical Assessment
Patient Appearance

- Height 5 feet 5 inches, weight 140 pounds, body mass index 23.3
- Posture: Samantha is in a reclining wheelchair for 4 hours a day and tolerates a recline of 70 degrees of the seat back angle

Cognitive Assessment

- Alert, oriented × 3

Cardiopulmonary Assessment

- Blood pressure 104/64 mm Hg, heart rate at rest 64 beats/min, respiratory rate 10 to 12 breaths/min, cough flows are ineffective (<360 L/min), vital capacity is reduced (between 1.5 and 2.5 L), and breathing pattern incorporates accessory muscles and upper chest wall only
- Patient has marked decrease in the anterior and lateral chest wall with a slight decrease in posterior wall expansion

Musculoskeletal and Neuromuscular Assessment

- Upper limb muscles are intact for key muscle groups C5, C6, C7, and C8 are 4/5
- Lower limb key muscle grades are 0/5
- Deep tendon reflexes 2+ in upper limbs and 0 in the lower limbs

Integumentary and Sensory Assessment

- Skin is intact throughout
- No drainage noted from halo pin sites
- Sensation is absent below C8 to all modalities; sensation is intact to light touch, deep pressure, temperature, and vibration

Range of Motion Assessment

- Passive ROM is within functional limits in both upper and lower limbs

Mobility and Activities of Daily Living Assessment

- Dependent in all mobility and transfers
- Dependent in all self-care activities

Equipment

- Multipodus boots, transfer board, reclining wheelchair and cushion, compressive stockings, abdominal binder, specialty bed

Evaluation of Clinical Assessment

Samantha Evans is a 62-year-old woman with a C8 tetraplegia, ASIA A diagnosis resulting from a motor vehicle accident. She underwent spinal surgery 2 weeks ago, which is being followed with halo traction. She has had no secondary complications and is medically stable. She is preparing for inpatient rehabilitation transfer.

Patient's Care Needs

1. Evaluation for ROM and strength of all limbs considering halo precautions
2. Evaluation for functional mobility with halo, such as transfers and low-level position changes
3. Evaluation of skin condition under halo vest
4. Education about bowl and bladder management
5. Evaluation of orthostatic tolerance to upright, sitting, or use of a tilt table
6. Evaluation for wheelchair propulsion and management
7. Evaluation of home to determine accessibility and needs for EADLs
8. Evaluation for psychological adjustment

Diagnosis and Prognosis

Diagnosis is C8 tetraplegia, ASIA A. Prognosis is for full independence in self-care activities after equipment setup with the exception of bowel and bladder management.

Preferred Practice Pattern*

Impaired Muscle Performance (4C), Joint Mobility, Motor Function, Muscle Performance, and Range of Motion Associated With Fracture (4G), Impairments Nonprogressive Spinal Cord Disorders (5H), Primary Prevention/Risk Reduction for Cardiovascular/Pulmonary Disorders (6A), Prevention/Risk Reduction for Integumentary Disorders (7A)

Team Goals

1. Team to develop goals for respiratory management and maintenance of pulmonary hygiene, including patient's ability to instruct caregivers about secretion removal and respiratory muscle strengthening
2. Team to help Samantha improve her tolerance of upright postures
3. Team to schedule Samantha to attend wheelchair seating clinic and assistive technology clinic to enable independence in wheelchair mobility and manipulation of environmental devices for home use
4. Team to establish an education plan for patient and caregivers stressing patient's ability to instruct others in bowel and bladder management, skin care, respiratory care including assisted cough techniques, weight shifts, home exercise program of exercises and stretches, wheelchair management, and wheelchair access on stairs and curbs
5. Team to consider psychological consultation to monitor adjustment to SCI

Patient Goals

"I want to return to teaching and be able to play with my grandchildren. I want to be active in the world around me!"

Care Plan
Treatment Plan & Rationale

- Complete a pulmonary assessment specific for PCF, vital capacity, and oxygen saturation during functional and wheelchair tasks and instruction in use of diaphragm with activity
- Initiate a patient and caregiver education plan for pulmonary hygiene and skin care, bowel and bladder management, and home exercise program that includes stretching and strengthening exercises
- Wean tolerance to upright postures in wheelchair, upright sitting, or on tilt table

CLINICAL CASE STUDY **Respiratory Care and Treatment Case 2—cont'd**

- Schedule a wheelchair seating evaluation to determine assistive technology device needs on the wheelchair for EADLs
- Schedule a home evaluation to determine assistive technology needs to enhance independence in management of home environment, accessibility, and needs for additional home modifications

Interventions

- Evaluate respiratory ability and manage respiratory restrictions related to halo device
- Instruct patient and family to manage respiratory care, including assisted cough techniques
- Instruct patient in and practice ROM management and strengthening exercises while considering halo precautions
- Instruct patient and family about pressure relief techniques when in bed and wheelchair
- Instruct patient and family in skin precautions, respiratory exercises, and secretion management
- Instruct patient to teach position changes to caregivers to prevent pressure ulcers, protect joints from pain and contracture, and use ideal seating and positioning in the wheelchair and the bed
- Monitor blood pressure and oxygen saturation during upright activities to improve orthostatic tolerance to upright
- Instruct patient in wheelchair use, functional mobility, and home exercise program
- Train patient and family to manage respiratory care, including education of cough technique
- Practice ROM and strengthening while considering halo precautions
- Practice functional mobility for low-level position changes including transfers and bed mobility
- Practice wheelchair mobility using reclining wheelchair; instruct patient in wheelchair propulsion and management, including wheelchair on stairs and curbs, considering halo precautions.

Documentation and Team Communication

- Team will document wheelchair prescription and communicate assistive technology goals for EADLs on wheelchair and at home
- Team will document short- and long-term goals and communicate these goals to the patient and family, including education, home modification, durable medical equipment, and assistive technology equipment
- Team will discuss patient's understanding of prevention of respiratory and skin complications, bowel and bladder management, and ability to instruct others in these prevention techniques
- Team will communicate and document patient's adjustment to SCI

Follow-Up Assessment

- Reassessment of team goals every 2 weeks
- Reassessment for consultations with other services

Critical Thinking Exercises

1. Identify which of Samantha's muscles remain intact for inspiration and expiration.
2. What muscles are not innervated for inspiration and expiration? What potential respiratory care complications may Samantha face?
3. What position puts the patient at a greater disadvantage for respiratory function?
4. Describe assistive cough techniques that would be appropriate for Samantha after her halo traction vest is removed and her cervical spine is stable without collar support.

Guide to physical therapist practice, rev. ed. 2, Alexandria, VA, 2003, American Physical Therapy Association.

SUMMARY

Addressing the respiratory status of a patient with SCI will allow the clinician to design a more comprehensive treatment program. All patients, especially those with neurological deficits, can benefit from a treatment plan that includes components that maximize pulmonary status. Sufficient knowledge of the pulmonary system anatomy and physiology is necessary to evaluate and plan a treatment program. Manual treatment techniques including postural drainage, percussion and vibration, assisted cough, deep breathing, and stretching must be learned and reviewed periodically to ensure proficiency. The therapist also should become proficient in the use of various respiratory equipment including forms of mechanical ventilation and secretion removal. A clinician who achieves these objectives can then provide a comprehensive treatment program, including education to the patient and his caregivers.

REFERENCES

1. Winslow C, Rozovsny J: Effect of spinal cord injury on the respiratory system, *Am J Phys Med Rehabil* 82:803-14, 2003.

2. Frownfelter D, Dean E: *Cardiovascular and pulmonary physical therapy: evidence and practice,* ed 4, St. Louis, 2006, Mosby Elsevier.

3. Lissoni A, Aliverti A, Molteni F, et al: Spinal muscular atrophy: kinematic breathing analysis, *Am J Phys Med Rehabil* 75:332-339, 1996.

4. Kendall FP, McCreary EK, Provance PG: *Muscles, testing and function: posture and pain,* ed 4, Baltimore, 1993, Williams & Wilkins.

5. Bach JR, Alba AS, Bodofsky E et al: Glossopharyngeal breathing and noninvasive aides in the management of post-polio respiratory insufficiency, *Birth Defects* 23:99-113, 1987.

6. Beachey W: *Respiratory care anatomy and physiology: foundations for clinical practice,* ed 2, St. Louis, 2006, Mosby Elsevier.

7. Shapiro BA, Kacmarek RM, Cane RD, et al: *Clinical application of respiratory care,* ed 4, St. Louis, 1991, Mosby.

8. Bach JR: Mechanical insufflation-exsufflation: comparison of peak expiratory flows with manually assisted and unassisted cough techniques, *Chest* 104:1553-1562, 1993a.

9. Oakes DF: *Clinical practitioner's guide to respiratory care,* Old Town, ME, 1996, Health Educator Publications.

10. Bach JR, Alba AS: Management of chronic alveolar hypoventilation by nasal ventilation, *Chest* 97:52-57, 1990.

11. Kirby NA, Barnerias MJ, Siebens AA: An evaluation of assisted cough in quadriparetic patients, *Arch Phys Med Rehabil* 47:705-710, 1966.

12. Braun SR, Giovannoni R, O'Connor M: Improving the cough in patients with spinal cord injury, *Am J Phys Med* 63:1-0, 1984.

13. Massery M: An innovative approach to assisted cough techniques, *Top Acute Care Trauma Rehabil* 1:73-85, 1987.

14. Sprague S, Hopkins P: Use of inspiratory strength training to wean 6 patients who were ventilator dependent, *Phys Ther* 83:171-181, 2003.

15. Dail C, Rodgers M, Guess V et al: *Glossopharyngeal breathing,* Downey, CA, 1979, Professional Staff Association, Ranchos Los Amigos Hospital.

16. Maitland GD: *Peripheral manipulation,* ed 2, London, 1984, Butterworths.

17. Bach JR: Inappropriate weaning and late onset ventilatory failure of individuals with traumatic quadriplegia, *Paraplegia* 31:430-438, 1993b.

18. Branson RD, Hess D, Chatburn RL: *Respiratory care equipment,* ed 2, Philadelphia, 1999, Lippincott Williams & Wilkins.

19. Reynolds JE: Noninvasive ventilation for acute respiratory failure, *J Emerg Nurs* 23:608-610, 1988.

20. Hoit JD, Shea SA, Banzett RB: Speech production during mechanical ventilation in tracheostomized individuals, *J Speech Hear Res* 37:53-63, 1994.

21. Dikeman KJ, Kazandijian MS: *Communication and swallowing management of tracheostomized and ventilator-dependent adults,* San Diego, 1995, Singular Publishing Group.

22. Eubanks D, Bone R: *Comprehensive respiratory care,* St. Louis, 1985, CV Mosby.

23. Bach JR: Update and perspectives on noninvasive respiratory muscle aids: 1, the inspiratory muscle aids, *Chest* 105:1230-1240, 1994.

24. Bach JR: Update and perspectives on noninvasive respiratory muscle aids: 2, the expiratory muscle aids, *Chest* 105:1538-1544, 1994.

25. Bickerman HA: Exsufflation with negative pressure: elimination of radiopaque material and foreign bodies from bronchi of anesthetized dogs, *Arch Int Med* 93:698-704, 1954.

26. Barach AL, Beck BJ: Exsufflation with negative pressure: physiological and clinical studies in poliomyelitis: bronchial asthma, pulmonary emphysema and bronchiectasis, *Arch Int Med* 93:825-841, 1984.

27. Pilbeam SP: *Mechanical ventilation: physiological and clinical applications,* ed 2, St. Louis, 1992, Mosby–Year Book.

28. Bach JR: *Pulmonary rehabilitation: the obstructive and paralytic conditions,* Philadelphia, 1996, Hanley and Belfus.

29. Bach JR, Alba AS, Saporito LR: Intermittent positive pressure ventilation via the mouth as an alternative to tracheostomy for 257 ventilator users, *Chest* 103:174-182, 1993.

30. Bach JR, Alba AS: Intermittent abdominal pressure ventilator in a regimen of noninvasive ventilatory support, *Chest* 99:630-636, 1991.

31. Peterson W, Charlifue W, Gerhart A et al: Two methods of weaning persons with quadriplegia from mechanical ventilators, *Paraplegia* 32:98-103, 1994.

32. Bach JR: A comparison of long-term ventilatory support alternatives from the perspectives of the patient and caregiver, *Chest* 104: 1702-1706, 1993c.

33. Blumenfeld L, Hahn Y, Lepage A et al: Transcutaneous electrical stimulation versus traditional dysphagia therapy: a nonconcurrent cohort study, *Otolaryngol Head Neck Surg* 135:754-757, 2006.

34. DiMarco AF, Onders RP, Ignagni A et al: Phrenic nerve pacing via intramuscular diaphragm electrodes in tetraplegic subjects, *Chest* 127:671-678, 2005.

35. DiMarco AF: Diaphragm pacing in patients with spinal cord injury, *Top Spinal Cord Injury Med* 5:6-20, 1999.

36. Glenn WW, Brouillette RT, Dentz B, et al: Fundamental considerations in pacing of the diaphragm for chronic ventilatory insufficiency: a multicenter study, *Pacing Clin Electrophysiol* 11: 2121-2127, 1988.

37. Bach JR, O'Connor K: Electrophrenic ventilation: a different perspective, *J Am Paraplegia Soc* 14:9-17, 1991.

38. Glenn WW, Phelps ML: Diaphragm pacing by electrical stimulation of the phrenic nerve, *Neurosurg* 17:974-984, 1985.

39. Krieger LM, Krieger AJ: The intercostals to phrenic nerve transfer: an effective means of reanimating the diaphragm in patients with high cervical spine injury, *Plast Reconstr Surg* 105:1255-1261, 2000.

40. Elefteriades JA, Quin JA, Hogan JF, et al: Long-term follow-up of pacing of the conditioned diaphragm in quadriplegia, *Pacing Clin Electrophysiol* 25:897-906, 2002.

SOLUTIONS TO CHAPTER 4 CLINICAL CASE STUDY

Respiratory Care and Treatment Case 1

1. The diaphragm, the primary muscle of respiration, is innervated by the phrenic nerve, C3 to C5. In Gary's injury, C3 and C4 should be intact, but the C5 portion of the phrenic nerve is compromised in this injury level resulting in a weakened diaphragm. The abdominal muscles for forced expiration (rectus abdominis, internal and external obliques, and transverse abdominis) are not innervated (T5 to T12) with this level injury. Gary must rely on suctioning by caregivers or CoughAssist insufflation-exsufflation and assistive cough techniques after he is weaned from the ventilator to clear secretions for effective pulmonary hygiene and prevention of pulmonary infection. Gary may also be taught glossopharyngeal breathing (GPB) or frog breathing during the weaning process.

The external intercostal muscles are innervated by T1 to T11 and are responsible for stabilizing the rib cage during inspiration. Without intercostal control, Gary's rib cage can move inward during inspiration because it is the external intercostals that move the ribs upward and outward. The internal intercostals are expiratory in function. Accessory muscles including the sternocleidomastoids (spinal accessory and C2 to C3) and upper trapezius (spinal accessory and C3 to C4) are both intact and can assist the impaired diaphragm by bringing the thoracic cage superior and anterior for expansion during inspiration. The scalenes can only partially assist in this capacity because they are innervated by C3 to C8. The pectorals (C5 to T1) and serratus anterior (C5 to C7) are not innervated and therefore cannot assist with respiratory functions. The intact erector spinae muscles can assist with stabilization and by stabilizing and extending the thoracic spine to help elevate the ribs with deep inspiration. Gary only is able to use the erector spinae muscles from C1 to C4, so he will be able to assist minimally with thoracic extension; upper cervical spinal muscles cannot assist with thoracic extension—only cervical extension when SOMI is removed.

2. Gary will need to maintain a vital capacity of greater than 10 ml/kg before weaning from the ventilator can be considered. Gary has an impaired vital capacity and cough. The potential respiratory complications he may face include atelectasis, pneumonia, and possible ventilatory failure.

3. Many treatment techniques are contraindicated at this time because of Gary's recent spinal surgery, his rib fractures, and his healing wound. Until Gary's condition is medically stable and he is cleared for therapy, percussion and vibration, assistive cough other than the Heimlich-type assisted cough, and any joint mobilization techniques are contraindicated. In some cases of recent rib fractures, even the Heimlich-type assisted cough may be contraindicated and medical clearance is required. Glossopharyngeal breathing (i.e., air stacking), measuring peak cough flow, spirometry evaluation, and diaphragmatic breathing exercises may be assessed.

4. Gary will not have sufficient inspiratory capacity for stage 1 of good cough mechanics because of his partial diaphragm innervation and absent intercostals. Although his ability for glottal closure has not been compromised, he will not be able to build up intrathoracic and intraabdominal pressure (stage 3). This means that Gary will not be able to capture air for stage 4—forceful expulsion.

5. Gary's rib fractures and an open wound contraindicate percussion and vibration.

6. When the ventilator high-pressure alarm sounds during patient treatment, it alerts the therapist that the ventilator has exceeded the high-pressure alarm limit. Possible causes that need to be checked include increased secretion buildup that requires removal, patient trying to speak or cough, possible kink in the tubing, or trunk spasm limiting thoracic expansion.

SOLUTIONS TO CHAPTER 4 CLINICAL CASE STUDY

Respiratory Care and Treatment Case 2

1. The abdominal muscles (rectus abdominis, internal intercostals, internal and external obliques, and transverse abdominis) would not be innervated (T5 to T12) for forced expiration with this level injury. Samantha must rely on assistive cough techniques to clear secretions for effective pulmonary hygiene and prevention of infection.

The external intercostal muscles are innervated by T1 to T11 and are responsible for expanding the rib cage during inspiration. Without this intercostal control, Samantha's rib cage can move inward during inspiration with diaphragmatic movement causing negative pressure because it is the external intercostals that move the ribs upward and outward and are not innervated. The internal intercostals are expiratory in function. Accessory muscles including the sternocleidomastoids (spinal accessory and C2 to C3), upper trapezius (spinal accessory and C3 to C4), and the scalenes (C3 to C8) are all intact and can assist during inspiration by bringing the thoracic cage superior and anterior for expansion. The pectorals (C5 to T1) are intact to C8, and the serratus anterior (C5 to C7) can also assist with inhalation, especially with fixed upper limbs. The intact erector spinae muscles can assist with stabilization and help extend the spine to assist with thoracic expansion.

2. Samantha has an impaired vital capacity and cough. Therefore, Samantha is at risk for several complications related to clearing secretions including infection, atelectasis, and pneumonia.

3. Upright position puts Samantha at a disadvantage for respiratory function because her abdominal muscles are not innervated, which leaves the diaphragm in a flattened position. An abdominal binder will help to keep the diaphragm in a more optimal mechanical position by positioning the abdominal contents up and under the rib cage.

While Samantha is in a halo vest, positional contraindications require modified postural drainage positions in which the patient leans laterally and forward. Samantha continues to be at risk for complications related to clearing secretions; after she has completed halo traction and her spine is stable, multiple techniques for assistive cough will be indicated.

4. Unless it cannot be tolerated because of halo precautions, the Heimlich-type assistive cough is the method of choice for the physical therapist and patient. When not tolerated, the costophrenic technique is used. With training, Samantha will be able to perform the tetra long-sit self-assisted technique and the short-sit self-assisted technique when seat-belted in her wheelchair after the halo traction vest is no longer needed.

CHAPTER FIVE

Psychological Adjustment to Spinal Cord Injury

Loran C. Vocaturo, ABPP(Rp), EdD

My spinal cord injury left me with two major areas in need of reconstruction: the physical and the psychological. The parameters of my physical limitations were more quickly realized and defined. After a time I became used to living within these parameters and could reasonably predict my capabilities from one day to the next. On the other hand my psychological framework is an ever-changing odyssey, which has no boundaries. No matter how hard I try not to dwell on it, my past life serves as a reminder that can affect my thoughts, moods, and outlook instantly in either a positive or negative way. This is the most difficult aspect of the injury to deal with for me.

Tom (C6 SCI)

Spinal cord injury (SCI) is a catastrophic injury that unexpectedly changes the manner in which a person is able to relate to the environment by suddenly thrusting him into a life challenged by disability. SCI is one of the most devastating injuries that an individual can experience. It results in physical changes that produce both an inability to feel and move body parts and the loss of control over internal organ functions; in severe cases, the ability to breathe independently is compromised.[1] Although normal cognitive function and intellectual facility may remain, the psychological, emotional, and social implications can significantly affect the patient's adaptation to the resultant disability.[2]

The psychosocial implications of spinal cord injury have changed over the years. Before the early 1940s, 80% to 90% of patients with SCI died within weeks of injury. At that time, the maximum life expectancy for survivors was considered to be 2 to 3 years. By the late 1940s, life expectancy rose to 10 years and in the 1950s to 20 years; by the 1970s major advances in medicine allowed patients to survive both the acute and chronic stages of the injury and attendant physical illnesses. Patients began to face a range of choices about how they might achieve independence, limited only by society's attitudes toward disabilities and inaccessible environments. Although the primary concern in the 1940s was survival, today's patients must work to achieve an acceptable quality of life and long-term psychosocial adjustment to disability.[3]

People with SCI are a fairly heterogeneous group with one thing in common: a disability that penalizes them by reducing their freedom. Strangers tend to avoid contact with them, so they must learn techniques to put others at ease and help them forget about their physical differences. Contending with the physical challenges resulting from SCI can tax coping skills and psychological adjustment. The psychosocial implications faced by patients with SCIs are many and extend past the completion of rehabilitation or physical adaptation to its imposed functional limitations.

Recently researchers are focusing more attention on the psychosocial adjustment after SCI and the social consequences of the long-term impairments associated with this disability. Psychological adjustment to disability varies and involves both physical and psychological domains. Adjustment to SCI was previously thought to be largely dependent on certain physical variables, including level of injury, age at injury, and time since injury, along with the long-term impairments associated with spinal cord injury.[4,5] Long-term impairments are characterized by the physical limitations imposed by the injury and physical and medical complications associated with SCI, including loss of bowel and bladder function, spasticity, chronic pain, sexual dysfunction, and variations in blood pressure. Although physical variables are still believed to play a role in adjustment to disability, psychosocial implications can be precipitated by physical and functional impairments and are thought to play a significant role in a patient's adjustment.[3] New efforts to understand the role of psychological variables on adjustment focus on examining individual variables such as self-perception, appraisals, locus of control, attribution of blame, premorbid coping, and personality styles along with psychosocial resources and support. These factors are also thought to play a role in determining quality of life and overall life satisfaction in patients with SCI.[4,6,7]

A patient's reaction and adjustment to SCI are predictable by both physical and psychological variables; however, it is important to note that adjustment and adaptation to SCI are unique to each patient.[8] Although there is no specific formula to determine how a patient will respond to an SCI, a discussion of the physical and psychological factors associated with SCI from the time of injury through the rehabilitation process is important in understanding the impact this trauma plays in the life of a patient (Figure 5-1). Social, psychological, and emotional implications play as an important and continuing role in the patient's adjustment, as does the physical injury.

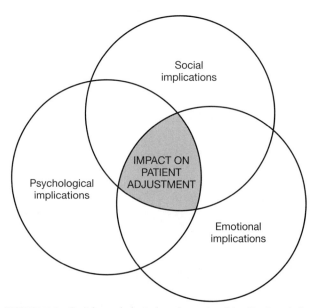

FIGURE 5-1 Social, psychological, and emotional implications influences overlap and affect patient adjustment to SCI.

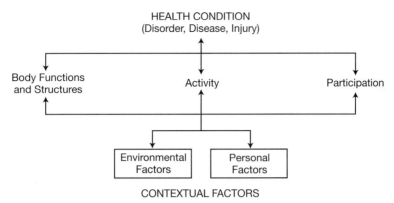

FIGURE 5-2 The *International Classification of Functioning, Disability, and Health* was developed and adopted by the WHO in 2001. Known as the ICF, the document represented by this algorithm provides a standard language and framework to describe health and health-related states and is useful in understanding and measuring health outcomes. (From WHO: *International classification of functioning, disability, and health [ICF]:* www3.who.int/icf/)

BOX 5-1 | Definitions of International Classification of Functioning, Disability, and Health Components

- **Health Conditions:** Diseases, disorders, and injuries
- **Body Functions:** Physiological functions of body systems (including psychological functions)
- **Body Structures:** Anatomical parts of the body such as organs, limbs, and their components
- **Impairments:** Problems in body function or structure such as a significant deviation or loss (both activity and participation)
- **Activity:** Execution of a task or action by an individual
- **Participation:** Involvement in a life situation
- **Activity Limitations:** Difficulties an individual may have in executing activities
- **Participation Restrictions:** Problems an individual experiences in involvement in life situations
- **Function:** Functioning of body part, the whole person, and the whole person in a social context

- **Disability:** Dysfunction at one or more levels (body part, the whole person, and the whole person in a social context) because of impairments, activity limitations, or participation restrictions
- **Contextual Factors:** The external environmental factors and internal personal factors interrelated to the health condition
- **Environmental Factors:** External factors including physical, social, and attitudinal environments in which people live and conduct their lives such as social attitudes, architectural characteristics, legal and social structures, climate, terrain
- **Personal Factors:** Internal factors including gender, age, coping styles, social background, education, profession, past and current experience, overall behavior pattern, character, and other factors that influence how disability is experienced by the individual

Adapted from World Health Organization: *International classification of functioning, disability, and health (ICF):* www3.who.int/icf/. Accessed November 2006.

During the same time period, realizing that diagnosis was not the sole predictor of health care needs and functional outcomes, the World Health Organization (WHO) developed a classification system that unifies and standardizes language concerned with the interrelationship of health and health-related states. Originally released as a trial document in 1980, the *International Classification of Impairments, Disabilities, and Handicaps* has evolved and developed over a 20-year period into a comprehensive second edition endorsed by the 54th World Health Assembly in 2001 as the *International Classification of Functioning, Disability, and Health,* known as ICF. [9]

The ICF model is based on a dynamic shift in emphasis from disability to health and functioning, which acknowledges the universal quality of disability and the continuing importance of levels of care that ensure the best functional outcomes. Just as caregivers and individuals with SCI consider a psychosocial model in the journey to adjustment, the new ICF synthesizes a biopsychosocial model that integrates the biological, individual, and social perspectives of health and care (Figure 5-2). This model was designed to clearly illustrate the interactions between health condition and contextual factors (environmental and personal factors).

Box 5-1 lists the specific terminology important to understanding the model.

ISSUES IN THE ACUTE PHASE
Hospitalization

The goal of hospitalization in the acute phase of injury is to achieve and maintain medical stabilization. Initially, the focus of the patient and his family is one of survival. Regardless of what the medical staff tells them about long-term prognosis, patients are often unaware of or do not fully appreciate the implications that SCI will have on daily life. Psychological symptoms may not be present in the early stages of treatment despite the existence of many acute stressors, including a physical traumatic injury, psychic stress, reactions of family, reactions of a larger social network, and hospitalization. [10] Once a patient is deemed to be medically stable, he is often transferred to a short-term rehabilitation hospital where he will learn how to function by the rules of his new body. Rehabilitation in the acute phase aims to stop or slow down the negative impact of the trauma. Although the rehabilitation setting is a safe, accessible environment where a patient is able to optimize his physical abilities, surrounded by

TASKS OF MOURNING

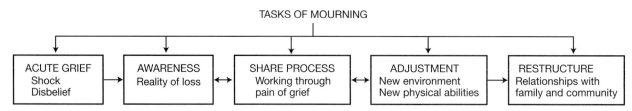

FIGURE 5-3 Tasks of mourning may help patients and their families move from the shock of acute grief to acceptance, adjustment, and restructuring of relationships.

a staff of professionals who offer positive support, these new rules can result in the onset of psychological symptoms and adjustment issues. Psychological intervention is critical at this time. Notably, studies show that the prevention of psychological syndromes through education and early intervention is a significant part of rehabilitation and critical to rehabilitation success.[11,12] The role of the rehabilitation psychologist has been characterized by the assessment of cognitive and psychological functioning and psychological interventions aimed to maximize the patient's rehabilitation and improve the patient's adjustment to his disability. Simply, the goal is to promote a sense of control out of a situation characterized by dependence.[10] For many patients, feeling dependent on others may be a foreign and oftentimes scary experience that can result in a number of emotional reactions.

Emotional Reactions

Stage theory of adjustment, originally developed to examine emotional responses to grief associated with death and dying, has been applied to early examinations of patients' emotional reactions and adjustment to SCI.[13,14] Stage theory posits that people who have experienced death or loss of personal or functional abilities often react in similar ways. Common emotional reactions include denial, anger, depression, and anxiety. According to this theory, patients work through a series of adjustment stages, including denial, anger, bargaining, depression, and acceptance. SCI researchers and clinicians have developed variations of stage theory in their effort to understand adjustment to SCI.[10,13] Although SCI research suggests that psychological adjustment does not predictably follow stages, it is important to understand the common emotional reactions through stages of adjustment after SCI. One model considers the tasks of mourning after loss and acute grief in which a patient moves from shock and disbelief through development of awareness and adjustment and finally to a restructured relationship with family and community (Figure 5-3). Table 5-1 outlines the stages of grief and adjustment, including an interpretation for a person with SCI, and the functional constructs.

Denial is defined as a rejection of the injury and resultant disability. Denial is a normal response and coping mechanism to a life-altering, tragic event. It may be a temporary phase, fluctuate over time, or become a long-term mechanism meant to maintain a premorbid sense of identity.[13] Because it is often misunderstood, denial can raise concerns among rehabilitation professionals who may perceive it as problematic. Denial, however, does not necessarily affect rehabilitation in a negative manner because it may be interpreted as a cognitive and emotional disavowal rather than a behavioral one. The clinical

TABLE 5-1	Interpretation of Stage of Grief Theory for Patients with Spinal Cord Injury	
Stage	Interpretation for SCI	Function
Denial	Hope of recovery and return to premorbid functioning	Maintain premorbid identity
Anger	Increased awareness; external expression of emotion	Control situation or destiny
Bargaining	Hope of improvement	Maintain motivation for treatment
Depression	Uncertainty of future; defeat	Grieving of losses; preparing for future
Acceptance	Willingness to do things differently	Regain quality of life

interpretation of denial is that it may arise from a patient's need to maintain hope of recovery.[3,10,13] Behaviorally, denial is seen in patients who refuse to try out adaptive equipment or perform activities of daily living. At times it may appear as a rigid and desperate attempt to maintain identity and refuse defeat. It becomes problematic when the denial of the permanence of the disability leads to self-neglect and the development of secondary conditions.[10] It is important to note that as the patient becomes aware of his limitations, the need for psychological and emotional support increases.[10,12] An increase in awareness may be manifested by psychological symptoms: anger, depression, or anxiety.

Anger is often understood to be a patient's acknowledgment or awareness of the physical magnitude and implications of his injury. It is an attempt to control his situation or destiny.[10,13] It is also the outward expression of frustration with self and situation and represents how the person is internally experiencing his disability. Through exhibiting anger, a patient is able to strike out at an environment that has ceased to cooperate. Anger or hostility is often misdirected to health professionals, rehabilitation staff, and family members. Many patients need to direct blame toward some specific force or entity as a way of understanding their injuries and making sense of the events that caused those injuries. Misdirected anger also allows a patient to displace self-blame or feelings of responsibility or guilt associated with the injury. Sometimes the patient's anger is with God. In such cases, a patient may experience a spiritual crisis as he questions his faith, beliefs, and potentially is unable to turn to a previous source of comfort and support.

Although it is a normal human reaction, anger often makes others uncomfortable. As a patient learns how to manage the

TABLE 5-2	**Signs and Symptoms of Depression**		
Mood	**Cognition**	**Behavior**
Depressed mood	Negative view of self	Tearfulness
Sadness or emptiness	Negative view of future	Insomnia or hypersomnia
Irritability	Decreased concentration	Psychomotor agitation or retardation
Apathy	Decreased ability to make decisions	Fatigue
Markedly diminished interest or pleasure in activities	Decreased ability to solve problems	Loss of energy
Feelings of worthlessness	Short-term memory loss	Significant unintentional weight loss or gain
Inappropriate guilt	Suicide ideation	Decreased or increased appetite
Helplessness		
Hopelessness		

Data from American Psychiatric Association: *Diagnostic and statistical manual of mental disorders*, Washington, DC, 1994, American Psychiatric Association; Calarco MM, Krone KP: An integrated nursing model for depressive behavior in adults: theory and implications for practice, *Nurs Clin North Am* 26:573-583, 1991; Fichtenbaum J, Kirshblum S: Psychologic adaptation to spinal cord injury. In Kirshblum S, Campagnolo DI, DeLisa JS, editors: *Spinal cord injury medicine*, Philadelphia, 2002, Lippincott Williams & Wilkins.

continuing frustrations of a body that no longer cooperates, he may become demanding or critical of the rehabilitation staff and family members. If untreated, the patient may continue to have difficulty relating to others and eventually alienate himself from a larger social network.

In an attempt to maintain a sense of control, motivation, and hope for the future, patients may engage in bargaining. Bargaining allows a patient to negotiate reality with tolerable outcomes.[13] It can be seen at different times during adjustment and can take many forms. An example of bargaining is seen when a patient with tetraplegia is reportedly willing to sacrifice the ability to walk with the hope of regaining the use of his hands. Other examples include the hope of gaining sensation without the ability to move. Patients with paraplegia bargain with the willingness to ambulate even with the use of adaptive equipment. One of the most common bargaining wishes is for the return of bowel and bladder functioning in exchange for the ability to ambulate. It is not surprising that the inability to control daily human functioning can lead to despondence.

A prolonged period of imposed helplessness with a gradual resumption of limited independent activities puts patients at risk for development of psychological symptoms in general and depression in particular.[15] As a patient becomes increasingly aware of his functional limitations and begins to grieve the associated losses, depression may ensue. Reported feelings of guilt for the effects injuries have on loved ones and the fear of becoming a burden to family members contribute to the development of depression. Emotionally, a patient may be unable to access the coping resources necessary to maintain motivation or may feel defeated by the consequences and implications of SCI.[16] Depression may be manifested by the patient's refusal to participate in treatment or to perform activities he can do independently. At times depressive symptoms are seen in a patient's refusal to participate because of his preoccupation with mild somatic complaints (e.g., nausea, headaches, dizziness, generalized pain symptoms). Although medical explanations for these symptoms may be present, this is often a sign that the patient feels psychologically defeated by his limitations. The refusal to participate in treatment, however, reinforces dependence and victimization and ultimately may contribute to the clinical depression.

Previous research and theories of adjustment to SCI suggested that depression was a normal and required part of adjustment.[10,13]

Few would argue that depression is not an understandable and appropriate reaction to this life-altering event; however, clinicians and researchers posit that most patients with SCI do not meet the diagnostic criteria for major depression as outlined by the *Diagnostic and Statistical Manual of Mental Disorders* (DSM-IV), in which five or more symptoms including depressed mood or loss of interest or pleasure must be present over a 2-week period of time. Many depressive symptoms are commonly seen throughout the adjustment process and are manifested by affective, cognitive, and behavioral symptoms[3,4,13,15] (Table 5-2).

Anxiety is also a common reaction that is precipitated by the patient's perception of fear and vulnerability. The fear might be in response to internal or external dangers that are real or imagined. For patients with SCI, fear may be the result of perceived loss of control of physical function, medical complications, or weaning from the ventilator. Anxiety symptoms can range from nervousness and sleep difficulty to panic or catastrophic reactions. It is the most common psychological symptom demonstrated by ventilator-assisted patients.[13] In patients who are ventilator dependent, anxiety is a response to the patient's fear of dying either by ventilator failure or choking on secretions. Because these patients demonstrate poor vocal quality, they may fear that medical personnel will not be able to hear and respond to their needs in the event of a medical crisis. Patients with anxiety symptoms can be demanding of medical personnel and family members for reassurance and security. Later, as a patient stabilizes, anxiety that represented a fear of dying is replaced by a fear of living with a disability.[13] The new anxiety can take the form of avoidance behaviors.

PHYSICAL SEQUELAE
Level and Severity of Injury
The physical sequelae after SCI include more than the inability for a person to use his arms and legs. There may be loss of motor skills and sensation and impairment in regulating body temperature, blood pressure, and internal organ functions, depending on the level and severity of the injury. For many patients the physical ramifications and medical complications can be more emotionally taxing than the paralysis itself because these issues can also be long term and often interfere with the patient's ability to function.[4,13,16]

Tetraplegia is characterized by impairment or loss of sensory or motor function in the cervical region as the result of an SCI. Injuries resulting in tetraplegia demonstrate impairment in the use of arms, trunk, legs, pelvic organs, and in some cases, the ability to breathe independently.[17] Mechanical ventilation is required by 41% of patients with SCI during the course of acute hospitalization.[13] Ventilator assistance not only impairs the patient's ability to breathe independently but also interferes with vocal quality and, early on, the ability to eat regular food. The majority of patients, however, are able to be weaned from the ventilator before discharge from rehabilitation.[13] Lesions at the thoracic level or lower result in paraplegia. Although the use of arms may be preserved, there is impairment of the trunk, legs, and pelvic organs depending on the level of injury.[17]

Early studies on the effects of SCI on emotional adjustment suggested that patients with higher-level injuries demonstrated poorer adjustment and higher levels of psychological distress because of the reduced independence associated with these level injuries.[3,16,18-20] Patients reported that the management of their bodies and the associated limitations are overwhelmingly difficult and therefore may choose not to participate in activities they are unable to perform independently. Recent studies have contradicted those earlier findings and have shown that level of injury is not a significant predictor of long-term adjustment.[13,20] Overall, patients with high-level injuries, including patients who are ventilator dependent, report similar life satisfaction as paraplegic patients. In sum, there is no evidence to suggest that the level of SCI or greater functional limitations result in poorer emotional adjustment.

Patients with incomplete injuries have partial preservation of sensory or motor function below the level of injury. Although these patients have better functional outcomes, many experience problems and complications similar to those of complete injuries.[3,17] Patients with incomplete lesions may continue to have bladder and bowel dysfunction, pain and spasticity, blood pressure abnormalities, temperature regulation problems, skin breakdown, sexual difficulties, depression, and the risk of unemployment because of severe physical disruptions. To a larger social community, these patients may not appear to be spinal cord injured because they might ambulate, sometimes without the use of adaptive equipment. These patients, however, continue to be faced with the challenges of disability. Often a patient with incomplete injuries is faced with adjustment difficulties as a result of his attempts to function "as if" the disability did not exist. When his body does not cooperate, he is left questioning his identity and abilities. His identity is hindered by a body that functions better than some patients'—those with complete lesions—but not as well as it functioned before injury, and not as well in comparison with able-bodied people.

Pain and Spasticity

Other consequences of SCI include chronic pain and spasticity. The initial pain that is associated with SCI usually resolves within weeks.[4] Some patients, however, are left with various forms of chronic pain, including paresthesias such as burning or tingling or hyperesthesias, which is described as increased sensitivity usually at or just below the sensory level of the lesion.[17] Patients also experience difficulty with muscle spasticity, which is reflexive

and involuntary in nature.[17,20,21] In the early stages of rehabilitation, patients confuse and possibly hope that the presence of pain symptoms and spasticity are indications of a return of functioning. The confusion associated with an inability to move and functionally use parts of the body yet feel pain is by itself disabling. As patients become aware that these symptoms do not lead to functional returns, they frequently find these symptoms to be intrusive and to interfere with daily functioning.

Somatic complaints may be a real consequence of SCI; however, pain is not strictly a physical phenomenon. The perception and response to pain involves a psychological component.[4] Psychological and social issues of SCI could have a serious impact on the resolution of somatic complaints. Researchers have argued the importance of taking the psychological, social, and biological aspects into consideration when treating patients with SCI chronic somatic complaints because chronic pain puts patients at risk for development of psychological symptoms (i.e., depression) and may lead to decreased independent behavior, less participation in daily activities, and social withdrawal.[20-23] Notably, depression is most often associated with chronic pain in patients with SCI.[20,21,24] The psychological and social consequences of SCI make management of somatic complaints more difficult for patients. Difficulty dealing with and managing pain issues can result in avoidance behaviors, decreased participation in daily activities, social withdrawal, and depression.[19,20,25] Studies have shown that psychosocial stress is directly related to reported severity of already existing pain symptoms.[24] Psychological treatment of pain is built on the premise that a patient has the ability to control his level of "suffering."[4] It has been argued that suffering is largely influenced by psychosocial variables in an individual's life; therefore, interventions need to be focused on addressing these psychosocial issues as well as the patient's emotional and behavioral reactions to pain.[21,24]

Bowel and Bladder

The inability of an individual to control his bladder and bowel function is one of the most difficult consequences of SCI.[3] Patients are not only unable to voluntarily control these functions but, depending on the level of injury, may not be able to perform management routines independently and may require the assistance of others. Performing bowel programs and learning catheterization techniques are often described as the most humiliating consequence of SCI. Patients may resist learning how to perform these practices independently and find it difficult to have family members learn how to assist them. Although many patients are able to develop a regular schedule for bladder and bowel management, incontinence is sometimes an unfortunate consequence and is extremely embarrassing for the individual. Fear of incontinence or finding an accessible bathroom can result in withdrawal from social activities and isolation. Urinary tract infections (UTIs) are a common occurrence after SCI. Over time most patients are able to identify the presence of a UTI; however, the somatic symptoms that are associated with these infections, especially in patients with chronic UTIs, may leave patients feeling discouraged and eventually cause them to withdraw from activities.[17,19]

Sexual Dysfunction

Sexuality is an important aspect of human activity and a frequent concern of patients after SCI. Many patients with SCI are at their developmental height of sexual activity and body image. Perception of body image is potentially damaged as the result of SCI. The rapid physical changes that result from spinal cord injury (e.g., atrophy, postural and positional changes) can drastically change an individual's perception from that of youth and vitality to aging and disabled.[3,13] A patient may be embarrassed by the way he looks because it may be considerably different from an able-bodied person. For some, the use of adaptive equipment (e.g., braces, canes, wheelchairs) is a concrete, daily reminder of how they are different from their peers and makes it difficult to hide from the public. Negative body image also represents a fear of judgment and rejection from the able-bodied world and can result in avoidance of social activities and isolation.

THE CLIENT'S PERSPECTIVE Sexuality

As a woman with SCI, dating was the last thing I chose to incorporate into my post-injury life. I had a boyfriend when I was injured, but the relationship only lasted for about a year because there was just too much change. I ended the relationship when it was no longer making me feel good about myself. Wheelchairs are not synonymous with women and sex in our culture.

When I started dating again, my attitude was I don't need any help from you! It's no wonder I had trouble. I didn't want to appear needy or vulnerable. But I did want to have a lasting relationship or at least give it a try. It was a confusing time for me.

I had several relationships before meeting my husband, some good and some bad, but they all contributed to making me who I am. I eventually learned that confidence and attitude are more important to being attractive than having nice legs or the perfect body, but I had huge hang-ups about this for a long time and have never owned a full-length mirror.

Sarah Everhart Skeels

Researchers have examined sexual functioning in patients with SCI to determine how patients are able to regain and maintain sexual satisfaction. Among men with SCI, sexual satisfaction was positively related to overall partner satisfaction, relationship quality, and sexual desire. Erectile functioning, level of genital sensation, and orgasm capacity have not been found to be related to overall sexual satisfaction.[26] In women with SCI, however, sexual satisfaction and drive tends to be lower than found in men with SCI. In women, both sexual satisfaction and drive continue to decrease with age, particularly in patients with comorbid psychological symptoms. More specifically, women with higher reported depressive symptoms and perceived isolation tend to report less sexual satisfaction and drive than women who demonstrate better overall adaptation to their injuries. It is important to note, however, that sexual drive and satisfaction in able-bodied women also tends to decrease with age, suggesting that sexual drive and satisfaction may be a function of age-related changes in hormone levels and body image.[27]

Overall, sexual satisfaction tends to be less a function of injury severity and more a representation of positive body image, relationship stability, and partner satisfaction. Patients who demonstrate the ability and willingness to expand their sexual repertoire to include nontraditional behaviors and means of sexual pleasure find their sex lives more satisfying.

Pressure Ulcers

Patients with SCI are at risk for development of pressure ulcers because of poor circulation along with their inability to voluntarily reposition themselves in their chairs and shift their weight.[3,17,19] The treatment for pressure ulcers requires decreased sitting time, which limits activities, opportunities for social interaction, and potentially leads to a regression of psychological states (e.g., depression) and poorer adjustment. It has been suggested that increased time in the hospital as a result of pressure ulcers and sitting restrictions can negatively affect quality of life.[3,17,19,28] In addition, psychological factors such as depression and substance abuse can lead to self-neglect and the increased risk for development of pressure ulcers.[29]

Traumatic Brain Injury

Researchers estimate that 50% of patients with SCI have cerebral insult.[3] The psychosocial issues that challenge patients with SCI are exacerbated by traumatic brain injury.[30] Complications associated with traumatic brain injury include cognitive deficits, potential seizure disorders, and personality changes. Patients who have a traumatic brain injury can show deficits in the areas of attention and concentration, learning and memory, judgment, planning, and personality changes. Deficits in learning and memory can interfere with the patient's ability to learn how to function independently from the wheelchair level or result in a patient forgetting to conduct regular weight shifts.[31] Changes in executive function may result in patients being less aware of the safety precautions needed for transfers or use of power mobility or in some cases contribute to difficulty with interpersonal relationships.

PSYCHOLOGICAL CONSEQUENCES AND ADJUSTMENT

Research designed to follow and explain psychological adjustment after SCI has attempted to define individual variables that might predict positive adjustment. Such literature suggests that adjustment to SCI may be largely predicted by psychological variables including self-perception, coping styles, and psychosocial resources.[32-37]

Self-Perception

Self-perception is defined as the way we see ourselves in relation to others and the world. Self-perception includes our self-defined identity and our perceived ability to protect or care for ourselves. It is not surprising that perception of the self can be significantly altered after SCI. Clinically, patients may perceive the person they used to be as having died. Most SCIs occur in young adulthood, although the average age of patients at the time of injury has increased over the last few years. Developmentally, patients are just learning who they are in the world and starting to become independent. They are securing their identity as adults through the completion of education, beginning a career, and forming a long-lasting romantic relationship.[3] The SCI thrusts them back into a life of dependence. The physical effects of SCI break all the rules and require patients to redefine who they are and how they are functioning. They must negotiate acceptance of themselves in relation to "as I am, who I was before the injury, and who I would have been without the SCI."[38] After injury, patients begin to learn everything they knew as if for the first time. Specifically, they must learn how to function differently on the basis of the rules of their new bodies. Learning how to do things differently requires patients to renegotiate their sense of self.[13] Self-perception is further damaged by a self-imposed thought pattern of overgeneralization that often translates as doing things differently is the same as not being able to do things as well as before the injury. Such overgeneralization is known as catastrophizing. Patients who hold this belief may conclude that not doing things as well is not worth the effort and thus choose not to participate in independent activities. Although avoidant behaviors may protect the patient from anticipated failures, these behaviors ultimately reinforce the damaged perception of self.

Researchers have also attempted to predict positive adjustment by examining age at the time of SCI along with time since injury.[5,13] Overall results indicate that younger patients tend to report a better quality of life and more life satisfaction than do older patients. Patients with SCI who were injured at an older age demonstrate higher levels of psychological distress and show more difficulty coping with and adjusting to the disability. One possible explanation for this finding is that older patients with SCI tend to perceive themselves in poorer health than younger patients with SCI and tend to be less active.[5] It has also been suggested that younger patients might demonstrate more positive adjustment because of more flexibility in coping styles or because of an ability to incorporate the limitations of their disability into their developing self-concept, whereas older patients with SCI are developmentally at a point in their lives where they may have begun assessing their purpose in life, successes and failures, and planning for the future.[13] Notably, older patients may not have the same opportunities for vocational retraining, social, and leisure opportunities as younger patients with SCI. Finally, it has been suggested that older patients with SCI who report positive adjustment may take the view that they have already lived their lives and can accept their limitations more easily than those who have not met their goals.[17]

Locus of Control

Some argue that a patient's attitude when faced with an unchangeable situation is the most important component for good outcomes.[39,40] Locus of control refers to the belief that the outcomes from experience are determined by either internal or external forces. Internal locus of control is characterized by the belief that the patient's health and recovery is based on his own behavior. It is related to self-efficacy or his ability to control the events in his life and manage a presented situation. Internally oriented patients are more likely not to perceive the injury as a great tragedy but as an adversity to be overcome. Patients who believe that they are responsible for their own health tend to have fewer symptoms of depression and more adaptive behavior than those who believe that their fate is controlled by external forces. Individuals with an internal health locus of control tend to lead more active and productive lives, tend to have fewer medical problems, and tend to demonstrate more positive adjustment.[13,41,42]

Patients with an external locus of control perceive the consequences of their injury as a disastrous event. Although externally oriented patients do well in the structured environment of the rehabilitation hospital, external locus of control has been associated with more perceived stress and limited coping.[13] On discharge, these patients may be at greater risk for development of secondary medical conditions. Finally, external locus of control among patients with SCI has been associated with a higher incidence of depression and learned helplessness and may be associated with an increased risk of suicide.[42]

Coping Styles

Individuals cope with traumatic events in different ways. Ditunno and Formal[17] suggest that, for patients to understand and accept their disabilities, there must be an attribution of blame or a place to direct their anger. Although other researchers have shown that an individual's response and adjustment to SCI is in part predicted by a patient's attribution of blame, attribution of blame either toward oneself or others for the injuries has not consistently been found to have a significant association with long-term outcomes in adjustment.[6,13]

Adjustment may be predicted by premorbid coping styles. Coping styles have been linked to adjustment to disability and are often examined in behavioral health literature. Increased stress and poor coping have been related to external locus of control, inadequate coping modes, and limited social support.[16,36,37,43] Individuals who experience a traumatic and life-altering event such as SCI are often burdened by overwhelming emotions and thoughts that result from their experience. Coping styles are cognitive and behavioral responses to these reactions. Some individuals respond by actively and extensively processing their emotions and thoughts through support seeking, problem solving, or venting. This is referred to as problem-focused coping. Other patients take a more avoidant approach or emotion-focused coping style. Emotion-focused coping is characterized by mental distancing and suppression of distressing emotions (e.g., blocking, ignoring, distracting). Studies indicate that both problem-focused and emotion-focused coping are useful in successful rehabilitation and adjustment. Fauerbach et al[44] suggest that problem-focused and emotion-focused coping promote mental control, allowing patients to experience a greater internal locus of control and predictability over the emotional implications of SCI. Consistent use of emotion-focused coping, however, has been associated with prolonged distress, psychological symptoms such as depression and anxiety, and poorer adjustment.[44]

Elfstrom et al[35] have attempted to predict psychological outcome (i.e., positive adjustment) to SCI through the development of a coping scale that addresses responses to illness and disability. This coping scale includes three factors: acceptance, fighting spirit, and social reliance (Figure 5-4). Acceptance of the injury and disability is defined by a re-evaluation of life values. Fighting spirit is characterized by efforts to behave independently and social reliance shows a tendency toward dependent behavior. The outcome scale is based on three levels of psychological response: helplessness, intrusion, and personal growth. Helplessness includes feeling perplexed, without control, and low self-esteem. Intrusion includes feelings of bitterness and a tendency toward

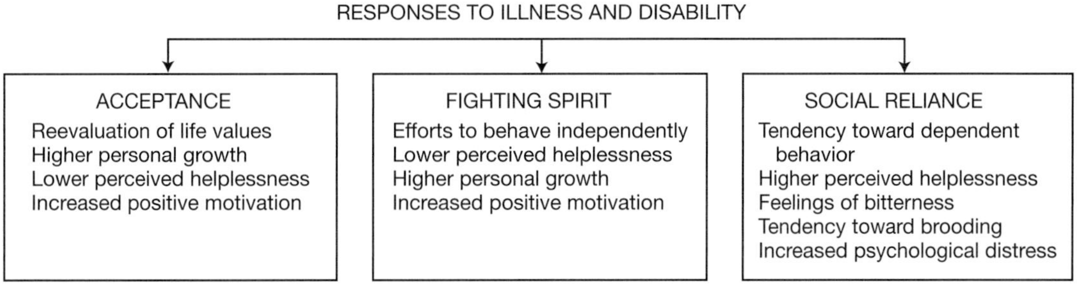

RESPONSES TO ILLNESS AND DISABILITY

ACCEPTANCE	FIGHTING SPIRIT	SOCIAL RELIANCE
Reevaluation of life values Higher personal growth Lower perceived helplessness Increased positive motivation	Efforts to behave independently Lower perceived helplessness Higher personal growth Increased positive motivation	Tendency toward dependent behavior Higher perceived helplessness Feelings of bitterness Tendency toward brooding Increased psychological distress

FIGURE 5-4 The Elfstrom Coping Scales attempt to predict adjustment to SCI on the basis of patient responses of personal growth, helplessness, and bitterness or brooding to illness and disability.

brooding. Personal growth is associated with perceived positive outcomes from a life crisis (e.g., SCI). Results of the study indicated that higher acceptance is associated with higher personal growth and lower perceived helplessness. Patients who perceive themselves with a "fighting spirit" tend to display less perceived helplessness and higher personal growth. Patients who report higher social reliance also tend to report higher helplessness and intrusion. Overall, higher levels of acceptance are associated with decreased psychological distress and increased positive motivation.[35] Patients' acceptance can be examined in relationship to the time elapsed since injury; patients injured 1 to 4 years report more helplessness, intrusion, and social reliance and less acceptance than those injured 5 or more years. This suggests that acceptance may improve over time as patients continue to participate in and regain a quality of life.

Personality Styles

Personality factors have consistently been linked to adjustment to SCI.[7,13,17,34,45] Rohe and Krause[7] have theorized that preinjury personality traits determine a patient's cognitive and behavioral responses to SCI and contribute to his adaptation to the limitations imposed by the injury. For example, patients with personality styles defined by excitement-seeking behaviors may be less conscientious than those who are characterized as assertive. They may display less energy, less determination, and less social participation and tend to engage in more catastrophizing than do more assertive patients. Patients who engage in catastrophizing tend to display more emotional difficulty and negative adjustment to SCI.[16,23,29]

Personality characteristics among recently injured patients with SCI are also predictive of positive adjustment that includes life satisfaction and negative adjustment as indicated by the development of psychiatric symptoms such as depression.[45] Table 5-3 lists negative and positive adjustment patterns.

PSYCHIATRIC DIAGNOSES

Increased psychosocial stress associated with trauma in general, and SCI in particular, puts patients at greater risk for the development of psychiatric symptoms.[15,38,46] Early difficulties in adjustment and the long-term implications and consequences of SCI can eventually lead to the onset of clinical syndromes and psychiatric diagnoses. Common psychiatric diagnoses found among the SCI population include mood disorders such as depression, anxiety disorders including acute stress and posttraumatic stress

TABLE 5-3	Individual Factors Associated with Adjustment	
Individual Factors	Positive Adjustment	Negative Adjustment
Self-perception	Who I am now?	Who I was then? Who I could have been?
Locus of control	Internal	External
Coping styles	Problem focused Emotion focused	Emotion focused
Personality styles	Assertive	Catastrophizing

disorder (PTSD), and substance use disorders.[13,29,47] Elliott et al[29] suggest that, along with psychiatric disorders, SCI patients might also be at greater risk for suicide.

Depression

Although most patients with SCI are not found to be clinically depressed, patients are at risk for and commonly display depressive symptoms. Research indicates, however, that 13% of patients will meet the DSM-IV diagnostic criteria for clinical depression[13,17,48] Calarco and Krone's[49] integrated model of depressive behavior shows the interactions of biological, cognitive, and interpersonal disruptions as related to the affect of acute and chronic stressors (Figure 5-5). These authors posit that an understanding of the interactions of "these dimensions constantly feed back and influence each other and cannot be separated," which helps clinicians individualize care to address the area of greatest need. It is important to note that biological factors may contribute to the development of depression, including the somatic effects of SCI such as fatigue, medications, and prolonged hospitalization, which may exacerbate sleep disturbance.[13]

Many studies have found that social support and coping strategies were the most significant determinants in preventing depression. For example, when the role of locus of control in the onset of depression was examined, patients with SCI who endorsed an external locus of control also reported a higher incidence of depression.[42] Similarly, Shnek et al[50] found that cognitive distortions, defined as perceived helplessness and low self-efficacy, were associated with depression among patients with SCI. It has also been argued that health, finances, and return to work deter from depression.[51] Not surprisingly, depression among patients with SCI has been associated with more days spent in the hospital and fewer functional gains in rehabilitation, along with a disruption in daily activities and social participation.[50] It is possible that the unpredictability of the onset of medical complications may be associated with cognitive distortion, which

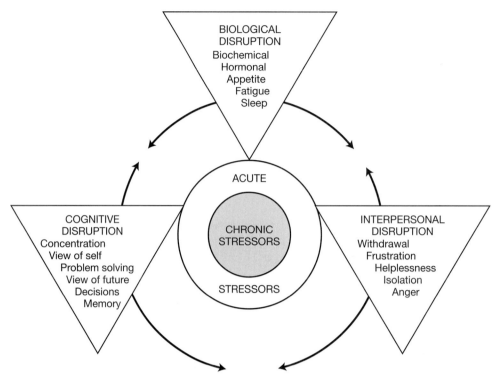

FIGURE 5-5 Calarco and Krone's Integrated Model of Depressive Behavior is based on evidence that depression is both a psychological and biological event. It conceptualizes a broad perspective where cognitive and interpersonal variables and biological response are interrelated with acute and chronic stressors.(Adapted from Calarco MM, Krone KP: An integrated nursing model for depressive behavior in adults: theory and implications for practice, *Nurs Clin North Am* 26:573-583, 1991.)

results in depression. Researchers and clinicians have also been concerned with the increase of depression levels over time. Aging and continuous medical complications associated with SCI may reduce the patients' freedom and independence, thereby contributing to an increased risk for development of depressive symptoms. In response to this concern, researchers and clinicians encourage psychological intervention to promote positive adjustment for recent patients with SCI who may be at risk for clinical depression.[13] Diagnostic criteria for a major depressive episode are outlined in the Clinical Note: Diagnostic Criteria for Major Depressive Episode.

Anxiety

Anxiety is a normal human response to the fear experienced as the threat of danger. Just as with depression, researchers and clinicians have attempted to understand the development of anxiety disorders among people with SCI. Anxiety reactions can form in response to the anticipation of perceived limitations and assumptions and overgeneralizations about an inaccessible world and rejection by the able-bodied community. Anxiety symptoms may be manifested by and range from inactivity and reduced social participation and isolation to the possible disabling effects of acute or PTSD.

Acute stress disorder and PTSD are anxiety disorders that result from an individual's experience with a traumatic event that is life threatening (Clinical Note: Diagnostic Criteria for Posttraumatic Stress Disorder). The prevalence of PTSD after SCI is questionable, with most studies suggesting an incidence of approximately 15%.[47] Patients who display symptoms of PTSD may depersonalize their injuries or may appear emotionally detached. They may have flashbacks and nightmares related to the accident that interfere with

CLINICAL NOTE **Diagnostic Criteria for Major Depressive Episode**

1. Five (or more) of the following symptoms including either depressed mood or loss of interest that are present during a 2-week period:
   - Depressed mood nearly every day on the basis of patient report or observation (tearfulness)
   - Markedly diminished interest or pleasure in almost all activities nearly every day
   - Significant change in weight; change in appetite
   - Trouble sleeping
   - Observed agitation or retardation of movement
   - Fatigue or loss of energy
   - Feelings of worthlessness or inappropriate guilt
   - Indecisiveness or inability to concentrate or solve problems by patient report or observation
   - Recurrent thoughts of death or suicidal ideation
2. Symptoms that do not meet the criteria for a mixed episode
3. Symptoms cause significant distress or impairment in social, occupational, or other important areas of functioning
4. Symptoms are not due to the direct physiological effects of a substance abuse or medication or general medical condition
5. Symptoms are not related to bereavement (symptoms last longer than 2 months and show marked functional impairments)

Data from the American Psychiatric Association: *Diagnostic and statistical manual of mental disorders*, Washington, DC, 1994, American Psychiatric Association.

both daily functions and sleep. In addition, in an attempt to control their symptoms, patients may refuse to discuss events related to the injury or fail to participate in activities that provoke their anxiety. PTSD symptoms can extend past the course of hospitalization and are often exacerbated by community re-entry activities such as driving. Psychological interventions focus on improving the patient's sense of safety and control. Psychopharmacological interventions (e.g., anxiolytics, antidepressants) can assist with PTSD-related sleep disturbance and management of anxiety symptoms that interfere with the patient's daily functioning.

CLINICAL NOTE Diagnostic Criteria for Posttraumatic Stress Disorder

1. Exposure to a traumatic event in which:
   - Actual or threatened death or serious injury or threatened injury was experienced or witnessed
   - Intense fear, helplessness, or horror were experienced or witnessed
2. Trauma is persistently re-experienced:
   - Recurrent and intrusive recollections of events, images, thoughts, or perceptions
   - Recurrent distressing dreams of trauma
   - Feeling traumatic events recurring (e.g., reliving, hallucinations, flashbacks)
   - Intense distress when exposed to cues of trauma
   - Physiological reactions to cues of trauma
3. Avoidance of everything associated with trauma:
   - Avoidance of thoughts, feelings, or conversations associated with trauma
   - Avoidance of activities, places, or people recollected with trauma
   - Inability to recall important aspects of trauma
   - Diminished interest or participation in significant activities
   - Detachment or estrangement from others
   - Altered emotions
   - Feelings of doom (shortened life)
4. Symptoms of increased arousal:
   - Sleep disturbances
   - Anger, irritability
   - Difficulty concentrating
   - Hypervigilance
   - Exaggerated startle response
5. Symptoms lasting more that 1 month
6. Symptoms cause significant distress or impairment in social, occupational, or other important areas of functioning

Data from the American Psychiatric Association: *Diagnostic and statistical manual of mental disorders*, Washington, DC, 1994, American Psychiatric Association.

Substance Abuse

The occurrence of substance abuse among patients with SCI is gaining investigative attention. Of particular interest is whether there is a risk for development of chemical addictions after SCI because of the medical and psychosocial implications associated with long-term adjustment. Research suggests that patients with SCI may be at greater risk for substance abuse problems.[52] Patients who have more difficulty coping and emotionally adjusting to their disabilities may turn to drugs and alcohol as a means of coping or emotional numbing. The use of drugs and alcohol, however, leads to more psychological difficulty and poor community reintegration.[16] Patients are also at greater risk for development of addiction to prescription pain and antispasticity medication (e.g., opioid analgesics and anxiolytics) because of the frequent occurrence of chronic pain after SCI. Drug and alcohol use by patients with SCI has been associated with lower safety judgment and emotional adjustment.[53]

Previous research suggested that patients with a premorbid history of chemical addiction may be at greater risk of having difficulty adjusting to their disabilities. Individuals with substance abuse problems have been found to spend less time in recovery and rehabilitation activities.[20] It has also been suggested that individuals with chemical addiction may have decreased investment in their health or engage in activities that interfere with self-care and potentially compromise their health.[29,53]

Patients with premorbid drinking or drug histories often revert to their patterns of use soon after they return to the community. Continuing use frequently leads to noncompliance with treatment and decreased participation in therapies and results in secondary physical complications and medical concerns. Research has also shown that patients who use drugs or alcohol are at greater risk for development of pressure ulcers after injury.[54] The long-term implications of these secondary medical issues are recurrent hospitalization, institutionalization, and revictimization.

Individuals who use alcohol and other substances as a means of coping with life stress also report a greater incidence of depression, anger, hopelessness, and anxiety soon after and during the first year after injury.[20,29,34,53] These patients also may be at greater risk for suicide than other patients with SCI.[13,51] Because patients with SCI are at greater risk of chemical addiction, substance abuse assessment and education are vital components of rehabilitation.

Suicide

Research shows that the suicide rate for disabled individuals is higher than for the general, able-bodied population. In 1996, Heinenmann[20] reported that the suicide rate for patients with SCI was two to six times greater than that of the able-bodied population.[20] Patients with SCI at higher risk of suicide include those with comorbid psychiatric diagnoses (e.g., depression, schizophrenia), previous suicide attempt(s), substance abuse, poor coping skills, and limited social support. Although it was once hypothesized, research has not consistently confirmed that the severity of injury puts patients at increased risk for suicide. SCI variables that are related to increased suicide risk include despondence, shame and guilt related to the injury, feelings of hopelessness, apathy, and family fragmentation. A suicide risk assessment is an important part of the clinical interview and is necessary on a patient's initial evaluation.[13] Suicidality can be assessed through measures, including the Beck Depression Inventory, the Beck Hopelessness Inventory, and the Beck Scale for Suicidal Ideation, all of which demonstrate a significant correlation with suicide risk.[55-58] Minimally, the clinician needs to ask patients about suicidal ideation, intent and plan and access to lethal means, prior suicide attempt(s), and comorbid substance abuse. Risk and assessment factors and warning signs associated with suicide are listed in Table 5-4.

Conclusions

Symptoms of depression and anxiety are normal and appropriate reactions to traumatic illness or injury. Such symptoms help to protect the patient from mental breakdown; they provide a signal to the patient and the therapist that the intrapsychic system is overwhelmed or that coping resources are limited. It is important not to interpret a patient's symptoms as a pathological failure in

TABLE 5-4 | Risk Factors and Warning Signs for Suicide

Risk Factors	Assessment Factors	Warning Signs
Multiple previous suicide attempts	Personal characteristics; membership in at-risk groups (e.g., gender, age, ethnicity)	Sudden changes in behavior (e.g., withdrawal, depressed mood, irritability, agitation)
Resolved plans and preparations; suicide desire	Dispositional factors (e.g., threshold for pain, self-control, problem-solving skills)	Changes in eating or sleeping habits
Isolation; limited or loss of family or social support; limited or loss of daily activities	Situational factors (i.e., support system, stressors, possible triggers)	Increased drug or alcohol use
Comorbid psychiatric diagnosis (e.g., depression, schizophrenia)	Current symptoms (e.g., increased pain, increased suicidal intent, desire and ideation, level of agitation and anxiety, problem-solving deficits, dysfunctional assumptions, capacity for reality testing, increased self-loathing)	Sudden changes in appearance (e.g., neglect)
Family history of child abuse; maltreatment		Hypersensitivity to criticism; overly self-critical
Poor coping skills; impulsive or aggressive tendencies		Inability to recover from loss; continuous and overwhelming feelings of grief, hopelessness
Barriers to mental health services		Increased isolation and withdrawal from activities
Physical illness		Drastic personality or behavioral changes; feelings of rage, revenge
Access to means of committing suicide		Increased impulsivity, recklessness, or risk-taking behaviors
Unwillingness to seek help (e.g., stigma, substance abuse)		Threatening to commit suicide, openly talking about death
Cultural and religious beliefs		Giving away personal belongings, making final arrangements
Local epidemics of suicide		Sudden and inexplicable improvements in behavior or appearance

Data from Centers for Disease Control and Prevention, National Center for Injury Prevention and Control: *Suicide: fact sheet—risk factors:* www.cdc.gov/ncipc/factsheets/suifacts.htm, accessed December 2006; National Suicide Prevention Lifeline, U.S. Department of Health and Human Services: *Suicide warning signs:* www.suicidepreventionlifeline.org, accessed December 2006; Packman WL, Marlitt RE, Bongar B et al: A comprehensive and concise assessment of suicide risk, *Behav Sci Law* 22:667-680, 2004; Wingate LR, Joiner TE Jr, Walker RL et al: Empirically informed approaches to topics in suicide risk assessment, *Behav Sci Law* 22:651-665, 2004.

coping and adjustment. Symptoms are problematic or become clinical syndromes when they cause significant impairment in the patient's functioning. On an inpatient level this is manifested in part by the patient's refusal to participate in therapies or educational programs or engage in self-care activities. In addition, it is better to reserve the use of psychotropic medications in managing and treating these disorders for situations in which the patient's ability to function has been significantly impaired or when psychological intervention alone does not produce desired effects.

PSYCHOSOCIAL IMPLICATIONS

Numerous psychosocial implications are associated with SCI, many of which contribute to a patient's quality of life. The psychosocial implications of SCI often become a focus of psychological treatment after re-entry into the community.[59-62] Indeed, these consequences may be more debilitating than the physical injury itself. Investigators have determined that quality of life can be characterized as either: positive, as reflected by high life satisfaction, or negative, as reflected by distress and depression.[62,63] This research has identified several themes, regardless of the level of injury or severity of impairment, that include the following[60]:

- Physical function and independence
- Accessibility
- Emotional well-being
- Stigma
- Relationship and social function
- Occupation
- Finances
- Physical well-being

Although these themes are similar for patients with paraplegia and tetraplegia, the quality of life for patients with tetraplegia is affected more by physical function, independence, and physical well-being (see Chapter 23).

Family Roles and Adjustment

One injured family member affects the entire family system.[1] The impact of SCI and the long-lasting effects of these injuries are not limited to the patient but extend to the patient's family and loved ones.[42,64] Just as an individual shows varying responses to SCI, family members may use different coping mechanisms and go through stages of adjustment at different times. Initially, patients and family members focus on surviving uncertainty and project recovery.[64] In some cases premorbid family functioning is exacerbated by SCI, whereas in others all the rules of family functioning can be broken. Sometimes rehabilitation professionals misunderstand family functioning and perceive family members as unsupportive when they do not go through the adjustment process at the same pace as the patient or when they refuse to learn how to care for all of the patient's needs. Quite simply, some family members are not emotionally capable of dealing with the necessary changes in family roles.

Drastic changes in family roles contribute to family stress and potential caregiver burden. Researchers and clinicians point out that caregivers of patients with SCI have levels of stress comparable to that of the injured patient.[42] Caregivers must learn new domestic roles at the same time that they are potentially learning how to physically care for their injured family member's health needs. Caregivers report that the most stressful situations concern the medical and health issues of their injured partners. For example, caregivers of patients who are ventilator dependent report increased stress and anxiety resulting from fear of medical complications and respiratory distress. This stress and imposed caregiving burden can lead to increased strain on family and marital interactions. Some have argued that these caregivers who perceive their roles as burdensome also tend to manifest higher levels of depression, caregiving burden, lower levels of life satisfaction, and marital adjustment problems.[41,64,65] Conversely, a recent study revealed that, although 79% of caregivers reported psychological distress, they were not found to be significantly depressed.[63] Symptoms of depression and distress are just as common in caregivers as in patients with SCI; however, such responses do not necessarily lead to clinical depression.

Premorbid family functioning plays an important role in successful family adjustment, just as family adjustment plays a significant role in a patient's adjustment and quality of life. Research consistently shows that families with cohesiveness, good communication, and low levels of conflict before the injury demonstrate better adjustment after SCI.[2] On the basis of these findings, it is important to include family members as part of the patient's treatment team and provide psychological support to the family during the progressive stages of rehabilitation.

Family and Social Support

Both researchers and clinicians argue that social and family support is the most significant predictor of positive adjustment after SCI.[17,19,45,59,66-68] Patients with strong family and social support tend to report lower feelings of helplessness and demonstrate greater participation in activities. Social reliance as characterized by an increased dependence on others to conduct activities that a patient is capable of performing independently, however, has been associated with heightened distress.[37] This apparent conflict can be explained as the difference between the patient's perception of dependence versus a premorbid belief in the value of independence, which is consistent with Western values of independence, privacy, and autonomy. For some patients, asking for and receiving assistance reinforces the perception of dependence.

Community Reintegration

Community reintegration after SCI continues to improve because of better acceptance by society, accessibility in the greater environment, and technology for building adaptations.[8,68] Clinicians frequently point out that before discharge patients require opportunities to explore the world outside the hospital. Although the rehabilitation hospital is accessible, it may provide the patient with a false sense of security. Patients need to learn how to navigate in an environment that is not structured for a disabled person's needs. Negotiating the environment outside the hospital is the first step toward community reintegration.

Adjustment issues are naturally triggered by the desire for independence and community reintegration coupled with the increased demands included in vocational and recreational goals. Employment opportunities may be narrowed by physical limitations, medical complications, and in some cases, cognitive deficits. Patients may require vocational retraining, which can be physically and emotionally difficult to sustain. Returning to work can also be limited by transportation and accessibility. Such increased demands and the frustration associated with restricted options can result in an exacerbation of psychological symptoms. The inability to successfully meet some of these demands can result in overgeneralizations in the patient's thought process and communications, such as "I can't do this."

Although social and recreational activities can be limited by transportation and accessibility, learning how to relate to others after SCI presents a significant challenge to many patients. Disabled individuals must learn how to develop a peer group that includes people who are able bodied as well as those who are physically challenged. Patients are concerned about how others will perceive them and whether their peers and strangers will accept them. They may find it difficult to relate to their able-bodied peers and, initially in an attempt to maintain their previous identities, they may be unwilling to develop a new group of peers with other disabled patients. Finally, dating and developing romantic relationships may be difficult because many patients feel that they are no longer desirable or have little to offer a partner.

Although life expectancy of patients with SCI has increased significantly, quality-of-life issues are influenced by the occurrence of chronic medical complications, including pressure ulcers, pain, fluctuation in blood pressure and body temperature, and difficulties with bowel and bladder management, which can prevent patients from maintaining consistent employment and can produce continuing financial hardship. This adds to the adjustments that patients and their families are required to make to their new circumstances.[4,17,52] Table 5-5 illustrates the psychological factors associated with positive and negative adjustment.

TABLE 5-5	Psychosocial Factors Associated with Adjustment	
Psychosocial Factors	Positive Adjustment	Negative Adjustment
Family support and adjustment	Positive family support	Limited or lack of family support; caregiver burden
Social and peer support	Participation in activities with existing peers and formation of new peers	Limited or lack of social/peer support; withdrawal from peer and social activities
Educational and vocational goals	Employment	Unemployment
Accessibility	Medical care Adaptive equipment Transportation	Lack of access or availability or resources

CLINICAL IMPLICATIONS AND INTERVENTIONS

In a medical rehabilitation setting, the theoretical basis of a therapist's work includes an understanding of the patient's illness or injury and its implication on psychological function. The premise of counseling patients with disabilities in general, and after SCI in particular, is based on the following notions[3]:

- It is the psychosocial issues of day-to-day living with a disability in the community environment, and not the physical aspects of disability, that determine or affect adjustment to such changes in life
- The disabled person must learn how to live in a world that is designed for and dominated by able-bodied people who may not easily accept or tolerate people with disabilities

Furthermore, counseling emphasizes the process of restoring balance among the psychosocial, biological-organic, and environmental factors in life to facilitate adjustment and to teach the individuals with disabilities to live in an environment structured for able-bodied people (Table 5-6).

After a patient is injured, he struggles to find meaning for the accident and the limitations that follow. He is challenged to develop a new identity and purpose in life.[10] One of the goals of counseling is to develop a patient's sense of control over dependence. This complements the process of rehabilitation by making the patient an active member in his treatment. Such an approach can be viewed as moving away from a medical model that focuses on underlying psychopathological processes (e.g., mental disease) as the cause of problems in adjustment. Adoption of a health care model that emphasizes maladaptive behaviors as the underlying problem can allow the patient and clinician to establish and work toward new behavioral solutions. In addition, rather than focusing on identification and elimination of disease-causing factors, counseling is focused on education and teaching adaptive behaviors to deal with the problems of living, specifically designed for a disabled person in an able-bodied community, and return to the world outside of the hospital.[3]

Recent research suggests that control promotes optimal adjustment to functional and emotional adaptation.[10,13] Patients need to master the new rules of their bodies and the emotional reactions that are associated with continuous challenges. Interventions that promote control include normalizing, empathizing, empowering, reframing, and reinforcement.[10] Patients and family members learn that they are not losing their sanity along with the physical challenges associated with SCI by normalizing the emotional reactions of shock, denial, anger, and grief. Empathizing communicates understanding of the patient's experience and allows the clinician to join with the patient and his family in their struggle for understanding and acceptance. Empowerment supports the patient's attempts to act both cognitively and emotionally. It gives the patient permission to think or act a certain way. Therapists also empower patients to use verbal communication, helping them to learn that power is not just a function of behavior or physical ability. Adjustment and coping are also affected by a patient's belief about his injury and disability. Reframing promotes control by allowing the patient to modify or change perspectives—essentially decatastrophizing—and to explain and understand life events and outcomes.

Specific strategies include the use of Socratic dialog, paradoxical intention, and humor.[39,41] Such interventions challenge the patient's tendency toward restrictive dichotomous thinking—independence versus dependence—and can help him redefine his struggle and respond differently. Reinforcement of emotional expressiveness and support-seeking behavior encourages positive behavior toward independence and mastery of self-care. It provides a sense of control by encouraging and supporting behaviors that lead to a sense of hopefulness and effectiveness.[10] It also enhances self-perception, self-efficacy, and self-worth and allows a patient to regain a purpose in life through self-control and independence (Clinical Note: Interventions to Promote Control and Independence).

CLINICAL NOTE | **Interventions to Promote Control and Independence**

- Normalize patient's emotional reactions
- Empathic understanding of the patient's experience
- Empower patient's ability to manage his care, disability, and life
- Reframe patient's potential negative perspective into a positive, constructive one
- Reinforce support-seeking behavior and expression

From Moore AD, Patterson DR: Psychological intervention with spinal cord injured patients: promoting control out of dependence, *SCI Psychosoc Process* 6:2-8, 1993.

TABLE 5-6 | Behavior as a Function of the Interaction of Psychosocial, Organic, and Environmental Variables

Psychosocial Variables	Organic Variables	Environmental Variables
Responsibility for oneself	Intelligence and cognition	Income
Coping skills	Physical impairment	Transportation
Social skills and support	Sensory abilities	Accessibility
Locus of control	General health	Education and vocationalresources
Self-confidence	Strength and endurance	Family and interpersonalsupport
Problem-solving ability	Bowel or bladder control	Availability of medical care
Belief system	Respiratory function	Availability of caregivers
Judgment	Pain	Role models

Adapted from Trieschmann RB: *Spinal cord injuries: the psychological, social, and vocational rehabilitation*, ed 2, New York, 1988, Demos Medical Publishing.

CLINICAL CASE STUDY   Psychological Adjustment to Spinal Cord Injury

Patient History

Natalie Lords is a 36-year-old woman referred to outpatient services with a T8 American Spinal Injury Association (ASIA) C paraplegia diagnosis resulting from a motor vehicle accident (MVA). She was a passenger in a car that was struck by a drunk driver; her husband, who was driving, had only minor injuries. She underwent a decompression laminectomy and fusion and wore a thoracolumbosacral orthosis for 4 weeks. Her hospital course was complicated by a right lower limb deep vein thrombosis after spinal stabilization surgery.

Natalie was moved to a rehabilitation hospital 14 days after her injury. She began to gain movement in both of her lower limbs and return of bowel and bladder function. Although she has movement in her legs, her strength is not sufficient for walking. She was discharged after 20 days and is attending outpatient therapy.

Patient's Self Assessment

Natalie is married and the mother of a daughter (age 6 years) and a son (age 8 years). Before her injury she was a physical education teacher in an elementary school. Her husband is a lawyer who works extremely long hours.

While in the acute hospital setting, Natalie would frequently make comments such as, "When I get home and everything is back to normal the children will be fine." Early in her rehabilitation, Natalie often commented about how lucky her husband was that he was not injured because he would never have been able to manage this; that he is really in love with his job. As time went on Natalie commented, "If only I could walk, I'd rather wear a diaper," which indicated her placing bowel and bladder control as a lower priority.

After her discharge from the rehabilitation hospital, Natalie was followed up as an outpatient at the same facility. During outpatient therapy, Natalie would discuss the changes in her home environment and the construction that was helping to make her home accessible. She was in the process of purchasing an adaptive car so she could have greater independence from her husband and be able to transport her children without relying on friends and family. Sometimes her children would come to therapy and watch what she was learning; her daughter often asked, "When are you going to walk Mommy?" And Natalie would respond saying, "Not now, dear."

Her husband did not accompany her to therapy and Natalie would comment that his plate was full and that help from her parents kept the house functioning because her husband's work hours continued to increase. She would also talk about her husband's lack of presence and the break down in their communication in their marriage. Natalie frequently came to therapy with complaints of nausea and requests for her therapist to assist her with transfers that she typically could perform independently.

Clinical Assessment
Patient Appearance
- Height 5 feet 2 inches, weight 108 pounds, body mass index 19.8

Cognitive Assessment
- Alert, oriented × 3

Cardiopulmonary Assessment
- Blood pressure 118/68 mm Hg, heart rate at rest 70 beats/min, respiratory rate 11 breaths/min, cough flows are ineffective (<360 L/min), vital capacity is reduced (2.5 L)

Musculoskeletal and Neuromuscular Assessment
- Motor assessment reveals T8 ASIA C motor score is 70, 5/5 all upper limbs and 2/5 all lower limbs, sensory score pinprick 112, light touch 112
- Deep tendon reflexes 3+ below the level of lesion

Integumentary and Sensory Assessment
- Skin is intact throughout; sensory intact to S5

Range of Motion Assessment
- Passive and active range of motion are within normal limits

Mobility and Activities of Daily Living Assessment
- Independent with bed mobility and transfers to all surfaces
- Independent with pressure relief and manual wheelchair maneuvering on all surfaces
- Independent in all self-care activities of daily living
- Passed driver's examination and is in the process of purchasing a vehicle

Equipment
Manual wheelchair and transfer board

Evaluation of Clinical Assessment
Natalie Lords is a 36-year-old woman referred to psychology with a T8 ASIA C paraplegia diagnosis resulting from MVA. She began attending outpatient physical therapy for 7 weeks post injury and is now 9 weeks post injury. She is seeking counseling to assist with her adjustment to her disability.

Patient's Care Needs
1. Evaluation for psychology services
2. Support services for adjustment to her disability

Diagnosis and Prognosis
Diagnosis is T8 incomplete, ASIA C paraplegia with a prognosis of full independence with all home- and work-related patient goals.

Preferred Practice Patterns*
Impaired Muscle Performance (4C), Joint Mobility, Motor Function, Muscle Performance, and Range of Motion Associated With Fracture (4G), Primary Prevention/Risk Reduction for Cardiovascular/Pulmonary Disorders (6A), Prevention/Risk Reduction for Integumentary Disorders (7A)

Team Goals
1. Team to use consistent encouragement to maintain or increase functional capacity to achieve independence and reduce reliance on the husband
2. Team to schedule a family visit with the husband to observe skill level so that there is better communication within the family and with the rehabilitation team
3. Patient to seek counseling with family difficulties or attend a peer support group

Patient Goals
"I want to get my life back in order. I want to take care of my children and return to work part time."

Care Plan
Treatment Plan and Rationale
- Schedule patient for psychology evaluation
- Assess the need for support group and vocational counseling referrals
- Continue functional retraining to gain independence

Interventions
- Outpatient one-on-one psychology counseling

Documentation and Team Communication
- Team consultation related to Natalie's adjustment to her disability focused on her ability to meet her goals biweekly
- Documentation/team consultation about physical rehabilitation goals

Continued

SUMMARY

SCI is a traumatic, life-altering event resulting in multiple physical and psychological consequences. Clinicians play an active role in promoting mental health, adjustment to disability, and achievement of community reintegration by patients after SCI. Psychosocial interventions aimed at helping individuals develop their coping strategies and expand social support can assist patients with SCI with positive adjustment.[35,37] Understanding the biological, psychological, and social implications of SCI is essential to treatment. Mental health professionals must be knowledgeable about these issues and be able to educate patients, family members and caregivers, and health care professionals about the psychological risks associated with the challenges facing patients with SCI as they work to regain their lives.

Premorbid psychological and social functioning contributes to a patient's ability to regain a satisfying life. Because the patient's perception of his identity is frequently damaged, part of the task is redeveloping a sense of self and control in the face of challenging physical limitations. Learning how to relate to others is crucial for family functioning, peer and social relationships, and vocational goals.

There are, however, no specific rules or time frames in understanding or achieving psychological adjustment and adaptation to spinal cord injury. Mental health professionals assist patients in psychological adaptation to their disabilities and as they strive to find a balance in their lives. This new balance will include developing and maintaining a purpose in life, securing their identities, and finding a place for their disabilities. When the disability is no longer the patient's dominant concern, adjustment and adaptation has been achieved.[20]

REFERENCES

1. Gill M: Psychosocial implications of spinal cord injury, *Crit Care Nurs Q* 22:1-7, 1999.
2. Glass CA, Jackson HF, Dutton J et al: Estimating social adjustment following spinal trauma, I: who is more realistic—patient or spouse? A statistical justification, *Spinal Cord* 35:320-325, 1997.
3. Trieschmann RB: The dimension of the problem. In Trieschmann RB, editor: *Spinal cord injuries: the psychological, social, and vocational rehabilitation,* ed 2, New York, 1988, Demos Medical Publishing.
4. Trieschmann RB: Long-term adjustment issues. In Trieschmann RB, editor: *Spinal cord injuries: the psychological, social, and vocational rehabilitation,* ed 2, New York, 1988, Demos Medical Publishing.
5. Krause JS: Aging and life adjustment after spinal cord injury, *Spinal Cord* 36:320-328, 1998.
6. Brown K, Bell MH, Maynard C et al: Attribution of responsibility for injury and long-term outcomes of patients with paralytic spinal cord trauma, *Spinal Cord* 37:653-657, 1999.
7. Rohe DE, Krause JS: The five-factor model of personality: findings in males with spinal cord injury, *Assessment* 6:203-214, 1999.
8. Stiens SA, Kirshblum SC, Groah SL et al: Spinal cord injury medicine, 4: optimal participation in life after spinal cord injury: physical, psychosocial, and economic reintegration into the environment, *Arch Phys Med Rehabil* 83(3 Suppl):S72-81, S90-S98, 2002.
9. World Health Organization: *International classification of functioning, disability and health (ICF):* www3.who.int/icf/. Accessed November 2006.
10. Moore AD, Patterson DR: Psychological intervention with spinal cord injured patients: promoting control out of dependence, *SCI Psychosoc Process* 6:2-8, 1993.
11. Lesky J: Needs of paraplegics with respect to psychological care during initial rehabilitation: a retrospective study, *Rehabilitation* 40:76-83, 2001.
12. Dewar AL: Challenges to communication: supporting the patients with SCI with their diagnosis and prognosis, *Spinal Cord Injury Nurs* 18:187-190, 2001.
13. Fichtenbaum J, Kirshblum S: Psychologic adaptation to spinal cord injury. In Kirshblum S, Campagnolo DI, DeLisa JS, editors: *Spinal cord injury medicine,* Philadelphia, 2002, Lippincott Williams & Wilkins.
14. Kubler-Ross E: *On death and dying,* New York, 1969, Macmillan.
15. Fullerton DT, Harvey RF, Klein MH et al: Psychiatric disorders in patients with spinal cord injury, *Arch Gen Psychiatry* 38:1369-1371, 1981.
16. Kennedy P, Marsh N, Lowe R et al: A longitudinal analysis of psychological impact and coping strategies following spinal cord injury, *Br J Health Psychol* 5:157-172, 2000.
17. Ditunno JF, Formal CS: Chronic spinal cord injury, *N Engl J Med* 330:550-556, 1994.
18. Marino RJ, Barros T, Biering-Sorenson F et al: International standards for neurological classification of spinal cord injury, *J Spinal Cord Med* 26:S50-S56, 2003.
19. Herrick SM, Elliott TR, Crow F: Social support and the prediction of health complications among persons with spinal cord injuries, *Rehabil Psychol* 39:231-250, 1994.
20. Heinemann AW: Spinal cord injury. In Goreczny AJ, editor: *Handbook of health and rehabilitation psychology,* New York, 1995, Plenum Press.
21. Matthew KM, Ravichandran G, May K et al: The biopsychosocial model and spinal cord injury, *Spinal Cord* 39:644-649, 2001.
22. Gerhart KA, Johnson RL, Whiteneck GG: Health and psychosocial issues of individuals with incomplete and resolving spinal cord injuries, *Paraplegia* 30:282-287, 1992.

23. Turner JA, Jensen MP, Warms CA et al: Catastrophizing is associated with pain intensity, psychological distress, and pain-related disability among individuals with chronic pain after spinal cord injury, *Pain* 98:27-134, 2002.

24. Widerstrom-Noga EG, Felipe-Cuervo E, Yezierski RP: Relationships among clinical characteristics of chronic pain after spinal cord injury, *Arch Phys Med Rehabil* 82:1191-1197, 2001.

25. Widerstrom-Noga EG, Felipe-Cuervo E, Yezierski RP: Chronic pain after spinal cord injury: interference with sleep and daily activities, *Arch Phys Med Rehabil* 82:1571-1577, 2001.

26. Phelps J, Albo M, Dunn K et al: Spinal cord injury and sexuality in married or partnered men: activities, function, needs, and predictors of sexual adjustment, *Arch Sexual Behav* 30:591-602, 2001.

27. Black K, Sipski ML, Strauss SS: Sexual satisfaction and sexual drive in spinal cord injured women, *J Spinal Cord Med* 21:240-244, 1988.

28. Krause JS: Skin sores after spinal cord injury: relationship to life adjustment, *Spinal Cord* 36:51-60, 1988.

29. Elliott TR, Kurylo M, Chen Y et al: Alcohol abuse history and adjustment following spinal cord injury, *Rehabil Psychol* 47:278-290, 2002.

30. Fee FA, Fee VC: Psychological consequences of concomitant spinal cord injury and traumatic brain injury, *SCI Psychosoc Process* 8:106-111, 1994.

31. Tun CG, Tun PA, Wingfield A: Cognitive function following long-term spinal cord injury, *Rehabil Psychol* 42:163-182, 1997.

32. Hicken BL, Putzke JD, Sherer JM et al: Life satisfaction following spinal cord and traumatic brain injury: a comparative study, *J Rehabil Res Dev* 39:359-365, 2002.

33. North NT: The psychological effects of spinal cord injury: a review, *Spinal Cord* 37:671-690, 1999.

34. Krause JS, Davis RV: Prediction of life satisfaction after spinal cord injury: a four-year longitudinal approach, *Rehabil Psychol* 37:49-59, 1992.

35. Elfstrom ML, Kreuter M, Ryden A et al: Effects of coping on psychological outcome when controlling for background variables: a study of traumatically spinal cord lesioned persons, *Spinal Cord* 40:408-415, 2002.

36. Galvin LR, Godfrey HP: The impact of coping on emotional adjustment to spinal cord injury (SCI): review of the literature and application of stress appraisal and coping formulation, *Spinal Cord* 39:615-627, 2001.

37. Elfstrom ML, Kreuter M, Ryden A et al: Linkages between coping and psychological outcomes in spinal cord lesioned: development of SCL-related measures, *Spinal Cord* 40:23-29, 2002.

38. Kennedy P, Duff J, Evans M et al: Coping effectiveness training reduces depression and anxiety following traumatic spinal cord injury, *Br J Clin Psychol* 42:41-52, 2003.

39. Thompson NJ, Coker J, Krause JS et al: Purpose in life as a mediator of adjustment after spinal cord injury, *Rehabil Psychol* 48:100-108, 2003.

40. Frankl VE: *Man's search for meaning*, Boston, 1962, Beacon Press.

41. Chan RC: Stress and coping in spouses of persons with spinal cord injuries, *Clin Rehabil* 14:137-144, 2000.

42. MacLeon L, MacLeod G: Control cognitions and psychological disturbances in people with contrasting physically disabling conditions, *Disabil Rehabil* 20:448-456, 1998.

43. Belciug MP: Coping responses in patients with spinal cord injury and adjustment difficulties, *Int J Rehabil Res* 23:157-159, 2001.

44. Fauerbach JA, Lawrence JW, Bryant AG et al: The relationship of ambivalent coping to depressive symptoms and adjustment, *Rehabil Psychol* 47:387-401, 2002.

45. Elliott TR, Herrick SM, Witty TE et al: Social support and depression following spinal cord injury, *Rehabil Psychol* 37:37-48, 1992.

46. Cook DW: Psychological adjustment to spinal cord injury: incidence of denial, depression, and anxiety, *Rehabil Psychol* 26:97-104, 1979.

47. Kennedy P, Duff J: Post traumatic stress disorder and spinal cord injuries, *Spinal Cord* 39:1-10, 2001.

48. American Psychiatric Association: *Diagnostic and statistical manual of mental disorders*, Washington, DC, 1994, American Psychiatric Association.

49. Calarco MM, Krone KP: An integrated nursing model for depressive behavior in adults: theory and implications for practice, *Nurs Clin North Am* 26:573-583, 1991.

50. Shnek ZM, Foley FW, LaRocca NG et al: Helplessness, self-efficacy, cognitive distortions, and depression in multiple sclerosis and spinal cord injury, *Ann Behav Med* 19:287-294, 1997.

51. Elliott TR, Frank R: Depression following spinal cord injury, *Arch Phys Med Rehabil* 77:816-823, 1996.

52. McKinley WO, Jackson AB, Cardenas DD et al: Long-term medical complications after traumatic spinal cord injury, *Arch Phys Med Rehabil* 80:1402-1410, 1999.

53. Bombardier CH, Rimmele C: Alcohol use and readiness to change after spinal cord injury, *Arch Phys Med Rehabil* 47:278-290, 1998.

54. Tate DG, Forchheimer MB, Krause JA et al: Patterns of alcohol and substance use and abuse in persons with spinal cord injury: risk factors and correlates, *Arch Phys Med Rehabil* 85:1837-1847, 2004.

55. Beck A: *Beck depression inventory II*, San Antonio, TX, 1996, Psychological Corporation.

56. Beck A: *Beck scale for suicide ideation*, San Antonio, TX, 1991, Psychological Corporation.

57. Beck A: *Beck hopelessness inventory*, San Antonio, TX, 1988, Psychological Corporation.

58. Packman WL, Marlitt RE, Bongar B et al: A comprehensive and concise assessment of suicide risk, *Behav Sci Law* 22:667-680, 2004.

59. Noreau L, Fougeyrollas P: Long-term consequences of spinal cord injury on social participation: the occurrences of handicap situations, *Disabil Rehabil* 22:170-180, 2000.

60. Gerhart KA, Weitzenkamp DA, Kennedy P et al: Correlates of stress in long-term spinal cord injury, *Spinal Cord* 37:183-190, 1999.

61. Manns PJ, Chad KE: Components of quality of life for persons with quadriplegic and paraplegic spinal cord injury, *Qual Health Res* 11:795-811, 2001.

62. Krause JS, Kemp B, Coker J: Depression after spinal cord injury: relation to gender, ethnicity, aging, and socioeconomic indicators, *Arch Phys Med Rehabil* 81:1099-1109, 2000.

63. Kemp BJ, Krause JS: Depression and life satisfaction among people aging with post-polio and spinal cord injury, *Disabil Rehabil* 21:241-249, 1999.

64. Kreuter M, Sullivan M, Dahllof AG et al: Partner relationships, functioning, mood, and global quality of life in persons with spinal cord injury and traumatic brain injury, *Spinal Cord* 36:252-261, 1998.

65. Sullivan J: Surviving uncertainty and projecting recovery: a qualitative study of patients' and family members' experiences with acute spinal cord injury, *Spinal Cord Injury Nurs* 18:78-86, 2001.

66. Manigandan C, Saravanan B, Macaden A et al: Psychological well-being among carers of people with spinal cord injury, *Spinal Cord* 38:559-562, 2000.

67. Fougeyrollas P, Noreau L, Bergeron H et al: Social consequences of long term impairments and disabilities: conceptual approach of assessment of handicap, *Int J Rehabil Res* 21:127-141, 1998.

68. Stiens SA, Bergman SB, Formal CS: Spinal cord injury rehabilitation: individual experiences, personal adaptation, and social perspectives, *Arch Phys Med Rehabil* 78(3 Suppl):65-72, 1997.

SOLUTIONS TO CHAPTER 5 CLINICAL CASE STUDY

Psychological Adjustment to Spinal Cord Injury

1. Natalie demonstrated various stages of adjustment, including denial and anger, during her early hospitalization; this response is not unusual or abnormal for an individual who has sustained a life-altering injury. She also began to exhibit coping mechanisms (e.g., bargaining) with her comments about a trade-off approach regarding walking versus bladder control. This coping technique helped Natalie to manage her adjustment to her disability within tolerable levels.

During her stay at the rehabilitation hospital she continued to exhibit anger. Her anger appeared to be related to her interaction and feelings with her husband. After her release, Natalie exhibits possible signs of depression when she comes for outpatient therapy, which are exemplified by her complaints of nausea and inability to perform transfers independently. Natalie is not yet at the stage of fully developing an awareness of the family's perception of her disability and therefore cannot fully adjust through resolution of this dilemma.

2. Stress is obvious in this family dynamic. The husband appears to have no experience with the caretaking role; he reportedly increases his work hours to avoid the family situation, although this may also be an effort to bring in more income to cover new expenses along with the loss of Natalie's income and an avoidance of guilt feelings because only his wife was injured in the accident. Their children were quite naturally in denial during the outpatient phase.

3. Team members can empathize with Natalie and the family throughout all phases of rehabilitation to help them gain understanding and acceptance of their changed life situation and to make successful adjustments to lifestyle. Both Natalie and her family will benefit from interventions that promote control. Empowerment through communication helps the patient to gain control and will give Natalie permission for emotional responses, including anger, as she works through her adjustment. In addition, empowering Natalie through tactful communication about the importance of bowel and bladder control instead of merely acquiescing to her bargaining comments about ambulation may help her to prioritize her goals without denying her the eventual goal of ambulation.

In addition to working on the physical challenges associated with SCI, team members can help Natalie and her family in understanding that they are not losing their sanity by normalizing the emotional reactions of shock, denial, anger, and grief. Early intervention focused on support, communication, and other marital issues would appear to be appropriate for this couple. Indeed, research supports the importance of including family members as part of the patient's treatment team and providing psychological support to the family during the progressive stages of rehabilitation. Family function plays an important role in successful family adjustment and a significant role in the Natalie's adjustment and quality of life. Thus, families with cohesiveness, good communication, and low levels of conflict before SCI demonstrate better adjustments.

Reframing and reinforcing conversations during Natalie's outpatient rehabilitation sessions will help to promote her and her family's control as they make positive steps toward adjustment (e.g., researching and buying an adapted vehicle, remodeling their home for accommodated access).

Reinforcing these steps is positive and will help Natalie gain independence and control of her life and restore her parental role within a new framework, which is critical during the outpatient period when she is exhibiting signs of depression.

The team should also refer Natalie and her family to the appropriate psychological expert and to outside resources that will assist them in the adjustment and acceptance of an altered lifestyle as a result of the SCI.

CHAPTER SIX

Evaluation

Sue Ann Sisto, PT, MA, PhD, and Kim Ratner, PT, BS

Despite all of our sophisticated tools, we must remember that we still can't measure the most important determinant of rehabilitation success, the human spirit. As a result, we should never underestimate what an individual is capable of achieving.

Trevor (C6 SCI)

A precise and comprehensive evaluation is fundamental to the rehabilitation of a patient with spinal cord injury (SCI). Daily evaluation of a patient's neurological status is necessary during the acute stage of care to monitor the rapid changes seen within the first few days and weeks after injury. The physician and rehabilitation team use components of their evaluations to determine when a patient is medically stable and ready to begin participation in physical and occupational therapy (see Chapter 1).

The initial evaluation sets the foundation for any therapeutic program. The data collected are used to identify the current physical and mental status, which are the basis for appropriate treatment intervention and the establishment of goals for the patient and caregivers. This initial baseline also sets a benchmark to which all future evaluations will be compared. Such comparisons allow the rehabilitation team to identify improvement or deterioration in status, the patient's response to treatment, and the need for goal modification. In addition, this evaluation begins the therapeutic interaction between the therapist and the patient. It is the first opportunity the therapist has to develop a rapport with the patient and learn about his expectations. It is also the first opportunity to educate the patient and his family about the SCI and the rehabilitation process.

Because of increasingly shorter hospital stays, it is imperative that the rehabilitation team initiate the patient and family education process as soon as possible while remaining sensitive to the psychological needs and learning readiness of those involved. The potential for negative consequences could result without proper education about skin care, weight shifts, passive range of motion (ROM) techniques, and safety considerations involved in mechanical ventilator troubleshooting. These components of care need to be explained, demonstrated, and practiced at the earliest stage possible to ensure optimal outcomes.

After the initial evaluation is complete and treatment is begun, varying components of the evaluation process are integrated into each treatment session. The therapist re-evaluates changes in the patient's signs and symptoms each session to assess the effectiveness of the treatment program, makes appropriate interventions modifications, and communicates with team members accordingly. Documentation of objective measurements within each progress note is the professional responsibility of the therapists and a requirement of most third-party reimbursement agencies.

A comprehensive evaluation is also performed just before the patient's discharge. This evaluation may be performed at discharge from the acute care hospital, acute rehabilitation hospital, or outpatient rehabilitation center. A patient is discharged to home care or to subacute care and may even be discharged to home while still wearing a halo traction orthosis device if he is functional in all other capacities. Regardless of discharge disposition, a thorough evaluation ensures the best continuity of care possible. This evaluation provides valuable information for the patient and his family or prospective caregivers regarding his current status and recommendations for continued care. The discharge evaluation also provides future caregivers with information about the effectiveness of initial treatment techniques and highlights areas that need further attention. In addition, the discharge summary documents treatment that can be used as the basis for outcome studies to illustrate the effectiveness of care practices. Current health care environments require efficiency and accountability. Outcome studies assist the rehabilitation team in identifying strengths and weaknesses of the therapeutic program as a whole.

EVALUATION PROCEDURES

The evaluation of a patient with an SCI includes both orthopedic and neurological components. The clinician must be competent in the standard techniques of evaluating musculoskeletal status and be able to modify those techniques when positions are limited or orthoses are present. For example, a patient may be limited to the side-lying position in an effort to facilitate healing of a sacral pressure ulcer. A patient may require a halo traction orthosis device for cervical stability, which limits positioning options and movement of the upper fourth of the body. Prone positioning is unlikely if not impossible, at least in the very acute stages after injury (see Chapter 2). Standard ROM and manual muscle testing (MMT) procedures are not possible in these situations in which the therapist must use problem-solving skills to develop alternative testing protocols that can still provide objective measures. Modified evaluation positions or conditions should be documented in detail so that they can be reproduced during future evaluations.

Guidelines established by the facility and the design of proprietary forms often direct the method a therapist uses to record information. An interdisciplinary assessment form includes evaluation information for physical therapy (Figure 6-1) and occupational therapy (Figure 6-2) along with nursing, speech, psychosocial, recreation, vocational, and case management data. Each member of the interdisciplinary team has an assigned section within this type of documentation. Therapists may gather more information than can be included in their designated sections, in which case they attach a separate progress note to the form so that all data remain a part of the official medical record. Greater detail in the documented evaluation findings will better support specific goals and improve the therapist's ability to monitor patient progress.

INTERDISCIPLINARY ADMISSION ASSESSMENT — PHYSICAL THERAPY

VITAL SIGNS	PAIN
Resting HR:	Intensity: 0 1 2 3 4 5 6 7 8 9 10
Resting BP:	Locations:
Premorbid Status:	Description:
Cognitive Status:	

FUNCTIONAL MOBILITY	STATUS	COMMENTS
Rolling Left		
Rolling Right		
Supine to Sit		
Sit to Supine		
W/C <-> Mat/Bed		
Sit <-> Stand		
Ambulation		
Stairs/Curbs		
W/C Propulsion		
W/C Parts Management		
Other		

Key: D=Dependent   Max A=Maximum Assist   Mod A=Moderate Assist   Min A=Minimum Assist   CG=Contact Guard
CS=Close Supervision   DS=Distant Supervision   TBA=To be assessed as appropriate   MOD I=Modified Independent

LOWER LIMB LIMITATIONS	RIGHT	LEFT
MMT/Motor Control		
ROM/Tone		
Sensation/Proprioception		

KEY: MODIFIED ASHWORTH SCALE (FOR SPASTICITY)	KEY: CLONUS
0 = No increase in muscle tone (normal or flaccid) 1 = Slight increase, catch and release or minimal resistant at end of ROM 1+ = Slight increase, catch followed by minimal resistance throughout remainder (<<<1/2) ROM 2 = More marked increase through mot of ROM, but affected part moves easily 3 = Considerable increase, passive ROM difficult 4 = Affected part rigid in flexion or extension	0 = No clonus 1 = 1 to 2 beats 2 = Moderate 3 = Sustained

BALANCE

Sitting: Static _____   Dynamic _____
Standing: Static _____   Dynamic _____

KEY: STATIC BALANCE	KEY: DYNAMIC BALANCE
1. Poor - Requires Max A to maintain static position 2. Poor Requires Mod A to maintain static position 3. Poor + Requires Min A to maintain static position 4. Fair - Requires CG to maintain static position 5. Fair Maintains static position with CS (< 2 min) 6. Fair + Maintains static position with CS (> 2 min) 7. Good - Maintains static position vs min resistance 8. Good Maintains static position vs mod resistance 9. Good + Maintains static position vs max resistance	1. Poor - Requires Max A to right; unable to move voluntarily from midline 2. Poor Able to move through 25%-50% range, requires Mod A to return 3. Poor + Able to move through 50% range, requires Min A to return 4. Fair - Able to move through 50%-75% range, requires CG to return 5. Fair Able to move through 75% range with CG, or 50%-75% with CS 6. Fair + Able to move through full range with CS, all directions 7. Good - Independent in basic dynamic balance activities 8. Good Independent in functional dynamic balance activities 9. Good + Independent in high level dynamic balance activities

Patient & Family Goals: _____

Patient Oriented to PT? ☐ YES ☐ NO **Assistive device(s) patient has access to:** _____
Patient & Family Education: _____
Assessment: _____
Short Term Goals: _____

DATE:	TIME	SIGNATURE:	LICENSE#:

FIGURE 6-1   Interdisciplinary Admission Assessment—Physical Therapy.

INTERDISCIPLINARY ADMISSION ASSESSMENT — OCCUPATIONAL THERAPY

SOCIAL HISTORY

Employed: __ | Unemployed: __ | Disability: __ | Retired: __ | Driving: __ Y, __ N | ADL Status Prior to Admission: __

Lives Alone: __ Y, __ N | Family Support: __ Y, __ N | Comments:

Home: ___ House; ___ Apt.; ___ # of Floors | Comments:

Entry: __ Steps; __ Railing? __ Y (L/R/B), __ N; __ Elevator Available? __ Steps Inside; __ Railing? __ Y (R/L/B), __ N

Patient's Bedroom: _____ Floor Location; Bathroom Locations: ____ 1/2 Baths (floor); ____ Full Baths (floor)

Bathroom Accessibility: Tub with Shower? ___ Y, ___ N; Grab Bars? ___ Y, ___ N; Shower/Tub Seat? ___ Y, ___ N;
Toilet Elevated? ___ Y, ___ N; Grab Bars? ___ Y, ___ N

HEARING
Within Functional Limits __; Comments _____ | Impaired __; Comments _____

VITAL SIGNS
Resting HR _____ | Resting BP _____

PAIN

0 1 2 3 4 5 6 7 8 9 10 | Location _____ | Description _____

SITTING BALANCE

Static _____ | Dynamic _____ (see Figure 6-1)

UPPER LIMB LIMITATIONS (ROM, Strength, Sensation, Coordination, Proprioception, Tone, see Figure 6-1)
Circle Dominant Hand

LEFT: | RIGHT:

VISUAL SCREENING

Vision: | Within Functional Limits ____ | Impaired ___ Y, ___ N | Glasses? ___ Y, ___ N

Acuity _____ | Visual Fields _____ | Oculomotor _____

Binocular Skills _____ | Inattention _____ | Visual Processing _____

COGNITION

Cognitive Function: | Intact ___ | Grossly Intact ___ | Impaired ___ | Arousal: | Not Impaired ___ | Impaired ___

Orientation: | Intact ___ | Grossly Intact ___ | Impaired ___ | Comments _____

Attention: | Intact ___ | Grossly Intact ___ | Impaired ___ | Comments _____

Behaviors Observed: _____

Short Term Memory:	Intact __	Grossly Intact __	Impaired __	Long Term Memory:	Intact __	Grossly Intact __	Impaired __
Problem Solving:	Intact __	Grossly Intact __	Impaired __	Flexibility:	Intact __	Grossly Intact __	Impaired __

FUNCTIONAL ACTIVITY	Status	Comments	Long-Term Goals	Key
Feeding				I=Independent
Grooming and Hygiene				Mod I=Modified Independent DS=Distant Supervision
Upper Body Dressing				CS=Close Supervision
Lower Body Dressing				CG=Contact Guard Min A=Minimal Assistance
Transfer to Toilet				Mod A=Moderate Assistance
Transfer to Tub/Shower				Max A=Maximum Assistance D=Dependent
Home Management				NA=Not applicable

Patient & Family Goals: _____

Patient Oriented to OT? ☐ YES ☐ NO Assistive device(s) patient has access to: _____

Patient & Family Education: _____

Assessment: _____

Short Term Goals: _____

DATE: | TIME | SIGNATURE: | LICENSE#:

FIGURE 6-2 Interdisciplinary Admission Assessment—Occupational Therapy.

The evaluation and examination process must consider federal laws, state practice laws, and insurance requirements for reimbursement. Each facility has procedures for ensuring that all documentation is accurate and current. The therapist can follow the American Physical Therapy Association's five elements of patient management: examination, evaluation, diagnosis, prognosis, and intervention.[1] These steps include the patient history, systems review, and tests and measures.

The history is a systematic gathering of past and current information related to the reasons for seeking care. The systems review is a brief examination of the anatomical and physiological status of the cardiopulmonary, integumentary, musculoskeletal and neuromuscular systems, and the communication ability, affect, cognition, language, and learning style. Tests and measures are the means of gathering data.[1]

The therapist uses the elements of the examination and critical thinking skills to formulate the evaluation. Each evaluation includes the following:

- A subjective (S) component, which includes a historical intake including a thorough chart review and a patient and family interview
- An objective (O) component, which includes a comprehensive systems review, including test measures of the neuromusculoskeletal systems and functional evaluation
- An assessment (A) of the information the clinician has gathered
- A plan (P), which includes the problem list along with short- and long-term goals

On the basis of the component letters, this form of documentation note is clinically referred to by the acronym SOAP. Regardless of the evaluation style specific to individual facility requirements, information about these same components is necessary to provide a full assessment of a patient.

Patient Historical Assessment
Chart Review

There are two components to a historical assessment: chart review and patient and family interviews. The chart review requires the therapist to gather information about the patient's medical and surgical histories, current diagnosis, current illness, medications, pulmonary function tests, laboratory and radiographic results, presence of secondary injuries or complications, and current response to treatment. Information regarding the emotional state of the patient and interactions between the patient and his family and between the family and health care team is also pertinent. When SCI is caused by ischemic lesions or tumors within the spinal canal, additional information about the onset and behavior of symptoms, when medical attention was sought, modifications made to the home, and who was assisting the patient and family before admission should be obtained. This enables a determination of the rate of deterioration leading to paralysis when not due to sudden trauma, as is the case with spinal cord disease.

Ideally, the documentation form or therapist worksheet includes a checklist to guide the chart review and to document medical findings. A checklist approach can help the therapist avoid overlooking pertinent information and allow the therapist

to note "NA" for not applicable or "NF" for not found as appropriate. Specific documentation on this level at the chart review supports the therapist's efforts when seeking appropriate medical information that in some cases may not yet be documented in the medical chart. The health care team should be mindful of confidentiality when medical information is displayed on a computer screen or copied and in public view. Because this information is protected health information (PHI), caution when sharing it with other staff or nonmedical personnel is important. PHI is governed by the Health Care Information Portability and Accountability Act (HIPAA). Box 6-1 outlines an overview of HIPAA.

Patient and Family Interviews

The next step is to interview the patient and his family. Therapists need to be active listeners and familiar with nonverbal traits of communication to recognize the emotional state of the person being interviewed and to guide the conversation. Understanding the meaning of silence, tone of voice, or physical cues helps the interviewer determine the congruency of the spoken words with the overall response (Clinical Note: Nonverbal Communication Behaviors). These skills are also important in cross-cultural communication.[2]

CLINICAL NOTE   Nonverbal Communication Behaviors

- Vocal cues: pitch, tone, and quality of voice, including moaning, crying, and groaning
- Action cues: posture, facial expression, and gestures
- Object cues: clothes, jewelry, and hair style
- Use of personal and territorial space: during interpersonal transactions and care of belongings
- Touch: involving the use of personal space and action

Adapted from Lapierre ED, Padgett J: How can we become more aware of culturally specific body language and use this awareness therapeutically? *J Psychosoc Nurs* 29:38-41, 1991.

SCI is usually a sudden and traumatic event with huge life-changing implications. Although it is important to gather as much information as possible during each interview, it is more important that the pace of the interview process is nonthreatening and that the therapist is sensitive to the needs of the patient. In a majority of cases, small amounts of information are gathered during each session. The ultimate goal is for the therapist to develop a partnership with the patient that allows his expectations to be melded with the therapist's knowledge and skills. The patient must feel free to share concerns, expectations, and fears. Developing a strong rapport sets the stage for the therapist to communicate the evaluation findings and their interpretation, making the process a learning experience for the patient. An interview can be greatly enhanced when the clinician pays close attention to the manner in which she asks the questions (Clinical Note: Ten Traps in Interviewing).

The therapist should learn to use open- and closed-ended or direct questioning techniques to gather information.[2] It is important to learn about the patient's medical history, including cardiac or pulmonary insufficiency, previous hospitalizations, cognitive

CLINICAL NOTE Ten Traps in Interviewing

- Providing false assurance or reassurance: instead acknowledge feelings and open the door for more communication
- Giving unwanted advice: instead take the time to involve the patient in the problem-solving process
- Using authority: instead talk to the patient rather than down to him
- Using avoidance language: instead use direct language to deal with frightening topics
- Engaging in distancing: instead use blunt specific terms to defuse anxiety
- Using professional jargon: instead use a vocabulary adjusted to the patient and avoid sounding condescending
- Using leading or biased questions: instead ask specific questions that the patient can answer honestly without fear of disapproval
- Talking too much: instead listen more, talk less
- Interrupting: instead concentrate on the patient's answer instead of appearing impatient or bored
- Using "why" questions: instead ask "who, what, and when" questions to elicit information without implying blame

Adapted from Jarvis C: *Physical examination and health assessment*, ed 4, Philadelphia, 2004, WB Saunders, pp 57-58.

impairments, smoking and alcohol history, and the presence of any premorbid orthopedic problems such as shoulder or back injuries. The therapist and patient should also discuss his current medical condition. This can be helpful in determining how much a patient understands about his injury. Taking notes during the interview diminishes eye contact and can interfere with the communication process, but it is important to accurately document the evaluation information from an interview. The notes can be used to capture this historical information in a summary form (Box 6-2).

Understanding the nature of how a person sustained his injury can provide the therapist with a wealth of additional information. This can be a very sensitive subject, however, that may be more appropriately addressed during a later therapy session. For example, a 23-year-old woman was injured in an automobile accident with her best friend when they were driving home after drinking at a bar. No one knows who was driving because both women were thrown from the car. The patient now has paraplegia and her best friend is dead. Instead of impeding the recovery process because of untimely interview queries, the basic accident information can be obtained during the chart review.

BOX 6-1 | Overview of Health Information Portability and Accountability Act (HIPAA)

Entities Covered
- The federal government (U.S. Department of Health and Human Services) requires that every individual who is employed by a covered entity must be educated in HIPAA
- A covered entity includes a health care providers who submits PHI electronically, health care clearinghouses, or business associates such as research organizations restricted by written agreements with the covered entity

Information Covered
- Protected health information (PHI)
  1. Information about past, present, and future physical or mental heath of a person, the provision of health care to a person, and payment for care
  2. Records, reviews, and clinical trials related to a person's care
- Individually identifiable health information: names; geographical subdivisions smaller than a state, address, city, county, precinct, zip code; dates except year related to date of birth or discharge date; phone and fax numbers; e-mail addresses; Social Security numbers; medical record numbers; health plan beneficiary numbers; account numbers; certificate or license numbers; vehicle identifiers such as license plate numbers; device identifiers and serial numbers; Internet universal resource locators; Internet protocol address numbers; biometrical identifiers including finger and voice prints; full-face photographic images and comparable media; any other unique identifying number, characteristic, or code

Requirements for Information Covered
- Requirements related to the standardization of certain electronic, administrative, and financial transmissions
- Requirements related to the security of electronic health information
- Requirements related to the privacy of individually identifiable health information

Patients' Rights
- Notice of Privacy Practices
  1. All designated entities must be in compliance by April 14, 2003, henceforth
  2. A covered entity must tell individuals how their PHI is used and disclosed by providing a privacy notice and a good faith effort to obtain a written receipt
- Authorizations
  1. Required to allow a person to agree or object for patient directories, informing family members, psychotherapy notes, fundraising, and within the context of research
  2. Not required for treatment, payment, health care operations; not required by law, abuse, neglect or domestic violence, judicial and administrative proceedings, public health activities, law enforcement activities, coroner or medical examiners to determine cause of death, cadaveric or eye tissue donation, health oversight agencies, and research when a waiver is approved
- A covered entity will not share PHI without express permission except with an institutional review board–approved waiver of authorization
- Individuals have a right to access their PHIs, request an amendment, receive a record of disclosures of PHI, request restrictions on uses and disclosures, revoke authorization, and request receipt of communication of PHI by alternative means or location

Minimum Necessary Standard
- Generally requires a covered entity to share the least amount of PHI necessary for a purpose
- Details exceptions as required by law (see HIPAA: www.hhs.gov/ocr/hipaa)

Data from American Physical Therapy Association: www.apta.org.

As the patient-therapist relationship develops, obtain additional details about the nature of the accident. Such details will help identify the possibility of secondary orthopedic complications, including injuries to the shoulder girdle, knee, or sacroiliac joint. For example, the therapist can guide the interview on the basis of the specific areas of the body injured as related to the mechanism of injury to ascertain whether potential secondary orthopedic or neurological conditions might have occurred. In the case described above, the therapist can ask whether the patient remembers hitting her head, twisting her shoulder, or the position she was lying in when found. It may be necessary to terminate the interview if the patient becomes agitated, emotional, or detached and continue at another time. It is important to document any disclosure of emotion, the patient's report of responses to current treatment, and his personal goals.

It is particularly important to learn about the patient's social background because it will help the therapist devise goals that are relevant to his previous lifestyle and may encourage the patient to become an active participant in his rehabilitation program. The therapist should note information regarding the patient's likes and dislikes, occupation, hobbies, cultural background, level of education, types of personal motivation, and role within his social circle. Often the hardest part of the therapeutic process is finding a way to help the patient become an active participant in his rehabilitation. Building a keen understanding of the patient's social history assists with this treatment goal.

A family interview allows the therapist to evaluate the family's knowledge level, attitudes and skills, involvement with the patient before his injury, and availability of family members to be involved in the rehabilitation process. Ryan et al[3] found that a therapist's perception of her patient's cognitive status was a factor that dictated the amount of family participation. The greater the cognitive or psychosocial limitations, the greater the amount of family intervention was needed. The interview process offers an ideal opportunity for therapists to tell families about formal and informal opportunities for family education and training through support groups and home visits. The advantages and benefits of an open policy on family visits, if the institution permits it, should be emphasized.

The historical interview is important on multiple levels:

- It clarifies and supplements the data gathered during the chart review.
- It helps the therapist establish rapport and trust with the patient by demonstrating attention to the patient's point of view.
- It provides insight into the patient and family's psychosocial background (see Chapter 5).
- It provides additional information that assists the therapist in determining the focus and sequence of the physical examination.

Curtis et al[4] found that families could be categorized on their willingness to help and their feelings of compassion on the basis of whether the patient was perceived to be responsible for his injury. In fact, families were more likely to overcompensate, creating patient dependence when he was not perceived as responsible for his injury.

Review of Systems Including Tests and Measures

The objective assessment of a patient with SCI begins with a standard neuromuscular evaluation. As part of the assessment, the therapist takes a few moments to observe the patient because a great deal of important information can be gained through such quiet observation. It is extremely important that the clinician understands the implication of four areas requiring specific precautions related to SCI before she continues: (1) spinal stability, (2) skin integrity, (3) ROM, and (4) blood pressure. This is because a patient with SCI is likely to have a spinal orthosis present or limited physical tolerance that prohibits the therapist from maneuvering him into different positions. To obtain the most objective and reproducible measurements possible, the therapist will need to be flexible and document her approach.

For example, if a patient is wearing a halo traction orthosis, prone positions are usually not feasible early on or, if there is a sacral wound, the supine position is to be avoided. These alternate positions affect some requirements of objective testing and should be documented for repeatability relative to later assessments. Halo precautions could be defined as follows:

- Patients with a halo apparatus must carry a wrench with them at all times in case of emergency (cardiopulmonary resuscitation)
- Patients with a halo apparatus will not try power mobility until the halo orthosis has been removed
- Patients with a halo apparatus will not perform upper limb active ROM, active-assisted ROM, or passive ROM greater than 90 degrees of shoulder flexion and abduction unless otherwise directed by the physician
- Patients with a halo apparatus will not perform bridging activities in the supine position, high-level position changes, pool therapy, or advanced wheelchair classes; prone activities are generally not permitted unless cleared by the physician

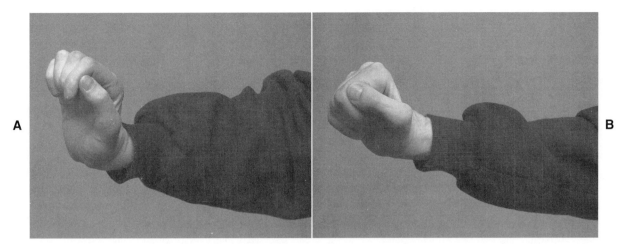

FIGURE 6-3 **A,** Tenodesis is the tension of the flexor tendons when the wrist is in extension. Tension in flexor tendons should be maintained and stretching of the flexor tendons when the wrist is in extension should be avoided in tetraplegia where grasp capacity must be maintained to assist in functional activities requiring grip. **B,** A patient's tenodesis in his hand has been enhanced after tendon transfer surgery (see Chapter 10) increasing grip function and lateral pinch.

- Manual muscle testing may be performed unilaterally up to 3+ resistance of the shoulder; all other muscle groups may be tested as usual
- Patients in a halo apparatus may perform upper limb exercise unilaterally up to 2 pounds and bilaterally up to 10 pounds; weights greater than 5 pounds should be avoided for shoulder abduction and horizontal flexion because increased cervical stress and upper body ergometer should be avoided unless otherwise directed by the physician
- Patients with incomplete lesions should avoid the following: isokinetics, ski track, car transfers (unless the vehicle is the appropriate size), bicycle (hip flexion should be kept below 90 degrees)
- Patients who are ambulatory must be guarded at the level of close supervision for ambulation, elevations, transfers, and balance activities

Always consult the physician to determine the patient's spine stability relative to antigravity versus resistive exercises before performing functional movements that require muscles attaching at or near the injured segment. Using or testing muscles that can pull on an unstable spine can be extremely dangerous. During the assessment process, listen for any sounds that might be attributed to untoward movement of spinal segments or to internal stabilization devices such as internal screws or spinal stabilization rods and immediately report such sounds to the physician. In addition, a sudden change in neurological status such as motor strength or sensory distribution must be reported immediately. A sudden deterioration may indicate either neurological compression from an unstable spine segment or the development or progression of a fluid-filled sac aligned longitudinally in the neurological canal, called a syrinx or posttraumatic cystic myelopathy (see Chapter 2).

Shearing of fragile skin sometimes occurs when patients are moved along any surface. This is a care concern with all patients who have fragile or healing skin and of particular importance with patients who cannot move themselves from one position to another. Take care to lift the body and avoid dragging the body weight over the surface. Skin is not tolerant of shear forces early after injury or when subjected to extended moisture, such as occurs with bladder or bowel incontinence. Where wounds are present, place foam supports under the patient on either side of a wound to form a bridge during the evaluation process (e.g., the sacrum, ischial tuberosities, greater trochanters, or heels). When a patient has a surgically repaired wound referred to as a flap graft, take extraordinary care to avoid shearing forces near the surgical site. Shearing forces can also occur during ROM of a joint that may overstretch the flap.

Again, before the evaluation begins, consult the physician to determine whether to restrict ROM testing. It is important not to overstretch the finger flexors, particularly when the wrist is in extension or if there has been surgical relocation of wrist flexor tendons, when evaluating hand and wrist ROM. Retention of tension in the wrist flexors is important for handgrip function (Figure 6-3, *A* and *B*).

Similarly, tightness in the low back is necessary to maintain sitting balance; therefore, the therapist must be careful not to overstretch these muscles when completing ROM exercises (Figure 6-4, *A*). Overstretching is contraindicated because it can result in lost independent sitting function. The clinician should ensure adequate hamstring length to allow for long-sitting balance capacity (greater than 90 degrees at the hip is needed to allow for long sitting) (Figure 6-4, *B*).

In addition, because of the potential pull of the muscles on the spine, the therapist should not flex or abduct the shoulders beyond 90 degrees during the shoulder ROM evaluation if the cervical spine is unstable (Figure 6-5).

Finally, during the evaluation, the patient may have occasional blood pressure fluctuations. Orthostatic hypotension can result when he is in a position where venous return is reduced such as in the upright position on a tilt table or a free-standing position when there is insufficient venous tension or muscle contraction to aid in venous return. Although patients usually will tell the examiner about visual symptoms such as lightheadedness, dizziness, and nausea, it is important to have a baseline sitting and supine blood pressure that was recorded before the evaluation began. This will allow an assessment of positional blood pressure changes as well.

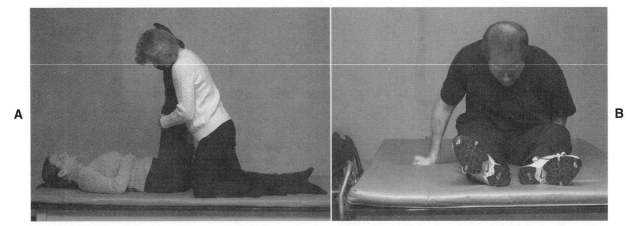

FIGURE 6-4 **A,** The therapist takes care when raising the patient's leg during ROM exercises not to overstretch back muscles. **B,** The patient moves forward on the mat using the long-sit position with hips flexed greater than 90 degrees and with weight bearing on upper limbs. Finger flexors are maintained in flexion to avoid overstretching and to maintain tenodesis.

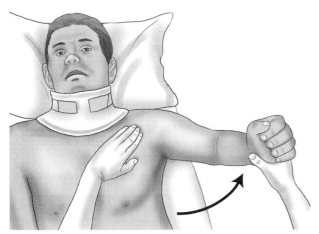

FIGURE 6-5 Therapists should avoid shoulder flexion above 90 degrees and rotation during ROM evaluation. The *arrow* indicates maximum movement restrictions.

If the patient's blood pressure drops, immediately sit him down or move him into a supine position and elevate his legs. In some cases, if sitting is not sufficient to relieve the blood pressure symptoms and moving to the supine position is not possible, tipping the patient's wheelchair back with the legs elevated is another option. This movement requires two people. When orthostatic hypotension pressure is a long-term problem, many tilt-in-space power wheelchairs have the option to recline and elevate the legs, which allows the patient to independently resolve the problem (see Chapter 11). Other options include the use of compressive stockings on the lower limbs or an abdominal binder to improve both venous return and blood pressure stability.

Conversely, autonomic dysreflexia (AD) can occur, resulting in a sudden elevation of blood pressure. It produces symptoms of headache, sweatiness, flushing above the injury level, and nausea. It is a very serious condition for patients with injuries above T6 and is usually brought on by some noxious stimulus such as a full bowel or bladder or excessive pressure on the skin. Immediately

bring the patient into an upright sitting position with his legs down and then remove the source of the problem (see Chapter 3). The patient's catheter should be checked to make sure it is not kinked. Other causes of AD include bladder infections and bowel impaction. Indeed, sometimes, patients and their caregivers are unable to determine the cause of the onset of AD.

Vital Signs

The therapist should evaluate and record the patient's heart rate, blood pressure, and respiratory rate before any other objective evaluations are made. In individuals with SCI, blood pressure is usually lower in sitting position and higher when the patient is supine. This is different than would be expected because a non-injured person normally has lower blood pressure in the supine position than when sitting. Such differences in blood pressure are usually dependent on the level and completeness of injury. In general, when the autonomic nervous system is involved at T6 and above, the cardiovascular system shows abnormal resting and exercise responses because of altered sympathetic outflow. The patient's vital signs must always be recorded so that in the event of a cardiac or respiratory crisis there will be baseline values that can be provided to the emergency team.

Respiratory Evaluation

Do not call specific attention to the technique when evaluating the patient's respiratory rate. A patient will frequently alter his respiratory rhythm when he realizes that it is being evaluated. By resting your hand on his chest or visually observing the rise and fall of his chest you can determine the breaths per minute. If a ventilator is assisting a patient, note whether he is receiving all his breaths by the ventilator or is able to initiate any breaths on his own (see Chapter 4).

Conduct a thorough respiratory evaluation as soon as possible to help prevent pulmonary complications. Adequate breathing capacity is essential for a patient to participate in the rigors of rehabilitation. There are a number of techniques specific to the evaluation of respiratory status for all patients with SCI including auscultation, measurement of chest expansion, palpation of bony

Respiratory Visual Inspection

- Facial expressions: look for distress, fear, sadness, lethargy
- Eyes: look for open or closed lids, visual scanning, maintenance or avoidance of eye contact, furrowed brows
- Breathing
- Flared nostrils: look for diaphragmatic breathing, the rise and fall of the chest; use of accessory muscles; shortness of breath; skin color
- Posture: look for head position, chest posture, scoliosis, rigidity of rib cage

and soft tissue elements related to proper respiration, measurement of vital capacity (VC), and assessment of cough function. In general, a respiratory visual evaluation includes careful observation of facial expression, the eyes, breathing, flared nostrils, and posture (Clinical Note: Respiratory Visual Inspection).

Auscultation

Auscultation is the act of listening for sounds, often with a stethoscope, to denote the condition of the lungs, heart, pleura, abdomen, and other organs.[5] The stethoscope does not magnify sound but rather blocks out extraneous room sounds. Of all the equipment used, the stethoscope quickly becomes a very personal instrument. Time should be taken to learn its features and make sure it is a good fit to the individual user. Auscultation is a skill that beginning examiners are eager to learn, but one that is difficult to master. First, the wide range of normal sounds must be learned. Once normal sounds are recognized, the clinician can begin to distinguish abnormal sounds.[2]

There are some general principles that apply to all auscultatory procedures. The environment should be quiet and free from distracting noises. The stethoscope should be placed on the naked skin because clothing obscures sound. The therapist should listen not only for the presence of sound but also its characteristics: intensity, pitch, duration, and quality. The sounds are often subtle or transitory, and intense listening is needed to hear the nuances. Closing the eyes may prevent distraction by visual stimuli and narrow the perceptual field to focus on the sound. The therapist should try to target and isolate each sound, concentrating on one sound at a time and taking enough time to identify all the characteristics of each sound.

One of the most difficult achievements in auscultation is learning to isolate sounds. Whether it is a breath sound or a heart beat in the sequence of respirations and heart beats, each segment of the cycle must be isolated and listened to specifically. After individual sounds are identified, they are put together in sequences. The clinician should not anticipate the next sound but rather concentrate on the one at hand.[6]

The patient should sit forward or, if this position is not possible, be placed in a side-lying position so that the upper and middle lung fields are exposed. The patient is reminded to breathe only through his mouth. First, he is asked to perform two repetitions of his normal breathing pattern: natural inspiration and expiration. Then systematically the stethoscope is placed over each of the auscultation landmarks (Figure 6-6), proceeding superior to inferior and evaluating at least one breath sound per pulmonary segment bilaterally.

The presence of abnormal breath sounds or the absence of breath sounds is noted and compared with the contralateral side. One or two repetitions of a maximal inspiration are taken at each landmark, again to note anything abnormal. Adventitious sounds such as crackles (rales) and wheezes (rhonchi) are also noted. Crackles may indicate the reopening of previously closed airways or, if nonrhythmic, may be a sign of fluid in the large airways. Wheezes are continuous and thought to be produced by air flowing through narrow airways at high velocities. Expiratory wheezes are associated with diffuse airway obstruction from extensive secretions in the airways (Figure 6-7).

Breath sounds are generated by air flow turbulence throughout the lung fields during inspiration and expiration. There are four types of breath sounds: tracheal, bronchial, vesicular, and bronchovesicular. Tracheal breath sounds are auscultated directly over the trachea. They are loud and high pitched with a pause of equal duration between inspiration and expiration. Bronchial breath sounds, which can be heard over the manubrium between the clavicles or posteriorly between the scapulae, are similar to tracheal breath sounds but the inspiration is shorter. Vesicular breath sounds can be heard over the peripheral lung fields and are identified by a long inspiration and short expiration with a faint, low-pitched sound and no pause between inspiration and expiration. Bronchovesicular breath sounds can be heard adjacent to the sternum or posteriorly between the scapulae and have a lower, medium-pitched sound with no pauses between inspiration and expiration; Table 6-1 illustrates and defines the difference.

Auscultation should be carried out last, after other techniques have provided information that will assist in interpretation. Too often the temptation is to rush right in with the stethoscope, thereby missing the opportunity to gather other data that might be useful. Auscultation is also used to determine the type of treatment and breathing retraining necessary for each patient's best respiration outcomes. It may provide feedback about the continuing effectiveness of pulmonary treatment.

Indeed, clinicians must always be open to what has been described as the "clinical pearl of unexpected findings"[7]: the key (one among many) to a successful physical examination is to respect your judgment and your instinct whenever you find that which you had not expected to find—that is, when your sense of the expected or of what you might call the normal has been violated. Pay attention when that happens even if it doesn't seem to make sense or you can't explain it easily.

Measuring Chest Expansion

Chest expansion should be measured to objectively document changes in thoracic mobility, determine loss of chest flexibility, and when re-evaluating the achievement of chest mobility goals. First, the circumference of the upper thorax is measured at the level of the third rib before inspiration and then measured again after a maximal inspiration has taken place while the patient continues to hold his breath. This process is repeated at the level of the xiphoid process of the sternum (the middle thorax) and at a point halfway between the xiphoid process and the umbilicus (the lower thorax). Scully and Barnes[8] documented an approximate increase in chest expansion from normal inspiration

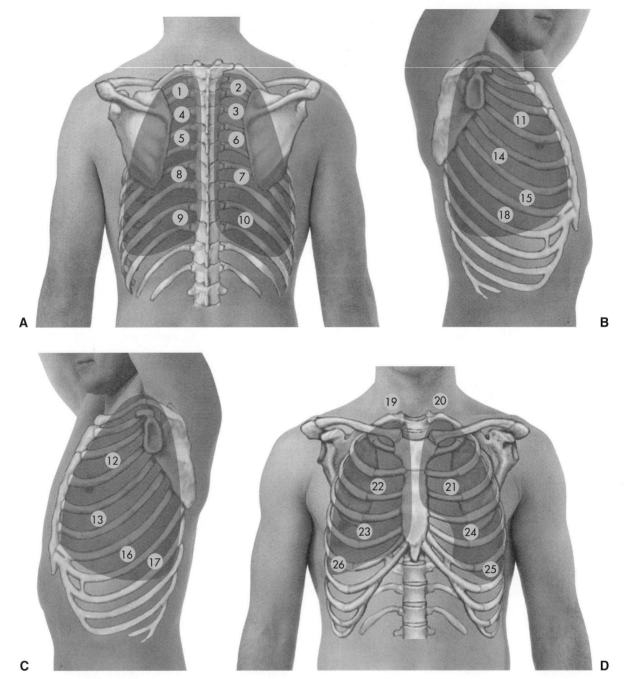

FIGURE 6-6 Auscultation landmarks for suggested sequence of systematic percussion and auscultation of the thorax. **A,** Posterior thorax. **B,** Right lateral thorax. **C,** Left lateral thorax. **D,** Anterior thorax. The pleximeter finger or the stethoscope is moved in the numerical sequence suggested; however, other sequences are possible. It is beneficial to be systematic. (From Seidel HM, Ball JW, Dains JE et al: *Mosby's guide to physical examination,* ed 5, St. Louis, 2003, Mosby.)

to maximal inspiration of approximately 2 to 4 inches in adult males.

Palpation

Manual palpation of the bony and soft tissue structures related to respiration is performed by palpating the sternum, clavicle, ribs, scapula, and spinal alignment as the patient is inhaling and exhaling (Figure 6-8). Any asymmetries between the right and left side are noted as are any hypermobile or hypomobile sections. Normal movement of the lower rib cage is often represented as of a bucket

handle with the lower ribs moving lateral and superior during inhalation; the upper ribs follow a pump handle movement moving anterior and superior (see Figure 4-2). Any difference in movement from one rib segment to the next should also be noted.

Next, the soft tissue structures involved in respiration are palpated including the muscles of respiration, quadratus lumborum muscle, paraspinal musculature, and the fascia and skin that envelop them. Any areas where hypermobility, hypomobility, or fascial restrictions exist are documented. Also noted are areas of increased muscle tone or spasm or places where palpation causes

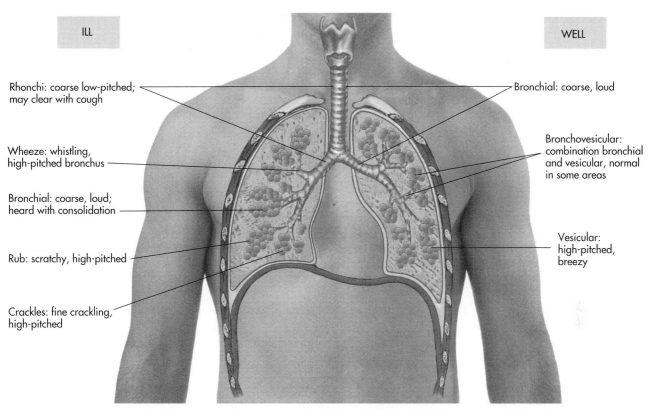

ILL

WELL

Rhonchi: coarse low-pitched; may clear with cough

Wheeze: whistling, high-pitched bronchus

Bronchial: coarse, loud; heard with consolidation

Rub: scratchy, high-pitched

Crackles: fine crackling, high-pitched

Bronchial: coarse, loud

Bronchovesicular: combination bronchial and vesicular, normal in some areas

Vesicular: high-pitched, breezy

FIGURE 6-7   Anatomical representations of adventitious breath sounds. (From Seidel HM, Ball JW, Dains JE et al: *Mosby's guide to physical examination,* ed 5, St. Louis, 2003, Mosby.)

TABLE 6-1 | Characteristics of Normal Breath Sounds

Type	Pitch	Amplitude	Duration	Quality	Normal Location
Bronchial (tracheal)	High	Loud	Inspiration < expiration	Harsh, hollow tubular	Trachea and larynx
Bronchovesicular	Moderate	Moderate	Inspiration = expiration	Mixed	Over major bronchi where fewer alveoli are located: posterior, between scapulae especially on right; anterior, around upper sternum in first and second intercostal spaces
Vesicular	Low	Soft	Inspiration > expiration	Rustling, like the sound of the wind in the trees	Over peripheral lung fields where air flows through smaller bronchioles and alveoli

From Jarvis C: *Physical examination and health assessment,* ed 4, Philadelphia, 2004, Saunders, Table 18-1, p 455.

pain when the musculature is being assessed. When palpating intercostal spaces, the therapist should not be surprised to find areas with very restricted movement or an area where the soft tissue is so restricted that palpation between two ribs is not possible. Palpation along the entire anterior, lateral, and posterior region of the thorax should be attempted. If the patient is wearing an orthosis that limits palpation, document as such and plan to complete the evaluation of those areas if and when the orthosis is removed.

Vital Capacity

VC is the maximal volume of gas that can be expelled from the lungs after a maximal inhalation or a full breath. An incentive spirometer is used to obtain this measurement (Figure 6-9, *A*). If the patient has a tracheostomy tube in place or has difficulty channeling air out of his mouth as opposed to his nose, assistance may be given to block the tracheostomy tube or close the nose shut while he exhales. Nose clips are also available that will gently pinch off the nose to avoid nasal air leakage when mouth expiration is required (Figure 6-9, *B*). It is important to note the patient's position and whether he is wearing an abdominal binder when testing VC. To get an accurate physiological measure, it is best to first measure the patient without the abdominal binder. Then another measure may be taken with the binder to determine if there is any improvement.

The resting position of the diaphragm is higher in supine position than it is in a short sit position (SSP); therefore patients with SCI will tend to have a higher VC in the supine position. The supine position allows for greater potential excursion of the diaphragm. In the SSP, the diaphragm is lower due to gravity (unless an abdominal binder is worn) and therefore has a small potential excursion distance. To ensure a good

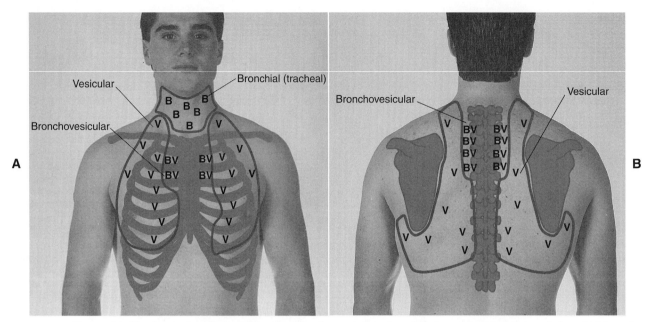

FIGURE 6-8 Topographical landmarks for palpation of the chest show the normal location of the three types of breath sounds: bronchial, bronchovesicular, and vesicular. **A,** Anterior. **B,** Posterior. (Jarvis C: *Physical examination & health assessment*, ed 4, St. Louis, 2004, WB Saunders.)

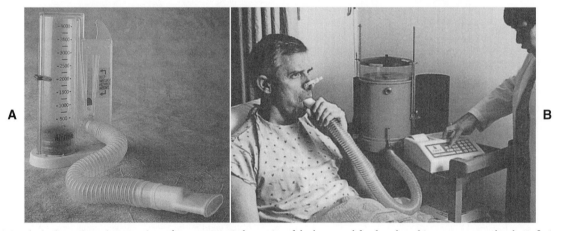

FIGURE 6-9 **A,** An incentive spirometer is used to measure vital capacity of the lungs and for deep breathing to promote alveolar inflation, restore and maintain lung capacity, and strengthen respiratory muscles. (From Black JM, Hawks JH: *Medical-surgical nursing: clinical management for positive outcomes*, ed 7, St. Louis, 2005, Elsevier Saunders; courtesy Baxter Healthcare Corporation, Round Lake, IL). **B,** Nose clips can be used during spirometry to gently pinch off the nose to avoid nasal air leakage when mouth expiration is required. (From Thibodeau GA, Patton KT: *Anatomy & physiology*, ed 6, St Louis, 2003, Mosby.)

test, the clinician needs to provide active forceful coaching until three acceptable maneuvers are obtained. An acceptable maneuver is defined as a quick and forceful start with no coughing, especially during the first second, no early termination of expiration, no variable flows, and good reproducibility and consistency of effort.[9]

Cough

A patient's ability to functionally cough must be evaluated to determine his ability to clear food, foreign objects, and secretions from his esophagus and trachea. To do this, the therapist must understand the mechanics of a normal cough so she can identify where the cough process is breaking down and set appropriate goals and treatment activities that will improve function (see Chapter 4). For example, a

patient may have an ineffective cough producing little to no sound and movement, thereby rendering it ineffective in clearing secretions.

In a patient with SCI, the ability to breathe and cough depends on the level of SCI and the innervation of the ventilatory muscles (Table 6-2). Coughs can be classified into three categories on the basis of force generation. A functional cough is strong enough to clear secretions, where the sound is loud and two or more coughs are possible per exhalation. A weak cough clears the upper airways, sounds less forceful, and can produce only one cough per exhalation. Small amounts of secretions are independently cleared but assistance is needed to clear larger amounts. A nonfunctional cough is ineffective in clearing bronchial secretions and sounds more like a sigh or clearing of

TABLE 6-2 | **Function, Care, and Spinal Cord Level Related to Innervation of Respiratory Muscles**

Function and Care	C1 to C3	C4	C5 to C8	T1 to T9	Below T10
Innervation of relevant muscles	Sternocleidomastoid, trapezius, cervical paraspinal, and neck accessory (provide superior expansion) muscles	In addition to C1-C3: Upper trapezius, diaphragm (provides inferior lateral/anterior expansion, also major muscle of passive respiration, effective coughing, concentric contractions to increase chest cavity, eccentric contractions aiding forced expiration/elongated phonation), and scalene (provide superior expansion) muscles	In addition to C1-C4: C5, Deltoid, biceps, brachialis, brachioradialis, rhomboids, and serratus anterior (partially) muscles C6, Clavicular pectoralis, serratus anterior, latissimus dorsi muscles C 7 to C8, Sternal pectoralis muscles	In addition to C1-C8: Internal and external intercostal (stabilize ribs, provide contractions—concentric for lateral/superior expansion for both quiet and forceful expiration and eccentric for exhalation and speech), and erector spinae muscles	In addition to C1-T9: Fully intact intercostal, external oblique, and rectus abdominis muscles
Outcomes related to respiratory muscle	Ventilator dependent; unable to clear secretions; dependent for assisted cough	May be able to breathe without ventilator	Low endurance and vital capacity; may require assistance to clear secretions and moderate assistance for independent self-assisted cough; paradoxical breathing in acute phase or longer	Compromised vital capacity and endurance; independent self-assisted cough aided by abdominal muscles builds up intrathoracic pressure for efficient cough	Intact respiratory function; able to clear secretions
Diaphragm	C1-C2, Diaphragm not innervated C3, Diaphragm partially innervated	Almost full use of diaphragm	Full use of diaphragm	Full use of diaphragm	Full use of diaphragm and abdominal muscles
Forced vital capacity*	Complete lesions: 25%-73% Incomplete lesions: 32%-82%	Complete lesions: 15%-74% Incomplete lesions: 49%-98%	Complete lesions: 22%-107% Incomplete lesions: 50%-116%	Complete lesions: 57%-114% Incomplete lesions: 79%-99%	Complete lesions: 61%-124% Incomplete lesions: 91%-114%
Respiratory equipment	Suction equipment; ventilators (bedside and portable); generator with battery backup	See C1-C3 if not ventilator free	None	None	None

Data from Consortium for Spinal Cord Medicine: *Traumatic spinal cord injury: clinical practice guidelines for health care professionals*, Washington, DC, 1999, Paralyzed Veterans of America; Lin VW, Cardenas DD, Cutter NC et al. *Spinal cord medicine: principles and practice*, New York, 2003, Demos; Massery M: The patient with neuromuscular or musculoskeletal dysfunction. In Frownfelter D, Dean E, editors: *Principles and practice of cardiopulmonary physical therapy*, ed 3, St. Louis, 1996, Mosby; Linn WS, Spungen AM, Gong H Jr et al: Forced vital capacity in two large outpatient populations with chronic spinal cord injury, *Spinal Cord* 39:263-268, 2001.
*Observed mean ranges.

the throat with an inability to cough with any expulsion force; assistance is needed with airway clearance in such instances.[10-13] This is important because secretion buildup occurs when the patient uses an artificial ventilator and a tracheostomy is present. If the patient cannot clear the secretions, document the assistance required along with its frequency, type, and the equipment required.

Integumentary Evaluation

The therapist can use the evaluation of a patient's skin integrity as a beginning forum for patient and family education. A starting point is to show the patient and his family the most common areas where skin breakdown occurs. Figure 6-10 illustrates areas that have a greater potential for breakdown because they are located over a bony prominence such as the occiput, scapula, elbow, spinous

processes, sacrum, coccyx, ischial tuberosities, greater trochanter, lateral and medial femoral epicondyles, lateral and medial malleoli, and heel. Potential causes for skin breakdown should be discussed including poor nutrition, smoking, swelling, incontinence, and lack of pressure relief mechanisms. Then the patient and his family may be shown the early warning signs of skin breakdown and how to prevent increased damage.

Areas where skin breakdown is present are documented including abrasions, incision sites, or pressure ulcers (see Chapter 3 and Figure 3-8). Stages of pressure ulcers should be documented and include the diameter of the wound, the presence of any odor, the color and type of tissue present (necrotic, eschar, epithelial), the amount and description of any drainage, and whether tunneling or a syrinx is present (Figure 6-11). The presence of drainage on a dressing should be described as fully saturated versus an

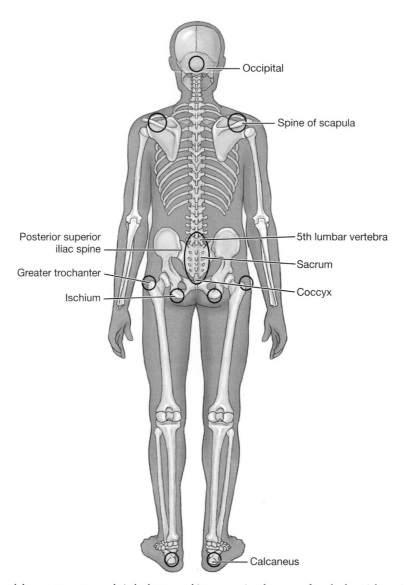

Occipital

Spine of scapula

Posterior superior
iliac spine

5th lumbar vertebra

Greater trochanter

Sacrum

Ischium

Coccyx

Calcaneus

FIGURE 6-10 Skin breakdown occurs commonly in body areas subject to continual pressure from body weight against bony prominences.

saturation over an area the size of a quarter because documenting the amount of drainage is not measurable. Taking a photograph of the wound or using a clear overhead transparency sheet that has been cleaned with alcohol to trace the size of the wound can also be helpful to objectively document the diameter and shape of the wound. The type of wound dressing and treatment being used to accelerate healing should be documented as well.

Skin with early signs of breakdown should be identified. These signs include skin with a papery appearance, no blanching, and a loss of hair growth. Palpation yields a boggy or perhaps a hard end feel unlike the surrounding area. Areas of previous scarring should also be documented; these areas are more susceptible to breakdown because of the lack of blood supply and tissue flexibility. A scar that results from a previous breakdown may indicate poor compliance with past skin care programs; therefore, identifying why that program was not working and involving the patient in structuring a new program that may be followed more rigorously is important to promoting improved wellness (see Chapters 2 and 3).

Range of Motion

Joint ROM is the physiological motion available at each joint. ROM can be limited by bony restriction or by the physiological characteristics of the connective tissue around the joint.[14] ROM involves the measurement of the available movement throughout all planes of motion (e.g., sagittal, coronal, transverse) at each joint. Assessment of ROM of neck, trunk, and the extremities should be done as permitted by the physician. Exceptions will include joints deemed unstable or limited by an orthosis.

Critical motions will include motions such as an elbow extension, forearm supination, and wrist extension needed to support the upper body when sitting on extended arms (see Chapter 7). Table 6-3 identifies the critical joints that need to be evaluated for a person with an SCI. Even a slight loss of motion in any of these areas can have significant implications on the patient's functional outcomes. For example, a reduction in full ROM into elbow extension would prohibit an individual from propping up on extended arms while sitting. The elbows could not lock into a

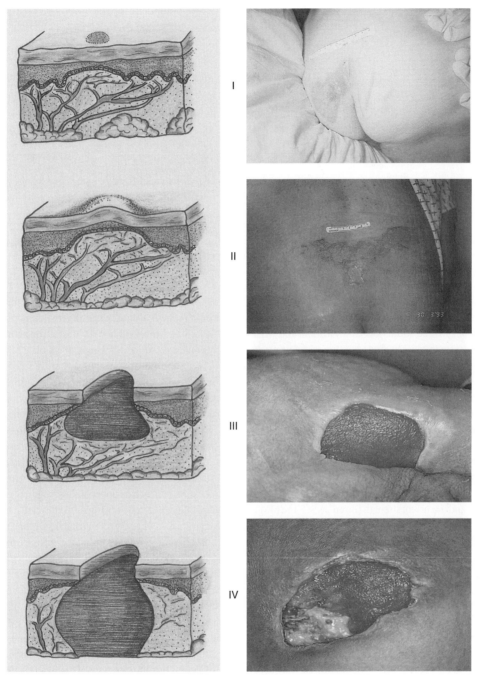

FIGURE 6-11 Staging of pressure ulcers: stage I, nonblanchable erythema of intact skin, heralding the lesion of skin ulceration; stage II, partial-thickness skin loss involving epidermis or dermis; stage III, full-thickness skin loss involving damage or necrosis of subcutaneous tissue that extends down to but not through the underlying fascia; stage IV, full-thickness skin loss with extensive destruction, tissue necrosis, or damage to muscle, bone, or supporting structures. (From Potter PA, Perry AG: *Fundamentals of nursing concepts, process and practice*, ed 4, St. Louis, 1997, Mosby.)

position without requiring excessive muscle contraction. These contractions are either fatiguing or altogether impossible because of paralysis of the triceps. Therefore, independent upright sitting would be impossible and a major functional deficit.

Muscle Evaluation

Manual Muscle Testing. A complete motor function assessment is part of an initial patient evaluation. The therapist, however, may choose to begin with a gross motor screen in some patients. A gross screen entails a brief break test of some of the patient's joint

motions. A break test is applied to a limb after it has completed its full ROM. Manual resistance (i.e., force acting in opposition to a contracting muscle) is applied in the direction of the line of pull of the muscle at the maximal point in the range of motion. The patient is asked to hold the limb at that point and not allow the examiner to break the hold with manual resistance.[15] This allows for consistency of procedure without estimating a midrange point where the examiner might reliably assess strength.

The active resistance test is an alternative to the break test, in which the examiner applies manual resistance against actively

TABLE 6-3	Range of Motion Evaluation of Critical Joints
Joint	Motion
Cervical	High cervical flexion
	Low cervical extension
Shoulder	Flexion
	Extension
	External rotation
Elbow	Extension
Wrist	Extension
Forearm	Supination
Trunk	Rotation
Pelvis	Neutral
Hip	Flexion
	Extension
	External rotation
Knee	Extension
Ankle	Dorsiflexion

BOX 6-3	Manual Muscle Testing Grading System

0 (Zero) = No visible or palpable contraction on palpation or visual inspection

1 (Trace) = Some muscle contraction is visual or palpable, but no limb movement

2 (Poor) = Limb has full range of movement with gravity eliminated (horizontal plane of motion)

3 (Fair) = Limb has full range of movement against only the resistance of gravity but no additional resistance is tolerated

4 (Good) = Limb has full range of movement with moderate resistance; yields under maximal resistance

5 (Normal) = Normal strength or the ability to complete a full ROM or maintain end-point range against maximal resistance

Adapted from Hislop HJ, Montgomery J: *Daniels & Worthingham's muscle testing: techniques of manual examination*, ed 8, St. Louis, 2007, Saunders Elsevier, pp 6-8.Use of plus (+) or minus (−) in addition to the MMT grade is discouraged except in three instances: Fair+, Poor+; and Poor−.

contracting muscle group (i.e., against the direction of movement as if to prevent that movement).[15] For instance, this test can be used with shoulder flexion and abduction, elbow flexion, and wrist extension. The gross screen quickly alerts the therapist to muscle areas that may be problematic and as to whether the patient will be able to assist with the first mobility activity attempted. Such assessment allows the therapist to better determine a focus and sequence for the evaluation and an opportunity to assess the patient's reaction to the results. It can be very discouraging for the patient to start the first session by evaluating all or many of the areas with minimal or absent innervation and it is usually not necessary.

The MMT uses a six-point grading system that includes clinical observation, palpation, and ROM movement to assess the viability of each muscle to work and its current strength (Box 6-3).[15,16] The MMT should be used to test all muscles above the neurological level of injury in a patient with a complete injury and to assess one muscle within each myotome below the level of the lesion. A complete MMT is performed on all muscle groups above and below the neurological level of injury in patients with incomplete injuries. Sometimes clinicians test movements such as shoulder abduction but do not identify the strength of specific muscles (e.g., supraspinatus versus middle deltoid). Treatment options will by better tailored to the patient and improved outcomes may result when a more specific evaluation is completed.

The ASIA Motor and Sensory Score is a standardized scale used to determine the neurological level and completeness of a patient's injury.[17] It should be available for review and updating during all assessments (Figure 6-12). Muscles with partial or full innervation should be tested at various points within their ROM, particularly as related to functionally simulated patterns. For instance, the shoulder external rotation will be tested with the arm in 0 degrees and 90 degrees of abduction. The clinician should not assume that when a patient demonstrates a particular strength grade at one point that it exists all the way through the available ROM; a patient may be able to lift his thigh up and offer minimal resistance when sitting in the wheelchair but it does not necessarily follow that his hip flexor strength is a grade 4 or that he can achieve full active motion in the side-lying position. Strength and motion should be verified by testing the patient in the side-lying position before assigning the MMT grade. Different results are frequently seen when the patient

is out of the wheelchair. Remembering such differences will allow the development of a more specific treatment plan.

In addition, muscles should be tested concentrically and eccentrically while the therapist attempts to simulate functional movement patterns. The strength of a muscle during an eccentric contraction is often the same as its limitation during a functional activity. For instance, a patient may be able to lift a cup to his mouth but may be unable to lower it to the table again in a controlled fashion.

The need for muscular substitution may limit complete MMT assessment just as a patient's impaired muscle tone, spasticity, orthoses, or a lack of trunk stability can interfere. Indeed, if a patient shows decreased trunk stability, it is imperative that support be provided to allow assessment of true upper limb strength. For example, when the anterior deltoid is tested through performance of shoulder flexion, a patient may not be able to withstand resistance because he cannot stabilize his trunk without losing his balance anteriorly rather than because of actual weakness of the anterior deltoid.

Muscular Substitution. Muscle substitution refers to the use of one or more muscles to compensate for the action of other muscles that are absent or weakened.[18,19] For example, the movement of the shoulder in external rotation can cause elbow extension, which may lead an observer to assume that the triceps muscle is actively contracting when this is not the case. Table 6-4 lists common muscular substitutions or compensations exhibited by patients with SCI.

Although muscle substitutions can assist function greatly, they make isolated muscle testing difficult. In addition, these substitutions grow stronger over time as the patient becomes more dependent on them for functional purposes and this can make MMT progressively more deceptive. To avoid inaccurate assessment results because of substitution, all muscles should be tested in the most supported position. The examiner should isolate the joint at which the muscle acts and palpate the muscle being tested. In addition, careful observation and palpation of the potentially substituting muscles can help achieve more objective results.

Muscle Tone and Spasticity. The term tone is often used as a description of the resting tension of a muscle or the degree of resistance to passive ROM. Attempts to define muscle tone more clearly or measure it quantitatively have not been successful.[8] Tone differs significantly from spasticity, which refers to the velocity-dependent muscle hypertonia or increased sensitivity and abnormally strong resistance of affected muscles to passive stretch.[20] Spasticity or reflexive contraction can occur when a muscle is being tested, which may make the muscle appear stronger than it actually is.

Although sudden and involuntary contractions of muscle fibers that cause a muscle spasm are often a symptom of spasticity, the two are not the same. The demonstrated changes in motor neuron activity that may occur in patients with SCI and other neuromotor dysfunctions—sometimes at rest and sometimes with various speeds of passive ROM—are discussed in Chapter 2. When documenting spasticity, the therapist should ask the patient to contract and relax the muscle on command on three consecutive attempts and should then use the MMT to reflect the patient's grade. If the patient is unable to relax the muscle on command, this may indicate the presence of spasticity. At this point, the therapist needs to identify differences in spasticity at variable speeds of passive motion and document her observations in detail by using the original Ashworth Scale or the Modified Ashworth Scale (see Box 2-1; Box 6-4).[21,22] Furthermore, documenting the influence of spasticity on functional activities is more descriptive than the Ashworth Scale indicates

in assessing resistance to passive stretch. For example, describing that there is an increase in hamstring muscle spasticity with subsequent inability to achieve full knee extension at heel strike provides the functional impact of spasticity.

Fluctuations in the degree of spasticity will occur throughout the patient's rehabilitation program, sometimes on a daily basis. Such fluctuations can be part of the normal postinjury course or can be indicative of a change in the patient's medical status. Increases in spasticity can result from a noxious stimulus below the neurological level of injury. For instance, spasticity may be seen in patients who have a urinary tract infection, fecal impaction, or an increase in severity of a pressure ulcer. The therapist is often the first person to recognize these changes and the information she provides to the physician is vital to prompt determination of treatment and care.

Increased spasticity is not always detrimental. A patient with SCI can use an increase in spasticity to assist in achieving functional movement with less assistance. For example, increased spasticity of a patient's trunk musculature can assist the patient with his sitting posture and balance during transfers. An increase in lower limb extensor spasticity in a patient with an incomplete

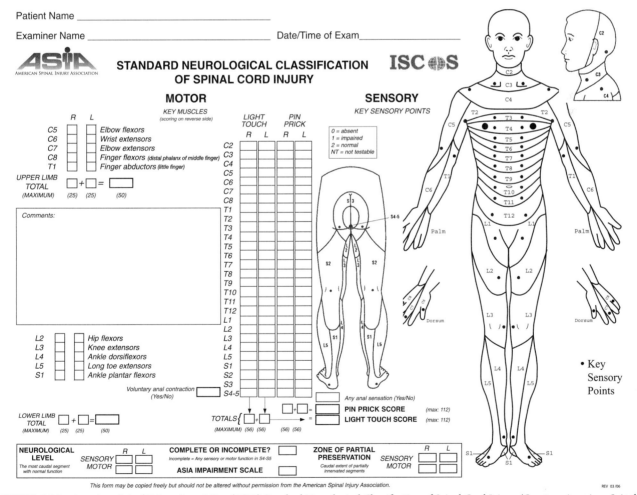

FIGURE 6-12 American Spinal Injury Association (ASIA) Standard Neurological Classification of Spinal Cord Injury. (Courtesy American Spinal Injury Association, Atlanta, GA, 2006.)

Continued

MUSCLE GRADING

0 total paralysis

1 palpable or visible contraction

2 active movement, full range of motion, gravity eliminated

3 active movement, full range of motion, against gravity

4 active movement, full range of motion, against gravity and provides some resistance

5 active movement, full range of motion, against gravity and provides normal resistance

5* muscle able to exert, in examiner's judgement, sufficient resistance to be considered normal if identifiable inhibiting factors were not present

NT not testable. Patient unable to reliably exert effort or muscle unavailable for testing due to factors such as immobilization, pain on effort or contracture.

ASIA IMPAIRMENT SCALE

☐ **A = Complete**: No motor or sensory function is preserved in the sacral segments S4-S5.

☐ **B = Incomplete**: Sensory but not motor function is preserved below the neurological level and includes the sacral segments S4-S5.

☐ **C = Incomplete**: Motor function is preserved below the neurological level, and more than half of key muscles below the neurological level have a muscle grade less than 3.

☐ **D = Incomplete**: Motor function is preserved below the neurological level, and at least half of key muscles below the neurological level have a muscle grade of 3 or more.

☐ **E = Normal**: Motor and sensory function are normal.

CLINICAL SYNDROMES (OPTIONAL)

☐ Central Cord
☐ Brown-Sequard
☐ Anterior Cord
☐ Conus Medullaris
☐ Cauda Equina

STEPS IN CLASSIFICATION

The following order is recommended in determining the classification of individuals with SCI.

1. Determine sensory levels for right and left sides.

2. Determine motor levels for right and left sides.
   Note: in regions where there is no myotome to test, the motor level is presumed to be the same as the sensory level.

3. Determine the single neurological level.
   This is the lowest segment where motor and sensory function is normal on both sides, and is the most cephalad of the sensory and motor levels determined in steps 1 and 2.

4. Determine whether the injury is Complete or Incomplete (sacral sparing).
   *If voluntary anal contraction = **No** AND all S4-5 sensory scores = **0** AND any anal sensation = **No**, then injury is COMPLETE. Otherwise injury is incomplete.*

5. Determine ASIA Impairment Scale (AIS) Grade:

Is injury **Complete**?   If **YES**, AIS=A Record ZPP
         NO ↓   (For ZPP record lowest dermatome or myotome on
                            each side with some (non-zero score) preservation)

**Is injury
motor incomplete?**   If **NO**, AIS=B
         YES ↓   (Yes=voluntary anal contraction OR motor
                         function more than three levels below the motor
                         level on a given side.)

**Are at least half of the key muscles below the
(single) neurological level graded 3 or better?**

NO ↓   YES ↓

AIS=C   AIS=D

If sensation and motor function is normal in all segments, AIS=E
Note: AIS E is used in follow up testing when an individual with a documented SCI has recovered normal function. If at initial testing no deficits are found, the individual is neurologically intact; the ASIA Impairment Scale does not apply.

FIGURE 6-12, cont'd American Spinal Injury Association (ASIA) Standard Neurological Classification of Spinal Cord Injury. (Courtesy American Spinal Injury Association, Atlanta, GA, 2006.)

TABLE 6-4 | Common Muscular Substitutions or Compensations

Joint Motion	Substitution or Compensation
Shoulder flexion or abduction	Shoulder shrug
Elbow extension	Shoulder external rotation, forearm supination, gravity
Wrist extension	Forearm supination, gravity
Wrist flexion	Forearm pronation, gravity
Hip flexion	Posterior pelvic tilt, hip hiking
Hip extension	Trunk extension
Hip abduction	Hip hiking
Knee flexion and extension	Can occur passively when performing hip flexion and extension in side lying

BOX 6-4 | Modified Ashworth Spasticity Scales

Grade	Description
0	No increased muscle tone
1	Slight increase in muscle tone, manifested by a catch and release, or by minimal resistance at end ROM when affected part is moved in flexion or extension
1+	Slight increase in muscle tone, manifested by a catch, followed by minimal resistance throughout the remainder (<50%) of ROM
2	More marked increase in muscle tone through most of ROM, but affected part is easily moved
3	Considerable increase in muscle tone, passive movement difficult
4	Affected part is rigid in flexion or extension

Data from Bohannon RW, Smith MB: Inter-rater reliability on modified Ashworth scale of muscle spasticity, *Phys Ther* 67:206-207, 1987.

SCI may assist with his ability to maintain a standing position. A patient may be able to trigger a hip flexor muscle spasm that will assist him with positioning his leg for dressing. For these reasons, it is important that the therapist be able to determine whether the intensity, duration, and frequency of the spasticity interferes with or assists with the patient's function. When spasticity interferes with functional activities, hygiene, or sleep, medications can be prescribed. The physician will often ask the therapist to assess whether the medication has improved these functional activities or reduced the spasticity so significantly that function is further impaired. Sometimes medication can cause a patient to become

very drowsy and fatigued. Regular documentation of spasticity assists communication within the rehabilitation team.

Sensation

The therapist needs to use light touch, deep pressure, pinprick, temperature, proprioception, and kinesthetic awareness to evaluate sensation. Because of the different neural pathways within the spinal cord, it is common to see preservation of different types of sensation at varying areas below the level of injury. The lateral spinothalamic tract responds to sharp-dull discrimination or pinprick and to deep pressure and temperature tests. The anterior spinothalamic tract is sensitive to light touch. The posterior columns in the spinal cord respond to proprioception or vibration tests. The dermatomes evaluated by these sensations are pictured in the ASIA Classification Form (see Figure 6-12). This illustration includes a dot within each dermatome (•) that represents the sensory distribution of the corresponding segmental level in the spinal cord.

The therapist documents the patient's intact, impaired, or absent sensory distribution on his ASIA examination form. The key areas are provided to complete the sensory testing efficiently unless there is skin scarring or another reason to alter the pattern. The same dermatome should be tested on both sides of the body in sequence, to enable the patient to report differences between sides. The therapist should always touch the patient's face in the same manner in which the sensory modality is tested (e.g., light touch, pinprick, deep pressure). This gives the patient a reference point for what he is expected to feel at other levels. The sensory levels often differ from the lowest intact muscle or myotome level; therefore report the lowest sensory level separately for each modality. In addition, right and left sides of the body may demonstrate different sensory levels and thus need to be reported separately. It is also important to test the trunk and all limbs in the event the injury is incomplete. It is also important to monitor the location of sensory patches below the injury level to determine neurological recovery. This can help guide decisions about wheelchair seating, positioning, and other potential threats to skin integrity. The zone of partial preservation is used for complete injuries only and describes sensory or motor sparing caudal to the neurological level (i.e., the most caudal level where both motor and sensory modalities are intact bilaterally).[17]

Pain is another sensation that needs to be assessed in patients with SCI. Determine pain pattern, duration, location, severity, relieving or provoking factors, and associated symptoms. Pain is multidimensional and may be referred to as a specific sensation other than touch, may result from every sensory stimulus reaching sufficient intensity, may be linked to abnormal reverberation of neural activity in the spinal cord or autonomic nervous system, or may be caused by a combination of physiological, cognitive, and psychological processes.[23] Patients should be examined for pain above, at, and below the neurological level of injury bilaterally. A body diagram, such as the one used in the McGill Pain Questionnaire[24] is a useful form of recording these symptoms (Figure 6-13).

Chronic pain or pain that persists long after the injury is referred to as neurogenic pain (see Figure 3-7). This pain results from damage to the spinal cord itself rather than the nerve roots. It can be constant or intermittent and can occur spontaneously or in response to a stimulus.[25] This type of pain consists of poorly localized complaints of numbness, tingling, burning sensations, and visceral discomfort. It is exacerbated by noxious stimuli such as urinary tract infections, spasticity, bowel impaction, or infection. Chronic and intense neurogenic pain is often very debilitating. Patients may seek pharmacological interventions for this pain, which may include nonsteroidal anti-inflammatory drugs, anti-inflammatory agents, tricyclic antidepressants, and anticonvulsants.

Another type of pain—upper limb pain—is musculoskeletal pain caused by overuse. Manual wheelchair propulsion,

transfers, or weight bearing through crutches during ambulation put continual and significant forces on the shoulder and wrist joints sufficient to produce pain symptoms that may be severe enough to produce pathological signs such as rotator cuff tears or carpal tunnel syndrome.[26,27] The incidence of these symptoms increases over time after injury.[28,29] Sometimes shoulder pain is exacerbated by poor wheelchair and sleeping postures. These postures can lead to other problems such as cervical radiculopathy resulting in referred pain into the upper limb.

The Wheelchair Users Shoulder Pain Index (WUSPI) is a good tool to quantify musculoskeletal shoulder pain when the patient uses a manual wheelchair. The WUSPI is a 15-item self-report instrument that measures shoulder pain intensity in wheelchair users during various functional activities of daily living (ADL), such as transfers, loading a wheelchair into a car, wheelchair mobility, dressing, bathing, overhead lifting, driving, performing household chores, and sleeping.[30] Each item is scored on a 10-cm visual analog scale (VAS) that is anchored at its beginning with no pain and at its end with worst pain ever experienced (Figure 6-14). A VAS can be used to measure other types and locations of pain as well.

Functional Assessment

The evaluation of a patient's functional abilities is the most important component of the evaluation process. Ultimately, it is where all the other evaluation procedures culminate. Function refers to the way in which a person carries out the physical demands of life. The other components of the evaluation, such as ROM and MMT, are important areas to evaluate, but it is their relation to function that is the key to the patient becoming as independent as possible in life skills.

When evaluating function, the rehabilitation team should take into account the amount of physical assistance; requirements for verbal, visual, or environmental cueing; and the kinds of assistive equipment that a patient needs. Decreased reimbursement and increased financial burdens to patients with SCI make it increasingly important for therapists to document very carefully and with great detail. For example, a patient with C4 tetraplegia may be dependent during transfers at initial evaluation and also expected to be dependent at discharge. If this is all the information documented, a third-party payer may request that the patient be discharged too soon because it does not appear that his status will change. What if that patient is actually learning how to tolerate a one-person dependent transfer over a two-person dependent transfer? What if he is learning to become independent in instructing caregivers about how to transfer him? What if he is being monitored during the first stages of receiving treatment for severe leg spasticity, a complication that could interfere with his safety and that of his caregiver(s)? Details related to function need to be carefully documented to justify the continued therapeutic intervention for the patient from skilled practitioners.

The Functional Independence Measure (FIM) instrument provides another way to characterize function.[31] The FIM is recognized by ASIA for the measurement of impact of SCI on function (Figure 6-15). The FIM allows for the assessment of self-care, sphincter control, mobility, locomotion, communication, and social cognition. Overall values are tallied in a total FIM score. Each rating is based on a seven-point scale that charts the amount

MEASUREMENT OF PAIN

McGill Pain Questionnaire

Patient's Name ______________________ Date____________ Time ________ am/pm

PRI: S ________ (1-10) A ________ (11-15) E ________ (16) M ________ (17-20) PRI(T) ________ (1-20) PPI ________

1 Flickering, Quivering, Pulsing, Throbbing, Beating, Pounding
2 Jumping, Flashing, Shooting
3 Pricking, Boring, Drilling, Stabbing, Lancinating
4 Sharp, Cutting, Laterating
5 Pinching, Pressing, Gnawing, Cramping, Crushing
6 Tugging, Pulling, Wrenching
7 Hot, Burning, Scalding, Searing
8 Tingling, Itchy, Smarting, Stinging
9 Dull, Sore, Hurting, Aching, Heavy
10 Tender, Taut, Rasping, Splitting
11 Tiring, Exhausting
12 Sickening, Suffocating
13 Fearful, Frightful, Terrifying
14 Punishing, Gruelling, Cruel, Vicious, Killing
15 Wretched, Blinding
16 Annoying, Troublesome, Miserable, Intense, Unbearable
17 Spreading, Radiating, Penetrating, Piercing
18 Tight, Numb, Drawing, Squeezing, Tearing
19 Cool, Cold, Freezing
20 Nagging, Nauseating, Agonizing, Dreadful, Torturing

PPI
0 No pain
1 Mild
2 Discomforting
3 Distressing
4 Horrible
5 Excrutiating

Brief	Rhythmic	Continuous
Momentary	Periodic	Steady
Transient	Intermittent	Constant

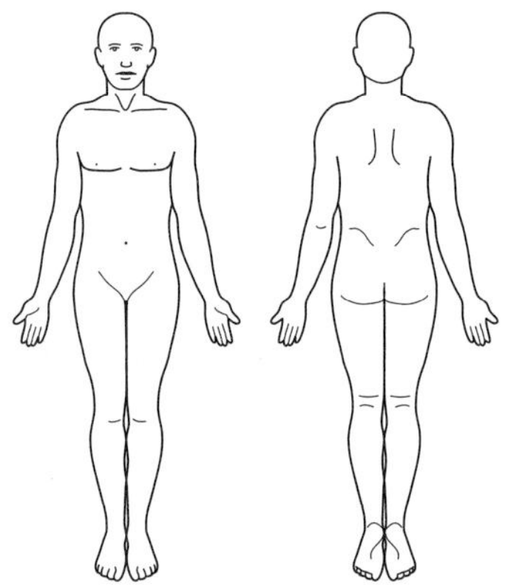

E = External
I = Internal

Comments:

FIGURE 6-13 McGill Pain Questionnaire. (From Melzack R, Katz J: The McGill Pain Questionnaire: appraisal and current status, In Turk DC, Melzack R, editors: *Handbook of pain assessment*, New York, 1992, Guilford Press.)

of assistance required. There are three categories under the heading of "Modified Dependence" with possible scores of 3 to 5 and two categories under the heading of "Complete Dependence." Although it is a standard tool, finer functional measures sometime show patient gains that are not reflected in the FIM scoring system and there are other important functional skills that are not part of this assessment system.

Another scale designed to measure the efficiency of rehabilitation treatment in patients with SCI is the Spinal Cord Independence Measure (SCIM) (Figure 6-16). Catz et al[32] have indicated that it is reliable and that it demonstrates greater sensitivity to changes in function than does the FIM. In addition, they found it rated functional achievements according to importance with patients with SCI, included ADL functions relevant to these

WHEELCHAIR USERS SHOULDER PAIN INDEX (WUSPI)

Place an **X** on the scale to estimate your level of pain with the following activities. Check box at right if the activity was **NOT** performed in the past week.

BASED ON YOUR EXPERIENCES IN THE PAST WEEK, HOW MUCH SHOULDER PAIN DO YOU EXPERIENCE WHEN:

1. Transferring from a bed to a wheelchair? ☐
No Pain _____ Worst Pain Ever Experienced

2. Transferring from a wheelchair to a car? ☐
No Pain _____ Worst Pain Ever Experienced

3. Transferring from a wheelchair to the tub or shower? ☐
No Pain _____ Worst Pain Ever Experienced

4. Loading your wheelchair into a car? ☐
No Pain _____ Worst Pain Ever Experienced

5. Pushing your chair for 10 minutes or more? ☐
No Pain _____ Worst Pain Ever Experienced

6. Pushing up ramps or inclines outdoors? ☐
No Pain _____ Worst Pain Ever Experienced

7. Lifting objects down from an overhead shelf? ☐
No Pain _____ Worst Pain Ever Experienced

8. Putting on pants? ☐
No Pain _____ Worst Pain Ever Experienced

9. Putting on a t-shirt or pullover? ☐
No Pain _____ Worst Pain Ever Experienced

10. Putting on a button down shirt? ☐
No Pain _____ Worst Pain Ever Experienced

11. Washing your back? ☐
No Pain _____ Worst Pain Ever Experienced

12. Usual daily activities at work or school? ☐
No Pain _____ Worst Pain Ever Experienced

13. Driving? ☐
No Pain _____ Worst Pain Ever Experienced

14. Performing household chores? ☐
No Pain _____ Worst Pain Ever Experienced

15. Sleeping? ☐
No Pain _____ Worst Pain Ever Experienced

FIGURE 6-14   Wheelchair Users Shoulder Pain Index (WUSPI). (From Curtis KA, Roach KE, Applegate EB et al. Development of the wheelchair user's shoulder pain index (WUSPI), *Paraplegia* 33:290-293, 1995.)

patients, and was organized to include scoring criteria on the evaluation sheet, increasing its usefulness in daily assessments.

Tolerance to Upright

Tolerance to upright is the only evaluation area where physical assistance and cueing measures are not noted. Tolerance to upright is the evaluation of a patient's physical ability to tolerate any degree of being upright, whether it is in a supine position with the head elevated, sitting, or standing. As discussed in Chapters 2 and 3, the presence of orthostatic hypotension is common in patients with SCI and is often the first hurdle that needs to be overcome.

Lack of an efficient skeletal muscle pump combined with an absent vasopressor response in the legs leads to venous pooling. This reduces the amount of circulating blood, decreasing

FIM™ Instrument

LEVELS	7 Complete Independence (timely, safely) 6 Modified Independence (device)	NO HELPER
	Modified Dependence 5 Supervision (subject = 100%) 4 Minimal Assistance (subject = 75%+) 3 Moderate Assistance (subject = 50%+) **Complete Dependence** 2 Maximal Assistance (subject =25%+) 1 Total Assistance (subject = less than 25%)	HELPER

	ADMISSION	DISCHARGE	FOLLOW-UP
Self-Care A. Eating B. Grooming C. Bathing D. Dressing - Upper Body E. Dressing - Lower Body F. Toileting			
Sphincter Control G. Bladder Management H. Bowel Management			
Transfers I. Bed, Chair, Wheelchair J. Toilet K. Tub, Shower			
Locomotion L. Walk/Wheelchair M. Stairs	W Walk C Wheelchair B Both	W Walk C Wheelchair B Both	W Walk C Wheelchair B Both
Motor Subtotal Rating			
Communication N. Comprehension O. Expression	A Auditory V Visual B Both A Auditory V Visual B Both	A Auditory V Visual B Both A Auditory V Visual B Both	A Auditory V Visual B Both A Auditory V Visual B Both
Social Cognition P. Social Interaction Q. Problem Solving R. Memory			
Cognitive Subtotal Rating			
TOTAL FIM™ RATING			

NOTE: Leave no blanks. Enter 1 if patient is not testable due to risk.

FIGURE 6-15 FIM Instrument. (From © 1997 Uniform Data System for Medical Rehabilitation (UDSMR), a division of UB Foundation Activities, Inc. (UBFA). Reprinted with the permission of UDSMR. All marks associated with FIM and UDSMR are owned by UBFA.)

SPINAL CORD INDEPENDENCE MEASURE (SCIM)

PATIENT NAME: _____ ID: _____ EXAMINER: _____

(The score attached to the relevant description of each function should be placed in the adjacent square below the relevant date.)

ACTIVITY	DATE AND SCORE				
SELF-CARE					
1. Feeding (cutting, opening containers, bringing food to mouth, holding cup with fluid)					
0 – Needs parenteral, gastrostomy, or dully assisted oral feeding					
1 – Eats cut food using several adaptive devices for hand and dishes					
2 – Eats cut food using only one adaptive device for hand, unable to hold cup					
3 – Eats cut food with one adaptive device, holds cup					
4 – Eats cut food without adaptive devices; needs a little assistance (e.g., to open containers)					
5 – Independent in all tasks without any adaptive device					
2. Bathing (soaping, manipulating water tap, washing)					
0 – Requires total assistance					
1 – Soaps only small part of body with or without adaptive devices					
2 – Soaps with adaptive devices; cannot reach distant parts of the body or cannot operate tap					
3 – Soaps without adaptive devices; needs a little assistance to reach distant parts of body					
4 – Washes independently with adaptive devices or in specific environmental setting					
5 – Washes independently without adaptive devices					
3. Dressing (preparing clothes, dressing upper & lower body, undressing)					
0 – Requires total assistance					
1 – Dresses upper body partially (e.g., without buttoning) in special setting (e.g., back support)					
2 – Independent in dressing and undressing upper body; needs much assistance for lower body					
3 – Requires little assistance in dressing upper or lower body					
4 – Dresses and undresses independently but requires adaptive devices or special setting					
5 – Dresses and undresses independently, without adaptive devices					
4. Grooming (washing hands & face, brushing teeth, combing hair, shaving, applying makeup)					
0 – Requires total assistance					
1 – Performs only one task (e.g., washing hands & face)					
2 – Performs some tasks using adaptive devices; needs help to put on or take off devices					
3 – Performs some tasks using adaptive devices; puts on or takes off devices independently					
4 – Performs all tasks with adaptive devices or most tasks without devices					
5 – Independent in all tasks without adaptive devices					
ACTIVITY	**DATE AND SCORE**				
RESPIRATION AND SPHINCTER MANAGEMENT					
5. Respiration					
0 – Requires assisted ventilation					
2 – Requires tracheal tube and partially assisted ventilation					
4 – Breathes independently but requires much assistance in tracheal tube management					
6 – Breathes independently and requires little assistance in tracheal tube management					
8 – Breathes without tracheal tube but sometimes requires mechanical assistance for breathing					
10 – Breathes independently without any device					
6. Sphincter Management – Bladder					
0 – Indwelling catheter					
5 – Assisted intermittent catheterization or no catheterization; residual urine volume > 100 cm^3					
10 – Intermittent self-catheterization					

FIGURE 6-16   Spinal Cord Independence Measure (SCIM). (From Catz A, Itzkovich M, Agranov E et al: SCIM—spinal cord independence measure: a new disability scale for patients with spinal cord lesions, *Spinal Cord* 35:850-856, 1997.)

Continued

15 – No catheterization required; residual urine volume < 100 cm^3						
7. Sphincter Management – Bowel						
0 – Irregularity, improper timing, very low frequency (less than once/3 days) of bowel movement						
5 – Regular bowel movements, with proper timing but with assistance (e.g., inserting suppository)						
10 – Regular bowel movements, with proper timing, without assistance						
8. Use of Toilet (perineal hygiene, clothes adjustment before/after, use of napkins or diapers)						
0 – Requires total assistance						
1 – Undresses lower body, needs assistance in all the remaining tasks						
2 – Undresses lower body and partially cleans self (after); needs assistance in adjusting clothes,						
3 – Undresses and cleans self (after); needs assistance in adjusting clothes, napkin, diaper						
4 – Independent in all tasks but needs adaptive devices or special setting (e.g., grab bars)						
5 – Independent without adaptive devices or special setting						

ACTIVITY	DATE AND SCORE					
MOBILITY (ROOM & TOILET)						
9. Mobility in Bed & Action to Prevent Pressure Sores						
0 – Requires total assistance						
1 – Partial mobility (turns in bed to one side only)						
2 – Turns to both sides in bed but does not fully release pressure						
3 – Releases pressure when lying only						
4 – Turns in bed and sits up without assistance						
5 – Independent in bed mobility; performs push-ups in sitting position without full body elevation						
6 – Performs push-ups in sitting position						
10. Transfers Between Bed–Wheelchair (locking wheelchair, lifting footrests, removing & adjusting arm rests, transferring, lifting feet)						
0 – Requires total assistance						
1 – Needs partial assistance or supervision						
2 – Independent						
11. Transfers Between Wheelchair–Toilet–Tub (if uses toilet wheelchair then transfers to and from; if uses regular wheelchair then locking wheelchair, lifting footrests, removing & adjusting arm rests, transferring, lifting feet)						
0 – Requires total assistance						
1 – Needs partial assistance or supervision, or adaptive device (e.g., grab bars)						
2 – Independent						

ACTIVITY	DATE AND SCORE					
MOBILITY (INDOORS & OUTDOORS)						
12. Mobility Indoors (short distances)						
0 – Requires total assistance						
1 – Needs electric wheelchair or partial assistance to operate manual wheelchair						
2 – Moves independently in manual wheelchair						
3 – Walks with a walking frame						
4 – Walks with crutches						
5 – Walks with two canes						
6 – Walks with one cane						
7 – Needs leg orthoses only						
8 – Walks without aids						
13. Mobility for Moderate Distances (10 to 100 meters)						

FIGURE 6-16, cont'd Spinal Cord Independence Measure (SCIM). (From Catz A, Itzkovich M, Agranov E et al: SCIM—spinal cord independence measure: a new disability scale for patients with spinal cord lesions, *Spinal Cord* 35:850-856, 1997.)

0 – Requires total assistance						
1 – Needs electric wheelchair or partial assistance to operate manual wheelchair						
2 – Moves independently in manual wheelchair						
3 – Walks with a walking frame						
4 – Walks with crutches						
5 – Walks with two canes						
6 – Walks with one cane						
7 – Needs leg orthoses only						
8 – Walks without aids						
14. Mobility Outdoors (more than 100 meters)						
0 – Requires total assistance						
1 – Needs electric wheelchair or partial assistance to operate manual wheelchair						
2 – Moves independently in manual wheelchair						
3 – Walks with a walking frame						
4 – Walks with crutches						
5 – Walks with two canes						
6 – Walks with one cane						
7 – Needs leg orthoses only						
8 – Walks without aids						
15. Stair Management						
0 – Unable to climb or descend stairs						
1 – Climbs 1 or 2 steps only in a rehabilitation environment						
2 – Climbs and descends at least 3 steps with support or supervision of another person						
3 – Climbs and descends at least 3 steps with support of handrail or crutch or cane						
4 – Climbs and descends at least 3 steps without any support or supervision						
16. Transfers Between Wheelchair–Car (approaching car, locking wheelchair, removing arm & foot rests, transferring to and from car, bringing wheelchair into & out of car)						
0 – Requires total assistance						
1 – Needs partial assistance or supervision or adaptive devices						
2 – Independent without adaptive devices						

FIGURE 6-16, cont'd Spinal Cord Independence Measure (SCIM). (From Catz A, Itzkovich M, Agranov E et al: SCIM—spinal cord independence measure: a new disability scale for patients with spinal cord lesions, *Spinal Cord* 35:850-856, 1997.)

stroke volume and cardiac output. The evaluation of tolerance to upright is essentially the same process for the treatment of the complication. The therapist assesses baseline blood pressure and heart rate and if both fall within accepted parameters then she slowly increases the elevation of the head by 5 to 10 degrees. Then she takes the blood pressure and heart rate again. If the patient is asymptomatic and vital signs are within an accepted range, the therapist can pause for a few minutes and then repeat the process. It should be noted that the process of orthostatic hypotension is a result of fluid pooling into the lower quarter and that it may take several minutes for an objective change in blood pressure to appear. Progressive increases in the degree of upright are undertaken with great caution to avoid syncope. These increases can be done on a mat table with a wedge under the head or on a tilt table where the angle is gradually increased while vital signs are monitored (Figure 6-17). The patient's blood pressure should not drop below 70/40 mm Hg because such a low pressure could result in cardiac arrest. The patient should never be left alone while the elevation of his head and body are being increased. Patient and family caregivers should be apprised about what symptoms might normally appear during the procedure. They should be encouraged to feel comfortable about notifying the therapist (see Chapter 7).

Bed Mobility

Evaluating bed mobility includes assessing how a patient moves within the bed, for instance, from side to side and head to foot of the bed. In addition, evaluating how he rolls from supine to the right and left and to prone and how he moves from supine to long sitting and from supine to short sitting at the edge of the bed. Often the patient is evaluated on a therapy mat and not in bed. This is a mistake because the two surfaces have a dramatically different resiliency and status. The mattress has a different surface environment from that of the mat on a wooden table.

The patient may not be able to perform a skill at all on the mat but is able to use the adjustments and side rails of a hospital bed to assist with greater independence. Document how the patient uses side rails and loops and responds to varying levels of bed firmness and to elevation of the head of the bed.

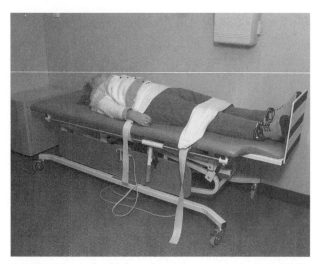

FIGURE 6-17 A tilt-table is used to evaluate a patient's physical ability to tolerate any degree of being upright through gradual adjustments from the supine position, to slight head elevation, to sitting, or to standing.

Transfers

There are multiple types of transfer techniques that can be performed between various types of surfaces (see Chapter 8). These transfers include transfer board transfers, lateral transfers, roll-out transfers, and dependent transfers. In the beginning, it is most important to evaluate transfers from bed to wheelchair, wheelchair to toilet or commode, and wheelchair to the shower or tub. Car transfers and floor transfers should also be evaluated. The details should be recorded to identify how the patient sets the wheelchair up at the transferring surface, whether the surfaces are even or uneven, whether the patient needs assistance with transfer board placement or lower limb management during the transfer, and whether verbal cueing is necessary. When transfers are difficult because of arm length, note the use of blocks to improve reach and elevation. It is vital that the status reported provides a true picture of what is occurring. For example, although a patient may be independent when transferring to a particular mat during the therapy session, he may require moderate assistance to every other surface. If it is documented that this individual is "independent with transfers," other members of the health care team may not realize the extent to which further rehabilitation is required for the patient to learn successful negotiation with other surfaces. Assess other characteristics such as level of fatigue, fear, balance awareness and ability to recover, pain, pressure ulcers, the presence of an orthosis or brace, and spasticity if it interferes with the transfer.

Wheelchair Management and Propulsion

Evaluation of wheelchair management and propulsion should focus on the patient's ability to manage the parts of a wheelchair or to instruct others to do so. These parts include the brakes, armrests, legrests, antitip bars, headrest, and power mobility components as needed (see Chapters 11 and 15). The patient needs to be able to get the parts on and off the chair and be able to store them within reach until they are needed again. For example, if a patient can take a legrest off and drop it to the floor but then cannot retrieve it from the floor to put it back on the chair, he is not independent in that skill. He may need to hook the removed legrest onto the outside wheel until he returns to the chair (see Chapter 8). Evaluation of wheelchair propulsion should involve the need for specialized components, such as rubberized push rims or lugs on push rims or power-assisted wheels (see Chapter 11).

Sitting and Standing Balance

Evaluating sitting balance includes evaluation of the patient in both the long-sitting position with the legs straight and the short-sitting position with the knees bent on various surfaces both statically and dynamically. Statically refers to a set position where all components are still versus dynamically where the patient is challenged to maintain his balance either while he is moving or the surface he is on is moving. The therapist can note the amount of assistance a patient requires, whether support with his upper limbs is needed, whether any external support is required, or whether the lower limbs are required to be in a particular position. Indicating how frequently balance is lost during a given time, the causes for the loss of balance, and what maneuvers are made to regain balance also should be documented.

Similarly to sitting balance, the patient's ability to maintain standing, for how long, with how much assistance, and with what assistive or orthotic equipment should be documented. Again the patient should be challenged to perform static standing and dynamic standing where he is asked to maintain standing while also having to move the trunk or upper limbs.

Ambulation

When the therapist is evaluating ambulation, assessment of the type of gait, the amount of assistance required, and the type of assistive devices or orthoses needed should be included. Details should be recorded to describe the walking surfaces (e.g., level or unlevel, grass, gravel), walking cadence, quality of the movement, and any motor control problems. In addition, the therapist should document the distance the patient can walk (e.g., outside in the community versus within the household distances), how long he needs to rest between intervals, and how many of each interval he can perform. Use of a heart rate monitor, such as a portable chest strap or wrist watch, may provide continuous recording of heart rate to determine the physiological level of difficulty and to better guide the use of gait training for a cardiovascular training effect. A patient who can walk 10 feet independently once or twice a day demonstrates more significantly reduced functional ambulation than a patient who can walk 10 feet independently at a normal rate four times an hour (see Chapter 16).

Stair Negotiation

The negotiation of stairs is important for ambulatory and non-ambulatory patients. For patients who are not ambulatory, stair negotiation should be evaluated in the wheelchair earlier rather than later, particularly if the patient plans to leave the facility on a pass before discharge. In addition, the ability of patients with paraplegia who are deemed able to bump up and down the stairs on their buttocks should be evaluated (with or without their wheelchair depending on whether someone will be assisting them) (see Chapter 15).

For patients who are ambulatory, stair negotiation should be evaluated on the basis of the type of technique used, variations between ascending and descending the stairs, the use of an assistive device or orthotic, and the need to access and use one or both handrails (see Chapter 16). Depending on the presence of a handrail, people with SCI who are ambulatory can ascend steps in either a forward or sideward position. In addition, the number, height, and surface of the stairs should be documented. Stairs are frequently the greatest obstacle to a patient with SCI when discharge to home is planned. Following the old adage that "practice makes perfect," practice should be initiated on stairs slowly but earlier rather than later so that preparation for discharge ensures a successful transition.

Designed as a generalized guideline, Table 6-5 summarizes functional mobility according to the SCI classification level.

TABLE 6-5 | Functional Expectations for Patients with Spinal Cord Injury

Level	Muscles Innervated	Bed Mobility	Transfers	Wheelchair Skills	Standing and Ambulation	FIM Score
C1-C4	C1-C3: Sternocleidomastoid, trapezius, cervical paraspinal, and neck accessory muscles C4: Above plus diaphragm	TA; full electric hospital bed with pressure relief mattress; verbalizes instructions for care	TA; transfer board or mechanical lift with body sling; verbalizes instructions for care	TA with manual wheelchair; Mod I with power wheelchair using head, chin, mouth, or breath control but TA for curbs; may be independent with pressure relief using a tilt-in-space wheelchair	TA: no functional ambulation; standing/tilt table use may improve circulatory hypokinesis and osteoporosis	1: Manual wheelchair 6: Power wheelchair
C5	Above plus deltoid, biceps, brachialis, brachioradialis, rhomboid, and serratus anterior muscles	I in control of electric bed, may use side rails and Mod A to Max A assist for bed mobility but verbalizes instruction for care	TA, may be able to assist with parts of transfer with a transfer board; other wise a mechanical lift is needed	Mod I in power wheelchair using hand controls; pressure relief may require a tilt-in-space wheelchair; I in use of manual wheelchair indoors, Mod I needed outdoors (e.g., curbs)	TA: no functional ambulation; standing/tilt table use may improve circulatory hypokinesis and osteoporosis	1: Ambulation and transfer 2-3: Bed mobility; 6: Wheelchair skills 6: Ambulation
C6	Above plus clavicular pectoralis, serratus anterior, latissimus dorsi, supinator extensor carpi, and radialis longus and brevis muscles	Min A and Mod I in hospital bed and Min A needed with a standard bed	Min A to Mod I, more assistance needed when surfaces are uneven, transfer board needed for some activities	Mod I in power wheelchair with standard arm controls on all surfaces; I in manual chair indoors and Mod A to Max A outdoors; I in pressure relief without equipment	TA; standing/tilt table use may improve circulatory hypokinesis and osteoporosis	4-6: Bed mobility and transfer 6: Power wheelchair and manual wheelchair indoors 1-3: Manual wheelchair outdoor 2: Ambulation
C7-C8	Above plus sternal pectoralis, triceps pronator, extensor, and flexor, carpi radialis, finger flexors, abductor pollicis, and partial lumbrical muscles	Mod I to Min A if surface is uneven with or without a transfer board	Mod I to Min A if surfaces are uneven	Mod I in all wheelchair activities, may need Mod A on uneven surfaces and curbs, TA assist on stairs	TA; standing/tilt table use may improve circulatory hypokinesis and osteoporosis	6: Except ambulation
T1-T9	Above plus full lumbrical and some trunk muscles	Mod I	Mod I	Mod I on level and uneven terrain except stairs	Mod I to Mod A with long leg braces	6
T10 and below	Above plus all trunk muscles	Mod I	Mod I	Mod I on level and uneven terrain	Mod I to Min A with long leg braces	6

Data from Atrice MS, Morrison SA, McDowell SL et al: Traumatic spinal cord injury. In Umphred DA, editor: *Neurological rehabilitation*, ed 4, St. Louis, 2001, Mosby; Consortium for Spinal Cord Medicine: *Traumatic spinal cord injury: clinical practice guidelines for health care professionals*, Washington, DC, 1999, Paralyzed Veterans of America; Lin VW, Cardenas DD, Cutter NC et al. *Spinal cord medicine: principles and practice*, New York, 2003, Demos; Pendleton HM, Schultz-Krohn W: *Pedretti's occupational therapy: practice skills for physical dysfunction*, ed 6, St. Louis, 2006, Mosby Elsevier.
TA, Total assistance; *I*, independent; *Mod I*, modified independent; *Min A*, minimal assistance; *Mod A*, moderate assistance; *Max A*, maximum assistance; *FIM Scale*, 1 = total assist, 2 = maximal assist, 3 = moderate assist, 4 = minimal assist, 5 = supervision, 6 = modified independence, 7 = complete independence.

There will be exceptions and, when the SCI is incomplete, the functional mobility changes drastically (see Chapter 2). Patients may also be asymmetrical, demonstrating a higher level of functional capacity on one side of the body as opposed to the other side. Equipment needed to enhance functional mobility is not included in this table but is described in detail throughout the textbook (see Chapters 12, 13, 14, and 16); ADLs, including dressing, grooming, hygiene, and feeding, are discussed in Chapter 9.

Cognitive Status

Cognitive status is an area in which interdisciplinary assessment and management are critical, and its assessment goes far beyond orientation to time, date, and place (see Chapters 5 and 22). Physical and occupational therapists play an active role in assessment of the patient's memory, judgment, problem solving, and safety awareness. When documenting these abilities, the clinician should give specific examples of patient behavior and avoid labeling or being judgmental. For example, documenting that the patient was tearful throughout the therapy session and stated "I want to kill myself" provides a lot more information than merely recording that the patient is depressed.

It is not uncommon during SCI trauma for brain injury to occur simultaneously. This can be seen as a result of trauma to the head during an automobile accident, a diving accident, or a fall. Clinically, the result may include behavioral changes or learning difficulties. It is important to consult with the family, colleagues, and friends to determine whether even subtle personality or memory difficulties were present before injury.

SETTING GOALS TO ACHIEVE THE BEST CLINICAL OUTCOMES

The *Guide to Physical Therapist Practice* recommends identifying patient goals and objectives during the initial evaluation to maximize outcomes.[1] Baker et al[33] found that, although goal setting was identified as important to therapists and patients, therapists did not take full advantage of patient participation in the goal-setting process. Goals should be patient centered. Randall et al[34] describe a six-step process for writing functional goals that are meaningful and measurable using and within the context of the *Guide to Physical Therapist Practice* (Box 6-5).

Patient-centered goals are defined as functional goals that involve the patient, significant other and caregivers in the plan of care.[1] Therapists need to establish goals that involve areas of work, leisure, and self-care. In other words, the patient should be asked what goals he would like to accomplish that are functionally meaningful to him and that will make a difference in his life.[35] Indeed, goals that address activities within the patient's environment

BOX 6-5 | Six Steps to Writing Patient-Centered Functional Goals

1. Collaborate with the patient and his family to identify the patient's desired outcomes of therapy
2. Focus all goals on the patient
3. Make sure the activities contained in the goal relate to the desired outcomes and are observable and repeatable with a beginning and an end
4. Structure conditions for patient achievement of the goal that include environmental variables and incorporate specific and relevant measures
5. Describe the amount or type of assistance, time, and number of attempts needed for the patient to achieve success
6. Set a target date for the patient to achieve the goal

Data from Randall KE, McEwen IR: Writing patient-centered functional goals, *Phys Ther* 80:1197-1203, 2000.

are more likely to result in independence after discharge. Writing patient-centered goals will help the therapist conform to a health policy in which health is defined as the potential to achieve goals or perform desired activities. In addition, establishing these goals will allow for better reimbursement, alignment with accreditation bodies, and aid in the patient's recovery.[34]

CLINICAL CASE STUDY Evaluation

Patient History

Richard Lingler is a 23-year-old man referred to physical therapy with a C6 incomplete tetraplegia, ASIA C diagnosis resulting from a motor vehicle accident. He had a left wrist fracture (scaphoid), which was in a cast for 6 weeks. Rich underwent a posterior cervical fusion procedure and was in halo traction for 8 weeks. In addition, his acute hospital care was complicated by an episode of pneumonia and a urinary tract infection. After removal of the halo traction device, Rich was placed in a Philadelphia collar for 1 week and a soft collar for 2 weeks.

Rich is a bachelor who was living with his parents while he paid off his college loans before the accident. His parents are completing a wheelchair-accessible bathroom on their first floor and they are converting their dining room into a temporary bedroom. Rich has one older brother, age 26 years, who was recently married.

Patient's Self-Assessment

Rich wants to return to his job as an accountant. He is uncertain about his living arrangements because he and his girlfriend were looking for an apartment before the accident.

Clinical Assessment
Patient Appearance

- Height 5 feet 9 inches, weight 140 pounds, body mass index 20.7

Cognitive Assessment

- Alert and oriented; Rich is a college graduate with a degree in accounting

Cardiopulmonary Assessment

- Blood pressure 108/63 mm Hg, heart rate at rest 64 beats/min, respiratory rate 11 breaths/min, cough flows are ineffective (<360 L/min), VC is reduced (between 1.5 and 2.5 L)
- Breathing pattern incorporates accessory muscles and upper chest wall only with marked decrease in the anterior and lateral chest wall with a slight decrease in the posterior wall expansion
- Auscultation reveals decreased breath sounds in the lower lobes bilaterally anteriorly and posteriorly while in supine with the head elevated 30 degrees
- Pulse oximeter reading is 98% SpO_2 in ambient air at rest

Musculoskeletal and Neuromuscular Assessment

- Posture: Rich initially presented in halo traction in a wheelchair recliner to 45 degrees; he progressed to a manual wheelchair with his low back and his abdominal muscle strength improved
- Motor assessment reveals C6 incomplete ASIA C motor score that improved from 20 to 34 in the upper limbs and from 0 to 14 in the lower limbs
- Sensory initially intact to C6 but improved to T10
- Deep tendon reflexes (DTRs) 3+ in the lower limbs
- Muscular substitution is present when flexing the shoulder by externally rotating the shoulder to avoid the elbow flexion resulting from absent triceps on the left
- Muscle spasticity was generally a 2 to 3 across all muscle groups of the lower limbs

Integumentary and Sensory Assessment

- Skin is intact throughout
- Sensation is impaired below T10

Range of Motion Assessment

- Passive and active ROM is within normal limits in both upper limbs and lower limbs
- Straight leg raise is 90 degrees bilaterally passively

Mobility and Activities of Daily Living Assessment

- Moderate assist in all self-care activities including dressing, grooming, and hygiene
- Dependent in bowel and bladder management
- Independent in wheelchair management and propulsion
- Nonambulatory

Equipment

- A tub bench has been ordered for home use

Evaluation of Clinical Assessment

Richard Lingler is a 23-year-old man referred to physical therapy with a C6 incomplete tetraplegia, ASIA C diagnosis resulting from MVA. He is being admitted for outpatient physical therapy at 11 weeks post injury.

Patient's Care Needs

1. Therapeutic interventions to maximize independence with mobility and return to work requirements
2. Evaluation of functional position changes for bed mobility, transfer to multiple surfaces, wheelchair use and management, and the potential for ambulation education for avoidance of pulmonary and urinary tract infections

Diagnosis and Prognosis

Diagnosis is C6 incomplete tetraplegia, ASIA C. Prognosis for Rich is excellent as a candidate who can attain independence with transfers and mobility for return to work.

Preferred Practice Pattern*

Impaired Muscle Performance (4C), Joint Mobility, Motor Function, Muscle Performance, and Range of Motion Associated With Fracture (4G), Impairments Nonprogressive Spinal Cord Disorders (5H), Primary Prevention/Risk Reduction for Cardiovascular/Pulmonary Disorders (6A), Primary Prevention/Risk Reduction for Integumentary Disorders (7A)

Team Goals

1. Team to instruct Rich in functional position changes over many surfaces including bed, tub, and toilet
2. Team to schedule consultation with wheelchair seating clinic to optimize wheelchair design for return to home and work
3. Team to consult with occupational therapist about home evaluation of parents' home and girlfriend's home
4. Physical therapist to consult with patient about ambulation goals and communicate with lower limb orthotic clinic team
5. Team to coordinate predriving and behind-the-wheel driving evaluation and lessons
6. Team to consult with vocational rehabilitation department to facilitate return to work

Patient Goals

"I want to go back to work and live with my girlfriend."

Care Plan
Treatment Plan and Rationale

- Initiate physical therapy evaluation for functional mobility training, strengthening and conditioning, stretching training to avoid contractures and prevent exaggerated spasticity, and evaluation for ambulation
- Initiate occupational therapy evaluation for home evaluation, technology needed for optimal work environment, and splinting needs for the upper limb
- Schedule a behind-the-wheel driver's test
- Initiate a consultation with the vocational counseling department

Continued

CLINICAL CASE STUDY   Evaluation—cont'd

- Organize a family visit with parent(s) and girlfriend to instruct them on tasks where their assistance is needed because Rich is not fully independent

Interventions
- Stretching exercises to prevent contracture and avoid excessive spasticity
- Strengthening exercises of all available musculature
- Functional training from bed mobility to the potential for ambulation
- Therapeutic exercises for strengthening the available shoulder girdle muscles to improve agonist and antagonist muscle balance to the rotator cuff, neuromuscular re-education, functional training of transfers and wheelchair propulsion to preserve the upper limb, modalities for reduction of pain, and aerobic exercises to increase aerobic fitness
- Instruct patient and family in strategies to relieve pain during healing and to preserve the upper limb during transfers and wheelchair propulsion

Documentation and Team Communication
- Team conference 1 week post admission for appropriate setting of team goals
- Team will refer patient to wheelchair seating clinic for evaluation of wheelchair alignment
- Team will refer to driver's training
- Team will refer to vocational rehabilitation
- Team will evaluate assistive technology needed for return to work
- Team will refer to lower limb orthotic clinic as appropriate
- Team will instruct patient and family in care needs as identified

Critical Thinking Exercises
Consider concepts discussed in this chapter that are associated with Rich's evaluation. The following questions will cover (A) the patient's initial evaluation when entering acute rehabilitation and while medically stable still in halo traction, and (B) the patient's initial evaluation after halo traction has been removed and he is out of cervical support and receiving outpatient therapy.

A. Initial evaluation in acute rehabilitation after an acute hospital stay:
   1. What critical information should you gather from the chart review and patient in addition to the information provided in the case study?
   2. List four pertinent areas to cover during your initial interview with the patient.
   3. Describe what should be included in the patient's respiratory evaluation while he remains in halo traction.
   4. How should you accommodate a patient in a halo traction device during your ROM and manual muscle testing examination? What positions are contraindicated?
   5. The patient in halo traction is limited to supported side-lying and supine positions with the head elevated. Related to integumentary evaluation, what areas are at risk for pressure ulcers and therefore require patient education?

B. Initial evaluation after halo traction device has been removed; Rich is out of cervical support and receiving outpatient therapy:
   1. What additional tests should be completed in the respiratory evaluation?
   2. How should the evaluation of ROM and muscle testing change?
   3. What functional tests should be performed that were prohibited in the halo traction device?
   4. What evaluations should be completed concerning equipment purchases for Rich to return to home and work?

*Guide to physical therapist practice, rev. ed. 2, Alexandria, VA, 2003, American Physical Therapy Association.

SUMMARY

Examination and evaluation involves the assessment of impairments, functional limitations, activity, and participation factors that contribute to the disablement process. It is essential to master the evaluation process of the patient with SCI. Strong evaluation skills will enable a well-directed therapeutic program and allow for a continuous comparison of new data with the original evaluation findings. Experienced clinicians make efficient evaluations a priority to avoid requiring the patient to undergo unnecessary maneuvers or position changes that can occur when an evaluation is disorganized. In addition, an efficient evaluation gives the patient confidence regarding the clinician's competence and willingness to become an active participant in his clinical care and progression.

A thorough evaluation includes a historical record of all events leading up to a patient seeking clinical care. The review of systems includes an objective assessment of vital signs, respiratory status, integumentary, range of motion, muscle performance, sensation, functional status, and cognitive status. The combined historical data and review of systems lead to a therapeutic estimation of the potential for functional gains, which in turn provides a foundation for the establishment of goals within a collaborative decision-making process between the patient and therapist. When establishing realistic goals, the clinician must take into account the resources available, discharge disposition, family help availability, home and community environments, and the potential level of recovery expected considering concomitant medical conditions. The next step is the implementation of a comprehensive treatment program, described in the following chapters.

REFERENCES

1. *American Physical Therapy Association: Guide to physical therapist practice*, ed 2, Alexandria, VA, 2001, American Physical Therapy Association.
2. Jarvis C: *Physical examination and health assessment*, ed 4, Philadelphia, 2004, WB Saunders.
3. Ryan NP, Wade JC, Nice A et al: Physical therapists' perceptions of family involvement in the rehabilitation process, *Physiother Res Int* 1:159-179, 1996.
4. Curtis KA, Davis CM, Trimble TK et al: Early family experiences and helping behaviors of physical therapists, *Phys Ther* 75:1089-1100, 1995.
5. Anderson MK, Hall SJ, Martin M: *Sports injury management*, ed 2, Philadelphia, 2000, Lippincott Williams & Wilkins.

6. Seidel HM, Ball JW, Dains JE et al: *Mosby's guide to physical examination*, ed 5, St. Louis, 2003, Mosby.

7. Lin VW, Cardenas DD, Cutter NC et al: *Spinal cord medicine: principles and practice*, New York, 2003, Demos.

8. Scully RM, Barnes MR: Respiratory analysis. In Scully RM, editor: *Physical therapy*, Philadelphia, 1989, JB Lippincott.

9. Wanger J: *Pulmonary function testing: a practical approach*, Baltimore, 1992, Williams & Wilkins.

10. Wetzel J: Respiratory evaluation and treatment. In Adkins HV, editor: *Spinal cord injury*, New York, 1985, Churchill Livingstone.

11. Rinehart M, Nawoczenski D: Respiratory care. In Buchanan L, Nawoczenski D, editors: *Spinal cord injury: concepts and management approaches*, Baltimore, 1987, Williams & Wilkins.

12. Wetzel J, Lunsford B, Peterson, M et al: Respiratory rehabilitation of the patient with spinal cord injury. In Irwin S, Tecklin J, editors: *Cardiopulmonary physical therapy*, ed 3, St. Louis, 1995, Mosby.

13. Irwin S, Tecklin J, editors: *Cardiopulmonary physical therapy: a guide to practice*, ed 4, St. Louis, 2004, Mosby.

14. Fletcher J: Range of motion. In Bandy WD, Sanders B, editors: *Therapeutic exercise: techniques for intervention*, Baltimore, 2001, Lippincott Williams & Wilkins.

15. Hislop HJ, Montgomery J: *Daniels and Worthingham's muscle testing: techniques of manual examination*, ed 8, St. Louis, 2007, Saunders Elsevier.

16. Kendall FP, McCreary EK: *Muscles testing and function*, ed 4, Baltimore, 1993, Williams & Wilkins.

17. American Spinal Injury Association: *International standards for neurological and functional classification of spinal cord injury worksheet*, Atlanta, GA, 2006, American Spinal Injury Association.

18. Massery M: The patient with neuromuscular or musculoskeletal dysfunction. In Frownfelter D, Dean E, editors: *Principles and practice of cardiopulmonary physical therapy*, ed 3, St. Louis, 1996, Mosby.

19. Frownfelter D, Dean E: *Principles and practice of cardiopulmonary physical therapy: evidence and practice*, ed 4, St. Louis, 2006, Mosby Elsevier.

20. Lundy-Ekman L: *Neuroscience: fundamentals for rehabilitation*, ed 2, Philadelphia, 2002, WB Saunders.

21. Ashworth B: Preliminary trial of carisoprodol in multiple sclerosis, *Practitioner* 192:540-542, 1964.

22. Bohannon RW, Smith MB: Inter-rater reliability on modified Ashworth scale of muscle spasticity, *Phys Ther* 67:206-207, 1987.

23. Bonica JJ: Evolution and current status of pain programs, *J Pain Symptom Manage* 5:368-374, 1990.

24. Melzack R, Katz J: The McGill Pain Questionnaire: appraisal and current status. In Turk DC, Melzack R, editors: *Handbook of pain assessment*, New York, 1992, Guilford Press.

25. Eide P: Pathophysiological mechanism of central neuropathic pain after spinal cord injury, *Spinal Cord* 36:501-612, 1998.

26. Sie I, Waters R, Atkins R et al: Upper extremity pain in post rehabilitation *spinal cord* injured patient, *Arch Phys Med Rehabil* 73: 44-48, 1992.

27. Boninger ML, Dicianno BE, Cooper RA et al: Shoulder magnetic resonance imaging abnormalities, wheelchair propulsion, and gender, *Arch Phys Med Rehabil* 84:1615-1620, 2003.

28. Pentland WE, Twomey LT: Upper limb function in persons with long term paraplegia and implications for independence: part I, *Paraplegia* 32:211-218, 1994.

29. Pentland WE, Twomey LT: Upper limb function in persons with long term paraplegia and implications for independence: part II, *Paraplegia* 32:219-224, 1994.

30. Curtis KA, Roach KE, Applegate EB et al: Development of the Wheelchair User's Shoulder Pain Index (WUSPI), *Paraplegia* 33:290-293, 1995.

31. Keith RA, Granger CV, Hamilton BB et al: The functional independence measure: a new tool for rehabilitation, *Adv Clin Rehabil* 1:6-18, 1987.

32. Catz A, Itzkovich M, Agranov E et al: SCIM—spinal cord independence measure: a new disability scale for patients with spinal cord lesions, *Spinal Cord* 35:850-856, 1997.

33. Baker SM, Marshak HH, Rice GT et al: Patient participation in physical therapy goal setting, *Phys Ther* 81:1118-1126, 2001.

34. Randall KE, McEwen IR: Writing patient-centered functional goals, *Phys Ther* 80:1197-1203, 2000.

35. Marvel MK, Epstein RM, Flowers K et al: Soliciting the patient's agenda: have we improved? *JAMA* 281:283-287, 1999.

SOLUTIONS TO CHAPTER 6 CLINICAL CASE STUDY

Evaluation

A. Initial evaluation in acute rehabilitation after an acute hospital stay:

1. In addition to the information provided, Rich's medical and surgical histories are reviewed. Current medications are recorded and their purpose noted. Any pulmonary function tests, laboratory reports, and radiographic results of both the cervical injury and left wrist are also reviewed. Additional information regarding the complications of urinary tract infection or pneumonia is noted. Information regarding the emotional state of the patient and interactions between the patient and his family and between the family and health care team are also pertinent.

2. It is critical to gather information by using open-ended questions during the initial interview in regard to the Rich's emotional state and a subjective report of his injury. Information about family should also be included regardless of whether the family is present. It is also important to get to know Rich as an individual by asking about his occupation, hobbies and interests, leisure activities, and social background. Knowledge about a patient's response to treatment during the acute hospital stay is valuable in planning a treatment approach and interventions. Finally, it is of utmost importance to include the patient's goals as the basis for designing interventions and therapeutic goals.

3. The respiratory evaluation includes auscultation, measurement of chest expansion, palpation of bony and soft tissue elements related to proper respiration, measurement of vital capacity, and assessment of cough function. Modifications of these procedures are necessary while the patient is in a halo apparatus because of both positional precautions and movement precautions. The medical stability of the patient's blood pressure dictates the position for each portion of the respiratory examination. Auscultation takes place in supine with the head of the bed in a position consistent with a stable blood pressure, usually between 30 and 60 degrees; supported semi-side-lying is also a possible position to listen to the lower lung lobes. The therapist is limited in all positions by how far the stethoscope can reach underneath the halo device. It is critical to note that the therapist must not hit the metal uprights of the halo traction device with her stethoscope because this sends an uncomfortable vibration through the client's skull.

It is important to document where the chest expansion measurements are taken because the halo device may limit the most optimal measure, restricting accessibility to a lower thoracic measure. Cough assessment is also important and must be documented. Rich will need effective cough with assistance because of his history of pneumonia and the level of his injury. Assistive cough technique positions will be limited because of halo precautions. Patient education regarding good pulmonary hygiene is critical to Rich's care. Recorded measurement of vital capacity should include both the instrumentation and the position of testing.

4. Prone and full upright positions will be contraindicated while Rich is in the halo device. The weight of the halo traction device moves the center of mass of the patient cephalad or he becomes top heavy; therefore, the fully upright position is unsafe. Rich does not have the muscular support to balance in the upright position.

All range of motion and manual muscle test values should include the position of testing. Supine on a wedge would provide adequate support for the patient and allow the therapist to modify traditional test positions and still gain sufficient information of strength and range of motion for designing treatment interventions and establishing goals. Manual muscle testing should be limited to 3+ at the shoulder unilaterally unless otherwise indicated by the physician.

5. Continuing assessment for prolonged pressure to any bony areas from the halo device is very important. These include any areas that the device may touch on bony areas on the trunk and spine. While Rich is in the supine position, the scapulae and spinous processes

may be at risk and in the side-lying position the ribs on the respective sides are susceptible to pressure ulcers. The top of the halo device must not create excessive pressure over the acromioclavicular joint to avoid the potential for pressure ulcers. Bony prominences are at risk for breakdown, including the elbows, sacrum, coccyx, greater trochanters, lateral and medial femoral epicondyles, lateral and medial malleoli, and heels. All these exposed bony prominences need to be supported for relief when possible and position changes need to occur in a timely fashion to avoid skin breakdown. Discuss the potential causes for skin breakdown, including poor nutrition, smoking, swelling, incontinence, and lack of pressure relief mechanisms, with the patient and family members or caregivers. Show the patient and his family the early warning signs of skin breakdown and how to prevent increased damage.

B. Initial evaluation after the halo device has been removed; Rich is out of cervical support and receiving outpatient therapy:

1. Auscultation is no longer limited by the halo device and upright positioning is now possible for any testing as long as blood pressure issues do not interfere. In addition, all chest expansion measurements can be taken. Vital capacity should be retested by the same method used as when the halo device was in place and also with additional instrumentation that could not previously be used for evaluation. The client can now be instructed in a full range of assistive cough techniques for self-care and family members or caregivers can be instructed in assistive techniques.

2. Accurate passive range of motion resulting from halo device precautions and limitations at the shoulder joint can now be reassessed because the device itself no longer restricts movement. The therapist can complete a thorough evaluation of joint integrity. Manual muscle testing can now be performed in full upright with trunk support for more accurate test position assessment. In addition, Rich was diagnosed with an ASIA C motor SCI and may have had changes in muscle strength because the lesion is incomplete and strength often improves over time. Even muscle strength of a grade 2 can significantly contribute to improved functional independence with activities of daily living and instrumental activities of daily living. The influence of muscle tone or spasticity will most likely have changed and should be evaluated, including the impact for assistance or restriction with function.

3. A comprehensive evaluation of bed mobility can now be completed; the patient can now be assisted to prone without contraindication (formerly because of the halo device). Full evaluation of transfers to all surfaces should be completed, including: bed to wheelchair, wheelchair to toilet or commode, and wheelchair to the shower or tub. Goals should include transfers to the car and floor transfers. Sitting balance in both short- and long-sit should be evaluated. Rich's control in these positions will affect independence in bed mobility and transfer levels. Depending on Rich's muscular return, evaluation of standing or ambulation with orthoses could also be a goal.

4. A comprehensive wheelchair evaluation and assessment of wheelchair propulsion needs to be completed. A work site assessment will help to establish what necessary equipment needs are warranted and what workplace adaptations are necessary. Assessment for a manual wheelchair, power wheelchair, or both, will need to be determined on the basis of considerations of future needs and possible functional changes. Proper selection of a wheelchair cushion related to the work ergonomic and skin care needs will also be considered. Prevention strategies for shoulder injuries from overuse or compensatory strategies with activities of daily living and instrumental activities of daily living are also important to patient and family or caregiver education. As driving progresses, the need for an adapted driving vehicle should be discussed.

CHAPTER SEVEN

Intervention Principles and Position Changes

Martha Macht Sliwinski, PT, MA, PhD, and Erica Druin, MPT

Remembering back to when I first got injured and entered rehab brings back some intense memories. There were feelings of frustration and lack of control over a body that seemed to have a mind of its own. I was overwhelmed, to say the least. Getting this body to do such simple things like rolling over in bed or simply sitting up without falling over was an enormous task. Things I took for granted my entire life had to be relearned.

Terri (T6 SCI)

Designing an intervention program for each individual with a spinal cord injury (SCI) presents the team of therapists with an enormous challenge. Each patient is different even when the injuries sustained are similar. Numerous physical variations are possible within each level of SCI (health condition) and psychosocial differences affecting health and care (contextual factors) (see Figure 5-2). The World Health Organization's *International Classification of Function* model for holistic medicine incorporates four components into treatment that address all aspects of an individual: the physical, the intellectual, the emotional, and the spiritual.[1] Considering these areas when developing a treatment design provides individualized programs with the potential to meet the needs and goals of the patient. An interdisciplinary team working closely together can address all four areas through their combined resources and expertise for the patient in a timely manner.

This chapter describes principles of effective treatment design and addresses specific methods of treatment intervention that meet the demands of functional position changes fundamental to the activities of daily living (ADL). Consideration of American Spinal Injury Association (ASIA) levels and functional goals are included for each training section.

INTERVENTION PRINCIPLES

Intervention programs incorporate functional training for position changes that meet the daily demands of the patient's lifestyle. To reach this end the therapist must examine fundamental principles of the treatment design. Principles of patient education, biomechanics, and range of motion (ROM), motor control, strength, and balance are fundamental to both the design and application of treatment programs. The expert clinician is capable of incorporating these principles for both the patient and therapist spontaneously during treatment sessions in a safe, efficient, and effective manner; however, this does not exclude adequate planning for care delivery. To achieve a seamless care plan, the clinician plans ahead, incorporating the individualized needs of the patient. The novice must therefore gain knowledge and practice skills in the above principles, to prepare to meet the challenges inherent in the treatment of individuals with SCI.

Patient Education

Clarity of instruction can be critical for optimal performance when a patient needs to learn new skills. Goals that have been established jointly between the patient and therapist set the starting point for functional training. The selection of functional training requires the therapist to identify the skills that are required for the task to be successful. Ultimately it is important for the patient to clearly understand what the components are for the task and to develop proficiency in completing each ingredient step for successful performance of the entire function. To this end, the therapist must deliver clear instructions considering individual learning style, language, educational background, cultural background, and life experiences (Clinical Note: Considerations for the Delivery of Instruction).[2-4] Instruction may include observing a demonstration of the activity, receiving verbal cues, or being manually assisted through the motion to develop a kinesthetic awareness of the functional task.

Throughout the process of acquiring the skill, the patient is learning through both structured regimen and trial and error. The therapist carefully sequences and delivers feedback and knowledge of results regarding performance while the patient learns each new skill (Clinical Note: Patient Learning Strategies). The therapist observes successful and unsuccessful performances while guiding the patient in modifying and practicing the component skills for functional tasks. She must have strong observational skills to detect the events that lead to success and failure of skills and immediately interject this feedback to the patient. Being aware of the proper timing and the amount of feedback are important skills that can optimize the patient's performance and facilitate his problem-solving skills (Clinical Note: Considerations for Feedback).[5] After a component skill leads to a functional task, the patient can benefit from performing the task again incorrectly and then correctly while describing what occurred that made the task successful. This reinforces problem-solving skills with the knowledge of results that are the key to progression of skill acquisition.

The patient continues through this process while the therapist provides timely feedback and offers alternative methods to complete the task. Methods for successful functional task completion vary from patient to patient. This chapter provides guidelines and suggested techniques. It is, however, a discovery process between the patient and the therapist. The role of therapist is to be the teacher and expert in instruction of new skills in a safe manner as the patient practices and learns his most efficient movement strategy. Special considerations must always be made for joint protection when new position changes are practiced. Success is noted when the patient can explain to the therapist how to do the skill, can teach others, and can repeat the functional tasks consistently over time.

Caregiver Education

Caregiver instruction is critical to ensure optimal fulfillment of established patient goals. Although the patient should be able to instruct a caregiver precisely, it is helpful for the caregiver to know the steps that require assistance for an activity to be completed and these instructions should emphasize how to complete the activity efficiently and safely. The physical therapist should demonstrate the proper techniques to caregivers while explaining what they are doing. Then the caregiver should perform the tasks with guidance until the therapist feels the caregiver has demonstrated the sequence using adequate safety precautions. The patient also can learn from observing caregiver education demonstrations and thus be able to instruct new caregivers and guide how assistance should be provided. Caregivers must also learn proper body mechanics for bending, lifting, pushing, and pulling so that they do not injure themselves. All these activities require adequate spinal stabilization for protection from injury.[6] Caregivers should stabilize the lower abdominals before all tasks that require effort to avoid putting the low back at risk for injury. The large muscles of the legs should be used primarily when lifting while the back and abdominal muscles stabilize the trunk.[6]

The proper lifting technique for safety should be used by caregivers during dependent transfers from wheelchair to bed or mat. The therapist begins with her center of mass (COM) close to the patient's (Figure 7-1, *A*) and then shifts the patient's COM closer as the actual lifting begins (Figure 7-1, *B*). Alternate methods need to be understood so that the therapist has many options to use during various clinical needs (Figure 7-1, *C*). Note the safe and protective position of the therapist's lower back throughout the lifting sequence.

Proper body mechanics is also important when transporting patients within the rehabilitation center. The therapist may need to push patients in both manual and power wheelchairs along flat surfaces and up and down ramps (Figure 7-2, *A*). Different arm

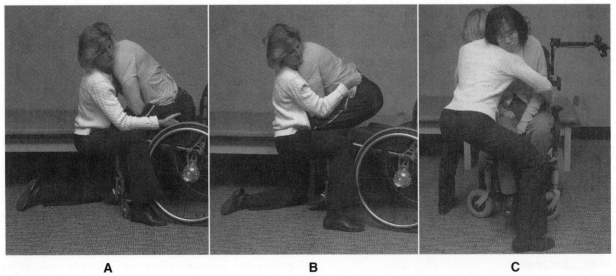

| A | B | C |

FIGURE 7-1 The caregiver demonstrates safe lifting techniques when assisting a patient in a dependent transfer from the wheelchair to the mat. **A,** Note that the caregiver must position herself with her COM close to the patient's COM. **B,** When the actual lift begins, the caregiver's arms are positioned on the patient's pelvis and the patient's COM is brought closer to the caregiver. In **A** and **B** the caregiver is positioned in half kneeling to perform the lift; an alternate method for performing the lift in a squat position demonstrated in **C.**

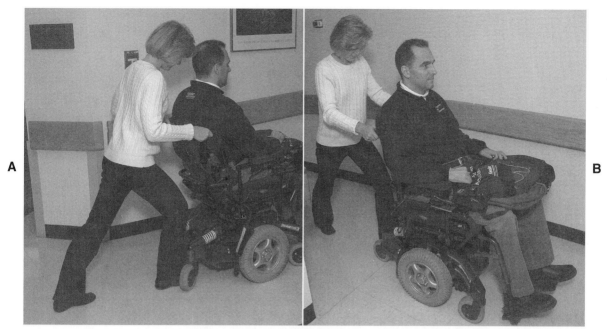

FIGURE 7-2 Caregivers need to practice safe pushing techniques to protect their backs and arms. **A,** The caregiver begins with elbows bent and one leg in front of the other to begin the ascent when pushing an individual with tetraplegia up a ramp. Note the position of the caregiver's legs, which will provide optimal safety for the caregiver's low back, and her stride, which will assist the push. **B,** When they reach the top of the ramp, the caregiver brings her COM close to the wheelchair to control its maneuverability at the top of the ramp.

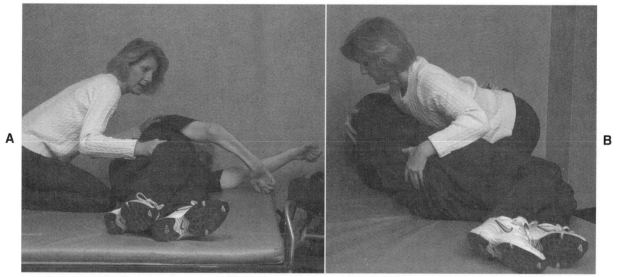

FIGURE 7-3 **A,** The caregiver first positions the patient's legs so that they are bent at the hips and knees. **B,** The caregiver must bring her COM close to the patient's COM and then pull from the pelvis and the scapula to move the patient to his side. It is critical that the caregiver maintain a neutral spine and keep the abdominal muscles engaged.

and body positions will be appropriate at the beginning and end of ramp negotiation (Figure 7-2, *B*).

Teaching dependent patients bed skills is another area where the therapist and caregiver need to practice good body mechanics and understand the role of the COM. After the patient is helped into the desired position (Figure 7-3, *A*), the therapist combines the power of her COM by placing it close to the patient's, which allows her to more readily roll the patient (Figure 7-3, *B*).

Biomechanics of Movement for Individuals with Spinal Cord Injury

The musculoskeletal system is composed of muscles with their tendon attachments to skeletal bones and the ligaments that stabilize bone to bone. Skeletal bones provide a framework to support the body and connect bones to one another to form joints that allow movement to occur through the action of the muscles.[7] The specialized physiology of the muscle organ builds on filaments, myofibrils, muscle fibers, fascicles,

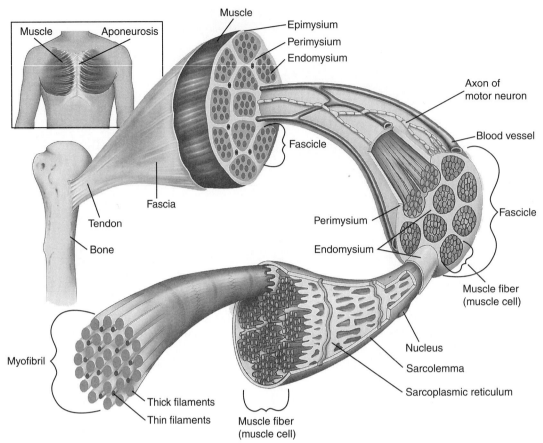

FIGURE 7-4 In a muscle, the connective tissue coverings, the epimysium, perimysium, and endomysium, are continuous with each other and with the tendon. Note that muscle fibers are held together by the perimysium in groups called fascicles. (From Thibodeau GA, Patton KT: *Anatomy & physiology*, ed 5, St. Louis, 2003, Mosby, Figure 10-3, p 281.)

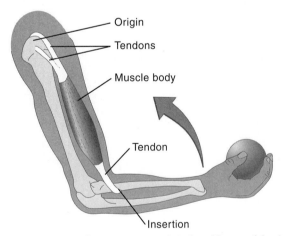

FIGURE 7-5 A muscle originates at a relatively stable part of the skeleton (origin) and inserts at the skeletal part that is moved when the muscle contracts (insertion). (From Thibodeau GA, Patton KT: *Anatomy & physiology*, ed 5, St. Louis, 2003, Mosby, Figure 10-4, p 282.)

and perimysium, which connect through tendons to the bone (Figure 7-4). Because the muscle organ is continuous with the tendons or aponeurosis that attach it to bone or other structures, it remains "firmly harnessed to the structures [it] pulls on during contraction."[7]

The level of the SCI and its ASIA score (see Chapters 1 and 6) dictates the alteration in the functional capability of the musculoskeletal system and therefore alters the related biomechanics for movement. The components that compose the musculoskeletal system have different mechanical properties. Mechanics explore the response of materials or objects to external forces. Muscle, bone, ligaments, and tendons each have their own unique properties, which relate to their ability to withstand forces. These characteristics are typically referred to as stress and strain responses of the tissue.

Physical laws of motion are also applied to the human body in describing movements. Rigid lever systems can be used to describe how joint motion occurs. The fulcrum of a lever is the point around which movement takes place and is often the joint center between two articulating bones in the human body. The lever also comprises two arms or distances from the fulcrum that work in opposition to one another as motion takes place. Combining movement principles and mechanical properties is what is referred to as biomechanics.[7-10]

Biomechanics applies the concepts of mechanics to the human body. The musculoskeletal system uses bones as levers with applied forces generated by the muscles to perform daily tasks. Human leverage systems are predesigned according to human anatomy because muscles have origins and insertions at given lengths from a joint center that cannot be altered (Figure 7-5). The internal lever arm is the distance of the muscles from the

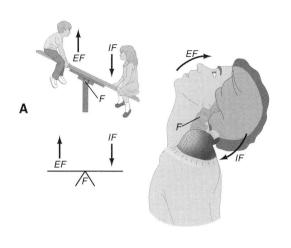

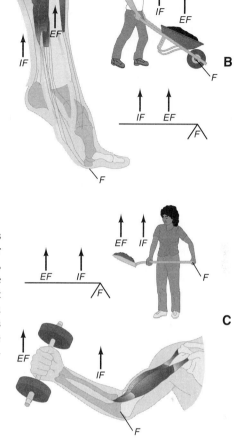

FIGURE 7-6 Understanding how first-, second-, and third-class levers work transfers to human body mechanics. **A,** First-class lever demonstrates the forces located on either side of the fulcrum. **B,** Second-class lever demonstrates the muscle or the internal force *(IF)* having greater leverage than the external force *(EF)* because it is further from the pivot than the external force but they are both on the same side of the fulcrum. **C,** Third-class lever demonstrates the muscle of internal force is closer to the axis of rotation than the external force.(From Thibodeau GA, Patton KT: *Anatomy & physiology*, ed 5, St. Louis, 2003, Mosby.)

joint center. Leverage or mechanical advantage of a muscle, therefore, from a joint center is preset. A second lever arm is the external force or load applied to the joint. The distance of an external force to the joint center can vary. If the internal force exerted by a muscle is equivalent to the external force, no movement will occur at the joint. Enhanced leverage occurs as the distance from the point of rotation or joint center is increased for the internal force to overcome the external applied force.[8-10] When the human body moves, it can change the leverage relationship of the internal and external force (e.g., fixing a limb to a surface versus moving the limb to a target).

Mechanical Advantage Through Levers

The human body is designed with first-, second-, and third-class levers. Each class of levers offers varying mechanical advantages. The first-class lever system is illustrated by the head on the neck, where the fulcrum for rotation is the axis (C2), the weight of the head or external force is on one side of the axis or fulcrum, and the neck extensors or internal force are on the other side (Figure 7-6, *A*). The neck extensor force keeps the head from falling forward. In this example the distance of the neck extensor muscles from the fulcrum is defined as the internal lever arm, and the external lever arm is the distance from the axis to the weight of the head.[7,9] The weight or force must be sufficient by either the muscle or the external load for motion to occur. A first-class lever can have

three types of mechanical advantage depending on the length of each lever arm. The mechanical advantage equals 1 when the distance between the fulcrum and the two lever arms is the same. The mechanical advantage is less than 1 when the internal lever arm is less than the external lever arm and greater than 1 when the internal lever arm is greater than the external lever arm.[8]

In functional situations the strength of the muscle must be strong enough to overcome the weight of the external force and the effects of gravity. Without our muscles counteracting the forces of gravity, a human body would collapse and be unable to maintain upright sitting or standing.[8] A paralyzed muscle, or muscles, adds to the external force that must be overcome to maintain upright stability or for movement to take place. Rolling is an example of this when an individual is paralyzed in the lower limbs; the force of the upper limbs must be sufficient to overcome the weight of the legs plus gravity. The fulcrum can be at any point along the spine depending on the available strength of intact trunk musculature. The external force includes the body below this point, including the paralyzed muscles and the force of gravity acting on the body. Although this example applies a first-class lever, ultimately, momentum is needed to assist the upper limbs when strength is insufficient or inefficient for the patient to roll. The use of momentum, however, should be applied with caution when excessive torque, or rotation, could be applied to joints.

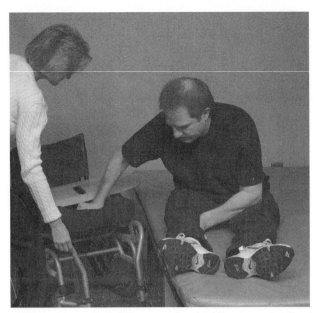

FIGURE 7-7 A patient demonstrates how his left wrist can be placed under his right leg as the fulcrum. The left wrist extensors generate wrist extension creating a lever arm that provides the mechanical advantage to initiate the lift of the weight of the leg.

Although rarely found in the human body,[8] a second-class lever system might feature the muscle or the internal force having greater leverage than the external force or imposed weight because it is further from the pivot and yields a longer lever arm. Both lever arms are on the same side of the fulcrum in this case (Figure 7-6, *B*). The imposed weight is placed distal to the muscle insertion to have this leverage system work. The ankle plantar flexors work in this fashion when the heel is lifted off of the ground. The fulcrum is the ball of the foot and the body weight (imposed weight) falls in front of the Achilles tendon.[7,9] Both lever arms are on the same side of the body fulcrum. In training individuals with SCI, the therapist who can apply the principles of a second-class lever during functional position changes will assist the patient in achieving greater mechanical advantage or leverage for function requiring less muscle force to generate motion. For example, when a patient moves from long-sitting position (LSP) to prone, the left wrist extensors can be used to assist in positioning the right lower leg to cross over the left foot. The left wrist serves as a fulcrum stabilized on the left lower leg (Figure 7-7). For example, when a patient begins to move from long sitting position to prone, he will first cross his right leg over the left. In this second class lever, the fulcrum is defined as the wrist, the external force is the weight of the leg, and the internal force is the wrist extensors (not seen under the right leg). The patient uses the wrist extensors to start the lift of the leg. Note also that the patient is supporting the weight of his trunk through his left elbow on his left thigh. He completes the task of crossing his right leg over the left using a weight shift to the left and a second class lever as the biceps are the internal force, lifting the weight of the leg and the elbow is the fulcrum.

The third-class lever is the most common in the musculoskeletal system. The biceps is an example of a muscle where the internal force (muscle force) is closer to the axis of rotation than

the external force, the weight of the forearm (imposed weight) (Figure 7-6, *C*). This is also accomplished by the deltoid muscle in reaching activities, where the deltoid must exert force to lift the humerus, forearm, and hand.

Application of Biomechanics

Application of the principle of mechanical advantage, or optimizing the length of the lever arm, is critical when teaching functional tasks to individuals with SCI. Over time, use of this increased mechanical advantage, learned by an individual with an SCI to compensate for weak musculature, can help prevent wear and tear on the muscles, bones, and joints because the muscles of the upper limbs are not designed to regularly lift the body weight through space in the manner that lower limbs do for individuals who walk as a means to transport their bodies. The reaction force, or force directed from the supporting surface up throughout the limb to lift the body weight, may contribute to wear and tear of the joints. This applies Newton's third law, where the force of the contacting surface is in equal magnitude to the force exerted downward to that surface by the body's muscle forces.[8] This disperses stresses throughout the weight-bearing joints. Factors influencing stress and strain on the musculoskeletal system include the structure of the tissue, the type and weight of load applied to the tissue, where along the length of the tissue the load is applied, the frequency of the load, the speed or velocity of the load, and how long the load is applied to the tissue.[8] Therefore, the smaller muscles of the upper limbs are subject to stress and strain when transporting the body and performing ADL. Patients need to be instructed in joint and muscle protection and prevention strategies to avoid repetitive stress conditions.

Range of Motion

Performance of functional position changes to complete daily self-care and to manage daily tasks requires that ROM remains maximal at most joints. Loss of ROM in the upper limbs or lower limbs can impair functional independence and require greater effort by the person with SCI or assistance from another individual. Cervical, thoracic, or lumbar ROM decreases may exist because of the nature of the injury and subsequent surgical interventions. Typically, the ROM of the spinal segments above and below the surgical site may increase in their mobility after healing, although the overall motion of that area of the spine is reduced compared to an able-bodied individual. Ideally, full ROM of the spine is desirable for functional position changes. Maintaining the trunk in a neutral alignment is critical for optimal wheelchair positioning, respiration, mobility, and balance. Mild tightness in the low back extensors is important for control of balance, particularly in the LSP to prevent falling from loss of balance during functional tasks performed in this position.

ROM exercises need to begin as soon as possible after injury and medical clearance is obtained. Precautions need to be taken in the acute phases of recovery when the spine is unstable (see Chapter 6). Cervical instability or a spinal orthosis may require limits to active and passive ROM in the upper limbs and with hamstring stretching. Joint mobilization used to maintain the motion of the bone-to-bone relationship and to stretch the joint capsule surrounding the joint can be performed within the precautions to prevent contracture of

TABLE 7-1 | **Range of Motion Requirements for Functional Position Changes and Wheelchair Management**

Joint Motion	Necessary ROM	Clinical Application
Cervical motions	Ideally full AROM all planes but may be limited secondary to surgical interventions	Assists with rolling, transfers, head-hips relationship for functional position changes
Trunk rotation	Ideally full AROM all planes but may be limited as a result of surgical interventions	Assists with rolling, transfers, head-hips relationship for functional position changes
Shoulder flexion	165 to 180 degrees	Assists with overhead functional activities and ADL
Shoulder extension	30 degrees	Functional position changes (supported LSP), wheelchair stabilization for ADL and skin relief, ambulation with crutches
Shoulder external rotation	80 to 90 degrees	Functional position changes (supported LSP), wheelchair stabilization for ADL and skin relief, ambulation with crutches
Elbow extension	0 degrees	Functional position changes (supported LSP), transfers, wheelchair stabilization for ADL and skin relief
Forearm supination	80 degrees	Functional position changes (supported LSP, head hips relationship), transfers, wheelchair stabilization for ADL and skin relief
Forearm pronation	80 degrees	Prone on elbows, transfers, lower limb leg management
Wrist extension	75 to 90 degrees	Functional position changes (supported LSP, head-hips relationship), transfers, wheelchair stabilization for ADL and skin relief
Pelvis	Neutral	Optimal seating position
Hip straight leg raise (hamstring length)	90 to 110 degrees	Functional position changes, ADL activities in LSP, ambulation with crutches
Knee extension	0 degrees	ADL activities in LSP, ambulation with crutches
Knee flexion	90 to 130 degrees	Optimal seating position, wheelchair to floor transfers
Ankle dorsiflexion	0 to 20 degrees	0 degrees for optimal seating position; 10 to 20 degrees for ambulation and elevation activities

Data from Clarkson HM: *Joint motion and function assessment: a research-based practical guide*, New York, 2005, Lippincott Williams & Wilkins; Norkin CC, White DJ: *Measurement of joint motion: a guide to goniometry*, ed 3, Philadelphia, 2003, FA Davis; Reese NB: *Muscle and sensory testing*, ed 2, St. Louis, 2005, Elsevier Saunders.
AROM, Active range of motion.

the joint capsule. Thoracic lesions are typically treated with spinal orthoses that restrict trunk motions in all planes and may require limits with hamstring stretching. Lumbar injuries may have spinal motion and hamstring stretching restrictions. The therapist is responsible for clarifying these restrictions with the physician. As precautions are removed and the individual no longer requires an orthosis, more aggressive ROM exercises and stretching is indicted to restore any loss of motion during the acute phase of recovery. Therapists must also be aware of the presence of open lesions because aggressive ROM may limit their healing. The location of the lesion will dictate the contraindicated motion. If the wound or a surgical suture can potentially be overstretched or reopened by stretching the joint that it crosses, then that direction of motion is contraindicated.

Muscle imbalances in the upper limb identified on evaluation can contribute to joint instability or have potential for joint contracture in the future. Patient instruction about proper positioning and care of joints at risk is critical to maintain his optimal functional performance. Table 7-1 defines the optimal ROM for each joint necessary for specific ADL, functional position changes, and wheelchair management.

Upper Limbs
Individuals with SCI use the upper limbs to perform all ADL and for transportation, unlike able-bodied individuals. Therefore, the shoulders are at risk for overuse injury. Cross-sectional studies

have reported the prevalence of shoulder pain in individuals with SCI to be between 31% and 73%.[11-15] In the large report on upper limb pain by Sie et al,[11] significant pain was present in 59% of individuals with tetraplegia and 41% of individuals with paraplegia. The shoulders, in particular, must be kept flexible to perform weight-shifting activities for skin relief in the wheelchair. Bilateral shoulder extension and external rotation ROM for the individual with tetraplegia, without triceps strength, must be adequate to hook onto the push handle to perform skin relief for each ischial tuberosity and the sacrum. These motions are also critical for bed mobility and self-care activities in the LSP. Shoulder flexion ROM is critical when any overhead equipment is used for functional mobility and overhead reaching activities. When overhead ROM and activities are performed, internal rotation of the humerus should be avoided to prevent impingement.[16]

Individuals with elbow flexion strength and unopposed triceps are at risk for elbow flexion contractures bilaterally as early as 1 to 2 months after injury.[11,17] Elbow extension ROM is critical for mechanical locking of the upper limb during long-sitting activities. When the upper limb is loaded in long-sitting, the anterior deltoid and upper pectoral muscles have been documented to extend the elbow in weight bearing by positioning the shoulder in external rotation to create the mechanically locked position.[18,19] These individuals need to be taught methods of daily stretching using the wheelchair tire for distal contact, with mechanical locking of the elbow and forward leaning of the trunk to stretch the elbow flexors and anterior chest muscles (Figure 7-8). Proper positioning in bed for stretching must also be reinforced (see Chapter 3).

Tenodesis is the passive shortening of the finger flexors as the wrist is extended to create a functional grasp for ADL activities and to enhance the use of equipment. The long finger flexors passively move into extension with wrist flexion for release. These muscles should not be stretched out passively because this inherent anatomical pulley system and functional independence could be lost. The tenodesis position of the wrist and hand should be maintained during all functional activities that require weight bearing through the arms (see Figure 9-2). The rehabilitation team needs to maintain clear communication regarding all ROM principles to provide optimal functional outcomes for the patient.

Prevention of pain and loss of ROM are critical for maintaining an active lifestyle and performing ADL. The Consortia for Spinal Cord Medicine suggests five guidelines for stretching (Clinical Note: Guidelines for Upper Limb Stretching).[16] Although all strategies should be used to avoid the incidence of pain, early management of pain is recommended. The Consortia for Spinal Cord Medicine also suggests guidelines for managing acute and chronic pain in the upper limb (Clinical Note: Management of Acute and Subacute Upper Limb Pain and Clinical Note: Management of Chronic Upper Limb Pain).

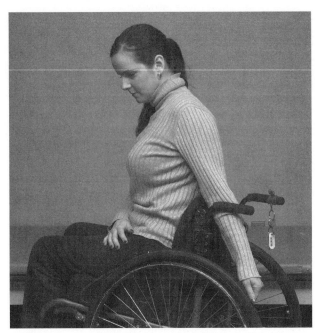

FIGURE 7-8 A patient holds her upper limb in tenodesis in contact with the tire while her shoulder is externally rotated on her fixed wrist, stretching the elbow flexors.

CLINICAL NOTE **Guidelines for Upper Limb Stretching**

- Perform stretching a minimum of two to three times per week
- Perform full ROM
- Stretch should be gentle and prolonged in the direction of tightness
- Avoid impingement using distractive forces along the long axis of the humerus
- Avoid internal rotation with overhead ROM

CLINICAL NOTE **Management of Acute and Subacute Upper Limb Pain**

- Follow guidelines of rest, pain management, ROM, modalities, splinting, injections, and surgery as with the general population
- Institute treatment to avoid chronic pain
- Gear treatment to rehabilitation first rather than surgical intervention
- Decrease regular use of the painful limb as much as possible by using home modification and resting night splints (those with limited resources may require admission to a medical facility)
- Emphasize optimal ROM
- Consider alternate techniques for ADL, transfers, and mobility
- Return gradually to normal activity
- Monitor closely treatment results and alter approach as needed
- Consider surgery with chronic pain
- Operate on fractures for early mobilization
- Plan for needed rehabilitation time after surgery

CLINICAL NOTE **Management of Chronic Upper Limb Pain**

Consider a multidisciplinary approach including:
- Etiology
- Pain intensity
- Functional capacities
- Psychological distress
Incorporate multiple modalities:
- Pharmacology
- Physical interventions
- Psychological interventions
- Monitor outcomes regularly for effective treatment
Consider a power wheelchair versus a manual wheelchair
Monitor psychological adjustment and provide treatment as necessary

---

because of the balance concerns described previously. Full ROM at the knee and ankle are also required for wheelchair positioning, ADL, and ambulation when applicable.

Therapists are encouraged to provide adequate limb and joint support while performing ROM exercises, joint mobilization, and muscle stretching techniques. Patients without sensation are unable to provide feedback during ROM exercises; therefore, extra care is important for joint safety. Therapists must make a decision on the "end feel" of the muscle and joint when sensation is absent to determine the maximal stretch point.[20] The end of the ROM may be limited by the ligaments, bone, or soft tissue structures, including muscle and connective tissue. The determination of the end point requires practice to determine what is normal to feel at a given point in the ROM versus an abnormal end feel; spasticity may present with a firm end feel.[20] When spasticity is present, the speed of performing ROM is critical; if done too quickly, spasticity will increase.[21]

Lower Limbs

Lower limb ROM needs to be maintained for optimal ADL and positioning. The hamstring muscles require 90- to 110-degrees rotation to perform ADL. When the hamstring muscles are stretched, the low back should not be stretched simultaneously

Self–Range of Motion Exercises

Self-ROM exercise is typically taught to individuals who can perform lower limb management for functional training. This training usually requires that the patient has an intact triceps so that the task becomes easier to perform with greater hand function. Although it is ideal to perform these exercises without equipment, leg lifters or loops can be used for assistance as necessary. A patient can demonstrate each motion in the series to be performed in an LSP beginning with hip motions and concluding with ankle ROM (Figure 7-9, A to E).

Strength Training

Strength is an important prerequisite for functional training. The manual muscle test evaluation will identify the muscles that can be trained (see Chapter 6). It is important to note that

individuals may demonstrate some weakness in fully innervated muscles as a result of deconditioning and bed rest. Muscle mass, morphology, and tone are altered after SCI, which influences the ability to sustain contraction for extended periods.[22] In addition, there is little published research validating effective methods for strength training individuals with SCI.[22] Circuit resistance training has demonstrated improvements in strength after a 16-week program.[23] A wheelchair circuit can also be used as a means to measure functional improvement during rehabilitation.[24] In other research, a 16-week program consisting of strength training by use of a circuit training method combined with wheelchair mobility skills and aerobic conditioning by arm crank training improved Functional Independence Measure scores, strength as measured by weight lifted, decreased time to perform wheelchair skills, and improved aerobic capacity.[25]

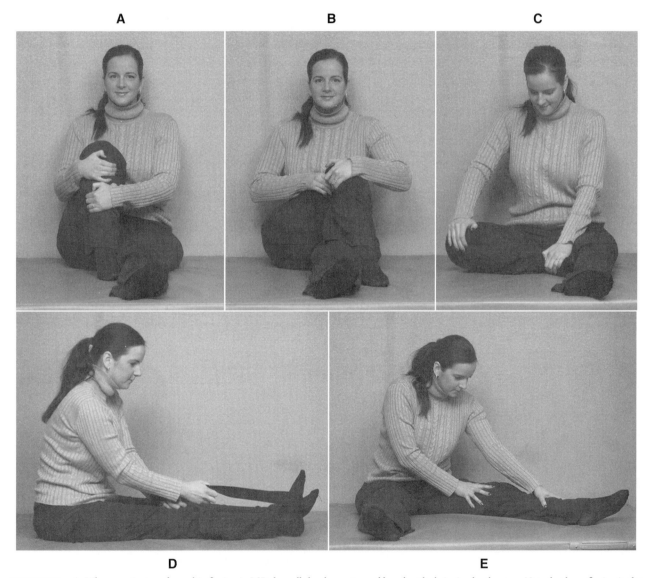

A   **B**   **C**

D   **E**

FIGURE 7-9 **A,** When a patient performs hip flexion in LSP, she pulls her leg up toward her chest by bringing her knee up. Note that knee flexion is also occurring at the same time. **B,** She brings her bent knee across the opposite thigh for hip internal rotation and out toward the mat for external rotation. From either position she can hook under her thigh for the next hamstring stretch. **C,** The patient performs ankle dorsiflexion when her knee is bent for the external rotation stretch and stretches the soleus in this position. **D,** The patient stretches the hamstrings and the gastrocnemius muscle using a strap under the metatarsals of the foot. Note that she must keep her lower back in a neutral position to avoid overstretching it, which could lead to instability with balance. **E,** The patient competes hip abduction in long sitting by bringing her leg out to the side while her knee is maintained in extension.

There have also been demonstrated improvements in objective measures of improved wheelchair skills performance, power output, and upper limb isometric strength after wheelchair skill training.[26,27] Therapists are encouraged to design strengthening programs consistent with the findings in literature emphasizing circuit resistance training with the consideration of level of injury, joint stability, and potential overuse that may lead to musculoskeletal pain. Details regarding exercise and fitness protocols can be found in Chapter 18.

It is important to be creative in designing strength training exercises and to interject variety in the program to keep patient interest and motivation high to increase improvement. Functional position changes provide the opportunity to add opportunities for strengthening into the practice of these skills. The component skills can be resisted or assisted by the therapist. Stabilization exercises for component skills can provide the avenue to address specific muscles that may need to be strengthened in a particular position. Therapists may want to incorporate principles of proprioceptive neuromuscular facilitation[28] when designing their treatment programs to address strength, mobility training, stability training, and component skills progression.

Motor Control Retraining

Individuals with SCI must learn how to perform functional tasks in entirely new ways because they no longer have the same choices of motor patterns to apply because of their level of injury. The ASIA classification is an extremely important factor when applying principles of motor learning to patient care. For example, a person classified with an ASIA A injury cannot receive physical information from the supporting surface regarding sensory input, whereas a person with a classification of ASIA B injury may. Therefore, even if two individuals have the same muscular strength, sensory feedback can influence motor learning of a task.[5,21,29]

Three principles must be considered when applying concepts of motor learning and motor control: the ASIA classification, the task being performed, and the environment in which the task is completed (Clinical Note: Principles for Applying Motor Learning Concepts). Each functional position change is accompanied by its own set of component skills that must be mastered for safe and successful completion of the task. The therapist must consider the level of injury and spasticity that may assist or hinder the method and the patient's goals when a patient performs each functional activity. The component skills of ROM, strength, and balance also need to be examined.[5]

CLINICAL NOTE **Principles for Applying Motor Learning Concepts**

- ASIA classification
- Functional task
- Environment of task performance

Bernstein[30] developed the concept of degrees of freedom on the basis of the study of dynamics and he applied these to human movement. Motor acquisition according to Bernstein can be acquired in three phases in which the way the individual controls degrees of freedom or variables changes as a skill is acquired. During the first phase there is freezing of degrees of freedom; therefore, the individual would have less to control as initial learning takes place. The second phase is characterized by a release of degrees of freedom, and the final phase is optimal performance of the acquired skill. Bernstein's concepts have been applied to biomechanical problems, and recent research questions whether this hierarchy of solving movement in his order of controlling degrees of freedom is applicable to all functional tasks and each joint that participates in a functional task.

Roux et al[31] examined wheelchair propulsion and did not find the freezing of degrees of freedom during early learning at various propulsion speeds. The dynamic systems theory and systems theory are an elaboration of Bernstein's original model and applicable to training individuals with SCI.[21,32] Application of these theories helps to guide the therapist as treatment interventions are designed to provide opportunities for optimal motor learning (Clinical Note: Application of Motor Control Concepts). Therefore, integration of motor control to treatment interventions should include consideration of degrees of freedom. Although the degrees of freedom are less relevant as the injury level becomes higher, the muscle exertion required by the remaining intact muscles becomes greater and therefore the movement is less efficient and often less stable. Stability and mobility component skills for each functional task should be assessed and practiced. For example, successful movement from the long-sitting to the short-sitting position (SSP) cannot occur without the ability to balance in the LSP both supported and unsupported by the upper limbs. Optimization of movement patterns to perform functional tasks therefore requires fundamental component skills. If sensation is present, then the individual can receive input from the periphery, such as that from the supporting surface, which will facilitate learning the task.

CLINICAL NOTE **Application of Motor Control Concepts**

- Resolution of degrees of freedom: learning varies depending on the characteristics of the learner and on the components of the task and environment
- Method to optimize movement: movements are specified to optimize a select cost function such as kinematic (spatial) or dynamic (force) factors that influence movement as an expense to the system
- Integration of sensory information: using sensory information pertinent to motor control from key sources—somatosensory (proprioceptive and tactile), visual, and vestibular processes

Data from Cech DJ, Martin ST: *Functional movement development: across the life span*, ed 2, Philadelphia, 2002, WB Saunders, p 89.

Instructional requirements additionally affect the overall success of the patient's motor control during functional activities. Previous life experiences, body awareness, and motivation must be considered. Initially the patient may be experimenting with a variety of methods to achieve a functional task and cognitive strategies to explore what methods are most efficient and successful.[5] The learner then moves to the associative phase, when strategies are refined on the basis of knowledge of results of previous performances and fine tuning for efficiency.[5] The final stage is the automatic stage in which less mental effort is required, thus allowing the patient to focus on environmental interaction.[5] This stage is an effective time to try similar skills in different locations or on different surfaces, such as transfers to a bed, car, or toilet, to determine whether the training can be generalized to new environments.

Incomplete lesions create additional challenges for the physical therapist as she assesses how a partially innervated muscle can contribute to function. A muscle grade of 2 out of 5 may help to partially assist the limb for positioning when gravity is not affecting the position of the limb, such as with lower limb management in the LSP. A grade 2 muscle may also act as a joint stabilizer for partial assistance, but such assistance will need to be evaluated with each functional task. Indeed, prevention of joint contracture because of muscle imbalances should be less likely when a grade of 2 out of 5 is possible. The muscle grade of 3 out of 5 will add significantly to function because the limb can now move against gravity and be participatory with all functional activities as required.

Balance Retraining

The concept of balance relates to the patient's ability to control his COM over the base of support.[33] During functional position changes, the base of support alters during dynamic movements to change a position but typically remains unchanged while the individual is learning stability within a position. For example, in the LSP the pelvis is in contact with the surface and the position of the legs provide the base of support for the patient to support the COM of the trunk and upper limbs (Figure 7-10, A). In the SSP the base of support is smaller because only the thighs are in contact with the surface; the lower limb below the knee is no longer contributing to the base of support. Short-sitting is therefore less stable and balance is more difficult (Figure 7-10, B).

Treatment interventions must include balance practice for the patient to gain an understanding of his own limits of stability in different positions. These activities can include the therapist guarding the patient from behind as he attempts to learn his COM (Figure 7-11, A) or guarding the patient from in front when he is practicing short-sit balance (Figure 7-11, B). The position of the legs may change because of spasticity, altering the base of support, or as the individual moves the upper limbs, shifting his weight. The most stable position is when the base of support does not change; however, while changing positions, the base of support changes during the activity. As the individual moves from the LSP to the SSP, the leg placement is changing, which requires the individual to continually adapt his balance strategy.

The level of injury significantly affects balance and recovery from a loss of balance. The higher the injury level, the higher the point from which the individual can move to prevent a loss of balance; therefore, the more difficult it is to control. Individuals with higher-level thoracic injuries do not perform as well as individuals with lower-level thoracic injuries when dynamic sitting balance is tested.[33] Individuals with a longer trunk length do not perform as well as individuals with a shorter trunk length when dynamic sitting balance is tested.[33] Lynch et al[34] explored the use of a modified functional reach test in a seated position for individuals with SCI and their results revealed high intratester reliability and functional reach differences between lesion levels of T10 through T12 from T4 or higher. Sparing of thoracic areas can significantly affect and improve the control of balance during functional position changes. It is critical that the therapist

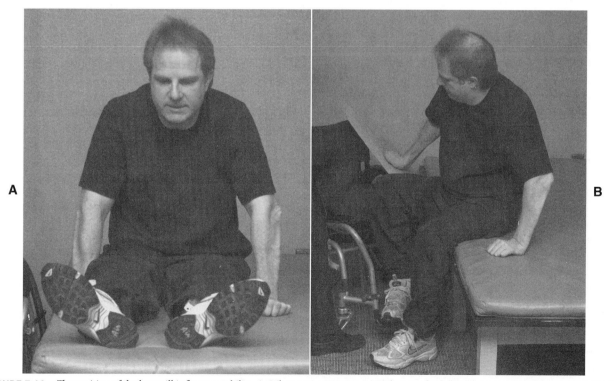

FIGURE 7-10 The position of the legs will influence stability. **A,** When patient practices LSP, keeping his legs wider apart provides more stability for his trunk. Additional support for his trunk is gained from his upper limbs. **B,** The same principles are important in the SSP.

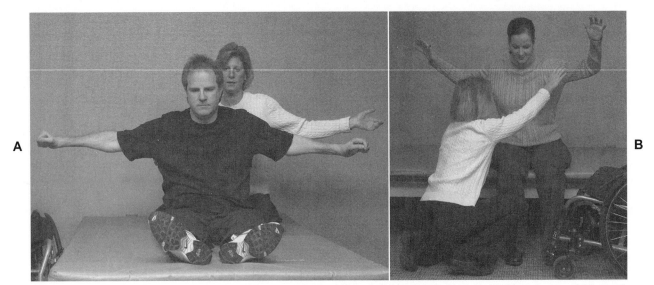

FIGURE 7-11 **A,** A patient can practice long-sitting balance with the therapist guarding from behind to protect from a backward fall. **B,** When a patient practices short-sitting balance, the therapist should guard in front to protect from a forward fall.

understand the optimal way to gain the most stable base of support for the patient given their level of injury and residual muscle strength for all variety of functional position changes.

Balance control in long-sitting, prone on elbows, short-sitting, during transfers, and in the wheelchair must be practiced. Recovery from a loss of balance and protective responses must also be taught with each activity. Body awareness and previous life experiences can be incorporated into balance training along with other individual factors (Clinical Note: Considerations for Balance Training). Therapists can use mental imagery to assist the patient during the process of learning new balance strategies. It is not unusual for the therapist and patient to spend an entire treatment session on balance activities.

Tolerance to Upright Retraining

During the acute stages of an SCI, medical stability takes priority over mobility. The patient's first hurdle for beginning mobility is to achieve a tolerance to sitting upright in a wheelchair and to overcome the effects of immobility while beginning functional retraining. Orthostatic hypotension can be a major obstacle during this process; it is most commonly a complication in individuals with lesions involving the sympathetic nervous system (see Chapter 2). Individuals with SCI may average a 15 mm Hg lower measurement of both systolic (SBP) and diastolic blood pressure (DBP) compared with able-bodied individuals.[35]

The use of a tilt table is a common clinical intervention in the management of orthostatic hypotension.[35] Initially patients will be reclined in the wheelchair to a level of tolerance determined by their blood pressure, or a tilt table can be used when orthostatic hypotension is considered severe. The lower limbs are typically elevated initially with the back reclined as well when a wheelchair is used. Incrementally, the lower limbs are lowered and the position of back recline is brought to upright. Prophylactic devices used to help prevent orthostatic hypotension are an abdominal binder, compressive stockings, or Ace wrap on the lower limbs (see Chapter 2). It is recommended that the patient's blood pressure be taken with each incremental change using a guide of

| CLINICAL NOTE | Considerations for Balance Training |

- Level of injury
- ASIA score
- Body type
- Previous life experiences
- Age
- Spasticity
- Medical complications
- Learning needs

15 degrees per angle of increase with a minimum of 4 minutes' adjustment.[35] Blood pressure recordings of 60 mm Hg SBP and 40 mm Hg DBP are considered acute hypotension, contraindicating an initial gradual tilting for upright tolerance. The progression of increased tilting should be terminated should SBP or DBP drop 20 mm Hg or with symptoms of hypotension perceived by the patient during a given treatment session.[35,36] The process of achieving upright tolerance may take several days to a few months.[35]

Tilt tables and wheelchairs with a standing function may be incorporated into treatment interventions (Figure 7-12, *A*) and used after discharge to enable the client to accomplish a wider variety of daily activities (Figure 7-12, *B*). Benefits include improved well-being, circulation, skin integrity, reflex activity, bowel and bladder function, digestion, sleep, pain, and fatigue.[37] Although these benefits of standing have long been identified, cost of the equipment is the most common preventive factor in achieving this activity.[37]

The use of functional electrical stimulation (FES) with the lower limbs in addition to an incremental rise in tilt table angulations has demonstrated less of a drop in both SBP and DSP with each increment of 15 degrees and a lower rise in heart rate and a longer tolerance to tilting in comparison with individuals receiving no stimulation.[35] Therefore, the addition of FES could be considered during the process of achieving upright tolerance.

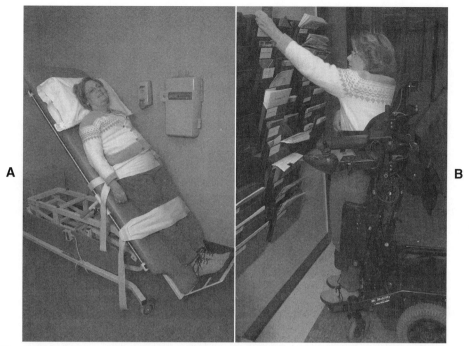

FIGURE 7-12 **A,** Tilt tables can be used to foster gradual tolerance to upright by increasing the position for supine to full upright in increments of degrees on the basis of objective data for position and time of tolerance related to blood pressure stability. **B,** When a patient can tolerate a full upright position, a standing wheelchair can help her reach for higher objects than would be obtainable from the seated wheelchair level.

CONSIDERATIONS FOR POSITION CHANGES

Rolling over, lying down, sitting up—these are just some of the position changes everyone performs daily without a second thought. For those with SCI, however, thought is not only required but relearning these activities using new techniques is often necessary. Various factors affect a patient's ability to perform position changes. These include the patient's level of injury, strength of innervated musculature, the presence of an orthosis, tolerance to upright, ROM, balance, level of spasticity, secondary diagnoses or complications (e.g., limb fractures, pain, skin breakdown, respiratory problems), age, body build, motivation, and cognitive status (Clinical Note: Considerations for Position Changes). In addition, the general principles discussed in Chapter 8

| **CLINICAL NOTE** | **Considerations for Position Changes** |

- Level of injury
- Strength of innervated musculature
- Orthosis
- Tolerance to upright
- ROM
- Balance
- Level of spasticity
- Fractures
- Pain
- Skin condition
- Respiratory problems
- Age
- Body type
- Motivation
- Cognitive status

concerning performance of transfers also apply to performance of position changes, such as using momentum and the head-hips relationship to facilitate movement (Figure 7-13).

Breaking position changes down into their component parts will help to facilitate successful training. Patients may more readily achieve success with small component parts of an activity and thus better maintain their motivation. When putting the component parts together, the patient should receive whatever assistance is needed. In this way, he will get a feel for the activity and as his strength improves more quickly incorporate the components and find greater success performing the entire activity. Balance becomes an important component with functional training. The base of support over which the patient controls his COM should be considered when training in sequences or an entire activity. The larger the base of support provided, the greater the distribution for COM and therefore increased limits of stability for the task. Weight-shift techniques also can be used by patients with SCI to avoid skin breakdown when sitting in their wheelchairs as well as strategies for performing low-level and high-level position changes.

Subsequent sections describe techniques to perform position changes. Patient progression with training in each activity is explained and illustrated as well as safe guarding strategies for various levels of dependency.

Weight-Shift Techniques

Pressure ulcers are a common complication after SCI (see Chapter 2). One of the primary techniques used to avoid skin breakdown is to perform weight shifts when seated to facilitate pressure relief (Table 7-2). There are four basic types of weight shifts: anterior, lateral, pushup, and tilt-back. The frequency of

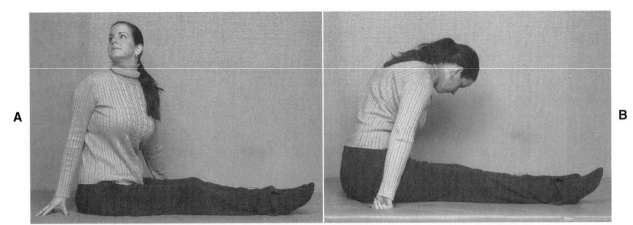

FIGURE 7-13 **A,** Learning to combine momentum with the head-hips relationship can facilitate movement of the body on the fixed upper limbs for multiple daily functional tasks. **B,** An individual with a higher injury level and less muscle strength will need to use principles of momentum while bringing her trunk into flexion over the thighs to clear her pelvis for movement. Note how her head and hips move in opposite directions.

CLINICAL NOTE **Skin Care Management**

Medical Risk Factors
- Complete injury
- Immobility
- Incontinence care (keeping the skin clean and free form moisture)
- Increased comorbidity

Psychological Risk Factors
- Psychological distress
- Cognitive impairment
- Substance abuse
- Written commitment to adherence

---

weight shifts must be based on the medical and psychological risks associated with the individual patient (Clinical Note: Skin Care Management).

Demographic variables such as age, duration of injury, sex, ethnicity, and marital status are controversial according to research about the relationship these factors to the development of skin ulcers.[38] Coggrave and Rose[39] posit that patients should be instructed to perform weight shifts for a duration ranging from 42 seconds to 3 minutes 30 seconds. The frequency of weight shifting should include the factors already discussed because these will influence how often the team educates the patient to perform a weight shift and for how long. The decision should be generated by the rehabilitation team and should be consistent among therapies. Instruction about the importance of pressure relief and weight-shift techniques should be emphasized during a patient's first therapy session and reinforced by all disciplines (see Table 7-2). If a patient is unable to perform weight shifts independently, he should learn how to instruct others to assist him, and for those who are ventilator dependent it is crucial to ensure that tubing is not pulled or kinked as the weight shift is performed. For patients who may be forgetful or who have documented cognitive deficits, carrying a timer set to go off every 30 minutes can be extremely helpful. In addition, documentation can travel with a patient so that team members who work with them or assist them can sign and date the log when weight shifts are performed.

THE CLIENT'S PERSPECTIVE Pressure Ulcers

Pressure ulcers are insidious and preventable secondary health conditions for people with SCI. Caring for our skin is vitally important to our health and well-being because after pressure ulcers develop, the chances of them recurring are enhanced. And the older we get, the thinner our skin becomes; the longer we are injured, the less muscle mass we have, which can make our skin increasingly prone to pressure ulcers.

Helpful hints:
- Remember—we are never immune to having a pressure ulcer
- Devote part of every daily routine to checking your skin
- Do plenty of pressure reliefs (e.g., weight shifts) or change position often
- Check clothing so you do not end up sitting on creases or folds
- Take back pockets off pants or buy pants without back pockets
- Do not have extra folds in socks
- Make sure shoes are not overly tight
- Eat a well-balanced diet with plenty of fruits, vegetables, and protein
- Drink plenty of water
- Exercise to increase blood circulation (if you cannot exercise, try to keep legs elevated)
- Try sleeping on your stomach to give your bottom free time from pressure, and stretch your hip flexors at the same time
- Stay off any red spots until they are no longer red—an ounce of prevention is worth a pound of cure!

Scott Chesney

Anterior Weight Shift

When performing an anterior weight shift, the patient must lean forward enough to take his weight off the ischial tuberosities. If a patient is wearing a spinal orthosis (e.g., a halo orthosis or thoracic lumbar sacral orthosis [TLSO]), medical clearance must be obtained before this technique is performed. Even if clearance is obtained, the presence of the orthosis may obstruct the patient's ability to lean far enough forward to make this the technique of choice. The push-up, with medical clearance, or tilt-back methods described later may be the more optimal techniques when

TABLE 7-2	Pressure Ulcer Prevention and Pressure Relief			
Therapy Prevention Strategy	Wheelchair Weight-Shift Techniques	Rolling	Prone on Elbows	LSP
Begin an interdisciplinary pressure relief program as early as possible	Communicate with team members the most effective technique	Communicate with team members the most effective technique for the patient for safety and participation in skin relief	Communicate with team members if and when the patient can assume this position for skin relief and instruct in risk of elbow shearing and pressure	Communicate with team members if and when the patient can assume this position and the ability to perform a push up in this position.
Avoid prolonged immobilization	Instruct the patient in frequency and duration of skin relief technique on basis of level of injury and individualized identified risk factors	Reinforce turning frequency for bed positioning and instruct the patient to educate family on appropriate level of assistance for rolling	Instruct the patient on appropriate use of prone-on-elbows position for skin relief and joint stretching; educate the patient on areas of risk for skin breakdown	Instruct the patient on guidelines to avoid friction and shear when moving in and out of this position and how to educate caregivers and family
Areas of daily skin inspections: ischii, sacrum, coccyx, trochanters, heels, malleoli, anterior knee, shoulder, side of head, elbow, occiput, rim of ear, dorsal thoracic spine	Inspection of ischii, sacrum coccyx, and trochanters for adequate seated skin relief daily and identifying seating positioning areas of risk	Inspection of trochanters, malleoli, anterior shoulder, side of head, elbow, ear for areas at risk with practicing this intervention	Inspection of elbows and anterior knee related to pressure, friction, and shear from interventions	Inspection of ischii, sacrum, coccyx, related to pressure, friction, and shear from interventions
Evaluate support surface	Monitor wheelchair seating support surfaces for optimal skin protection	Identify hazards of support surfaces during interventions Provide appropriate bridging for skin relief	Identify hazards of support surfaces for optimal protection and prevention	Identify hazards of support surfaces for optimal protection to prevent surface shear and surface friction
Pressure relief program	Perform and educate on weight shift in upright every 15 to 30 minutes allowing adequate oxygen replenishment	Educate on the application of rolling as pressure relief	Educate on the application of prone on elbows as pressure relief	Educate on the application of long sitting as pressure relief
Mobility program training for prevention of deconditioning	Educate on the importance of mobility for decreasing the incidence of pressure ulcer development and why wheelchair skin relief is critical for this	Educate on the importance of maintaining rolling mobility for optimal skin relief with bed positioning and sleeping	Educate on the importance of prone on elbows positioning as a lifetime skin relief and joint stretching position	Educate on the importance of LSP for ADL functioning and overall mobility
Individualized patient education program	Consider learning styles of the patient and family Assess understanding with questions Clarify and give explanations considering psychosocial issues			

a spinal orthosis is present. When the anterior technique is performed, the wheelchair brakes should be engaged. The casters should be facing forward and the wheelchair's leg rests should be placed in a lowered position to decrease the risk of the chair tipping forward.

To move his trunk forward into the anterior position, the patient first lowers his elbows onto his thighs and then slides his hands down toward his feet (Figure 7-14). To return to the upright position, the patient positions his hands on his thighs and pushes up. If the patient has weak triceps, he may still be able to perform this function by using momentum gained by extending his head and neck (also as cleared by his physician) and by using the strength of his anterior deltoid and pectoralis muscles (Figure 7-15, A and B). Adducting and externally rotating the shoulders with the hands fixed produces elbow extension, which is an alternative method when the triceps are weak. Another option for regaining the upright position is to hook the push handle by using wrist extensors and then pull up by using the biceps. If a patient has difficulty reaching his push handle, a loop may be placed on one or both sides of the chair. After the patient leans anteriorly, it may be difficult for him to reach the loops, so it should be recommended that he position his arms through the loops before lowering into the anterior position.

When guarding a patient performing an anterior weight shift, the therapist may be positioned either in front of or to the side of the patient. When helping the patient lean forward and then resume upright, the therapist should place her hands at the anterior aspect of his shoulders. For a new patient who may be nervous about leaning so far forward or for a patient who is dependent in performing an anterior weight shift, it is recommended that the therapist guard from the front to reassure the patient and to best control the patient's upper body.

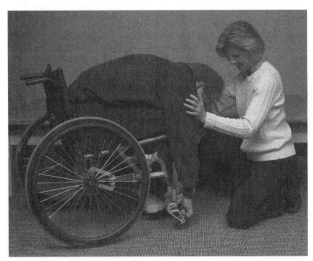

FIGURE 7-14   To accomplish an anterior weight shift, the patient first rests his elbows on the thighs and relieves pressure on his sacrum. He then continues to slide his hands down his anterior tibias, maintaining stabilization, and to his feet for relief of the ischial tuberosities. Notice that the physical therapist guards in front of the patient to protect from an anterior fall. The wheelchair caster wheels should be facing forward to provide maximal stability and avoid tipping the chair.

Lateral Weight Shift

When a lateral weight shift is performed, the wheelchair should be locked before the patient leans to each side for the predetermined time, making sure to lean far enough to adequately clear each side of the buttocks. To ease himself into the weight-shift position, he may hook his arm around his armrest, push handle, or through a loop attached to the chair on the side opposite from which he is leaning (Figure 7-16, A). To get maximal excursion, the armrest should be removed from the side of the chair toward which he is leaning. The patient may need to cross his lower limbs, bringing one lower limb over the other on the side he is leaning toward to achieve adequate pressure relief. Initially the patient may be fearful about leaning so far to the side when he is unable to support himself in this position. In such cases, the patient should park his wheelchair next to a mat or bed (Figure 7-16, B). He may then lean onto one elbow resting on the mat or bed and then turn the chair around and repeat the lean toward the other side. Alternate weight-shift maneuvers include a lateral lean using a slight twist of the trunk to help elevate the buttocks (Figure 7-16, C).

To regain an upright position, the patient may push off the arm on which he is leaning while pulling up with his other arm from the armrest, push handle, or loop. Ventilatory strategies have been shown to effectively assist with recovery to upright from a lateral weight shift and should therefore be considered during weight-shift instruction.[40]

When a therapist is guarding a patient performing this technique, she should provide support laterally at the patient's trunk. A patient who is dependent can be taught how to instruct others in this technique, with an emphasis on the caregiver controlling and supporting the patient's trunk.

Push-Up Weight Shift

The push-up weight shift is performed, after the caster wheels are aligned forward and the wheelchair is locked, by performing elbow extension and shoulder depression to lift the buttocks (Figure 7-17). The patient's hips should be positioned slightly

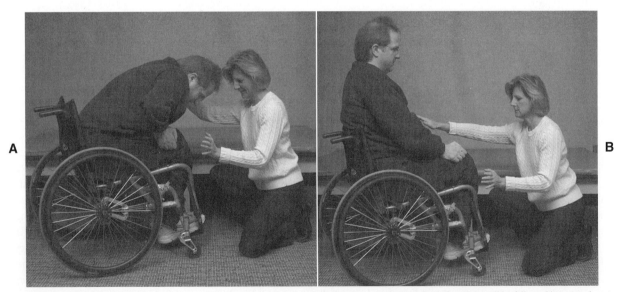

FIGURE 7-15   A, The wrist extensors may be needed to begin recovery to upright from an anterior weight shift and, B, will be followed by using the triceps or momentum as seen in this example. Note the therapist's guarding position to assist the upper limbs or trunk as needed for optimal joint protection.

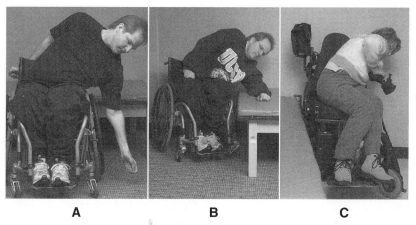

A   **B**   **C**

FIGURE 7-16   **A,** When initiating a lateral weight shift, the patient should lock the wheelchair's brakes and make sure the caster wheels are facing forward to provide maximum wheelchair stability. The patient can use the push rim or chair handle for stability while he leans over the opposite side of the chair. **B,** The height of the bed will determine whether the armrest needs to be removed or swung away to allow the patient to lean onto the mat. **C,** The lateral weight shift also can be done with the patient leaning against her armrest with a slight twist in a power wheelchair. Placing both upper limbs on the armrest will afford an easier push back to upright when the triceps are weak.

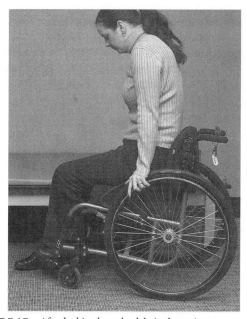

FIGURE 7-17   After locking her wheelchair, the patient can use a push-up weight shift using her wheelchair tires as the contact point; the height of the push-up may not be as great with this technique as using armrests; however, the most important issue is complete tissue relief without shear and the least amount of strain for the patient. Notice that the patient uses her triceps and gains optimal leverage with the hands positioned directly below the shoulder and that the buttock is not in contact with the posterior wall of the wheelchair, which avoids shearing.

anterior in the wheelchair when he starts to perform the push-up to avoid shearing his sacral region against the back of the wheelchair as he lifts his body up. The patient's hands may be on the wheels of the chair or on the armrests when performing this maneuver. The casters face forward to increase the base of support of the wheelchair. A higher lift may be obtained if the patient positions his hands on the armrests. This, however, should not be done if the patient has tubular armrests because they are not designed to withstand weight-bearing forces. To execute this technique

independently, a patient must have sufficient sitting balance and should perform it for the predetermined time established by the team.

In individuals without innervated triceps, the push-up technique requires an altered approach in which the elbows are locked first before lifting. The contact forces on the glenohumeral joint have been shown to be as much as 25% higher in individuals with tetraplegia than paraplegia during this weight shift.[41] In addition, the activity level in the rotator cuff muscles was higher in individuals with tetraplegia than paraplegia.[41] Alternate weight-shifting techniques as previously described should be selected for an individual without triceps strength as a means to avoid musculoskeletal injury and pain.

Tilt-Back Weight Shift

Newly injured patients and those dependent in performing weight shifts will find the tilt-back technique helpful. When this technique is performed, the wheelchair should be locked and the antitip bars removed or rotated upward to prevent obstruction during the tilting maneuver. The caregiver then sits in a sturdy chair positioned behind the patient and leans the wheelchair back so it is resting on her lap. After holding the weight shift for the predetermined time established by the team, the wheelchair is gently set back into its upright position. It is important to remember to reposition the antitip bars. Patients also may perform this maneuver independently by using a tilt-in-space power wheelchair (Figure 7-18). Because the tilt-back weight shift may not sufficiently relieve pressure from the sacral region, a patient with a sacral pressure ulcer should also perform an anterior weight-shift, which will allow the patient to further unweight the sacral region.

Low-Level Position Changes

Teaching a patient with SCI how to move his body into various positions is a vital component of his therapy program. There are numerous techniques that will help a patient best use his strength and enable him to actively participate in changing positions. If he is unable to actively participate, or needs assistance in doing

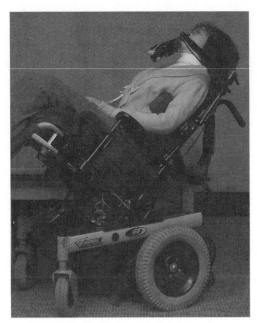

FIGURE 7-18 An individual also can use her tilt-in-space wheelchair to perform a tilt weight shift.

so, he should be taught to clearly instruct others how to change his position safely and efficiently. As mentioned previously, the techniques described here can be broken down into their smaller component parts to allow the patient to achieve success sooner. In patients with increasing strength as a result of neurological recovery or improved conditioning or who have an incomplete injury, functional training for each position can change throughout the rehabilitation process. A patient may eventually rely less on the original techniques and be able to progress to less complex strategies. Because every patient is unique, it is strongly recommended that clinicians be creative and try variations of a technique to solve individual problems: there is no right or wrong way to perform an activity as long as the patient is safe.

When guarding patients during position changes, the therapist must consider what body part may be most at risk during the intervention. For example, if the patient could lose his balance forward, the therapist must be positioned adequately to protect his head. Shoulder joints become particularly vulnerable during position changes and should be adequately protected because the weight-bearing requirements through the joint may be high. It is recommended that the therapist not support directly under the axilla secondary to the potential pressure to the brachial plexus. Rather, it is recommended that the therapist use a broad hand support over the upper ribs to distribute the supporting forces through bone as opposed to soft tissue.

It is also critical to note that patients without sensation are at greater risk for skin injury during training. The therapist must be particularly careful regarding pressure and length of time that the patient maintains a position. For example, prone on elbows can create skin breakdown if frictional forces and duration are too high, affecting tolerance of the patient's elbow skin. The therapist becomes an excellent example to the patient and his caregivers when she is fastidious about monitoring and visually inspecting the skin during training.

Lower Limb Management

To move from SSP from LSP and back again, a patient must learn to bring his lower limbs onto and off the mat.

Techniques

One technique for doing this is to hook the lower limbs. Hooking the lower limbs to lift them onto the mat requires sufficient upper limb strength and sitting balance. Completion of this task independently requires innervation of the wrist extensors at a minimum and becomes more stable with triceps innervation.

The patient positions himself in SSP with his knees angled toward the direction he wishes to raise his lower limbs. He accomplishes this by using the heads-hip relationship as described previously and in Chapter 8. For example, twisting the shoulders to the left will facilitate moving the right hip anteriorly and thus angle the knees to the left. The patient may already be in this position after completing a transfer from the wheelchair to the mat. When he is in position, the patient is ready to lift his lower limbs onto the mat. It may be easier to first try this with the shoes off to lighten the limb, avoid getting it caught on the edge of the mat, and allowing it to slide on the mat more easily. When lifting his lower limbs toward the left, the patient should lean on his left elbow or left hand, depending on his strength and balance, and lift his left leg with his right upper arm (Figure 7-19, *A*). While the patient is lifting with his right arm, he shifts his weight to the left onto his hand or elbow to have better leverage and to prevent falling to the right. It may be beneficial to move the lower limb in small increments, rocking to the left and using momentum to help move the lower limb. If the patient has sufficient hand strength, he can lift his lower limb by grabbing it at the thigh, knee, or calf or pulling on loose-fitting clothing. If he does not have sufficient hand strength, he can hook his forearm under his thigh and use his biceps strength to lift his lower limb (Figure 7-19, *B*). Alternatively, if he has wrist extensor strength, he should keep his forearm pronated and his wrist extended to assist in controlling the lower limb as he lifts it. After his left lower limb is on the mat, the patient needs to continue moving it to the left to make room for his right lower limb (Figure 7-19, *C*). He may need to reposition himself at this time, scooting his hips to the left so that when he leans down to lift his right lower limb, he will not lose his balance and fall toward the right. The right lower limb is then lifted in the same manner as the left (Figure 7-19, *D*), ending in a supported LSP on the mat (Figure 7-19, *E*).

Another option is for the patient to bring both lower limbs onto the mat at once rather than one at a time. This method requires greater patient strength because the balance requirements are greater when positioning the upper limbs under both of the lower limbs to lift them. To do this, the patient hooks under both thighs with his arm and throws his upper body back and toward the left, simultaneously bringing his lower limbs onto the mat. The hooking technique to bring the lower limbs onto the mat may be made easier by using equipment to assist with the lifting. The patient may use loops fastened with Velcro around his thighs to grab or hook his forearms under. A stiff leg lifter or a series of cloth loops also may be used to lasso the ball of the foot and lift the limb. When these techniques are used, it is recommended that the limb be lifted in an extended position rather than flexed because there will be less chance of catching the foot on the edge

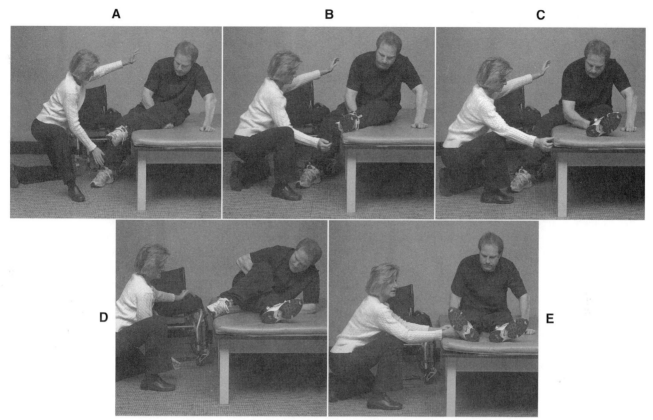

FIGURE 7-19 A patient can learn to manage his lower limbs when moving from SSP to LSP by moving one leg at a time. **A,** The patient lifts his left lower limb with the right upper limb using the wrist extensors and biceps. Notice that his left upper limb provides stabilization for balance and can be positioned to create the most beneficial base of support for trunk control during the actual lifting of the lower limb. **B,** After the patient's left lower limb is on the mat surface, **C,** he continues to use his right upper limb to move his left lower limb across the mat and gain momentum for the next step. **D,** The patient uses his right upper limb, lifting under the thigh by his posterior knee, to bring his right lower limb onto the mat. The left upper limb now is positioned with his elbow on the mat to improve stability while his right upper limb performs the work. **E,** The task is completed after both limbs are on the mat with the patient assuming LSP. The therapist provides guarding in front to prevent a forward fall and to assist in the movement of the lower limbs as needed.

of the mat. If both lower limbs are lifted simultaneously, soft loops or a strap may be placed under the thighs to provide the patient an easier hold on his lower limbs.

These techniques are done in reverse when a patient wants to bring his lower limbs down off the mat. For example, if the patient wishes to bring his right lower limb off the mat first, he can lean onto his left hand or elbow and bring his right limb off the mat with his right arm. He also can use the hook method, loops around the thigh, or a stiff leg lifter.

Considerations for Spasticity and Incomplete Lesions

A patient with flexor or extensor spasms may be able to use them to his advantage to bring his lower limbs up onto the mat. When his knees are angled to the left, as in the previous example, he may be able to trigger extensor spasms to straighten his legs. He then can continue to bring his limbs onto the mat by shifting his left hip posteriorly while scooting to the left. In the same manner, flexor spasms may become an asset by providing hip flexion to lift the lower limbs. The patient will need to be leaning left as much as possible so that the flexor spasm will bring the limbs on the mat sideways without his lower leg catching under the mat. When reversing the process, he may use extensor spasms to straighten his knees and then scoot and twist to the right.

A patient with asymmetrical or recovering strength will deviate from the techniques described in minor ways. For example, a patient with stronger upper limbs may be able to lift with or use them as stabilizers for balance while bringing his lower limbs to the surface. The most effective methods will result from the patient's ability to solve problems and through trial-and-error practice focusing on the safest strategies. As always, the patient should be taught to examine his skin if he suspects excessive shear or a damaging surface when moving his lower limbs.

Guarding

When guarding a patient who is moving from SSP to LSP, the therapist should be positioned in front of the patient and to the side opposite the direction the lower limbs are being moved. In this way the therapist may provide support at the patient's trunk to ensure that he does not fall off the surface and to provide assistance with lifting and moving his lower limbs but without getting in his way.

Caregiver Assistance

A patient who requires total assistance should learn how to instruct others clearly about how to move him safely and efficiently. One method for moving a dependent patient requires the therapist or caregiver to support the patient's trunk while bringing one or both legs onto the mat so that the patient can assume an LSP. The patient may then be lowered into a supine position. The therapist needs a long reach and strength to fulfill this maneuver, which may not be feasible if the patient is much larger than the therapist. A second option is for the therapist to simultaneously cradle the trunk and lower it to the mat with one arm while lifting the lower limbs onto the mat with her other arm. Another option is for the therapist to first lower the patient's upper body onto the mat and then lift his lower limbs up onto the mat; however, this method can cause the patient a significant amount of spinal rotation and must only be used when there is no restriction or danger of injury.

To move back to an SSP, a patient who is dependent should instruct his assistant to support his trunk with her left arm and bring his lower limbs off the mat with her right arm. As the patient becomes stronger and his balance improves, he may progress through different techniques, requiring less assistance.

Rolling

For a patient with decreased or absent lower limb and trunk strength, rolling from supine to side lying can be a very challenging activity. It can be made even more difficult when performed on a soft surface such as a bed. A patient will achieve greater success in a shorter period of time on a firm surface such as a therapeutic mat. Once the patient has practiced on the mat and understands the technique, it can then be applied to rolling in bed. Because most component skills for rolling involve segmental rolling, it is contraindicated to practice rolling if a patient's orders exclude such activity because of orthopedic instability. Only log rolling should be practiced in these cases.

Before training it is advisable to evaluate the direction in which the patient prefers to move his head: flexion, extension, or neutral with rotation. If the patient prefers extension, it may be advisable to move in that direction when training for the first technique and then progress to the other directions should extension not be effective.

Techniques

In the absence of sufficient lower limb and trunk strength, a patient can achieve rolling by using his upper limbs to create enough momentum to pull his lower body over. One technique involves swinging the upper limbs side to side simultaneously to build momentum and bring the upper body into the side-lying position with the lower body following along (Figure 7-20, *A*). After the patient swings the arms a number of times with increasing velocity and ROM, a final vigorous thrust of the upper limbs is given in the direction that the patient wishes to turn (Figure 7-20, *B*). Turning the head in the direction the arms are moving can contribute significantly to the effort of rolling the body because the body will tend to follow where the head goes (Figure 7-20, *C*).

The therapist can use diagonal patterns to maximize muscle recruitment. The diagonal of choice should be determined by which one the patient can best perform. Some patients will do best starting with the arms at the side and reaching up as they swing their arms, whereas others may do better by starting with their upper limbs in flexion and reaching down as they swing. Another technique that may contribute to successful rolling is to incorporate breathing into the motion, especially with the diagonal patterns where the patient may inhale with an extension diagonal and exhale with a flexion diagonal.

A patient without strong triceps needs to be protected from inadvertently hitting himself in the face when he swings his arms but is unable to maintain his elbows in extension. If a patient has triceps strength in one arm, he may interlock his extended wrists to help keep his weaker elbow from flexing. A patient with bilaterally weak triceps will need to keep his arms positioned low enough to allow gravity to maintain his elbows in extension or he may choose to keep his arms bent throughout the activity. It is, however, more difficult to gain enough momentum to successfully roll when having to use these techniques.

Training Progression

Several positioning techniques can be used to assist the patient to achieve side lying. If the patient is rolling to the right, it will be helpful if the therapist bends his left lower limb up into hip flexion, internal rotation, and knee flexion (Figure 7-21). Now, in essence, his lower body is practically in side lying and he just needs to get his upper body over without worrying about generating enough momentum to bring the lower body along. As the patient achieves success with this, the therapist gradually decreases the amount of left lower limb internal rotation until it is in a neutral position (although still flexed). The next step further increases the challenge; the left lower limb is brought into less flexion until it is fully extended and crossed over the right at the ankle. The ultimate goal is for the patient to be able to roll from a supine to the side-lying position without the crossing his lower limbs.

Another rolling sequence that the therapist can practice with the patient is to place a pillow or wedge under one side of the patient's upper body. By starting with a quarter turn of the upper body, he may be better able to turn and see results sooner. The size of the pillow or wedge can be decreased so that the amount of effort required to roll is increased. It may also be beneficial to actually start in side lying and then work back and forth out of this position in small increments. Other equipment also can be used to assist patients when rolling:

- Air splints may hold the patient's elbows straight as he swings his arms
- Cuff weights can be placed on a patient's arms to increase his momentum as he swings them
- Bed rails or loops at the side of the bed can help the patient to pull himself into side lying

A patient can also be instructed to lower into side lying from the LSP. This is especially useful for a patient wearing a TLSO who must not roll segmentally (Figure 7-22). When performing this technique, the patient should cross his right lower limb over his left when still in the LSP so that his lower limbs will be in a better position after he has lowered himself into the left side-lying position.

Considerations for Spasticity and Incomplete Lesions

Spasticity may help or hinder the patient to accomplish rolling. The therapist must evaluate what positions are most strongly influenced by the patient's flexor or extensor patterns. For example, if extensor spasticity is strong in supine the therapist may need to reduce the influence of the spasticity by flexing

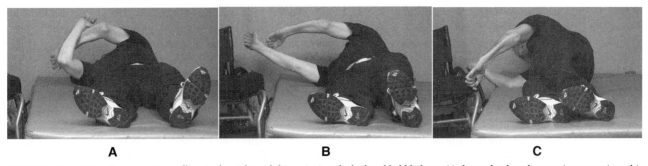

A   **B**   **C**

FIGURE 7-20 **A,** A patient practices rolling to the right with his wrist interlocked and held below a 90-degree level so that gravity can assist at his shoulders. This positioning also helps him avoid hitting his head as momentum is gained by swinging his upper limbs from side to side. **B,** His momentum helps him to come into a side-lying position. **C,** The patient also can use his wheelchair as a fulcrum to assist him in pulling over.

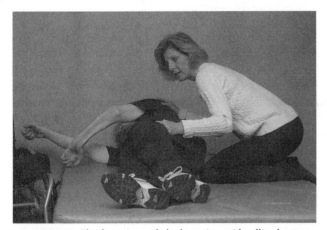

FIGURE 7-21 The therapist can help the patient with rolling by prepositioning his lower limbs and then providing assistance with contacts at both the scapula and thigh. As the patient gains control of the activity, the therapist will provide less assistance.

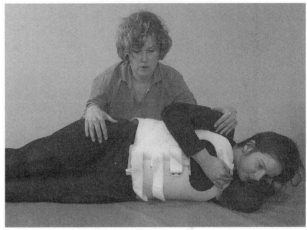

FIGURE 7-22 When the patient is using a TLSO, spinal rotation is contraindicated. The therapist assists the patient movement to side lying with hand contacts on the patient's shoulder and hip.

the patient's lower limbs. Throughout training the patient must learn how to effectively alter his position or avoid certain positions to successfully complete position changes without the interference of spasticity. Individuals with incomplete lesions should be assessed for the participation of partial innervation that may assist with rolling. For example, trunk innervations of the intercostal muscles may be patchy and not identified on the ASIA assessment but can assist with rolling. The therapist can palpate to assess the contribution of partial innervations with the patient side lying while he moves forward and back. Identified areas of strength can be incorporated into training.

Caregiver Assistance

A patient who cannot roll independently should be taught to instruct others to help move him safely and efficiently. If his orders contain the precaution of log rolling only, he should instruct his caregiver to move him into the side-lying position by moving his shoulders and hips simultaneously. If he is allowed to roll segmentally, he should instruct his caregiver to bend his opposite lower limb up into flexion and internal rotation as previously described to assist with the roll. In either case, the important points of control for the caregiver are at the patient's hips and shoulders.

Supine to and from Prone and Prone on Elbows

Medical clearance should be obtained before having a patient move into prone position because of possible orthopedic precautions. Before practicing supine to prone, the therapist may want to place the patient in prone to test his tolerance of the position. Initially, the patient may be placed over a wedge to lessen the weight bearing on the shoulders (Figure 7-23) or a prone pillow can be used to rest the neck musculature. If the patient tolerates weight bearing on his elbows or can turn his head to lie prone without upper limb support, he is ready to practice assuming the position. The therapist should be aware that many patients with cervical injuries have undergone spinal surgery with fusion and these patients will not be able to rotate their heads sufficiently in prone lying.

When moving from supine to prone, a patient uses a rolling technique as described previously, and the therapist's challenge is to devise a way for the patient to move from side lying to prone. After achieving the side-lying position, the patient needs to continue the momentum to bring his body toward the prone position (Figure 7-24, *A*). This may be accomplished if he will roll over the arm that he is rolling toward; when rolling from a right side-lying position, he will place his left arm next to his body (Figure 7-24, *B*) or in as much flexion as possible. When in prone, a patient may achieve prone on elbows by weight shifting side to side to work his arms underneath him and onto his elbows (Figure 7-24, *C*).

The order of upper limb for weight acceptance in prone is often predetermined by the limb the patient is rolling over, flexed, or extended over his head. The level of the lesion and strength of the upper limb will also influence the technique. Trial-and-error practice is required to devise the most efficient and safe technique. Shoulder pain needs to be avoided when selecting which method works for the patient. A dependent patient can instruct his caregiver to lift him below his axilla on his ribs and place him in prone and, if necessary, instruct a second person to guide the hips into prone from side lying.

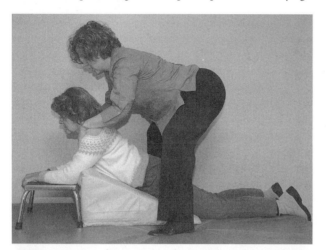

FIGURE 7-23 A wedge to support the patient's trunk and shoulders can be used when the patient is first learning to tolerate prone positioning but finds weight through the shoulders is too painful or she is too weak. Notice the therapist's position for guarding and the use of the stool to support the patient's arms. Hand contacts along the pectoral muscle will avoid pressure to nerves or vessels.

Therapeutic activities can be performed in prone on elbows to work on balance and stability as a prerequisite for other skills, including crawling on elbows (Figure 7-25, *A*) and moving from supine to LSP (Figure 7-25, *B*). The higher the level of the lesion, the greater the pressure will be felt on the shoulders in the prone-on-elbows position. The therapist must monitor the patient carefully to avoid any pain during prone-on-elbows activities. In addition, skin monitoring is critical because the skin of the elbows is at high risk for breakdown in the insensate patient.

To return to supine from prone, one arm is placed at the patient's side or up in flexion and the patient rolls back into side lying and then supine by pushing off with the other arm and assisting with upper trunk rotation as much as possible with the head moving into extension.

Supine to and from Long Sitting

Long sitting is an extremely important position for a patient to learn because he achieves independence through balance control, statically and dynamically with and without upper limb support. Long sitting serves as the following:

- A transition position for moving in and out of bed
- A safe position to perform dressing
- A position to reposition the body
- A position for strengthening

It is a position that has been shown to have a different pattern of pressure under the buttocks and is less stable with individuals with SCI in comparison to able-bodied individuals.[42] A patient may need to use his upper limbs throughout various transitions in long sitting to optimize his balance and to control position changes safely.[42] Therefore, it is important that he learn a method

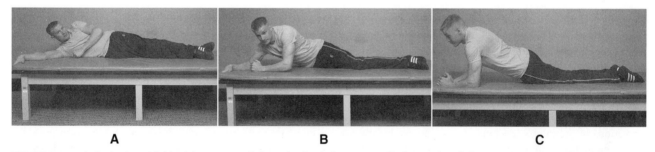

A	B	C

FIGURE 7-24 **A,** Beginning with his right arm extended over his head, the patient rolls from right side lying to, **B,** prone on elbows. **C,** Because the patient has good upper body strength, he is now able to push up on his elbows. Pain, ROM, and strength will determine optimal methods for this technique.

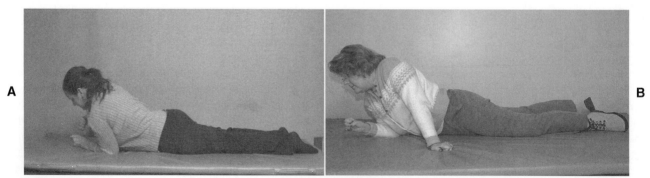

FIGURE 7-25 **A,** The prone-on-elbows position facilitates a patient's work on weight shifting. **B,** The same position can be the basis for a patient to perform weight shifts, reaching and extending the opposite upper limb.

to achieve long sitting from supine as part of his position changes training.

The therapist should be aware that a patient must work on activities to improve stability and balance both in supported and unsupported LSPs (Figure 7-26, *A*). These activities often precede moving from supine to long sitting. A patient without triceps acquires skill in supported long sitting on extended elbows. He locks his elbows into extension by externally rotating his shoulders. To obtain this position, the patient must throw each upper limb back (Figure 7-26, *B*), which takes practice and requires the use of momentum and proper placement for stability (Figure 7-26, *C*).

Techniques for Supine to Long Sitting

The therapist can teach the patient to move from supine to long sitting by rolling into side lying and then onto his elbows, as described in assuming prone on elbows (Figure 7-27, *A*). On one elbow or two, the patient next starts walking his hands toward his legs (Figure 7-27, *B*). Shifting his weight side to side will allow him to walk his upper limbs closer to his lower limbs. Some patients

crawl around until the trunk is directly over the lower limbs and then push up into long sitting. Another option is to weight bear on one elbow and hook the other forearm around the thigh (Figure 7-27, *C*). The patient then pushes off the one upper limb while pulling with the other to assume an upright position (Figure 7-27, *D* to *F*). The patient may opt to hook under both lower limbs keeping them in more knee flexion to bring the trunk over the thighs (Figure 7-28). Hamstring and arm length can play critical rolls in this method; if the hamstrings are tight, the activity becomes more difficult and balance throughout the task is compromised as the trunk is forced posteriorly because of short hamstring length.

Another method the patient can use to move from supine to long sitting starts with the patient's elbows at his sides. He works up into a supine-on-elbows position by weight shifting to the right and left. He may find it beneficial to hook his thumbs through his belt loops or place his hands under his buttocks to enable him to better use elbow flexors and shoulder extensors while positioning his elbows. Initially, the therapist may need to assist the patient under the axillary region on the ribs bilaterally, lifting as the patient shifts

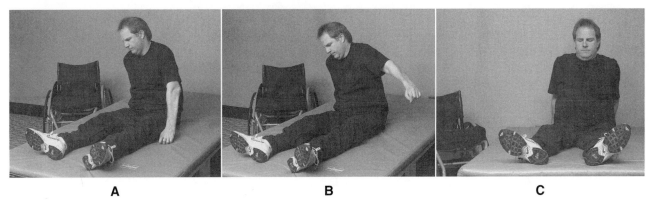

FIGURE 7-26 **A,** The patient steadies his balance when preparing to assume LSP on extended locked elbows. **B,** He uses his head to assist momentum as his arm is extended back behind his body. **C,** He achieves a long-sit with elbows locked into extension by externally rotating his shoulders.

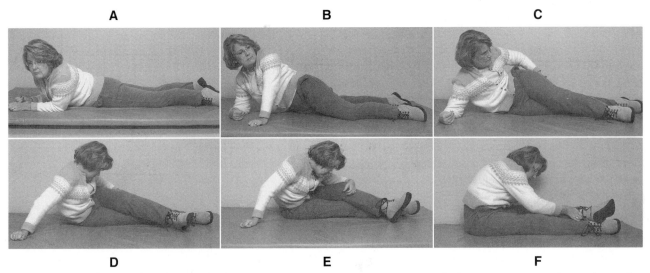

FIGURE 7-27 **A,** A patient begins top move from prone to side lying. **B,** She pushes up on her upper limbs, gaining momentum by straightening her left arm. **C,** Hooking her left upper limb over her hip, she begins to pull up from the side-lying position. **D,** When the patient is able to reach a lower limb, she continues by hooking onto her thigh with her forearm by using her elbow flexors or wrist extensors. **E,** Holding onto her knee and using head momentum, she brings her right hand forward. **F,** Finally, with both arms her legs, she can straighten her hips and pull on her calves and ankles to assume the LSP.

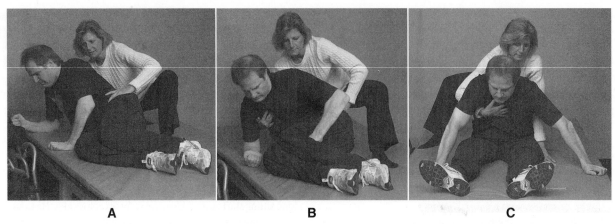

FIGURE 7-28 **A,** A dependent patient can move from side lying to LSP with the therapist assisting from behind and using contact points on his trunk to prevent a fall out in any direction. **B,** The therapist lifts while the patient shifts and brings his right elbow underneath him. He now shifts his weight to one side and off weights the other arm, which allows him to move it behind into an elbow extension position. **C,** Then the patient shifts his weight onto his extended arm, which will allow him to place his other arm into the extended position.

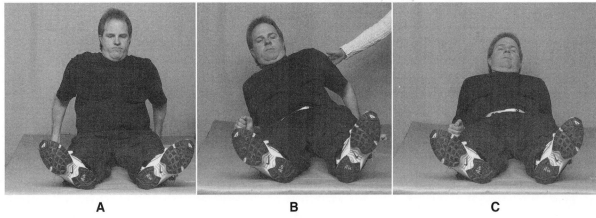

FIGURE 7-29 **A,** The patient begins to move down from long sitting to supine on elbows by unlocking each elbow one at a time. **B,** He then bends his left elbow and shifts his weight to his right elbow for a controlled descent. **C,** He bends his left elbow and equalizes his balance to assume supine on elbows.

and brings his elbows underneath him. From supine on elbows, the patient now shifts his weight to one side and off weights th e other arm, which allows him to move it behind into an elbow extension position. Then he shifts his weight onto his extended arm, which allows him to place his other arm into this position. After he is weight bearing on his upper limbs posteriorly in SLP, he can walk his arms forward until he achieves long sitting without upper limb support.

Techniques for Long Sitting to Supine

A patient can assume supine from LSP in a controlled fall. Supported on both upper limbs in long sitting, the patient unlocks one elbow at a time. After moving to supine on elbows, the patient shifts his weight off one upper limb to unload it from weight bearing and then off the second limb (Figure 7-29, *A, B,* and *C*). An alternate method is for the patient to lower into side lying and then roll back. If an individual has triceps he can control, he can descend through an eccentric contraction of the triceps.

Considerations for Spasticity and Incomplete Lesions

The manner in which spasticity is influenced by the patient's position will affect the way the therapist selects the optimal training techniques. For example, if strong extensor spasticity

is present when the patient is in supine, the optimal technique may be to move to side lying because coming up from supine may be too difficult. Breathing techniques may be used to assist in movement because exhalation may relax the spasticity, but this must be evaluated with each patient. A patient with an incomplete lesion or recovering strength may find that various modifications to the previously described techniques help to incorporate the energy of his partial innervations. For example, if the patient has partial innervation of the triceps sufficient to stabilize the elbow, he may be able to avoid walking around on his elbows while improving the safety and efficiency of moving from supine to LSP.

Guarding

When guarding a patient moving from supine to long sitting, the therapist should be located behind him to provide support laterally at the trunk to make sure he does not collapse back into side lying. The caregiver can also assist the patient who has intact biceps into long sitting by hooking onto the patient's forearm while the patient pulls up as the caregiver assists the pull as needed. The caregiver must make sure that her back is stabilized during this assist (Figure 7-30).

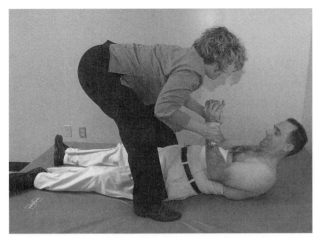

FIGURE 7-30 The caregiver assists the patient into LSP. Notice how her low back is stabilized as she uses her abdominal muscles during the lift.

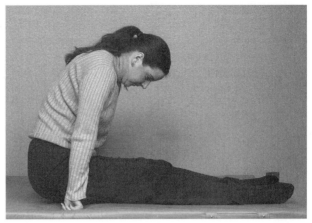

FIGURE 7-32 To scoot up on the mat or in bed, the patient extends her neck and then moves her neck and trunk into flexion. As she pushes into the mat's surface, her hips will move in the direction opposite her head's position.

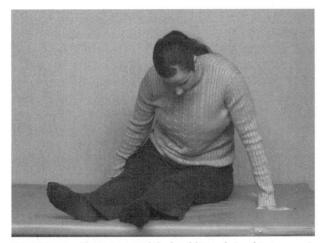

FIGURE 7-31 The patient used the head-hips relationship to move in the lateral direction as she scoots from side to side.

Caregiver Assistance

A patient who is dependent in position changes from supine to long sitting and back must be able to explain to his caregiver that she should place both hands at the scapular region and lift him directly from supine to LSP while maintaining good body mechanics herself. The caregiver may need to position one or both of her legs on the mat to bring herself closer to the patient and thus better protect her back while lifting (see Figure 7-28, B). The bed environment may not provide enough space for this option; therefore, the caregiver must understand how to adjust techniques to provide the safest of these methods.

Scooting

Accomplishing independent balance both statically and dynamically in the LSP is an important achievement because many individuals with SCI perform upper and lower body dressing and self-care activities in this position. The patient will also need to learn how to scoot or move in this position up and down as well as side to side. Performance of these movements will vary depending on the level of the lesion and on whether the triceps are innervated.

Scooting side to side requires that the patient apply the head-hips relationship in combination with an accompanying lift of the body off the contact surface. For example, when the patient moves to the left, his head and trunk are first shifted to the left and then quickly shifted to the right as the body is lifted and the hips move to the left (Figure 7-31). A weaker patient may exaggerate the head-hips relationship more when using it to assist with a shift. An individual without triceps will fix his upper limbs distally and his shoulders will be held in external rotation to maintain the mechanical lock at the elbow. An individual with triceps may choose to perform a series of lifts by using a push-up technique. In either case, to reposition the body, the lower limbs will need to be repositioned before or after the hips are moved.

Scooting forward and back also will require the patient to use an alternate head-hips relationship because the direction of movement is different. When scooting in bed, the patient first extends the head, neck, and upper trunk and then flexes the head as the hips are lifted (Figure 7-32). This pattern of movement facilitates the movement of the hips toward the head of the bed. The upper limbs may be locked without triceps innervation, as described previously. The individual with triceps will use a push-up technique with the head motion.

A patient can use the reverse motion to move down in bed: first the head, neck, and upper trunk are flexed and then extended (Figure 7-33). The downward direction is a greater challenge because the lower limbs create resistance and friction as a result of the direction of movement. Often the lower limbs flex while trying to move. An individual who cannot clear the surface of the bed during the lifting phase is subject to shearing forces on the buttocks, which places his skin at risk for breakdown. A patient can use the alternative method of moving in the prone-on-elbows position to move up and down the bed, which may minimize his risk for skin abrasions. In this position, he can use an army crawl to move up or down in bed (Figure 7-34). He also may choose to use one upper limb at a time or dig into the mat's surface with both simultaneously. His head and neck can use a rocking motion of head flexion and extension to assist with the direction

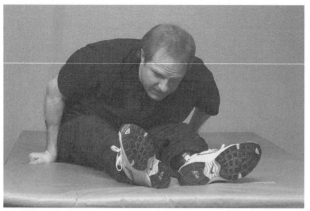

FIGURE 7-33 The patient scoots down the mat or bed by first flexing his head, neck, and upper trunk and then extending with momentum. As his buttocks lift up, they will move in the direction opposite his head. Note his transition from flexion to extension as his head begins the direction shift.

of movement. His elbows will be at risk for shear and pressure when this technique is used.

Therapists are encouraged to try variations of these techniques with their patients to establish the safest and most efficient methods for movement. For example, if an individual has tight hamstrings, his hips and knees can be bent to accommodate for the tightness and facilitate successful scooting. Scooting can also be applied as a treatment intervention to strengthening muscles and lead up to many ADLs and transfers. Push-up blocks can be used to assist individuals with triceps innervation. The therapist can add resistance at the shoulders, pelvis, and distal ankles to increase the difficultly of the task. Finally, the contact surface on which these skills are practiced will significantly affect performance (e.g., a bed will be much more difficult to negotiate than a mat table). When performing the activities in bed, additional equipment may be needed, such as an overhead trapeze or loops or loops on the legs to facilitate movement.

Special Considerations

As mentioned previously, it is easiest to practice the position change techniques described on a firm surface such as a mat. When the patient understands the basic principles of low-level position changes and has practiced sufficiently on a mat, it is important to apply these techniques to more functional surfaces such as a bed where balance is further challenged and motions may require more force to overcome the soft surface. Modification to techniques learned on the mat may be needed when moving in a bed. For example, a patient who does not need leg straps to assist repositioning of the lower limbs while on a mat may require them while moving in a bed. In addition, if the patient will use a hospital bed, use of the side rails may be incorporated to assist with position changes. The patient who is equipped with a basic level of knowledge and the ability to solve problems will be better able to handle these more difficult situations.

High-Level Position Changes

Two examples of high-level position changes that a therapist may teach her patients are assuming and maintaining the quadruped and tall-kneeling positions. These positions can further challenge

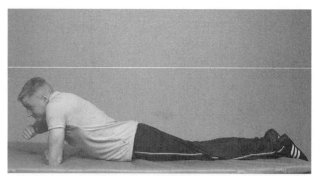

FIGURE 7-34 The patient scoots in prone on his elbows, demonstrating the army crawl in which one forearm moves over the other in front.

a high-functioning patient's strength, balance, and problem-solving skills. They also are component skills for floor transfers and excellent choices to teach patients control of the lower body through movement of the upper body. Medical clearance regarding spinal precautions and weight bearing through the lower limbs should be obtained before high-level position changes are practiced. High-level position change will require a minimum of triceps innervation in most cases, but caution must be taken to recognize the lack of trunk innervations and stability as these positions are practiced. The therapist must provide adequate stabilization and guarding to compensate for the patient's lack of trunk and pelvis control.

Quadruped

A patient may assume the quadruped position by beginning in the prone position with his hands in the push-up position. The therapist is positioned over him to provide assistance at his hip and pelvis (Figure 7-35, *A*). The patient can then walk backward on the elbows or push up into a straight arm position and walk back on the hands while the therapist helps to lift the pelvis off the mat. Another option is to have the patient move from a side-sitting position into quadruped with the therapist assisting at the hips. After the patient has achieved quadruped, he needs to immediately center his weight equally on both his upper and lower limbs. Assistance at the pelvis should gradually be eliminated until the patient is able to maintain this static position. He may need to frequently adjust the position of his hips with shoulder motions. For example, if the patient's hips are falling to the left, he can twist his shoulders to the left to move his hips to the right. A Swiss ball or bolster may be positioned under the patient's abdomen to provide additional support if he exhibits an excessive lumbar lordosis. A patient may be further challenged in this position by having him perform push ups while maintaining his balance. A patient with an incomplete injury may also work on balance by raising an upper (Figure 7-35, *B*) or lower limb or a combination of each. He may even work on crawling forward, backward, or sideways.

Tall Kneel

The therapist may instruct a patient to first assume quadruped and then sit back into a kneeling position when working on a tall kneel position. Care should be taken that the patient does not sit

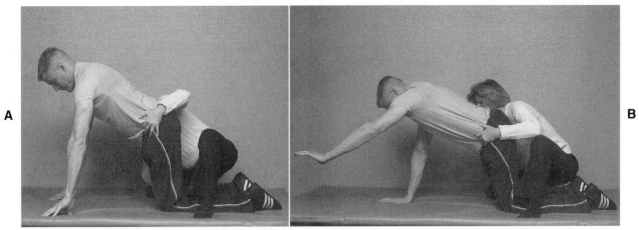

FIGURE 7-35 **A,** The patient assumes the quadruped position by controlling his upper body push up while the therapist guards and lifts his lower body with hand contacts at the pelvis. **B,** The patient can then perform balance training in quadruped stretching out with his upper limb.

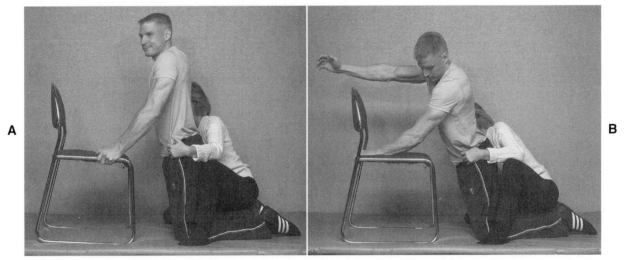

FIGURE 7-36 **A,** The patient assumes the tall kneeling position with the therapist guarding and supporting his pelvis from behind. **B,** The patient secures both upper limbs on a chair when in tall kneeling. The therapist guards from behind to protect him in the event of loss of trunk balance while the patient performs balance training reaching exercises with his upper limb. This activity is used as a lead-up to pre–gait training to increase trunk and hip control.

back onto his heels because this may compromise skin integrity and circulation. A pillow should be placed between the heels and the buttocks or a prayer bench used. After sitting back, the patient can walk his hands back to bring his trunk into an upright position. The therapist may be positioned behind the patient to provide assistance and support at the trunk. Another option is for the patient to push himself into an upright position with upper limb support provided by the therapist in front of the patient or by placing a chair or bolster in front of the patient (Figure 7-36, *A*).

When the patient has achieved the tall kneel position, various activities may be performed to further challenge the patient's balance, such as playing catch, lifting weights, or reaching for various objects. Achieving tall kneel with full hip extension is difficult with insufficient trunk and lower limb strength, yet it may be achieved by allowing the patient to support himself with his upper limbs on a chair placed in front of him (Figure 7-36, *B*). The tall kneel is a good lead-up to standing in the parallel bars with long leg splints or performing a floor-to-wheelchair transfer.

CLINICAL CASE STUDY — Intervention Principles and Position Changes Case 1

Patient History

Phil Adams is a 30-year-old man with a T12 paraplegia, ASIA A diagnosis resulting from a fracture dislocation sustained in a motor vehicle accident. His fracture was stabilized 1 day after injury by surgical decompression laminectomy and fusion of spinal levels T9 to L2. He wore a TLSO for 4 weeks after surgery. Phil's acute care course was complicated by a grade 2 pressure ulcer of his sacrum, which required 2 weeks of bed rest to heal. After discharge from the acute care hospital, Phil completed 4 weeks of inpatient rehabilitation where he gained independence in all ADL. Phil has been discharged and is now attending outpatient therapy where he is concentrating on improving his movement skills and advanced wheelchair skills.

Phil lives in a wheelchair-accessible loft. He travels a great deal by car and plane to supervise architectural sites and has been fitted in a lightweight wheelchair with quick response and agility, which is easily maneuverable on a variety of terrain. Phil also has a passion for outdoor sports and recreation activities.

Patient's Self-Assessment

Phil wants to improve his mobility skills to facilitate access in the community, at work, and for recreational outings.

Clinical Assessment
Patient Appearance

- Height 5 feet 10 inches, weight 150 pounds, body mass index 21.5
- Posture: Phil exhibits a mild kyphotic posture in the wheelchair

Cognitive Assessment

- Alert, oriented × 3

Cardiopulmonary Assessment

- Blood pressure 112/65 mm Hg, heart rate at rest 76, respiratory rate 12 breaths/min, vital capacity is within normal limits

Musculoskeletal and Neuromuscular Assessment

- Upper limb muscle strength is 5/5, trunk is 4/5, and lower limbs are 0/5
- Deep tendon reflexes are 2+ in the upper limbs and 0 in the lower limbs

Integumentary and Sensory Assessment

- Skin is intact throughout; sacral region is completely healed
- Sensation is absent below T12

Range of Motion Assessment

- Passive and active range of motion is WNL in both upper limbs and lower limbs, SLR is 105 degrees bilaterally passively

Mobility and ADL Assessment

- Is independent in all self-care activities including dressing, grooming, hygiene, bowel and bladder management, wheelchair management and propulsion, and driving; Phil is nonambulatory
- Nonambulatory

Equipment

- Tub bench, rental manual wheelchair, two-door sedan adapted with hand controls

Evaluation of Clinical Assessment

Phil Adams is a 30-year-old man with a T12 paraplegia, ASIA A diagnosis resulting from a motor vehicle accident. He is 10 weeks post injury and is being admitted for outpatient physical therapy for high-level position changes, ROM and strengthening, and pressure relief techniques.

Patient's Care Needs

Functional training for high-level position changes for independence in the home, work, and sports and recreation; education on pressure-relief techniques for prevention of pressure ulcers; and ROM and strengthening for improving community and sports and recreation participation

Diagnosis and Prognosis

Diagnosis is T12 paraplegia, ASIA A. Prognosis is for full mobility independence with high-level position changes, strengthening and capacity for home, work, and sports and recreation participation.

Preferred Practice Pattern*

Impaired Muscle Performance (4C), Joint Mobility, Motor Function, Muscle Performance, and Range of Motion Associated With Fracture (4G), Impairments Nonprogressive Spinal Cord Disorders (5H), Prevention/Risk Reduction for Integumentary Disorders (7A)

Team Goal

1. Discuss high-level position changes for home, work, and sports
2. Discuss strengthening and conditioning needs for Phil's active lifestyle
3. Discuss body mechanics and ergonomics to manually lift the chair in the car
4. Educate in pressure relief techniques
5. Discuss ROM limitations and impact on functional position changes and ADLs

Patient Goals

"I want to be comfortable getting into different positions, to get around in the wheelchair independently and avoid another wound."

Care Plan
Treatment Plan and Rationale

- Educate in stretching techniques for lower limbs to improve independence in high-level position changes
- Identify strengthening and conditioning approaches that lead to independence in high level position changes for home and sports/recreational activities
- Establish educational plan for pressure relief techniques
- Determine impact of lower limb ROM limitations on ADL e.g. bowel and bladder management

Interventions

- Practice in stretching techniques for lower limbs to improve independence in high-level position changes
- Perform strengthening and conditioning approaches that lead to independence in high-level position changes for home and sports/recreational activities
- Review and educate in pressure relief
- Practice and educate on stretching exercises for the lower limbs
- Practice car transfers teaching the use of good body mechanics

Documentation and Team Communication

- Team will communicate regarding progress on independence in high-level position changes
- Team will discuss progress on learning ROM and strengthening exercises
- Team will review knowledge of pressure relief techniques
- Team will document level of independence in all wheelchair skills and car transfers with use of optimal body mechanics

CLINICAL CASE STUDY Intervention Principles and Position Changes Case 1—cont'd

Follow-Up Assessment
- Follow-up on high-level position changes when at home, at work, and in the community in sports and recreation activities
- Follow-up on ROM and strength maintenance for ADL and position changes

Critical Thinking Exercises
Consider factors that will be affected by Phil's level of injury and trunk control as he regains mobility. Also consider the position the therapist or assistant will assume for guarding during training activities and techniques.

1. Describe an optimal weight-shifting technique that Phil can practice.
2. Describe how ROM and strength limitations restrict functional position changes.
3. Describe the best way for Phil to change position from prone to quadruped.
4. Describe how you would teach Phil to achieve the kneeling position.

Guide to physical therapist practice, rev. ed. 2, Alexandria, VA, 2003, American Physical Therapy Association.

CLINICAL CASE STUDY Intervention Principles and Position Changes Case 2

Patient History
James Winter is a 60-year-old male with the diagnoses of C6 tetraplegia AISA A. He sustained his injury 20 years ago secondary to an MVA. He is a retired banker. He has a wife and two children. His daughter, 38, has two young children ages 3 and 5, and his son, 35, has two children ages 8 months and 4 years. His children live nearby, but his son has just been transferred and will be moving 200 miles from his current location.

James's wife is 55 and is still working as an elementary school teacher. James has recently had right shoulder tendonitis and is not able to propel his wheelchair or drive his van. He also has a small left ischial decubitus, which is healing. He has started a course of physical therapy for his shoulder.

Patient' Self Assessment
James feels he has been fortunate since his injury at age 40. His career was not altered significantly, and he continued to be able to provide for his family and supported both children through college. He has an aide that comes 2 hours daily to help with bathing, bowel and bladder care, and dressing in the mornings. Overall his health has been good, and he has had to battle only minor issues such as urinary tract infections, one sacral decubitus that required 2 weeks of hospitalization, and a couple of bouts of the flu with pneumonia. He has some growing concerns with his shoulder pain and is considering a power wheelchair. He is also sad that his son will be moving because he enjoys having his grandchildren nearby, usually seeing them three to four times a week. He enjoys editing on photography at his computer and reading biographies.

Clinical Assessment
Patient Appearance
- Height 5 feet 10 inches, weight 178 lb, body mass index 25.5.

Cognitive Assessment
- Retired banker

Cardiopulmonary Assessment
- BP 126/80, heart rate at rest 74, respiratory rate 13 breaths/min, cough flows are ineffective (<360 L/min), VC (vital capacity) is reduced (between 1.5 and 2.5 L).

Musculoskeletal and Neuromuscular Assessment
- Motor assessment reveals C6 ASIA A, sensory C6
- DTR's 3+ below the level of lesion

Integumentary and Sensory Assessment
- Left ischial decubitus 3 × 3 × 2 cm, sensory intact to C6

Range of Motion Assessment
- Passive and active motion is within normal limits in the left upper limb, the right shoulder is limited as follows:

	Active range of motion (degrees)	Passive range of motion (degrees)
Flexion	112	116
Abduction	92	96
Internal rotation	52	55
External rotation	32	39

- Straight leg raise is 80° in both lower limbs and dorsiflexion is 2°; all other motions in the lower limbs are within functional limits.

Mobility and ADL Assessment
- James requires minimal to moderate assist with bed mobility and transfers to all surfaces.
- James is independent with pressure relief.
- James is currently dependent in manual wheelchair maneuvering on all surfaces.
- James is dependent in all self-care ADL.
- James is currently unable to drive.

Evaluation of Clinical Assessment
James Winter is a 60-year-old male with a C6 tetraplegia ASIA A diagnoses. He sustained his injury 20 years ago from an MVA. He began attending outpatient physical therapy 1 week ago for his shoulder pain and decreased functional ability.

Patient's Care Needs
1. Interventions for physical therapy to restore pain-free right shoulder movement and return to his prior level of function
2. Assess need for seating clinic referral
3. Education regarding prevention of worsening of wound
4. Evaluation for psychology services

Diagnosis and Prognosis
Diagnosis is C6 complete tetraplegia, ASIA A with a prognosis of full recovery of his right shoulder to his prior level of pain free function.

Preferred Practice Pattern*
Impaired Muscle Performance (4C), Joint Mobility, Motor Function, Muscle Performance, and Range of Motion Associated with Localized Inflammation (4E), Joint Mobility, Motor Function, Muscle Performance, and Range of Motion Associated with Fracture (4G), Impairments Nonprogressive Spinal Cord Disorders (5H), Primary Prevention/Risk Reduction for Cardiovascular/Pulmonary Disorders

Continued

CLINICAL CASE STUDY Intervention Principles and Position Changes Case 2—cont'd

(6A), (7A) Impaired Integumentary Integrity Associated with superficial skin involvement (7B).

Team Goals

1. Team to improve patient's right shoulder pain-free range of motion and strength
2. Team to educate patient on prevention of future pressure ulcers and current wound care
3. Team to return patient to prior level of function with a pain-free right shoulder

Patient Goals

"I want to be able to drive again without any shoulder pain and control my own wheelchair again, even if it is a power chair."

Care Plan
Treatment Plan and Rationale

• Initiate physical therapy interventions for the reduction of pain in client's right shoulder and restoration of function to prior level
• Educate patient about prevention strategies and pressure relief strategies to avoid future pressure sores
• Schedule patient for psychology evaluation

Interventions

• Outpatient physical therapy therapeutic exercise, neuromuscular re-education, therapeutic activities training and modalities for reduction of pain; wound prevention education

Documentation and Team Communication

• Team consultation for adjustment to life changes and probable wheelchair clinic consultation.

Follow-Up Assessment

• Biweekly team conferences for timely attainment of goals
• Re-assessment for consultation with other services

Critical Thinking Exercises

Consider factors that will influence patient education, physical therapy, and team care decisions unique to James's level of injury and trunk control at this level. Also consider the position of the therapist or of an assistant during activities.

1. Describe one weight shifting technique for James.
2. Describe one method of rolling for James.
3. Describe one position change method from supine to long sitting for James.

Guide to physical therapist practice, rev. ed. 2, Alexandria, VA, 2003, American Physical Therapy Association.

SUMMARY

Early in their therapy, patients may find working on basic actions such as rolling or coming to a sitting position overwhelming and frustrating. Therapists, however, can offer techniques to address mobility concerns and to help patients develop confidence in their abilities. It is beneficial to be open minded and consider combining technique components or developing variations on the techniques described in this chapter because every patient is unique in his injury and the attendant challenges that he faces in achieving movement. Two patients with the same neurological level injury will do well using very different techniques. Teaching patients basic movement patterns and emphasizing problem-solving skills will help them learn to adapt techniques to the unique situations in which they may find themselves.

REFERENCES

1. Davis CM: *Complementary therapies*, ed 2, Thorofare, NJ, 2004, Slack.
2. Davis CM: *Patient practitioner interaction: an experiential manual for developing the art of health care*, ed 3, Thorofare, NJ, 1998, Slack.
3. McManus CA: *Group wellness programs: for chronic pain and disease management*, St. Louis, 2003, Butterworth Heinemann.
4. Shepard KF, Jensen GM: *Handbook of teaching for physical therapists*, ed 2, St. Louis, 2002, Butterworth Heinemann.
5. Cech DJ, Martin ST: *Functional movement development: across the life span*, ed 2, Philadelphia, 2002, WB Saunders.
6. Richardson C, Hodges P, Hides J: *Therapeutic exercise for lumbo-pelvic stabilization: a motor control approach for the treatment and prevention of low back pain*, ed 2, New York, 2004, Churchill Livingstone.
7. Thibodeau GA, Patton KT: *Anatomy & physiology*, ed 5, St. Louis, 2003, Mosby.
8. Levangie PK, Norkin CC: *Joint structure and function: a comprehensive analysis*, ed 3, Philadelphia, 2001, FA Davis.
9. Neuman DA: *Kinesiology of the musculoskeletal system: foundations for physical rehabilitation*, St. Louis, 2002, Mosby.
10. Oatis CA: *Kinesiology: the mechanics & pathomechanics of human movement*, New York, 2004, Lippincott Williams & Wilkins.
11. Sie IH, Waters RL, Adkins RH et al: Upper limb pain in the post rehabilitation spinal cord injured patient, *Arch Phys Med Rehabil* 73:44-48, 1992.
12. Pentland WE, Twomey LT: The weight-bearing upper limb in women with long term paraplegia, *Paraplegia* 29:521-530, 1991.
13. Gellman H, Sie I, Waters RL: Late complications of the weight-bearing upper limb in the paraplegic patient, *Clin Orthop* 233:132-135, 1988.
14. Bayley JC, Cochran TP, Sledge CB: The weight-bearing shoulder: the impingement syndrome in paraplegics, *J Bone Joint Surg [Am]* 69:676-678, 1987.
15. Wylie EJ, Chakera TM: Degenerative joint abnormalities in patients with paraplegia of duration greater than 20 years, *Paraplegia* 26:101-106, 1988.
16. Consortium for Spinal Cord Medicine: *Preservation of upper limb function following spinal cord injury: a clinical practice guideline for health-care professionals*, Washington, DC, 2005, Paralyzed Veterans of America.
17. Bryden AM, Kilgore KL, Lind BB et al: Triceps denervation as a predictor of elbow flexion contractures in individuals with C5-C6 tetraplegia, *Arch Phys Med Rehabil* 85:1880-1885, 2004.
18. Maricello MA, Herbison GJ, Cohen ME et al: Elbow extension using the anterior deltoids and upper pectorals in spinal cord-injured subjects, *Arch Phys Med Rehabil* 76:426-432, 1995.
19. Zerby SA, Herbison GJ, Marino RJ et al: Elbow extension using the anterior deltoids and upper pectorals, *Muscle Nerve* 17:1472-1474, 1994.

20. Norkin CC, White DJ: *Measurement of joint motion: a guide to goniometry*, ed 3, Philadelphia, 2003, FA Davis.

21. Shumway-Cook A, Woollacott MH: *Motor control theory and practical applications*, ed 2, Philadelphia, 2001, Lippincott Williams & Wilkins.

22. Nash MS: Exercise as a health promoting activity following spinal cord injury, *J Neurol Phys Ther* 29:87-103, 2005.

23. Jacobs PL, Nash MS: A comparison of 2 circuit exercise training techniques for eliciting matched metabolic responses in persons with paraplegia, *Med Sci Sports Exerc* 33:711-717, 2001.

24. Kilkens OJ, Post MW, van der Woude LH et al: The wheelchair circuit: reliability of a test to assess mobility in persons with spinal cord injuries, *Arch Phys Med Rehabil* 83:1783-1788, 2002.

25. Durán FS, Lugo L, Ramírez L et al: Effects of an exercise program on the rehabilitation of patients with spinal cord injury, *Arch Phys Med Rehabil* 82:1349-1354, 2001.

26. Kilkens OJ, Dallmeijer AJ, Nene AV et al: The longitudinal relation between physical capacity and wheelchair skill performance during inpatient rehabilitation of people with spinal cord injury, *Arch Phys Med Rehabil* 86:1575-1581, 2005.

27. Dallmeijer AJ, van der Woude LH, Hollander PAP et al: Physical performance in persons with spinal cord injuries after discharge from rehabilitation, *Med Sci Sports Exerc* 31:1330-1335, 1999.

28. Knott M, Voss DE: *Proprioceptive neuromuscular facilitation: patterns and techniques*, ed 2, New York, 1968, Harper and Row.

29. Carr J, Shepard R: *Neurological rehabilitation: optimizing motor performance*, New York, 1998, Butterworth Heinmann.

30. Bernstein N: *The coordination and regulation of human movements*, New York, 1967, Pergamon Press.

31. Roux L, Hanneton S, Roby-Brami A: Shoulder movements during the initial phase of learning manual wheelchair propulsion in able-bodied subjects, *Clin Biomech (Bristol, Avon)* 21(1 Suppl 1): S45-S51, 2006.

32. Thelan E: Motor development: a new synthesis, *Am Psychol* 50: 79-95, 1995.

33. Chen CL, Yeung KT, Bih LI et al: The relationship between sitting stability and functional performance in patients with paraplegia, *Arch Phys Med Rehabil* 84:1276-1281, 2003.

34. Lynch SM, Leah P, Barker SP: Reliability of functional reach test in individuals with spinal cord injury, *Phys Ther* 78:128-133, 1988.

35. Chao CY, Cheing GL: The effects of lower limb functional electric stimulation on the orthostatic responses of people with tetraplegia, *Arch Phys Med Rehabil* 86:1427-1433, 2005.

36. Sidorov E, Townson A, Dvorak MF et al: Orthostatic hypotension in the first month following acute spinal cord injury, *Spinal Cord* Apr 10, 2007. Epub ahead of print.

37. Eng JJ: Use of prolonged standing for individuals with spinal cord injuries, *Phys Ther* 81:1392-1399, 2001.

38. Consortium for Spinal Cord Medicine: *Pressure ulcer prevention and treatment following spinal cord injury: a clinical practice guideline for health-care professionals*, Washington, DC, 2000, Paralyzed Veterans of America.

39. Coggrave MJ, Rose LS: A specialist seating assessment clinic: changing pressure relief practice, *Spinal Cord* 41:692-695, 2003.

40. Henderson CE: Application of ventilatory strategies to enhance functional activities for an individual with spinal cord injury, *J Neurol Phys Ther* 29:107-111, 2005.

41. van Drongelen S, van der Woude LH, Janssen TW et al: Glenohumeral contact forces and muscle forces evaluated in wheelchair-related activities of daily living in able-bodied subjects versus subjects with paraplegia and tetraplegia, *Arch Phys Med Rehabil* 86:1434-1440, 2005.

42. Shirado O, Kawase M, Minami A et al: Quantitative evaluation of long sitting in paraplegic patients with spinal cord injury, *Arch Phys Med Rehabil* 85:1251-1256, 2004.

SOLUTIONS TO CHAPTER 7 CLINICAL CASE STUDY

Intervention Principles and Position Changes Case 1

1. Because Phil has normal (5/5) strength in bilateral upper limbs and trunk, he will be required to strengthen his upper limbs and trunk. After that is accomplished, he will be able to perform push-up pressure relief. Education on timing of weight shifting and skin risks related to shearing will be critical for this individual. Phil also will be able to perform an anterior weight shift with relative ease. His T12, ASIA A injury should allow him to combine a push-up and anterior weight shift for sacral relief by performing a push-up to bring the body away from the backrest, followed by an anterior weight shift. Care with engaging brakes and forward position of the casters to prevent chair tipping is important to remember with these position changes.

2. Phil's passive ROM at the hamstrings and ankles plantar flexion prevent him from proper positioning in the wheelchair, resulting in possible risk for skin breakdown on the sacrum and plantar foot because of poor position on the footrests. Importantly, the ROM limitations prevent him from doing his bowel and bladder routine independently because he is unable to flex his trunk forward enough without falling backward. These ROM limitations also prevent the assumption of a tall kneeling position as a result of hip flexor and hamstring tightness. This position is important to Phil because he would like to get out of his chair onto the floor or beach during his recreational activities and tall kneeling is an important position to return to his wheelchair (see Solution 4).

3. From the prone position, Phil can come up on his elbows and crawl backward toward his knees while at the same time pushing up extending his elbows to obtain the quadruped position. If assistance is needed, Phil may begin his movement to quadruped in the prone position with his hands in the push-up position. The therapist is straddled over him providing assistance at his hip and pelvis. He can then walk backward on his elbows or push up into a straight arm position and walk back on his hands while the therapist helps to lift his pelvis off the mat.

Another option is to maneuver from a side-sit position into quadruped with the therapist assisting at the hips. After he has achieved the quadruped position, he needs to immediately center his weight equally on his legs and arms. Assistance at the pelvis should gradually be eliminated until the patient is able to maintain this static position.

4. Phil can be taught to move from quadruped to kneeling through a transitional phase of sitting back on his heels and then pulling up from a stable structure such as a wheelchair or couch to lift and rotate back into the desired seated position. Another option might be to reach up with one arm onto the wheelchair or couch, load that arm sufficiently to allow the possibility of the other arm to come up onto the elevated surface to achieve the tall kneeling position. This is generally feasible when the arms are quite strong, the knees may not be flexible enough, or the body size may be too large to sit back on the heels. If Phil uses an indwelling catheter, it would be important not to have him sitting back on heels in such a way as to kink the catheter tube.

SOLUTIONS TO CHAPTER 7 CLINICAL CASE STUDY

Intervention Principles and Position Changes Case 2

1. The length of the individual's arms will affect the variations for weight shifting, particularly with the recovery process. James would most commonly perform a lateral weight shift, but his age must be considered during any weight shift or position change training. Using the push handle or armrest for support on the leaning side will provide for stability to compensate for the lack of trunk control. The opposite arm may need to be hooked on the push handle with wrist extension when using the arm rest because this injury level may not be able to recover from the weight-shift position. Another option would be to use the opposite arm rest to assist with resuming upright after the weight shift. The anterior weight shift may or may not be feasible. The use of loops with the anterior weight shift may be considered for James and should be tried for efficiency, safety, and any decrease in shoulder strain while performing a weight shift. The tilt-back technique can serve as a backup for James performed by another individual should the shoulder injury require this secondary to pain. Therefore James must be well versed in educating others with the technique.

2. James uses momentum of the upper limbs to roll because of the extent of paralysis. The patient with this level of injury can hook both wrists and externally rotate at the shoulders to avoid elbow flexion. This must be practiced, and the therapist needs to guard the patient from hitting his head during acquisition of this skill. Consideration as to whether or not James has a preference for flexion or extension should be evaluated before teaching the skill: simply observe the direction James moves his head when asked to roll. It is typical to begin training patients in their preferred direction, flexion or extension, first, and if this is not successful, attempt the opposite or neutral position. The techniques described in this chapter should be applied with lower extremity positioning as the patient is learning the task, pillows should bel used to support the trunk in varying degrees of partial side-lying until the patient is successful without these assists. Additionally, breathing and level of spasticity may affect the task of rolling and need to be evaluated.

3. James is 60 years old, and therefore decreasing shoulder strain must be considered with all position changes. The position change from supine to supine on elbows could place a great deal of anterior shoulder strain on him. It is therefore recommended that James assume the on-elbows position from side-lying and walk the elbows around to his knees until he is stable enough to throw one extremity behind him into the locked elbow position and then the second one. The therapist must constantly guard the patient during this training to prevent shoulder injury or pain and support of his trunk if his balance is compromised.

CHAPTER EIGHT

Transfer Techniques

Alicia Koontz, RET, ATP, PhD, and Erica Druin, MPT

When I first started working on transfers in therapy it seemed like something I'd never be able to do but as I got stronger it got easier. Once I was home I also found that I could modify the techniques I had learned to work better for me. As I come across new situations I find myself able to figure out how to handle them based on the basic techniques I learned back in therapy.

Marco (C8 SCI)

Throughout the course of a day an individual with a spinal cord injury (SCI) is required to move or transfer between his wheelchair and various surfaces including the bed, chair, tub, commode, and car. Therefore, learning to perform transfers is a vital component in the rehabilitation of any patient with an SCI. A variety of techniques may be used whether a patient performs a transfer independently or with assistance. This chapter provides an overview of transfer techniques and includes important items to consider: patient characteristics, risks associated with patient transfers, transfer ergonomics, wheelchair management, positioning for transfers, and types of transfers. For ease of discussion, transfers are described as they are performed between the wheelchair and mat; special considerations for various functional surfaces are discussed at the end of the chapter.

PATIENT CHARACTERISTICS

The ability to perform transfers varies considerably from patient to patient. Individual patient characteristics need to be considered when determining the most appropriate transfer techniques for that patient to use as well as the appropriateness for independent versus assisted transfers (Box 8-1).

Physical Considerations
Level of Spinal Cord Injury

The level of SCI has been traditionally used to predict the level of independence during transfer tasks.[1] Patients with thoracic and lumbar spinal injuries are usually expected to achieve competence in all types of transfers, and studies have shown that 80% to 85% actually do on discharge from a rehabilitation facility.[2,3] There is great variability in performance among persons with

---

BOX 8-1	Patient Considerations When Learning Transfer Techniques

- Level of spinal cord injury
- Strength of innervated musculature
- Muscle imbalances
- Fatigue
- ROM
- Spasticity
- Presence of an orthosis or brace
- Tolerance to upright
- Sitting posture and balance
- Secondary diagnoses or complications
- Excessive body mass and pregnancy
- Age
- Cognitive ability
- Motivation and fear

---

tetraplegia, with one study showing that 58% (31/53) with incomplete tetraplegia and 16% (12/75) with complete tetraplegia were able to perform wheelchair transfers independently 3 years after discharge.[2] Individuals with tetraplegia may not be able to lift their weight if greater flexion is needed at the elbow as needed when transferring uphill.[4] The higher the level of injury, the lower the physical capacity of the patient. Patients with tetraplegia have been shown to have higher levels of physical strain while performing transfers than do their counterparts with paraplegia.[5] Transfer-assist devices, such as transfer boards and mechanical lifts, can help with performing transfers for individuals with decreased muscle strength and weakness.

Strength of Innervated Musculature

Muscle strength is an important consideration for independent transfers. The upper limbs must be strong enough to lift and support the weight of the trunk and pelvis as the body is transported from one surface to another. Performing transfers uphill requires more strength than performing downhill or level transfers.[6] Muscle strength is also a function of level of SCI. Individuals with high-level injuries place an increased demand on their muscles during transfers in comparison to individuals with some trunk innervation.[7] Using a transfer assist device, such as a transfer board, will reduce the amount of force needed for lateral movement and may enable the patient to perform transfers independently.[8]

Muscle Imbalances

Individuals with SCI are predisposed to muscle imbalance in the shoulders as a result of functional strengthening during routine activities such as wheelchair propulsion, transfers, and overhead reaching. Muscle imbalance is also a risk factor for rotator cuff conditions. Individuals who routinely perform independent transfers and in whom muscle imbalance develops should consider assisted transfers and engaging in an exercise program to stretch the anterior shoulders and chest musculature and strengthen the posterior shoulder muscles.[9]

Fatigue

Transfers and wheelchair propulsion are high-stress activities and thus muscles are susceptible to fatigue. Fatigue is related to risk of injury. Dugan and Frontera[10] provide a review in this important area. Fatigue decreases the ability to protect the joint, especially the shoulder, which requires muscle activation for stability.[11] If a patient feels tired, he needs to seek assistance for transfers.

Range of Motion

Assess upper limb and trunk joint range of motion (ROM) to determine whether any limitations are present that would interfere with the patient's ability to perform transfers of different heights and to various surfaces (Table 8-1, also see Table 6-4). Restricted ROM can lead to pain, injury, and reduced activity.[12,13]

Spasticity

The act of performing a transfer may trigger spasticity in a paralyzed limb, for example, clonus in the lower limbs. Clonus can impede proper alignment for transfers or make it more difficult to finish a transfer once it is started. Evaluate patients for their ability to safely complete a transfer if spasticity occurs during the performance of the transfer task. If a patient has the potential to lose control of balance or stability while transferring because of spasticity, it is recommended that he perform assisted transfers.

Tolerance to the Upright Position

A patient who has orthostatic hypotension, or a low tolerance to an upright position, could become dizzy or lose his sense of position in space when attempting a transfer (see Chapter 7). Instruct such patients about the need for safety in assisted transfers and teach them how to avoid falls until their tolerance to upright has improved.

Secondary Diagnoses or Complications

Take secondary diagnoses or complications into consideration when assessing a patient's ability to perform transfers. These include but are not limited to upper limb repetitive strain injuries (such as carpal tunnel syndrome (CTS), shoulder impingement, and rotator cuff tendonitis and tears), upper or lower limb fractures, pain, skin breakdown, and respiratory or cardiovascular deficits. A patient needs to avoid independent transfers if an upper or lower limb injury or fracture is present or accompanied by significant pain. If only one side of his body is affected, a patient may continue to perform independent transfers remembering to use the unaffected limb as the trailing arm because the forces and work performed with the trailing arm are greater than that of the leading arm.[14] A patient with pressure ulcers needs to get assistance or learn how to perform a transfer in a manner that avoids applying excessive pressure or shear to the affected area. Performing independent transfers can be straining on the respiratory and cardiovascular systems,[5,15] so if these systems are compromised, patients need to obtain assistance from a caregiver.

Excessive Body Mass or Pregnancy

A patient with excessive body mass has increased difficulty with independent transfers. Not only must he bear more weight through his upper limbs but transfers can be stressful to his respiratory and cardiovascular systems. Individuals with excess body mass and diminished upper limb strength because of higher levels of SCI need to use greater muscular effort to perform transfers.[7] Excessive mass around the abdomen, such as in pregnancy, inhibits hip flexion during transfers, thereby leading to poor placement of the hands and subsequently poor shoulder alignment. To compensate for this alignment problem, always consider the use of assisted transfers and devices with individuals with a high body mass index and with bariatric and pregnant patients.

Psychosocial Considerations

Age

Older adults face additional challenges because of sensory, vision, and hearing changes as well as decreases in bone density and muscle strength that accompany increasing age.[16] In addition, seniors with SCI are at a particularly high risk for skin breakdown.[17] A patient and his caregivers need to be aware of these issues and how each might influence his ability to transfer safely.

Cognitive Ability

Patients with SCI and a traumatic brain injury or chronic illness such as dementia or Alzheimer's disease will have a more difficult time with performing ADLs as a result of impaired memory, judgment, and decision-making skills. Therapists should evaluate the patient's cognition to ensure his ability to comprehend the steps involved in transfer activities and perform them safely.

Motivation and Fear

Therapists may increase the patient's motivation by providing a safe and nonthreatening environment for transfer training and by making transfers as easy as possible to learn. Therefore, it is advisable to begin training with transfers between level, firm surfaces (e.g., between the wheelchair and the mat) and then

| TABLE 8-1 | Muscles Exhibiting Moderate or High Activity During a Depression (Lateral) Transfer |

	Preparation Phase	Lift Phase	Descent Phase
Leading upper limb	Sternal pectoralis major Subscapularis Biceps long head	Sternal pectoralis major Serratus anterior Latissimus dorsi Infraspinatus Biceps long head	Sternal pectoralis major Latissimus dorsi
Trailing upper limb	Sternal pectoralis major Infraspinatus	Serratus anterior Sternal pectoralis major Latissimus dorsi Infraspinatus Supraspinatus Anterior deltoid	Serratus anterior Sternal pectoralis major

Adapted from Perry J, Gronley JK, Newsam CJ et al: Electromyographic analysis of the shoulder muscles during depression transfers in subjects with low-level paraplegia, *Arch Phys Med Rehabil* 77:350-355, 1996.

progress to functional surfaces that are more difficult to negotiate. Give patients plenty of opportunity to practice, demonstrate skills, and refine transfer techniques. This will help each patient overcome his fears and acquire the confidence necessary to apply his new knowledge to different situations as they arise.

Environmental Considerations
Presence of an Orthosis
A hand, wrist, or elbow orthosis may inhibit the patient's ability to bear weight on the upper limbs or may inhibit proper placement of the hands. Spinal orthoses create limitations that have a significant effect on a patient's ability to transfer. Depending on the type of spinal orthosis a patient is using, the apparatus will limit cervical or trunk motion. Educate each patient about the precautions he and his caretakers need to be aware of so he can in turn reinforce them with other caregivers who may be assisting him to transfer. It is imperative that these precautions be followed at all times to ensure optimal spinal healing, and always remember when assisting a patient in an orthosis, the orthosis is not to be used as a hand-hold to assist the patient. Spinal orthoses are discussed in more detail in Chapter 2.

Once a patient is no longer wearing a spinal orthosis or when the type of orthosis changes (e.g., from a halo brace to a Philadelphia collar), his transfer techniques may be quite different and require relearning. This is because the patient's balance and center of gravity will change. He may now be cleared for increased forward flexion, which can affect his posture during the transfer. When he no longer needs to use the device, he can use the head-hips relationship (discussed later in this chapter). The head-hips relationship allows the patient to take advantage of momentum and principles of biomechanics during his transfer (see Chapter 7). Carefully screen any patient with an orthosis or brace or whose spinal stabilization device has been recently changed, for his ability to perform independent transfers and provide or modify assistance as necessary (Clinical Note: Important Considerations for Caregivers About Patients in Spinal Orthoses).

CLINICAL NOTE	Important Considerations for Caregivers About Patients in Spinal Orthoses

- Maintain spinal precautions to facilitate optimal healing
- Never use the orthosis as a hand-hold during transfers
- Educate patient regarding his spinal precautions to promote carryover
- Identify how orthosis or spinal precautions will affect transfer
  - Balance or center of gravity
  - Posture
  - Ability to use head-hips relationship or momentum
- When the orthosis is changed or no longer needed, reassess and modify transfer techniques as appropriate

---

Sitting Posture and Balance
Posture and balance directly affect transfer performance.[18] Appropriate seating and trunk support are crucial to provide a stable base of support for the upper limbs. Balance is also related

---

BOX 8-2	Optimal Seating for Pressure Relief and Function

Pelvic Positioning
- Neutral to slight anterior tilt of the pelvis
- Equal weightbearing through the ischial tuberosities

Lower Limb Considerations
- Thighs fully supported
- Hips in neutral to slight abduction and neutral rotation
- Ankles in slight dorsiflexion
- Heels and balls of feet in contact with footplates

Trunk Position
- Promote lumbar extension
- Prevent kyphosis and scoliosis

---

to the level of SCI, with patients who have high-level injuries demonstrating decreased balance.[19,20] Chapter 11 provides general principles to follow so that the patient is seated properly for pressure relief and function (Box 8-2). It is, however, important to be aware that certain wheelchair adjustments made to improve posture can affect a patient's ability to transfer. For example, seat dump—a situation in which the rear of the seat is lower than the front—can make transfers more difficult because the transfer from surface to surface becomes an uphill battle.

TRANSFER RISKS
Transfers are not without risk to the patient or to the caregiver who is helping him with the transfer. Transfers can be partly responsible for the development of upper limb pain, pressure ulcers, and wheelchair-related accidents. Caregivers are at risk for low back injuries from improper transfer and lifting techniques. It is important for patients and caregivers to learn and always use ergonomically sound transfer techniques that are based on the anatomic, physiological, and mechanical principles that influence the efficient use of human energy (see Chapter 7).

Upper Limb Pain and Injury
Transfers, along with pressure relief and wheelchair propulsion, are the primary sources of upper limb pain among individuals with SCI. Dalyan et al[21] surveyed 130 patients with varying levels of SCI about the presence and severity of pain in the shoulders, elbows, wrists, and hands and whether upper limb pain interfered with 10 functional ADLs. Of the 130 patients who were surveyed, 76 (59%) had upper limb pain. Respondents recorded their perceived impact of pain on functional activity with one of the following: never or rarely, sometimes or usually, and always. Of the 10 activities, pain was more likely to be associated with transfers, wheelchair mobility, ambulation, pressure relief, and upper body dressing.

Bayley et al[22] found 33% (31/94) of individuals with paraplegia in their study had pain while transferring and 16% had a rotator cuff tear. Nichols et al[23] reported that 51% of 538 individuals with SCI had shoulder pain and that 92% of these individuals noted wheelchair propulsion and transfers as the primary reasons. Curtis et al[24] reported that activities requiring high levels of upper limb strength such as ascending a ramp in a wheelchair, overhead reaching, washing your back, and transfers between surfaces that are not level were most closely associated with intense shoulder pain.

Women with SCI may be at higher risk for development of upper limb pain and injury than are their male counterparts. Pentland and Twomey[25] studied upper limb pain and mobility (transfers and wheelchair propulsion), self-care ADLs, and other general activities in 11 women with paraplegia. The percentages of women experiencing pain during bed transfers was 73%, car transfers 64%, toilet transfers 55%, and bath transfers 55%. They also found that 89% of the women had pain when propelling outdoors and 75% had pain while loading their wheelchairs into a car. The women in this study reported shoulder pain more often than reports of pain by men with paraplegia. Boninger et al[26] investigated shoulder magnetic resonance imaging abnormalities in a longitudinal study of 14 persons with paraplegia and found significantly more advancement of shoulder injury during follow-up in seven persons, six of whom were women. Women were noted to push with higher propulsion forces than men. The study concluded that women with paraplegia who use wheelchairs are more susceptible than men to shoulder injuries, underscoring the importance of educating women about the risks of repetitive strain injuries and using preventive strategies such as those discussed later in the chapter.

Scientific evidence exists that repetitive weight bearing during transfers can lead to upper limb injury. Bayley et al[22] inserted pressure transducers in pain-free shoulders of five patients with paraplegia and measured intra-articular pressure while patients performed ROM activities, pressure reliefs, and lateral transfers. Pressure measurements recorded during transfers were 2.5 times higher than that recorded when the shoulder was not bearing weight. The increase in pressure is likely due to the shift in body weight from the trunk through the clavicle and scapula and across the subacromial tissues to the humeral head. The increased pressures stress the vasculature of the rotator cuff and can contribute to tendon degeneration, inflammation, and tears.

Structural changes in the shoulder may or may not be associated with pain symptoms. Lal's[27] research found that 72% of individuals with paraplegia and tetraplegia (38/53) showed x-ray–confirmed degenerative changes in the shoulder, mostly involving the acromioclavicular joint, but impingement, spur formation, and necrosis were also common. Only six subjects (11%) in this study reported pain. Boninger et al[28] conducted magnetic resonance imaging and radiographs on 28 individuals with paraplegia and found that 68% had confirmed shoulder abnormalities (e.g., coracromial thickening, acromioclavicular joint degeneration, distal clavicle osteolysis), whereas only 32% reported pain. If an individual has upper limb pain or concomitant injury, his ability to continue to perform independent transfers will be greatly compromised.[29] To avoid injury to a patient's upper limbs when providing assistance during a transfer, it is vital to avoid pulling on a weak or unstable upper limb when lifting or repositioning the patient.

Pressure Ulcers

Pressure ulcers occur in up to 80% of individuals with SCI, and of those individuals, 30% have more than one pressure ulcer.[30] Avoid transfer techniques that allow excessive sliding movements

of the buttocks because pressure ulcers can develop in areas exposed to large shear forces. Encourage older adults with SCI or individuals with recurring pressure ulcers to take extra precautions and consider using transfer-assist devices that reduce or eliminate shear forces during transfers. Techniques to minimize shearing forces are discussed in more detail throughout the chapter (Clinical Note: Techniques That Minimize Shearing Forces During Transfers).

CLINICAL NOTE **Techniques That Minimize Shearing Forces During Transfers**

- Transfer using a closed fist with wrist in neutral for increased vertical excursion
- Depress shoulders for additional height
- Begin transfer in forward flexed position to help off-weight buttocks and pivot on feet
- Use a transfer board or mechanical lift

Wheelchair-Related Accidents

Transfers are responsible for many wheelchair-related accidents. Of the 770 wheelchair-related accidents leading to death that were reported to the U.S. Consumer Products Safety Commission between 1973 and 1987, more than 8% were caused by falls during transfers.[31] Between 1986 and 1990, 17% of the estimated 36,559 wheelchair-related accidents that were serious enough to necessitate a visit to an emergency department were falls during transfers.[32] Many accidents are caused by parking the wheelchair too far away from the surface the patient is transferring to, failure to adequately move the footrests out of the way, failure to activate the wheel locks, loose brakes (e.g., caused by tire deflation or wear), attempting to transfer to an unstable surface, or carelessness.[33] The case report by Kirby and Smith[33] also discusses an incident in which the fall was related to mismatched wheel locks. Thus the patient's ability to properly manage the components of his wheelchair is essential to avoiding falls (see Wheelchair Management).

Caregivers

Caregivers, including family members, nurses, therapists, and others who assist patients in transfers are at an extremely high risk for development of low-back pain and injuries.[34,35] The greatest risk has been associated with one-person transfer techniques; however, some studies have shown that two-person techniques result in high spinal loads and low-back pain risk as well.[36-38] In terms of ease for the caregiver, there is a consensus that pulling techniques using assistive devices (e.g., gait belt, patient handling sling) are easier than lifting the patient. The shearing involved in pulling the patient, however, places him at high risk for skin breakdown and therefore is not the ideal technique to use. Using a mechanical lift whenever possible maximizes ease for the caregiver while protecting the patient's skin integrity.

With two-person lifts, it is important to have both helpers working in unison when moving the patient because they can actually fight each other's movements and add to the risk of back injury. Repositioning a patient in a wheelchair, discussed in more detail later, is also associated with high spinal compressive and shear forces and warrants consideration for mechanical assistance.[34,39] When manual assistance is the only option available, practicing good body mechanics to protect the lower back is paramount (see Chapter 7).

TRANSFER ERGONOMICS

The Guide to Physical Therapist Practice defines ergonomics as "the relationships among the worker, the work that is done, the tasks and activities inherent in that work, and the environment in which the work is performed. Ergonomics uses scientific and engineering principles to improve the safety, efficiency, and quality of movement involved in work."[40] Modification of task performance on the basis of ergonomic principles has proven to reduce the incidence of pain and cumulative trauma disorders of the upper limb in various work settings.[41-47] The same approaches used in these studies can be used to prevent upper limb pain and injury in persons with SCI. Key ergonomic approaches for persons performing independent transfers are highlighted in this chapter. It is also important for the caregivers and professionals who are providing assistance with the transfer to practice ergonomic principles of lifting and moving patients (see Chapter 7).

Using ergonomically sound transfer techniques and reducing the number of transfers performed each day can help minimize joint loading, lower injury risk, and preserve upper limb function (Box 8-3).

BOX 8-3 | Ergonomic Tips for Patients Performing Transfers

- Use head-hips relationship or momentum
- Transfer between level surfaces whenever possible
- Avoid a position of impingement when possible
- Ensure appropriate hand placement
- Use forward flexed trunk position
- Consider demands on leading versus trailing upper limbs during transfer
- Use transfer assist devices as needed

Head-Hips Relationship

Because patients with SCI must compensate for weak or absent muscle strength, emphasize the controlled use of momentum during transfer training. The head-hips relationship involves using the body to generate momentum to move from one surface to another and can be illustrated with the use of a pen. As the top of the pen is moved to the right, the bottom of the pen consequently swings to the left and vice versa (Figure 8-1). The same principle applies when moving the body. As the head and shoulders swing to the right, it will promote the hips to move left and vice versa. As the head and shoulders move forward, it will assist the hips in moving backward and vice versa. Taking advantage of this principle will make the performance of transfers considerably easier.

It is important to teach each patient how to best use the head-hips relationship to his advantage to obtain clearance of the buttocks (Figure 8-2). Patients with strong triceps, however, may not need to generate momentum to move their body so may find it more efficient to move the head, shoulders, and hips in the same direction.[48] A patient with tetraplegia will likely need to exaggerate the head-hips relationship. To maximize the benefit from the head-hips relationship, the patient can first move his head in the direction he wants to move and then quickly move it in the opposite direction. This will allow him to move his head through a greater excursion and gain increased momentum.

Surface Heights

Teach the patient to perform level transfers whenever possible. Transfers across two surfaces that are not level impose increased demands on the arm muscles.[6] Transferring uphill requires increased muscle activation of the triceps. The triceps and posterior shoulder muscles work harder to maintain control of the body during downhill transfers versus level transfers. Another potential problem with nonlevel transfers, in addition to higher muscle forces, is that alignment of the wrist and shoulder joints may be less than optimal. An evaluation of each patient's environment where transfers are routinely performed can help identify when

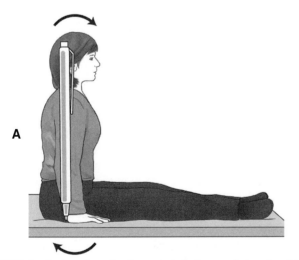
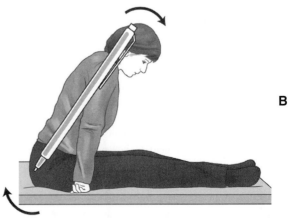

FIGURE 8-1 **A,** A pen is used to demonstrate the leverage that can be achieved when a patient uses the head-hips relationship to move her head forward and down while keeping her back straight, thereby facilitating the movement of her hips in the opposite direction. **B,** As the patient's hips rise up off the mat, it is easier for her to move from side to side or back and forth. This concept can be applied to training for transfers and functional position changes.

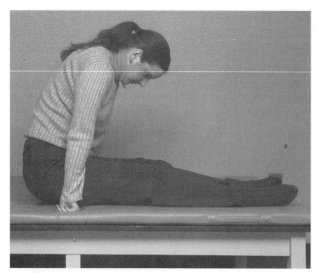

FIGURE 8-2 When the patient combines shoulder depression and pushing up from a closed fist with the wrist in neutral and momentum generated by throwing her head forward, she can achieve greater lift of the buttocks and subsequent improved clearance during transfers.

and where to intervene. For example, adapted bath equipment such as height-adjustable tub benches can be used to achieve level transfers. If a power wheelchair is being recommended, an elevating seat feature may be considered to enable level transfers from the wheelchair to the desired surface. In the past, seat elevation added seat height to the wheelchair, making transfers back into the wheelchair more difficult and making it difficult to fit under tables. Newer wheelchairs with seat elevation have lower seat heights, which helps alleviate this concern.

Teach patients to minimize the number of nonlevel transfers performed each day. On average, individuals with SCI transfer between six and 32 times a day, which can be a risk factor for repetitive strain injury at the wrists and shoulders.[25,49] Although performing a large number of transfers a day may be essential, reducing the number of nonlevel transfers each day will reduce the muscular effort needed, thereby lowering the risk of injury. Using adaptive equipment that allows for height adjustability and multiple tasks, for example, bathing and bowel and bladder care, can decrease the number of nonlevel transfers required.

Shoulder Alignment

The classic position of shoulder impingement is with the arm internally rotated and abducted.[50] If the arm is in this position, the rotator cuff tendon insertions at the greater tuberosity of the humerus are in closer proximity to the undersurface of the acromioclavicular joint. In a normally functioning shoulder, this will not necessarily cause impingement; however, in the presence of pain or rotator cuff impairment, impingement may occur. It is often difficult to avoid these positions during transfers. Using transfer techniques that avoid extreme positions of impingement will reduce the load on the shoulders because the forces borne by the shoulder depend on the position of the joint. For example, when an object is pushed down with the arm at the side, forces are transmitted directly through the elbow and wrist to the shoulder.[4]

There is a tendency for joint rotation at the shoulder if the arm is abducted or forward flexed. This leads to higher forces in the muscles around the shoulder. Higher forces are correlated with injuries or pain at the wrist[51-53] and shoulder.[36,54] Forces defined as high in these studies are almost always exceeded during transfers and pressure relief.[4,14,55] When reaching is necessary for certain transfers (e.g., into a car or truck), position the body as close as possible to the transfer surface, trapeze, or other transfer assist device so that abduction and internal rotation of the arm is minimized. This concept is further supported by Nawoczenski et al.[56] Their research found a reduction in the subacromial space in healthy individuals while performing a push up and transfer. They identified that the scapula was tipped anteriorly, with decreased upward rotation and increased internal rotation, and the shoulder showed a reduction in external rotation. It is therefore important that the therapist minimize these positions that may lead to impingement by examining the position of the shoulder and scapula during transfers and all functional activities.

Locking Elbows

For individuals without triceps, mechanical locking of the elbow must occur. Full elbow extension ROM is critical for mechanical locking of the upper limb during transfers and functional activities. The anterior deltoid and upper pectoral muscle have been documented to extend the elbow in weight bearing[57,58] and position the shoulder in external rotation to create the mechanical lock position for lifting the body weight during transfers and when upper limb support is required for balance and functional tasks.

Hand Placement

Forces associated with transfers are transmitted through the wrist and hand. Applying force through an extended wrist and flat palm can increase the pressures in the carpal canal, thereby compressing the median nerve. A number of studies have documented the association between wrist posture and CTS, with greater flexion and extension linked to injury, more so in the presence of high forces.[52,53,59-62] One study on the association between wrist postures and CTS specific to individuals with SCI found that individuals with paraplegia, both with and without CTS, had higher pressures in wrist extension than did unimpaired individuals with CTS.[63] In a cadaver study, Keir et al[64] found that hydrostatic carpal tunnel pressure was greatest in extension and in ulnar deviation with the palmaris longus loaded. This is a common position for transfers when the hand is resting on a flat surface.[4] In addition, it has been observed that with excessive wrist extension carpal hypermobility may occur over time with this maneuver.[65] When possible, encourage the patient to place his hand in a position that allows it to avoid extremes of wrist extension (e.g., allows the fingers to drape over and grasp the edge of the transfer surface) (Figure 8-3). Transferring by using closed-fist maneuvers with the wrist in neutral may reduce the pressures in the carpal tunnel and increase vertical excursion and therefore improve clearance of the buttocks; however, the impact on the metacarpal joints is unknown. In addition, transfers performed with the wrist in extension should maintain the fingers in flexion to preserve tenodesis for individuals who use tenodesis (see Chapter 7).

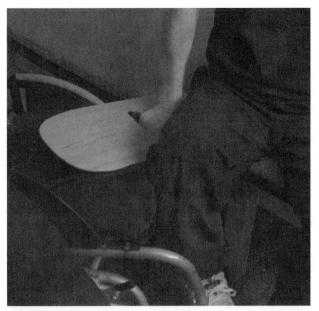

FIGURE 8-3 It is important to encourage the patient to place his hand in a position that allows it to avoid extremes of wrist extension such as allowing his fingers to drape over and grasp the edge of the transfer surface.

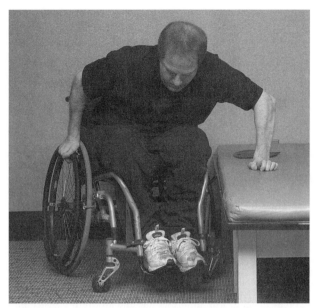

FIGURE 8-4 The patient performs a forward trunk lean in his wheelchair by leaning forward toward his thighs to improve his ability to unweight his pelvis for transfers.

Trunk Flexion

Another transfer technique to consider involves flexing the trunk forward while protracting and depressing the scapula and elevating the trunk when moving the buttocks over to the mat. Elevating the trunk during the lifting part of the transfer requires significant effort from sternal pectoralis major and latissimus dorsi muscles, which in turn helps to transfer the body weight between the trailing arm and leading arm with less loading of the glenohumeral joint.[7,14] This may protect the rotator cuff muscles against potential impingement between the head of the humerus and acromion when the arm is in a loaded position. The lower serratus muscle (scapular protractor) helps to resist the upward thrust on the scapula during weight-bearing.[14] With forward positioning of the trunk an even higher demand is placed on this muscle to hold the scapula against the thorax. The stabilizing action of serratus anterior muscle may enhance the patient's ability to transfer the weight of the body between the hands. In addition, shoulder depression plays an important role in enabling patients with SCI to bear weight on their upper limbs.[55]

In a forward-flexed position, the vertical distance between the shoulders and buttocks is reduced.[4] The reduced distance helps to ensure that elbow extension will result in clearing the buttocks off the surface. In addition, a patient with tetraplegia may actually begin his transfer in an exaggerated forward-flexed position providing he does not have an orthosis that limits this kind of movement (Figure 8-4). This posture will help to take weight off off his buttocks and allow him to clear the wheel or side guards and pivot with weight on his feet.

Leading and Trailing Upper Limbs

During a transfer, the shoulders must support the weight of the body as in a push-up pressure relief and also shift the trunk mass between the outreached hands. Perry et al[14] examined the specific activity of key shoulder musculature during depression

(lateral) transfers in subjects with low-level paraplegia. They found that different demands were placed on the shoulders during the various phases of the transfer and that these demands differed in the leading and trailing arms. Their findings are summarized in Table 8-1. Differences in trailing and leading arm biomechanics during transfers have been found in a study of unimpaired individuals as well.[56,66] When the ultimate goal is improving a patient's ability to transfer, the data of Perry et al[14] can be used to develop the appropriate strengthening program. It can also serve as the basis for a problem-solving tool when assessing a patient exhibiting difficulty with transfers. For example, a patient with a right rotator cuff tendonitis or tear could potentially decrease his pain during transfers if he uses the right arm as the leading arm. When initiating transfer training with a patient, always emphasize that he should alternate the arm used to lead the transfer. Ideally this will help prevent future shoulder problems. Nawoczenski et al[56] found a decrease in the subacromial space in healthy individuals during the final phase of transfers: when the hips were positioned, the leading arm showed that the scapula was tipped anteriorly with decreased upward rotation, and the shoulder showed a reduction in external rotation. They advise therapists to use the nonpainful limb as the leading limb. The therapist must therefore use her observational skills to assess at what point in the transfer the patient is at greatest risk for injury and problem solve with the patient. Patients should be encouraged to evaluate the compression that they feel in the shoulder with the different phases of the transfer.

Transfer Assist Devices

Consider the use of transfer assist devices by all individuals with SCI because assistive devices have the potential to reduce forces in the upper limbs during transfers and, therefore, may be effective at preventing and treating upper limb injuries. Inform each patient about the various transfer assist devices available and

TABLE 8-2	**Transfer Assist Devices and Indications for Use**
Assistive Device	Indication for Use
Transfer board	Enable transfer to be accomplished in small steps rather than one large movement
	Bridge gap between surfaces
	Use during transfer requires less upper limb muscle work
Lifting sling	Provide hand-hold for caregiver(s) during transfer
Mechanical lift	Need for significant assistance during transfer that will put patient or caregiver(s) at risk for injury

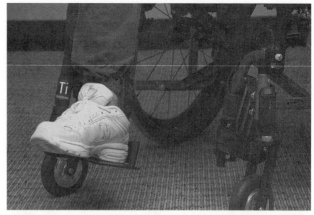

FIGURE 8-5 It is important to remove or move the wheelchair footrest closest to the mat out of the way before the patient transfers to ensure that it does not get in his way during the transfer. Some wheelchairs have footrests that can be moved to the outside or underneath the chair.

instruct him along with his caregivers on how and when to use such devices. Medical status can change and individuals with SCI may be faced with unforeseeable and awkward transfer situations that are eased with assistive devices. As mentioned earlier, individuals with higher-level SCI place a higher demand on their muscles during transfers.[7] Using a transfer board, for instance, will reduce the amount of force needed for lateral movement. In addition, transferring across surfaces of different heights increases the demands on the muscles,[6] so use of a transfer assist device can make it easier and safer for the patient (Table 8-2).

WHEELCHAIR MANAGEMENT

Wheelchair management to aid transfer techniques encompasses adjustments made to the wheelchair or its components (e.g., footrests and armrests) that will allow the patient to safely clear the wheelchair and provide for a stable wheelchair surface to transfer out of or back into. When transferring from a wheelchair with swing-away footrests to the mat, the footrest closest to the mat needs to be moved out of the way before the wheelchair is placed in its final position. To efficiently do this, teach the patient first to park his chair parallel with or with the rear wheels angled slightly away from the mat and engage his wheel locks. The caster wheels should be facing forward or forward and symmetrically angled (approximately 45 degrees) because the wheelchair base is most stable in this position. The lower limb closest to the mat is then removed from the footrest. It is recommended that it be placed over the opposite foot. In this way, possible injury caused by the foot getting caught on the floor or in the casters may be avoided.

The footrest closest to the mat is then moved out of the way. It can be swung out to the side, or to ensure that it does not get in the patient's way during the transfer, it may need to be removed. Whenever a footrest is removed from a wheelchair, make sure it is placed within easy reach to replace it when the patient transfers back into the wheelchair. Many patients will have difficulty reaching the footrest if it is lying on the floor, particularly if they have decreased balance or limited trunk flexion caused by the presence of an orthosis. To ensure that the footrest remains within easy reach, hook it onto another part of the wheelchair (e.g., the opposite armrest). Some wheelchair footrests are designed to swing underneath the chair, eliminating this concern (Figure 8-5). The wheel lock farthest from the mat is then disengaged with the

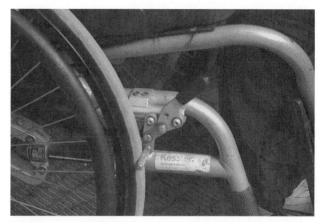

FIGURE 8-6 Wheel locks play an important role in helping the patient maneuver his chair as close as possible to the point to which he will be transferring. After the chair is in place, the patient makes sure both wheel locked are engaged.

closer one remaining engaged. The unlocked wheel is propelled forward to position the wheelchair next to and angled slightly in toward the mat, minimizing the gap between the wheelchair seat and mat. The wheel lock is again engaged (Figure 8-6). The foot closer to the mat is placed on the floor, the other leg is removed from its footrest and placed on the floor, and that footrest is swung out to the side.

Sometimes a patient finds it difficult to maintain his balance when he is removing his legs from the footrests and then swinging the footrests out of the way. He may compensate for this by hooking one upper limb around the back of his wheelchair, holding on to an armrest, or leaning on an arm placed on his thighs. Various techniques may be used to move his lower limbs off the footrests, including grasping the leg with one or both hands, hooking the leg by using elbow flexors and wrist extensors, or incorporating the assistance of loops or a stiff leg lifter. Lower limb management techniques are discussed in more detail in Chapter 7.

A patient who uses a wheelchair with a rigid front or who chooses not to swing his footrests out of the way because of the time and difficulty involved can pull directly up to the mat and into position for his transfer. He may leave his feet on the chair's footplates but may find that in doing so he gets tangled during the transfer. To avoid this, some find that placing the foot closer to the mat on the floor in front of the footplate and leaving the other on the footplate is sufficient. Others may need to place both feet on the floor in front of the wheelchair footplates. When leaving his feet on the footplates during the transfer, a patient may find that the wheelchair has a tendency to tip forward. To avoid this, instruct the patient to position his wheelchair with the casters pointing forward for increased wheelchair stability as previously described.

Once the lower limbs are in position, swing the armrest closest to the mat out of the way or remove it. Again, if a piece of the wheelchair is removed, place it within easy reach. The last step in setting up for a transfer is removal of the seatbelt. These steps are then reversed when the patient returns to the wheelchair. Sometimes a patient is unable to achieve independence in wheelchair management and then must learn to accurately instruct others in providing the assistance he requires.

Independent Positioning in the Wheelchair

Once the wheelchair has been set up, the patient needs to position himself properly in the chair in preparation for actually moving from the wheelchair to the mat. This involves maneuvering

his buttocks forward in the chair with the hip closer to the mat being farther out so he is angled away from the mat. This will allow him to pass in front of the rear wheel of the wheelchair during the transfer. It will also limit potential shearing at the thighs and buttocks and avoid bumping into the wheel, thereby protecting the patient's skin integrity.

The head-hips relationship described previously can be used to assist in attaining proper positioning in the wheelchair. A patient with good upper limb strength may lift his buttocks by performing a press-up with his hands on the wheels of his chair and simultaneously swinging his head and shoulders in the direction opposite of where he wants his buttocks to move. A patient without sufficient upper limb strength to lift his buttocks may use a strong twisting motion (unless prohibited because of spinal instability) to position himself in the wheelchair. For example, to move his right hip forward, a patient can hook the left arm behind the wheelchair and lean left to off weight the right hip. Then he can forcibly swing his head and right arm to the left to take advantage of momentum to move his right hip forward in the seat. A variation of this technique is for the patient to use his right arm to pull on the left armrest and then twist to bring his left hip forward (Figure 8-7, *A* and *B*). To return to the wheelchair, the patient may use the same techniques for lifting his buttocks and then following with head-hips relationship or off weighting the hip while

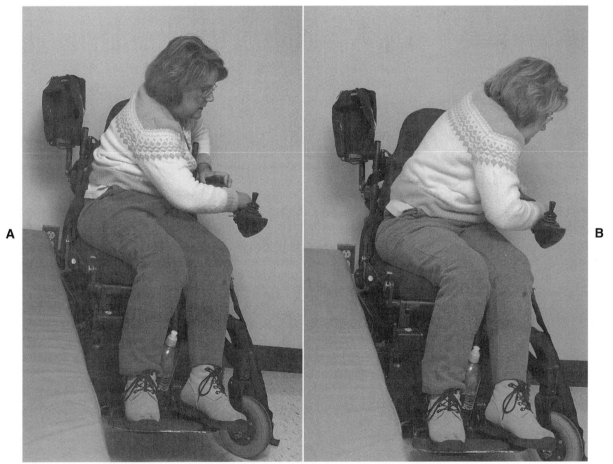

FIGURE 8-7 A patient with tetraplegia performs pelvic positioning in preparation for transfer (**A**) by using both arms to pull and twist her trunk toward the left chair arm, which helps her position her right pelvis forward in the wheelchair in preparation for transferring. **B,** She increases the pull force to give more momentum to raise her buttocks higher.

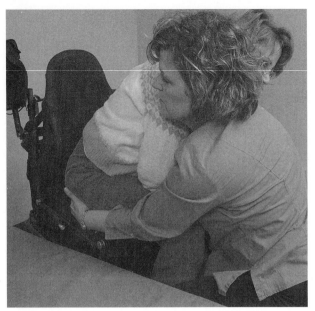

FIGURE 8-8 The therapist is positioning a patient with tetraplegia in preparation for a dependent transfer. Note that the therapist's hand placement is under the patient's ischial tuberosity to ensure stability of the patient's pelvis.

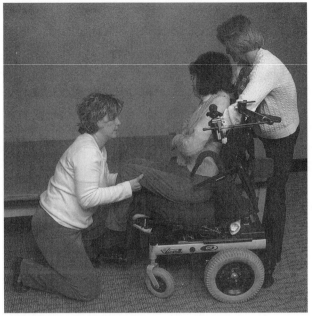

FIGURE 8-9 Two therapists take care to ensure that the patient's weight is distributed evenly on both ischial tuberosities when repositioning a patient with tetraplegia back into her wheelchair.

channeling momentum to twist and properly position his buttocks back into the wheelchair.

Dependent Positioning in the Wheelchair

A patient who is dependent on others to adjust his position in the wheelchair must learn to instruct his caregivers about how to maneuver him. When one person is assisting a dependent patient in preparation for a transfer, that caregiver positions herself in front of the patient. Support the patient with a hand placed at the lateral aspect of the trunk with him leaning away from the mat to off weight the side of the buttocks closest to the mat. Then place the other hand under the off-weighted ischial tuberosity and move it forward (Figure 8-8). Next, lean the patient in the opposite direction to off weight and move that side of the buttocks. Lean the patient alternately from side to side, thereby maneuvering the buttocks forward in the chair with the hip closest to the mat ultimately being farthest forward in the chair.

This same technique of leaning the patient to the side to allow the buttocks to be moved can be used when a patient is transferred to his wheelchair and his hips need to be moved back in the chair. When moving the buttocks back into the seat, there are several other options that also may be used. Lean the patient to the side as previously described, but instead of placing a hand under the buttocks, put it at the front of the knee. By pushing back through the knee, the off-weighted buttocks can be moved back into the wheelchair. Another option is to stand behind the patient, with him either leaning forward or resting back on your arms, and then lift his buttocks back into the wheelchair. This option is more easily performed with a second person standing in front of the patient (Figure 8-9). The caregiver in front lifts the patient from under the thighs or the person in front can support the patient's trunk in a forward position while the person in back lifts the buttocks into

the proper position. For a patient in a tilt-in-space wheelchair, gravity may be used to assist with positioning his buttocks in the wheelchair. This is done by tilting the wheelchair back, standing to the side of the chair, and lifting the buttocks to adjust appropriately.

TYPES OF TRANSFERS

The simplest place to begin describing types of transfers is with those between the wheelchair and mat because the therapy mat is a firm surface and, typically, is approximately wheelchair height. Patients can then learn the techniques before applying them in the more difficult transfers to functional surfaces.

Transfer Board Transfers

A transfer board is a commonly used piece of equipment for patients with SCI. It is a thin, smooth board that allows a patient to perform a transfer in a series of moves rather than in one large movement. Transfer boards are made of wood or plastic and are typically rectangular, although they can come in various shapes and sizes, depending on a patient's needs (Figure 8-10). Transfer boards are particularly useful for patients with weak upper limbs or poor balance or those who cannot achieve good transfer ergonomics as described in the previous sections for reasons that are not modifiable (e.g., excessive body mass). A transfer board bridges the gap between two surfaces and enables the transfer to be performed in smaller steps and with less muscular work of the upper limbs. Transfer boards, however, are not suitable for transfers occurring across two surfaces that vary greatly in height, for example, from a wheelchair to a truck seat or sport utility vehicle.

Unfortunately, the term "sliding board" is often used interchangeably with the term "transfer board." This is not recommended because when the term "sliding board" is used it may

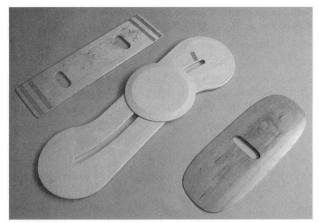

FIGURE 8-10 Numerous types of transfer boards are available to make transferring easier, including BeasyTrans (shown in the middle) and more traditional wooden transfer boards with a variety of hand cutouts.

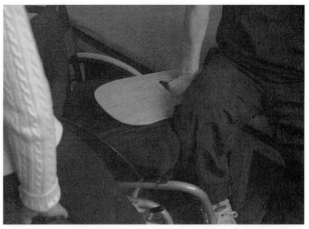

FIGURE 8-11 Three criteria for proper transfer board positioning include (1) placing the leading edge of the board forward of the rear wheel, (2) placing the trailing end of the board under the buttocks of the patient's leading side, and (3) angling the board toward the back corner of the wheelchair farthest from the mat.

encourage patients and caregivers to allow the buttocks to be dragged across the board. Shearing forces can significantly contribute to skin breakdown, so sliding the buttocks will result in a greater chance of skin injuries that are difficult to heal. It is important that the buttocks be lifted rather than slid during transfers. If this is not possible, several types of transfer boards are available that are designed to help decrease the shearing forces that occur when a patient slides during a transfer. One such transfer board (BeasyTrans) consists of a board with an attached disk that the patient sits on. The disk then slides through a channel in the board. Because the disk moves through the board, the patient avoids the shearing that would have been created by the patient having to slide along the board. Another option is a transfer board made up of a series of rollers (Roll Easy) that the patient moves across, thus decreasing the shearing forces. If sliding does occur during transfers, it is imperative that the skin be monitored closely. Transfers that involve any sliding must be discontinued immediately at the first sign of possible skin breakdown.

A properly placed transfer board is placed on an angle passing in front of the rear wheel of the wheelchair pointing from the mat toward the back seat corner farthest from the mat (Figure 8-11). Placement of the board is easier when the side of the buttocks that the board is to be placed under is off weighted. This may be achieved in several ways. For example, if the patient is transferring toward the right, he can lean toward the left to off weight the right side of the buttocks. This may be combined with crossing the right leg over the left, lifting the right leg by holding it under the thigh, or placing the right foot up on the wheelchair footrest. Once the side of the buttocks is off weighted, the transfer board is placed in position. When placing the board, the patient or caregiver aims it downward to avoid accidentally pinching the skin. For patients with compromised hand function, cutouts in the board can make placement easier by allowing the patient to use his tenodesis to hook the board and then wiggle it back and forth to work it under the buttocks (Figure 8-12). The use of wheelchair pushing cuffs or gloves may also be helpful because they allow the patient to use friction to push the board underneath himself (Figure 8-13).

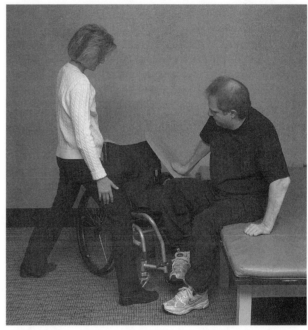

FIGURE 8-12 A patient with tetraplegia makes use of his tenodesis (reflex grip) by placing his hand through the cutout in the transfer board to achieve proper placement of the board under his buttocks. He can then wiggle the board back and forth until it is placed sufficiently under his buttocks. He aims the board in a downward direction to avoid accidentally pinching his skin.

Short-Sit Position

Once the transfer board is appropriately placed, the patient uses the previously described head-hips relationship to move across it (Figure 8-14, *A* and *B*). The patient performs a press-up and simultaneously swings his head and shoulders in the direction opposite of where he wants his buttocks to move. The weaker the patient, the more he will need to rely on momentum and the more exaggerated the head-hips relationship will need to be. A patient with weak or absent triceps may find it easier to lock out his upper limbs when performing his press-up (see Chapter 7). In addition, instruct the patient to fully depress his shoulders during the push-up. This can give him extra height in his lift and help to ensure his buttocks clears the board during the transfer.

When performing the transfer, the patient needs to be aware of the position of his feet. Having his feet flat on a surface, whether it be the floor or on one or both footrests, will provide him with increased stability during the transfer. Once he begins to move across the board, his feet may not maintain this proper positioning and he may need to stop and adjust his feet during the transfer.

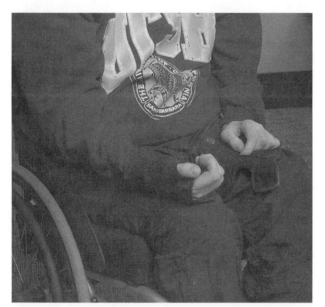

FIGURE 8-13 A patient can use wheelchair pushing cuffs or gloves to add friction when pushing a transfer board underneath himself.

When guarding a patient during this type of transfer, the therapist typically stands in front of him. In this way, if a patient is fearful of falling forward, his fear may be alleviated. The therapist may place her knees in front of the patient's knees (being careful to avoid the excessive pressure of having her patellas directly against the patient's patellas) to prevent the patient from sliding forward. The therapist then holds the patient at his hips or under his buttocks to assist him in moving across the board. Variations of this technique that may be appropriate; for stronger patients, the therapist guards the patient with one hand at the buttocks and one laterally at the trunk or uses both hands at the patient's scapular region. In this way she assists the patient in maintaining his balance and facilitates the head and shoulder movement required to use the head-hips relationship in moving the buttocks. Another option is to guard the patient from behind. This allows the patient to lean further forward to facilitate increased clearance of the buttocks without the therapist being in the way. This, however, is not recommended for new patients. Although the therapist may assist the patient in moving across the board from this position, it may be more difficult to prevent the patient from falling forward and the therapist will be unable to block the patient's knees or help him adjust his foot positioning, if necessary. A patient who requires significant help during the transfer may need to have two people guarding him, one in front and one from behind.

Long-Sit Position

The transfer described above can also be performed in a long-sit position. This entails putting the lower limbs onto the mat before moving across the transfer board and leaving them on the mat when moving back into the wheelchair (Figure 8-15). Various techniques for lower limb management are described in Chapter 7. A long-sit

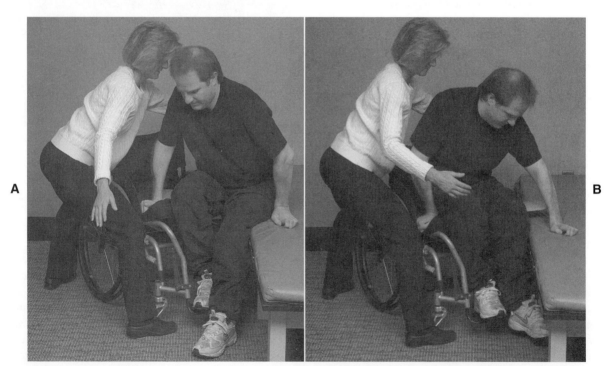

FIGURE 8-14 A patient with tetraplegia uses the head-hips relationship to increase his momentum (A) when performing a transfer board transfer from the mat to wheelchair in the short-sit position and (B) to position himself correctly as far back as possible in his wheelchair.

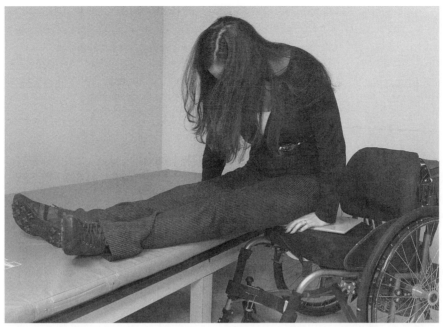

FIGURE 8-15 A patient with paraplegia performs a long-sit position transfer from wheelchair to mat. She has placed her lower limbs on the mat before moving across the transfer board. It is important to note that with this type of transfer the patient may be at risk for losing her balance backward, particularly if the surface she is transferring to is higher than the wheelchair.

position transfer provides the patient with a greater base of support than does a transfer using the short-sit position. Thus it may be easier for a patient to maintain his balance when transferring in a long-sit position as long as his hamstring length is sufficient to not to shift his center of mass backward and compromise balance. In addition, during this transfer the lower limbs are lifted on and off the mat while in a supported sitting position in the wheelchair. This can be much easier than performing leg management in the usual unsupported short-sit position at the edge of the mat. Although appropriate for transferring on and off a mat or bed, this technique is not an option for other functional surfaces such as a tub seat or automobile.

Guarding for this type of transfer is done in a manner similar to that described previously with a transfer in a shortsit position. In this position, however, it is less likely that the patient will fall forward. In addition, it is difficult for the therapist to position herself in front of the patient because the patient's legs are extended onto the mat. The therapist may be more likely to guard the patient from behind for this transfer technique.

Prone Push or Pull Transfer

For patients who rely on locking their elbows during a transfer board transfer because of weak or absent triceps, a prone push or pull transfer may be a good alternative. This technique may be easier to perform because it eliminates the need to maintain elbow extension. When performing this type of transfer, the patient rotates at the trunk and leans laterally onto his elbows. Transferring between the wheelchair and mat, he may rotate toward the mat and lean his elbows on the mat. He then pulls himself across the surface, relying on the momentum gained from a rocking motion along with the strength in his shoulder extensors and adductors (Figure 8-16).

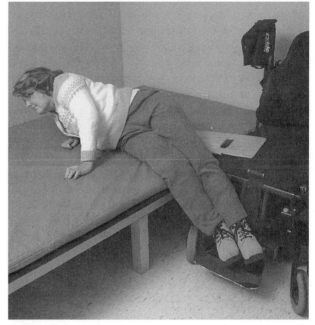

FIGURE 8-16 A patient with tetraplegia performs a prone-pull transfer by rotating her body toward the mat and with both upper limbs on the mat pulling the rest of her body from the transfer board onto the mat.

Another option is for the patient to rotate away from the mat, putting his elbows first against the wheelchair armrest and then on the seat of the wheelchair and then push his body across to the mat by using a rocking motion encouraged by shoulder flexion strength. Similarly, when transferring from the mat to the wheelchair, the patient may rotate toward the chair and pull himself into it or rotate away from the wheelchair and push himself into it. Obviously, when rotated away from the surface he is transferring

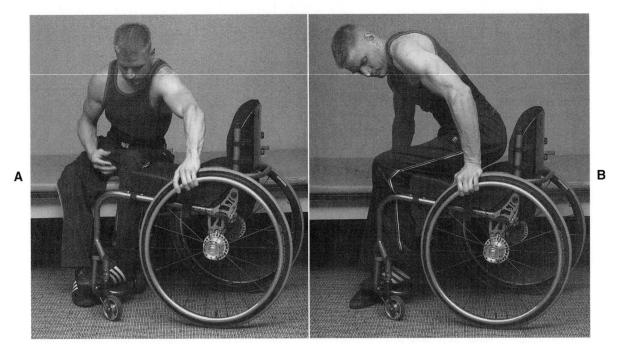

FIGURE 8-17 A patient **(A)** prepares for and **(B)** performs a lateral transfer from the mat to his wheelchair. Notice the clearance and distance of movement achieved.

to, the patient will not be able to see where he is going. Therefore, good body awareness is required. Because the prone push and pull techniques require sliding the buttocks across the transfer board, the considerations discussed earlier about sliding must be kept in mind to make maintenance of skin integrity the highest priority.

After the patient has moved across the board onto the mat, he may remain leaning to the side to lift his lower limbs onto the mat. If assuming an upright position once on the mat, he may walk his upper body around to the front so he is leaning anteriorly rather than laterally. Then, lifting his head while pushing up on his arms (using his anterior chest and shoulder musculature), he can assume an upright position. Another option is for the patient to use his elbow flexors to hook the lower limb he is leaning away from and pull with that arm while pushing up with the other arm. For many patients, assuming the upright position on the mat can be the most difficult part of the transfer. Assuming the upright position in the wheelchair is easier because the patient can hook an upper limb behind the wheelchair and then pull himself into the upright position.

When guarding a patient performing a prone push or pull transfer, the therapist stands in front of the patient. She then guides the patient's hips as he pulls or pushes across the transfer board. During initial training, a patient may also require support at the trunk to assist him in maintaining the prone-on-elbows position. In addition, he will typically require verbal cueing regarding his positioning, especially in cases where he is facing the direction opposite to which he is transferring.

Lateral Transfer

A lateral transfer is basically a transfer board transfer without the board. It requires good upper body strength and balance. The patient uses the head-hips relationship, leaning forward and

performing a press-up while twisting his head and shoulders away from the surface to which he is transferring. This helps him to lift his buttocks and perform the transfer in one large movement (Figure 8-17, *A* and *B*). Guarding during this transfer is done in the same way described for transfers with a transfer board, but with extra attention given to achieving adequate clearance and distance of movement.

Roll-Out Transfer

A roll-out transfer is only appropriate for a patient transferring onto a mat or bed, but it is often very useful for these specific transfers, especially with a large patient. The preparation for a roll-out transfer is the same as that for a long-sit position transfer. Once in position, the patient leans laterally onto the mat resting on his elbow or outstretched arm. He then reaches for the mat with his other arm and, relying on the momentum this creates, rolls into a prone position on the mat (Figure 8-18). During this type of transfer, the therapist stands at the patient's side and assists him as needed at his hips. Once on the mat, the patient remains prone or continues to roll into a supine position.

Dependent Transfers

When initiating dependent transfers with a patient, even when performing a one-person technique, it is always best to have a second person standing by in case the patient unexpectedly has orthostatic hypotension or strong spasms. In addition, when transferring a patient who is ventilator dependent, it is recommended to have a third person available to make sure that no lines or tubes are accidentally pulled or disconnected. If a patient is able to tolerate it and he has physician clearance, he may be disconnected from the ventilator during the transfer and then immediately reconnected afterward. Ideally the long-term goal

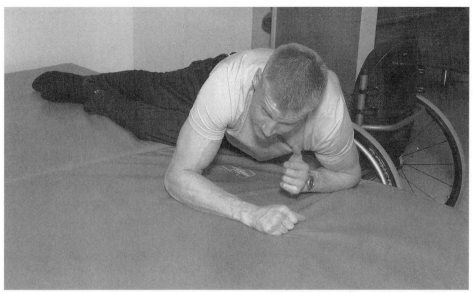

FIGURE 8-18 A patient with paraplegia performs a roll-out transfer from his wheelchair to the mat. First both lower limbs are placed on the mat, next the patient leans his elbow onto the mat, and follows by rolling to prone. This technique can be used with a large patient or when a patient is fatigued.

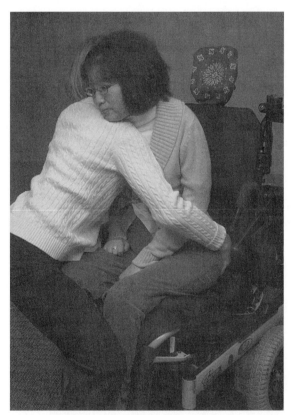

FIGURE 8-19 The therapist performs a dependent pivot transfer with patient. Note stabilization of the patient's spine is important when a therapist is performing this type of one-person lift.

for any dependent patient is to be able to be transferred by one person, whether by a manual technique or a mechanical lift. Achieving this goal may help facilitate a patient's return to home on discharge.

One-Man Lifts

Various versions of a pivot technique can be used to help a dependent patient transfer. Set the wheelchair up and position the patient as previously described; then stand in front of the patient. The therapist holds the patient's legs between her legs, the patient's arms are placed in his lap, and the patient is leaned forward and away from the mat. In this way the therapist has a clear view of the surface to which she is transferring the patient. The patient may be supported in this forward position by leaning against the therapist's shoulder or chest (Figure 8-19). If the patient has a tracheostomy, it is imperative that the therapist positions herself off to the side and low enough to avoid hitting it during the transfer.

Another option is to lean the patient forward and away from the wheelchair or mat with his shoulder resting against the therapist's hip. This can be a very useful technique when transferring a patient who tends to have extensor spasms because this flexed position can help break up the extension pattern. For a patient with short legs that do not easily reach the floor or for a patient who, because of his spasticity, would benefit from being in even further flexion, a bucket transfer may be performed. In this type of transfer, the patient leans forward against the therapist's hip and, with the therapist holding the patient's knees high between hers, the patient's feet remain off the floor during the transfer (Figure 8-20).

For a patient who tends to have lower limb flexor spasms, place a transfer board in front of the wheelchair casters. This will prevent the patient's feet from getting caught under the wheelchair in case of a sudden flexor spasm. It is, however, important to protect the patient's heels when they are up against the board. Therefore, make sure the patient is wearing shoes or place a pillow between the board and the patient's heels. If the patient has a rigid front wheelchair, his feet may be left on the footrests and a strap across the uprights of the footrests will help limit the effects of a sudden flexor spasm.

Once the patient is leaning forward onto the therapist, the therapist cups her hands under the patient's ischial tuberosities

(ITs) (see Figure 8-8). If she is unable to hold the patient under the ITs, his clothing may be held instead, although this is not an option for transfers to or from a shower chair. If it is necessary to hold the patient's clothing, avoid holding the back of his pants because doing so will cause the pants to ride up and put excessive pressure on the groin and buttocks areas. Instead, hold the sides of the pants, first taking up the slack. In this way the pants can

act as a sling from which to lift the patient. Various commercial slings are also available for this purpose.

Continue by rocking the patient forward, shifting his weight anteriorly onto his feet, and pivoting him to the mat (Figure 8-21, *A*). To avoid injury, it is important that the therapist pivots her entire body rather than twisting at her back during the transfer (Figure 8-21, *B*). Use a transfer board to avoid having to perform the entire transfer in one movement, especially with a heavy patient. In this manner, a patient can be moved in a series of lifts. In addition, a second person can be positioned behind the patient to provide assistance lifting him at the hips if necessary.

Two-Man Lifts

In addition to the pivot type of transfer with two people that is described above, there are various other two-man dependent lift techniques. A common one positions one person behind the patient while the other stands alongside his lower limbs on the side farthest from the mat. The person at the rear holds the patient under his ITs, at the sides of his pants or a lifting sling, or under his arms when his arms are crossed over his chest. Do not lift the patient under his arms unless he has the muscle strength to depress and stabilize his shoulders while being lifted. Otherwise his shoulders may be jammed during the transfer, which can result in a potential injury. For the person in the back to get a proper hold on the patient, the caregiver in front can lean the patient forward. After the person in the rear is in position, the front person leans the patient back so he is resting on the arms of the person behind him. The person in front then faces the mat and places one arm as high as possible under the patient's thighs to ensure that she is sharing the work of lifting the patient's body weight with the caregiver in the rear. The other arm is placed under the patient's calves to ensure that his feet do not get caught on the edge of the mat during the lift.

Another option for a two-man lift is to park the patient's wheelchair perpendicular to the mat. Both lifters stand next to the patient on the side closer to the mat. The caregivers reach

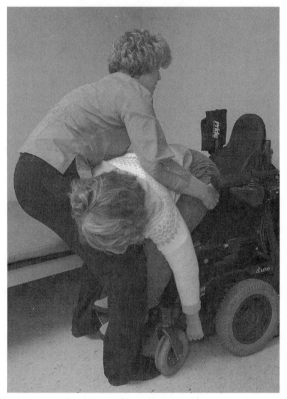

FIGURE 8-20 The therapist leans the patient forward and away from the wheelchair so that the patient's shoulder rests against the therapist's hip to perform a bucket transfer.

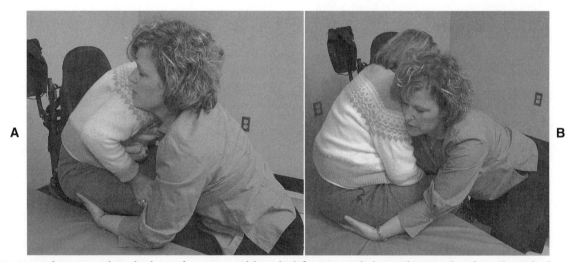

FIGURE 8-21 A therapist can dependently transfer a patient with lower limb flexor spasms by having the patient lean forward onto the therapist, who then cups her hands under the patient's ischial tuberosities (see Figure 8-8). The therapist continues by rocking the patient forward, shifting her weight anteriorly forward, and pivoting her to the mat **(A).** To avoid injury, it is important that the therapist pivots her entire body **(B)** rather than twisting at her back during the transfer.

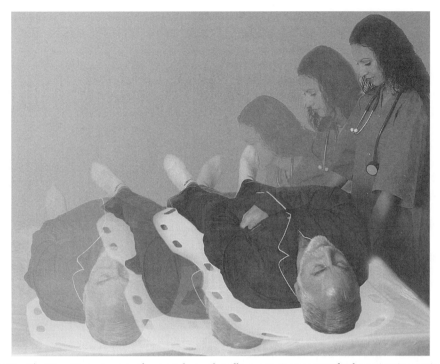

FIGURE 8-22   The MoveMaster is a transfer assist device that allows caregivers to transfer the patient in a supine position.

under the patient, the person near the top of the wheelchair places one arm behind the patient's back and one at his pelvis, the other person places one arm as high as possible at the patient's thighs and the other under his calves. Then they lift the patient and hold him as close to their bodies as possible. The lifters follow through by turning and placing the patient on the mat. If a patient is heavy or has poor head control, three people can use this scoop-and-turn technique with one person at the head and trunk, one at the pelvis and buttocks, and the third at the legs.

The Mover Master is yet another option for transferring a dependent patient. This large flexible board can be particularly helpful for very heavy patients or patients who have poor tolerance to the upright position. It is placed under the patient by rolling the patient onto his side. The board and patient are transferred together onto the other surface and the board is then removed (Figure 8-22). The number of people needed to perform this type of transfer depends on the size of the patient.

Mechanical Lifts

In some cases it is difficult to manually transfer a patient, so a mechanical lift may be the appropriate choice. There are numerous mechanical lifts on the market that offer manual hydraulic or power-driven systems. Medical equipment suppliers can serve as resources to learn about the best options for the particular patient.

In general, mechanical lifts are either mobile, meaning they can be moved from one place to another to be used in different locations (e.g., Hoyer Lift, Transaid Lift) or stationary, meaning use is limited to a specific designated area depending on the range of a mounted tracking system. The principle behind both

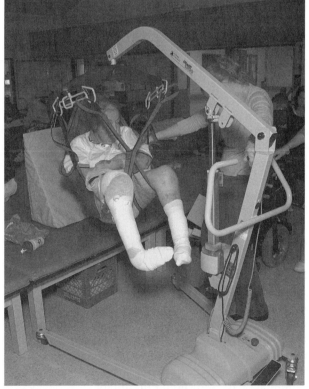

FIGURE 8-23   A mechanical lift makes it easier for a caregiver to transfer a patient who is large or has limited ability to assist in his transfer.

systems is the same. A sling is placed under the patient and then is attached to the mechanical lifting device. The patient can be raised and moved from surface to surface while the caregiver is careful to keep his buttocks from bumping into anything (Figure 8-23).

Once the patient is positioned over the new surface, he is lowered, and the sling is removed. When transferring a patient into a manual wheelchair by using a mechanical lift it is recommended that the caregiver stabilize the wheelchair against a sturdy surface, such as a wall, to ensure that the wheelchair does not tip.

SPECIAL CONSIDERATIONS FOR SPECIFIC SURFACES

After a patient begins to understand the basic transfer techniques described above, he needs to adapt them to a variety of functional surfaces. This involves the use of considerable problem-solving skills by both the therapist and the patient. The following suggestions are based on clinical experience and have been found to be helpful with this process.

Wheelchair to Bed

Although not all beds are adjustable to the same height as the wheelchair, a bed with adjustable height controls certainly makes transfers easier because it can be moved up or down as needed so transfers to or from it are performed between even surfaces. It may even permit the patient to transfer downhill, thus allowing gravity to assist him. When setting up for a transfer to a bed, park the wheelchair at the head of the bed with the patient facing toward the foot of the bed. This will properly position the patient to lie down without having to scoot up or down in the bed after the transfer. In addition, the wheelchair will not be in the way when the patient is bringing his legs up onto the bed.

Transfers to a bed closely resemble those to the mat. Depending on the softness of the mattress, however, a patient may find it more difficult to maintain his balance and to move once on the bed. It may be helpful to have a patient with an air mattress deflate it during transfers. In this way he will have added stability provided by the firm foam base below. It is, however, vital that the patient remember to reinflate the mattress after the transfer so that skin integrity is not compromised (see Chapter 14).

Wheelchair to Couch

Transfers between the wheelchair and a couch are easier if some simple techniques are followed. When transferring the patient onto or off of a couch, start from its end, rather than in the middle. This way the patient can use the arm at the end of the couch for assistance (Figure 8-24). When on the couch, a patient can pile pillows next to him to provide a higher surface to push off from. In addition, extra cushions may be added to the seat of the couch, so it is not such a low surface to transfer back to the wheelchair, or the cushions can be added to the back of a deep couch to discourage a patient's slumped posture.

Wheelchair to Bathroom Equipment

Transfers to bathroom equipment are typically practiced with the patient clothed in the clinic. It is important, however, to also practice bathroom transfers as they will be performed at home, unclothed, because this can certainly make the transfer more challenging. Always remember to use appropriate drapes when this training takes place to protect and respect the patient's modesty. When performing a transfer unclothed, extra care must be

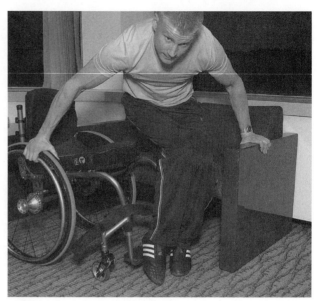

FIGURE 8-24 A patient can use the arm at the end of the couch for assistance in getting a higher lift and consequently improved clearance during his transfer from wheelchair to couch.

taken to protect the skin. If the patient is using a transfer board, place a towel over the board to decrease the risk of shearing in case the patient's buttocks are accidentally dragged.

Because bathrooms are typically small, there may not be much room for maneuvering a wheelchair inside it. Therefore, it may be helpful for the patient to enter the bathroom with one leg crossed over the other and one wheelchair footrest already removed. Depending on the bathroom setup, there may not be space to position the wheelchair next to the commode in preparation for transferring. In this case, park the wheelchair perpendicular to the commode with the front of the seat lined up with the middle of the commode. Given such space constraints, this will provide the smallest gap possible between the wheelchair and the commode.

When transferring onto a tub seat or bench, the patient positions his lower limbs into the tub before moving from the w/c. In this way, lower limb management is performed while still having the support of the wheelchair. When balance is not an issue, a patient can begin to move from the wheelchair to the tub seat before placing his legs in the tub. Approximately halfway through the transfer, however, he will probably need to place one leg into the tub so he is positioned properly to continue transferring (Figure 8-25). After he is fully on the tub seat or bench, he can place his other leg in the tub.

A patient with adequate balance and upper limb strength may choose to not use a tub seat or bench but rather to transfer to the floor of the tub. It is important, however, that the patient sits on a cushion (e.g,. Jay Protector with the cover removed) to protect his skin from the hard acrylic or porcelain tub surface. To transfer into the tub, the patient parks his wheelchair beside the tub. First he puts his feet into the tub and then he performs a lateral transfer to the edge of the tub before transferring to the tub floor by using the lateral floor transfer technique described in Chapter 15. Another option is to park the wheelchair so it is facing the tub.

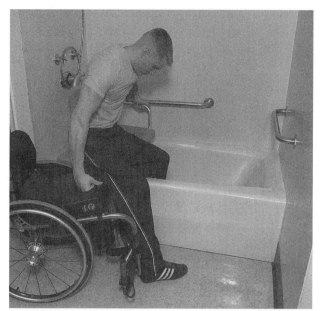

FIGURE 8-25 Notice that midway through a transfer from wheelchair to tub, the patient places one leg into the tub to increase his leverage before continuing the transfer.

After placing his feet into the tub, the patient scoots forward onto the edge of the tub. He then turns as he transfers down into the tub. A grab bar on the wall behind the tub can be very helpful in performing these transfers. A bath-lift will allow a patient who is unable to perform these types of transfers to get into a tub for bathing. The patient transfers onto the bath-lift just like he would to a tub seat and, by hydraulics, is lowered to the floor of the tub. If the patient has a shower stall rather than a tub, he may transfer from his wheelchair onto a seat positioned in the stall (Figure 8-26).

Transfers into a shower chair are typically performed from the bed. If a mechanical lift is used, the shower chair is positioned against a wall to prevent it from tipping while the patient is lowered into the chair. A mesh sling is recommended for use when transferring a patient into a shower chair. A mesh sling need not be removed during showering (see Chapter 14).

Wheelchair to Automobile

When initiating transfers into an automobile with a patient who was injured in a car accident, it is important to be sensitive to how the patient may feel about being back in a car. If a patient appears to be having a difficult time with this transition, call on the psychologist to help address the patient's needs.

Keep these basic principles in mind when performing car transfer training with patients. Two door cars allow more room to perform transfers and the subsequent loading of the wheelchair than four door cars. Always remember to move the car seat back as far as possible to maximize the room available. Bench seats are easier for transfers than bucket seats although a cushion may be added to a bucket seat to raise the surface for an easier transfer. If head clearance is an issue, slightly recline the car seat. Reclining the seat also helps prevent patients with poor trunk control from falling forward. A chest strap placed around the patient and car seat in addition to the standard chest and

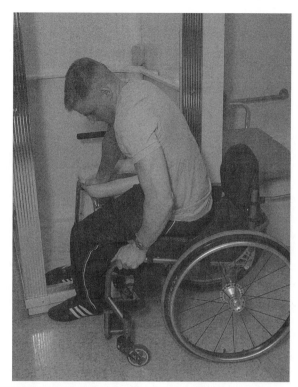

FIGURE 8-26 A patient transfers from his wheelchair to a seat positioned in his shower stall.

lap belts already present in the car can be used to protect the patient. It is a good idea to put the window down when performing a car transfer. This gives the patient the door jam to push off from. Additionally, it will ensure that he will not hit his head against the window when leaning forward, especially in the case of dependent transfers.

The patient uses the lateral or short sit position transfer board techniques previously described to perform the transfer (Figure 8-27). When sitting in the car, the patient can fasten his seat belt and lean back on the car seat to provide increased stability when lifting his legs into and out of the car as well as when loading and unloading his wheelchair.

When transferring a dependent patient into a car, use a long transfer board to bridge the gap between the wheelchair and car seat. Perform the car transfer in much the same way as the pivot technique for a dependent transfer previously described. If one person is performing the transfer, she stands in front of the patient. She lifts the patient's buttocks into the automobile first, then his upper body is leaned back against the car seat while the caregiver is careful not to bump his head, and finally his legs are moved into the car, with care that his trunk is adequately supported when doing so. If a second person is available to assist with this transfer, she starts off positioned behind the patient. In this way, she can help guide the patient's buttocks into the car and ensure that the transfer board does not accidentally move during the transfer. After the patient's buttocks have been transferred onto the passenger seat, the second person positions herself in the driver's seat. From this position she can help scoot the patient's buttocks further back on the car seat, guide the patient's head as he is being leaned back into the car, and provide support when the patient's legs are being positioned. After the patient is positioned inside the automobile, he can be readjusted as needed by having one person positioned on each side to lift the patient's buttocks. Another option for readjusting the patient is to recline the patient's seat and, with one person in the back seat behind the patient and the other alongside the patient, perform the two-man lift described in the section on positioning in the wheelchair.

After the patient is in the car, his wheelchair will need to be loaded into the car. When a patient is performing car transfers with assistance, the person assisting him may place the wheelchair into the back seat or trunk of the car. When a patient performs car transfers independently, an important part of this activity is learning to load the wheelchair himself. Depending on where the wheelchair will be placed (e.g., behind the driver's seat or on the front passenger seat), various parts of the wheelchair may need to be removed so the chair will fit the space and is not too heavy to lift. Parts that need to be removed and can be removed before transferring (e.g., armrests, footrests) are placed into the car first. It could be difficult for the patient to maintain his balance when reaching for these parts if this is not done until after he has transferred to the car.

When the patient is in the automobile with his seatbelt on, he can remove his wheelchair seat cushion and any other additional parts that require removal before loading (e.g., rear wheels, antitips) and place those in the car. Before loading the frame of the chair, the patient makes it as compact as possible: lifting up on the seat to fold a folding chair, folding down the seat back, if possible, of a rigid chair (Figure 8-28, *A*). In the case of a folding wheelchair, the frame of the chair (either with the rear wheels on or off) usually fits behind the driver's seat. This may not be possible in a four-door car, in which case the chair may need to be loaded much like a rigid-frame wheelchair. When loading a rigid wheelchair, the patient will need to lift the frame of the wheelchair across his body and onto the front passenger's seat or back to the rear seat. He will need to recline the driver's seat to provide increased balance and

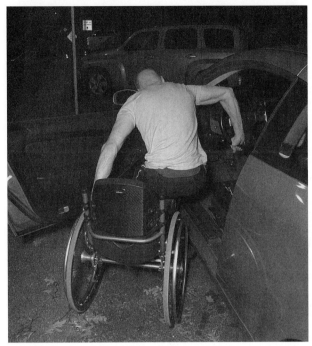

FIGURE 8-27 A patient performs a lateral transfer from his wheelchair into his car.

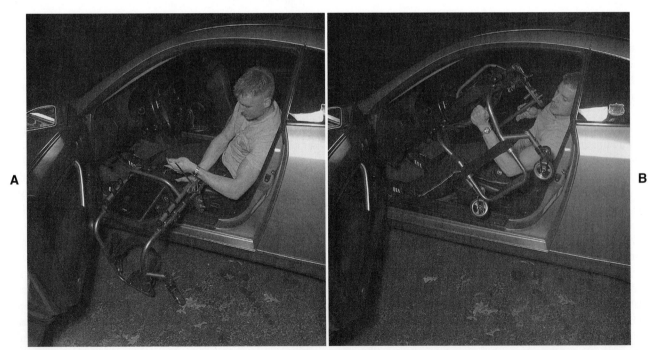

FIGURE 8-28 Preparing to load his rigid wheelchair into the car, **(A)** a patient makes the wheelchair as compact as possible by removing the rear wheels and folding down the seat back. Then **(B)** he loads the wheelchair frame by lifting it across his body into the front passenger seat. Notice that the driver's seat is reclined to assist the patient with his balance and to maximize the space between the patient and the steering wheel.

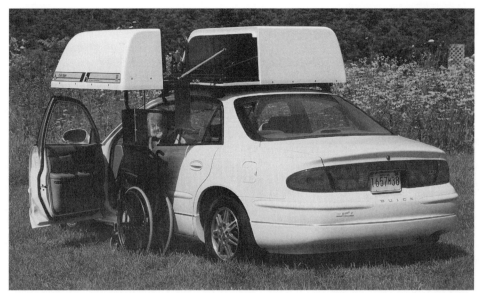

FIGURE 8-29 Developed to assist wheelchair users who are able to independently transfer, the ChairTopper automatically folds and stores a wheelchair into the carrier on top of the sedan. (Photo courtesy Braun Corp.)

increased clearance room between him and the steering wheel so that the frame can be lifted across his body (Figure 8-28, *B*). For a patient who uses a car with a front bench seat, another option is to transfer into the car on the passenger side and then pull the wheelchair into the car as he moves across into the driver's seat.

Another option for loading a wheelchair is a ChairTopper (Figure 8-29). This device mechanically lifts the wheelchair and places it in a storage bin on top of the car. Most ChairToppers can only be used with a folding wheelchair, although there are now some versions that will provide power loading for a rigid wheelchair.

When transferring a dependent patient out of a car, put the transfer board in place before positioning the patient for the transfer. Otherwise it may be difficult to adequately support the patient when placing the board. After the board is in place and while the patient is still leaning back on the car seat, remove the legs from the car and place the feet on the ground. Lean the patient forward, being careful not to let him hit his head, so he is facing out of the car. He is then ready to be lifted across the transfer board into his wheelchair.

CLINICAL CASE STUDY | Transfer Training

Patient History
Joseph Mainer is an 18-year-old man referred to physical therapy with a C6 ASIA A diagnosis as the result of being hit by a car while riding his bike. He was wearing a helmet at the time of injury and therefore did not have a brain injury. He underwent an anterior fusion procedure from C5 through C7 and was placed in a halo orthosis for 12 weeks. After the halo device was removed, he was placed in a Philadelphia collar for 2 weeks, followed by a soft collar for an additional 2 weeks. His acute care hospital course was complicated by a sacral pressure ulcer, which healed 5 weeks after injury. He is now 22 weeks after injury and has been readmitted to outpatient physical therapy because of a tendonitis in his right rotator cuff.

Patient's Self-Assessment
Joe wants his shoulder to heal so that his transfers can be painless. He was expecting to go away to college but has chosen to attend the local community college in the fall for his first year. He is undecided about a major now, although originally he wanted to be an engineer. He lives with his parents and two younger sisters. The first floor den has been converted to a bedroom and a bathroom next to his room is fully accessible. He also has wheelchair access to the garage from his bedroom. He has passed his driving test with a vehicle with hand controls and is in the process of selecting an accessible van. He is currently using a lightweight manual wheelchair.

Clinical Assessment
Patient Appearance
- Height 5 feet 11 inches, weight 165 pounds, body mass index 23
- Posture: Joe has a mild slouched posture in the wheelchair

Cognitive Assessment
- Joe is a high school graduate who graduated second in his class. He was home schooled after his injury.
- Joe reports good grades before his injury without any known learning disabilities.

Cardiopulmonary Assessment
- Blood pressure 112/65 mm Hg, heart rate at rest 68 beats/min, respiratory rate 12 breaths/min, cough flows are ineffective (<360 L/min), vital capacity is reduced (between 1.5 and 2.5 L), and breathing pattern incorporates accessory muscles and upper chest wall only; there is marked decrease in the anterior and lateral chest wall with a slight decrease in the posterior wall expansion

Musculoskeletal and Neuromuscular Assessment
- Motor assessment reveals AISA A motor and sensory C6
- Pain on rotator cuff impingement tests
- Deep tendon reflexes 4+ in the lower limbs

Continued

CLINICAL CASE STUDY Transfer Training—cont'd

Integumentary and Sensory Assessment
- Skin is intact throughout; sacral region is completely healed
- Sensation is absent below C6

Range of Motion Assessment
- Passive ROM is within normal limits in both upper limbs; however, pain is produced on the right during passive internal and external rotation; straight leg raise of the lower limbs is 110 degrees bilaterally passively, but otherwise all other lower limb pivots are within normal limits

Mobility and ADL Assessment
- Joe is dependent in self-care activities including lower body dressing and bowel and bladder management; he requires moderate assistance with bathing
- Joe is independent in self-care activities including upper body dressing, grooming, eating, wheelchair management and propulsion, and driving but is experiencing pain with all of these activities
- Joe is nonambulatory

Equipment
- Tub bench, manual wheelchair

Evaluation of Clinical Assessment
Joseph Mainer is an 18-year-old man referred to physical therapy with a C6 ASIA A diagnosis resulting from being hit by a car while riding his bike. He is 22 weeks post injury and is currently being admitted for outpatient physical therapy because of a right shoulder tendonitis.

Patient's Care Needs
1. Interventions for therapeutic exercise to restore pain free functional use of the right upper limb for body transport in the wheelchair and transfers to all surfaces
2. Review skin precautions and the importance of maintaining or improving of aerobic fitness

Diagnosis and Prognosis
Diagnosis is C6 tetraplegia ASIA A. Joe is an excellent candidate for attaining independence with transfers, with pain-free prognosis in both upper limbs.

Preferred Practice Pattern*
Impaired Muscle Performance (4C), Joint Mobility, Motor Function, Muscle Performance, and Range of Motion Associated With Localized Inflammation (4E), Joint Mobility, Motor Function, Muscle Performance, and Range of Motion Associated With Fracture (4G)

Team Goals
1. Team to improve patient's right shoulder pain-free ROM and strength
2. Team to educate patient on prevention of future pressure ulcers and current wound care
3. Patient to improve cardiopulmonary capacity

Patient Goals
"I want my shoulder to heal and be able to perform my transfers without pain."

Care Plan
Treatment Plan & Rationale
- Initiate evaluation for shoulder impairments interfering with optimal pain free functional use
- Initiate physical therapy interventions for restoration of functional activities limitations
- Initiate physical therapy interventions for return to community participation without shoulder pain
- Educate patient on wound prevention and cardiopulmonary fitness exercises that preserve the upper limb from future injury

Interventions
- Therapeutic exercises for strengthening the available shoulder girdle muscles to improve agonist/antagonist muscle balance to the rotator cuff, neuromuscular re-education, functional training of transfers and wheelchair propulsion to preserve the upper limb, modalities for reduction of pain, and aerobic exercises to increase aerobic fitness
- Patient and family will receive training for strategies to relieve pain during healing to preserve the upper limb during transfers and wheelchair propulsion

Documentation and Team Communication
- Team will complete the Wheelchair Users Shoulder Pain Index (WUSPI) biweekly
- Team will refer patient to wheelchair seating clinic for evaluation of wheelchair setup (alignment) to remove potential causes of shoulder pain from poor wheelchair seating

Critical Thinking Exercises
Consider factors that will influence physical therapy therapeutic exercises, patient and family education, transfer progression, and team care decisions associated with Joe's shoulder tendonitis and preventive practices going forward when answering the following questions:
1. What is the safest type of transfer that the rehabilitation team can perform from the hospital bed to the wheelchair while Joe was in halo orthosis traction and had the sacral pressure ulcer?
2. After removal of the halo orthosis, describe the progression of Joe's transfer training first in the Philadelphia collar and then in the soft collar from the wheelchair to an even level mat surface. How would the therapist change the transfer from bed to wheelchair after the sacral pressure ulcer had healed?
3. Describe the expected outcome of the transfer technique from his wheelchair to his bed when at home.
4. What type of assistance would this client need at home with transferring to various surfaces (e.g., bed, shower chair, car)?
5. List three considerations when training Joe's family or caregiver in transfer techniques.
6. What key muscle group is Joe lacking that would improve the ease of his transfer?
7. Joe developed a tendonitis in his right shoulder (his dominant side) week 22 post injury. How would this affect his transfer technique? What accommodation needs to be made regarding his transfer techniques?

*Guide to physical therapist practice, rev. ed. 2, Alexandria, VA, 2003, American Physical Therapy Association.

SUMMARY

There are many considerations that are involved in how an individual with SCI will transfer from one place to another. There are risks to avoid and proper ergonomic techniques to teach and encourage with the patient and his caregivers. Before the actual transfer can take place, the wheelchair must be set up and the patient positioned appropriately. It is impossible to simulate each transfer a patient may need to perform after his discharge from a rehabilitation program. Therefore, it is important that all patients learn a variety of basic transfer techniques as well as being exposed to various options for adapting those techniques. Each patient should be encouraged to use problem-solving skills when practicing transfers rather than always relying on input from the therapist. In this way the patient learns to assess each new situation as it arises and develops his own personal resources for the best way to handle each new challenge.

REFERENCES

1. Garret AL: Functional potential in spinal cord injury, *Clin Orthop Relat Res* 112:60-65, 1975.

2. Yarkony GM, Roth EJ, Heinemann AW et al: Functional skills after spinal cord injury rehabilitation: three-year longitudinal follow-up, *Arch Phys Med Rehabil* 69:111-114, 1988.

3. Yarkony GM, Roth EJ, Meyer PR Jr et al: Rehabilitation outcomes in patients with complete thoracic spinal cord injury, *Am J Phys Med Rehabil* 69:23-27, 1990.

4. Harvey LA, Crosbie J: Biomechanical analysis of a weight-relief maneuver in C5 and C6 quadriplegia, *Arch Phys Med Rehabil* 81:500-505, 2000.

5. Janssen TW, van Oers CA, van der Woude LH, et al: Physical strain in daily life of wheelchair users with spinal cord injuries, *Med Sci Sports Exercise* 26:661-670, 1994.

6. Wang YT, Kim CK, Ford III HT et al: Reaction force and EMG analyses of wheelchair transfers, *Percept Motor Skills* 79:763-766, 1994.

7. Gagnon D, Nadeau S, Gravel D, et al: Biomechanical analysis of a posterior transfer maneuver on a level surface in individuals with high and low-level spinal cord injuries, *Clin Biomech (Bristol, Avon)* 18:319-331, 2003.

8. Grevelding P, Bohannon RW: Reduced push forces accompany device use during sliding transfers of seated subjects, *J Rehabil Res Dev* 38:135-139, 2001.

9. Curtis KA, Tyner TM, Zachary L et al: Effect of a standard exercise protocol on shoulder pain in long-term wheelchair users, *Spinal Cord* 37:421-429, 1999.

10. Dugan SA, Frontera WR: Muscle fatigue and muscle injury, *Phys Med Rehabil Clin North Am* 11:385-403, 2000.

11. Voight ML, Hardin JA Blackburn TA et al: The effects of muscle fatigue on and the relationship of arm dominance to shoulder proprioception, *J Orthop Sports Phys Ther* 23:348-352, 1996.

12. Ballinger DA, Rintala DH, Hart KAL: The relation of shoulder pain and range-of-motion problems to functional limitations, disability, and perceived health of men with spinal cord injury: a multifaceted longitudinal study, *Arch Phys Med Rehabil* 81:1575-1581, 2000.

13. Waring WP, Maynard FM: Shoulder pain in acute traumatic quadriplegia, *Paraplegia* 29:37-42, 1991.

14. Perry J, Gronley JK, Newsam CJ et al: Electromyographic analysis of the shoulder muscles during depression transfers in subjects with low-level paraplegia, *Arch Phys Med Rehabil* 77:350-355, 1996.

15. Hagiwara A, Kanagawa K: Cardiovascular responses during bed-to-wheelchair transfers in frail elderly subjects living at home [in Japanese], *Nippon Ronen Igakkai Zasshi* 39:296-302, 2002.

16. Cech DJ, Martin ST: *Functional movement development across the life span*, Philadelphia, 2002, WB Saunders.

17. Krassioukov AV, Furlan JC, Fehlings MG: Medical co-morbidities, secondary complications, and mortality in elderly with acute spinal cord injury, *J Neurotrauma* 20:391-399, 2003.

18. Bolin I, Bodin P, Kreuter M: Sitting position—posture and performance in C5-C6 tetraplegia, *Spinal Cord* 38:425-434, 2000.

19. Lynch SM, Leahy P, Barker SP: Reliability of measurements obtained with a modified functional reach test in subjects with spinal cord injury, *Phys Ther* 78:128-133, 1998.

20. Chen CL, Yeung KT, Bih LI et al: The relationship between sitting stability and functional performance in patients with paraplegia, *Arch Phys Med Rehabil* 84:1276-1281, 2003.

21. Dalyan M, Cardenas DD, Gerard B: Upper extremity pain after spinal cord injury, *Spinal Cord* 37:191-195, 1999.

22. Bayley JC, Cochran TP, Sledge CB: The weight-bearing shoulder. The impingement syndrome in paraplegics, *J Bone Joint Surg [Am]* 69:676-678, 1987.

23. Nichols PJ, Norman PA, Ennis JR: Wheelchair user's shoulder? Shoulder pain in patients with spinal cord lesions, *Scand J Rehabil Med* 11:29-32, 1979.

24. Curtis KA, Roach KE, Applegate EB et al: Development of the Wheelchair User's Shoulder Pain Index (WUSPI), *Paraplegia* 33:290-293, 1995.

25. Pentland WE, Twomey LT: The weight-bearing upper extremity in women with long term paraplegia, *Paraplegia* 29:521-530, 1991.

26. Boninger ML, Dicianno BE, Cooper RA et al: Shoulder magnetic resonance imaging abnormalities, wheelchair propulsion, and gender, *Arch Phys Med Rehabil* 85:1615-1620, 2003.

27. Lal S: Premature degenerative shoulder changes in spinal cord injury patients, *Spinal Cord* 36:186-189, 1998.

28. Boninger ML, Towers JD, Cooper RA et al: Shoulder imaging abnormalities in individuals with paraplegia, *J Rehabil Res Dev* 38:401-408, 2001.

29. Nyland J, Quigley P, Huang C et al: Preserving transfer independence among individuals with spinal cord injury, *Spinal Cord* 38:649-657, 2000.

30. Klebine P, Lindsey L, Oberheu AM: Prevention of pressure sores through skin care. In *Spinal cord injury info sheets*, Birmingham, AL, 2000, University of Alabama, Board of Trustees.

31. Calder CJ, Kirby RL: Fatal wheelchair-related accidents in the United States, *Am J Phys Med Rehabil* 69:184-190, 1990.

32. Ummat S, Kirby RL: Nonfatal wheelchair-related accidents reported to the National Electronic Injury Surveillance System, *Am J Phys Med Rehabil* 73:163-167, 1994.

33. Kirby RL, Smith C: Fall during a wheelchair transfer: a case of mismatched brakes, *Am J Phys Med Rehabil* 80:302-304, 2001.

34. Marras WS, Davis KG, Kirking BC et al: A comprehensive analysis of low-back disorder risk and spinal loading during the transferring and repositioning of patients using different techniques, *Ergonomics* 42:904-926, 1999.

35. Zelenka JP, Floren AE, Jordan JJ: Minimal forces to move patients, *Am J Occup Ther* 50:354-361, 1996.

36. Frost P: Lifting patients poses high risk for back injuries, Ohio State University, *Reports on News Coverage*, 2003: http://researchnews.osu.edu/archive/resthome.htm. Accessed September 25, 2007.

37. Garg A, Owen B, Beller D et al: A biomechanical and ergonomic evaluation of patient transferring tasks: bed to wheelchair and wheelchair to bed, *Ergonomics* 34:289-312, 1991.

38. Garg A, Owen B, Beller D et al: A biomechanical and ergonomic evaluation of patient transferring tasks: wheelchair to shower chair and shower chair to wheelchair, *Ergonomics* 34:407-419, 1991.

39. Varcin-Coad L, Barrett R: Repositioning a slumped person in a wheelchair: a biomechanical analysis of three transfer techniques, *AAOHN J* 46:530-536, 1998.

40. American Physical Therapy Association: *Guide to physical therapist practice,* ed 2, Alexandria, VA, 2001, American Physical Therapy Association.

41. Herberts P, Kadefors R, Hogfors C et al: Shoulder pain and heavy manual labor, *Clin Orthop Relat Res* 191:166-178, 1984.

42. Hoyt W: Carpal tunnel syndrome: analysis and prevention, *Prof Saf* 16-21, 1984.

43. McKenzie F, Storment J, Van Hook P et al: A program for control of repetitive trauma disorders associated with hand tool operations in a telecommunications manufacturing facility, *Am Ind Hyg Assoc J* 46:674-678, 1985.

44. Beck L: Your company needs an ergonomics program, *Modern Materials Handling* 62-68, 1987.

45. Drury C, Kleiner B, Zahorjan J: How can manufacturing human factors help save a company: intervention at high and low levels. In *Proceedings of the Human Factors Society 33rd Annual Meeting,* pp 687-689, Denver, 1989, The Society.

46. Chatterjee DS: Workplace upper limb disorders: a prospective study with intervention, *Occup Med* 42:129-136, 1992.

47. Carson R: Reducing cumulative trauma disorders: use of proper workplace design, *AAOHN J* 42:270-276, 1994.

48. Allison GT, Singer KP, Marshall RN: Transfer movement strategies of individuals with spinal cord injuries, *Disabil Rehabil* 18:35-41, 1996.

49. Sinnott KA, Milburn P, McNaughton H: Factors associated with thoracic spinal cord injury, lesion level and rotator cuff disorders, *Spinal Cord* 38:748-753, 2000.

50. Neer CS II: Impingement lesions, *Clin Orthop Relat Res* 173:70-77, 1983.

51. Silverstein BA, Fine LJ, Armstrong TJ: Occupational factors and carpal tunnel syndrome, *Am J Ind Med* 11:343-358, 1987.

52. Roquelaure Y, Mechali S, Dano C et al: Occupational and personal risk factors for carpal tunnel syndrome in industrial workers, *Scand J Work Environ Health* 23:364-369, 1997.

53. Werner RA, Franzblau A, Albers JW et al: Median mononeuropathy among active workers—are there differences between symptomatic and asymptomatic workers, *Am J Ind Med* 33:374-378, 1998.

54. Andersen JH, Kaergaard A, Frost P et al: Physical, psychosocial, and individual risk factors for neck/shoulder pain with pressure tenderness in the muscles among workers performing monotonous, repetitive work, *Spine* 27:660-667, 2002.

55. Reyes ML, Gronley JK, Newsam CJ et al: Electromyographic analysis of shoulder muscles of men with low-level paraplegia during a weight relief raise, *Arch Phys Med Rehabil* 76:433-439, 1995.

56. Nawoczenski DA, Clobes SA, Gore SL et al: Three-dimensional shoulder kinematics during a pressure relief technique and wheelchair transfer, *Arch Phys Med Rehabil* 84:1293-1300, 2003.

57. Maricello MA, Herbison GJ, Cohen ME et al: Elbow extension using the anterior deltoids and upper pectorals in spinal cord-injured subjects, *Arch Phys Med Rehabil* 76:426-432, 1995.

58. Zerby SA, Herbison GJ, Marino RJ et al: Elbow extension using the anterior deltoids and upper pectorals, *Muscle Nerve* 17:1472-1474, 1994.

59. Tanzer RC: The carpal-tunnel syndrome, *J Bone Joint Surg [Am]* 41A:626-634, 1959.

60. Armstrong TJ, Chaffin DB: Carpal tunnel syndrome and selected personal attributes, *J Occup Med* 21:481-486, 1979.

61. Gelberman RH, Hergenroeder PT, Hargens AR et al: The carpal tunnel syndrome. A study of carpal canal pressures, *J Bone Joint Surg [Am]* 63:380-383, 1981.

62. Lundborg G, Gelberman RH, Minteer-Convery M et al: Median nerve compression in the carpal tunnel—functional response to experimentally induced controlled pressure, *J Hand Surg [Am]* 7: 252-259, 1982.

63. Gellman H, Chandler DR, Petrasek J et al: Carpal tunnel syndrome in paraplegic patients, *J Bone Joint Surg [Am]* 70:517-519, 1988.

64. Keir PJ, Wells RP, Ranney DA et al: The effects of tendon load and posture on carpal tunnel pressure, *J Hand Surg [Am]* 22: 628-634, 1997.

65. Schroer W, Lacey S, Frost FS et al: Carpal instability in the weight-bearing upper extremity, *J Bone Joint Surg [Am]* 78:1838-1843, 1996.

66. Papuga MO, Memberg WD, Crago PE: Biomechanics of sliding transfer: feasibility of FES assistance. In *Proceedings of the Second Joint EMBS/BMES Conference,* pp 2382–2383, Houston, 2002, The Conference.

SOLUTIONS TO CHAPTER 8 CLINICAL CASE STUDY

Transfer Training

1. The rehabilitation team must perform a two- or three-man lift for precautions with an orthosis. The patient must never be lifted by use of the halo vest because it serves as the counterpressure to support the uprights screwed into the skull to maintain cervical traction for healing (see section on orthotic precautions).

2. Joe should continue to be transferred by a two-man lift technique after the halo device is removed until the sacral wound is healed. Once the wound is healed, a transfer board with the technique for locking out the elbows (see Chapter 7) can be initiated. This technique must be performed by using a series of lifts with the therapist assisting the lift at the ischial tuberosities and guarding in front while Joe is in both the Philadelphia and soft collar. He cannot initiate the head-hips relationship technique to facilitate the transfer until after the soft collar is removed. When the soft collar is removed, Joe should begin using the head-hips relationship technique to move himself across the transfer board.

3. There are several transfer techniques that could be attempted to and from the bed for the outcome requiring the least amount of assistance from another individual. The long-sit transfer, push-or-pull transfer, or the transfer board techniques are good options.

4. Joe may not achieve full independence in transferring to all surfaces. His lack of triceps innervation places him at a disadvantage for lifting his body mass and he will be more susceptible to shoulder injury and impingement. Careful consideration should be given during training to reinforce optimal shoulder position. Keeping the shoulder in external rotation during closed chain lifting techniques provides biomechanical efficiency and avoids impingement. Alternating the leading limb should be emphasized because the trailing limb does absorb more of the force during transfers.

Joe is tall and does not have a high body mass index. The length of his trunk in relationship to his legs and the length of his arms will all influence the biomechanical solutions to each transfer surface that he encounters and should be considered by the therapist. Individuals with longer arms in proportion to their body have an advantage, individuals with shorter arms may need to use a neutral wrist position to gain more arm length. Individuals with longer trunks may have greater difficulty with balance as they reposition their upper limbs during the transfers. Body mass is also a consideration because the heavier the patient the more difficult the transfer will be in most cases, especially if the weight is most concentrated in the pelvis.

Other factors that may limit transfer independence for patients with limited muscle strength include tone or spasticity, poor body sense with nonfunctional sitting balance, age, motivation, fear of falling, and heterotrophic ossification of the hip with joint mobility restrictions. A prediction of independence for Joe is uncertain considering the influence of the above factors. The therapist should, however, project a goal of independence on the basis of the most optimal outcomes associated with the considerations discussed above.

5. It is vital that the caregivers receive education for back safety and proper lifting techniques. The therapist should use a variety of education tools to assist in demonstrating for and evaluating the caregivers' transfer techniques.

Skin considerations related to shearing forces with transfer surfaces and types of clothing should be discussed with the caregivers. Areas for potential skin breakdown and positions placing the patient at risk in these areas should be reviewed with the patient and caregivers.

The relationship of the transfer surface height to the wheelchair must be reviewed because it influences the level of assistance required by the caregiver and may also influence the type of transfer attempted and performed.

Guarding position and leverage advantages and disadvantages should be reviewed with the caregivers regarding how they affect the types of transfer.

Last, individual differences regarding precautions and considerations such as fluctuations with tonal influence by position should be reviewed with the caregivers.

6. The triceps is the key muscle group that Joe is lacking and inhibits the ease of his transfer techniques.

7. Joe's new secondary diagnosis of right shoulder tendonitis needs to be treated. This might involve the use of pain/swelling relieving modalities and therapeutic exercises to increase the shoulder muscle balance. Functional training should guide him to use his right upper limb as the leading limb with transfers. Joe and his caregivers should be instructed in proper positioning to avoid internal rotation of the humerus on the glenoid, which could cause impingement. Avoidance of forces driving the humerus into the glenoid during wheelchair propulsion should be practiced. These principles should be carried over during pressure relief techniques while in the wheelchair to prevent pressure ulcers and during aerobic exercise.

CHAPTER NINE

Activities of Daily Living

Paula M. Ackerman, OTR/L, MS, Sarah Broton, OTR/L, Amanda Gillot, OTR/L, MS, Julie Hartrich, OTR/L, and Polly Hopkins, OTR/L

I rolled up my new ramp for the first time…How would I cook? Clean? Reach the cabinets? Pay the mortgage? Tuck my kids in at night? "Time heals all wounds," says it all. It was striving to do these things that helped me recuperate. In just two years I have the pleasure of doing all the things I thought I would never do again. My life is more complete than before my injury because I truly value everyday accomplishments that I once so hated. My children no longer see me as a mom in a wheelchair but just plain mom.

Linda (T11 SCI)

A spinal cord injury (SCI) not only affects an individual's strength, motor control, and sensation but also the ability to complete activities of daily living (ADL) and instrumental activities of daily living (IADL). ADLs are generally considered basic skills and may include self-care, mobility, and communication, whereas IADLs are more complex and require advanced problem solving skills. Home management and community living skills are examples of IADLs.[1] ADL and IADL retraining are accomplished through adaptive techniques, assistive devices, and assistive technology.[2]

The role of the therapist when addressing ADL and IADL begins with an evaluation (Box 9-1) to establish appropriate therapeutic interventions.[2,3]

A thorough history will help to determine necessary background information and pertinent medical precautions specific to each patient. Evaluations of the physiological and anatomical status, communication, affect, cognition, language, and learning style need to be reviewed.[3,4] The International Standards for American Spinal Injury Association (ASIA) should be used for the specific neurological examination (see Figure 6-12). Specific manual muscle testing, range of motion (ROM) assessments, and shoulder or other orthopedic assessments should also be completed.

In addition, a complete functional assessment needs to be performed. Myriad tools exist to assess functional skills,[5] including the Functional Independence Measure (FIM) (see Figure 6-15) and the Spinal Cord Independence Measure (SCIM).[6]

After the assessments and input from the patient, functional goals should be determined on the basis of premorbid roles and daily routine. For example, cooking should not be a primary area of focus for a patient who is not responsible for any meal

preparatory activities in his home. Areas such as makeup application or inserting contact lenses may be overlooked when an individual is hospitalized because it may not be part of the patient's routine during this time. These activities, however, may be important to the patient on return home and should therefore be addressed. Initial and continuing evaluations should be thorough and comprehensive to address all the patient's roles. This chapter describes categorical ADL skills with considerations for training with appropriate adaptive equipment that considers the level of injury for each ADL category.

LEVEL OF INJURY

The functional outcomes of a patient with SCI are largely dependent on the level of injury and the extent or completeness of the injury. Consideration of the level of injury is helpful in identifying potential goals and setting an appropriate treatment regimen. An overview of injury level, innervated muscles, and functional outcomes for ADL performance is described in Table 9-1. The use of appropriate adaptive equipment is paramount in maximizing a patient's independence. An overview of adaptive equipment is presented in Table 9-2.

An individual with C1 to C4 level injuries has use of his neck and facial musculature. A person with this level of injury will be dependent for self-care activities such as feeding, grooming, dressing, bathing, and bladder and bowel management. Despite an inability to physically perform these skills, it is crucial that the individual is able to clearly and specifically verbalize all self-care needs. This skill will help ensure health and safety and give him more control in achieving his comfort level. A broad range of adaptive equipment from no technology to high technology is available to assist with many daily activities from reading to communication to hygiene (Figure 9-1) and is described later (also see Chapters 9 and 13).

A person with a C5 level injury has use of his deltoid and biceps muscles, but lacks nerve innervation to his trunk, wrist, and hand musculature. Individuals with C5 level injury can perform many tabletop activities including feeding, grooming, and communication with setup assistance. At this injury level, proper body positioning is critical to increase independence. A chest strap is required to maintain an upright position in a wheelchair. In addition, the wheelchair should be adjusted to as close to a 90-degree upright position as possible to allow for gravity-assisted muscle substitutions to compensate for the lack of triceps innervation. This upright posture

---

BOX 9-1	**Components of an Activities of Daily Living and Instrumental Activities of Daily Living Evaluation**

- History
- Medical precautions
- Physiological and anatomical status
- Assessment of communication, affect, language, and learning style
- Cognition
- Neurological examination (e.g., ASIA assessment)
- Manual muscle test
- ROM
- Orthopedic assessment
- Functional assessment (e.g., FIM, SCIM)

TABLE 9-1	**Overview of Functional Outcomes Related to Level of Injury**	
Neurological Level	Muscles Innervated	Functional Skill and Related Functional Outcome
C4	Neck accessories Diaphragm Trapezius	Communication: setup Feeding: verbalizes Grooming: verbalizes Bathing: verbalizes Dressing: modified independent Weight shifts: verbalizes Bladder management: verbalizes Bowel management: verbalizes Home management: verbalizes Child care: verbalizes
C5	Deltoids Biceps	Communication: setup Feeding: setup Grooming: minimum assist and setup Bathing: maximum assist to dependent Dressing: maximum assist to dependent Weight shifts: modified independent Bladder management: verbalizes Bowel management: verbalizes Home management: maximum assist to dependent Child care: verbalizes

C6	Wrist extensors
	Clavicular pectoralis
	Serratus anterior
	Pronator teres
		Communication: modified independent
		Feeding: modified independent
		Grooming: modified independent
		Bathing: modified independent
		Dressing: modified independent
		Weight shifts: modified independent
		Bladder management
		  Male: modified independent
		  Female: maximum assist to dependent
		Bowel management: moderate assist to modified independent
		Home management: moderate assist to modified independent
		Child care: moderate assist to modified independent

C7 to C8	Triceps brachii
	Extensor carpi radialis
	Flexor digitorum Superficialis and profundus (C7 to C8, T1)
	Extensor digitorum (C6 to C8)
	Extensor pollicis longus
	Extensor pollicis brevis
	Abductor pollicis longus
		Communication: modified independent
		Feeding: modified independent
		Grooming: modified independent
		Bathing: modified independent
		Dressing: modified independent
		Weight shifts: modified independent
		Bladder management
		  Male: modified independent
		  Female: maximum assist to dependent
		Bowel management: modified independent
		Home management: moderate assist to modified independent
		Child care: moderate assist to modified independent

C8 to T1	Pronator quadratus
	Flexor carpi ulnaris
	Lumbricals
	Dorsal and palmar interossei
	Flexor pollicis longus and brevis
	Adductor pollicis
	Opponens digiti minimi
	Opponens pollicis
		Communication: modified independent
		Feeding: modified independent
		Grooming: modified independent
		Bathing: modified independent
		Dressing: modified independent
		Weight shifts: modified independent
		Bladder management
		  Male: modified independent
		  Female: moderate assist to dependent
		Bowel management: modified independent
		Home management: moderate assist to modified independent
		Child care: minimum assist to modified independent

Data from Adler C: Spinal cord injury. In Pendleton HM, Schyultz-Krohn W, editors: *Pedretti's occupational therapy: practice skills for physical dysfunction*, ed 6, St. Louis, 2006, Mosby Elsevier; Atrice M, Morison S, McDowell S et al: Traumatic spinal cord injury. In Umphred D, editor: *Neurological rehabilitation*, ed 5, St. Louis, 2005, Mosby Elsevier; Martin ST, Kessler M: Spinal cord injuries. In Martin ST, Kessler M, editors: *Neurologic interventions for physical therapy*, ed 2, St. Louis, 2007, Saunders Elsevier.

Continued

TABLE 9-1	**Overview of Functional Outcomes Related to Level of Injury—cont'd**	
Neurological Level	Muscles Innervated	Functional Skill and Related Functional Outcome
Paraplegia	All muscles of the upper extremities	Communication: modified independent Feeding: modified independent Grooming: modified independent Bathing: modified independent Dressing: modified independent Weight shifts: modified independent Bladder management: modified independent Bowel management: modified independent Home management: minimum assist to modified independent Child care: modified independent

Data from Adler C: Spinal cord injury. In Pendleton HM, Schyultz-Krohn W, editors: *Pedretti's occupational therapy: practice skills for physical dysfunction*, ed 6, St. Louis, 2006, Mosby Elsevier; Atrice M, Morison S, McDowell S et al: Traumatic spinal cord injury. In Umphred D, editor: *Neurological rehabilitation*, ed 5, St. Louis, 2005, Mosby Elsevier; Martin ST, Kessler M: Spinal cord injuries. In Martin ST, Kessler M, editors: *Neurologic interventions for physical therapy*, ed 2, St. Louis, 2007, Saunders Elsevier.

will allow the patient to rotate his shoulders so that gravity creates elbow extension through eccentric contraction of the biceps. Because of an inability to hold the wrist in neutral, a wrist splint will assist the patient to engage in functional activities.

At a C6 level injury, an individual can become much more independent with ADLs and IADLs than those with previously described levels of injury. The use of adaptive equipment and proper caregiver setup for an accessible environment will still be necessary. A person with a C6 level injury also has use of his deltoid, biceps, brachialis, brachioradialis, clavicular portion of the pectoralis major, serratus anterior, and wrist extensor muscles. The presence of the wrist extension with C6 to C7 level injuries allows an individual to use a tenodesis grasp for functional tasks.

Tenodesis, the mutual action between the fingers and wrist, occurs because of passive extension of the finger flexors as the wrist is flexed (Figure 9-2, *A*) and the passive flexion of the finger flexors as the wrist is extended (Figure 9-2, *B*). These actions can create an automatic grasp because finger muscle tendon units have a resting length and cross multiple joints before inserting on to the phalanges. This anatomical alignment allows the tendons to affect the position of several joints without any contraction or length change required of the muscles. Therefore, tenodesis contributes to the passive actions of the digits in association with wrist extension and flexion.[7] Depending on the patient's muscle strength regained after SCI, or when used in conjunction with adaptive equipment, tenodesis allows for more functional use of the hand leading to greater independence with self-care tasks.[3] Grasp for some individuals with tetraplegia can be enhanced by a surgical tendon transfer (see Chapter 10), which can allow greater hand and thumb function such as holding a water bottle by its cap (Figure 9-3, *A*) or preparing to take a drink (Figure 9-3, *B*).

When the SCI is at the C7 level, the patent's triceps muscles are innervated and he can perform self-care tasks, including transfers, with greater ease because he has the ability to perform a push-up by using the triceps, whereas an individual with a C6 SCI does not. The adaptive equipment and techniques used by individuals with C6 and C7 level injuries are very similar because functional hand use also is limited at the C7 level. People with

injuries at the C8 and T1 spinal levels exhibit weak, partially innervated hand and finger musculature, which again increases the ease with which self-care tasks are performed. Techniques and adaptive equipment vary for those with C8 and T1 level injuries as will be described later.

An individual with paraplegia has full function of the upper limbs and does not require adaptive techniques or equipment to compensate for decreased upper limb function. The level of injury will affect trunk control and balance, which are important for ADL and functional activities. People with high thoracic injuries may still require additional trunk support or balance techniques if working outside their base of support to increase ADL performance. The use of stabilization techniques with one upper limb while manipulating with the other is one way to compensate for the lack of trunk control.

Depending on the presentation of the SCI, patients will achieve varying levels of independence with ADLs and IADLs. The following sections describe the general functional expectations in commonly addressed ADLs by individuals with complete, bilaterally equal levels of injury. Actual functioning can vary extensively as a result of concomitant issues, body type, age, goals, cognition, type, and extent of injury.

FEEDING

Individuals with C1 to C4 level injuries require total assistance with feeding. People with injuries at these levels should be active in menu planning with regard to diet and become proficient in instructing a caregiver on how they would like to be fed. At the C5 level, setup is required for feeding and the meal will need to be cut into bite-sized pieces. At this level, a wrist splint may be required to use an eating utensil. An individual can don the splint by pushing the volar portion of the wrists together and fastening the straps with his mouth. He can position the silverware by grasping it in the same manner as the splint and using his mouth to place the silverware in the cuff or splint. Individuals with C5 tetraplegia sometimes prefer to lift small cups for drinking with the volar aspects of the wrists, instead of using a long straw.

It is uncommon for a patient with C5 tetraplegia to present with functional shoulder strength while in an inpatient

TABLE 9-2 | Overview of Adaptive Equipment

Adaptive Equipment	Purpose	Level of Injury
Bent fork or spoon	For use with U-cuff; to compensate for the lack of forearm pronation during feeding and to assist with scooping food	C5, C6
Button aid with U-cuff	Assists with buttoning with absent or impaired finger function	C6, C7, C8
5-in-1 connector	Makes connecting catheter to tubing for intermittent catheterization possible with absent or impaired finger function	C6, C7, C8
Digital bowel stimulator splint	Holds digital bowel stimulator during digital stimulation bowel program for individuals with absent or impaired finger function	C6, C7, C8
Digital bowel stimulator	Increases functional reach for individuals who perform digital stimulation bowel programs	Any level
Dycem	Holds plate steady during feeding	C5, C6
Household (Flexlife Medical, Kingwood, Tex.)	Holds penis in accessible position during intermittent catheterization	C6, C7, C8
Labia spreader	Holds labia apart during female intermittent catheterization	C6, C7, C8
Lap tray	Offers accessible surface for mouthstick activities and ECU equipment	C1 to C4
Lever-type faucet	Allows manipulation of faucet with absent or impaired finger function	C5, C6, C7, C8
Liquid soap dispenser	In shower, can be mounted on wall to eliminate the need to handle soap/shampoo bottles	Any level
Long-handled sponge	Increases functional reach in shower. Cuff can be added for use with absent or impaired finger function	Any level
Long straw/straw holder	Offers access to beverages without requiring the individual to handle a cup	C1-C5
Magazine holder	Holds book or magazine open for mouthstick users	C1 to C4
Mobile arm support	Decreases the demands of gravity on the shoulder during functional activities	C5
Mouthstick	May feature a rubber stop or an implement holder; allows individuals with absent arm function to interact with environment	C1 to C4
Mouthstick holder/ docking station	Offers accessible resting place for mouthstick	C1 to C4
Pants holder	Holds pants open during male IC	Any level
Plate guard	Provides a surface against which to scoop food and prevents food from falling off plate during feeding	C5, C6
Push gloves	With Dycem palms, offers increased friction for clothing manipulation during lower body dressing	C6, C7
Right angle pocket	Option for writing with absent or impaired finger function; holds writing implement in U-cuff	C5, C6, C7, C8
Scald guard	Can be purchased at home supply store; helps to decrease the chances of scalding in the shower	Any level
Skin mirror	Available for use with full or absent hand function; allows individual to inspect skin, especially in the sacral and ischial areas	C6 and lower
Spring loaded scissors	Cut without requiring the handles to be squeezed; used with the side of the hand	C5, C6, C7, C8
U-cuff	Part of a wrist support or a single strap, offers a slot at the medial and lateral aspects of the palm to hold utensils, including a fork or toothbrush.	C5, C6, C7, C8
Wanchick	Option for writing with absent or impaired finger function; holds writing implement and can provide wrist support	C5, C6, C7, C8
Wash mitt	Can be secured over hand to allow assistance with bathing despite absent or impaired finger function	C5, C6, C7, C8
Wrist support	Splint that holds the wrist in neutral during functional activities	C5
Zipper loops	Allow manipulation of zippers with absent or impaired finger function	C5, C6, C7, C8

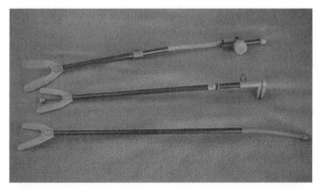

FIGURE 9-1 Three examples of commercially available mouthsticks, which may be used by an individual with C1 to C4 tetraplegia to aid in a variety of tasks that require fine motor skills including turning book and magazine pages, playing cards, and practicing dental hygiene.

rehabilitation program after injury. Participation in ADL during inpatient rehabilitation, therefore, is difficult to achieve without overfatiguing the individual or promoting unbalanced shoulder movement. To help the patient gain strength and participate in ADL (e.g., feeding) while maintaining proper shoulder alignment and muscular balance, therapists often fit the patient for a mobile arm support (MAS), also known as a ball-bearing feeder (Figure 9-4) (see Chapter 14).

The MAS clamps to the patient's wheelchair or table and minimizes the effect of gravity on the shoulder during functional tabletop activities. Muscles that are not strong enough to maneuver and control the arm safely without the device are able to do so during activities requiring endurance, including feeding, oral care, and typing or writing. The patient is typically

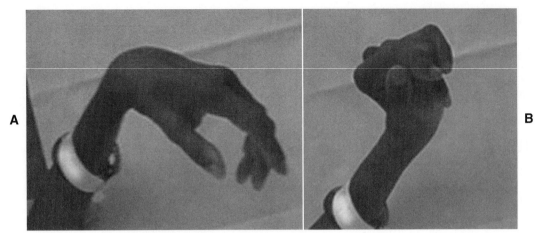

FIGURE 9-2 The tenodesis grasp affects **(A)** passive finger extension that results from active wrist flexion, and **(B)** passive finger flexion that results from active wrist extension.

weaned from the MAS when shoulder strength and alignment are appropriate for participation in tabletop activities. It is important for the therapist to monitor the patient's progress closely because premature weaning from the MAS can result in unbalanced strengthening and set the patient up for shoulder pain in the future. Research conducted by van Drongelen et al[8] studied upper limb musculoskeletal pain during and after rehabilitation in wheelchair-using subjects with SCI and its relation to lesion characteristics, muscle strength, and functional outcome in eight rehabilitation centers in The Netherlands. Testing occurred on four occasions during rehabilitation and again 1 year after rehabilitation. Upper limb pain decreased over time (30%) during the latter part of inpatient rehabilitation and individuals with tetraplegia showed more musculoskeletal pain than did subjects with paraplegia. This supports special consideration and monitoring of shoulder pain when weaning from patients from MAS.

Functional expectations for persons with a C6 level SCI require setup assistance or their achievement of modified independence with feeding. Adaptive equipment or a tenodesis brace may be used (Figure 9-5).

Utensils can be held in the hand with use of a universal cuff (U-cuff) with a cutout for the utensil. A person can don this cuff with modified independence by using his teeth or thumb of his opposite hand. If the individual's tenodesis is tight enough to hold a utensil that has been built up with foam, a U-cuff may not be needed for feeding. Cutting may require the use of a rocker knife (Figure 9-6) or a right-angle knife that can be adapted with a U-cuff. Commercial cutting boards that will hold food in place during cutting are available.

For drinking, the tenodesis grasp may be used to pick up a cup in one hand while the other hand supports the cup from underneath. A U-shaped handle on a cup can give the hand more support when the tenodesis grip is used (Figure 9-7).

Containers, including those commonly used for condiments, chips, and beverages can be opened with the teeth or with spring-loaded scissors (Figure 9-8), and beverage cans can be opened with a U-cuff and a utensil. Setup may be required for cutting tough foods and opening containers that involve increased dexterity.

Individuals with C7 to C8 level injuries can achieve modified independence to independence with feeding. With enough finger strength, built-up handles can be woven between fingers for a firm hold. Packets and containers may be opened with the fingers, if able, or with the teeth.

GROOMING

According to the FIM, grooming encompasses multiple activities (Clinical Note: Grooming Activities). This section discusses numerous types of adaptive equipment available to assist with grooming (Figure 9-9). To facilitate personal care, patients learn to suck toothpaste out of the tube and develop good spitting skills; benefit from flip-top containers and use sports bottles for liquids such as mouthwash; use long straws and cup holders, lever faucets, and U-cuffs to attach to a variety of implements such as electric razors, hair brushes, and hair dryer holders; and learn to maneuver nail clippers mounted on a board.

CLINICAL NOTE **Grooming Activities**

- Oral care
- Washing hands and face
- Combing hair
- Shaving
- Applying makeup

Modifying the environment can also increase an individual's independence with grooming activities. Environmental modifications include an accessible sink that gives clearance for a chair to fit beneath it and that has lever on-off handles on the faucets. All metal piping under sinks should be insulated to protect the user from burning his lower limbs.

It is important that individuals with C1 to C4 level injuries be able to verbalize grooming needs because they will be dependent on other people for these tasks.

Oral Care

Brushing the teeth requires use of a wrist support with a utensil holder for the person at a C5 level injury (Figure 9-10, *A*) or a U-cuff without wrist support for people with C6 to C7 SCI

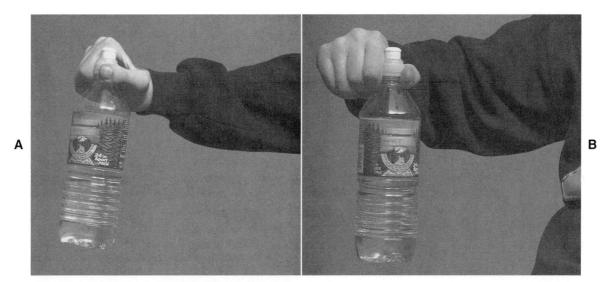

FIGURE 9-3 **A,** An individual with tetraplegia, who has had successful tendon transfer surgery to increase thumb and hand function through tenodesis action, demonstrates a tenodesis grip sufficient to easily hold a water bottle at arms length. **B,** He continues to hold the bottle against gravity as he moves it to a forward position when preparing to take a drink.

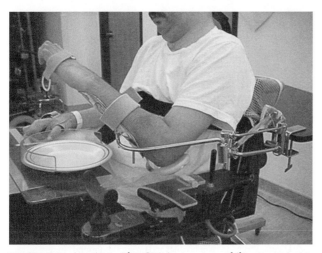

FIGURE 9-4 A patient with a C5 injury uses a mobile arm support to maintain proper shoulder alignment and muscular balance while working on prefeeding skills.

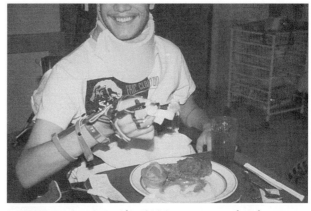

FIGURE 9-5 A patient with a C6 injury uses a tenodesis brace to enhance finger grasp when he feeds himself.

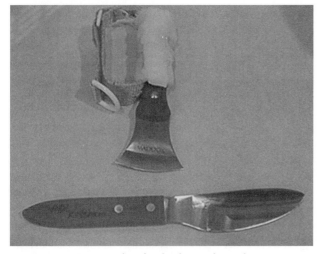

FIGURE 9-6 Two examples of rocker knives that make cutting easier for individuals with limited hand function.

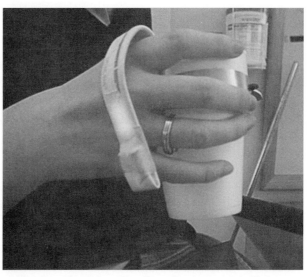

FIGURE 9-7 The U-shaped handle on this cup provides added support for an individual relying on her tenodesis grasp.

(Figure 9-10, *B*). An individual with C7 to C8 or T1 level injuries should have enough dexterity to hold the toothbrush with a built-up handle or without using any adaptive equipment. Flossing can be achieved through the use of a prethreaded floss applicator. The handle can be built up for a better grasp or a cuff can be used to hold the applicator.

Patients often purchase electric toothbrushes; however, the handles on these units are often too bulky to fit into a U-cuff. In addition, it can be very difficult for an individual with C5 tetraplegia to control the on-off switch on an electric toothbrush. Therefore, a standard narrow-handled toothbrush is recommended for optimal independence at a C5 injury level. People with C6 to C8 level injuries can hold the larger handle of an electric toothbrush with a tenodesis grasp or a grasp with finger dexterity. Turning the toothbrush on and off can be achieved with the teeth or by sliding the toothbrush against a counter.

There are a variety of ways to extract the toothpaste from the dispenser. An individual can use his teeth to open the flip-top and squeeze the toothpaste directly into his mouth. A pump dis-

penser secured to a counter or toothpaste tubes taped securely to the edge of the sink are additional ways to access toothpaste. Mouthwash can be accessed by using a long straw and cup holder or by placing mouthwash in a sports bottle. Regardless of the techniques chosen, replacing items in an accessible fashion for the next use is imperative.

Facial Hygiene

A person with a C5 level injury can wash his face by holding a washcloth in both hands by using wrist supports or by using a wash mitt with D-ring closures. At the C6 level, an individual may be able to use his tenodesis grasp to hold the washcloth. At the C7 to C8 levels, a person may have enough dexterity to hold

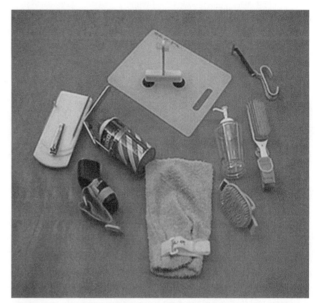

FIGURE 9-9 Various examples of low-technology adaptive equipment make grooming easier for individuals with limited hand function. These include U-cuffs attached to hair brushes and razors, flip-top and plunger-activated containers, terry cloth hand mitts, and nail clippers mounted to a board.

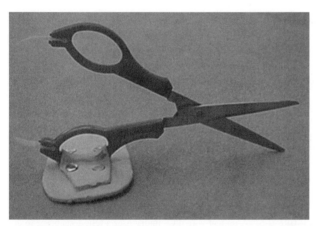

FIGURE 9-8 An individual with tetraplegia can use the side of his hand to cut with these adapted spring-loaded scissors.

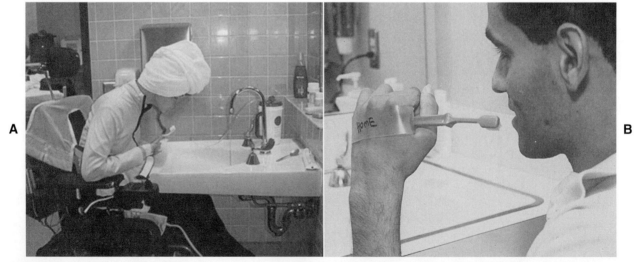

FIGURE 9-10 **A,** A commercially available dorsal wrist extension support or splint with a U-cuff is used by an individual with a C5 injury to brush her teeth. **B,** An individual with C6 tetraplegia uses a U-cuff with an inserted toothbrush as an aid to his weak or absent handgrip. This cuff enables him to brush his teeth independently.

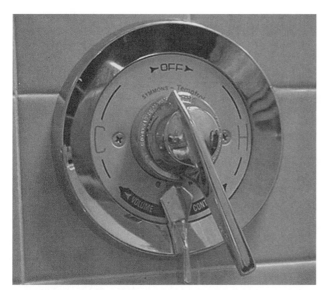

FIGURE 9-11 People with limited dexterity find lever faucet handles easier to turn on and off.

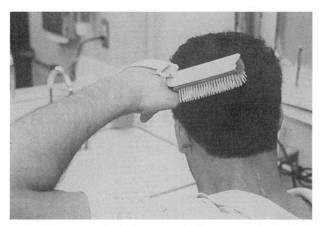

FIGURE 9-12 An individual with tetraplegia uses a U-cuff with a brush handle inserted to enable independence in hair brushing. For individuals who have sufficient tenodesis strength, a built-up handle can be used to enhance an in-hand grip and independence with hair brushing.

the washcloth in his hands. Pump soap dispensers can be used if there is limited finger dexterity because using a bar soap requires increased finger function. Again, lever faucets (Figure 9-11) will be easier to turn on and off for a person with limited dexterity. Finally, a sink that is open underneath and permits an individual to roll his chair under will provide optimal access.

Hair Care

An individual can comb or brush his hair by using a U-cuff attached to a comb or brush handle (Figure 9-12) or by using a built-up handle to support a tenodesis grasp. A strong tenodesis grasp or a two-handed technique can be used when drying hair with a blow dryer. Commercial adaptive devices can assist with drying and styling hair, such as a hair dryer that sits on a stand or attaches to a wall. Safety must be considered when using commercial devices because they may not be designed for the unique needs of a person with SCI who will need to avoid burns or electric shock.

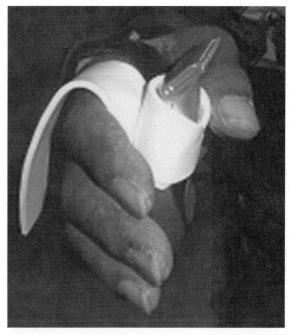

FIGURE 9-13 An individual with tetraplegia uses an adapted electric shaver.

Shaving

People with C5 to T1 SCI can achieve modified independence with shaving. To avoid accidental laceration, electric razors or trimmers are recommended for individuals with decreased motor control or for those who are taking blood-thinning medication. Electric razors can be adapted with a U-cuff, or a cuff made of splinting material can be affixed to the electric razor or trimmer (see Figure 9-9). At the C5 to C6 level injuries, some prefer to hold the razor or trimmer with the volar aspects of both wrists because this often offers more movement of the razor or trimmer (Figure 9-13). People with C7 to C8 level injuries should be able to hold an electric razor because the handle is usually wider, allowing it to be held with a relatively weak tenodesis grip. The on-off button can be moved with the teeth or by sliding the razor against a counter or the armrest.

Standard razors can be held in a cuff; however, changing the direction of the razor may require some assistance. There are safety concerns when a person with an SCI shaves with a standard razor. Involuntary spasms can cause the hand to slip, resulting in skin cuts and abrasions. It is important to clear the use of a standard razor with a physician for patients on blood-thinning medication because excess bleeding could occur from any cut.

Makeup Application

Applying makeup generally requires fine motor skills and therefore will require some creativity for individuals with C5 to C6 level injuries, but it can be achieved by adapting the materials and the environment (Figure 9-14).

It is very difficult for a person without finger function to open containers, including makeup packages.[9] Removing the clasp from compact cases allows a person to flip open the case with her teeth, fingernail, or thumb with ease. Long cotton swabs can be built up with tape (Figure 9-15, *A*) and held in a U-cuff to apply eye makeup and lipsticks (Figure 9-15, *B*).

Lipstick and eye pencils can be adapted to fit in the cuff as well (Figure 9-16). Mascara tubes can be firmly attached to a counter and opened with both hands as long as the top is loosely screwed. A tongue depressor can be attached to the mascara top or foundation sponge and fit into a U-cuff during application (Figure 9-17).

Other modifications include bases in which to secure items to a table or to a wall (a patient can put her face to the makeup item as opposed to bringing the item to the face). Assistance is required for setup of all materials and the environment for those at C5- to C6-level injuries. Some individuals with a C6 injury choose to use a tenodesis brace to help achieve the pinch reflex often required for makeup application. With C7 to C8 injuries, the shafts of the makeup pencils, mascara, and lipsticks can be built up with foam or tape to allow for an in-hand grasp (Figure 9-18).

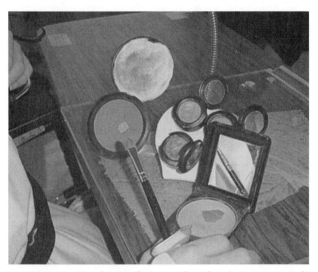

FIGURE 9-14 By adapting the materials and environment, an individual with tetraplegia can apply her makeup. This is an example of a makeup setup for an individual with a C5 level injury.

Nail Care

Adapted nail cutters, brushes, and emery boards are available from commercial vendors for people with limited hand dexterity (see Figure 9-9). It is recommended that a person get assistance with nail care because it has the potential for cuts and abrasions to the skin. Nail polish can be applied by securing the brush to a right-angle pocket with tape. A tenodesis brace might be used for cotton ball manipulation during polish removal.

Contact Lens Management

When applying contact lenses, a person with a C6-level injury can open his contact lens container with his teeth and use his knuckles to remove the lens from the case. Once the lens is removed from the case, he can place the lens on the outside of his first digit or on a knuckle. He can use a thumb to hold his lower lid open while he inserts the lens into his eye. This task requires a counter that the individual can use to prop his elbows on for balance, a mirror at eye level, and steady hands. At C7- to C8-level injuries, the patient may have the motor control to place the contact on his fingertip and then insert it into his eye.

BATHING

Bed baths are an option for individuals with SCI. This method of cleaning is generally sufficient for health; however, most people prefer to occasionally shower. People with SCI require adaptive durable medical equipment for showering (see Chapter 14). Various kinds of bathroom equipment exist to meet individuals' multiple needs. Most pieces of equipment have features that address skin integrity, positioning, and safety. For example, all bathroom equipment recommended for individuals with SCI include padded seats to reduce the effects of pressure on the individual's buttocks (see Figures 14-10 and 14-18).

Safety in the shower is always a primary concern for individuals with SCI (Clinical Note: Tips to Prevent Scalding During Bathing). Because of diminished sensation, water temperature should be monitored closely and tested on an area of the person's skin that has normal sensation. To decrease the chance of scalding, water heaters should be set to temperatures of 120° F or less. In addition, scald guards (available at home supply stores) can

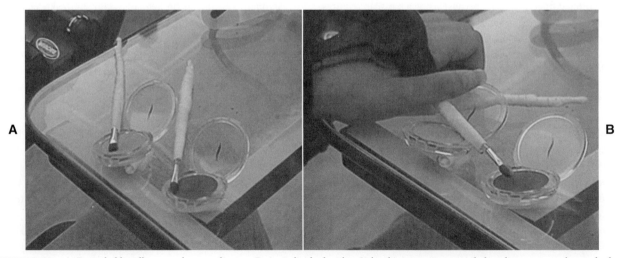

FIGURE 9-15 **A,** Extended handles on makeup applicators. **B,** An individual with a C5 level injury using extended applicators to apply eye shadow.

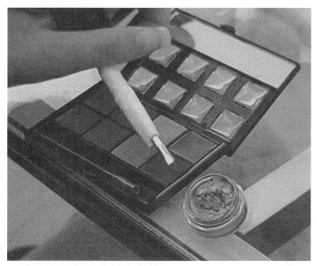

FIGURE 9-16   An individual with a C5 level injury uses an extended applicator in a U-cuff to apply lip gloss.

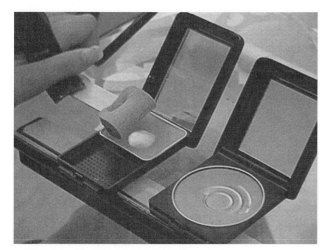

FIGURE 9-17   A sponge applicator attached to a tongue depressor is held in a U-cuff and used to apply makeup foundation.

CLINICAL NOTE   Tips to Prevent Scalding During Bathing

- Closely monitor water temperature
- Test water temperature on area of skin with normal sensation
- Set water heater to 120° F or below
- Install scald guards in faucet plumbing
- Do not rest hand-held shower head in a position where water is falling on an area of decreased sensation
- Do not position feet directly under the faucet

be installed on the faucets. Hand-held shower heads should be placed so that water does not fall on an area of the body with decreased sensation. An individual should ensure that his feet are not positioned directly under the faucet because dripping hot water could burn the skin. By incorporating these safety techniques, unintended water temperature changes will not cause harm. If doing a transfer without clothing from a wheelchair, a

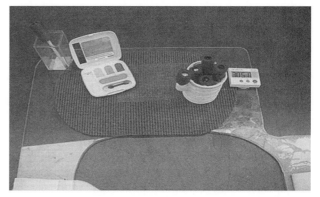

FIGURE 9-18   A makeup setup on a tray table that is attached to a wheelchair or standing table uses a hatched mat (Dycem pad) to provide traction for the items placed on top. A container holds a variety of built-up foam handles to use for independent application of makeup.

towel, pillowcase, or gel pad should be placed over the wheelchair tire to decrease the effects of shearing to the buttocks.

Individuals with SCI at the C1 to C4 level are generally dependent for showering and need to be able to verbalize all the steps of care. Recommended home modifications will often include a roll-in shower, and a tilting roll-in shower chair is often prescribed (see Chapter 14). The ability of the chair to tilt is important for these individuals because this feature allows caregivers to easily perform weight shifts for the client. In addition, the tilt feature may be used if the individual regularly experiences orthostatic hypotension. The tilting roll-in chair is usually equipped with armrests that cradle the person's arms to help keep them in place. An opening, or cutout, in the seat portion of the chair is usually present to allow the caregiver access to the perineum for cleaning and possibly for bowel care management.

A mechanical lift can be used to transfer an individual into a roll-in shower chair (see Figure 14-8, *A*). If the person requires a ventilator, two caregivers are required to assist with bathing: one to provide manual ventilation with a valve mask resuscitator (Ambu bag) while the person is off the ventilator and the other to bathe the individual. Spouses or partners who bathe individuals with SCI often report showering with them to increase efficiency and sometimes to provide intimacy. It is prudent for the therapist to recommend that the caregiver wear nonskid shoes to prevent slips or falls during bathing.

Individuals with a C5 SCI also are usually dependent for bathing because splints providing wrist support necessary for functional activities are not typically worn in the shower. The patient, family, and rehabilitation team must choose between a tilting roll-in shower chair and an upright roll-in shower chair. The upright chair may be the most cost-effective and appropriate if the individual is able to tolerate an upright position in the chair. A chest strap for balance is recommended. Often individuals with C5 tetraplegia choose to have bed baths between shower days to decrease the work required for hygiene. Wrist supports can be worn during bed baths so that the individual can assist with upper body bathing if he so chooses.

With C6 level injury, individuals may be prescribed a roll-in shower chair if this will provide the most independence with bathing. Strong individuals can achieve a high level of independence using a chair in the tub that features a seat cutout, armrests, a back, and a ledge that rests on the edge of the tub for increased ease with transfers. Because of lack of finger function, individuals with C6 tetraplegia usually require several adaptations to increase safety and independence with bathing. Basic shower adaptations include a hand-held shower head. A U-shaped cuff purchased commercially or fabricated from splinting material can be applied to the shower head to allow manipulation without finger function. Environmental adaptations should include lever-type faucet controls and securely mounted grab bars.

Soaps and shampoos can be kept in bottles that the person finds easy to use, or liquid soap dispensers can be mounted in the shower. A bar of soap can be more easily handled by slipping it into the toe of an old pair of pantyhose and tying the hose to the grab bar so that dropped soap can be retrieved without difficulty; drilling a hole into the bar of soap and looping a rope through the hole so that the rope can be tied to the grab bar or bench; or slipping the bar of soap inside a pocket that is made by sewing three sides of two washcloths together. Sometimes individuals with C6 level injury use a wash mitt (see Figure 9-9) instead of handling a regular washcloth. One drawback to the wash mitt is that it can be difficult to move from one hand to the other while wet.

Washing hair can be a challenge for an individual with a C6 level injury because of the lack of functional triceps strength. Often a person with this level injury will lean over his lap while washing his hair and use gravity to help with his elbow extension. To wash his feet and lower legs, an individual with C6 SCI can lift one leg to cross his foot over his opposite knee. If he is not yet proficient with leg management, leaning forward over his lap offers access to his feet and lower legs, though the bottoms of his feet will be difficult to manage. The cutout in the seat of the bathroom equipment offers access to the individual's perineum.

Keeping towels within reach of the inside of the tub will eliminate the need for a caregiver's assistance. It is important for the individual to place a towel on the wheelchair cushion after transferring to the bathroom equipment and before beginning the shower. This will help to keep the cushion and cushion cover dry in case of accidental splashes as well as when transferring back to the chair.

Individuals with SCI at the C7 level will have triceps function and at the C8 to T1 level will begin to have finger function. The adaptations necessary for the person with C6 tetraplegia also may apply to individuals with C7 to T1 SCIs. In addition, wrapping rubber bands or nonskid strips around the shower head and soap containers can assist with manipulation of these items when an individual's grip is weak. A standard tub bench may be appropriate, depending on the individual's balance, body type, strength, and endurance.

People with paraplegia are typically able to achieve modified independence with bathing by using a tub bench without a cutout in a standard tub-shower. Full hand and arm function eliminates the need for many of the adaptations mentioned previously; however, grab bars and a hand-held shower head are still recommended. Perineum hygiene can be achieved by leaning side to side, although this method can prove dangerous and less than adequate. Perineum hygiene can also be performed after bowel management on the raised toilet seat instead of in the shower. Transferring to the bottom of the tub to bathe is an advanced skill for an individual with paraplegia. It is important that he protect his skin if bathing in the bottom of the tub by sitting on a cushion prescribed by a therapist for that purpose. Testing the temperature of the water before entering the tub is an important safety precaution.

DRESSING

Individuals with SCI at levels C1 to C4 will be dependent for dressing. The therapist should train caregivers in proper body mechanics during dependent dressing. By placing a knee up on the bed or onto a step stool next to the bed during dressing, the caregiver will decrease the amount of stress imposed on her back. It is important for the caregiver to raise or lower the bed to a level comfortable for her and to constantly be aware of the stress that her back is under. If the caregiver begins to feel too much stress, she should stop the activity, reassess the situation, and resume in a manner that is comfortable for her back.

It is possible for individuals with C5 tetraplegia to achieve modified independence with upper body dressing. This activity can require a lot of energy, and most individuals with injuries at the C5 level are dependent for lower body dressing. People with a C5-level injury may choose to have a caregiver perform upper body dressing so that time and energy can be saved for IADL. A person with C5 function who chooses to perform upper body dressing will require wrist support splints but otherwise will use the same techniques as an individual with C6 tetraplegia.

People with C6 tetraplegia can achieve modified independence with upper and lower body dressing. Especially while learning the skills, dressing takes much time and energy.[10] It is important that the therapist help the individual assess the importance of independence with these skills because the time and energy might be more meaningfully spent elsewhere.

An individual with C6-level injury can be independent donning a T-shirt from the wheelchair level. One technique used for this is to place one arm into the shirt, then the head, and then the other arm; in this way the individual keeps one arm free at all times to assist with balance (Figure 9-19). Getting the shirt down in the back is often the most difficult part of this activity, but it can be achieved by leaning forward in the chair to "shimmy" the shirt down.

The tradeoff between time saved by accepting assistance with dressing and psychological motivation and self-image achieved by an individual's own accomplishment is sharp edged. Each successful accomplishment leads to another challenge, which in turn leads to a greater sense of independence. The therapist is able to assess a person's special needs and provide training that pinpoints the most efficient techniques for that particular individual. Steps for upper extremity dressing that will help the individual save time and energy when putting on a polo shirt (Figure 9-20, A to D) or removing a sweatshirt may be learned (Figure 9-21, A to F). Once accomplished, these sequences allow an individual to choose whether to seek help with a process or to take care of his needs on his own; and when alone he is able to move on with appropriate care needs independently, whether the weather is hot or cold or he is just getting cleaned up.

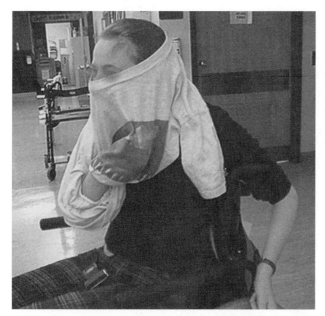

FIGURE 9-19 An individual with a C6 level injury dons a t-shirt; she keeps one upper limb free to hook over the wheelchair's push handle to assist with balance.

It is important that people with tetraplegia who use manual wheelchairs are able to put on wheelchair gloves (Figure 9-22, *A* to *C*). These gloves, sometimes referred to as flexion mitts, generally with Dycem palms and Velcro straps, protect the hands and fingers, which may be insensitive and therefore subject to blisters, lacerations, and abrasions. The gloves also provide a greater level of friction for those unable to grasp sufficiently to propel the wheel unassisted and may be used in a variety of tasks that require aids to dexterity.

Because of decreased finger dexterity, adaptive equipment is useful in helping people with tetraplegia facilitate buttons and zippers (Figure 9-23). A button aid attached to a U-cuff can be used for buttoning shirts. The individual should button up the shirt while it is placed in the lap, leaving the top two buttons open. At this point the shirt can be donned the same as a pullover shirt. Some people may find it easier to keep shirts buttoned even during laundering. Zippers can be adapted for a person with limited hand function by placing a key ring through the zipper or tying a small loop of fishing line through the zipper. Other options are to replace zippers and buttons with Velcro fasteners.

The patient with a C6 injury should have the following for lower body dressing: a double bed to provide room for rolling,

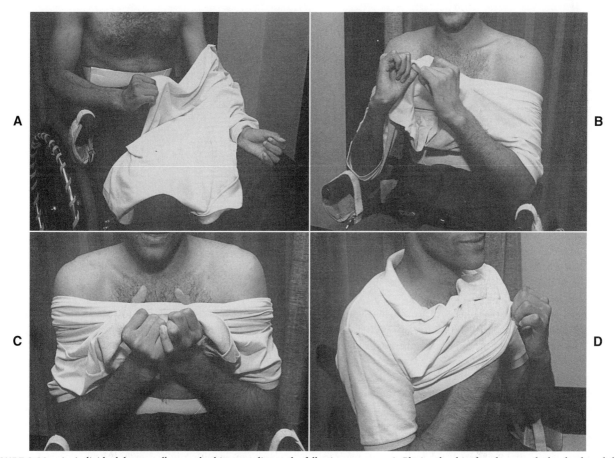

FIGURE 9-20 An individual dons a pullover polo shirt according to the following sequence: **A,** Placing the shirt face down on the lap, he threads his arms through the arm holes. **B,** He works the shirt as high as possible up the arms. **C,** He uses his thumbs to grab the shirt back material through the collar to bring it over his head. **D,** After the shirt is over his head, he pulls the front of the shirt down by using one hand inside and one outside the shirt to maneuver the material over his chest.

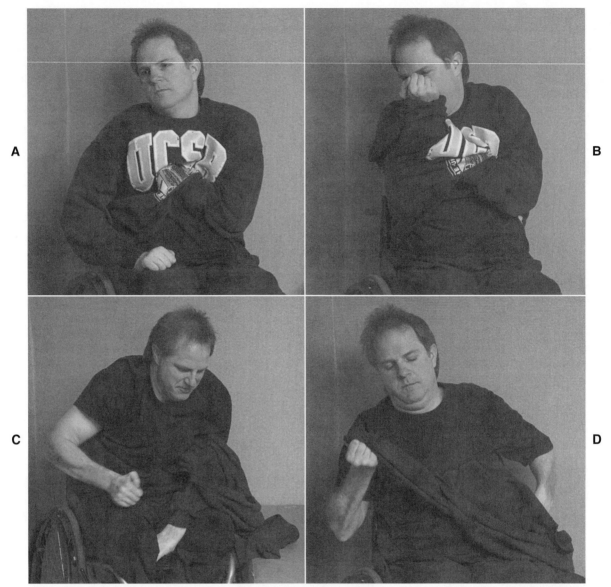

FIGURE 9-21   A different sequence demonstrates the skill needed to take off a sweatshirt. **A,** A person with tetraplegia first lifts his sweatshirt from underneath to pull out his right arm. **B,** He then grabs the end of the sleeve with his teeth and pulls his arm out from the sleeve while pulling the sweatshirt sleeve off with his left hand. **C,** After his right arm is out of the shirt, he pulls it over his head with his right hand. **D,** He pulls the shirt off of his left arm. Pulling a sweatshirt over the head can be very challenging for trunk balance and requires practice in stabilizing with the opposite arm not needed for overhead removal.

push gloves with Dycem in the palms to assist with managing the clothing, at least 90 degrees of hip flexion, and clothing within reach. There are many ways in which individuals with C6 injuries can perform lower body dressing. In a common technique the individual (1) comes to sit in the long-sitting position, (2) crosses his feet (one at a time) to lift his heels off the bed (Figure 9-24, *A*), (3) works the pants over his feet by using a tenodesis grasp and Dycem gloves, (4) pulls the pants up to the hips using hands in the pockets, fingers in the belt loops, tenodesis grasp, or the Dycem gloves, and (5) works both hands into the pants to avoid slipping and lies down. Then, he rolls to one side, placing a hand in the front of the pants and rotating the arm to get the hand in the back. Friction from the Dycem on the glove can be used to manipulate the pants and bring them over his bottom. An

individual may also use his wrist extensors to hook onto the waistband of the pants to pull them up (Figure 9-24, *B*). This procedure may require rolling several times.

Donning socks is also a difficult task for individuals with C6 tetraplegia. Some individuals think that ankle socks are easier to put on, and most prefer to do this task in bed rather than in the wheelchair. Again, wearing gloves with Dycem palms will make this task easier. Another option is to sew loops to the sides of the socks or make an adaptive tool out of splinting material.

Shoes can be put on in bed or in the wheelchair. Some prefer donning shoes in bed to protect their feet during the transfer and to give them more stability. Others think leg management is more difficult on the bed with shoes. Either way, crossing the foot over the opposite knee will lift the heel off the bed or footplate of

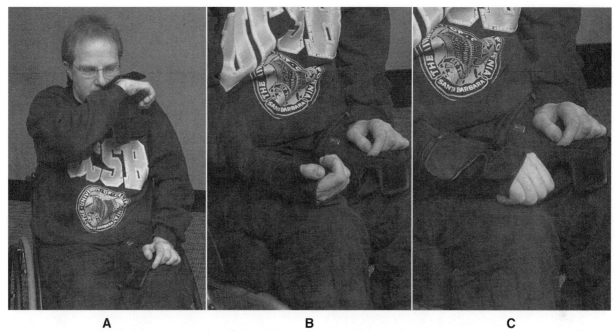

FIGURE 9-22   A person with tetraplegia dons his wheelchair gloves. **A,** First he pulls the thumb through the glove opening with his teeth. **B,** Then he places his hand and glove unit on his lap to maintain glove on hand until, **C,** the dorsal Velcro attachment can be closed with the opposite hand.

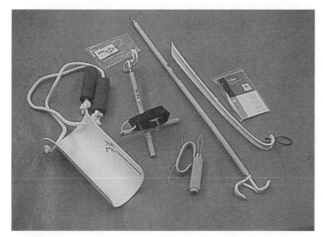

FIGURE 9-23   Various types of adaptive equipment used for dressing includes sock aid, adapted dressing stick, button aids, economy dressing stick, shoe horn, and elastic laces.

the chair. The shoe is grasped between the volar portions of both hands, placed over the toes, and is then pushed over the heel. Care should always be taken to avoid wrinkles in socks or shoes that are too tight, particularly if the feet swell. Because the feet have numerous bony prominences, they are susceptible to pressure ulcers with improper sock and shoe wear because of lack of sensation.

Individuals with paraplegia are expected to be independent with upper body dressing in a regular bed or wheelchair. The techniques for an individual with a C6 level injury and an individual with paraplegia are very similar when dressing in the bed, although the individual with paraplegia more easily masters the task. Finger dexterity makes tasks such as putting on shoes an easier operation (Figure 9-25, *A* to *C*). It is important to remember that there are many ways to achieve lower body dressing.

When bathing is performed before dressing, an individual may consider dressing in the wheelchair to decrease the number of transfers required. The ability to dress in a wheelchair is beneficial because it allows for clothing adjustments that enable bowel and bladder management and increased independence with dressing in the community (for example, when trying on clothing at a store). To don pants, socks, and shoes over the feet, an individual can either cross one ankle over the other, or lean forward with ankles crossed. When pulling pants over hips and buttocks, an individual may scoot forward and lean side to side to pull the pants over each hip; do a depression lift with the heels of his hands, walking the pants up the hips with his fingers; or scoot his hips forward into the pants by placing the hands in the sides of the pants, lifting, and pushing the hips forward.

SKIN CARE

Loss of sensation, increased moisture, and shearing forces all combine to increase the chance of pressure ulcers in individuals with SCI. Skin checks, weight shifts, and padding and positioning are three ways in which individuals with SCI must care for their skin.

Skin Checks

Skin checks involve inspecting the skin where there is decreased sensation, especially over bony prominences (see Figure 6-10). An individual or his caregiver looks for red or dark pressure spots, rashes, bruises, or marks from moisture or shearing. Skin checks should occur in bed in the morning and evening. Individuals with C1 to C5 level injuries are typically dependent for skin checks and must instruct caregivers in the correct way to complete a skin check.

Individuals with C6 to C8 level injuries can complete skin checks by using a mirror held with a tenodesis grasp or with a U-cuff handle that wraps around the hand (Figure 9-26). The back

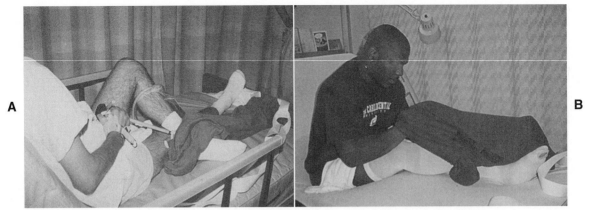

FIGURE 9-24   **A,** An individual with a C6 level injury crosses his foot over his opposite leg to lift his heel off the bed and gain access to his pointed foot to don his pants by using a modified dressing stick. **B,** A person uses his wrist extensors to hook onto the waistband of the pants to pull them up.

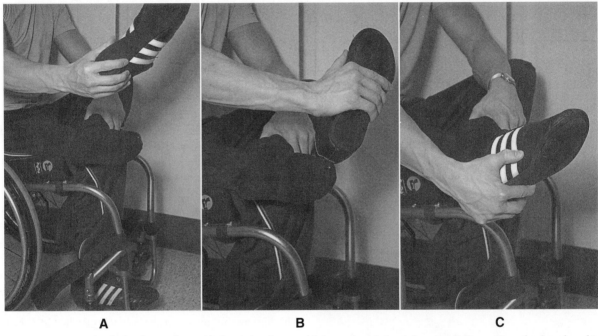

FIGURE 9-25   **A,** An individual with paraplegia with shoe in hand crosses his leg so that his foot is hanging. **B,** He positions the shoe above his toes and, **C,** slides the shoe over his toes and up onto his heel.

and buttocks are checked with the mirror when the person is in side lying or propped on one elbow. The sacral area is a common area for skin breakdown to occur and is a difficult area to see with a mirror. A full-length mirror can be mounted next to the bed and can be used with the hand mirror to increase skin visibility. Individuals must be able to sit up and complete leg management with adequate balance in a hospital or regular bed to effectively check the lower extremities. An individual with paraplegia also completes skin checks with a hand-held mirror by using these techniques.

Weight Shifts

Weight shifts are done when an individual is sitting upright by changing position in the wheelchair to prevent continuous pressure on parts of the body that are susceptible to development of pressure sores. The performance and frequency of weight shifts is

discussed in detail in the Chapter 7. According to Coggrave and Rose[11] patients should be instructed to perform weight shifts for a duration ranging from 42 seconds to 3 minutes 30 seconds. The frequency of weight shifting will be specific to the individual and the rehabilitation team will educate each patient on his best care practices, following consistent parameters among therapies. People with C1 to C5 level injuries can be independent with weight shifts in a power wheelchair by using a head or pneumatic control or switch or sip-n-puff control to tilt back the wheelchair (see Figure 11-44, *A*). If the individual does not have a power wheelchair, he must instruct the caregiver about when and how to complete weight shifts. A digital timer is a useful tool to remind him when a weight shift should be done.

Individuals with C6 to C8 injuries can also be independent with weight shifts. In a power chair, a switch to tilt the chair back will perform a weight shift. In manual chairs, an individual can lean

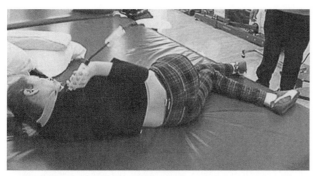

FIGURE 9-26   An individual with a C6 level injury practices performing skin checks with a long-handled mirror.

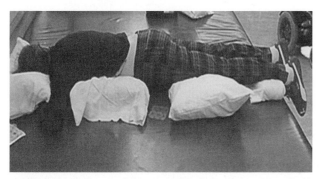

FIGURE 9-27   Pillow can be positioned under and around an individual with SCI that will float bony prominences to reduce pressure when she is lying prone.

forward so his chest rests on his lap or lean side to side to complete a weight shift. It is important for the patient to practice weight shifts and be able to come back to an upright position independently. In addition, it is important that weight is being sufficiently unloaded from the ischium during weight shift. Individuals without use of their fingers can use a knuckle or the eraser end of a pencil held in a splint or U-cuff to set a timer with buttons.

Patients with a C7 level or lower injury may be strong enough to do push-up weight shifts by lifting their buttocks off their cushion independently. If an individual is not strong enough to do this technique or needs to conserve energy, he can effectively complete any of the previously mentioned techniques independently.

Padding and Positioning

Padding and positioning include correct positioning in the wheelchair or bed to prevent skin breakdown and to maximize function. Pillows need to be placed above and below the bony prominences so that these areas are floating over rather than touching unyielding surfaces (Figure 9-27). Bony prominences must be padded with pillows in bed when an individual is lying on his back, side, and stomach to prevent skin breakdown. Specific areas that need padding include heels, toes, ankles, knees, and elbows. Individuals with C1 to C5 level injuries are dependent for padding and positioning; they must instruct their caregivers in these care needs. Those with a C6 injury and below can achieve independence with these skills.

It is also crucial that individuals with SCI are properly positioned in their wheelchairs to effectively complete ADLs

and IADLs. Improper positioning can negatively affect balance and thoracic, upper extremity and cervical ROM, and strength, thus limiting an individual's ability to engage in functional activities. In addition, sitting in the chair with a posterior pelvic tilt, also called sacral sitting, can cause tissue breakdown over the ischium, sacrum, and spinal processes. See Chapter 11 for additional information about wheelchair seating and positioning.

BLADDER MANAGEMENT

After SCI, normal bladder function is typically impaired but may be managed in several ways (see Chapter 3). According to Yavuzer et al,[12] the patient's family should be involved in decisions regarding a bladder program. The technique chosen, however, should reflect the preference of the patient.

For those individuals who have sustained C1 to C5 SCI, bladder management requires caregiver assistance. The individual should be able to instruct caregivers in all steps clearly and concisely and he should take responsibility for making sure the caregiver uses proper technique.

Bladder Management for Men

To be independent with intermittent catheterization (IC), the patient must be independent with clothing management in the wheelchair. Men master this task more easily than women because of anatomical differences. If elastic-waist pants are worn, a commercially available metal pants holder can be purchased or a bungee cord adapted with finger loops may be used to hold the pants down during the IC.

Those who choose to wear pants with an elastic waistband may have trouble keeping the penis upright for catheter insertion. Some individuals find propping the penis up with antibacterial wipes or a washcloth is sufficient. Others may find that using the HouseHold tool (Flexlife Medical, Kingwood, Tex.) is necessary to prop up the penis. Adler and Kirshblum[13] reported that using the HouseHold device was an easily learned means to promote independent IC for individuals with tetraplegia who otherwise would require an alternative method of neurogenic bladder management.

Many individuals choose to wear pants with zippers; adapted zippers can be easily managed and the penis can be pulled through the opening. Men with a C6 level injury or lower can be independent in the community and at home performing IC. Learning how to perform IC by using a clean technique allows the individual to be more independent and to be more flexible with his daily activities.[14] It also decreases the stigma associated with the physical appearance of a leg bag.[14,15]

Men who leak between IC or who have a reflexive bladder may choose to wear a leg bag attached to a condom catheter. The reflexive bladder schedule is more flexible, and an electric leg-bag emptier can be used by individuals with C5 to C6 injuries. Men who use a leg bag can unhook straps adapted with loops without finger dexterity. These loops also can be placed on the device that holds the condom in place. In addition, leg bags with flip levers are easier to open with limited finger function. Donning the condom can be a very difficult task; it can be done with the palm of the hands if an erection is

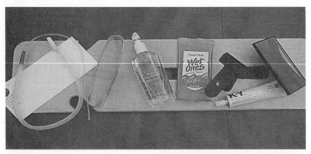

FIGURE 9-28 Supplies commonly used for intermittent catheterization include an envelope that can hold a Christmas tree connector already attached to the catheter, pants holder, hand sanitizer, antibacterial wipes, water-based lubricant, and mirror.

stimulated. For those who have a more difficult time with erection, a HouseHold tool can be used to prop and hold the penis in place.

Supplies should be kept in an accessible place in the home and in a traveling container with the person when he is away from home (Figure 9-28 and Table 9-3). Some individuals use a wheelchair bag for storage of IC items when traveling. The key to performing clean IC is to maintain a clean environment. Catheters must be handled as little as possible before insertion. Because of limited hand function, attaching tubing to the catheter can be a challenge in the community. To cut down on contamination, these attachments can be connected at home and both the tubing and catheter can be placed in an envelope or a brown paper sack. Use of 5-in-1 connectors can also make attachments easier to complete. Tubing management is another issue that frequently complicates community IC. To eliminate this, Velcro can be placed around the tubing and around the leg rest of the chair so that the tubing can be held in the correct position when urine is being eliminated. Another option is to place the tubing underneath the seat of the toilet to hold the tubing in place.

Bladder Management for Women

A woman with normal hand function can be independent with bladder management. A woman with tetraplegia, however, may choose not to do IC because of decreased hand function and the challenges female anatomy presents.[12] For a woman to perform IC with a clean technique, the labia must be spread to eliminate catheter contamination. For an individual with absent or limited hand function, a labia spreader can be fabricated out of splinting material to assist holding the labia away from the meatus. The spreader must be custom made to fit each individual. Practice and persistence is then necessary to achieve success with standard IC for women with limited hand function.

For women to be independent with IC, they typically need to reposition their hips and legs. In a wheelchair, a woman must scoot her hips forward on the seat cushion and place her legs either on the outside of the wheelchair frame and foot rests or up on a toilet seat or bed. Her pants need to be lowered far enough to allow for adequate positioning. To save time and energy, women may want to wear long skirts or adapt their pants by adding a placket that opens with Velcro or snaps. Care must be taken to prevent skin breakdown when the pants are adapted with hard snaps. Women will typically begin performing IC in bed by using

TABLE 9-3	Adaptive Equipment and Supplies for Catheterization	
Supplies for IC	Properties
Catheter	Can be reused for up to 1 week if washed with soap and water and stored in an envelope after each use
Tubing	Used to guide the urine from the catheter to the commode
5-in-1 connector	Attaches to the catheter and the tubing. Allows for an easier connection during task
Water-based lubricant	Reduces friction during insertion of the catheter
Antibacterial wipes or hand sanitizer	Used for cleaning penis and hands before and after IC. Can be stored in sandwich bag for easy accessibility with absent or limited finger function; however, should not be left in the bag, to avoid mildew
Pants holder	Holds the pants down during male IC
Mirror	May assist a female during IC

a mirror. Eventually a touch technique may be used, which eliminates the need to rely on a mirror.[3]

It is easier for a caregiver to perform clean intermittent IC dependently when an individual is in bed versus a wheelchair. IC must be completed several times throughout the day, and it is often not feasible for someone to get back into bed several times a day to accommodate bladder care assistance, especially if she plans to return to school or work. For such people, a tilt-space wheelchair may make bladder management easier when out in the community. Women may also consider surgery for suprapubic catheterization. Suprapubic catheterization allows access to the bladder through the abdomen; leakage between IC also can be controlled. In this way, a woman can use a leg bag and decrease the number of ICs necessary each day. There are additional surgical options for women who need flexibility and control over bladder care regimens, Individuals with tetraplegia should work closely with their physicians to establish the best bladder care methods for their lifestyles.

BOWEL MANAGEMENT

As with bladder management, bowel function is also affected by SCI (see Chapter 3). Bowel management programs should be initiated and patient and caregivers trained early in the rehabilitation process.[16] The most common bowel programs include digital stimulation and manual evacuation.[17] According to Kirshblum et al,[18] bowel problems can limit a person's ability to be independent. Educating the family and the patient on daily fiber and fluid intake is important, as well as performing the program consistently and at the appropriate time. Kirshblum et al also found that most acute-care hospitals performed bowel programs in the evening, but after discharge individuals performed their programs in the morning.[18] Therefore, interviewing the patient about premorbid voiding routines and including him in planning the rehabilitation schedule can help prepare him for seamless postdischarge bowel management because bowel programs are most effective when performed at the same time every day. If the patient or caregiver is considering changing the time or type of bowel program, care should be taken to prevent accidents or constipation.

Individuals with C1 to C5 level injuries are dependent with bowel management but should be able to instruct caregivers in all steps of the process. Bowel programs can be performed in the bed or a shower chair over the commode. Bowel programs are often more successful and less time consuming when the program is performed in the upright sitting position because gravity assists with elimination. The individual and caregiver should decide together the most desirable method. Regardless of this choice, it is important for an individual and his caregiver to discuss and plan daily routines that will optimize efficiency. For example, a caregiver and individual with SCI may decide to perform the bowel program before bathing in the roll-in shower.

Depending on the type of bowel management program, an individual with a C6 level injury or below can be independent with his bowel management. Two types of bowel management programs are (1) digital stimulation and (2) suppository with manual evacuation. These programs are based on the presence of a bulbocavernosus reflex (BCR) and an individual's rectal sensation. For those with BCR and little to no rectal sensation, a digital stimulation program is performed. A person with limited grasp will need a digital bowel stimulator and splint to perform this program independently (Figure 9-29). Splints can be fabricated or purchased from commercial vendors. An individual with paraplegia will not need a digital bowel stimulator as long as he has sufficient reach to perform the program with his gloved finger. For those without sufficient reach, a digital bowel stimulator can be used without a splint.

For those individuals without BCR or who have rectal sensation, a suppository program can be initiated.[19] A person must have functional pinch dexterity to hold a suppository and intact sensation and proprioception of the hand. A commercial suppository inserter can be purchased for those without finger function. Few individuals are independent with this program at C6 to C8 level injuries because optimal response is associated with the rectal vault being emptied of stool before the insertion of the suppository. Individuals without finger function often choose to have the caregiver perform the rectal clearance and insert the suppository. Adequate rectal tone is also necessary to keep the suppository from falling out. Individuals with inadequate rectal tone may want to insert the suppository in bed and allow enough time for the suppository to dissolve before transferring to the toilet.

An individual with paraplegia should be able to perform rectal clearance and insert a suppository without assistance. For a person with paraplegia who has an areflexive bowel, rectal clearance may need to be performed after every meal to prevent bowel accidents. It is important to achieve this skill in the community so the individual is not confined to the home for meals.

COMMUNICATION

Writing, typing, and accessing phones, computers, and call systems are all means of communicating with others. Individuals with SCI can retain independence in communication tasks by using adaptive equipment, computer technology, and environmental control units (see Chapter 13). A lap tray provides an accessible surface for someone to reach communication devices with a mouthstick or with the upper limbs. The therapist often works with individuals to setup a lap tray to optimize interaction with the environment. For instance, applying Velcro to the tray and devices including cellular phone, television remote, or personal digital assistant will prevent the devices from sliding off the tray during weight shifts (Figure 9-30).

Writing and Typing

With good oral structure and enough cervical ROM and strength, individuals with C1 to C4 level injuries can complete writing, typing, or page-turning activities with minimum setup assistance. The therapist can prescribe appropriate mouthsticks for different activities (see Chapter 13). A variety of mouthsticks are commercially available to meet a patient's goals: a standard mouthstick with a rubber end may be used to turn pages or play cards, whereas a mouthstick with an implement holder can hold a pen or pencil for writing. It is especially important that individuals with C1 to C4 injuries maintain good oral hygiene because they will use mouthsticks to access their environment.[20,21] Without good dental health, the use of adaptive equipment for communication will be limited.

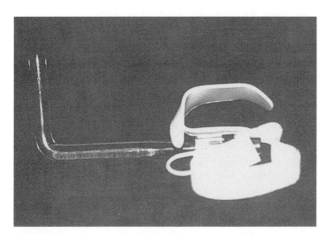

FIGURE 9-29 An example of a digital stimulator modified with a splint for use in a bowel management program.

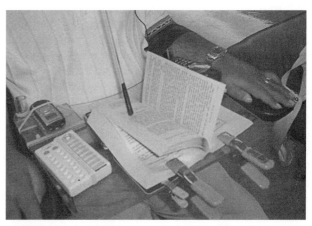

FIGURE 9-30 An individual with a C4 level injury uses a lap tray setup for independent work.

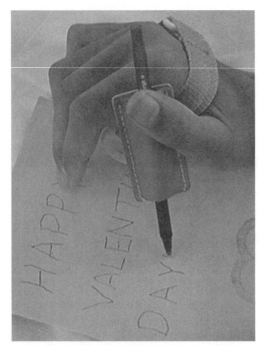

FIGURE 9-31 An individual with a C6 level injury uses a U-cuff and a right-angle pocket for a writing activity.

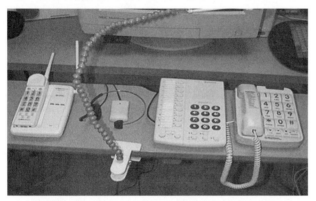

FIGURE 9-32 Examples of several home phone systems.

Setup and positioning of equipment is also crucial to maximize independence for individuals with C1 to C4 tetraplegia. For example, a magazine and book holder can be positioned, along with a mouthstick holder, to allow page turning with modified independence.[22] Individuals with a C5-level injury are able to use their upper limbs to interact with the environment and do not need a mouthstick. With proper support of his wrists, an individual with a C5 SCI can write with devices such as a long Wanchick hand-based writer tool or a right-angle pocket (Figure 9-31). Page turning can be achieved by placing a pencil in the wrist support cuff with the eraser extending medially from the palm. The friction of the eraser against the paper allows the individual to flip through pages with modified independence. Donning splints with pencils placed bilaterally will allow an individual to type.

People with C6 to C7 level injuries will use the same techniques described previously but will not require a wrist splint. Because these individuals have wrist extension, a U-cuff may be all that is needed to assist with grasp. A tenodesis brace can assist someone

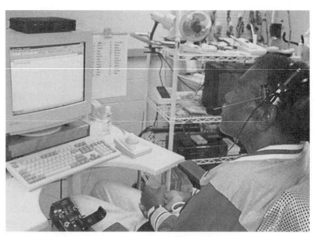

FIGURE 9-33 An individual with tetraplegia uses voice recognition software to increase his independence with school, work, or home computer activities.

with C6 to C7 injuries to strengthen and improve tenodesis grasp for activities such as writing. Tenodesis braces may be constructed of splinting material or fabricated by an orthotist. The finger function present for individuals with C8 to T1 level injuries will allow the use of a pen or pencil, possibly built up with foam.

Phone Access

It is advisable that all individuals with tetraplegia have access to a telephone for safety. In the home, a speakerphone allows an individual with C1 to C4 injuries to use a mouthstick to independently dial or hit preprogrammed memory buttons. Telephones with pneumatic controls can also provide access for an individual with limited upper limb function. A mobile phone with larger buttons allows a person to easily dial and answer the phone. Some cellular phones come standard with hands-free technology and are excellent options for anyone with tetraplegia.

People with C5 to C8 injuries may use a cuff on the earpiece of a regular phone or use their tenodesis grasp to handle the phone. The phone can be dialed either by using the eraser end of a pencil in a wrist support or U-cuff or by using a knuckle. The therapist can explore all the options and assist the patient in determining the most appropriate system for his access to the phone (Figure 9-32).

Computer Access and Electronic Aids for Daily Living

Access to and knowledge about computers allows an individual with tetraplegia to perform tasks in school or work settings, participate in leisure activities, and communicate through e-mail and computerized phone systems. There are a number of software programs available that provide hands-free technology such as switches or voice recognition (Figure 9-33) (see Chapter 13). Sometimes these systems require direct keyboard access through the use of a mouthstick.[23]

An individual with an SCI also may rely on an environmental control unit (ECU), more currently called electronic aids to daily living (EADLs), to access a call system, which allows him to call caregivers for assistance when needed. EADLs also let him operate electrical devices such as telephones, TVs, lamps or other lighting, radios, and even drapes and doors through infrared or

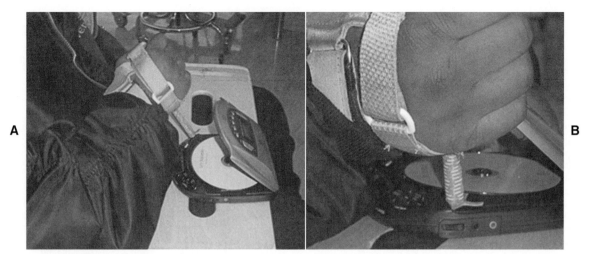

FIGURE 9-34 An individual with limited hand function (**A**) uses an eraser tip end of a pencil to operate a CD player's buttons to (**B**) change the CD.

other technology.[24] When the electrical device is plugged into a unit, a master remote can be operated with voice activation, mouthstick, an eraser end of a pencil in a splint, or the patient's knuckle. The device offers some control over the home environment and the call system permits a person and his caregivers to feel safe when he is alone in a room for short periods.

Because software, computer programs, and ECUs change and improve constantly, an assistive technology specialist should prescribe the appropriate systems for individuals with tetraplegia to enable them to be as independent as possible (see Chapter 13).

Indeed, no- and low-technology solutions are often used with electronic equipment in rehabilitation and home settings. As already mentioned, an eraser end of a pencil on a splint can provide individuals with cervical injuries with limited hand function to control button-operated equipment. Such an interface between a patient and electronics can offer enjoyment and be a potent motivational tool that helps him increase dexterity as he relearns a variety of daily skills (Figure 9-34, *A* and *B*).

The future holds great promise with new technology such as the BrainGate Neural Interface System, which consists of a sensor implanted on the brain's motor cortex with a wireless link to a device that interprets the brain's signals. Neurotechnology innovator Cyberkinetics is currently partnering with three leading rehabilitation centers in clinical trials for patients with SCI, stroke, muscular dystrophy, and amyotrophic lateral sclerosis.[25] The system operates on the principle that intact brain function can generate brain signals that when received will mimic cursor movements and allow the individual to control a computer with thought in the same way that able-bodied people use their hands to access the mouse or keyboard.

HOME MANAGEMENT

The former and current roles of the individual in the home setting should be considered before home management tasks are addressed.[1] Home management activities include cooking, washing dishes, general cleaning, and laundry. Individuals with C1 to C5 injuries are typically dependent with most home management tasks. Those with C6 to C8 injuries may gain some independence with meal preparation and light home management tasks. Individuals with paraplegia should be able to complete both light and heavy home management activities (Box 9-2). Independence can be enhanced at all levels of SCI by rearranging the home environment to allow the individual to reach necessary objects and by using long-handled cleaning tools.

Cooking

For an individual with SCI to increase independence with cooking, the kitchen should be reorganized to permit him to reach items needed for cooking (see Chapter 9). Heavy objects, such as pots and pans, should be placed within arm reach, typically in lower cabinets. Lighter objects, such as spices and pantry items, can be placed in higher cabinets because they can be retrieved with a long-handled reaching tool. A side-by-side refrigerator and freezer can provide a person with access to both refrigerated and frozen foods (Figure 9-35).

Working with hot items is the primary safety concern for a person with decreased sensation. An individual should never carry a hot object on his lap because it will burn his skin. A rolling cart can be used to decrease the risk of burns. Transfer boards or wooden trays also can be used to transport multiple light items to increase efficiency while working in the kitchen and around the house (see Figure 9-35). Sliding items along the counter and using a rolling cart also makes moving items around the kitchen easier and safer.

People who spend a lot of time cooking may consider modifying the kitchen significantly to promote efficiency. Free-standing ovens elevated off the floor are easier to reach and decrease the chance of burns. A roll-under range allows easier use of the stovetop. Lazy Susan shelving and pull-out cabinets provide greater access to kitchen items.

Washing Dishes

Roll-under kitchen sinks make it possible for an individual in a wheelchair to wash dishes. Just as in the bathroom, however, an individual with SCI must be protected from burns because of decreased skin sensation by having all exposed pipes insulated. Lever faucets let an individual without finger function manipulate

BOX 9-2 | Light and Heavy Home Management Tasks

Light Home Management Tasks
- Laundry, dusting
- Tidying up around the home
- Bed making
- Emptying and loading the dishwasher
- Light cleaning

Heavy Home Management Tasks
- Cleaning bathrooms
- Scrubbing bathtubs
- Washing floors
- Vacuuming
- Stripping and remaking the entire bed
- Cleaning baseboards

the faucet. A person may also consider elevating a dishwasher so that he may more easily reach the bottom rack.

General Cleaning

An individual with paraplegia should be independent with general cleaning. He should be able to lean forward or to the side to pick items off the floor. Sweeping can be accomplished by several different techniques, such as leaning forward and holding a dust pan in one hand and a hand-held broom in the other while propelling the wheelchair across the floor with the hands. Other options for sweeping include using a regular broom and long-handled dust pan or using a commercially available lightweight sweeper. A variety of cordless and lightweight vacuum cleaners are available. Long-handled dusters and window washers can be used to clean out-of-reach areas while conserving energy.[3]

Laundry

Front-loading washers and dryers are ideal for all people completing laundry tasks from a seated position. If a top-loading machine is the only option, an individual with paraplegia can use a mirror mounted to the inside of the lid to see the clothes and a long-handled reacher to retrieve the clothes. Economy dressing sticks and reachers also can be used to access controls that are out of an arm's reach. Clothes may be stored on shelves, lowered closet rods, or in drawers so that an individual with SCI can be independent in putting his clothing away.

CHILD CARE

Individuals with any level of SCI should be encouraged to participate in child care whether in decision making, discipline, or playing an active role in the child's care. Every activity will help to strengthen the bond between parent and child. According to Palmer et al,[26] most published research focuses on parents with disabilities, adaptive equipment, and resources for social support. Through the Looking Glass is an Internet resource center for parents with disabilities, which has found that adaptive equipment helps parents with disabilities better care for their child while minimizing their need for physical assistance.[27] Adaptive equipment can allow a parent to have close interactions with his child by decreasing the physical demands of child care (Table 9-4).

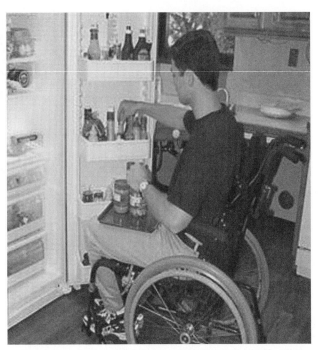

FIGURE 9-35 An individual with paraplegia working in the kitchen efficiently accesses both refrigerator and freezer in this side-by-side unit while using the transfer board in his lap to transport light items.

TABLE 9-4 | Adaptive Equipment to Use with Child Care

Product	Use	Level of Injury
Cosleeper	Reduces transfers during nighttime hours	All levels
Baby slings	Keeps child close to the individual's body; helpful for decreased upper limb strength or while propelling a manual wheelchair	All levels
Adapted diapers	Cloth diapers can be adapted with loops and Velcro for decreased hand function	C6, C7, C8
Adapted bibs and clothing	Commercially available or items may be adapted with loops and Velcro for decreased hand function	C6, C7, C8
Telephone clip holders	May be added to bottles to assist with limited hand function	C5, C6, C7, C8
Bath washing centers	All in one centers that can be filled with water and placed in an accessible location for bathing	All levels

A variety of commercially equipment appropriate for different levels of injury is available that can increase child care participation for an individual with an SCI. Fanny pack baby carriers or lap free carriers can be used to free a parent's hands for functional activities and are designed specifically for wheelchair users. There are also baby seat attachments for power chairs, which give parents with limited upper limb function the ability to play with their child. This seat can be rotated to maximize accessibility and to permit the parent to have close physical contact with the child. Lifting harnesses are also available for individuals with limited fine motor coordination, grasp strength, or trunk instability to lift a child more independently. For older children, climb-up steps let a child climb up a power or manual wheelchair into the parent's lap.

Feeding

Adapted high chairs may increase a parent's independence in feeding his child. When selecting an adapted high chair, it is important to look at features such as adjustable seat height and wide base of support that will allow for wheelchair access. Swing-away trays also offer better accessibility. Adaptations of equipment, such as using a phone cuff for the baby bottle, let the individual with limited or absent hand function hold the bottle. Tenodesis braces or U-cuffs may be used for feeding infants solid foods.

Bathing and Dressing

Clothing adaptations can be made to the infant's clothes so that a parent with SCI can be more independent with dressing the child. Similar to his own clothing, loops for zipper management, clothes with fewer snaps or adapted with Velcro closures help a parent with limited upper limb function dress his children. Selecting larger clothing and pullover tops will also promote ease when dressing children.

Adapted bath tubs that are height adjustable allow a parent in a wheelchair to safely bathe a child. Other adaptations can be made to bathing equipment such as adapted clothes washer, pump soap dispensers, and hand-held shower heads to promote ease with the child's bath time.

CLINICAL CASE STUDY **Activities of Daily Living Case 1**

Patient History
Perry Jacobs is a 29-year-old man with a C5 tetraplegia, ASIA A diagnosis resulting from a motor vehicle accident. He is 3 months post injury and medically stable. His injury did not require surgery. He has completed acute care and inpatient rehabilitation and has been attending outpatient therapy for 1 week. He is using a power tilt-in-space wheelchair. He has improved in using his residual strength and ability to compensate. Perry is now attending outpatient physical and occupational therapy to optimize his self-care.

Perry is a computer programmer. He lives with his wife and their home has been modified to meet his needs. He has an attendant who comes 6 days a week for 2 to 3 hours a day.

Patient's Self-Assessment
Perry wants to achieve the greatest independence with as little equipment as possible.

He hopes to return to work at his office 2 to 3 days a week and work from home on the other days. His employer is willing to work toward this outcome and will help with modifications needed in the workplace.

Clinical Assessment
Patient Appearance
- Height 5 feet 9 inches, weight 150 pounds, body mass index 22.1

Cognitive Assessment
- Alert, oriented ×3

Cardiopulmonary Assessment
- Blood pressure 110/62 mm Hg, heart rate at rest 68 beats/min, respiratory rate 14 breaths/min, cough flows are ineffective (<360 L/min), vital capacity is reduced (between 1.5 and 2.5 L)

Musculoskeletal and Neuromuscular Assessment
- Motor assessment is intact to the C5 level
- Deep tendon reflexes 3+ below the level of lesion

Integumentary and Sensory Assessment
- Skin is intact throughout; sensory is intact to C5

Range of Motion Assessment
- Passive and active ROM is within normal limits in both upper limbs except shoulder external rotation, which is limited to 75 degrees on the left and 78 degrees on the right

- Straight leg raise is 90 degrees in both lower limbs and dorsiflexion is 0 degrees; all other motions in the lower limbs are within functional limits

Mobility and ADL Assessment
- Dependent with bed mobility
- Semidependent, requiring maximal assistance in bed transfers using a transfer board; dependent in shower chair and toilet transfers
- Independent with pressure relief in power wheelchair
- Independent in power wheelchair maneuvering on all surfaces
- Dependent in bowel and bladder care
- Dependent in upper body dressing and in lower body dressing
- Dependent in driving

Equipment
- Transfer board to assist family and caregiver in providing help with transfers; shower chair

Evaluation of Clinical Assessment
Perry Jacobs is a 29-year-old man with a C5 tetraplegia, ASIA A diagnosis as a result of a motor vehicle accident. He is 3 months post injury and medically stable. He has attended outpatient therapy for 1 week. Perry is using a power tilt-in-space wheelchair and has improved in using his residual strength and ability to compensate. He is now being evaluated for ADL equipment needs for optimal self-care with minimal setup and for return to work needs as a computer programmer.

Patient's Care Needs
1. Evaluation for adaptive equipment for self-care and occupational therapy evaluation for night splints for positioning of hands
2. Evaluation by wheelchair seating clinic for cushion needs and potential for backup manual wheelchair in the event the power wheelchair is in need of repair
3. Evaluation by occupational therapist for adaptive equipment for workspace needs
4. Evaluation by physical therapist for optimal functional strategies for work and home transfers and positional control for functional ADL strategies
5. Evaluation of home with assessment to determine home modifications and durable medical equipment to ease caregiver requirements

Continued

CLINICAL CASE STUDY Activities of Daily Living Case 1—cont'd

Diagnosis and Prognosis
Diagnosis is C5 complete tetraplegia, ASIA A, with a prognosis of improved ADL function with efficient use of equipment to maximize Perry's functional potential with as little assistance as possible.

Preferred Practice Patterns*
Impaired Muscle Performance (4C), Impairments Nonprogressive Spinal Cord Disorders (5H), Primary Prevention/Risk Reduction for Cardiovascular/Pulmonary Disorders (6A), Primary Prevention/Risk Reduction for Integumentary Disorders (7A)

Team Goals
1. Team to evaluate for adaptive equipment to achieve self-care and to provide greatest independence
2. Team to evaluate for adaptive equipment to provide greatest independence and efficiency with daily home and office needs
3. Team to provide optimal use of selected adaptive equipment during interventions
4. Team to evaluate home modifications and durable medical equipment needs on the basis of the home visit

Patient Goals
"I want to be as independent as possible at home and work."

Care Plan
Treatment Plan and Rationale
- Initiate evaluations for optimal adaptive equipment
- Initiate application of interventions that provide optimal use of adaptive equipment for home and office needs
- Reinforce patient and caregiver instruction for pulmonary hygiene, skin care, bowel and bladder management, and ROM maintenance for home and work environments
- Initiate physical therapy interventions for restoration of functional activities limitations
- Evaluate for driving skills and vehicle modifications to enable independent transportation to work environment

Interventions
- Practice functional position changes, transfers to all surfaces, and strengthening exercises to increase available musculature
- Provide workspace modifications to enhance independence at home and office
- Order necessary home and office durable medical equipment to enhance independence in ADL (e.g., toileting, bathing)
- Instruct patient and family to manage respiratory hygiene, skin care, bowel and bladder management, and ROM maintenance
- Instruct patient to manage his care including weight shifts, home exercise program, passive ROM, transfers, wheelchair management on flat surfaces, stairs, curbs, and in the community
- Initiate driver's training

Documentation and Team Communication
- Team meeting once a week to discuss updates in functional goals, ADL skills, especially transfers to all surfaces and strengthening goals
- Communicate about workspace needs and demands on upper limbs for strengthening and endurance emphasis
- Discuss assistive technology needs regarding workplaces at home and office
- Communicate regarding driver's training and transportation needs

Follow-Up Assessment
- Monthly team meetings and reassessments of identified team and patient goals

Critical Thinking Exercises
Consider factors that will influence Perry's therapeutic exercises and ADL training, patient and family education, and transfer and mobility progression associated with his desire for an independent lifestyle and return to work when answering the following questions:
1. What equipment and positioning will Perry need for optimal independence when eating?
2. What considerations and equipment are applicable to Perry's needs for daily grooming and dressing?
3. Describe the types of adaptations that will be necessary for Perry to type on his computer in the home or office?

*Guide to physical therapist practice, rev. ed. 2, Alexandria, VA, 2003, American Physical Therapy Association.

CLINICAL CASE STUDY Activities of Daily Living Case 2

Patient History
Lisa Adams is a 36-year-old woman with a C6 tetraplegia, ASIA B diagnosis. She was injured in a motor vehicle accident 4 months ago. Her acute-care course was complicated with a urinary tract infection and a deep vein thrombosis that prolonged her acute stay. She underwent a spinal fusion and wiring and wore a sternal occipital mandibular immobilizer for 6 weeks and Philadelphia collar for 3 weeks. She was discharged from inpatient therapy at 14 weeks post injury and has been attending outpatient therapy for 2 weeks.

Lisa is a stay-at-home mom and lives in a fully accessible ranch house. Her three children are ages 5, 7, and 9 years. Her husband is a dentist and his office is attached to their home. Lisa uses both a lightweight manual and a power wheelchair. She has recently passed her driver's test and uses her power wheelchair for access in the community and when driving her van. The van has a power lift for ease of entry. Lisa is assisted by an attendant 2 hours each morning and a housekeeper three times a week.

Patient's Self-Assessment
Lisa wants to be able to improve her self-care and feel better about her appearance overall. She is concerned about her adequacy as a mother and wife.

Clinical Assessment
Patient Appearance
- Height 5 feet 3 inches, weight 119 pounds, body mass index 21.1

Cognitive Assessment
- Alert, oriented ×3

Cardiopulmonary Assessment
- Blood pressure 108/60 mm Hg, heart rate at rest 66 beats/min, respiratory rate 12 breaths/min, cough flows are ineffective (<360 L/min), vital capacity is reduced (between 1.5 and 2.5 L)

CLINICAL CASE STUDY Activities of Daily Living Case 2—cont'd

Musculoskeletal and Neuromuscular Assessment
- Motor assessment reveals C6 ASIA B, sensation is intact throughout
- Deep tendon reflexes 3+ below the level of lesion

Integumentary and Sensory Assessment
- Skin is intact throughout; sensory is intact throughout

Range of Motion Assessment
- Passive and active motion are within normal limits in both upper limbs except shoulder abduction 170 degrees on the left and 172 degrees on the right
- Straight leg raise is 100 degrees in both lower limbs and dorsiflexion is 5 degrees; all other motions in the lower limbs are within functional limits

Mobility and ADL Assessment
- Minimal assistance in bed mobility
- Independent in bed transfers with a transfer board
- Dependent in shower chair and toilet transfers
- Independent with pressure relief in both her power and manual wheelchairs
- Independent in power wheelchair maneuvering on all surfaces
- Independent with her manual wheelchair maneuvering in her home
- Dependent in bowel and bladder management
- Independent in upper body dressing
- Dependent in lower body dressing
- Independent with minimal assistance with grooming
- Independent in transportation needs; has passed driver's test

Equipment
- Power and manual wheelchair; wheelchair-accessible van; transfer board

Evaluation of Clinical Assessment
Lisa Adams is a 36-year-old woman with a C6 tetraplegia, ASIA B diagnosis. She was injured in a motor vehicle accident 4 months ago. She was discharged from inpatient rehabilitation at 14 weeks post injury and has been attending outpatient therapy for 2 weeks.

Patient's Care Needs
1. Evaluation for occupational therapy adaptive equipment to enable self-care and home management
2. Evaluation for physical therapy optimal functional strategies for home transfers and positional control for functional ADL strategies

Diagnosis and Prognosis
Diagnosis is C6 incomplete tetraplegia, ASIA B. Lisa's prognosis is for improved ADL function with efficient use of equipment to maximize her functional potential with as little assistance as possible.

Preferred Practice Patterns*
Impaired Muscle Performance (4C), Impairments Nonprogressive Spinal Cord Disorders (5H), Primary Prevention/Risk Reduction for Cardiovascular/Pulmonary Disorders (6A), Primary Prevention/Risk Reduction for Integumentary Disorders (7A)

Team Goals
1. Team to evaluate patient for adaptive equipment for self-care and daily home needs to provide greatest independence and efficiency
2. Team to provide interventions that teach and provide optimal use of selected adaptive equipment
3. Team to instruct family, including children, regarding pressure relief, wheelchair maneuverability, grooming, and hygiene needs

Patient Goals
"I want to be the best mother and wife that I can."

Care Plan
Treatment Plan and Rationale
- Initiate evaluations for optimal use of adaptive equipment for home
- Initiate application of interventions that provide optimal use of adaptive equipment for home
- Initiate physical therapy interventions for restoration of functional activities limitations
- Schedule a home evaluation to determine assistive technology needs to enhance independence in the management of the home environment

Interventions
- Evaluate outpatient occupational and physical therapy treatment to include strengthening, position changes, transfers to all surfaces, and practice with adaptive equipment for independent grooming and hygiene
- Instruct patient and family to manage her care including weight shifts, skin care, bowel and bladder management, home exercise program, passive and active ROM, transfers, wheelchair management, and mobility at home and in the community

Documentation and Team Communication
- Team meeting 1 week after team evaluations to discuss use of assistive technology for independence at home with minimal setup
- Team communication regarding patient and family knowledge of prevention of pressure ulcers, bowel and bladder management, and wheelchair safety during transport

Follow-Up Assessment
- Monthly team meetings and reassessments of identified team and patient goals

Critical Thinking Exercises
Consider factors that will influence the therapeutic exercises, patient and family education, transfer and mobility progression, and team care decisions associated with Lisa's desire for an independent lifestyle and specific ADL considerations when answering the following questions:
1. Describe the optimal setup for makeup application and nail care for Lisa.
2. Describe the optimal bathing routine for Lisa.
3. What considerations should the team chart to help Lisa in managing her home environment and family care?
4. How can the team help Lisa implement strategies for meal preparation for her family?

*Guide to physical therapist practice, rev. ed. 2, Alexandria, VA, 2003, American Physical Therapy Association.

THE CLIENT'S PERSPECTIVE   Managing Day-to-Day Activities

After rehabilitation, we need to apply all the new skills we've learned. Hopefully a major dose of critical thinking and problem-solving activity was part of that training because there we'll face lots of practical challenges along the way. Some of the keys for success include the following:

- Retain our perspective as individuals rather than patients
- Focus on what we are still able to do as a starting point
- Work on the interrelationship of mind, body, and spirit as well as ADL skills
- Learn how our bodies function in every way possible
- Set daily routines to manage body care: skin checks, stretching, bowel programs are imperative
- Learn what foods and beverages are best for our bodies
- Have the courage to test our wings

Sarah says, "Graduate school was the first time I was with a large group of people who did not know me before my injury, which let me test my newly found self. Could I still make friends who knew nothing about me even though I had to catheterize and manage my bowels differently, even though I couldn't keep up with walking pace when going up hill, even though I was so different and the first wheelchair-using student the George Washington School of Public Health had ever had? Could I manage all of the activities of daily living that are necessary to be independent, including cooking, which was hardly my forte? The only way to know was to try, and thankfully, the answer was a resounding yes. Not that it was always easy, mind you, but it was what I needed to prove to myself that I could continue to lead the same sort of life I had wanted before my SCI, the difference was that I was doing it using a wheelchair.

Scott Chesney and Sarah Everhart Skeels

SUMMARY

ADLs and IADLs are an integral part of functional independence for individuals with SCI, and this chapter addressed how therapists guide, educate, and retrain patients with varying levels of injury so that they may make choices about how to continue important life roles after a physical disability.

Functional outcomes for patients with SCI are largely dependent on the level and completeness of the injury. Therapists play a crucial role in training people to regain an optimal level of functional independence after SCI. Occupational therapists introduce their patients to the numerous devices and their use for feeding, grooming, oral care, facial hygiene, hair care, and other ADLs, which enhance independence. Although individuals with high-level cervical injuries may be completely dependent on others for ADLs, therapists provide a pivotal role in teaching patients to become proficient in instructing caregivers about their individual needs. This training is important to the patient's safety and psychological well-being.

ADL and IADL training also include communication needs such as writing, typing, and computer use; home management; and child care. Among the specific skills discussed in this chapter, hygiene care including bathing, skin care, and bowel and bladder management becomes tantamount to continuing skin integrity, health, and feelings of personal daily cleanliness and freshness. The therapist works to empower her patients because loss of privacy during personal hygiene can be one of the most disturbing aspects of functional dependence when patients with greater disability need continual caregiver assistance.

REFERENCES

1. Foti D, Kanazawa LM: Activities of daily living. In Pendleton HM, Schultz-Krohn W, editors: *Pedretti's occupational therapy: practice skills for physical dysfunction*, ed 6, St. Louis, 2006, Mosby Elsevier.
2. Adler C: Spinal cord injury. In Pendleton HM, Schultz-Krohn W, editors: *Pedretti's occupational therapy: practice skills for physical dysfunction*, ed 6, St. Louis, 2006, Mosby Elsevier.
3. Atrice M, Morison S, McDowell S et al: Traumatic spinal cord injury. In Umphred D, editor: *Neurological rehabilitation*, ed 5, St. Louis, 2005, Mosby Elsevier.
4. Hammell KR: Psychological and sociological theories concerning adjustment to traumatic spinal cord injury: the implication for rehabilitation, *Paraplegia* 30:317-326, 1992.
5. Hamilton BB, Laughlin JA, Granger CV et al: Interrater agreement of the seven level functional independence measure (FIM), *Arch Phys Med Rehabil* 72:790-801, 1991.
6. Catz A, Itzkovich M, Agranov E et al: The spinal cord independent measure (SCIM): sensitivity to functional changes in subgroups of spinal cord lesion patients, *Spinal Cord* 39:97-100, 2001.
7. Lashgari D, Yasuda L: Orthotics. In Pendleton HM, Schultz-Krohn W, editors: *Pedretti's occupational therapy: practice skills for physical dysfunction*, ed 6, St. Louis, 2006, Mosby Elsevier.
8. van Drongelen S, de Groot S, Veeger HE et al: Upper extremity musculoskeletal pain during and after rehabilitation in wheelchair-using persons with a spinal cord injury, *Spinal Cord* 44:152-159, 2006.
9. Fisher JM, Hunter J: Adapted make-up kit for persons with C5 and C6 quadriplegia, *Can J Occup Ther* 59:268-274, 1992.
10. Weingarden SI, Martin C: Independent dressing after spinal cord injury: a functional time evaluation, *Arch Phys Med Rehabil* 70: 518-519, 1989.
11. Coggrave MJ, Rose LS: A Specialist seating assessment clinic: changing pressure relief practice, *Spinal Cord* 41:692-695, 2003.
12. Yavuzer G, Gok H, Tuncer S, et al: Compliance with bladder management in spinal cord injury patients, *Int Med Soc Paraplegia* 38:762-765, 2000.
13. Adler US, Kirshblum SC: A new assistive device for intermittent self-catheterization in men with tetraplegia, *J Spinal Cord Med* 26:155-158, 2003.
14. Sutton G, Shah S, Hill V: Clean intermittent self-catheterization for quadriplegic patients-a five year follow-up, *Int Med Soc Paraplegia* 29:542-549, 1991.
15. Gray M, Rayome R, Anson C: Incontinence and clean intermittent catheterization following spinal cord injury, *Clin Nurs Res* 4:6-21, 1995.
16. Han TR, Kim JH, Kwon SB: Chronic gastrointestinal problems and bowel dysfunction in patients with spinal cord injury, *Spinal Cord* 36:485-490, 1998.

17. Lynch AC, Wong C, Anthony A, et al: Bowel dysfunction following spinal cord injury: a description of bowel function in a spinal cord-injured population and comparison with age gender matched controls, *Spinal Cord* 38:717-723, 2000.

18. Kirshblum SC, Gulati M, O'Conner K et al: Bowel care practices in chronic spinal cord injury patients, *Arch Phys Med Rehabil* 79:20-23, 1998.

19. Gender AR: Bowel elimination and regulation. In Hoeman SP, editor: *Nursing: process, application, and outcomes*, ed 3, St. Louis, 2000, Mosby.

20. Lancashire P, Janzen J, Zach GA et al: The oral hygiene and gingival health of paraplegic inpatients—a cross sectional survey, *J Clin Periodontol* 24:198-200, 1997.

21. Spratley MH: A toothbrushing aid for a quadriplegic patient, *Spec Care Dent* 11:114-115, 1991.

22. Schmeisser G: Low cost assistive device systems for a high spinal-cord-injured person in the home environment—a technical note, *Bull Prosthetics Res* 217-218, 1979.

23. Riley JK: Assistive technology and spinal cord injury, *SCI Nurs* 17:179-180, 2000.

24. McDonald DW, Boyle MA, Schumann TL: Environmental control unit utilization by high-level spinal cord injured patients, *Arch Phys Med Rehabil* 70:622-626, 1989.

25. Cyberkinetics Neurotechnology SystemsL www.cyberkineticsinc.com. Accessed March 2007.

26. Palmer S, Kriegsman KH, Palmer JB: Children of parents with spinal cord injuries: adjusting, learning, coping, *Spinal Cord Inj* 134-136, 2000.

27. Vensand K, Rogers J, Tuleja C et al: *Adaptive baby care equipment: guidelines, prototypes, and resources*, Berkley, CA, 2000, Through the Looking Glass.

SOLUTIONS TO CHAPTER 9 CLINICAL CASE STUDY

Activities of Daily Living Case 1

1. Perry has a C5 level of SCI. He has use of his deltoids and biceps but lacks trunk musculature. Therefore a chest strap is recommended for optimal upright positioning in his wheelchair and to assist his balance while performing various ADL tasks. He will require wrist splints to maintain his wrists in neutral position. The occupational therapist will most likely use a MAS to minimize the effect of gravity on Perry's shoulders during initial training. In this way he may work on strengthening his upper body/limbs and participate in ADLs such as eating while maintaining proper shoulder alignment and muscular balance. Perry gradually will be weaned off the MAS when his shoulder strength and alignment are appropriate for participation in various tabletop activities. The eventual goal will be to ensure that the upper limb musculature has sufficient endurance so that he is able to maintain workspace activities without excessive fatigue.

2. Perry will need to use assorted equipment for independent grooming care, including a wrist support with a utensil holder or a U-cuff when brushing his teeth. He will be able to wash his face by holding a washcloth in both hands with use of wrist supports or by using a wash mitt with D-ring closures. He can comb his hair with a U-cuff attached to a brush handle. An electric razor can be adapted with a U-cuff or a cuff made of splinting material that can be fitted to the electric razor or trimmer.

3. Perry can wear bilateral wrist splints with pencils attached that will enable him to type. The computer and keyboard will need to be set up to provide for eccentric control of the biceps for striking the keys. The team will need to evaluate the keyboard size and angle to provide optimal positioning for muscular efficiency and proper posture for balance and stability. Perry will receive training in how to use sticky keys to enhance efficiency in typing.

SOLUTIONS TO CHAPTER 9 CLINICAL CASE STUDY

Activities of Daily Living Case 2

1. The presence of wrist extension at a C6 level of injury allows Lisa to use a tenodesis grasp for functional tasks. Assistance is required, however, for setup of all materials and the environment for individuals with a C6 level of injury. Lisa may choose to use a tenodesis brace to help achieve the finger pinch often required for makeup application. Clasps should be removed from compact cases to enable her to flip the cases open with ease with her teeth, fingernail, or a thumb. Long cotton swabs can be built up with tape and held in a cuff to apply eye makeup and lipsticks. Lipsticks and eye pencils can be adapted to fit in the cuff as well. Mascara tubes can be firmly attached to a counter and opened with both hands as long as the top is loosely screwed onto the tube. A tongue depressor can be attached to the mascara applicator or foundation sponge and fit into a U-cuff during application.

Other modifications include attaching bases that can secure items to a table or to a wall, which can allow Lisa to touch her face to the makeup item as opposed to bringing the item to her face. Adapted nail cutters, brushes, and emery boards are available commercially. Because Lisa has limited hand dexterity, safety is the deciding factor on her independent performance of nail cutting because there is the potential for cuts and skin abrasions. Nail polish can be applied by securing the brush to a right-angle pocket with tape. A tenodesis brace might be used to manipulate cotton balls during polish removal.

2. Lisa may choose a roll-in shower chair to provide independence with bathing. Because of her lack of finger function, she will need a variety of adaptations to increase her safety and independence when bathing. A hand-held shower head may be one adaptation. A U-shaped cuff purchased commercially or fabricated from splinting material can be applied to the shower head to enable manipulation without finger function. Lever-type faucet controls should be installed and grab bars securely mounted with enough clearance from the wall to allow for wrist extensor or bicep hooking if stabilization is needed during bathing.

Continued

SOLUTIONS TO CHAPTER 9 CLINICAL CASE STUDY

Activities of Daily Living Case 2—cont'd

Liquid soaps, body washes, and shampoos can be kept in pump bottles and mounted in the shower. Bar soap can be more easily handled if it is slipped into the foot of an old pantyhose leg and the hose is tied to a grab bar or a hole is drilled into the bar and a rope is looped through so it can be tied to a grab bar or shower bench.

Lisa may choose a wash mitt instead of handling a regular washcloth. One drawback to the wash mitt is that it can be difficult to move from one hand to the other while wet. To wash her feet and lower legs, Lisa will need to lift her leg to cross her foot over the opposite knee or lean forward over her lap. The cutout in the seat of the shower chair offers access to her perineum. Keeping towels within reach while inside the tub will decrease the need for a caregiver's assistance. She will need to place a towel on the wheelchair cushion before entering the shower. This will help to keep the cushion and cushion cover dry in case of accidental splashes as well as when transferring back to the chair.

3. Lisa may gain some independence with light home management tasks, such as laundry, dusting, and light cleaning. Sweeping can be accomplished by propelling across the floor (most likely in the power wheelchair) by using an adapted broom and long-handled dust pan or a commercially available lightweight sweeper. She may prefer to use a lightweight vacuum cleaner with an appropriate handle adaptation designed for hard surfaces.

A front-loading washer and dryer are ideal for all individuals who complete laundry tasks from a seated position. Economy dressing sticks and reachers can also be used to access controls that are out of an arms reach. Lisa will most likely require assistance when folding the laundry, although a table at the appropriate height for her to fold small items may help facilitate this activity. This is an excellent activity for family interaction and will give her three young children a sense of accomplishment as well. Lisa will most likely need assistance from her family when retrieving clothes to launder and putting clean clothes away.

4. Meal preparation and cooking will require that the kitchen is organized so that Lisa can reach the items she is able to manipulate with her tenodesis within her balance control. Control of heavy objects, such as pots and pans, will need to be evaluated. A side-by-side refrigerator and freezer will enable Lisa to access both refrigerated and frozen foods. Transfer boards or wooden trays can be used to transport many light items to increase efficiency while working in the kitchen and around the house. Also, sliding items along the counter or using a rolling cart makes moving items around the kitchen easier and safer. Lisa will probably need assistance to use the oven but a roll-under range may allow easier use of a stovetop. Cabinets with a lazy Susan and pull out shelves provide easier access to kitchen items. A roll-under kitchen sink with lever faucets will provide her easier wheelchair access to the sink.

CHAPTER TEN

Management of the Upper Limb in Individuals with Tetraplegia

Mary Jane (M.J.) Mulcahey, OTR, PhD

*I admire your patience with both me and my arm, you pick the most complex individuals
to give us the little independence that we all value so greatly.*

Molly (C4 to C5 SCI)

Although it is one of the greatest challenges in spinal cord injury (SCI) rehabilitation, restoration of arm and hand function remains central in working with individuals with tetraplegia. After upper limb capability is restored, maintenance of pain-free, spontaneous, and effortless function is equally challenging. Traditional rehabilitation of the upper limb after SCI focuses on strengthening muscles, re-education of motor patterns to restore compensatory function, and orthotic intervention. Contemporary management of the upper limb considers traditional therapies but also recognizes the advantages of surgical reconstruction and neuroprostheses. Moreover, rehabilitation today anticipates new medical and scientific discoveries for individuals with SCI and therefore protects the limb from irreversible changes and eliminates factors that may interfere with future treatment.

This chapter discusses important clinical considerations in the evaluation of individuals with tetraplegia and provides recommendations about what standardized outcome measures may be best suited to build evidence in support of upper limb therapies. The indications for orthotic intervention are described and the outcomes and current status of neuroprostheses are reviewed. In addition, a treatment algorithm for surgical reconstruction of the upper limb is presented, rehabilitation protocols and outcomes of tendon transfers for arm and hand function are discussed, and serial casting is described.

EVALUATION OF THE UPPER LIMB IN INDIVIDUALS WITH TETRAPLEGIA

The neurological and functional evaluations of individuals after SCI have been discussed elsewhere[1,2] and are reviewed in Chapter 6. There are subtle yet critical considerations in the evaluation of the upper limb and upper limb performance in individuals with tetraplegia, however, that are often unrecognized (Clinical Note: Critical Considerations in the Evaluation of the Upper Limb).

CLINICAL NOTE Critical Considerations in the Evaluation of the Upper Limb

- Paralytic progressive scoliosis and kyphosis
- Scapulothoracic instability
- Strategies used for postural stability

Paralytic Spine Deformity

Although there are other contributing variables,[3] the most significant factor influencing the development of paralytic scoliosis is the age of the person at injury onset.[4] Almost all children injured before puberty,[5,6] approximately 25% of youth between 10 and 16 years, and 17% of those older than 17 years will have a progressive paralytic scoliosis.[3] There is also an increasing trend in paralytic spine deformities in older adults. Although wearing a thoracolumbarsacral orthosis may slow the rate of curve progression,[7] many individuals with progressive paralytic scoliosis require spinal fusions with instrumentation to stop the curve from progressing to a degree that compromises breathing.

When evaluating upper limb function or considering restorative interventions for the arm and hand, clinicians must consider the degree to which the paralytic spine deformity assists in function. For example, and as illustrated in Figures 10-1 and 10-2, once present, paralytic spine deformity enables many with C5 and weak C6 tetraplegia and poor shoulder strength the ability to get their feeding utensils to their mouth by using a compensatory mouth-to-hand function. Although this compensatory strategy is often effective, curve progression may eventually compromise pulmonary function, and a spinal fusion may be needed. Spine fusions with instrumentation result in a rigid spine and prevent active or gravity-assisted thoracic flexion. After a spine fusion, individuals with tetraplegia lose their thoracic flexibility and therefore may no longer have the compensatory ability to perform mouth-to-hand functions. Although alternative surgical procedures to correct progressive paralytic scoliosis without fusing the spine are under investigation,[8,9] evaluation of compensatory strategies should be a core component in evaluation of upper limb function. Box 10-1 summarizes key questions therapists can ask to determine the degree to which the paralytic spine deformity acts as a compensatory strategy for function.

Scapulothoracic Instability

Scapulothoracic instability is a result of paralysis of the primary stabilizers of the thoracoscapular joint[10] and, as shown in Figure 10-2, can contribute to the challenges of restoring pain-free and effortless use of the arm and hand. Also, with extensive paralysis about the shoulder and with lower motor neuron changes, the inferior corners of the scapula can overlap and cause skin breakdown. Surgical stabilization of the scapula has been reported with varying degrees of success.[5,10] Preventing secondary complications of shoulder paralysis is the best treatment and may be achieved by exercise and proper positioning while in bed and upright. Evaluation of shoulder function has been discussed elsewhere[10] and the clinical practice guidelines published by the Consortium for Spinal Cord Medicine[11] provide treatment recommendations for exercise and prevention.

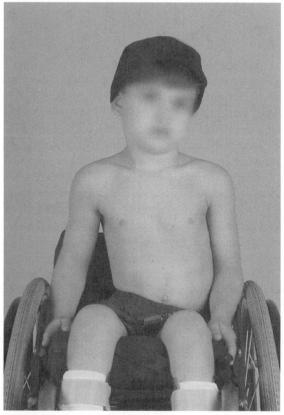

FIGURE 10-1 Typical clinical presentation of paralytic spine deformity. Appreciate the potential for the curve to act as a compensatory method to achieve independent eating for those who are unable to bring the hand to the mouth.

Mechanisms Used for Postural Stability

A hallmark of performance by those with SCI is the use of strategies to achieve postural stability. In fact, during activities of daily living (ADL) training, such as dressing and bed mobility, therapists often teach patients how to hook their elbow or hook their wrists around bed rails. Other strategies, such as leaning and hooking arms and wrists around wheelchair features, are commonly taught to individuals with SCI. Although these strategies undoubtedly promote independence, they may also violate a primary principle in upper limb management in SCI, that is, to prevent factors that may interfere with future treatment paradigms such as functional electrical stimulation (FES) (see Chapters 7 and 9).

With the clinical deployment of FES systems in the late 1900s, an appreciation for lower motor neuron (LMN) integrity below the level of injury was developed. FES systems rely on intact LMN pathways for successful stimulation. Although the injuries are subclinical to non-FES clinicians, repeated hooking of the arm and wrist and leaning on the outer arm for balance can result in peripheral nerve damage in paralyzed muscles and therefore interfere with successful application of FES. Evaluation of LMN in SCI has been described[12,13] and, to protect the LMN of paralyzed

---

BOX 10-1 | **Assessment Questions Used to Determine the Degree to Which Paralytic Spine Deformity Acts as a Compensatory Mechanism**

- What is the muscle strength of shoulder forward flexion and adduction?
- What is the muscle endurance of shoulder forward flexion and adduction? Can the patient maintain the same function throughout a 30-minute meal?
- Is the patient able to bring the hand to the mouth while the trunk is held upright?
- Is the patient slouching and actively moving the head down toward the hand during meal time?
- If the patient is placed in the temporary thoracolumbosacral orthosis, is he able to bring his hand to his mouth?

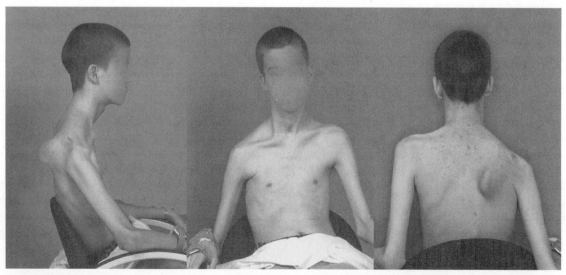

FIGURE 10-2 Young adult with adolescent-onset tetraplegia. Note the paralytic spine deformity and scapula instability.

muscles for future FES and other restorative therapies, training in strategies for postural stability warrants reexamination.

Standardized Outcome Measures for Upper Limb and Hand Function

The challenges to evidence building in support of upper limb interventions are many,[14] the primary one being a lack of sensitive and valid outcomes measures.[10,15] The strengths and limitations of available measures have been reviewed elsewhere[16,17] and include poor sensitivity to the small but significant gains in hand and arm function that can be made in tetraplegia. Although the standard assessment of the upper limb for clinical decision making includes measures of muscle strength, range of motion, sensation, tone, and function,[1,14,18] the Grasp and Release Test (GRT),[19] the Capacity of the Upper Extremity (CUE),[20,21] and the Canadian Occupational Performance Measure (COPM),[22,23] which is a patient-perceived measure of outcomes, are more useful measures to build evidence in support of upper limb interventions.

Among the greatest strengths of the GRT is that it was designed specifically for the tetraplegic hand; it measures pinch strength, grasp strength, and hand function. Stroh-Wuolle et al[19] first reported on the psychometrics of the GRT, which were further established by Mulcahey et al.[24] The GRT has been used to build evidence in support of neuroprostheses and tendon transfers.[25-27] The CUE, also designed specifically for the tetraplegic hand, is a 17-item questionnaire in which patients are asked to rate their ability to perform functional tasks with their arms by using a seven-point ordinal scale. The questionnaire separates proximal arm function from hand function and has been shown to be effective in measuring outcomes after surgery to improve upper limb function.

Unlike the GRT and CUE, the COPM considers outcomes from a broader perspective and has emerged as the recommended evaluation to measure changes in function.[10,16,18,28] The COPM uses an interview process to identify goals that are rated by the patient; performance and satisfaction are rated on a scale between 1 (cannot perform, not satisfied) to 10 (performs well, very satisfied). Ratings on the same goals are repeated after intervention to obtain a patient-perceived score on the outcomes of performance of and satisfaction with self-selected goals. The COPM has been endorsed by those centers specializing in tendon transfer reconstruction and is available at the CanChild Web site (www.canchild.ca).

ORTHOTIC INTERVENTION

The indications for orthotic prescription for individuals with SCI are summarized in Clinical Note: Considerations for Upper Limb Orthotic Intervention and have been reviewed by Hentz and LeClercq,[1] Malick and Meyer,[29] Mulcahey et al,[15] and Mulcahey.[30] Generally, for those with poor or absent wrist extension, forearm-hand orthoses are needed. Conversely, for those with against-gravity wrist extension strength, shorter hand-based orthoses are usually sufficient. Functional hand splinting is indicated for those with C6 and C7 tetraplegia, which is based on the principles of the tenodesis hand in which, with gravity-assisted wrist flexion (Figure 10-3, *A*) and with volitional wrist extension (Figure 10-3, *B*), the fingers and thumb passively open and close, respectively.

CLINICAL NOTE **Considerations for Upper Limb Orthotic Intervention**

- Prevention of deformity
- Stabilization of joints
- Maintenance of a functional hand

Acute Tetraplegia

Early protective splinting is important in acute tetraplegia (Clinical Note: Benefits of Early Protective Splinting). Regular skin checks are necessary and, because of changing neurological status and edema, frequent modifications to the splint should be anticipated.

Range of motion exercises and proper bed positioning techniques are also critical components of upper limb management in acute tetraplegia and are described elsewhere.[1,11,30-32] In addition

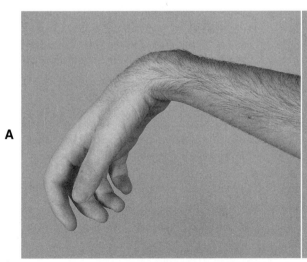
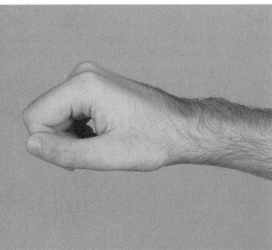

FIGURE 10-3 Fundamental principle of tetraplegia hand function. **A,** With gravity-assisted wrist flexion the fingers and thumb passively open for grasp. **B,** With volitional wrist extension, the thumb and fingers passively close for grasp. The tenodesis hand function provides sufficient force for light objects.

Benefits of Early Protective Splinting

- Prevents over stretching of the ligaments
- Maintains a functional hand position
- Prevents deformity
- Protects and stabilizes flaccid joints

to preventing deformity, static splinting promotes a functional hand.[33] Except for the controversy about tenodesis splinting that can facilitate effective tenodesis hand function but be detrimental to hand function if done incorrectly,[1,15] there are practice guidelines for splinting regimens during acute stages of injury that are generally agreed on.[1,30,31,33]

High-Level Tetraplegia

The clinician's goals of upper limb intervention for individuals with high-level tetraplegia—those patients with C1 to C4 lesions—bear close scrutiny (Clinical Note: Goals of Upper Limb Intervention for Individuals with High-Level Tetraplegia). During waking hours, a long opponens wrist-hand-orthosis should be used to support the proximal and distal transverse arch and the longitudinal arch (Figure 10-4). The wrist should be positioned

Goals of Upper Limb Intervention for Individuals with High-Level Tetraplegia

- Prevent and control development of paralytic deformities
- Protect insensate areas from injury
- Prevent or reduce edema
- Maintain a supple hand for human contact
- Protect the limb from irreversible changes and preserve it for future treatment paradigms

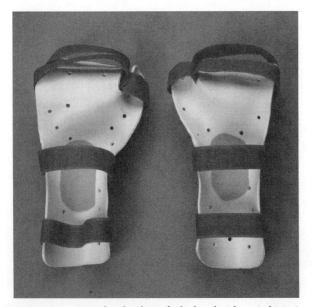

FIGURE 10-4 Wrist-hand orthosis for high and mid cervical injuries.

in 30 degrees of extension and the thumb placed in full abduction (carpometacarpal joint) and extension (metaphalangeal joint). Nighttime splinting also supports the arches and holds the thumb in full abduction-extension but places the hand in an intrinsic plus posture.

For those with C4 tetraplegia, mobile arm supports (MAS) and suspension slings are available for hand-to-mouth and table top activities. MAS, such as the one shown in Figure 10-5, are mechanical devices that support the arm and forearm and assist with shoulder and elbow movement through a linkage of ball bearing joints,[30,34-36] whereas suspension slings are kinetic devices that support the upper limb.[36] Other assistive technologies such as augmentative communication devices, control sources for power mobility, computer interfaces for access, and others, as described in Chapter 13, serve an important role in replacing arm and hand function resulting from extensive paralysis associated with high tetraplegia.

Midcervical Injuries

Individuals with midcervical injuries can be separated into two distinct functional groups: those with gravity-eliminated wrist extension strength and those with against-gravity wrist extension strength. A person with C5-level tetraplegia typically has adequate or good elbow flexion but poor or no wrist extension, placing him at a disadvantage for tenodesis hand function (Figure 10-6, A). The flexor hinge orthosis (Figure 10-6, B) is the functional orthosis of choice for those with C6 tetraplegia and, despite conflicting findings of continued use after discharge,[32,37-39] should be offered as an option for independent performance of activities.

Rehabilitation with the wrist-driven flexor hinge orthosis encompasses training in activities such as self-catheterization, feeding, toothbrushing, writing, and other instrumental ADL (Figure 10-7) and training in donning and doffing the orthosis.

Because there are no commercially available functional orthoses that fit young pediatric hands, custom-made splints are required. Light material and frequent modifications are needed to accommodate constant growth, but, as illustrated, with adequate design children as young as 8 months of age are able to engage in developmentally important activities (Figure 10-8, A to D).

Low technology and simple devices are considered a mainstay in the rehabilitation of individuals with midcervical tetraplegia.[34,40] The universal cuff is the single most important assistive device for those with midcervical injuries because it offers versatility and accommodates many types of objects such as a toothbrush, pen, utensil, or razor. Essential considerations in the provision of assistive devices can be found in the Clinical Note: Essential Considerations in the Provision of Assistive Devices.

Essential Considerations in the Provision of Assistive Devices

- Independence in donning
- Low weight and profile
- Pleasing appearance

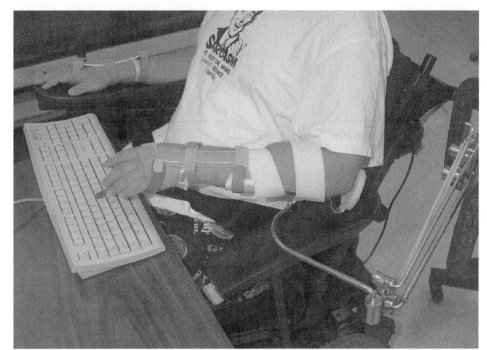

FIGURE 10-5   Individual with a newly acquired C4-C5 SCI tries out MAS unit. After optimal positioning is determined and the individual receives his permanent wheelchair, the MAS bracket will be mounted directly onto the wheelchair for daily use.

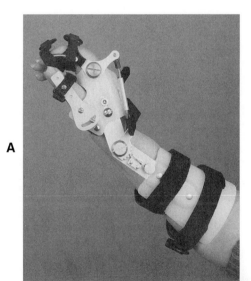

A

FIGURE 10-6   Wrist-driven flexor hinge splint augments the force provided by tenodesis (**A**) hand grasp and (**B**) release.

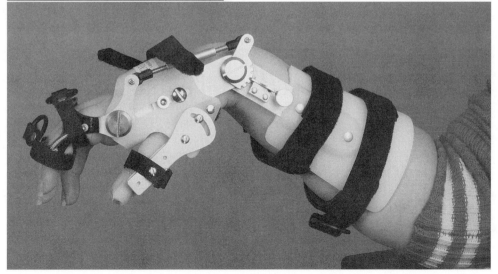

B

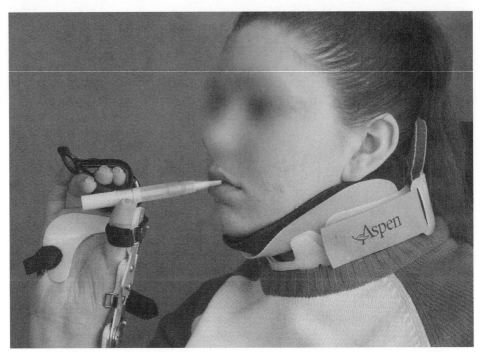

FIGURE 10-7 An individual with C6 tetraplegia uses a wrist-driven flexor hinge splint.

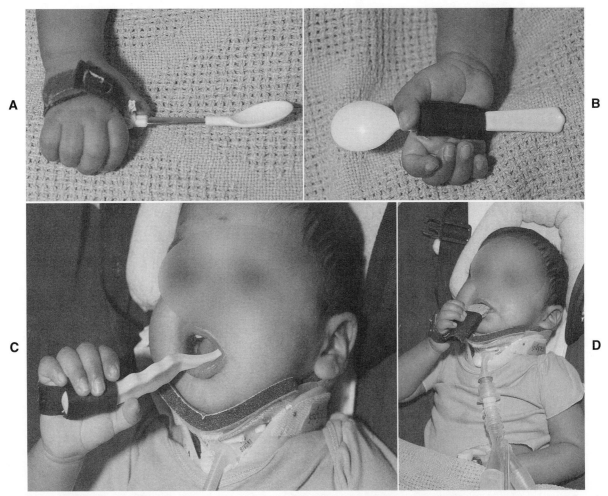

FIGURE 10-8 Adult principles of hand function can be applied to children. Here, (**A** and **B**) an 8-month-old infant uses a custom-made universal cuff to hold a spoon, (**C**) hold a toothbrush, and (**D**) hold a toddler biscuit.

NEUROPROSTHESES FOR THE UPPER LIMB IN TETRAPLEGIA

In cases of SCI, FES is the coordinated stimulation of two or more muscles to achieve a functional outcome.[41] The primary purpose of FES is to restore functional abilities with stimulated hand and arm function. This is different from therapeutic electrical stimulation, which is delivered in rote and automatic fashion for therapeutic purposes such as muscle strengthening and range of motion. Neuroprosthesis is a term used to describe bracing of the limb by means of FES. Early upper limb work with percutaneous FES restored palmar and lateral grasp and release to individuals with midcervical impairments[42,43] and demonstrated restored capabilities in ADL.[26,27,44,45] Successful outcomes of percutaneous work led to the development of an implantable neuroprosthesis[9,46] marketed under the name Freehand System. Despite the evidence in the form of functional outcomes[47-50] and reduction of costs associated with disability as a result of FES,[51] marketing of the Freehand System was stopped in 2001.[52] Next-generation implantable neuroprostheses systems are under development[9,52] and are anticipated in this century to be a treatment of choice for restoring upper limb function in individuals with tetraplegia.

The NESS H200 (Bioness Inc., Santa Clara, Calif.), formerly known as the Handmaster, is now commercially available. The NESS H200 consists of an arm-hand orthosis and a control box. Five surface electrodes are contained within the orthosis and deliver stimulation to the long extensor and flexor tendons of the fingers and thumb and to intrinsic thenar muscles.[53] Preliminary reports of 10 consecutive patients were positive[53] and, although there have been no prospective studies with large numbers of individuals using the system, Alon and McBride[54] have demonstrated positive outcomes of the NESS H200 with a series of patients with midcervical SCI. Chapter 17 provides additional information on FES as it relates to SCI rehabilitation.

SURGICAL RECONSTRUCTION FOR RESTORATION OF ARM AND HAND FUNCTION

After almost 40 years of surgical refinement, technical development and analysis of outcomes, surgical management of the upper limb in individuals with cervical-level SCI has culminated in a well-defined algorithm of evaluation and rehabilitation.[55-72] Without exception, presurgical assessment of the upper limb in tetraplegia should be approached from a comprehensive perspective[10,16] with the International Classification of Surgery of the Hand in Tetraplegia (ICSHT),[73] which is outlined in Table 10-1. This advocates the evaluation of each arm separately, assessment of two-point discrimination, and determination of muscle strength.

Tendon Transfers to Restore Elbow Extension

Up to 70% of individuals with tetraplegia can benefit from tendon transfer surgery to restore active and noncompensatory elbow extension strength (Figure 10-9). The deltoid-to-triceps transfer remains the most common procedure to restore elbow extension. Several surgical techniques for the deltoid-to-triceps transfer have been reported[60,61,69-73] and complications, including elongation of the tendon transfer from rapid and early mobilization,

TABLE 10-1	International Classification for Surgery of the Hand in Tetraplegia		
Classification	ASIA	Key Muscle	Surgical Options
O[CU]:0	C5	No grade 4 muscle below elbow	1. Possible deltoid to triceps or biceps to triceps
O[CU]:1	C5	BR	1. Deltoid to triceps or biceps to triceps 2. BR to ECRB 3. FPL tenodesis 4. FPL split tendon transfer
O[CU]:2	C6	BR + ECRL	1. Deltoid to triceps or biceps to triceps 2. BR to ECRB and FPL tenodesis OR BR to FPL 3. FPL split tendon transfer
O[CU]:3	C6	Above + ECRB	1. Deltoid to triceps or biceps to triceps 2. BR to FPL 3. ECRL to FDP 4. FPL split transfer 5. Intrinsic tenodesis
O[CU]: 4	C6	Above + PT	1. Deltoid to triceps 2. (A) BR to FPL and PT to ABPB and EDC/EPL tenodesis or (B) PT to FPL and BR to EDC/EPL 3. ECRL to FDP 4. FPL split transfer 5. Intrinsic tenodesis
O[CU]:5	C6	Above + FCR	As above
O[CU]: 6	C7	Above + EDC	Elbow extension typically not indicated (as above without finger extension transfer)
O[CU]: 7	C7	Above + EPL	Elbow extension typically not indicated (as above without thumb extension transfer)
O[CU]: 8	C8	Above + finger flexion	1. Transfer for thumb flexion 2. Intrinsic tenodesis
O[CU]: 9	C8-T1	Lacks intrinsics	Intrinsic tenodesis

BR, Brachioradialis; *FPL*, flexor pollices longus; *ECRB/L*, extensor carpi radialis brevis/longus; *PT*, pronator teres; *FCR*, flexor carpi radialis; *EDC*, extensor digitorum communis; *EPL*, extensor pollicis longus.

attenuation over time, graft failure, elbow flexion contractures,[71] biceps spasticity,[60] and the inability of the patient to tolerate the demands of the postoperative course including the lengthy period of immobilization, have been recognized.[66, 70-72]

The biceps tendon has also been transferred to the triceps to restore elbow extension but until recently, only when the clinical picture involved an intact brachialis and supinator, severe biceps spasticity, and an elbow flexion contracture of more than 20 degrees.[64, 73-77] Recent reports,[28,76] however, suggest that the

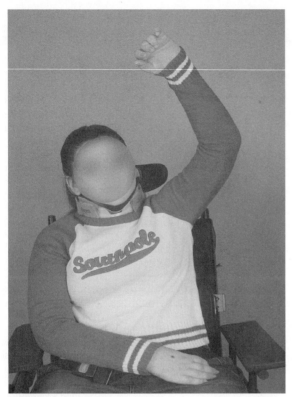

FIGURE 10-9 A biceps-to-triceps transfer resulted in against-gravity elbow extension strength. Appreciate this individual's ability to extend her elbow without the compensatory shoulder external rotation that typically is used by people with tetraplegia and absent triceps muscle.

biceps to triceps may provide superior strength and isolated motor activity outcomes compared with the deltoid-to-triceps transfer.[77] Mulcahey et al[28] found that the biceps-to-triceps transfer provided against-gravity elbow extension strength (grade 4 and 5) in all but one arm compared with the deltoid-to-triceps transfer, which provided elbow extension strength in only one arm. Further benefit of the biceps-to-triceps transfer[76] involves the degree to which isolated motor activity is possible after the biceps tendon transfer.

Because the postoperative rehabilitation after the biceps-to-triceps transfer is far less demanding to the patient than that of the deltoid-to-triceps transfer and, because the surgical procedure is easier than the deltoid-to-triceps surgery, continued research on the outcomes of both surgical techniques is under way. Detailed surgical techniques to restore elbow extension are described elsewhere.[1,69,77,78]

Tendon Transfers to Restore Hand Grasp and Release

Wrist extension is the fundamental movement for hand function.[69,79,80] Active wrist extension and gravity-assisted wrist flexion provide passive tenodesis and a primitive grasping mechanism. An individual without wrist extension (ICSHT motor groups 0 and 1) has no means to produce tenodesis and is therefore unable to acquire, grasp, or release objects. Those with C5 tetraplegia with ICSHT motor group 0 do not have any muscles available for transfer but have benefited by using neuroprostheses.[49,81] Although patients with C5 tetraplegia with ICSHT motor

group 1 also do not have voluntary wrist extension, they do have all three elbow flexor muscles, including the brachioradialis muscle that is available for tendon transfer to restore voluntary wrist extension.

After transfer of the brachioradialis to radial wrist extensor, tenodesis hand function is restored and can be augmented by the wrist drive flexor hinge orthosis,[1] flexor pollicis longus tenodesis,[70] or by a neuroprosthesis.[52] If voluntary wrist extension is preserved, such as the case in C6 tetraplegia, restoration of pinch (Figure 10-10, *A*) and, if sufficient muscles are available for transfer, grasp can be restored (Figure 10-10, *B*).[80] As described in Table 10-1, for those with C6 tetraplegia and motor group 3, the brachioradialis can be transferred to the flexor pollicis longus for active pinch; passive finger flexion by voluntary wrist extension positions the index finger for active pinch. For those with C6 tetraplegia in ICSHT motor group 4, the brachioradialis can be transferred to the flexor pollicis longus for active pinch and one of the two radial wrist extensors under voluntary control can be transferred to the flexor digitorum, usually the profundus, for active finger flexion.[68,73,79,82]

Although typical grasp that uses synchronous activity between the intrinsic and extrinsic hand muscles is not achieved, restoration of volitional pinch and gross grasp restores unilateral and bilateral hand function (Figure 10-11).

Hand opening for acquisition of objects is typically dependent on gravity-assisted wrist flexion and passive finger and thumb extension. Active finger extension is obtainable when there are sufficient muscles available for transfer (ICSHT group 4 or greater). Isolated tendon transfer to the extrinsic finger extensors produces metacarpophalangeal joint extension with minimal interphalangeal joint extension.[77,83] A passive intrinsic reconstruction to limit intrinsic minus posturing is typically necessary.[77] Restoration of both finger flexion and extension requires a two-stage reconstruction because the postoperative precautions and mobilization protocols conflict.[14,61,68] Detailed surgical technique to restore pinch, grasp, and release is described elsewhere.[1,64-66,79,82]

Rehabilitation Guidelines for Tendon Transfer Rehabilitation and Re-education

Tendon transfer rehabilitation begins preoperatively[84,85] and involves mobilization and strengthening activities, education about surgery and postoperative restrictions, and evaluation for equipment that may be needed during the immobilization period.[14] Although rehabilitation guidelines vary,[1,14] there are general principles that are important. During the immediate postoperative stage, immobilization of the arm and hand is obtained by using a bulky soft dressing or well-padded fiberglass or plaster casts. During this time the limb should be elevated to reduce or prevent edema and any early active mobilization activities should be initiated; passive range of motion is provided to the shoulder; the therapist should remain cognizant of any postoperative range limitation precautions as required after elbow extension transfers.

After the cast is removed, static splints that position the hand and arm in the postoperative position are removed only during therapy sessions; the primary purpose of the postoperative splint is to protect the tendon transfer from attenuation or unwanted

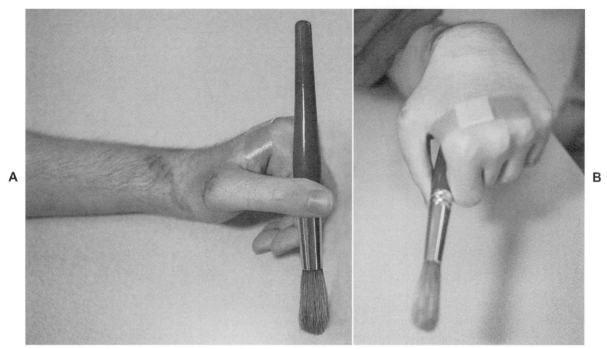

FIGURE 10-10   After transfer of the brachioradialis to the flexor pollicis longus and transfer of one radial wrist extensor to the finger flexors, the ability (**A**) to pinch and (**B**) to grasp a paintbrush is achieved.

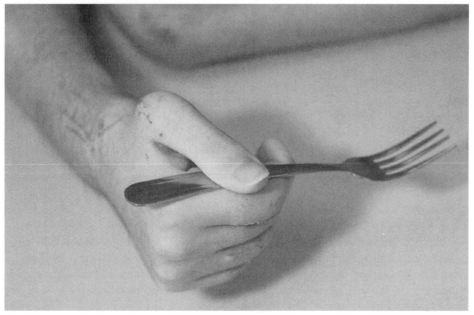

FIGURE 10-11   The ability to pinch a fork is demonstrated after transfer of the brachioradialis to thumb flexor.

movement from spasticity or accidental range. If needed, retrograde and scar massage[14] are provided to reduce edema and to minimize scarring, respectively. Active or active-assisted movement of the transferred tendon is initiated in a gravity-eliminated position, and over the course of several therapy sessions active movement is increased to eventual use of the new movement for light ADL. During retraining of tendon transfers, the primary role of the therapist is to ensure that the transferred tendon is being used for function as opposed to compensatory strategies. For example, while retraining elbow extension, the therapist must ensure that the shoulder is internally rotated and locking the elbow is avoided. The therapist should, however, be aware of the potential for impingement at the shoulder with internal rotation and be aware of activities that could create pain such as transfers (see Chapter 8). Likewise, while retraining the brachioradialis for active thumb pinch, the therapist must have an appreciation of force provided by natural tenodesis and that provided by the transferred muscles.

TABLE 10-2 | **Postoperative Protocol for Biceps-to-Triceps Transfer for Elbow Extension**

Phase	Action
Immobilization phase (1 to 3 weeks postoperatively)	Patient is immobilized in long arm cast with elbow in full extension
	Avoid shoulder flexion above 90 degrees and extension of shoulder beyond 0 degrees
	ROM of uninvolved joints, edema control
Mobilization phase (3 to 4 weeks postoperatively)	Cast removed:
	Avoid shoulder flexion above 90 degrees and extension of shoulder beyond 0 degrees
	No passive elbow flexion
	Active elbow flexion and extension is progressed in increments of 15 degrees elbow flexion each week
	Do not progress elbow flexion if extension lag is present
	No resistive exercises
	Fabricate and provide elbow extension splint for night
	Fit with Bledsoe: to be worn during the day; set elbow flexion block at 15 degrees
	Active elbow flexion to 15 degrees, active extension to full
	Edema control and scar management
Mobilization phase (4 to 5 weeks postoperatively)	Avoid shoulder flexion above 90 degrees and extension of shoulder beyond 0 degrees
	No passive elbow flexion
	Active flexion is progressed in increments of 15 degrees to 20 degrees each week
	Must monitor for extension lag; do not progress if lag is present
	Continue elbow extension night splint
	Continue Bledsoe Brace for daytime use
	Adjust Bledsoe in increments of 15 degrees of flexion as patient progresses; do not increase range in brace if extension lag is present
	Active elbow flexion and extension
	Initiate exercises in an antigravity plane, blocking external rotation
	Progress active elbow flexion in increments of 15 degrees to 20 degrees/week
	Assess for extension lag
	Decrease amount of flexion if extension lag is present; if lag is present focus on end range extension
	Light functional training or activities may begin in allowed elbow ranges (pending time frame and assessment of allowed amount of elbow flexion) only after the therapist is sure the transfer is firing with the activity
Strengthening and functional retraining phase (6 to 12 weeks)	No passive elbow flexion before 3 months
	Adjust Bledsoe as flexion is gained.
	Continue Bledsoe until the patient has achieved 90 degrees elbow flexion
	Continue nighttime extension splint until postoperative week 12
	Active range of motion: progress flexion as able
	Strengthening
	Initiate light elbow extension at week 10

Strength of movement provided by tendon transfers will continue to increase throughout the first year after surgery[25,28] and, as such, a person may benefit from therapeutic services throughout the first year after surgery to integrate tendon transfer function into performance of work, leisure, school, and self-care activities. Rehabilitation protocols for the most commonly performed tendon transfers for individuals with tetraplegia involve specific guidelines for action from the immobilization phase through strengthening and functional retraining (Tables 10-2 to 10-5).

Outcomes of Tendon Transfers for Elbow Extension and Hand Grasp

Outcomes of upper limb reconstruction in individuals with tetraplegia are overwhelmingly positive. Tendon transfers for active grasp have shown to increase pinch force,[60,63-65,71,82] improve performance on hand function tests,[25,82] facilitate independence in ADL,[14,25,65,81] and improve social, emotional, and vocational status.[14,25,65,82] In addition to these common outcomes,

spontaneity is realized for the first time since injury because of no longer needing multiple pieces of adaptive equipment for the many activities performed throughout the day and the effort required for activity performance is reduced (Box 10-2).

For those with C5 tetraplegia, motor group 1 and 2, surgically restored passive pinch or active thumb flexion provides the ability to manipulate small light objects without adaptive equipment. Both the surgical passive and active pinch provides slightly stronger forces than nonsurgical natural tenodesis hand function. Importantly, regardless of what type of pinch (natural or surgically restored), individuals with C5 tetraplegia remain obligatory two-handed individuals (most tasks require two hands to complete). In contrast, for individuals with C6 tetraplegia (motor groups 3 to 6) tendon transfers restore unilateral and bilateral hand function when performed on both hands.

A reoccurring outcome of upper limb reconstruction concerns the pivotal role of elbow extension (Box 10-3). For all individuals with tetraplegia, restoration of elbow extension is considered

TABLE 10-3	Postoperative Protocol for Brachioradialis to Radial Wrist Extensor with Flexor Pollicis Longus Tenodesis (Moberg Tenodesis)	
Phase	**Action**
Immobilization phase (1 to 3 weeks postoperatively)	Tendon immobilized in a shortened position to protect transfer
	Upper limb immobilization position in cast: wrist 20 to 30 degrees extension and thumb: in adduction against index finger
	Range of motion of uninvolved joints
	Edema control of uninvolved digits
Mobilization phase (3 to 6 weeks postoperatively)	No wrist flexion beyond neutral
	No thumb extension or abduction
	No resistive exercises
	Volar wrist splint with wrist in 20 to 30 degrees extension, thumb in adduction on at all times with exception for home program, bathing, and therapy sessions.
	Active range of motion: active wrist extension through exercise or activities to facilitate tendon recruitment; stabilize forearm to ensure that patient does not rotate it; this will promote excursion for wrist extension vs. forearm rotation/gravity assisted extension
	Initiate scar massage; use of silicone gel sheet or elastomere as indicated
	Educate patient and family about postoperative precautions, scar management, and splint wear/care.
Strengthening and functional retraining phase (6 to 12 weeks postoperatively)	No passive wrist flexion or thumb extension
	Avoid resistive activities until 8 weeks postoperatively
	Splint wearing schedule week 6 to 8: off for nonresistive functional tasks; on all night
	Splint wearing schedule week 8 to 12: off all day; on all night
	Splint wearing schedule week 12: discontinue use of splint
	Active range of motion: wrist flexion and extension (which will promote thumb tenodesis release/pinch); elbow flexion and extension; passive digit flexion and extension
	Stabilize forearm to ensure that patient does not rotate it: this will promote excursion for wrist extension vs. forearm rotation/gravity-assisted extension
	Initiate light resistive exercises at week 8
	Continue scar massage; use of silicone gel sheet or elastomere as indicated
	Educate patient and family on changes with postoperative precautions, splint wear, and care, and incorporate strengthening into home program

TABLE 10-4	Postoperative Protocol for the Brachioradialis to the Flexor Pollicis Longus for Active Pinch	
Phase	**Action**
Immobilization phase (1 to 3 weeks postoperatively)	Tendon immobilized in a shortened position to protect transfer
Mobilization phase (3 to 6 weeks postoperatively)	Avoid overextension of thumb
	No passive wrist extension and no passive elbow extension
	Avoid resistive exercises
	Splint: dorsal forearm–based splint with thumb adducted; wrist in neutral; elbow free
	Splint wearing schedule: on at all times with exception for home program, bathing, and therapy sessions
	Active range of motion: lateral pinch, gravity-assisted wrist flex, wrist extension to 20 degrees, to 30 degrees, elbow flexion and extension, passive digit flexion and extension; stabilize forearm to ensure that patient is able to pinch in various forearm and elbow positions
	Initiate scar massage; use of silicone gel sheet or elastomere as indicated
	Educate patient and family on: postoperative precautions, scar management, and splint wear and care
Strengthening and functional retraining phase (6 to 12 weeks postoperatively)	Avoid overextension of thumb and passive elbow extension
	Avoid resistive exercises
	Splint wearing schedule week 6 to 8: off for nonresistive functional tasks; on at night
	Splint wearing schedule week 8 to 12: off all day; on all night
	Splint wearing schedule week 12: discontinue use of splint
	Active range of motion: lateral pinch, gravity-assisted wrist flexion and extension, elbow flexion and extension, passive digit flexion and extension
	Stabilize forearm to ensure that patient is able to pinch in various forearm and elbow positions
	Initiate light resistive pinch exercises at week 8
	Continue scar massage; use of silicone gel sheet or elastomere as indicated
	Educate patient and family on changes with postoperative precautions, splint wear and care, and incorporate strengthening into home program

TABLE 10-5	Postoperative Protocol for the Radial Wrist Extensor Transfer to the Flexor Digitorum Profundus for Active Finger Flexion	
Phase	**Action**
Early mobilization phase (day 1 to 3 weeks postoperatively)	Tendon immobilized in shortened position to protect transfer
	Upper limb immobilization position in a dorsal blocking cast with elbow 90 degrees, wrist neutral, MCPs flexed to 70 degrees, and IPs extended
	Strap may be used at night to position IP joints in extension to prevent flexion contractures
	Active range of motion: active composite digit flexion place and hold digit extension
Mobilization phase (3 to 6 weeks postoperatively)	No passive or active MCP extension past position of resting tension of transfer
	No passive or active wrist extension past position of resting tension of transfer
	No passive or active composite extension
	No resistive exercises
	Dorsal block splint with wrist in neutral; MPs flexed 70 degrees and IPs extended
	Splint wearing schedule: on at all times with exception for home program, bathing, and therapy sessions
	Active range of motion: protected active range of motion—composite digit flexion
	When performing this exercise, stabilize the wrist in 30 degrees extension and work on active digit flexion, active digit IP extension to protected position only wrist flexion and extension to neutral—tendon placed in shortened position (i.e., digits fully flexed manually) during this exercise passive digit flexion: composite flexion and individual joints as indicated
	Initiate scar massage; use of silicone gel sheet or elastomere as indicated
	Educate patient and family on: postoperative precautions, scar management, and splint wear and care
Strengthening and functional retraining phase (6 to 12 weeks postoperatively)	No composite extension stretching
	No resistive exercises until postoperative week 8
	Splint wearing schedule week 6 to 8: off for nonresistive functional tasks; on at night
	Splint wearing schedule week 8 to 12: off all day, on all night
	Splint wearing schedule week 12: discontinue use of splint
	Active range of motion: composite flexion, composite digit extension to end range (avoid extrinsic flexor stretch)
	Remove splint for light ADL at 6 weeks
	At 8 weeks, begin using limb to perform body transfers with digits in a fisted position (not with composite wrist and digit extension)
	Initiate light strengthening at 8 weeks
	Educate patient and family on changes with: splint wear and care and incorporate strengthening into home program

MCP, Metacarpophalangeal; *IP*, interphalangeal; *MP*, metaphalangeal.

BOX 10-2	Outcomes of Tendon Transfers for Active Grasp

- Increased pinch force
- Improved performance on hand function tests
- Increased independence in ADL
- Improved social, emotional, and vocational status
- Increased spontaneity in task performance
- Eliminated need for multiple pieces of adaptive equipment
- Reduced effort required for activity performance

BOX 10-3	Benefits of Elbow Extension Restoration

- Restores reachable work space
- Eliminates reliance on shoulder external rotation and locking the elbow joint
- Restores proximal control for efficient distal hand function
- May provide the necessary upper limb strength required to use walkers and crutches for those with incomplete tetraplegia who are ambulatory

fundamental because it restores reachable work space, against-gravity elbow extension without reliance on shoulder external rotation and locking the elbow joint, and proximal control for efficient distal hand function.* In addition to these important goals, elbow extension has provided the necessary upper limb strength required to use walkers and crutches for upright mobility by those with incomplete tetraplegia who are ambulatory.

---

*References 28, 56, 58, 64-66, 72, 73, 76.

SERIAL CASTING OF THE UPPER LIMB IN TETRAPLEGIA

Understanding the potential impact of upper motor neuron and LMN changes after SCI provides insight into joints prone to developing tightness and contracture.[12,13,34,86] Joint tightness or contracture can result as a secondary consequence of muscle imbalance, abnormal tone, and sensory alterations.[2,86] Additional predisposing factors to tightness include stresses imposed by the use of mechanical devices (flexed posturing in sitting from long-term wheelchair use), failure or inability to comply with positional programs (repetitive side lying while sleeping), and inability to implement a routine preventive program.[2,86] Johansen and Murray[12] provide an excellent review of anatomy and biomechanical changes of the upper limb after SCI.

Serial casting is the application of low-load prolonged stretch to shortened tissue with the objective of remodeling tissue in the lengthened positions.[87,88] It has been shown to be an effective intervention to enhance passive range of motion (PROM) in patients with SCI with secondary joint tightness or recent contracture.

Serial casting is indicated when there is limited joint PROM with a soft or capsular end feel.[87,89] In cases of a suspected bony or empty end feel, radiographic imaging can be performed to examine the joint and bone quality proximal and distal to the joint being casted.[89] In general, patients with recent onset of tightness tend to regain PROM quicker than patients with long-standing involvement.[90] In cases of long-standing tightness, a trial period of serial casting can be introduced to assess for any increases in PROM. When no appreciable change in ROM is measured, alternative treatment options may be considered (e.g., surgical lengthening).[91]

An important delineation in patients with SCI is an appreciation of the functional consequences of structures that cross the joint.[34] For instance, before any intervention, those with C5 complete SCI rely on the tenodesis function.[12] If the long finger flexor tendons are fully lengthened through stretching or casting, loss of tenodesis function is likely to occur. Serial casting therefore is indicated for a person with SCI when soft tissue structures that cross a joint are limiting PROM and flexibility and functional ability. When joint PROM is normal but flexibility is limited, a program of stretching, splinting, or casting is performed in positions that elongate the target tissue. In cases of more severe tightness, surgical lengthening may be necessary. Whichever form of treatment is introduced, the extent of lengthening must be weighed against the functional needs. In patients with typical PROM and tissue flexibility with awkward posturing or joint proprioception, alternative treatments to serial casting such as medication management and inhibitive casting are indicated.[89]

The presence or absence of volitional movement in the presence of limited PROM can warrant serial casting.[89] After serial casting, the individual with absent volitional control of the antagonist muscle may require dynamic functional splinting or a more permanent solution to restore balance to the joint, such as tendon transfer. For example, after serial casting of an elbow flexion contracture, the biceps can be transferred to the triceps to prevent reoccurrence of the contracture and to facilitate active elbow extension. An understanding of the functional implications of potentially elongating a tight joint in a patient with SCI is important to assess. Some patients may rely on that passive limitation for enhancing functional performance. Conversely, patients may not understand the activities available to them if they had a more pliable hand. It is important to weigh the functional benefits against potential losses when considering serial casting in these cases.

TABLE 10-6	Advantages and Disadvantages of Casting Material	
Type of Cast	Advantages	Disadvantages
Plaster of paris	Easily molded	Not water resistant
	Strong	Heavy, bulky
	Inexpensive	Long drying time
	Easily removed	Long time to weight
	Smooth surface	bearing
Fiberglass	Lightweight	Rough edges
	Water resistant	Difficult to mold
	Durable	More expensive
	Stronger	Fiberglass/latex
		exposure
	Faster set-time	Possible skin
	Faster time to weight	maceration with
	bearing	water immersion
Fiberglass free and latex free	Same as fiberglass	Same as fiberglass
	Latex and fiberglass free	
	Improved moldability	

Casting Procedure

The types of cast materials used for serial casting include plaster of paris, fiberglass, or fiberglass-free, latex-free casting tape.[92] The advantages and disadvantages of each material are summarized in Table 10-6.

To maximize range of motions, tissue warming can be performed through the application of hot packs, ultrasound, or an endurance activity followed by several minutes of stretch. Afterward, the limb is maintained in a stretched position, ensuring a low-load pull. After the joint is preconditioned, stockinet is placed over the limb with 1 inch extra length cut both proximally and distally to cover the distal ends of the final layer of cast material. The limb is wrapped with web roll using approximately two layers, avoiding wrinkles. All bony prominences are padded and pressure relief pads are created for excessively bony areas. The cast material is applied in distal to proximal direction. Proper wrapping uses a half overlap of the material, avoiding pulling because some shrinkage is anticipated during the drying process. The lengthened position is maintained during casting to avoid undue pressure spots during the casting process. After application of casting, the material can be gently rubbed to facilitate the drying process.

Casting Follow-Up

After casting, the cast should be evaluated for a smooth contour, adequate proximal and distal rim spaces, and avoidance of rough edges. Skin checks should be done to assess appropriate skin color, temperature, pulses, and adequate capillary refill. Emergency and cast care instructions are reviewed with the patient and family with instructions on cast removal, if necessary, at the local emergency department.

Cast changes are typically scheduled anywhere from 3 to 5 days.[92] Cast cutting is done by using a sinusoidal motion along bisected lines. After the cast is successfully cut, separators are used and the cast is removed. After stockinet removal, skin checks and skin care are performed while the arm is maintained in an extended position. The limb is maintained in the lengthening position and another session of warming and stretching ensues followed by repeat casting.

CLINICAL CASE STUDY Recovery of Upper Limb Function

Patient History

Justin Harrison is a 33-year-old man with a C6 tetraplegia, ASIA A diagnosis resulting from a motor vehicle accident He did not have secondary medical complications after injury and completed his inpatient and outpatient rehabilitation. Justin works full time as a lawyer and is now 4 years post injury. He is considering tendon transfer surgery to improve his elbow extension and grip function to aid with transfers and ADL tasks. Justin is medically stable for surgery.

Justin has a health care aide assist him with bowel and bladder care, bathing, and dressing every morning before he leaves for work. He drives himself to work independently in a van equipped with a power lift. Justin frequently travels from his office to the courthouse and so uses a power wheelchair at work because he has determined that his manual wheelchair would be less efficient. Justin is right handed and he needs to improve his independence in transfers and other ADLs. His home is fully accessible. He and his wife are considering having a child and are currently undergoing fertility counseling.

Patient's Self-Assessment

Justin feels he has adjusted well to his injury. He is satisfied with his work and thankful that he was able to complete his law degree. Now he would like to decrease the level of assistance he requires from his part-time aide (2 hours each morning) as well as from his wife in the evenings. Justin believes the tendon transfer surgery will decrease the amount of time it takes for him to perform daily tasks and the level of dependence he feels he places on his wife. He thinks the surgery will also improve his quality of life by allowing him more opportunities for recreation. Justin would like to be involved in fitness activities. His goal is to return to playing tennis using a grip glove attached to the tennis racquet; he was an avid tennis player before his injury.

Clinical Assessment
Patient Appearance
- Height 5 feet 9 inches, weight 160 pounds, body mass index 23.6

Cognitive Assessment
- Alert, oriented × 3

Cardiopulmonary Assessment
- Blood pressure 118/64 mm Hg, heart rate at rest 68, respiratory rate 14 breaths/min, cough flows are reduced (<360 L/min), vital capacity is reduced (between 1.5 and 2.5 L)

Musculoskeletal and Neuromuscular Assessment
- Motor assessment reveals C6 ASIA A, sensory C6
- Deep tendon reflexes 3+ below the level of lesion

Integumentary and Sensory Assessment
- Skin is intact throughout, sensory intact to C6

Range of Motion Assessment
- Passive and active range of motion is within normal limits in both upper limbs
- Straight leg raise is 100 degrees in both lower limbs and dorsiflexion is 0 degrees; all other motions in the lower limbs are within functional limits.

Mobility and ADL Assessment
- Independent with bed mobility
- Independent in wheelchair-to-bed transfers
- Requires moderate assistance to transfer to the shower chair
- Independent with pressure relief
- Independent in manual wheelchair maneuvering on level surfaces

- Independent in power wheelchair maneuvering on all surfaces
- Dependent in bowel and bladder care
- Independent in upper body dressing and dependent in lower body dressing
- Independent in driving

Equipment

Transfer board, manual and power wheelchairs, driving vehicle adapted with hand controls, and shower chair.

Evaluation of Clinical Assessment

Justin Harrison is a 33-year-old man with a C6 tetraplegia, ASIA A diagnosis. He sustained his spinal cord injury 4 years ago as the result of a motor vehicle accident. He is scheduled for a consultation for tendon transfer surgery.

Patient's Care Needs
1. Consultation for tendon transfer surgery
2. Education regarding functional outcomes post surgery

Diagnosis and Prognosis

Diagnosis is C6 complete tetraplegia, ASIA A, with a prognosis of improved functional abilities after rehabilitation after tendon transfer surgery.

Preferred Practice Patterns*

Impaired Muscle Performance (4C), Impairments Nonprogressive Spinal Cord Disorders (5H), Primary Prevention/Risk Reduction for Cardiovascular/Pulmonary Disorders (6A), Primary Prevention/Risk Reduction for Integumentary Disorders (7A)

Team Goals
1. Team to educate patient on postsurgical precautions including demonstration of a sample splint or cast, provide a sample of the surgeon's structured exercise progression program, and prepare patient for alternative technologies that will be needed during the early recovery period when weight bearing and range of motion will be restricted.
2. Team to improve patient's functional mobility and ability to perform ADLs after tendon transfer surgery

Patient Goals

"I want to be able to do more of my care independently and participate in fitness activities again."

Care Plan
Treatment Plan & Rationale
- Tendon transfer surgery consultation
- Presurgical education by physical and occupational therapists

Interventions
- Outpatient physical therapy and occupational therapy services as indicated for postsurgical rehabilitation

Documentation and Team Communication
- Team consultation for optimal tendon transfer surgery
- Documentation of patient's current functional activities that require the use of the target surgical limb and consult regarding postsurgical functional alternatives

Follow-Up Assessment
- Reassessment for consultation with other services

CLINICAL CASE STUDY Recovery of Upper Limb Function—cont'd

Critical Thinking Exercises

Consider factors that will influence patient education, therapy, and team care decisions unique to Justin's spinal cord injury associated with his recovery of upper limb function and alternative options to enhance function when answering the following questions:

1. On the basis of the information provided in the chapter, what type of tendon transfer surgery is indicated in this case?
2. What information should be provided to Justin regarding immobilization of his limb after surgery? What information should be provided to Justin regarding remobilization of his limb after surgery?

3. What functional gains should Justin anticipate when considering a successful outcome?
4. What are some considerations related to rehabilitation after surgery and the impact on Justin's work and home life and schedules?

*Guide to physical therapist practice, rev. ed. 2, Alexandria, VA, 2003, American Physical Therapy Association.

SUMMARY

Upper limb management of individuals with SCI requires expertise in assessment and treatment. Traditional noninvasive therapies remain a mainstay in upper limb rehabilitation; however, there is strong evidence in support of more invasive procedures such as tendon transfers. New restorative therapies such as implantable FES technology are being developed and care must be taken to protect the limb for these and other treatment paradigms that will emerge in the future as a result of continuing research.

REFERENCES

1. Hentz VR, Leclercq C: *Surgical rehabilitation of the upper limb in tetraplegia*, Philadelphia, 2002, WB Saunders.
2. Kirshblum S, Campagnolo DI, DeLias JA: *Spinal cord medicine*, Philadelphia, 2002, Lippincott Williams & Wilkins.
3. Renshaw TS: Spinal cord injury and posttraumatic deformities. In Weinstein SL: *The pediatric spine: principles and practice*, ed 2, Philadelphia, 2001, Lippincott Williams & Wilkins.
4. Renshaw TS: Paralysis in the child: orthopedic management. In Bradford DS, Hensinger RM, editors: *The pediatric spine*, New York, 1985, Thieme.
5. Betz RR: Orthopaedic problems in the child with spinal cord injury, *Top Spinal Cord Inj Rehabil* 3:9-19, 1997.
6. Lubicky J, Betz R: Spinal deformity in children and adolescents after spinal cord injury. In Betz RR, Mulcahey MJ, editors: *The child with spinal cord injury*, Rosemont, IL, 1996, American Academy Orthopaedic Surgeons.
7. Mehta S, Betz RR, Mulcahey MJ et al: Effect of bracing on paralytic scoliosis secondary to spinal cord injury, *J Spinal Cord Med* 27 (1 Suppl):S88-S92, 2004.
8. Guille JT, Betz RR, Balsara RK et al: The feasibility, safety, and utility of vertebral wedge osteotomies for the fusionless treatment of paralytic scoliosis, *Spine* 28:S266-S274, 2003.
9. Peckham PH, Gorman P: Functional electrical stimulation in the 21st century, *Top Spinal Cord Rehabil* 10:126-50, 2004.
10. Landi A, Mulcahey MJ, Caserta G et al: Tetraplegia: update on assessment, *Hand Clinics* 18:377-389, 2002.
11. Consortium for Spinal Cord Medicine: Preservation of upper limb function following spinal cord injury: a clinical practice guideline for health care professionals, *J Spinal Cord Med* 5:433-470, 2005.
12. Johansen ME, Murray WM: The unoperated hand: the role of passive forces in hand function after tetraplegia, *Hand Clinics* 18:391-398, 2002.
13. Mulcahey MJ, Smith BT, Betz RR: Evaluation of lower motor neuron integrity of the upper extremity muscles in high level tetraplegia, *Spinal Cord* 37:585-591, 1999.

14. Mulcahey MJ: Rehabilitation and outcomes of upper extremity tendon transfer surgery. In Betz RR, Mulcahey MJ, editors: *The child with spinal cord injury*, Rosemont, IL, 1996, American Academy Orthopaedic Surgeons.
15. Mulcahey MJ, Hutchinson D, Kozin S: Assessment of the upper limb in tetraplegia: considerations in evaluation and outcomes research, *J Rehabil Res Dev* 44:91-102, 2007.
16. Bryden A, Sinnott KA, Mulcahey MJ: Innovative strategies for improving upper extremity function in tetraplegia and considerations in measuring functional outcomes, *Top Spinal Cord Inj Rehabil* 10:75-93, 2005.
17. van Tuijl JH, Janssen-Potten YJM, Seelen HAM: Evaluation of upper extremity motor function tests in tetraplegics, *Spinal Cord* 40:51-64, 2002.
18. Wukich DK, Motko J: Safety of total contact casting in high-risk patients with neuropathic foot ulcers, *Foot Ankle Int* 25:556-560, 2004.
19. Stroh-Wuolle K, Thrope G, Keith M et al: Development of a quantitative hand grasp and release test for patients with tetraplegia using a hand neuroprosthesis, *J Hand Surg* 19A:209-218, 1994.
20. Marino RJ: Upper extremity capabilities in SCI, *Arch Phys Med Rehabil* 79:1512-1521, 1998.
21. Marino RJ, Shea JA, Stineman MG: The capabilities of upper extremity instrument: reliability and validity of a measure of functional limitation in tetraplegia, *Arch Phys Med Rehabil* 79:1512-1521, 1998.
22. Law M, Baptiste S, McColl M et al: The Canadian occupational performance measure: an outcome measure for occupational therapy, *Can J Occup Ther* 57:82-87, 1990.
23. McColl MA, Paterson M, Davies D et al: Validity and community utility of the Canadian occupational performance measure, *Can J Occup Ther* 67:22-30, 1999.
24. Mulcahey MJ, Smith BT, Betz RR: Psychometric rigor of the Grasp and Release Test for measuring functional limitation of persons with tetraplegia: a preliminary analysis, *J Spinal Cord Med* 27:41-46, 2004.
25. Mulcahey MJ, Betz RR, Smith BT et al: A prospective evaluation of upper extremity tendon transfers in children with cervical level spinal cord injury, *J Pediatr Orthop* 19:319-328, 1999.

26. Smith BT, Mulcahey MJ, Betz RR: Quantitative comparison of grasp and release abilities with and without functional neuromuscular stimulation in adolescents with tetraplegia, *Paraplegia* 34:16-23, 1996.

27. Smith BT, Mulcahey MJ, Triolo RJ et al: The application of a modified neuroprosthetic hand system in a child with C7 spinal cord injury: case report, *Paraplegia* 30:598-606, 1992.

28. Mulcahey MJ, Lutz C, Kozin S et al: Prospective evaluation of biceps to triceps and deltoid to triceps for elbow extension in tetraplegia, *J Hand Surg* 28A:964-971, 2003.

29. Malick MH, Meyer CM: *Manual on management of the quadriplegic upper extremity*, Pittsburgh, 1978, Harmerville Rehabilitation Center.

30. Mulcahey MJ: Upper extremity orthoses and splints. In Betz RR, Mulcahey MJ, editors: *The child with spinal cord injury*, Rosemont, IL, 1996, American Academy Orthopaedic Surgeons.

31. Consortium for Spinal Cord Medicine: *Outcomes following traumatic SCI: clinical practice guidelines for health care professionals*, Washington, DC, 1999, Paralyzed Veterans of America.

32. Knox CC, Engel WH, Siebens AA: Results of a survey on the use of a wrist-driven splint for prehension, *Am J Occup Ther* 25:109-111, 1971.

33. Krajnik S, Bridle M: Hand splinting in quadriplegia: current practice, *Am J Occup Ther* 46:149-156, 1992.

34. Kirsblum S, O'Conner K, Benevento B et al: Spinal and upper extremity orthotics. In DeLisa J, Gans B, editors: *Rehabilitation medicine: principles and practice*, ed 3, Philadelphia, 1998, Lippincott-Raven.

35. Landsberger S, Leung P, Vargas V et al: Mobile arm supports: history, application and work in progress, *Top Spinal Cord Inj Rehabil* 11:74-94, 2005.

36. Lathem PA, Gregorio TL, Garber SL: High level quadriplegia: an occupational therapy challenge, *Am J Occup Ther* 39:705-714, 1985.

37. Allen VR: Follow-up study of the wrist-drive flexor hinge splint use, *Am J Occup Ther* 25:398-401, 1971.

38. Martin C: Functional hand orthosis for quadriplegia: long term use, *Am Spinal Inj Assoc Abstr Digest* 372, 1987.

39. Shepherd CC, Ruzicka SH: Tenodesis brace use by persons with spinal cord injuries, *Am J Occup Ther* 45:81-83, 1990.

40. Garber SL, Gregorio TL: Upper extremity assistive devices: assessment of use by spinal cord patients with quadriplegia, *Am J Occup Ther* 44:126-131, 1990.

41. Mulcahey MJ, Betz RR: Upper and lower extremity applications of functional electrical stimulation: a decade of research with children and adolescents with spinal injuries, *Pediatr Phys Ther* 113-122, 1997.

42. Peckham PH, Marsolais EB, Mortimer JT: Restoration of key grip and release in C6 tetraplegic through functional electrical stimulation, *J Hand Surg* 5:462-469, 1980.

43. Peckham PH, Mortimer JT, Marsolais EB: Controlled prehension and release in the C5 quadriplegic elicited by functional electrical stimulation of the paralyzed forearm musculature, *Ann Biomed Eng* 8:369-388, 1980.

44. Davis SE, Mulcahey MJ, Smith BT et al: Outcome of functional electrical stimulation in the rehabilitation of a child with C5 tetraplegia, *J Spinal Cord Med* 22:107-113, 1999.

45. Mulcahey MJ, Smith BT, Betz RR et al: Functional neuromuscular stimulation: outcomes in young people with tetraplegia, *J Am Paraplegia Soc* 17:20-35, 1994.

46. Peckham PH, Kilgore K, Keith MW et al: An advanced neuroprosthesis system for restoration of hand and upper arm control employing an implantable controller, *J Hand Surg* 27A:265-276, 2002.

47. Davis SE, Mulcahey MJ, Betz RR: Freehand their hand: the role of occupational therapy in implementing FES in tetraplegia, *Technol Disabil* 11:29-34, 1999.

48. Kilgore KL, Peckman PH, Keith MW et al: An implanted upper-extremity neuroprosthesis: follow-up of five patients, *J Bone Joint Surg Am* 79:533-541, 1997.

49. Mulcahey MJ, Betz RR, Smith, BT et al: Implanted functional electrical stimulation hand system in adolescents with spinal injuries: an evaluation, *Arch Phys Med Rehabil* 78:597-607, 1997.

50. Stroh-Wuolle K, Van Doren C, Bryden A et al: Satisfaction with and usage of a hand neuroprosthesis, *Arch Phys Med Rehab* 80:206-213, 1999.

51. Creasy GH, Kilgore KL, Brown-Triolo D et al: Reduction of costs of disability using neuroprostheses, *Asst Technol* 12:67-75, 2000.

52. Keith MW, Hoyden H: Indications and future direction for the upper limb neuroprostheses in tetraplegic patients: a review, *Hand Clin* 18:519-528, 2002.

53. Snoek GJ, Ijzerman MJ, Groen T et al: Use of the NESS handmaster to restore hand function in tetraplegia: clinical experiences in ten patients, *Spinal Cord* 38:244-249, 2000.

54. Alon G, McBride K: Persons with C5 or C6 tetraplegia achieve selected functional gains using a neuroprosthesis, *Arch Phys Med Rehabil* 84:119-124, 2003.

55. Beasley R: Surgical treatment of hands for C5-C6 tetraplegia, *Orthop Clin North Am* 14:893-904, 1983.

56. Bryan RS: The Moberg deltoid-triceps replacement and key-pinch operations in quadriplegia: preliminary experiences, *Hand* 9:207-214, 1977.

57. Coyler RA, Kappelman B: Flexor pollicis longus tenodesis in tetraplegia at the sixth cervical level: a prospective evaluation of functional gain, *J Bone Joint Surg* 63A:376-379, 1981.

58. DeBenedetti M: Restoration of elbow extension power in the tetraplegia patient using the Moberg technique, *J Hand Surg* 4A:86-89, 1979.

59. Freehafer AA: Tendon transfers in patients with cervical spinal cord injury, *J Hand Surg* 16A:804-809, 1991.

60. Freehafer AA, Kelly CM, Peckham PH: Tendon transfer for the restoration of upper limb function after a cervical spinal cord injury, *J Hand Surg* 9A:887-893, 1984.

61. Freehafer AA, Kelly CM, Peckham PH: Planning tendon transfers in tetraplegia: Cleveland technique. In Hunter JM, Schneider LH, Mackin EJ, editors: *Tendon transfer surgery in the hand*, St. Louis, 1987, CV Mosby.

62. Freehafer AA, Peckham PH, Keith MV: New concepts in the treatment of the upper limb in tetraplegia: surgical restoration and functional neuromuscular stimulation, *Hand Clin* 4:563-574, 1988.

63. Freehafer A, Vonhaam A, Allen V: Tendon transfers to improve grasp after injuries of the cervical spinal cord, *J Bone Joint Surg* 56A:951-959, 1974.

64. Hentz VR, Brown M, Keoshian LA: Upper limb reconstruction in quadriplegia: functional assessment and proposed treatment modifications, *J Hand Surg* 8A:119-131, 1983.

65. Hentz VR, Hamlin C, Keoshian L: Surgical reconstruction in tetraplegia, *Hand Clin* 4:601-607, 1988.

66. Hentz VR, House J, McDowell C et al: Rehabilitation and surgical reconstruction of the upper limb in tetraplegia: and update, *J Hand Surg* 17A:964-967, 1992.

67. James M: Surgical treatment of upper extremity: indications, patient assessment and procedures. In Betz RR, Mulcahey MJ, editors: *The child with spinal cord injury,* Rosemont, IL, 1996, American Academy of Orthopaedic Surgeons.

68. McDowell CL, House JH: Tetraplegia. In Green DP, Hotchkiss RN, Pederson WC, editors: *Operative hand surgery*, ed 4, New York, 1999, Churchill Livingstone.

69. Moberg E: Surgical treatment for absent single-hand grip and elbow extension in quadriplegia: principles and preliminary experience, *J Bone Joint Surg* 57A:196-206, 1975.

70. Moberg E: Surgical rehabilitation of the upper limb in tetraplegia, *Paraplegia* 28:330-334, 1990.

71. Moberg E: The new surgical rehabilitation of arm-hand function in the tetraplegic patient, *Scand J Rehab Med* 17(Suppl):131-132, 1998.

72. Mohammand K, Rothwell A, Sinclair S et al: Upper limb surgery for tetraplegia, *J Bone Joint Surg* 74B:873-879, 1992.

73. McDowell CL, Moberg EA, House JH: The second international conference on surgical rehabilitation of the upper limb in tetraplegia, *J Hand Surg* 11A:604-608, 1986.

74. Ejeskar A: Upper limb surgical rehabilitation in high level tetraplegia, *Hand Clin* 4:585-599, 1988.

75. Revol M, Brian E, Servant JM: Biceps to triceps transfer in tetraplegia, *J Hand Surg* 24B:235-237, 1999.

76. Stackhouse C, Mulcahey MJ, Duffy T et al: Biomechanical measures of elbow extension following biceps to triceps tendon transfer surgery. In *Proceedings of the 51st Annual Conference of the American Paraplegia Society*, Las Vegas, September 2005.

77. Kozin SH, Schloth C: Bilateral biceps to triceps to salvage failed bilateral deltoid to triceps transfer: a case report, *J Hand Surg* 27:666-669, 2002.

78. Kuz J, Van Heest A, House J: Biceps to triceps transfer in tetraplegia patients: report of the medical routing technique and follow-up of three cases, *J Hand Surg* 24:161-72, 1999.

79. House J, Gwathmey FW, Lundsgaard DK: Restoration of strong grasp and lateral pinch in tetraplegia due to cervical spinal cord injury, *J Hand Surg* 1:152-159, 1976.

80. Paul SD, Gellman H, Waters P et al: Single-stage reconstruction of key pinch and extension of the elbow in tetraplegic patients, *J Bone Joint Surg Am* 76:1451-1456, 1994.

81. Peckham PH, Keith MW, Kilgore KL et al: Efficacy of an implanted neuroprosthesis for restoring hand grasp in tetraplegia: a multicenter study, *Arch Phys Med Rehabil* 82:1380-1388, 2001.

82. House JH, Camadoll J, Dahl AL: One stage key pinch and release with thumb carpal-metacarpal fusion in tetraplegia, *J Hand Surg* 17A:530-538, 1992.

83. Kozin SH, Clark P, Porter S et al: The contribution of the intrinsic muscles to grip and pinch strength, *J Hand Surg [Am]* 24:64-72, 1999.

84. Reynolds CC: Preoperative and postoperative management of tendon transfers after radial nerve injury. In Hunter JM, Schnieder LH, Mackin EJ, editors: *Rehabilitation of the hand: surgery and therapy*, ed 3, St. Louis, 1990, CV Mosby.

85. Riordan DC: Rehabilitation and re-education in tendon transfers, *Orthop Clin North Am* 5:445-449, 1974.

86. Zancolli E: Functional restoration of the upper limbs in traumatic quadriplegia. In Zancolli E, editor: *Structural and dynamic bases of hand surgery*, ed 2, Philadelphia, 1979, Lippincott.

87. Bell-Krotoski JA: Plaster cylinder casting for contractures of the interphalangeal joints, In Hunter JM, Mackin EJ, Callahan AD, editors: *Rehabilitation of the hand*, ed 5, St. Louis, 2002, Mosby.

88. Flowers KR, LaStayo P: Effect of total end range time on improving passive range of motion, *J Hand Ther* 7:150-157, 1994.

89. Leahy P: Precasting work sheet—an assessment tool: a clinical report, *Phys Ther* 68:72-74, 1988.

90. Bonutti PM, Windau JE, Ables BA et al: Static progressive stretch to reestablish elbow range of motion, *Clin Orthop Relat Res* 303:128-134, 1994.

91. Tynan M: Joint contractures in children with spinal cord injuries. In Betz RR, Mulcahey MJ, editors: *The child with spinal cord injury*, Rosemont, IL, 1996, American Academy of Orthopaedic Surgeons.

92. Adkins LM: Cast changes: synthetic versus plaster, *Pediatr Nurs* 23:425-427, 1997.

SOLUTIONS TO CHAPTER 10 CLINICAL CASE STUDY

Recovery of Upper Limb Function

1. Optimal surgery indicates the biceps to triceps for restoration of elbow extension.

2. Immobilization after tendon transfer surgery lasts from 1 to 3 weeks with a long arm cast in full elbow extension. Shoulder flexion is limited to 90 degrees and extension to 0 degrees for the biceps-to-triceps transfer. Edema control is used. The cast is replaced by a splint that prevents accidental range of motion and is only removed in therapy (see Table 10-2).

3. Remobilization after the cast is removed takes from 3 to 12 weeks (see Table 10-2 for details). No passive range of motion for elbow flexion should be performed until 3 months after surgery. No strengthening exercises should be preformed until 6 weeks after surgery.

4. Justin should be able to anticipate an improved ability in all transfers to all surfaces and increased ease with bed mobility, ADLs, and skin relief techniques after surgery and rehabilitation.

5. Rehabilitation after tendon transfer surgery is very lengthy. The impact from the loss of upper limb use for functional mobility and job tasks as a lawyer needs to be considered and discussed thoroughly. The arm chosen for surgery should be carefully considered as well because of limb dominance issues and the related needs for ADL before and immediately after surgery and for postsurgical outcomes.

CHAPTER ELEVEN

Seating and Positioning

Kim Davis, MSPT, David Kreutz, PT, ATP, Chris Maurer, ATP, MPT, and Stephen H. Sprigle, PT, PhD

I was very discouraged with my first wheelchairs. It took me a couple of years to figure out that your chair is part of your attire. A chair should fit you like a well-tailored suit and its design blend with your personality. When all this works together you hardly know it's under you!

Frank (T12 SCI)

Many factors can influence a client's choice of wheelchair and his positioning in the chair. These include spasticity, range of motion (ROM), surgical stabilization of the spine, muscle strength, muscle imbalance, the effects of gravity, orthopedic deformities, balance, functional status, environmental issues, transportation status, and lifestyle. A thorough evaluation can provide information about each of these areas. Each client will have different goals and priorities, and determining the relative importance of these goals will help to determine the features of the seating and mobility system that are most appropriate and important to that particular client. Often there are conflicting goals and trade-offs, which make a thorough seating evaluation process vital to achieving optimal outcomes. Wheelchair selection is best performed with the help of a client-centered team.[1]

The team should include, but not be limited to, the client, family or significant others, physician, physical and occupational therapist, nurse, assistive technology specialist who specializes in seating and wheeled mobility, adaptive driving specialist, case manager or social worker, and rehabilitation technology supplier (RTS). Not all these people need to be present at the time the seating and mobility system is selected, but their input can be extremely beneficial and, at times, essential to a successful outcome. For example, if a wheelchair is recommended without considering transportation needs, a client may end up with a wheelchair that he cannot load into his car or a wheelchair that he cannot tie down properly. The goal of maximizing functional mobility would thus not be achieved. Generally, individuals who are newly injured and receiving their first wheelchairs rely more heavily on the input of multiple team members; those seeking replacement wheelchairs often have a very good sense of what has and will best suit their needs.

COMPONENTS OF A COMPREHENSIVE SEATING AND WHEELED MOBILITY EVALUATION
Client Information

As with any therapy evaluation, basic client-identifying data, such as name, date of birth, referral date, height, and weight should be collected. What is somewhat unique to a wheelchair evaluation is the predictive data that must be gleaned from this intake process. The nature of this predictive quality is related to the length of time that this equipment is expected to serve the client's needs. This in turn is largely related to the funding source for the equipment. The guidelines for third-party payers vary, whether private insurance or a federal (i.e., Medicare) or state program (i.e., Medicaid). Some private insurance companies may have an annual allowable amount

for durable medical equipment or a cap, whereas other insurance companies or federal-state programs may expect equipment to last a minimum of 5 years. Such guidelines can be ever changing and the RTS is often the key team member to research this information.[1]

In addition to a person's weight, a clinician should note whether it is stable or if there is any trend in weight loss or gain. This information can be figured into the equipment recommendation with regard to dimensions and weight capacity. If the client is newly injured and has had a significant weight loss since the injury, it is helpful to note a premorbid weight; if there is a current trend of regaining weight, using the premorbid weight as a target can be helpful as a rough guide in predicting equipment dimension needs. If the client is young enough to still be growing in height, especially if of an age where a growth spurt is occurring or soon anticipated, this should also be factored into the equipment dimensions. It must be noted, however, that factoring in growth does not mean that the client should be expected to grow into the equipment. Equipment must meet the needs at the time of delivery and may have the ability to accommodate growth by reconfiguring the setup or by replacing certain components, both of which are less costly than replacing the entire system. Again, the RTS is usually best suited to provide guidance with these options.[1]

As previously suggested, noting the client's goals is crucial to a successful match of person and technology. If these goals are not considered, there is a greater chance of dissatisfaction as well as technology abandonment. Such negative outcomes are compounded if the guideline of the particular funding source includes an expectation that equipment will be used for a minimum of 5 years. Equally important, this equipment should be an extension of self-expression of the user. A newly injured individual, especially, is getting accustomed to a new body image; the equipment features, whenever possible, should have a positive impact on his self-image. In the case where a client may require assistance to use the equipment (e.g., an individual with C5 tetraplegia), it is important to also note the input of the caregiver. The caregiver must be comfortable with, and capable of, the supportive role required for successful use of the equipment. The evaluation period is the time to work through any issues of incongruence, rather than after the equipment arrives.

Pertinent Medical History

In addition to the primary, and secondary if applicable, diagnosis, medical history that is pertinent to the wheelchair and seating recommendation should be recorded. Funds for the wheelchair itself and its particular components are reviewed by medical funding sources on the basis of medical necessity. Therefore, the medical history, in combination with the physical findings and functional status of the client, must support the recommendation. Pertinent items include sensory status, visual status, past or present pressure ulcers, cardiac or pulmonary disease, bowel and bladder status, history of arthritis, recent or planned surgeries (i.e., orthopedic procedures, Baclofen pump insertion), presence of heterotopic ossification, and peripheral vascular disease or edema. It is not uncommon for individuals with spinal cord injury (SCI) to have also sustained a concurrent traumatic brain injury, often mild. If this is the case, any impairment in judgment or safety awareness should be noted.

Equipment History

In the case of a first wheelchair, the client and primary therapy team can provide input regarding the pros and cons of the equipment tried during his inpatient rehabilitation. If the client is seeking a replacement wheelchair, providing input on past equipment success and failures helps to ensure that successful features will be resought and that equipment feature failures will not be repeated. In addition, any other equipment that will be used in conjunction with the new wheelchair and seating must be reviewed to make sure it will interface effectively.

Environment

The primary environments, including home and community, where the wheelchair will be used should be reviewed. If possible, having a team member perform an on-site home accessibility evaluation is preferable. Important items include accessible entrance, secondary emergency egress, adequate door widths, and adequate space for turning—especially on landings and in hallways. The clinician should also inquire whether the client has any immediate plans to move. It may behoove the team to delay ordering the equipment until accessibility in the new home can be reviewed. Secondary environments, such as school, workplace, or recreation areas should also be discussed. Keep in mind that most medical insurance plans are primarily concerned with equipment features that fulfill medical necessity. Thus, a feature that primarily meets a recreational, academic, or work-related need may not be funded by medical insurance. Alternative funding may need to be sought.

Activities of Daily Living and Transfer Status

Knowing the independence levels and techniques used for the client's various activities of daily living (ADL) will help to ensure that the equipment facilitates independence wherever possible. Likewise, transfer status should be reviewed. Choosing incorrect footrests, inappropriate seat height or tilt, or a cushion with the wrong firmness or contour could negatively affect transfer techniques. These issues are discussed later.

Transportation

It is important to review current method(s) of transportation as well as any plans for future changes. Generally, wheelchair users either enter a vehicle while seated in their wheelchairs or transfer into the vehicle and stow their wheelchairs. Furthermore, those who enter the vehicle while in a wheelchair may drive or ride as a passenger and may do so from the wheelchair or after transferring to a vehicle seat. All these transportation approaches are related to the type of wheelchair and seating system being used. These and other transportation issues are discussed in Chapter 20.

Considerations in Selecting Power Versus Manual Wheelchairs

The level of SCI is not the only consideration when choosing between a power and manual wheelchair recommendation. Medical and environmental factors all contribute to the decision.

Age, level of injury, concurrent injuries, and secondary complications are medical issues that need to be examined. People who are injured later in life may not have the strength or endurance to propel a manual wheelchair functionally, regardless of the level of injury. Even people with the same level of injury vary in their functional skill levels. Some people with a C7 level of injury may be able to propel over all terrain and others may not be able to negotiate over a door threshold. The strength and endurance of the intact musculature and the symmetry of strength, especially around the scapula, can dictate how well someone can propel a manual wheelchair. Successful manual wheelchair use depends on appropriate scapular mobility and stability while propelling. Concurrent injuries, such as upper limb or clavicular fractures and peripheral nerve injuries, and upper limb pain also contribute to the success of propulsion. In addition, the impact of secondary complications such as arthritis, carpal tunnel syndrome, cardiopulmonary issues, spasticity, head injury, and postural issues must be assessed to determine the most safe and functional means of mobility.

The evaluation of the home, school, and work environments is crucial to the proper equipment recommendation. Power wheelchairs are heavy pieces of equipment and the integrity of the building structures the person will encounter need to be able to handle the weight of the person in addition to the power mobility device. Terrain around a home and community environments vary widely. Extremely rough or unpaved terrain may not be conducive to manual wheelchair use. A student may be able to propel a manual wheelchair at home but may not be able to negotiate the terrain around the school campus or be fast enough to get to classes on time. A supervisor of a warehouse has different mobility requirements that may require different equipment recommendations than someone who works in an office cubicle. Because power wheelchairs typically require the use of a van for transportation, lack of transportation options for a power wheelchair may affect the final decision on whether a power or manual chair should be prescribed. Obtaining funding for both power and manual wheelchairs can overcome this potential obstacle and provide a backup means of mobility.

Physical Assessment and Mat Evaluation

The primary focus of the physical assessment is to determine whether there are any barriers to achieving a functional, comfortable, upright seated posture. Anthropometric neutral seated postures are illustrated in Figure 11-1; these are ideal positions to use as a reference comparison for recording actual postural and anatomical measurements.

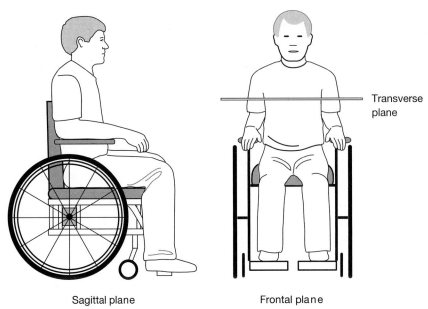

Transverse plane

Sagittal plane   Frontal plane

FIGURE 11-1 Anthropometric neutral seated reference positions show the body's sagittal, frontal, and transverse planes.

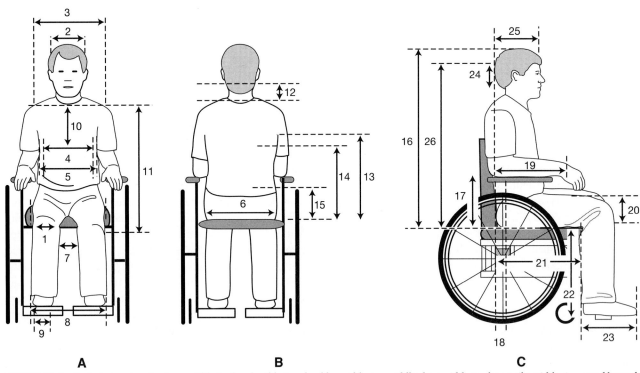

A   **B**   **C**

FIGURE 11-2 **A,** Anterior view; 1 = knee width, 2 = head width, 3 = shoulder width, 4 = middle chest width, 5 = lower ribs width, 6 = seated buttock width (posterior view), 7 = interknee width, 8 = bilateral seated width, 9 = unilateral foot width, 10 = sternal height. **B,** Posterior view; 11 = seat to shoulder height (anterior view), 12 = cervical length, 13 = seat to axilla height, 14 = seat to inferior angle of the scapula, 15 = seat to posterior ilium. **C,** Lateral view; 16 = seat to top of head, 17 = seat to elbow height, 18 = vertical orientation from floor past posterior occiput, 19 = forearm length, 20 = thigh or lap height from seat, 21 = axle to posterior leg, 22 = footrest to seat height, 23 = foot length, 24 = posterior occiput to superior cervical height, 25 = head length.

The postural assessment is done with the client in supine with gravity eliminated and in sitting (i.e., noting the effects of gravity). Important areas to address in supine and side-lying positions include skin integrity (e.g., noting both current pressure ulcers and scar tissue), spine and pelvis mobility,

presence of orthopedic deformities and whether each is flexible or fixed, presence of abnormal tone, adequate joint ROM for the seated posture, and adequate ROM and strength for the mode of propulsion or drive control. In sitting, areas to be addressed include static and dynamic balance, the presence of asymmetries

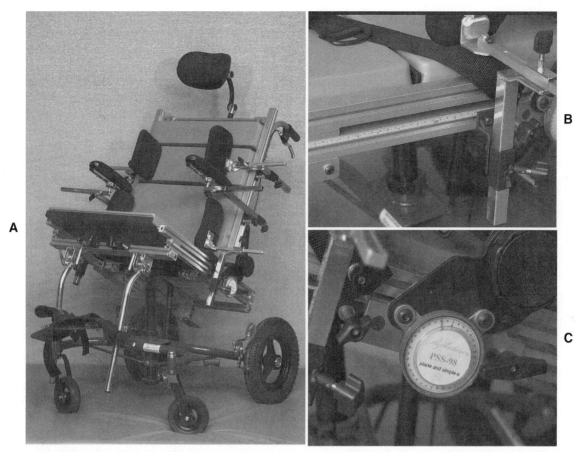

FIGURE 11-3 **A,** The Prairie Seating Simulator is used to determine planar alignment for clients such as lateral trunk curvatures, pelvic obliquities, or thigh adduction while providing head support. **B,** Close-up view of the adjustability of the hip pads through the lateral mounting bracket. **C,** Laterally placed angle dial to quantify the seat back angle of trunk flexion that can vary between 60 and 180 degrees. {Prairie Seating Simulator No. 2845, 2848, and 2850.}

and orthopedic deformities, how these may differ in sitting under the influence of gravity, and the amount of force required to correct or reduce the deformity, if flexible. If abnormal tone is noted in supine, this should also be reassessed in sitting because there are often positional differences. Anatomical dimensions that are used to choose wheelchair and seating product dimensions should also be taken in sitting (Figure 11-2), but it is crucial that the client is supported in the posture that will be assumed in the wheelchair. For this reason, for clients who do not have independent sitting balance, it is useful to take anatomical measurements with the client in a Prairie seating simulator, if available (Figure 11-3).

If measurements are taken with the client seated on the edge of a mat table and proper support is not provided, two of the most common measurement errors are underestimated shoulder height and overestimated thigh length (Figure 11-4). The former occurs if the client has a flexible scoliosis or kyphosis and collapses into gravity versus being supported to minimize the deformity. This could lead to ordering a backrest, intended to provide full posterior trunk support, that would be too low to accommodate the actual condition. The latter occurs if the client has a flexible pelvis and can achieve a neutral to slight anterior pelvic tilt (i.e., the goal for optimal sitting posture) but instead is slouched in a posterior pelvic tilt during measurement. This could lead to ordering a seat frame or cushion depth which is too long, which may end up forcing the client into a posterior tilt.

Seating Simulation and Mock-Up

The physical assessment findings guide determination of what product features are needed for the seating system and wheelchair. Seating and postural needs are determined first, before moving onto the mobility system. It is helpful to go through this intermediate step of listing features, which the RTS can then use to identify specific commercial options that will best meet the needs. If the team jumps straight from physical findings to specific product, it may lead to trying to force a product to fit the client when that product may not have been the best match to the client's array of needs. Especially in the case of a client with complex postural needs, use of a seating simulator helps to cement the product feature list, including the desired location of postural support components. Seating simulators are highly adjustable with respect to the seat and back surfaces (including tilt and recline) and the postural support components (see Figure 11-3, *B* and *C*). They are used to verify how to best set up a seating system to provide the necessary postural support with respect to optimizing balance, comfort, visual orientation, correcting flexible orthopedic deformity, or accommodating fixed deformity. They can be used by sitting the client directly on the planar seat surface as well as by placing a cushion atop the seat surface. If a simulator is not available, this step can be accomplished with use of a wheelchair that has similar adjustability. High-functioning individuals with paraplegia who do not have significant postural

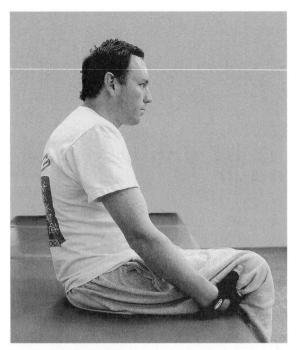

FIGURE 11-4 A client sitting without back support shows gravitational influences producing a posterior pelvic tilt, kyphotic thoracic spine, and absence of lumbar curve that will cause overestimation of seat depth if not properly corrected before measurement. (From Pendaleton HMcH, Schultz-Krohn W: *Pedretti's occupational therapy: practice skills for physical dysfunction,* ed 6, St. Louis, 2006, Mosby Elsevier, F 11-08 C, p 213.)

problems are not as likely to need to go through the step of using an actual seating simulator. Their postural needs are best determined with a properly configured wheelchair based on specific measurements (Figure 11-5, *A*) so that postural support can be assessed in conjunction with effective propulsion.

Equipment Trial

After the client's postural needs are determined by simulation, the next step is equipment trial, where the seating components are married to the mobility base, whether a manual or power wheelchair. It is preferable for the team, lead by the RTS, to provide multiple options for trial and comparison. This contributes significantly to a good match of person to technology. Ordering equipment without benefit of trial is strongly discouraged. The wheelchair is set up according to the simulation findings with regard to seat-to-back angle, system tilt (i.e., angle of the seat with respect to the horizontal), seat depth, back height, and arm-leg-foot rest position. The seating is configured with respect to postural support pad location (i.e., lateral trunk support, lateral pelvic support, or medial-lateral thigh support) and positioning strap angle and location (i.e., anterior pelvis or chest strap). Of course, the types and number of different postural components are unique to each individual. As stated previously, there are always trade-offs. For example, more supports may mean less freedom of movement. Every wheelchair recommendation is a delicate balance of the two. Most high-functioning individuals with paraplegia will require only a well-configured manual wheelchair, a low profile backrest, and an appropriate cushion. A minimalist approach should be implemented to address the goal of seeing

the individual first and foremost, not the equipment. Additionally, in the case of manual wheelchairs, keeping the weight to a minimum is key to efficient propulsion and aids in prevention of shoulder injury.

One additional comment is warranted at this time. Because of decreasing lengths of stay in inpatient rehabilitation, some clinicians may feel the need to initiate wheelchair trials when clients are still in halo devices or thoracolumbosacral orthoses (TLSOs). This should be done only with direct supervision because of the lack of peripheral vision and balance. Additionally, it will be difficult to assess the client's balance and comfort when he is in a halo device or TLSO. Therefore the final determination of a client's wheelchair prescription should not be done until the client is no longer limited by the orthosis.

Wheelchair Prescription

After the wheelchair and seating are selected by the trial process, the specific equipment recommendation is completed by the primary team, consisting at minimum of the client, therapist, assistive technology specialist, and the RTS. Each manufacturer provides order forms that are used by the team to select specific dimension, configuration, and component options. The therapist or assistive technology specialist is responsible for writing a letter of medical justification that supports the recommendation and must be approved by the physician. This is submitted by the RTS to the funding source, together with the quote and any additional supportive documentation. When funding approval is obtained, which can vary from days to months, the equipment is ordered by the RTS.

Delivery

When delivery of the equipment occurs, the primary team should gather to ensure the best quality outcome. The RTS verifies that the equipment was correctly configured and ordered, the therapist ensures that the setup is optimal to meet the client's needs, especially if there have been any changes in condition since his evaluation, and the client confirms that the equipment is as was expected. The RTS reviews maintenance and operational features with the client; the therapist reviews clinical items such as cushion setup, seating component setup, confirms wheelchair configuration with respect to wheelchair skills and transfers, and reviews driving specifications in the case of power wheelchairs. The client should not leave the delivery appointment without knowing how to safely operate and oversee the maintenance of the equipment. It may be determined that additional training sessions are needed to optimize use of the equipment.

Follow-Up

The technology team should be available for follow-up to address any concerns that may arise after the client has had a chance to use the equipment. Examples of follow-up needs include power wheelchair electronics may need to be reprogrammed to optimize driving; cushion setup may need to be readdressed to optimize balance, postural stability, or skin integrity; or rear axle position may need to be fine-tuned to optimize propulsion or balance point for wheelies. In addition, the RTS must provide maintenance or repair services as needed throughout the life of the equipment.

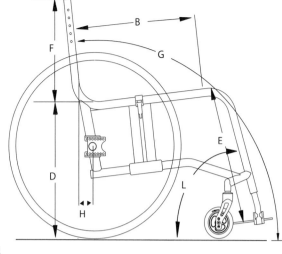

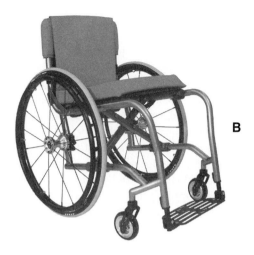

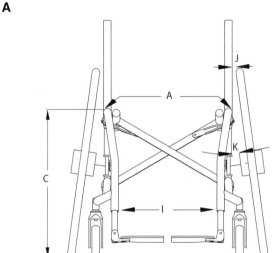

FIGURE 11-5 The TiLite TX wheelchair is designed (**A**) to incorporate the latest folding chair technology while meeting customer demands for a chair (**B**) that is stronger, lighter, and supports better energy transfer and efficient propulsion. *A,* Seat width; *B,* seat depth; *C,* front seat height; *D,* rear seat height; *E,* seat to footrest; *F,* seat back height; *G,* seat back angle; *H,* center of gravity; *I,* footrest width; *J,* rear wheel spacing; *K,* camber angle; *L,* front angle. (Courtesy TiLite, Kennewick, WA.)

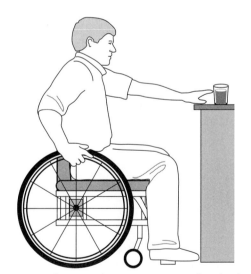

FIGURE 11-6 Proper seating support promotes functional posture.

POSTURAL CONSIDERATIONS

Correct seating and positioning play a pivotal important role in the ability of an individual with SCI to function safely and independently. Proper seating provides an individual with sufficient stabilization to allow optimal functioning and control

(Figure 11-6). With improper seating, an individual may be forced to use valuable energy to simply maintain an upright position. The ultimate goal of proper seating is to provide support that enables the client to achieve his highest level of functional independence. This generally equates to providing adequate proximal or core stability to afford the greatest functional mobility.

Pelvic Positioning

The pelvis is the keystone to a stable seated posture. When the pelvis, legs, and feet are supported, they become the foundation for positioning the spine, upper limbs, and head. The pelvis moves in three planes: transverse, frontal, and sagittal (see Figure 11-1).

In the transverse plane, or top view, which divides the body into upper and lower segments, the pelvis can rotate left or right. In the ideal position, both anterior superior iliac spines (ASISs) face directly forward (Figure 11-7, *A*). In the sagittal plane, or side view, which divides the body into left and right segments, the pelvis can rotate forward (i.e., anterior pelvic tilt) or backward (i.e., posterior pelvic tilt). In the ideal position, both ASISs are level with or slightly lower than the posterior superior iliac spines (PSISs). In other words, the goal is a neutral pelvic position (Figure 11-7, *B*) or a slight anterior tilt (Figure 11-7, *C*). In the frontal plane, or front view, which divides the body into front and back segments, the pelvis can rotate so that one ASIS is higher than the other (i.e., a pelvic obliquity) (Figure 11-7, *D*).[2] In the ideal position, the ASISs are level, which translates to equal weight bearing through the ischial tuberosities.

Intrinsic factors that can affect the position of the pelvis include muscle contractures, spasticity or muscle tone, limited hip ROM or lumbar mobility, surgical stabilization of the spine, surgical ischiectomy, and hip instability (i.e., subluxation or dislocation). Extrinsic factors include the type of seat, back, and cushion used on the wheelchair; angle of the wheelchair seat and back; use of pelvic positioning straps; and proper support of the feet. These extrinsic factors can be manipulated to improve pelvic position and support within the client's tolerance and flexibility. Wheelchair seats are typically either upholstery or solid. Seat upholstery is made of fabric that extends from one seat rail to the other, allowing ease of folding for folding frame manual wheelchairs. Use of upholstery contributes to keeping the overall weight of the wheelchair to a minimum and combined with certain cushions can yield the best pressure distribution for some individuals. Over time, however, the upholstery tends to stretch or sling. Some types of upholstery can be tightened by its attachment to the seat rail, and upholstery can be replaced to regain

tautness. If not addressed, stretched out upholstery can encourage a pelvic obliquity, posterior pelvic tilt, or internal rotation of the hips.[3] Pelvic obliquities occur if the pelvis is positioned off center on the sling, such that one side of the pelvis is supported higher than the other (Figure 11-8, *A*). Internal hip rotation can increase the risk of subluxation or increase pressure at the greater trochanters, compromising skin integrity (Figure 11-8, *B*).

As stated previously, the position of the pelvis dictates the position of the spine. Consequently, if the wheelchair back does not provide adequate support, the spine will tend to curve into scoliosis or round into kyphosis. A solid seat used under the cushion, which can be made of wood, plastic, or a composite material or steel or aluminum in power wheelchairs, can provide the pelvis with a firm, level base of support, thus ensuring the client with increased stability. It is important to note that there could be an impact on pressure distribution and this must be addressed on an individual basis. Likewise, solid backrests (Figure 11-9, *A* to *C*) or tension-adjustable backrest upholstery (Figure 11-10) provide posterior pelvic and lumbar support to encourage neutral pelvic positioning.

In addition to the wheelchair seat and back, the cushion plays a major role in pelvic positioning and support. The depth of the cushion can influence pelvic position, postural stability, and pressure

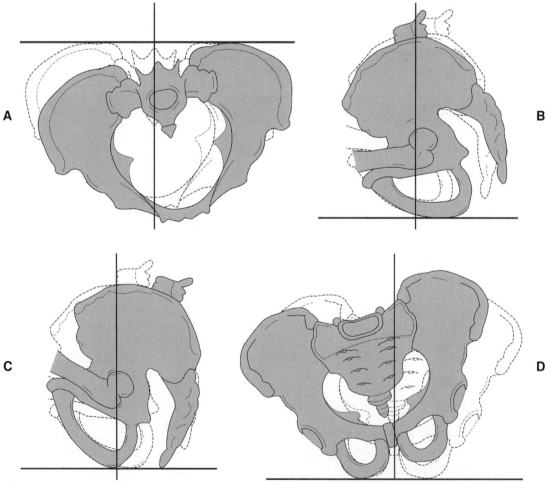

FIGURE 11-7 A, Transverse view of pelvic rotation of the right hemipelvis with respect to the left. **B,** Sagittal view of anterior pelvic rotation (ASISs move anteriorly). **C,** Sagittal view of posterior pelvic tilt (ASISs move posteriorly) showing how the coccyx abuts the seat surface. **D,** Frontal plane view (from the posterior perspective) of lateral pelvic tilt to the left. (Courtesy Stephen H. Sprigle, PhD, © Georgia Tech Research Corporation, Atlanta, GA.)

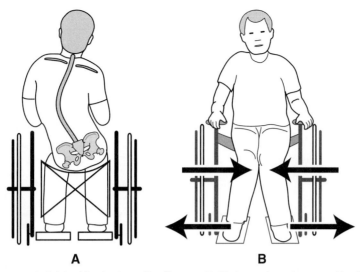

FIGURE 11-8 **A,** Pelvic obliquity created by sling seat. **B,** Hip internal rotation created by sling seat.

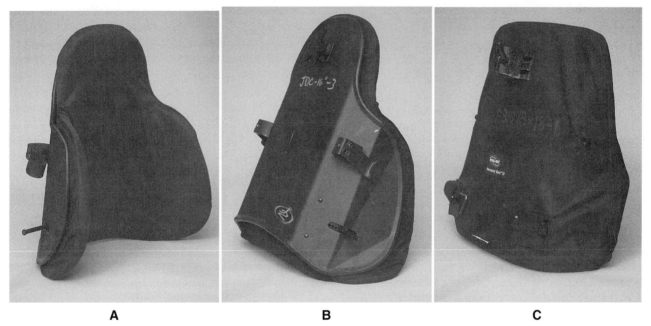

A **B** **C**

FIGURE 11-9 Examples of solid backrests. **A,** Rigid padded back with depressions to clear the scapulae for full upper limb movement without obstruction. **B,** View of rigid back indicating curved support for thoracic spine and ribs and mounting brackets. **C,** Rectangular rigid back with cover that does not have scapular clearances and thus is not used for clients who manually propel their chairs because it would not provide adequate clearances for full upper limb movement and it is also heavier than that in view **B.**

distribution. A cushion that is too deep (e.g., exceeds the distance from the posterior buttocks to the popliteal space) promotes a posterior pelvic tilt, which can further cause a rounded, kyphotic spine and forward head posture (i.e., cervical flexion with capital extension). Full support along the thigh may be needed to adequately distribute pressure on the buttocks and provide thigh stability. In this case, a cushion that extends to within 1 to 2 inches of the popliteal space may be warranted. However, trade-offs occur: a 1- to 2-inch space behind the knee does not allow ample space for hooking under the distal thigh, which is a functional skill used in transfers and lower limb management. Also, a longer cushion may dictate the need for a longer wheelchair seat frame, which creates a larger turning radius

and thus negatively affects maneuverability. As stated previously, prioritizing goals for each client is crucial to a successful outcome. Seat cushions are discussed in detail later in the chapter.

An anterior pelvic positioning strap is used to provide pelvic stability. Positioning straps should be padded if skin integrity is of concern and location should be carefully assessed. The direction of pull determines the forces on the pelvis. To discourage a posterior pelvic tilt, the belt should be positioned perpendicular to or at an acute angle to the seat and should pull across the most proximal portion of the thigh. To control an anterior tilt, the direction of pull should be almost parallel to the seat with the padded strap inferior to the ASISs.[4]

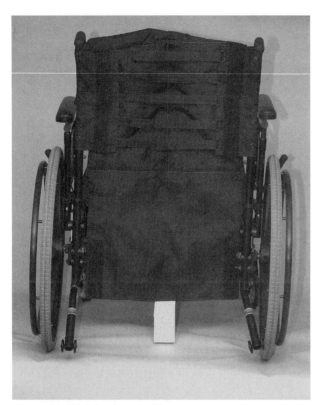

FIGURE 11-10 A folding wheelchair with adjustable tension upholstery allows the clinician to adjust the degree of support to the thoracic spine depending on whether there are rigid or flexible kyphotic deformities. This type of upholstery is commonly used with folding wheelchairs to ease the chair's collapsibility. The cover that attaches with Velcro is flipped down for viewing.

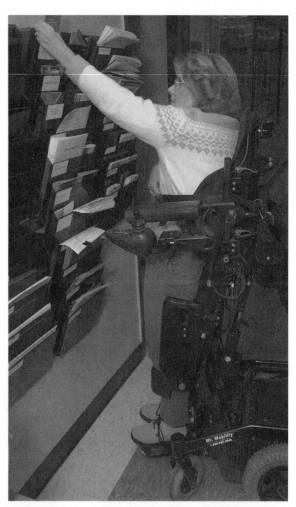

FIGURE 11-11 A standing wheelchair shows lateral knee and thigh supports for control of lateral thigh movement during standing and when sitting.

Lower Limb Considerations

Support of the lower limbs is important for stability, pressure distribution, and sitting balance. Generally, the thighs should be level with the seating surface and fully supported. (The clinician should be aware of the trade-offs mentioned previously.) The hips should be in a position of neutral to slight abduction and neutral rotation. The simplest way to achieve this is by using a solid seat, a cushion of the appropriate depth, and a footrest at the appropriate height. If a footrest is too high, the inferior thigh is unsupported and increased pressure is created at the ischial tuberosities. If a footrest is too low, it will result in undue pressure on vascular and neural structures running through the popliteal space, which could lead to lower leg or foot edema or nerve compression and could promote a posterior pelvic tilt.[2] Occasionally, external supports are required to maintain neutral hip abduction, especially when the chair has the capacity to change configuration (e.g., tilt, stand) (Figure 11-11). Medial and lateral thigh supports should be padded and placed as distal as possible to control alignment. Although the size of the support pad should be minimized, the same guideline applies for distribution of pressure as with seat cushions. A pad that is too small may cause skin irritation. Transfers and other functional activities may require these positioning devices to swing out of the way or be removable.

If lower limb ROM has been lost as a result of heterotopic ossification or a muscle contracture, then the seating system must be set up to accommodate these limitations. Loss of hip flexion must be accommodated through the seating system while a neutral pelvic position is maintained. A bilateral hip flexion limitation that is symmetrical, or nearly so, can be accommodated with an appropriate seat-to-back angle. The seat-to-back angle should never be set more acutely than client's hip flexion ROM. If this is inadvertently done, the buttocks or posterior pelvis will not reach the back of the seat cushion or backrest, which will negatively affect postural control or pressure distribution. In the case of a slight right-left discrepancy in hip flexion ROM, the angle chosen favors the side with the greatest limitation. With a unilateral limitation, accommodation can be achieved through modifying (e.g., scooping out or cutting down) the front section of the cushion that supports the thigh on the limited side (Figure 11-12).

Limitations in joint ROM at the knee are less common. Hamstring tightness or flexor spasticity can cause a limitation in knee extension; heterotopic ossification may result in a limitation of knee flexion. It is important to remember that the seating system should not be used to stretch contractures or attempt to correct any fixed deformity. Attempting to force the knees into extension

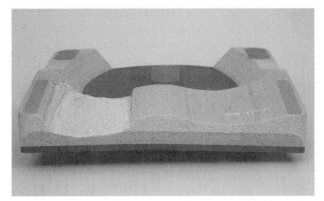

FIGURE 11-12 Modified cushion with increased thigh trough accommodates unilateral hip flexion limitation such as might occur with heterotopic ossification.

generally causes the pelvis to slide forward on the seat and into a posterior pelvic tilt. In these cases, the leg posture must be accommodated by the position of the seat and legrests.[4]

Ideally, the ankles should be positioned in slight dorsiflexion, with the heel and ball of the foot in contact with the footplate (Figure 11-13). Proper positioning early on can help to prevent footdrop. Padded ankle straps may be required to maintain foot and ankle support and alignment when severe lower limb spasticity is present. Care should be taken to ensure that pressure from these straps does not compromise skin integrity and circulation. Limitations in joint ROM at the ankle can be accommodated with the use of angle adjustable footplates. Some footplates offer adjustment for dorsiflexion and plantarflexion, whereas others additionally offer adjustment for inversion and eversion.

Trunk Position

As stated previously, pelvic position dictates trunk position. Wheelchair backrest characteristics will affect pelvic position and trunk position. Characteristics include shape, length, mounted height, angle and depth adjustment, postural support components, and material. The mobility of the spine, position of the scapula, sitting balance, and posture should be assessed to determine the most appropriate backrest. If the client has lumbar extension range and pelvic mobility, the backrest must provide support while concurrently affording optimal functional mobility. Thus, the placement of the lumbar and pelvis support is critical. Generally, the lumbar pad is placed at or just above the PSISs. A lumbar support placed too high can result in poor balance and an increased kyphosis, whereas one that is placed too low may push the pelvis into a posterior pelvic tilt. If the client does not have lumbar mobility, this fixed position must be accommodated to distribute pressure and achieve balance. Angle adjustability of the backrest is useful for improving anterior-posterior balance and promoting a more horizontal field of vision.

A kyphotic spine is one of the most common postural deformities observed in clients with SCI (Figure 11-14, *A*). If the spine is flexible, this posture can be corrected. Providing support beginning at the level of the PSISs to promote lumbar extension will facilitate thoracic extension and improve postural alignment for function, such as upper limb tasks (Figure 11-14, *B*). However, some clients

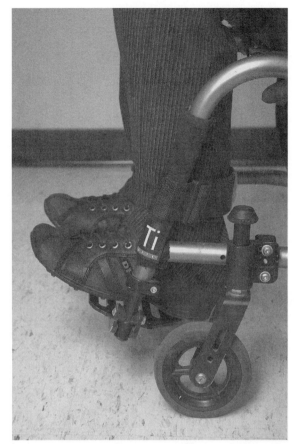

FIGURE 11-13 Ideally, when the foot is compensated on the footrest, the ankles should be positioned in slight dorsiflexion, with the heel and ball of the foot in contact with the footplate.

seek stability through a slouched posture. Therefore changing posture by increased spinal extension will almost definitely change their balance points so that a decreased sense of functional balance could occur. Often a concurrent rearward shift in the system tilt of the wheelchair can regain a functional balance point. Interventions for achieving this posture include tension-adjustable back upholstery, biangular backs, pneumatic inserts, contoured foam inserts, and a variety of precontoured backs.

Fixed (i.e., nonflexible) kyphotic postures require an angle-adjustable and concave-shaped back to accommodate the spinal curve. These backs may be custom contoured, on-site foam contoured, or modular foam. Pressure over the sacrum, spinous processes, and inferior angle of the scapula must be assessed. Custom contouring may provide adequate pressure distribution. If not, sacral, scapular, and spinal reliefs may be necessary. These cutouts may be left void or filled with a pressure distribution medium. Regardless of which material is used, the back support must address the issues of comfort, function, balance, and skin integrity.

Interventions to prevent scoliotic deformities should include the cushion, lateral pelvic supports, and lateral thoracic supports. The cushion must support the pelvis in a stable position; it may need to be custom ordered to achieve symmetrical pressure distribution through both ischia. Lateral pelvic supports center the pelvis on the cushion. They may be a part of the cushion or

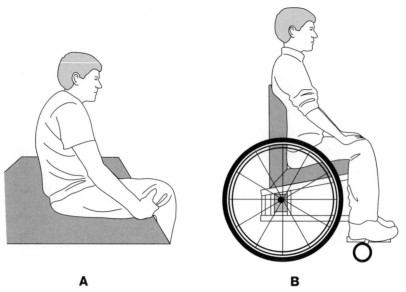

A **B**

FIGURE 11-14 **A,** Client with SCI sitting with back poorly supported results in posterior pelvic tilt, kyphotic thoracic spine, and absence of lumbar curve. **B,** Same client seated with rigid back support and pressure-relief seat cushion, resulting in erect thoracic spine, lumbar curve, and anterior tilted pelvis. (Adapted from Pendaleton HMcH, Schultz-Krohn W: *Pedretti's occupational therapy: practice skills for physical dysfunction*, ed 6, St. Louis, 2006, Mosby Elsevier, F 11-08 C-D, p 213.)

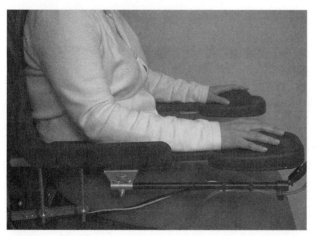

FIGURE 11-15 Cone type modular hand pad with channel forearm pad.

attached to the solid seat or backrest. Lateral thoracic supports should be height-, width-, and angle-adjustable. Measurement of the desired height of the lateral supports and chest width-depth is important to ensure an appropriate fit and posture. The thinner the trunk support, the less likely it will interfere with upper limb function and positioning.

Three points of contact are necessary to correct a spinal curvature.[5,6] The lateral thoracic support on the convex side of the scoliotic trunk should be set to push against the ribs, corresponding with the apex of the vertebral curve. The contralateral thoracic support should be placed as high as possible without interfering with upper limb function or causing pressure in the axillary region. The lateral pelvic support on the side of the high thoracic support acts as the third point of pressure for the curvature correction. A substitute for lateral thoracic supports is a corset with postural stays, which provides both postural and abdominal

support for improved respiratory function. Young children and adolescents at risk for development of scoliosis as they grow often receive spinal stabilization through an orthosis.

Upper Limb Positioning

Ideally, when the individual is seated in a wheelchair the upper limbs are positioned at the sides of the body with the elbow flexed and the forearm supported. Armrests that are too high cause the shoulder to be elevated and can lead to shoulder and neck pain and a scoliotic sitting posture. Armrests that are too low can contribute to a thoracic kyphosis, trunk instability, and shoulder subluxation, depending on the client's level of SCI.

Muscle strength, joint integrity, muscle tone, edema, and contractures are among the factors that influence armrest shape and position. Upper limb support may range from no support for an active individual with paraplegia to a fully contoured arm support for the client with little or no volitional movement. Optimal arm supports allow for a great degree of adjustment and positioning. Armrests may be angled to match limitations in shoulder rotation or to allow for improved function within the person's limited ROM. For clients with severe tone and contractures, a padded lap tray may provide better support and pressure distribution. Some armrests have cone-shaped extensions to help decrease finger flexor spasticity (Figure 11-15). Also, a variety of styles of armrests are available to give full support to the flaccid upper limb.

Head Positioning

The head should be positioned in midline with neutral rotation and with a horizontal field of vision. Spasticity, muscle imbalance, and alignment after surgical stabilization often hinder the ideal head position. There are many headrests available commercially to help with head positioning. Each of these headrests

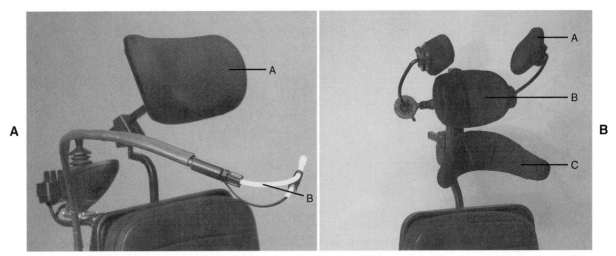

FIGURE 11-16 **A,** Standard headrest with occipital pad (A), and sip-n-puff control (B). **B,** Headrest with temporal swing-away pads (A), occipital pad (B), and suboccipital pad (C).

provides some combination of the following points of control: posterior, occipital, lateral, or anterior (Figure 11-16, *A*). Occipital and posterior supports are the most commonly used type for clients with SCI. If additional support is required, lateral head supports may also be incorporated, but care should be taken to ensure that they do not interfere with hearing or obstruct the client's visual field (Figure 11-16, *B*). An anterior strap should be used only as a last resort, and when it is used the client's skin integrity should be carefully monitored.

MANUAL WHEELCHAIRS

Choices of manual wheelchair frames and components continue to increase. Upright, tilt-in-space, reclining, and standing wheelchair frames are available. Choosing the right frame style depends on the functional and postural requirements of the client. The wheelchair components, such as armrests, legrests, wheel locks, and tire type, also must be chosen carefully with each client's needs considered individually. Configuring the wheelchair to maximize the user's ease of propulsion, stability of the user and the chair, and pressure distribution as well as the functional ability of the user is vital to the health and performance of a person after SCI.

Frame Materials

Steel, aluminum, and titanium are the three most common materials used for wheelchair frames, with increasing usage of composite materials. Each material has different strengths and weaknesses.

Steel is the heaviest of the three materials but is inexpensive and easy to work with. Steel alloys can be configured to have high strength but the strength-to-weight ratio is less than other materials. Aluminum is lighter than steel and has good strength for a wheelchair frame. It is noncorrosive and able to be manufactured with different colors and appearances. Titanium is the lightest and most expensive of these three materials and has the best strength-weight ratio. However, it is the hardest to machine and fabricate into a frame. Titanium is a very durable, strong, and noncorrosive material. Composite materials, such

as carbon fiber, are being used for frame members, joints, and fasteners. Composite materials are the most expensive but can be fabricated into many shapes, sizes, strengths, and appearances.

It is difficult to relate wheelchair performance directly to frame material. All the components, including frame design (e.g., rigid or folding), wheel and caster size, and tire type (e.g., solid or pneumatic) make a significant contribution to the weight and ride comfort of a wheelchair. Steel, aluminum, and titanium frames have been around for many years and manufacturing issues have been adequately addressed, so good durability can be expected from any frame tubes.

Frame Types

Manual wheelchairs are available with rigid or folding upright frame options (Figure 11-17, *A*). Rigid frames do not have moving parts and therefore are more durable than a frame with a cross-brace, which allows the frame to fold for storage or transport. Rigid frames are generally lighter than folding frames, which makes lifting the chair for transportation easier (Clinical Note: Advantages Versus Disadvantages of Rigid and Folding Wheelchair Frames). Indeed, the way a person loads or stores the wheelchair in his vehicle may dictate the type of frame chosen. Folding frames fit more easily into car trunks and can be stored behind the driver's seat, but that limits the number of people who can be transported in that vehicle (Figure 11-17, *B*). To load a rigid frame chair, the wheels are typically removed and the frame is then lifted into the car. Many people who load the wheelchair from the driver's seat find that a rigid frame chair is easier to fit between their lap and the top of the door frame (see Figure 8-28).

Manual tilt-in-space and manual reclining frames are options for people who cannot weight shift on their own or who require gravity-assisted positioning. These frames are heavier than traditional upright frames and are more difficult to transport. Each may be used early in a rehabilitation program to allow for gradual progression of vertical sitting tolerance to accommodate for postural hypotension and impaired sitting balance.

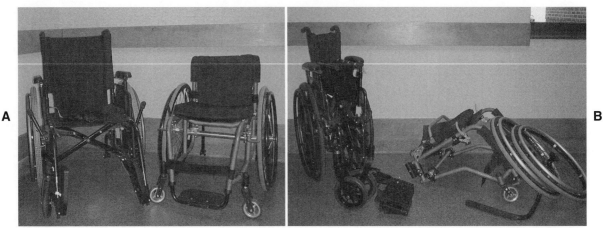

FIGURE 11-17 **A,** Manual folding wheelchair *(left)* and manual rigid wheelchair *(right).* **B,** Folding-frame wheelchair *(left)* and rigid frame wheelchair *(right)* disassembled for transport. (From Pellerito JM Jr: *Driver rehabilitation and community mobility: principles and practice*, St. Louis, 2006 Elsevier Mosby, Fig 9-2 A&B, pp 203-204.)

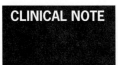 **CLINICAL NOTE** Advantages Versus Disadvantages of Rigid and Folding Wheelchair Frames

Rigid Wheelchair Frames
Advantages
• More durable
• More efficient
• Generally lighter
• Adjustable

Disadvantages
• Transportation considerations

Folding Wheelchair Frames
Advantages
• Easier to transport
• Can propel with lower limbs

Disadvantages
• Less durable
• Generally weighs more
• Generally less adjustable

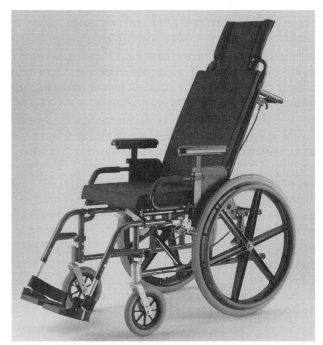

FIGURE 11-18 Manual reclining wheelchair on a folding base. (From Pendaleton HMcH, Schultz-Krohn W: *Pedretti's occupational therapy: practice skills for physical dysfunction*, ed 6, St. Louis, 2006, Mosby Elsevier, Fig 11-4 A, p 208.)

Tilt-in-space frames maintain fixed seating angles while allowing the whole system to tilt backward to provide a weight shift. Most tilt-in-space frames are rigid, although a few folding frames exist. Most systems tilt back 45 to 55 degrees. Tilt-in-space systems are usually recommended over those that recline when moderate to severe spasticity affects the person's positioning. The fixed position of the limbs afforded by tilt eliminates sensory input and reflexive muscle spasms. Power tilt units can be added to some manual tilt-in-space frames to allow the user to independently tilt the system with a switch.

Manual reclining frames have a folding frame configuration (Figure 11-18). If the standard upholstery back is used, reclining frames are easier to fold for transport than are tilt-in-space frames. Antitip bars are essential to prevent rearward tipping, especially when the back is reclined. The user or caregiver should be instructed about

rearward instability, effects of shear, reflexive muscle spasms, and increased pressures over the sacrum when a reclining back is used.

Standing manual wheelchair frames allow a person to move from sitting to standing, thereby profiting from the medical benefits of weight bearing, improved interaction with others from the standing positioning, and improved vertical reach to access objects at heights above the seated reach.

Dimensions and Components

Wheelchair selection usually begins by determining which frame design best addresses the majority of a person's functional needs. Selecting a frame design, however, is only part of the prescriptive process. Prescribing a functional wheelchair requires assembling appropriate dimensions and component parts, such as armrests, front riggings (i.e., leg supports), footrests, wheels, wheel locks, and tires, that ensure optimal independence and safety.

Dimensions and Orientation

Width and depth dimensions of the wheelchair are important considerations in the person with SCI in relation to proper propulsion, posture, and pressure distribution. The width of the manual wheelchair for a person with SCI needs to be as narrow as possible to assist him in maintaining midline pelvic positioning if he no longer has voluntary trunk or lower extremity control and to enable the drive wheels of the chair to be positioned near the shoulder joint for efficient propulsion. The seat depth needs to be long enough to support the thighs to ensure neutral positioning and to distribute pressure adequately to minimize excessive pressure on the ischial tuberosities. Some wheelchair frames come in sequential sizing (e.g., 15 inch, 16 inch, 17 inch, 18 inch) and others come in even sizes (e.g., 16 inch, 18 inch, 20 inch). Frame growth for children is available from some manufacturers, which will allow the frame to be widened or replaced for a lower cost than replacing the whole chair.

Seat-to-floor height adjustability varies according to each manufacturer's make and model. The height off the floor depends on the user's lower leg length and mode of propulsion. A minimum of 2 inches of ground clearance under the footplates is required when the person is properly positioned in the wheelchair. A compromise to adequate ground clearance and leg positioning is made in chairs for users who propel with one or both lower limbs. The distance from the floor to the top of the wheelchair cushion needs to be equal to the person's lower leg length to allow for an adequate purchase on the ground to propel the chair. For instance, many people with hemiplegia propel with one upper and one lower limb while the contralateral lower limb rests on a footplate (Figure 11-19, *A* and *B*). In another example, the footplate has to be raised higher than normal to allow for ground clearance. Using a lower ground clearance will most likely cause the footplates to scrape the ground during uneven transitions of the ground surface (e.g., ascending or descending a ramp onto level ground) (Figure 11-20).

The orientation of the wheelchair seat can also be adjusted on some frames. A rearward slope of the seat can be achieved by lowering the rear seat to floor height in comparison to the front seat to floor height, usually through a vertical wheel axle adjustment. Different wheelchair frames offer different amounts of vertical adjustment of the rear axle. Opening the back angle in conjunction with sloping the seat will result in a static tilt to allow gravity-assisted positioning (Figure 11-21, *A*). Maintaining the same back angle relative to the ground (i.e., a more upright backrest) while sloping the seat, which is termed squeeze, may allow individuals with poor trunk control to sit up in a more erect posture without loss of balance (Figure 11-21, *B*). Lowering the rear seat to floor height also may improve a person's access to the wheel.

Ideally, the elbow flexion angle between the upper arm and the forearm should be between 100 and 120 degrees when the hand is placed at the top dead-center position on the pushrim to permit the best propulsion dynamics (Figure 11-22).[7]

Back height, angle adjustability, and push handle style are additional features to explore when choosing a manual wheelchair. Back heights can be adjustable within a certain range or of a fixed height. Certain frames provide an adjustable back angle that is static once set or a reclining back that can easily be moved forward and back. Push handles can be integrated as part of the back cane if necessary. Obviously, push handles assist a caregiver in dependently maneuvering a wheelchair user. Stroller handles are available on some frames to achieve the necessary height from which to comfortably push the wheelchair. Push handles also serve a functional purpose for some users. Users can hook an arm around a push handle for stability while performing upper limb tasks (Figure 11-23). If push handles are used for hooking, choosing the proper height so the user can access the push handle is essential. Push handles can be bolted onto the rigidizer bar of rigid frame wheelchairs. These handles are typically used for dependent propulsion and can be removed when no longer needed. Both types of push handles increase the depth of the wheelchair when folded for transport, which increases the space needed for storage (Clinical Note: Advantages Versus Disadvantages of Integrated and Bolted-On Push Handles).

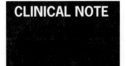

CLINICAL NOTE — **Advantages Versus Disadvantages of Integrated and Bolted-On Push Handles**

Integrated (Folding Frame)
Advantages
- Allows safe dependent handling
- Can hook for stability
- Can pull chair up stairs

Disadvantages
- Increases depth of chair
- More difficult to load
- May interfere with propulsion

Bolted-On (Rigid Frame)
Advantages
- Removable
- Allow for dependent propulsion

Disadvantages
- Can't easily hook
- Can loosen easily if set screws are used
- May not be safe to pull up stairs
- Increases depth of chair

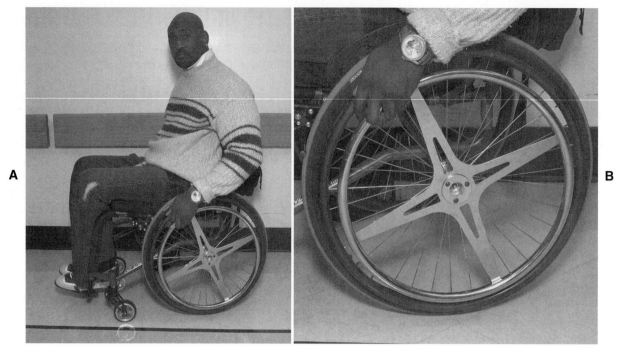

FIGURE 11-19 Hemi propulsion wheel. **A,** Client pushes outer rim versus inner rim to turn and both pushrims to move straight ahead. **B,** Close-up of wheel shows outer and inner pushrims.

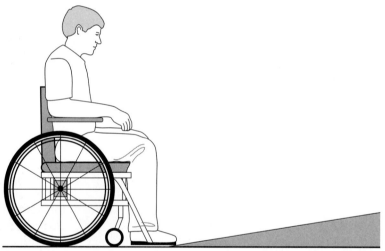

FIGURE 11-20 When the wheelchair footrests are adjusted too low, the client will not be able to negotiate all surfaces, particularly over rough terrain or up ramps.

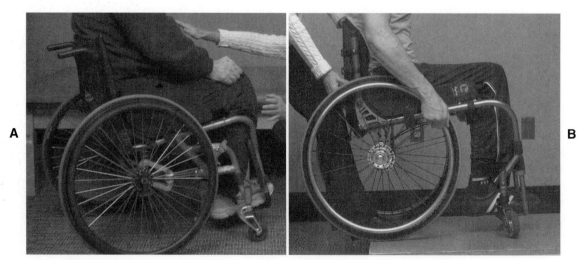

FIGURE 11-21 **A,** In a tilted seating system both the backrest and the seat tilt. **B,** In a squeeze orientation, the backrest is more upright, whereas the wheelchair seat tilts up from a lower back to higher front.

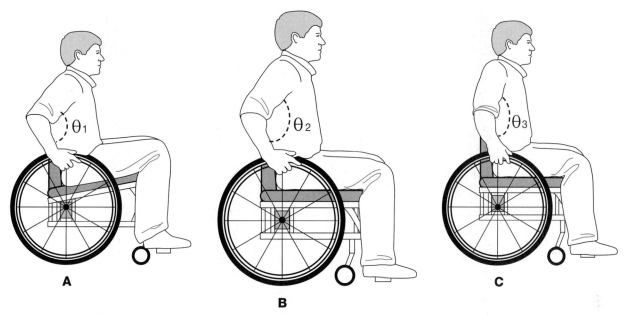

FIGURE 11-22 Elbow flexion at wheel contact. **A,** Back of the seat height is too low causing excessive elbow angle, **B,** Seat height correctly adjusted to allow for ideal elbow angle of 110 degrees to 120 degrees, **C,** Seat height is too high placing the elbow in an extended position, which does not optimize propulsion forces and reduces contact with the pushrim.

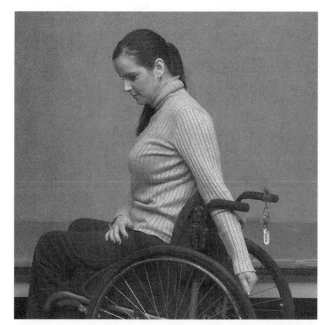

FIGURE 11-23 Hooking on the push handle is useful to counterrotate the opposite pelvis or to use as an anchor to reach forward when the trunk does not have muscular support

Armrests

Numerous styles of armrests are available in full or desk lengths and fixed or adjustable heights. Typically, the armrest height should be adjusted at the elbow height or an inch higher. In addition, many different types of armpads and arm troughs of varying lengths and widths are available from numerous manufacturers. Different attachment options for the armrest to the frame also are possible. For example, there are dual-post and single-post attachments, removable or fixed armrests, and flip-back and swing-away features (Figure 11-24). The type of armrest attachment depends of the functional ability of the user to manipulate the armrest and how the person transfers as well as the setting in which he transfers.

Legrests and Footplates

Rigid front hangers are available on rigid frame chairs (Figure 11-25, *A*), although some models offer swing-away or swing-behind legrests (Figure 11-25, *B*) or flip-up footplates. Rigid hangers do not allow for foot propulsion. In addition, the footplate of a rigid hanger may interfere with using a stand or squat-pivot transfer method. Folding frame chairs typically have removable legrests. Some folding frames offer nonremovable legrests. Manually elevating legrests are also an option on folding frame chairs. Assessing the user's ability to raise and lower the legrests and evaluating accessibility with the increased chair length required for elevating legrests are important. The angle of the legrests and front rigging also can be chosen among predetermined options (Clinical Note: Advantages Versus Disadvantages of Hanger Angle of Legrests).

Footplates come in a variety of options. Composite footplates are typically a standard chair feature. Angle- and depth-adjustable footplates allow accommodation of various foot deformities and slight knee flexion limitations. After-market footplates are available that can rotate in any direction to accommodate severe deformities.

Wheels, Pushrims, Wheel Locks, and Tires

Several different types of wheels and wheel sizes exist for manual wheelchairs. Rear wheels range from 12 to 26 inches depending on method of propulsion and height of user. Dependent mobility users and users who use their lower limbs for propulsion require smaller wheels, whereas 24- and 26-inch wheels are mainly used by upper limb propellers.

The main types of rear wheel options are spoke (Figure 11-26, *A*) and mag (Figure 11-26, *B*). Within these categories are

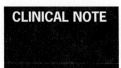

Advantages Versus Disadvantages of Hanger Angle of Legrests

60-Degree Angle
Advantages
- Increases foot/ground clearance
- Allows for larger casters/lower seat-to-floor heights
- Accommodates decreased knee flexion

Disadvantages
- Increases overall length and turning radius of chair

70-Degree Angle
Advantages
- Increases knee flexion
- Reduces overall length compared with 60-degree hanger

Disadvantages
- Increased overall length compared with 90-degree hanger

90-Degree Angle
Advantages
- Accommodate knee flexion contractures
- Decreases chair length and turning radius

Disadvantages
- Limited caster size options
All are available with straight and tapered design and swing-away or fixed.

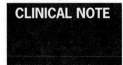

Advantages Versus Disadvantages of Spoke or Mag Wheelchair Wheels

Spoke
Advantages
- More shock absorbing
- Lighter
- Example: Standard, Spinergy, Twister

Disadvantages
- Most require maintenance
- Can get fingers caught

Mag
Advantages
- Minimal to no maintenance
- Example: Standard, Xcore, Spider

Disadvantages
- Less shock absorbing
- Wheel bearings may work loose from hubs
- Most are heavier than standard spoke wheels

CLINICAL NOTE **Advantages Versus Disadvantages of Caster Sizes**

Smaller
Advantages
- Easier to turn
- More foot clearance
- Smaller turning radius

Disadvantages
- Harder to maneuver over obstacles and negotiate uneven or soft surfaces

Larger
Advantages
- Less rolling resistance
- Easier to negotiate uneven or soft terrain

Disadvantages
- Less foot clearance
- Harder to turn

several versions of each type (Clinical Note: Advantages Versus Disadvantages of Spoke and Mag Wheelchair Wheels). Wheel axles can either be bolted onto the frame or quick release. Quick-release axles are available in button or pin styles or quad release, which does not require finger dexterity to operate (Figure 11-27, *A*). Quad-release axles also are available without quick release for those with good hand function (Figure 11-27, *B*). Spoke guards are available to protect fingers from getting caught in the spokes and can assist in preventing damage to the spokes. Care must be taken to ensure that the spoke guards do not interfere with the tie-down system being used for transport.

Front casters range from 3 to 8 inches. Larger front casters can maneuver over obstacles easier but require a larger turning radius (Clinical Note: Advantages Versus Disadvantages of Caster Sizes). The front caster size is sometimes dictated by the specific front seat height that is being requested. Front casters can also come with a quick-release option that decreases the amount of space necessary for storage of the frame when the casters are removed.

Anodized, foam-coated, plastic-coated, and projection pushrims are available. The type of handrim chosen typically depends on the strength of the user's upper limbs, the amount of finger function available, and the user's preference. Coated handrims may benefit those with limited hand function because the coating provides increased friction during propulsion, but caution must be used because friction on the handrim is also used for stopping and a coated handrim can abrade skin more easily. Projection pushrims provide a lever against which a user can push to propel and can allow people with extremely weak upper limbs to

maneuver a manual wheelchair. The number of projections and the angle of projections also can be chosen.

Wheel locks are an important feature to consider when recommending a manual wheelchair. The ability to safely operate the wheel locks can assist in preventing injury during transfers. Wheel locks can be configured as push to lock (Figure 11-28, *A*), pull to lock, scissor lock, or hub lock (Clinical Note: Advantages Versus Disadvantages of Wheel Lock Types). Depending on the frame style, wheel locks can be high mounted, low mounted, or as an attendant feature, such as a foot lock. When locked, the axle can no longer turn (Figure 11-28, *B*).

CLINICAL NOTE Advantages Versus Disadvantages of Wheel Lock Types

Push to Lock
Advantages
• Can engage without finger use

Disadvantages
• May catch thumb while propelling
• May hit transfer surface and unlock

Pull to Lock
Advantages
• Can engage without finger use
• Will not hit transfer surface

Disadvantages
• May interfere with transfer clearance
• May catch thumb while propelling

Scissors
Advantages
• Out of way during propulsion

Disadvantages
• More difficult to engage
• May require hand function

CLINICAL NOTE Advantages Versus Disadvantages of Tire Options

Pneumatic
Advantages
• Shock absorbing
• Light
• Most tread for outdoor mobility

Disadvantages
• Maintenance of tire pressure
• May get flats

Solid Urethane
Advantages
• Maintenance free
• Tread lasts longest

Disadvantages
• Less shock absorbing
• Less tread
• Heavier

Primo (High Pressure Pneumatics)
Advantages
• Lightest
• High performance
• Example: Standard, Kenda

Disadvantages
• Tread wears easily
• Prone to flats
• Higher maintenance

Performance and maintenance are two main considerations when choosing tires. Caster tires are typically solid, whereas drive wheels can be solid or pneumatic. There are specific advantages and disadvantages of pneumatic-urethane and primo (i.e., high-pressure pneumatic) tires (Clinical Note: Advantages Versus Disadvantages of Tire Options). Pneumatic tires are available with different tread options from standard to knobby. Flat free inserts can be requested with pneumatic tires; they eliminate maintenance while maintaining the tread option but decrease shock absorption and increase rolling resistance. Solid, polyurethane tires come in high or low profiles and typically have less tread than pneumatic tires. In general, solid tires have a higher rolling resistance and less shock absorption than do properly inflated pneumatic tires.[8,9]

Accessories

There are numerous storage options and carrying accessories available for wheelchairs. Common storage options are backpacks, under-chair nets, and under-seat pouches. Ventilator trays, oxygen holders, crutch holders, IV carriers, impact guards, and travel wheels are also available.

It is important to work closely with a variety of manufacturers' representatives to stay abreast of the various wheelchair components and how they work. There are often minor differences in how a component looks or works among different manufacturers and these differences may have an impact on a person's function.

User Interface

When the frame style and components have been chosen, attention must shift to addressing the configuration of the frame to match the needs of the user. The importance of choosing the appropriate frame width and depth and seat-to-floor height was

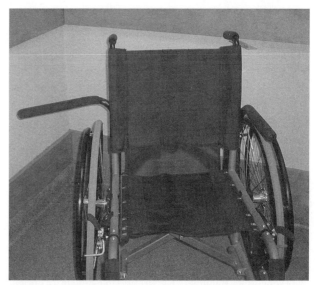

FIGURE 11-24 Tubular armrest in a swing-away position. (From Pellerito JM Jr: *Driver rehabilitation and community mobility: principles and practice*, St. Louis, 2006 Elsevier Mosby, Fig 9-8, p 208.)

addressed in the previous section. How the frame is configured can affect postural stability that affects the functional ability of the user; pressure distribution that affects the potential for development of skin breakdown; and vital organ capacity such as breathing and swallowing.

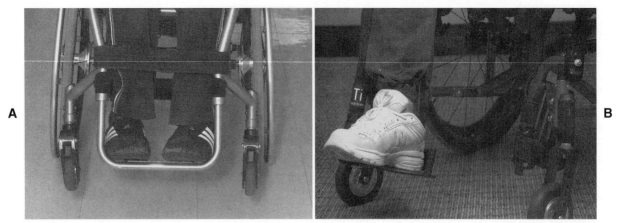

FIGURE 11-25   A, Rigid footrests with front strap to limit forward slippage of legs and feet off the footrest during rough or downhill terrains, and a strap behind legrests prevents the knees from flexing and pulling the feet backward off the footrests in the case of flexor spasms or spasticity. **B,** Swing-away footrest that swings underneath wheelchair to avoid widening the wheelchair width or catching the footrest on the transfer surface as is the case when the footrest swings outward.

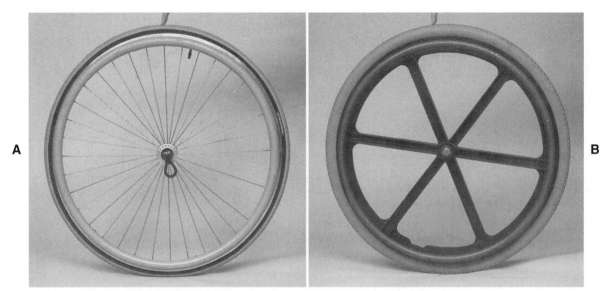

FIGURE 11-26   A, Spoke and **B,** Mag wheel options.

Postural Stability

Maximizing postural stability in the wheelchair improves the ability to perform functional daily activities/wheelchair propulsion without loss of balance. Options within wheelchair frames to address postural stability for people with SCI include height of the chair back, gravity-assisted positioning, and lowering the rear seat height with respect to the front while closing the back angle (i.e., squeezing the seating system; see Figure 11-21, *B*).

The proper height of the backrest depends on the trunk control and functional ability of the user. Some people require total trunk support for stability. Others are able to maintain an upright position and prefer a very low back support for maximum function and ability to rotate the trunk and reach in any direction.

Gravity-assisted positioning is achieved in two ways: tilting or reclining. Tilting the seating system maintains the seat angles while allowing the whole system to be moved rearward or forward (Figure 11-29, *A*). Opening the seat-to-back angle reclines the seat (Figure 11-29, *C*). Each method positions the force of gravity in front of the user's head, which decreases the effort required to maintain an

upright head and trunk posture for those with limited muscle control. Research by Janssen-Potten et al[10] has reported that tilting the wheelchair seat 7 degrees and 12 degrees and reclining the back 22 degrees improved sitting balance and reach and required less muscle activity for people with low SCI than did a standard chair with a 10-degree backrest recline. People with high SCI also demonstrated decreased muscle activity with the same configuration. Tilting or reclining the system can improve the visual field for people with a fixed kyphosis as well. Opening the back angle can accommodate such postural deformities as limited hip flexion less than 90 degrees.

Care must be taken when deciding the degree to which the seating system will be tilted or reclined. Each option moves the center of gravity rearward and makes the chair more unstable, depending on the rear axle position. If the user is a self-propeller, access to the wheels for propulsion can be affected by the amount of tilt or recline of the system.

Squeezing the seating system is another option commonly used to improve balance while maintaining an upright trunk posture to maximize use of upper limbs. Squeezing the seat lowers

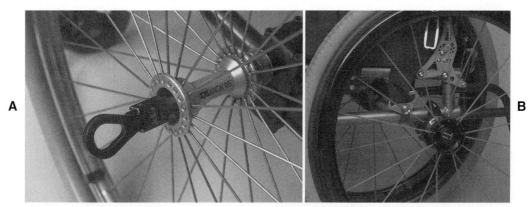

FIGURE 11-27 **A,** Quick release axle with quad loop extended outward for grabbing. **B,** Quad release axle without quick release for those with good hand function.

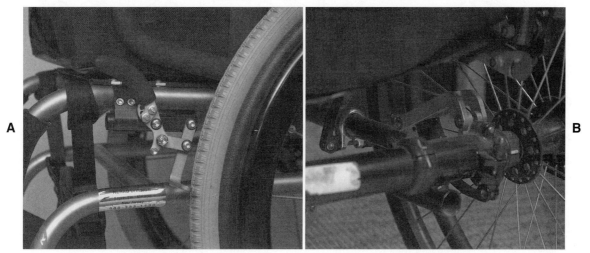

FIGURE 11-28 **A,** Wheel lock, **B,** Undercarriage view shows the locking mechanism.

the person in the system, thereby improving access to the rear wheels for propulsion. Squeezing has been found to improve posture and reach[11] while not increasing seated pressures under the ischial and sacrococcygeal area.[12]

Pressure Relief

People with SCI have varying degrees of sensory loss and mobility that place them at risk for skin breakdown (see Table 7-2). Those who do not have the functional ability to weight shift while sitting up in the wheelchair require an external means of redistributing the weight off of the ischial tuberosities at consistent intervals throughout the day to decrease potential for development of pressure ulcers. In addition to careful selection of seating system components such as backrests and cushions, tilt-in-space and reclining wheelchair frames offer a means of weight shifting. Most frames are meant for dependent weight shifts, and adding a power tilt option on some manual tilt-in-space frames is available. A combination of manual tilt and recline option is also offered.

Vital Organ Capacity

People who have severe trunk deformities, such as kyphosis and scoliosis, may have difficulty with breathing, swallowing, or digestion. The influences of gravity can exacerbate those issues. Positioning in a tilted or reclined position can decrease the effects of gravity for people with severe deformities. The effects of tilting the seating system with subjects with multiple sclerosis and symptoms of fatigue, poor sitting posture, and decreased voice projections was studied by Chan and Heck.[13] They found that respiratory measures of forced vital capacity and chest expansion improved with tilt, whereas kyphosis and forward head posture was decreased. A clinically significant voice volume increase of 2 decibels for most subjects and a reduction of perceived effort for breathing and speaking were also documented.

System Configuration

The configuration of the wheelchair system as a whole to maximize performance and self-propulsion is a crucial part in the evaluation and equipment recommendation process. Rolling resistance and inertia are the biggest influences on performance of a manual wheelchair. The less rolling resistance, the more maneuverable a wheelchair becomes. Rolling resistance is a function of overall mass of the user and wheelchair, ground characteristics, weight distribution over the wheels, and rear wheel, tire, and caster characteristics.[9,14]

Wheelchair propulsion is more difficult the greater the overall mass of the system, with added resistance from uneven terrain.

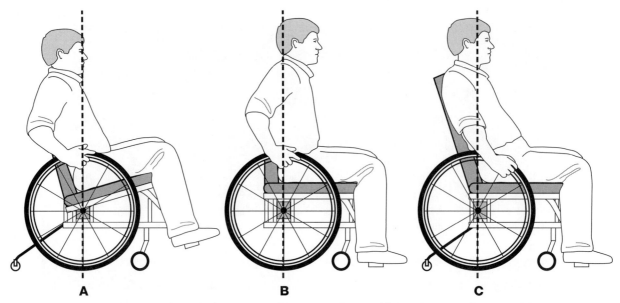

FIGURE 11-29 **A,** Tilting wheelchair. **B,** Upright posture ready to propel wheelchair. **C,** Reclining wheelchair.

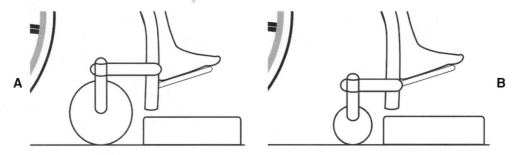

FIGURE 11-30 The size of the forward wheel influences obstacle clearance. **A,** A larger wheel is harder to raise up curbs but is less likely to get caught in ruts. **B,** A smaller wheel is easier to lift over obstacles (e.g., wheelie maneuver). (Courtesy Stephen H. Sprigle, PhD, © Georgia Tech Research Corporation, Atlanta, GA.)

Rolling resistance is the least when propelling over a smooth, flat surface. Unfortunately, most people are required to propel over many different surfaces, indoor and outdoor, during their daily activities. It is important to keep in mind the types of terrain a person typically encounters when choosing an appropriate mobility device or the adjustability required. Rolling resistance propelling on carpet is five times that of linoleum,[15] which may make the difference between independent and dependent propulsion for some individuals or justify the need for an adjustable rear axle on the recommended wheelchair.

A conflict between system stability and maneuverability arises in attempting to create an efficient but safe system for a user. The location of the rear axle with respect to the center of mass affects stability. Moving the rear axle forward increases the weight on the drive wheels with respect to the front casters (see Figure 15-1). Increasing the relative weight on the drive wheels will decrease rolling resistance and increase maneuverability but makes the chair more susceptible to tipping rearward. Because a forward axle position shortens the wheelbase, the overall length of the chair is reduced. Clinicians must assess the stability of the system to ensure safety of the user. Ways to compensate for decreased stability are to train the user in proper wheelchair skills and appropriately position antitip bars and added loads on the wheelchair (e.g., backpacks).

Mastering wheelie performance is an important functional skill. Wheelies can enhance successful negotiation over a variety of terrain and obstacles and also help the user to compensate for a less stable chair by leaning the trunk forward and rearward to change the balance point of the chair. When an individual leans forward while propelling his wheelchair up inclines, his position will assist in decreasing the chair's tendency to tip backward. Antitip bars serve to prevent the wheelchair from tipping backward. If antitip bars are used, they must extend just beyond the tire outline and not too high from the ground to be effective (see Figure 15-2). Properly adjusted antitip bars do not increase the overall length of the wheelchair.

Adding a heavy backpack on the push handles can also reduce stability. To minimize this impact, loads can be distributed between the backrest, on the person's lap, or under the seat.[16] Anytime heavy loads are carried on the wheelchair, the user must understand that stability can be compromised, either in the forward or rearward direction. The choice of rear wheel diameter is dictated by access to the handrim or ground to facilitate propulsion. The general principle to remember when choosing wheel size is that, as the diameter of the wheel increases, the greater its ability to climb obstacles and the less its rolling resistance (Figure 11-30, *A*). The smaller wheel reduces the ability to climb obstacles and has greater rolling resistance. (Figure 11-30, *B*). This relationship holds true for both the front casters and rear drive wheels.

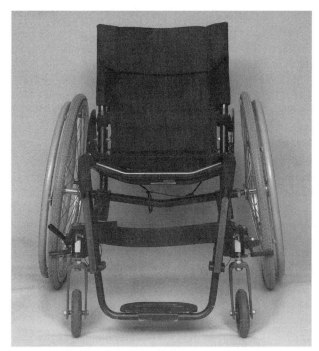

FIGURE 11-31 Wheel camber is important to improve mediolateral stability and turning radius and brings the pushrim closer to the client but widens the wheel base.

Rear wheel camber is also a common feature among adjustable manual wheelchairs. Camber is created by positioning the rear wheels in such a way that the top of the wheels are closer together than the bottom (Figure 11-31). Camber improves lateral roll stability and turning responsiveness as the wheelbase is widened. Wheel camber in chairs used for everyday mobility ranges typically from 0 to 6 degrees and within this range does not appreciably change rolling resistance.[17,18] The disadvantage of camber is that it increases the overall width of the chair, which may affect accessibility. With 24-inch-diameter rear wheels, chair width is increased by 0.42 inch for every degree of camber.

As discussed previously, rolling resistance is an important aspect of manual wheelchair propulsion and performance and is influenced by many components and wheelchair configurations in addition to the weight of the wheelchair and its occupant. Rolling resistance is less with use of pneumatic versus solid tires, larger-diameter versus smaller-diameter wheels, and a forward axle versus rear axle because of increased weight distribution over the rear wheels. The differences in rolling resistance between configurations often are small at slow speeds and increase with increasing speed. The entire system configuration needs to be taken into consideration with an understanding of the component trade-offs. This reinforces the need for a comprehensive evaluation of the person with SCI and the general use of the wheelchair before a final equipment recommendation is made.

Propulsion

Efficiency, defined as work per metabolic energy, of wheelchair propulsion is only 5% to 10%,[19] which is low compared with an activity such as cycling, which has an efficiency of 20% to 25%. Therefore,

paying attention to how a wheelchair is configured and propelled is worth the effort to maximize the performance of the user.

Wheelchair propulsion consists of propulsion and recovery phases. Propulsion is the application of torque on the handrim or wheel. Muscle strength, upper limb ROM, and access to the handrims influence the amount of torque and, therefore, the ability to propel.

An effective stroke is one that applies torque over a large portion of a wheel revolution. This requires the ability to reach behind to contact the handrim and bring the arms forward until they are nearly fully extended (see Figure 15-3). Decreased upper limb strength and ROM will limit the ability to contact and push on the handrim. Almost all movements and muscles of the upper limb are involved with the propulsion and recovery phases; therefore, weakness or limited range of any joint will affect the ability to efficiently propel the wheelchair. Adequate training and supervision is needed to ensure that new wheelchair users adopt long, smooth strokes during propulsion.

Axle position and seat height affect access to the handrims, thereby influencing propulsion. Axle placement that is forward of the backrest canes will permit the user to reach back and contact the handrims behind the center of the wheel, which allows for a longer stroke. A seat that is too high or too low will also prevent a person from contacting the handrim. A general rule of thumb is to configure the wheelchair so the user has about 100 to 120 degrees of elbow flexion when his hand is resting on the top of the handrim. This permits a long propulsion stroke without the need to put the shoulder and wrist in extreme ROMs.

The recovery stroke is needed to get the upper limb back in a position to contact the handrim again. The arm needs to be moving forward at the wheel speed as it contacts the handrim to avoid slowing the wheel down. In general, people use many different techniques for propelling a wheelchair. Clients should strive to achieve long, smooth strokes with a consistent rhythm. Rolling to a stop requires the user to overcome inertia with each push, which is very inefficient and increases stress on the upper limbs.

Repetitive Strain Injuries and Vibration
Manual wheelchair users are at high risk for development of pain and repetitive stress injuries at the shoulder and wrist.[20-24] Myriad factors contribute to upper limb problems in people with SCI, including wheelchair propulsion, transfers, and performance of ADLs.

High-repetition, high-force activities contribute to the development of a repetitive strain injury. Wheelchair propulsion is a very repetitive task, which cannot be avoided for manual wheelchair users. However, decreasing the force exerted and the impact transmitted to the upper limb from contacting the handrim can be influenced. As discussed previously, decreasing the rolling resistance of the system through appropriate component choices and configuration of the wheelchair will decrease the force necessary to propel the wheelchair. Longer and smoother strokes limit high forces and rate of loading at the pushrim. Longer strokes decrease the frequency of pushes to reach a destination.

Proper assessment of the user and the user's needs are only the beginning of the recommendations for a manual wheelchair prescription. The choice of frame style, components, and configuration influences mobility and independence in many ways, including the ability to propel the wheelchair, rolling resistance, stress on the upper limbs, vibration transmitted to the user, the user's postural stability, and performance of functional activities from the wheelchair.

POWER WHEELCHAIRS

Prescribing power wheelchairs for individuals with SCI has become more complex because of the number of options and factors that must be considered to achieve functional independence and client satisfaction. Power wheelchair technology continues to evolve and improve. Development of the power base has increased options for different drive configurations, maneuverability, and performance. The modular construction of the power base wheelchairs also allows for different styles of seating systems and the ability to change these over time. The development of pushrim-activated power assist wheels allows for conversion of a manual wheelchair into a power assist device. Midwheel drive scooters have significantly improved the maneuverability of scooters indoors. Power add-on units can be used to convert manual wheelchairs to transportable power chairs. In addition to these advances, manufacturers are also developing power wheelchairs with the ability to manage rough terrain and climb stairs. This section will cover power mobility options, related considerations, input devices for controlling the power wheelchair, and power mobility training.

Wheelchair Selection

Understanding how the person intends to use the wheelchair on a daily basis is one of the most important considerations in prescribing a power wheelchair.[25] Accessibility and function are key to the user's acceptance of the device. To ensure that the wheelchair can be used in the home and community environment, it is important to review house plans and environmental barriers that the person may encounter on a daily basis. Reviewing this information will help to determine the maneuverability requirements, overall size limitations, and performance requirements of the power wheelchair.

The prescription for a power wheelchair must include the client's accurate dimensions to achieve an appropriate fit and specifications for the type of seating system. Every power wheelchair seating system has a specific weight capacity. The weight of the user must not exceed the weight capacity of the wheelchair. The RTS and therapist must present a client with options that are appropriate for his given weight. Seat dimensions also must be considered. Dimensions for seat system will affect posture, balance, and function. One of the advantages of power base design is that it can accept a relatively large range of seat widths and depths. Modular seating systems are adjustable to accommodate growth and weight changes. Certain manufacturers make it possible to have a seat width that is different from a back width to achieve a more customized fit for a given body type.

Configuration of a seating system will depend on the client's balance, postural support needs, and function. Power wheelchair seating varies considerably. Basic power wheelchairs may offer nonadjustable (van style) seating for an individual with good balance and trunk control. Power base wheelchairs offer semi-adjustable seating with seat angles and back angles that can be adjusted to improve balance and posture. In addition, an array of power seating is available for those individuals who are unable to change positions and are fully dependent in balance or have a medical condition that requires frequent position changes. Power seat functions include power tilt, power recline, power tilt and recline, power stand, power seat lift, and power elevating legrests. These features will be discussed in more detail, but first it is important to be aware that certain power seat functions are compatible with only certain power wheelchair bases and electronics. Compatibility varies from one model to the next. The RTS, manufacturer's representative, or customer service representative from the manufacturer would be the best source for confirming compatibility of power seat functions with a specific power base wheelchair.

Assessment of the strength, function, and endurance for input device operation and placement is another consideration. The input device is used to drive the wheelchair and control power seat functions, if prescribed. Input device options for driving and controlling necessary seat functions will be discussed in more detail, but the initial decision is whether a standard proportional joystick or specialty control is needed. Specialty input devices require a more advanced control module and programming features not found on more basic power wheelchairs.

Transportation of a power wheelchair is another consideration that influences and narrows choice decisions. Determining whether the person intends to drive or be a passenger in a vehicle while seated in a wheelchair will limit the wheelchair options. Although transferring to the vehicle seat is always recommended, it is not always feasible. If the person is unable to transfer, consideration must be given to the type of mobility base, securement system, restraints, and positioning that will be required (see Chapter 20).[26]

Additional considerations include the need to carry life support systems such as a ventilator, oxygen concentrator, or suction machines. This equipment may require support trays or mounting hardware to accommodate the device and there may be requirements for orientation of the device and battery support. Consideration must be given to how this equipment will affect the performance and size of the wheelchair.

Cost, warranty, and durability also factor into the selection of a mobility system. Cost varies significantly. Typically scooters are the least expensive, whereas power base wheelchairs with multiple power seating functions and respiratory support systems are the most expensive. Discussion regarding cost, copayments, and authorization of equipment must take place between the client, family, RTS, and case manager. Information about the warranty and service are the responsibility of the rehabilitation technology supplier. In prescribing a power wheelchair, the therapist also must consider the durability of the product. A durable product will provide years of reliable service and decreased service calls and expenditures. Consultation with the RTS is one source for information on durability of power wheelchairs. The American National Standards Institute/Rehabilitation Engineering Society of North American Wheelchair Test procedures are another source of information on power wheelchair performance and durability.[27]

The selection of an input device primarily depends on identifying the client's most consistent volitional movement. The input device allows the client to control the chair's speed and direction as well as stop it. Input devices may be proportional, where the response is directly proportional to the user's input (i.e., similar to the accelerator in an automobile) or nonproportional, in which switches are either on or off and do not allow the user to vary the speed. A proportional joystick is the most common input device and gives the user the greatest degree of control, but it requires eye-hand coordination. Nonproportional multiswitch input devices are harder to use because the user can select only preset speeds. Digital input devices include pneumatic, touch switches, proximity switches, and certain head control switches. Most power wheelchair electronics are compatible with a variety of different input devices and this compatibility gives users more options when it comes to selecting an input device. Some of the less expensive power wheelchairs, however, combine the joysticks and control module in one unit, which prevents easy exchange of input devices.

The control module, or controller, is the one component that is seldom discussed during the wheelchair selection process, but it is critical to the operation of the wheelchair. The control module receives input signals from the input device and converts this signal into electric output to run the motor. The module also receives feedback from the motor and compares it with the input signal and adjusts the speed and direction accordingly. A good example of a controller at work can be felt when descending or ascending a steep incline. The controller maintains a constant speed despite the variation in terrain. In addition to relaying information back and forth, the controller also allows for adjustments to the wheelchair so that it can be fine tuned to each client. The clinical indications for these adjustments are discussed later.

The controller may also allow a client to use other assistive technology through the same input device. Power seating systems, environmental control units, and augmentative communication devices are just a few examples of assistive technology devices that can be operated through the wheelchair input device if they interface with the controller (see Chapter 13). It is important to keep in mind that all wheelchairs come with a controller and to check that the controller on a particular wheelchair will accept a specific input device, allow for parameter adjustments for safe mobility, and be compatible with other assistive technology.

When the seating components, dimensions, input device, and controller parameters have been determined, it is time to present the client with options for power mobility bases. Power mobility technology has advanced tremendously over the past few decades. Frame designs, digital controllers, batteries, motor efficiency, and input options are just some of the improved components. Power mobility systems may be grouped into the following categories: power add-on-units, scooters, conventional cross-frame wheelchairs, power base wheelchairs, and specialty power wheelchairs.

Power Add-On Units

Power add-on units can be mounted on certain manual wheelchairs to convert them to power wheelchairs (Figure 11-32). The purpose of the power add-on unit is to provide both manual and powered mobility in a unit that can be transported without a van. Power add-on units have the motors incorporated into the hub of the wheel, a battery pack to power the wheelchair, and a joystick for the input device. The power add-on unit allows the client to have a manual wheelchair for household distances and a power device for community mobility. For example, a power add-on unit manual wheelchair may be very functional for an individual returning to school or work, who cannot push a manual wheelchair long distances but does not have any means of transporting a power wheelchair. The weight of the wheels, disassembly for transport, range on a single charge, and cost are a few of the factors that should be discussed when considering a power add-on unit.

Pushrim-Activated Power Assist Wheels

Pushrim-activated power assist wheels are similar to a power add-on unit in the conversion of a manual wheelchair into a power wheelchair. This device is controlled by the amount of force on the pushrims. It does not use a joystick. The motors in the wheels magnify the force that the user applies to the pushrim (Figure 11-33, *A*). The power assist pushrim is unique in that it reduces the amount of effort that the client must exert to propel the wheelchair. Pushing is similar to that of a manual wheelchair but requires less effort and a reduced stroke frequency. When the motor is activated by pushrim contact, it propels the chair forward. The power assist makes it possible for people with weak upper limbs or impaired endurance to ascend ramps and push longer distances with less effort (Figure 11-33, *B*). Discussion with the client should include system cost, battery cost, disassembly, range per charge, and compatibility with specific wheelchair mobility bases.

Scooters

Scooters (i.e., power-operated vehicles) may be prescribed for individuals with incomplete SCIs who are able to sit with good balance, walk short distances, and perform stand-pivot transfers. In general, these devices are not commonly prescribed for people with SCI. Both three- and four-wheel scooters are available. Three-wheel scooters are smaller and more maneuverable but less stable (Figure 11-34). Four-wheel scooters are more stable but tend to be longer and wider and require more space to maneuver. In addition, the four-wheel versions are much safer on rough terrain. A four-wheel scooter is more appropriate when there is a need for increased weight capacity or to accommodate a very tall individual.[28]

Steering and acceleration are separate functions on most scooters. Steering is done with a tiller, whereas acceleration is controlled with thumb levers or finger triggers. The client must have good sitting balance, proximal stability, and shoulder mobility to use a tiller. Fine motor control is necessary to operate the accelerator.

Because scooters are lighter than power wheelchairs, they are easier to transport. One option for transporting a scooter is to use a power lift mounted inside of a van, sport utility vehicle, or the trunk of a car. A power lift platform mounted to a class three hitch is another option. Such options depend on the dimensions of the scooter, the size of the vehicle, and available lift options.

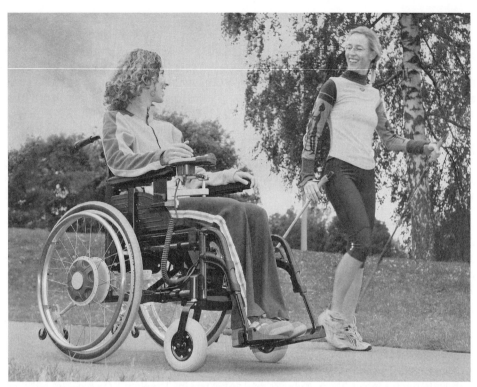

FIGURE 11-32 The E-Fix wheelchair system with power add-ons includes the joystick, battery, and E-Motion power wheels. (Courtesy Frank Mobility Systems, Inc., Oakdale, PA.)

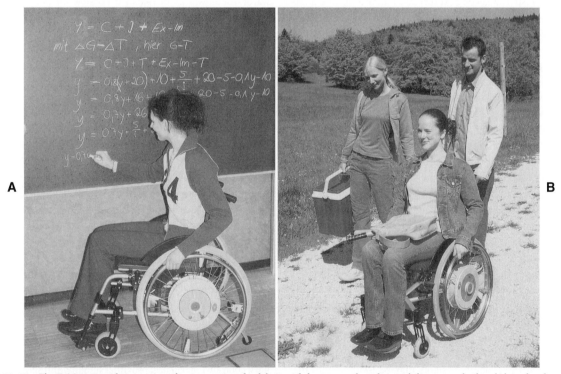

FIGURE 11-33 The E-Motion pushrim-activated power-assist wheelchair with battery pack makes mobility easy whether **(A)** in the classrooms or **(B)** out and about on a picnic. (Courtesy Frank Mobility Systems, Inc., Oakdale, PA.)

Transportable Power Wheelchairs

Lightweight transportable power wheelchairs were designed to disassemble and fold for transport. Being able to transport a power wheelchair is a boon for individuals who cannot afford a van and lift to accommodate a power wheelchair. This design emphasizes a lightweight collapsible wheelchair, which can be disassembled into two or three component parts: battery pack, power base, and seat unit (Figure 11-35, *A*). The seating unit disconnects from the mobility base and collapses flat. Clients and caregivers must be instructed in the process and given practice time to perform the task so that they have a clear understanding of what is involved to assemble and disassemble the wheelchair.

Transportable wheelchairs are the least expensive of the power wheelchairs (Figure 11-35, *B*). Operation of these wheelchairs is limited to a joystick. The controller has minimal programming capability. Folding styles vary from a traditional cross-frame design to a lawn chair–type design. Most chairs are equipped with 12-inch rear wheels. Armrest and legrest designs also vary. Transportable power wheelchairs do not accept power seating systems and have very limited adjustability. Seat dimensions and weight capacity are also limited.

Power Base Wheelchairs

The basic concept of power base wheelchairs has been around for a number of years. The power base wheelchairs offer a modular design (i.e., a power mobility base and separate seating system). The

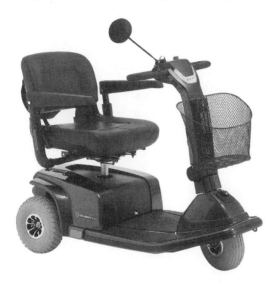

FIGURE 11-34 Three-wheel scooter. (Courtesy Pride Mobility Products Corp., Exeter, PA.)

advantage of the modular design is that the seating system can be changed over time to address different functional needs without having to replace the power base. Seating options include basic captain's chairs (Figure 11-36, *A*), standard rehabilitation seating frames (Figure 11-36, *B*), and an array of power seat functions.

Mounting of the seating system on the power base allows for angle adjustment of the seat, different seat height options, and forward or aft adjustment of the seating system on the base. Moving the seating system forward will improve stability and caster wheel clearance. Moving it rearward will allow for easier turning and improved tracking but reduce stability. Power seat functions compensate for a client's physical impairment(s). The addition of a power tilt or recline seating system to the power base allows the client to independently perform a weight shift to redistribute sitting pressures (Figure 11-37, *A*). A power seat elevator allows the client to raise and lower the seat to assist with transfers or to gain access to high objects (Figure 11-37, *B*). Power standing can also be added to certain power bases for its therapeutic and accessibility benefits (Figure 11-38, *A*). The Independence Technology iBot takes power mobility one step further by using a patented balance system that relies on the integration of gyroscopic sensors and software components that are custom programmed to the user's center of gravity, ensuring that the chair responds to the user's movement but stays balanced over smooth and rough terrain, up and down stairs, or when elevating to reach objects or look another person in the eye (Figure 11-38, *B*). It is important to check for potential compatibility before selecting a power base, especially if changes in condition over time are anticipated. A short frame length or specific frame design may prevent integrating a particular seating system.

Power base wheelchairs are designed with three different drive wheel locations: front wheel drive, mid wheel drive, and rear wheel drive (Figure 11-39). Front wheel and mid wheel drive systems tend to offer better maneuverability in tight spaces.[29] Mid wheel drive wheelchairs have the smallest turning radius. The disadvantage of the mid wheel and front wheel drive wheelchairs

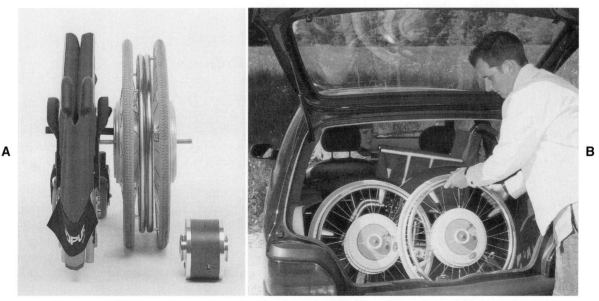

FIGURE 11-35 The transportable power-assist E-Motion wheelchair. **A,** Disassembled for transport. **B,** Snugly packed in the car. (Courtesy Frank Mobility Systems, Inc., Oakdale, PA.)

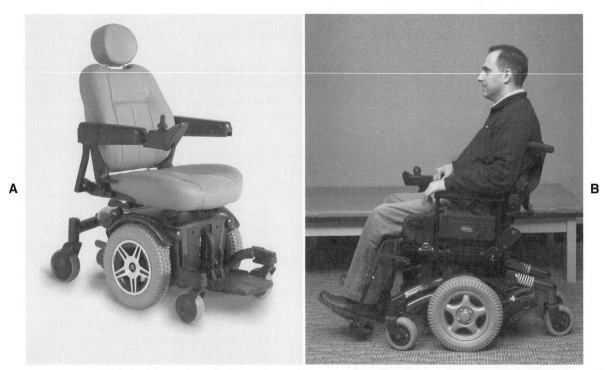

FIGURE 11-36 **A,** Power base wheelchair with standard captain's seat. (Courtesy Pride Mobility Products Corp., Exeter, PA.) **B,** Power base wheelchair with conventional rehabilitation seat and joystick control.

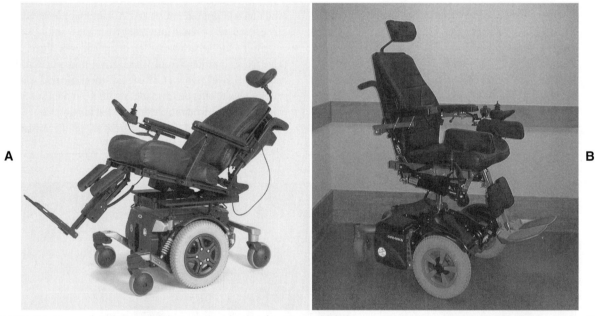

FIGURE 11-37 Power wheelchairs with (**A**) power tilt and recline functions and (**B**) elevator seat. (**A,** Courtesy Pride Mobility Products Corp., Exeter, PA. **B,** From Pellerito JM Jr: *Driver rehabilitation and community mobility: principles and practice*, St. Louis, 2006 Elsevier Mosby, Fig 9-22, p 217.)

is associated with tracking or maintaining a straight line. Programming the wheelchair's turn acceleration response or adjusting the weight distribution over the drive wheels can improve the tracking on a mid wheel drive chair.

Mid wheel drive wheelchairs are equipped with six wheels, two drive wheels and four swiveling casters. All six wheels are in contact with the ground, and some users report more vibration while traversing some surfaces. Conversely, front wheel drive

wheelchairs have a long wheel base because of the trailing position of the casters. This reduces the vibration and smoothes the transitions for a more comfortable ride. The large drive wheels in the front also improve obstacle negotiation. Certain front wheel drive wheelchairs are able to climb a 6-inch curb.

Rear wheel drive systems are easier to control and track better than front and mid wheel drive wheelchairs. The disadvantage of a rear wheel drive wheelchair is its large turning radius. Power base

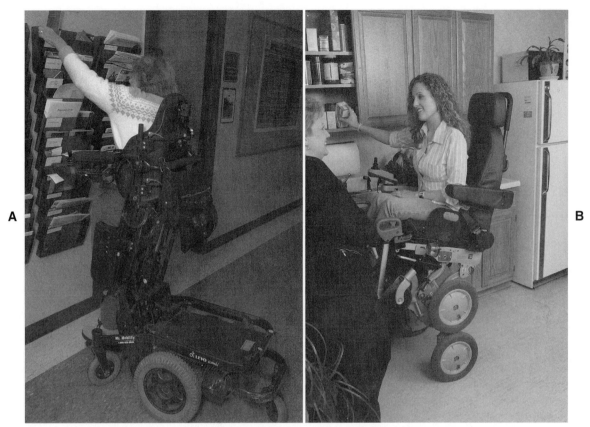

FIGURE 11-38 Some power wheelchairs can provide ease of mobility in reaching high objects. **A,** Power standing chair allows occupant to reach a vertical magazine rack. **B,** The i-BOT makes access to high cupboards a breeze. (Courtesy Independence Technology, LLC, Trenton, NJ.)

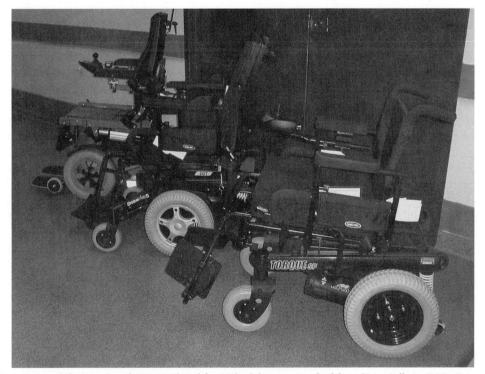

FIGURE 11-39 From right to left, examples of a rear, mid, and front wheel drive power wheelchair. (From Pellerito JM Jr: *Driver rehabilitation and community mobility: principles and practice,* St. Louis, 2006 Elsevier Mosby, Fig 9-16, p 213.)

TABLE 11-1 | **Power Seating Components**

Power Seating Component	Functional Benefits	Considerations
Power tilt	Weight shift Gravity-assisted positioning Postural alignment Reduce triggering of spasticity during weight shifts/position changes Postural hypotension	Is degree of tilt adequate for pressure distribution? Is client's vertical sitting tolerance adequate to allow safe operation of the wheelchair?
Power recline	Pressure distribution Gravity-assisted positioning Intermittent catheterization Postural hypotension	Is degree of recline adequate for pressure distribution? Does shear or loss of position occur during recline and does it negatively affect function? Does client have necessary ROM?
Power stand	Pressure distribution Physiological benefits of lower extremity weight bearing Accessibility	Does client have available ROM? Is bone density adequate to allow standing without lower extremity fracture? Does angle of stand achieve goal of accessibility and reach?
Vertical seat elevation	Transfers Accessibility	Is lowest available seat height adequate for transfers and knee/head clearance? Does range of elevation achieve access goal?
Power elevating legrests	Reduction of edema Provide clearance over uneven terrain	Does legrest lengthen as elevated to maintain proper alignment? In combination with power tilt or recline, is edema reduced? Will power legrests raise seat height or overall length of the seating system?

wheelchairs may have adjustable drive motor positions, adjustable seat positions, and programming features that can be adjusted to improve the performance of the power wheelchair for a specific user.

The modularity of a power base wheelchair design allows the seating system to be angled, its dimensions adjusted, and, if need be, switched to a power seating system. Compatibility with power seating systems, switch options, and tie down systems will vary and should be carefully assessed before ordering a power base wheelchair.

Power Seating Technology

Power seating options include tilt, recline, standing, vertical seat elevation, elevating legrests, and power footrests. Power seating systems enable a person with an SCI to change his position to redistribute pressure, to address postural hypotension, and improve his sitting balance or postural alignment. Certain power seating functions can be combined (e.g., tilt and recline; tilt, recline, and elevate; stand and recline). The manufacturer of the power seating system determines the compatibility of combining systems. The development of the weight shifting tilt (i.e., a seating system that slides forward on the base as the seating system tilt backwards) allows for a power tilt system to be installed on relatively small mobility bases.

Some power seating systems are manufacturer specific, whereas others can be installed on different manufacturers' mobility bases. Each power seat component adds a specific benefit and function. Occasionally more than one component is needed to address a specific goal or variety of goals. Table 11-1 briefly describes each component and its functional benefits.

Specialty Power Wheelchairs

Specialty power wheelchairs focus on a specific niche function. Examples include power wheelchairs with variable seat heights, all-terrain wheelchairs, or stair climbing units. Variable seat height wheelchairs are designed for pediatric clients and provide for access under tables and desks, assist with picking objects up off the floor, and allow children to explore and interact with other children by access to the floor. In addition, through lowering the seat to the floor the user gains increased stability on ramps and increased maneuverability.

All-terrain power wheelchairs enable active users to explore areas where a standard power wheelchair would not be able to function safely (Figure 11-40). There are different approaches to solving this problem. Designs include using four oversized wheels, larger more powerful motors, power steering casters, power wheel base length adjustment, and increased ground clearance. Because of the size, large turning radius, and raised seat to floor height many of these chairs cannot be used indoors and are difficult to transport. Usually, these chairs are prescribed for a person to gain independence on rough and off-road terrain. An individual returning to employment in the areas of farming, forestry, or construction may find these devices beneficial.

Stair climbing units can be divided into three categories: units that attach to a manual wheelchair for attendant operation, units that attach to a manual wheelchair that are jointly operated, and independently operated power units. The unit that attaches to a manual wheelchair has controls on the back and an attendant will operate the mechanism for stair climbing (see Figure 14-7). The jointly operated system is controlled by the user and an attendant. The reason for the jointly operated unit is that less training is required on the part of the caregiver. Therefore, it allows the user, who may not have an attendant, to instruct anyone available to assist him. The independent iBot unit described previously does not require an attendant to traverse stairs. The user would select a mode for accessing steps and the chair would then maneuver the stairs (see Figure 11-38, *B*).

Power Wheelchair Components

Power wheelchairs have many components that are similar to those previously described in the section about manual wheelchairs (Figure 11-41, *A* and *B*). In fact, some manufacturers

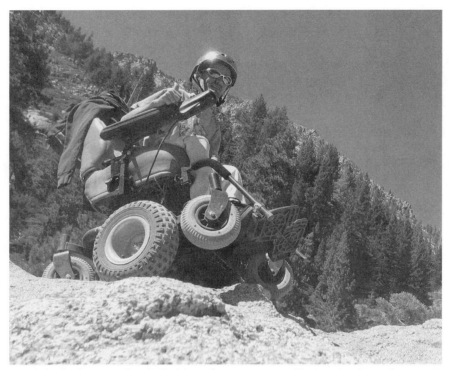

FIGURE 11-40 The Extreme 4×4 off-road wheelchair takes on any terrain. (Courtesy Vestil Manufacturing, Angola, IN.)

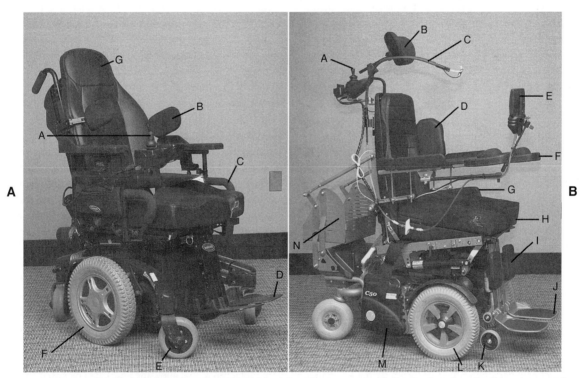

FIGURE 11-41 **A,** Power wheelchair with captain seat and mid wheel drive features. *A,* Standard joystick; *B,* lateral trunk supports; *C,* hip guides; *D,* footplates; *E,* front casters; *F,* mid wheel drive; *G,* captain seat. **B,** Front wheel drive wheelchair with additional components. *A,* Attendant controller; *B,* standard occipital headrest; *C,* pneumatic controller; *D,* lateral trunk supports; *E,* electronic display; *F,* arm trough with palmar piece; *G,* hip guide; *H,* Jay 2 deep contour cushion; *I,* calf pads; *J,* angle-adjustable footplates; *K,* antitip wheels; *L,* front wheel drive; *M,* battery box; *N,* articulating ventilator tray.

make components interchangeable between power and manual wheelchairs. Manufacturers list many different options and components for each model of power wheelchair; a basic mid wheel drive chair offers different options (Figure 11-41, *A*) than a front wheel drive chair designed to be operated with sip-n-puff technology or caregiver assistance (Figure 11-41, *B*). Items include different wheel sizes, flat free tire inserts, mechanical wheel locks, transit option, seating components, heavy-duty upgrades,

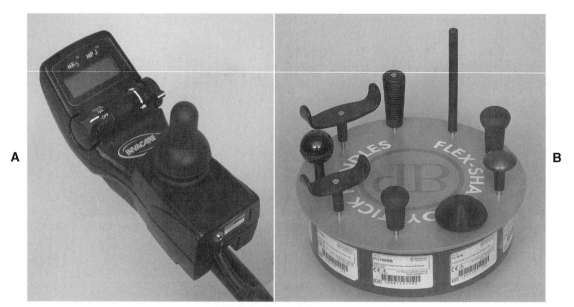

FIGURE 11-42 A, Standard joystick. **B,** Various joystick options.

front and rear suspension systems, motor speed options, and different battery sizes.

The rehabilitation team and client should review the available options on the order form and discuss each component's purposes. The RTS or manufacturer can provide more detailed information about a particular option. Recently, independent rehabilitation Web sites have emerged that provide evaluation forms, specific information about products, and product options. These sites can be very beneficial for identifying a list of manual or power wheelchair options in a specific category.

Joysticks and Specialty Controls

Joysticks and specialty controls are the input devices (i.e., switch) that allow a client to drive a power wheelchair, activate its seat functions, and control electronic accessories that are connected to the controller or module. Selecting the appropriate input device involves identifying the optimal site for consistent and efficient switch activation and determining the type of switch. Postural stability is a critical component when assessing a person's ability to use a particular switch. For example, a person with C5 complete SCI with trunk muscle spasticity will require lateral pelvic and trunk supports to maintain good control of the input device. In addition to assessing the person's ability to drive the wheelchair over various terrain, it is also important to assess his ability to operate the switch throughout the range of any prescribed power seat functions. Gravity can have a detrimental effect on a person's ability to access a switch when in a tilted or reclined position.

Selecting the optimal switch and site for operation of the wheelchair can mean the difference between dependent and independent mobility. When choosing an input device, the clinician and client must determine the ideal input device and the best location for its optimal use. If a decline or improvement in function is anticipated, then it is important to prescribe a wheelchair controller or module that is capable of accepting a variety of input devices. A person with C4 incomplete tetraplegia may progress

from using a specialty control device (e.g., pneumatic, chin, or head control) to a joystick if he regains upper limb strength. This same person may be able to control the joystick on smooth level surfaces but lack control to use the same interface on rough terrain or slopes. Nearly all third party-payers recognize that a person's function may change. The key to cost containment and function is to prescribe a wheelchair base and controller that accepts multiple switch systems. Options for input devices are divided into two categories, proportional and nonproportional (i.e., multiswitch) input devices.

Proportional Input Devices

Therapists and clients must be aware that not all joysticks are proportional; nonproportional joysticks result in a fixed speed on their deflection. Still, the joystick is the most common proportional input device (Figure 11-42, *A*). It is called proportional because the speed of the wheelchair is directly related to the amount of deflection of the joystick. In addition to controlling the wheelchair speed, the joystick is also used to control the direction and braking (i.e., release of the joystick). Joysticks are typically controlled by the user's upper limb and mounted on the outside of one of the wheelchair's armrests. The shape, size, and number of additional functions can vary considerably. Modifications to the joystick knob are available to support a paralyzed hand or adapt to forearm contractures (Figure 11-42, *B*).

Mounting options and adjustments are available from specialty manufacturers that allow the joystick to be raised and lowered, swing away, mounted midline between the armrests, or adjusted in special configurations for a person with limited active ROM. Driving a power wheelchair with a joystick requires good upper limb coordination and proprioceptive awareness. The client must have upper limb strength and range of motion in four directions. He must be able to get his hand on and off the joystick independently. Although this may sound easy, it can be very difficult for an individual with C5 tetraplegia and increased upper limb tone to externally rotate the shoulder to place his hand on the joystick.

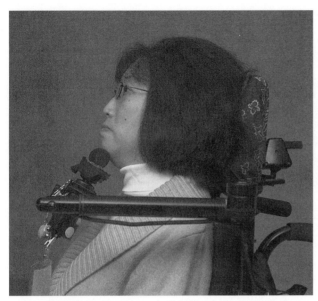

FIGURE 11-43 Power wheelchair with chin control.

Mounting the joystick in midline and at a position midway within the client's greatest active ROM in all directions will offer the best opportunity for success.

A joystick can be mounted to allow foot control, arm control, chin control, and head control. These examples use a standard or remote joystick attached to an extremity interface. For example, a foot-controlled joystick uses a swivel footplate that moves freely into plantarflexion and dorsiflexion for controlling forward and reverse. Internal and external rotation control directional turns. A remote on-off or standby switch is necessary for periods of rest if the person cannot remove the limb from the interface platform. This type of foot platform control can work extremely well for clients with C4 central cord injuries with impaired upper limb function and limited function in their lower limbs.

Chin control can be very functional for weak clients with C4 and C5 injuries. Mounting a remote or minijoystick in front of the chin allows the client to maneuver the wheelchair with his chin (Figure 11-43). A small chin cup may be used instead of the standard joystick knob to improve operation.

Proportional head control is achieved through several different systems. Some use a standard joystick attached to a horseshoe-shaped interface that can be controlled by extension and rotation of the neck and head. Other systems sense the position of the head and require head and neck flexion to control forward-reverse and speed. Lateral flexion of the head is needed to steer the chair. Any limitations in a client's head and neck ROM should be noted because it will affect the client's ability to operate a head control input device. Some of the chin and head control systems are proportional, whereas others are digital and the difference in varied speed control is notable. Generally, proportional input devices are more responsive and simpler to operate.

Nonproportional Input Devices

Individuals with high SCIs who are unable to use one of the previously discussed proportional switch systems because of their physical impairments may achieve independence by using a nonproportional or multiswitch input device. These input devices are useful when a person lacks the gross and fine motor skills needed to operate a proportional input device. Proximity switches, pneumatic (e.g., sip-n-puff) switches, and tongue switches are just some examples of nonproportional input devices. Switches are either on or off and do not allow the user proportional speed control. Advancement in controller technology, however, allows the user to step up and step down the speed by giving commands in sequence or selecting a higher speed option. The end result is better control of the wheelchair. One means of improving efficient operation of a switch input is to be able to latch forward and reverse commands. With latched control, when a command is initiated the wheelchair will continue to move forward until a reverse command is given. This differs from the momentary control seen in proportional input devices where continuous input is required to keep the wheelchair in motion.

Contact or Proximity Switches

Contact or proximity switches are single switches that are mounted so that the user can activate the switch with head movement or some other consistent motion. Contact switches require direct contact and vary in the amount of pressure needed to activate the switch. Proximity switches are activated by the user moving his head or other body part within the range of detection of the switch. The sensitivity of these proximity switches can be adjusted to improve user activation. The most common placement site is within the headrest. In a three-switch array both forward and reverse directions are activated by head extension, whereas steering is controlled by lateral flexion or rotation of the head to activate switches in the right and left lateral pads of the headrest. A fourth switch is used to toggle between forward and reverse and may be mounted in the headrest or in some other location. An audible beep or visible display verifies the direction selected. Many individuals find that using the head to drive is very natural and can be learned fairly quickly provided they have good head and neck strength and ROM.

Pneumatic Input Device

A pneumatic input device is activated by commands that the individual initiates; when using sip-n-puff technology the commands are breath puffs through a straw positioned in front of the mouth (Figure 11-44, A). The user must be able to differentiate between soft and hard commands. Hard puffs result in forward motion (Figure 11-44, B). A hard sip is used to stop the wheelchair. A sustained soft sip or soft puff will result in a left and a right turn, respectively. A hard sip while the chair is stationary will cause the chair to move in reverse. A hard puff will stop the reverse movement. Forward is usually latched. Care should be taken with latched reverse because the client cannot usually see where the wheelchair is headed and an uncontained latch command could lead to an accident. With any switch that is latched the user must have a second switch that acts as a safety or reset switch, which will enable the user to stop the wheelchair should he ever lose control of the primary drive switch.

A pneumatic input device is an appropriate option for a person with a complete SCI at C4 or above. If head or neck ROM is

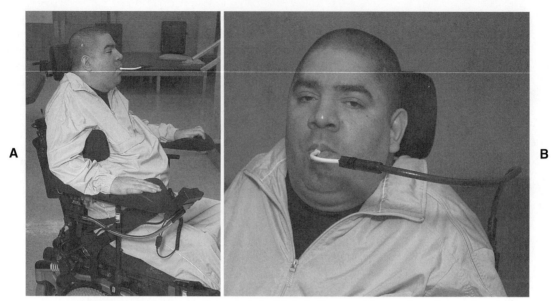

FIGURE 11-44 **A,** Sip-n-puff–operated wheelchair. **B,** Close-up of sip-n-puff mouth control.

limited or very weak, pneumatic controls become a very viable option to achieve independent mobility. Some manufacturers of specialty switches can actually combine pneumatic and proximity switches to allow the client to steer the chair with right and left lateral flexion of his head. This is very beneficial for the client who has difficulty discriminating between hard and soft commands.

Programming the Controller

Once an input device has been selected, the next step is to program it and fine tune the wheelchair for a particular user. Programming the controller is necessary so that the client knows how the wheelchair will respond to his commands. The controller deciphers the information from the input device and converts it into motor output. Programming allows the clinician and supplier to adjust different performance parameters to ensure safe mobility for a variety of driving conditions. In addition, the controller may allow a port for interfacing one or more power seating components. Power seating systems may be activated through the same switch that is used to drive the wheelchair.

Manufacturers differ on their definitions of some of the terms, so it is very important to understand how these adjustments will alter the performance of a wheelchair before any adjustments are made. When the adjustments are complete, the clinician must drive the wheelchair before the client to ensure that the wheelchair is safe.

Training for Power Mobility

Simulation and training in the prescribed equipment is necessary to ensure adequate postural support and safe operation of the device (see Chapter 15). Before the client is trained to use the equipment, the therapist and supplier must become familiar with the controls and performance settings of the wheelchair. Then they will be able to instruct the client, beginning with how to turn the chair on and off or access a reset switch if applicable. The on-off switch or reset switch act as safety stop switches in the event that the wheelchair would behave erratically for unexplained reasons.

Training usually begins with the use of any power seat functions. This allows the client to orient the seating system to his needs for optimal balance and function. Assessment of the client's ability to access the seat function switches throughout the available range is necessary to ensure safe operation. Next, instruction about the drive lock-out feature must be reviewed so that the client understands that he must return the seating system to a certain orientation before it will drive. A drive lock-out feature prevents operation or reduces the available speed when a power seat function is not within the range for safe operation of the wheelchair.

When power mobility training is initiated, it should be in an open area free of barriers so that the client is comfortable and can become accustomed to the input device and the wheelchair's response. Progression should include hallways, narrow spaces, doorways, and ascending and descending ramps that meet Americans With Disabilities Act accessibility guidelines. Advanced progression might include elevator access, ascending and descending steeper inclines, van lifts, and obstacles. Use of a seat belt, chest belt (if necessary), and leg support is always recommended for safety during power mobility training.[30] The client's posture, ability to drive and steer, and ability to stop the chair should be carefully assessed throughout the training period. Programming adjustments may need to be altered to improve efficiency or operation or responsiveness of the wheelchair as the user becomes more skilled.[31] Clinician instruction and spotting will allow the client to gain experience in a safe environment while he learns to understand the performance limits of the wheelchair.

WHEELCHAIR CUSHIONS

When the rehabilitation team and client have selected the type of manual or power wheelchair and its components, the next important part of any wheelchair prescription process is the determination of an appropriate wheelchair cushion. More than 250 cushions are commercially available, so many choices exist. Because no single clinician can know every product, a basic understanding of materials, design, and performance can assist

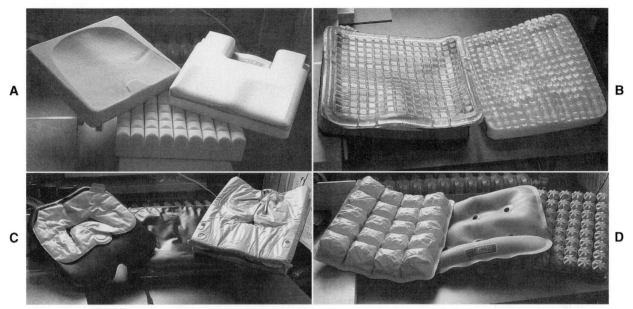

FIGURE 11-45 Various types of wheelchair cushions. **A,** Foam cushions. **B,** Gel cushions. **C,** Viscous fluid cushions. **D,** Air cushions. (Courtesy Stephen H. Sprigle, PhD, © Georgia Tech Research Corporation, Atlanta, GA.)

in selecting an appropriate cushion for wheelchair users. The most important thing to remember is that no one cushion is best for all people!

Cushions affect many aspects of function during everyday activities, including posture, upper limb function, comfort, transfers, heat and moisture of the cushion interface, and a host of other factors. In addition, the environment of use, amount of use, and activity level of the user all will influence cushion selection. A person who sits in his wheelchair for 16 hours a day and travels outdoors over a variety of surfaces has different needs than a person who sits in his wheelchair for 4 hours a day because he is able to independently transfer into other chairs or surfaces.

In a general sense, cushions are designed to provide skin protection or positioning for the user. The design and construction of a cushion should be appropriate to its purpose. A cushion's mechanical properties are reflective of the cushion's materials and overall construction. Wheelchair cushions are made from a variety of materials and are available in many designs. Four material types can be defined: foam or flexible matrix (Figure 11-45, A), gel (Figure 11-45, B), viscous fluid (Figure 11-45, C), and air (Figure 11-45, D). Most cushions are fabricated from a combination of materials with the intent of maximizing cushion performance by managing the good and poor features of each material. Cushion performance is affected by several material properties, including load deflection, friction, heat capacity, loaded contour depth, recovery, and impact damping. This chapter discusses the first three properties, but clinicians should not ignore the others. An International Wheelchair Standards Working Group is developing standards to describe test methods and clinical implications for these and other properties of cushions.

Load Deflection

Stiffness is a measure of deflection under a given load. For a wheelchair cushion, stiffness defines how much a person immerses into the cushion. Different materials deflect and deform in different manners as the buttocks impart load. Foam and air compress under load; the volume of the material decreases, thereby contouring around the body. Gel and viscous fluid displace under load because they are essentially incompressible. Cover materials act in tension and can also affect the load distribution properties of a cushion.

The optimal stiffness of cushion materials is not easy to determine clinically. Body weight, body type, tone, and posture combine to influence how much a person sinks into a cushion.[32,33] If a cushion is too stiff, the body will not be supported well and high pressures and instability can result (Figure 11-46, A). Conversely, if not stiff enough, the cushion will bottom out, a condition that also increases pressure on the body (Figure 11-46, B).

Foam comes in various levels of stiffness and has a very evident cushioning ability, which explains its popularity as a wheelchair cushion material. Many cushions incorporate foams of varying stiffness with the softest material as the top layer. No best stiffness can be defined because the thickness of the foam is also an important factor. For instance, a very soft foam will not bottom out if it is thick enough and a relatively stiffer foam can be used in contoured cushions because they are not expected to deflect as much as flat cushions do.

Air cushions also compress under load but, unlike foam, are very dependent on bladder design and inflation level (Figure 11-46, C). The stiffness of an air cushion changes according to how the bladder is designed and how much air is contained in the bladder. The bladder of a single-compartment cushion cannot deflect in the same manner as a multisegmented cushion (Figure 11-46, D) because of the surface tension of the bladder material, a fact that helps explain why the latter design tends to be thicker. Regardless of design, proper inflation of air cushions is needed to provide the proper stiffness in the same manner as foam cushions.

The stiffness of viscous fluid material is reflected in its viscosity. Some fluids have a viscosity very close to water, whereas

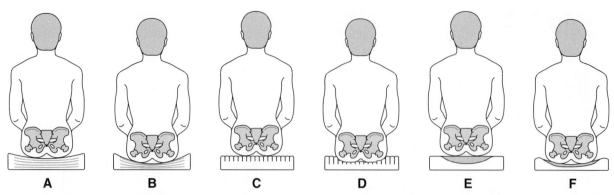

FIGURE 11-46 High seating pressures can result from **(A)** a cushion that is too stiff and does not offer adequate immersion and **(B)** cushion that is too soft leading to bottoming out. **C** and **D**, Air cushions with multisegment designs. **E** and **F**, Both immersion and envelopment are provided by a viscous fluid cushions. (Adapted from illustrations courtesy Stephen H. Sprigle, PhD, © Georgia Tech Research Corporation, Atlanta, GA.)

others are much thicker. Gels can also vary in stiffness, a measure designated by the durometer of the material. Viscous fluid and gel materials are most often used in combination with other materials to accommodate their incompressible nature (Figure 11-46, *E*). Foam, either contoured or flat, is most often used to provide contouring while the viscous fluid or gel wraps around and envelops the buttocks (Figure 11-46, *F*).

Tension

A tight, nonstretch fabric will adversely affect cushion performance. Loose covers and those made from a stretch material are better suited to let the cushioning material deform as intended. Bladder covers, used in air and viscous fluid cushions, can also act in tension and affect the deflection and displacement of the material. The best cover materials are those that protect the cushioning material(s) without affecting their action(s) as a cushion.

Skin Protection

Skin protection is obviously very important for the person with SCI. Decreased mobility and lack of sensation are the most significant contributing factors for pressure ulcer development. Because of these sequelae, clinicians must always assess skin protection needs when selecting a cushion for a person with spinal injury. Cushions designed for skin protection target loading on the skin, the management of temperature, and moisture at the buttock-cushion interface.

Forces on Tissues

In the seated posture, loading on the buttocks represents the greatest risk for tissue damage. Cushions attempt to redistribute pressures away from bony prominences such as the ischial tuberosities and sacrum-coccyx. Two general techniques are followed: (1) envelopment and (2) redirection or off-loading.

Envelopment is defined as the capability of a support surface in deforming around and encompassing the contour of the human body.[34] An enveloping cushion should encompass and equalize pressure about irregularities in contour resulting from buttock shape, objects in pockets, and clothing. Cushions that target envelopment must deflect and deform to immerse the buttocks in the material. Flat cushions must deflect more than precontoured cushions that incorporate a concave sitting surface. The design

of the pelvis requires about 2 inches of immersion to adequately encompass the buttocks because of the inferior position of the ischial tuberosities.

Some cushions are designed to purposely redirect forces away from bony prominences. Off-loading parts of the body is a common approach used on prosthetics and orthotics, and the concept used by cushions is similar. Cushions accomplish this by cutouts or reliefs in the cushion surface. Some cushions are customized or individualized to the user as a way to ensure that the person fits properly (see Figure 11-12). Because the goal is to redirect load away from bony prominences, these cushions generally require the person to sit on the cushion in a specific manner. This requirement should be discussed with the client and followed by training to ensure that he understands the proper use of the cushion.

Interface Pressure

Interface pressure measurement is an increasingly common tool used to judge a cushion's ability to manage pressure on the buttocks. The most common interface pressure measurement systems comprise a series of sensors configured into a mat that interface into a computer, which then produces a digital profile of the client's seated pressure distribution, highlighting areas of high pressure that require load reduction (Figure 11-47). Although a discussion of interface pressure measurement is beyond the scope of this chapter, two important points must be made: no one cushion offers the best interface pressure for all people and no pressure value has been determined to be harmful for all people.

Shear and Friction

Shear and friction are often discussed together as risk factors for pressure ulcers, but they are not the same thing. Friction is a force that opposes the movement of two bodies in contact, such as the sliding of the buttocks on the cushion surface. The term shear can refer to either shear stress (i.e., the force acting tangentially on an area of an object) or shear strain (i.e., the deformation of an object in response to shear stresses). In seating, shear strain results from all the forces that cause the deformation of buttock tissues, including normal forces from gravity, shear forces, and frictional forces at the buttock-cushion interface. Research has shown that

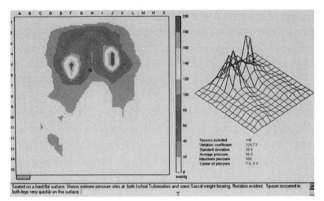

FIGURE 11-47 Commercial pressure measuring systems produce a profile of the client's seated pressure distribution. The display allows the clinician to easily spot areas of high pressure and apply options for relief that will reduce mechanical load under varying conditions. (From Cook AM, Hussey SM: *Assistive technologies: principles and practice*, ed 3, St. Louis, 2008, Elsevier Mosby, Fig 10-25B.)

the presence of shear stresses on tissues reduces the tissues ability to withstand normal loads.[35-37] In other words, tissues are more at risk for damage in the presence of shear.

Cushions manage friction in different ways but cannot completely eliminate it. Friction is needed for postural stability just as friction is needed to walk or to drive a car. Certain materials and cushions have a higher horizontal stiffness, meaning that they prevent sliding but can increase shear strain on the tissues as a result. Consider a highly contoured foam cushion. This cushion would have a high horizontal stiffness, so it should keep a person from sliding forward better than a cushion with lower horizontal stiffness. However, this feature may also impede the user from sliding forward during transfer. Therefore, consistent with other performance features, a design trade-off can be identified.

Clinicians can help reduce shear strain resulting from sliding by ensuring a stable seating system that does not encourage the person to slide forward on the seat. When a person slides forward in his chair, the pelvis rotates posteriorly, thereby exposing the sacrum and coccyx to damaging loads. Moreover, sliding forward or the resistance to sliding also induces shear strain throughout the buttocks. Reducing the sliding tendency may be done by attention to the seat-to-back angle of the wheelchair and to the proper sizing of the wheelchair seat. A backrest that is too vertical and seats that are too long or short are contributors to postural instability.

Heat and Moisture

As discussed in Chapter 2, many individuals with SCI lack the ability to regulate their body temperatures. They may be hot and perspire regularly or they may be habitually cold. The cushion may have an impact on comfort as well as on tissue integrity. The ability of the cushion to dissipate heat affects the temperature and moisture of the buttock tissues. Increasing evidence suggests that a rise in tissue temperature exacerbates the tissue's susceptibility to pressure ulcers.[38,39] Furthermore, any increase of moisture, whether from sweating or another source, will increase the coefficient of friction of the skin.[40,41] Excessive moisture can

also macerate tissue, resulting in a reduced ability to withstand external forces. Therefore, temperature and moisture are often linked when assessing cushion performance. Until a definitive test for heat and moisture dissipation is developed, an understanding of material characteristics and features can help differentiate performance.

Cushions handle heat dissipation with varying abilities. Foam is an insulator, so the temperature of the buttocks-cushion interface can rise well beyond the optimal temperature when sweating occurs. Viscous fluid and gel materials have a high thermal mass, meaning they conduct and absorb heat. Cushions topped with an adequate amount of gel of viscous fluids have a lower buttock-cushion interface temperature than foam cushions. Air cushions are hard to judge without testing. Their impermeable cover has a huge impact on temperature. Some designs are better able to allow air flow than others, which helps reduce the interface temperature. A person's activity on a cushion also affects temperature. Regular unweighting by using pressure relief or leaning activities helps dissipate heat from the cushion's surface. Alternatively, very active users will have a higher workload, which can lead to sweating. A judicious clinical guideline is, if a person regularly sweats on a particular cushion, other cushion options should be investigated.

Moisture can result from sweating and many other sources. Cushions and their covers have a huge impact on how this moisture is managed. Cushions that permit airflow with a breathable cover and cushioning material are better able to dissipate moisture than are cushions that do not. Some incontinence covers are breathable because they are made from fabric that prevents water passage but allows air flow and thus have skin care advantages over covers that block both air and water flow.

Positioning

Postural support is an important factor in cushion selection because a wheelchair user must perform myriad activities while seated. Cushions offer a range of positioning features that can enhance postural stability. If positioning is a problem, the clinician should determine whether alignment, accommodation, or correction is needed. Cushions that provide alignment are designed to support the body in a certain position and may include one or all of the following: contouring for the buttocks, lateral pelvic supports, and lateral or medial thigh supports. Postural accommodation is needed when a client cannot achieve a stable and symmetrical posture, so the cushion is configured to accommodate a deformity. Conversely, if an asymmetry is correctable, a cushion can be used to position a client into a symmetrical posture. Evaluation should include ROM, tone, and functional assessment in the effort to determine what type of positioning is needed.

Foam components are most often used for the positioning features in cushions. These foams may be stiffer than the foam used on the cushion surface because they are designed to push on the pelvis or leg to provide support. Some cushions offer adjustability to achieve positioning capability. Foam, gel, or viscous fluid inserts can be placed in location to accommodate a pelvic obliquity or to create a wedge to increase stability. Some air cushions are also designed to permit adjustable inflation in ways that address postural alignment, correction, or accommodation.

The positioning features of cushions often need to be individualized to the user. This also results in a cushion surface that is site specific, meaning that the user must sit on the cushion correctly. For example, sitting too forward on a cushion may result in the individual sitting on the medial thigh support or pommel. This not only eliminates the positioning ability of the support, it can also adversely affect the cushioning and functionality of the cushion. Clinicians should discuss and instruct their clients in the correct sitting and proper positioning of their cushions to ensure proper use. In addition, positioning cushions may have certain features that can hinder transfers.

A contoured cushion with a pommel may be needed, but if the user is independent in transfers, assessment must be made to ensure that these positioning features do not pose a barrier to that independence.

Ensuring the Best Fit

Many wheelchair cushions are commercially available. Having myriad choices can empower clinicians and clients, but choice can also be confusing. By reflecting on the seating goals with respect to cushion materials and designs, an informed decision can be made.

CLINICAL CASE STUDY | Seating and Positioning Case 1

Patient History
Carl Miller is a 62-year-old man with a C6 tetraplegia, American Spinal Injury Association (ASIA) A diagnosis resulting from a fall down his basement stairs. He underwent 1 week of spinal traction followed by a sternal occipital mandibular immobilizer collar for 4 weeks. His acute care course was complicated by pneumonia. He was discharged to inpatient acute rehabilitation 3 weeks after his injury and received inpatient therapy for 6 weeks. Carl began outpatient physical therapy 2 weeks after his discharge with an expected 2-month therapy program. He completed 1 month of outpatient therapy and then had family visitors for 2 weeks. He is now returning to the outpatient therapy program at 17 weeks post injury. He has a mild right thoracic C structural scoliosis.

Carl is a general contractor and owns his own company. His son is a certified CPA and works with him as the chief financial officer of the company. His company health coverage does not provide for long-term disability; however, he will most likely receive coverage for half the cost of a power wheelchair. Carl is in the process of receiving both power and manual wheelchair prescriptions during his outpatient therapy program and has authorization for 1 more month of outpatient therapy. He has been using a loaner power wheelchair donated through his church, which he will return when his chair arrives. Home modifications for accessibility were completed by his employees.

Carl lives with his wife Gwen, age 63 years, who is a retired bank manager. She is a former marathon runner and in excellent health. Gwen is collecting a pension and is able to support their regular monthly expenses. She is currently the primary caretaker of her husband. Their church recently sponsored a fundraiser and raised $3000 toward Carl's wheelchair order. Carl already owned a van; a power lift and hand controls have been installed. He has passed his written and hand control driver's test.

Patient's Self-Assessment
Carl intends to return to his job, which includes both office work and on-site supervision at his construction sites.

Clinical Assessment
Patient Appearance
- Height 6 feet 2 inches, weight 228 pounds, body mass index 29.3 with a mild right thoracic C structural scoliosis

Cognitive Assessment
- Alert, oriented × 3

Cardiopulmonary Assessment
- Blood pressure 125/80 mm Hg, heart rate at rest 72 beats/min, respiratory rate 12 breaths/min, cough flows are ineffective (<360 L/min), vital capacity is reduced (between 1.5 and 2.5 L), and breathing pattern incorporates accessory muscles and upper chest wall only

- Patient has marked decrease in the anterior and lateral chest wall with a slight decrease in posterior wall expansion

Musculoskeletal and Neuromuscular Assessment
- Motor assessment reveals AISA A and sensory to the C6 level
- Deep tendon reflexes 3+ below the level of lesion

Integumentary and Sensory Assessment
- Skin is intact throughout
- Sensory intact to C6

Range of Motion Assessment
- Passive and active ROM is within normal limits except bilateral hip flexion contractures of 10 degrees

Mobility and ADL Assessment
- Partially dependent with bed mobility and transfers; requires minimal assistance
- Independent with pressure relief and power wheelchair maneuvering on all surfaces
- Independent with upper body dressing but dependent with lower body
- Independent with eating and grooming after equipment setup
- Dependent in bowel and bladder management

Evaluation of Clinical Assessment
Carl Miller is a 62-year-old man with a C6 tetraplegia, ASIA A diagnosis from a fall. He is 17 weeks post injury and attending outpatient physical therapy for further rehabilitation of functional training, wheelchair prescription, and wheelchair skills management.

Patient's Care Needs
1. Evaluation for manual and power wheelchair prescription including support for scoliosis and seating surface
2. Evaluation of independence with selected manual and power wheelchair mobility on level and uneven surfaces, ramps, and curbs
3. Evaluation for compatibility of wheelchairs with equipped van

Diagnosis and Prognosis
Diagnosis is C6 tetraplegia, ASIA A. Prognosis is for full independence in power wheelchair mobility and management on even and uneven surfaces.

Preferred Practice Pattern*
Impaired Muscle Performance (4C), Joint Mobility, Motor Function, Muscle Performance, and Range of Motion Associated With Fracture (4G), Primary Prevention/Risk Reduction for Cardiovascular/Pulmonary Disorders (6A), Prevention/Risk Reduction for Integumentary Disorders (7A)

CLINICAL CASE STUDY Seating and Positioning Case 1—cont'd

Team Goals

1. Team to draft a manual and power wheelchair prescription and review with patient and wife
2. Team to discuss seating options relative to cost and functionality during transfers and van use and review with patient and wife
3. Team to review advanced wheelchair training skills needed to negotiate home and community environments with patient

Patient Goals

"I want to get my own wheelchair and be able to use it properly. I also want to be able to perform pressure relief independently."

Care Plan

Treatment Plan and Rationale

- Schedule patient for wheelchair seating clinic
- Provide a variety of seating options to try out for support of scoliosis and pressure relief
- Initiate wheelchair management and mobility training in selected wheelchair
- Practice van access with final wheelchair, including safety features for himself and his wheelchair

Interventions

- Instruct and practice wheelchair management, maintenance, and propulsion
- Instruct and practice taking apart wheelchair components and reinstating
- Instruct and practice advanced wheelchair skills on all surfaces in both power and manual wheelchair and review how to instruct a caregiver to assist on difficult terrain
- Practice pressure relief techniques and review the importance of proper seating and cushions during all seating activities, including driving

Documentation and Team Communication

- Team will document wheelchair prescription for scoliosis and proper pressure relief
- Team consultation for seating and positioning for wheelchair propulsion on multiple surfaces and for driving
- Team will document Carl's knowledge of wheelchair management, maintenance, and safety during driving

Follow-Up Assessment

- Reassessment of team goals weekly
- Check status of wheelchair prescription weekly
- Evaluate effectiveness of scoliosis and pressure relief options weekly

Critical Thinking Exercises

Consider intrinsic and extrinsic factors that will influence Carl's seating and positioning prescriptions, including his physical needs, anticipated lifestyle, and the types of environments to be encountered, along with patient and family education regarding his mobility when answering the following questions:

1. What physical assessment considerations (client physical limitations or characteristics) are important to Carl's wheelchair prescription process?
2. List seating components that can be manipulated in Carl's wheelchair prescription process. What evaluations are important related to Carl's scoliosis?
3. Carl wants a power wheelchair. Select the wheelchair components including the type of control that will be most appropriate.
4. What type of manual wheelchair would provide Carl with optimal mobility? What are the handrim considerations? Describe two safety additions that will benefit Carl relative to wheelchair propulsion and mobility?

*Guide to physical therapist practice, rev. ed. 2, Alexandria, VA, 2003, American Physical Therapy Association.

CLINICAL CASE STUDY Seating and Positioning Case 2

Patient History

Sharon Jacobs is a 30-year-old woman with a T10 paraplegia, American Spinal Injury Association (ASIA) A diagnosis. She was injured in a company plane crash and is the only survivor. She also had multiple internal injuries, which prolonged her acute stay to 4 weeks. She underwent a posterior decompression, fusion, and wiring 1 week after injury and was in a thoracic body jacket for 6 weeks. She received 4 weeks of inpatient therapy and was discharged to home. All orthopedic restrictions were lifted at 9 weeks after injury. She is 10 weeks post injury and has just begun outpatient physical therapy.

Sharon is a fashion designer. She worked for a large company that provided a long-term disability insurance option in which she was enrolled, so funding for her wheelchair will be covered in full. She is currently in the process of ordering her permanent wheelchair as an outpatient.

She is married and has an 18-month-old daughter. Her husband works for the same company in its finance division. They own a ranch home, which has been modified to accommodate her wheelchair. They also have a full-time live-in caretaker who cares for the baby and does the cooking and cleaning.

Patient's Self Assessment

Sharon lifestyle has always been very active. She was an avid tennis player and cycled three times a week. She hopes to return to work and to her sports regimen.

Clinical Assessment

Patient Appearance

- Height 5 feet 4 inches, weight 110 pounds, body mass index 18.9

Cognitive Assessment

- Alert, oriented × 3

Cardiopulmonary Assessment

- Blood pressure 100/62 mm Hg, heart rate at rest 72 beats/min, respiratory rate 10 breaths/min, cough is effective, vital capacity is normal (approximately 4.8L), and breathing pattern is diaphragmatic

Musculoskeletal and Neuromuscular Assessment

- Motor assessment reveals ASIA A motor and sensory T10.
- Deep tendon reflexes 1+ below the level of lesion

Integumentary and Sensory Assessment

- Skin is intact throughout, sensory intact to T10.

Range of Motion Assessment

- Passive and active ROM is within normal limits.

Mobility and ADL Assessment

- Independent with all ADLs and bowel and bladder care
- Independent with pressure relief and manual wheelchair maneuvering on level surfaces and is using a loaner wheelchair

Continued

CLINICAL CASE STUDY | Seating and Positioning Case 2—cont'd

Evaluation of Clinical Assessment
Sharon Jacobs is a 30-year-old woman with a T10 paraplegia, ASIA A diagnosis resulting from a plane crash. She is attending outpatient physical therapy to acquire high-level wheelchair skills and obtain a wheelchair prescription.

Patient's Care Needs
1. Evaluation for wheelchair prescription
2. Instruction in wheelchair mobility and high-level wheelchair skills
3. Evaluation for knowledge of wheelchair maintenance and optimal wheelchair alignment for propulsion efficiency.
4. Evaluation for participation of wheelchair sports

Diagnosis and Prognosis
Diagnosis is T10 paraplegia, ASIA A. Prognosis is for full independence in wheelchair propulsion, management, and high-level wheelchair skills.

Preferred Practice Pattern*
Impaired Muscle Performance (4C), Joint Mobility, Motor Function, Muscle Performance, and Range of Motion Associated With Fracture (4G), Primary Prevention/Risk Reduction for Cardiovascular/Pulmonary Disorders (6A), Prevention/Risk Reduction for Integumentary Disorders (7A)

Team Goals
1. Team to discuss optimal wheelchair prescription
2. Team to plan for wheelchair skills training and carryover on all surfaces
3. Team to review wheelchair maintenance and propulsion skills
4. Team to discuss possible sports options

Patient Goals
"To get my wheelchair and be independent in it and begin wheelchair sports."

Care Plan
Treatment Plan & Rationale
• Schedule patient for wheelchair seating clinic.
• Initiate wheelchair management, maintenance, propulsion, and high-level wheelchair skills training in the selected wheelchair. Discuss driving options and car transfers.
• Provide sports options.

Interventions
• Evaluate wheelchair propulsion skills with a variety of manual wheelchair components and cushions.
• Instruct and practice wheelchair management, maintenance, propulsion, and high-level wheelchair skills training on all terrains.

Documentation and Team Communication
• Team consultation for seating and positioning for wheelchair prescription
• Team to discuss wheelchair cushion needs for pressure relief
• Team consultation regarding optimization of skills needed to cover a variety of terrain
• Team to discuss transportation of wheelchair
• Team to discuss wheelchair sports options

Follow-Up Assessment
• Reassessment weekly on status of wheelchair prescription
• Follow-up on wheelchair breakdown and ability to repair and maintain wheelchair parts
• Reassess new needs for high-level wheelchair skills on the basis of home, community, and work sessions.

Critical Thinking Exercises
Consider intrinsic and extrinsic factors that will influence Sharon's seating and positioning prescriptions, including her physical needs, anticipated lifestyle, and the types of environments to be encountered, along with patient and family education regarding her mobility when answering the following questions:
1. What type of manual wheelchair would you recommend for Sharon?
2. Describe two features that would be important to Sharon's wheelchair prescription.
3. What future wheelchair(s) may be applicable if Sharon returns to an active lifestyle?

*Guide to physical therapist practice, rev. ed. 2, Alexandria, VA, 2003, American Physical Therapy Association.

SUMMARY

A thorough evaluation to determine seating and mobility needs is just the beginning component when determining a client's wheelchair and cushion prescription. Because of the many options, the prescriptive process for manual and power wheelchairs has become more complicated over the years. Multiple factors have contributed to this complexity, which has been driven by the explosion of technology options. Most wheelchair manufacturers offer many types and styles of wheelchairs. Within a single wheelchair design, there are an overwhelming number of choices for component parts, optional features, and even color. The same situation exists in wheelchair cushions.

Differences among insurance carriers and policies along with shortened lengths of hospital stays can further complicate the process of prescribing and delivering appropriate equipment. Although these factors have made the process more difficult, it remains the role of the team to help individuals identify their needs and understand the factors that will play a role in narrowing the list of appropriate mobility options. Setting specific goals and priorities will help decipher what equipment features are necessary. Prioritizing these goals will also help identify the relative importance of a specific feature when looking at equipment options. Although the process may seem complicated, good organization, goal setting, simulation, and trial of the equipment can simplify the prescription process.

REFERENCES

1. Crane B, Cohen L: Clinician task force, correspondence to CMS, evaluation and documentation recommendations for MAE: 2005. Available from: http://www.cliniciantaskforce.org. Accessed August 11, 2006.

2. Trefler E, Douglas DA, Taylor SJ et al: *Seating and mobility for persons with physical disabilities*, Tucson, AZ, 1993, Therapy Skill Builders.

3. Zacharkow D: *Posture: sitting, standing, chair design and exercise*, Springfield, IL, 1988, Charles C Thomas.

4. Zollars JA: *Special seating: an illustrated guide*, Minneapolis, MN, 1996, Otto Bock.

5. Letts RM: *Principles of seating the disabled*, Boca Raton, FL, 1991, CRC Press.

6. Bergen AF, Presperin J, Tallman T: *Positioning for function: wheelchairs and other assistive technologies*, Valhalla, NY, 1990, Valhalla Rehabilitation Publications.

7. Brubaker CE: Ergonometric considerations, *J Rehabil Res Dev Clin Suppl* 2:37-48, 1990.

8. Sawatzky BJ, Denison I, Kim WO: Rolling, rolling, rolling, *Rehab Manag* 15:36-9, 2002.

9. Thacker J, Sprigle S, Morris B: *Understanding the technology when selecting wheelchairs*, Arlington, VA, 1994, Rehabilitation Engineering Society of North America.

10. Janssen-Potten YJ, Seelen HA, Drukker J et al: Chair configuration and balance control in persons with spinal cord injury, *Arch Phys Med Rehabil* 81:401-408, 2000.

11. Hastings JD, Fanucchi ER, Burns SP: Wheelchair configuration and postural alignment in persons with spinal cord injury, *Arch Phys Med Rehabil* 84:528-534, 2003.

12. Maurer CL, Sprigle S: Effect of seat inclination on seated pressures of individuals with spinal cord injury, *Phys Ther* 84:255-261, 2004.

13. Chan A, Heck C: The effects of tilting the seat position of a wheelchair on respiration, posture, fatigue, voice volume and exertion outcomes in individuals with advanced multiple sclerosis, *J Rehabil Outcomes Meas* 3:1-14, 1999.

14. Brubaker CE, McLaurin CA, McClay IS: Effects of side slope on wheelchair performance, *J Rehabil Res Dev* 23:55-58, 1986.

15. Glaser RM, Sawka MN, Wilde SW et al: Energy cost and cardiopulmonary responses for wheelchair locomotion and walking on tile and on carpet, *Paraplegia* 1981;19:220-6.

16. Kirby RL, Ashton BD, Ackroyd-Stolarz SA, et al: Adding loads to occupied wheelchairs: effect on static rear and forward stability, *Arch Phys Med Rehabil* 77:183-186, 1996.

17. Veeger D, van der Woude LH, Rozendal RH: The effect of rear wheel camber in manual wheelchair propulsion, *J Rehabil Res Dev* 26:37-46, 1989.

18. Thacker J, Foraiati KT: Ride comfort: task 9. In Thacker JG, editor: *Improved wheelchair and seating design: summary of activities February 1, 1991–January 31 1992, Charlottesville, VA*, 1992, Rehabilitation Engineering Center (University of Virginia).

19. van der Woude LH, Hendrich KM, Veeger HE et al: Manual wheelchair propulsion: effects of power output on physiology and technique, *Med Sci Sports Exerc* 20:70-78, 1988.

20. Boninger ML, Towers JD, Cooper RA, et al: Shoulder imaging abnormalities in individuals with paraplegia, *J Rehabil Res Dev* 38:401-408, 2001.

21. Nichols PJ, Norman PA, Ennis JR: Wheelchair user's shoulder? Shoulder pain in patients with spinal cord lesions, *Scand J Rehabil Med* 11:29-32, 1979.

22. Sie IH, Waters RL, Adkins RH et al: Upper extremity pain in the postrehabilitation spinal cord injured patient, *Arch Phys Med Rehabil* 73:44-48, 1992.

23. van der Woude LH, Veeger HE, Dallmeijer AJ et al: Biomechanics and physiology in active manual wheelchair propulsion, *Med Eng Phys* 23:713-733, 2001.

24. Veeger HE, Rozendaal LA, van der Helm FC: Load on the shoulder in low intensity wheelchair propulsion, *Clin Biomech (Bristol Avon)* 17:211-218, 2002.

25. Cooper RA: *Wheelchair selection and configuration*, New York, 1998, Demos.

26. Buning M, Manary M: Wheelchair transportation safety workshop. In *Proceedings of the Rehabilitation Engineering Society of North America 1996 Conference*, Atlanta, GA, The Society.

27. American National Standards Institute/Rehabilitation Engineering and Assistive Technology Society of North America: *American National Standard for wheelchairs*, Arlington, VA, 1998, The Society.

28. Boyd B: Unlocking the facts about scooters, *Paraplegia News* 49:30-38, 1995.

29. Babinec M: *Rear v/s mid v/s front wheel drive power wheelchair*, New Orleans, 2001, Medtrade.

30. Cooper RA, Dvorznak MJ, O'Connor TJ et al: Braking electric-powered wheelchairs: effect of braking method, seatbelt, and legrests, *Arch Phys Med Rehabil* 79:1244-1249, 1998.

31. Rentschler AJ, Cooper RA, Boninger ML et al: A comparison of power wheelchair stability using ANSI/RESNA standards. In *Proceedings of the Rehabilitation Engineering Society of North America 1999 Conference*, Long Beach, CA, 1999, The Society.

32. Garber SL, Krouskop TA: Body build and its relationship to pressure distribution in the seated wheelchair patient, *Arch Phys Med Rehabil* 63:17-20, 1982.

33. Sprigle S, Chung KC, Brubaker CE: Factors affecting seat contour characteristics, *J Rehabil Res Dev* 27:127-134, 1990.

34. Sprigle S, Press L, Davis K: Development of uniform terminology and procedures to describe wheelchair cushion characteristics, *J Rehabil Res Dev* 38:449-461, 2001.

35. Bennett L, Kavner D, Lee BK et al: Shear vs pressure as causative factors in skin blood flow occlusion, *Arch Phys Med Rehabil* 60:309-314, 1979.

36. Goldstein B, Sanders J: Skin response to repetitive mechanical stress: a new experimental model in pig, *Arch Phys Med Rehabil* 79:265-272, 1998.

37. Bennett L, Lee BY: Pressure versus shear in pressure sore causation. In Lee BY, editor: *Chronic ulcers of the skin*, New York, 1985, McGraw-Hill.

38. Patel S, Knapp CF, Donofrio JC et al: Temperature effects on surface pressure–induced changes in rat skin perfusion: implications in pressure ulcer development, *J Rehabil Res Dev* 36:189-201, 1999.

39. Kokate JY, Leland KJ, Held AM et al: Temperature-modulated pressure ulcers: a porcine model, *Arch Phys Med Rehabil* 76:666-673, 1995.

40. Egawa M, Oguri M, Hirao T et al: The evaluation of skin friction using a frictional feel analyzer, *Skin Res Technol* 8:41-51, 2002.

41. Buchholz B, Frederick LJ, Armstrong TJ: An investigation of human palmar skin friction and the effects of materials, pinch force and moisture, *Ergonomics* 31:317-325, 1998.

SOLUTIONS TO CHAPTER 11 CLINICAL CASE STUDY

Seating and Positioning Case 1

1. Carl's physical characteristics, including age, weight, height, muscle strength, contractures, spasticity or muscle tone, joint ROM, lumbar mobility, sensory status, skin condition and integrity, and postural deformities (i.e., scoliosis), should be evaluated and considered when the wheelchairs are prescribed. Bowel and bladder continence, perspiration, nutritional status, medications, and cognitive status of user and caregiver should be noted as needed. Considerations for power seating components should also include the client's ability for independent weight shift. Balance, function, and transfer technique are factors that influence which wheelchair will provide the greatest independence possible while maintaining comfort and functional ability for work and social needs. Insurance coverage affects choices as well. In this case the fundraiser will help substantially, but what about future wheelchairs?

2. Extrinsic factors include the type of seat, back, and cushion chosen for the wheelchair; angle of the wheelchair seat and back; system tilt; use of pelvic belts; lateral supports; and support of the feet. Interventions to prevent further scoliotic deformity should include evaluation of lateral supports and the chair cushion. The cushion must support the pelvis in a stable position because pelvic position is the key to postural stability. Carl may need a custom cushion to achieve symmetrical pressure distribution through both ischia and the cushion must have the appropriate depth. A cushion in conjunction with the wheelchair seat that is too deep will allow the client's posture to slide into a posterior pelvic tilt.

Lateral pelvic supports will center the pelvis on the cushion, whether provided as part of the cushion or attached to the solid seat or backrest. Lateral thoracic supports must be height, width, and angle adjustable. Measurement of the desired height of the lateral supports and chest width and depth is important to ensure an appropriate chair fit that maintains Carl's posture. The thinner the trunk support, the less likely it will interfere with upper limb function and positioning. Three points of pressure may be necessary to contain the spinal curvature; however, a comprehensive evaluation must be done to explore what will be appropriate in this particular case. If three points of pressure are recommended on the basis of Carl's evaluation and a simulation of the seating options, then the lateral thoracic support on the right convex side of the scoliotic trunk should be set to push against the ribs, corresponding with the apex of the vertebral curve. The contralateral thoracic support should be placed as high as possible without interfering with upper limb function or causing excessive pressure in the axillary region. The lateral pelvic support on the side of the high thoracic support acts as the third point of pressure for the curvature correction. A substitute for lateral thoracic supports is a corset with postural stays, which provides both postural and abdominal support for improved respiratory function. Carl's upper limb function must be carefully considered because he will require maximum use of his shoulder girdle with all functional activities. The length of his trunk given his height is also important because maximized respiratory function with aging is critical. Accurate back height is crucial here and should be simulated with practice using different trunk support options because miscalculation causes frequent errors in wheelchair prescription. Regardless of whether a lateral support or supports are needed, provision for their eventual addition is advisable.

3. Carl's mobility needs for home and work must be examined carefully. Accessibility and function are critical along with his ability for independent weight shift. Typically an individual with a C6 lesion can weight shift adequately; however, shear may occur with repositioning. Therefore, repositioning after a weight shift needs to be carefully evaluated. If this client cannot weight shift adequately or his skin is fragile, then a power tilt or power recline wheelchair may be indicated. In addition, Carl's age and overall health status must be considered when deciding whether tilting or reclining will allow for greater independence for a longer period of time.

Transportation of a power wheelchair is also a consideration. Carl has passed his written and behind-the-wheel driver test and may operate a van. Every power wheelchair seating system has a specific weight capacity that should be included in the decision-making process. The input device selection, such as a joystick device, will depend on the seating system and should be proportional to Carl's upper limb ability. The controller may also allow him to use other assistive technology through the same input device. Adjustable swing-away footrests are necessary to ease Carl's transfers. His footrests on a reclining power wheelchair should be elevating; the armrests should be two-point flip back for ease during transfers. Casters and tires should be pneumatic because of the type of terrain that Carl may encounter. However, maintenance increases when pneumatic tires are used on both front and rear wheels because of the need to maintain tire pressure and the possibility of getting tire punctures. Swing-away or retractable joystick mounts allow the joystick to be moved out of the way for access, which may be necessary at various job sites. Vertical seat elevation could be important for Carl to ease transfers or to reach surfaces higher than standard table heights. Momentary control would also be more practical for job sites because Carl could then maneuver stops and starts more easily.

4. A fully adjustable manual wheelchair is ideal for this client because seat and axle adjustment can assist ease of propulsion. Carl's method of propulsion may change over time as he becomes more efficient with his strokes and improves his balance through increased body awareness along with functional compensations for ease of function. Carl's degree of independence should be evaluated to optimally prescribe equipment that allows him to meet his mobility needs. Because these may change over time, power add-ons should be considered. Plastic-coated handrims should be chosen because Carl does not have hand function; vertical or oblique projections should be considered as well. Grade aids can be used to prevent the wheelchair from rolling backward while being propelled uphill and antitip devices designed to prevent rearward tipping are also advised. Type of armrest should be considered for its relation to home life and work. Carl will require push handles for assistance when another individual needs to push his wheelchair. Again with the manual chair, pneumatic tires will be more suitable to accommodate the variety of terrain that Carl will encounter on the job site.

SOLUTIONS TO CHAPTER 11 CLINICAL CASE STUDY

Seating and Positioning Case 2

1. A lightweight, durable titanium frame would be best for Sharon because she is young and petite, works outside the home, and is a mother. The chair should also be fully adjustable to allow seat and axle adjustment that can assist with efficient propulsion. Careful measurement for optimal seat width and back height should be simulated with a cushion that will meet Sharon's home and work needs. When the ideal position for ease of propulsion, including the type of handrim and functional parameters for ADLs, child care, and work, is fully known, a rigid wheelchair with quick release wheels may be considered and financially would most likely be plausible. A folding frame should not be eliminated, however, because her vehicle needs to be evaluated for wheelchair access (i.e., ease of loading and unloading).

2. Swing-away legrests are appropriate initially to ease function with child care, transfers, and ADLs unless she chooses a rigid frame without swing-away footrests. Armrests should be desk arms for ease at work unless the tubular swing away options do not interfere with her workstation. The type of tires on Sharon's chair may be important because of maintenance issues. The wheelchair's color and fabric may have particular bearing in this case because of Sharon's occupation as a designer. Her occupation may also influence her decisions about other wheelchair parts because of her perceptions about the importance of appearance. In addition, the weight of the wheelchair is critical because she is a small-framed individual.

3. A custom nonadjustable, most likely a rigid, model may provide Sharon with the postural support and maneuverability in the lightest weight wheelchair available. Front and rear seat heights, seat width and depth, seat angle, back angle, back height, rear wheel camber, and position of the rear axle will be specified at the time the wheelchair is ordered. If all of these factors were known, this would be the most durable product for Sharon's active lifestyle. Considerations for rear wheel camber adjustment should be included in the prescription if Sharon will be involved in wheelchair sports that involve more than one camber for optimal performance. Optimally, two wheelchairs—one for everyday use and another for sports—may be the best solution for this client.

CHAPTER TWELVE

Assessment and Match for Effective Assistive Technology

Marcia J. Scherer, PhD, and Phil Parette, EdD

Without today's modern electronics it would be hard for me to have self-respect or the energy to want to continue with life's daily chores. My environmental control unit allows me to do things without assistance from other people. This has given me independence, dignity and mental strength.

(Keith C4 SCI)

Technology plays an increasingly important role in the lives of everyone in our society. From the time we wake up in the morning until retiring in the evening, our awareness and use of technological applications is constant. Each successive generation becomes more influenced by or acculturated to the presence and need for technology.[1] Not too many years ago, self-checkout counters in grocery stores, voice-activated telephone menus, and touch screen information kiosks in public buildings would have been unimaginable, although now they are commonplace technologies. Admittedly, such an increased presence of technology in our lives has markedly changed our quality of life in virtually all facets of human functioning. These facets include living independently, self-determination, making choices, pursuing meaningful careers, and enjoying full inclusion and integration in the economic, political, social, cultural, and educational mainstream of American society. For many individuals who have disabilities, particularly those with spinal cord injuries (SCI), assistive technology (AT) plays an even more important role in ensuring both maintenance and quality of life on a daily basis.

DEFINING ASSISTIVE TECHNOLOGY DEVICES AND SERVICES

AT has been defined as any item, piece of equipment, or product system, whether acquired commercially, modified, or customized, that is used to increase, maintain, or improve functional capabilities of individuals with disabilities.[2] These devices cover a range of product categories that include mobility, sensory assistance, communication, personal care, and recreation (Box 12-1). AT devices include hardware, software, and other technology solutions that are required by people with SCI to perform specific tasks, improve their functional capabilities, and become more independent. Specialized AT devices are currently available from a variety of vendors and manufacturers (e.g., Abledata, www.abledata.com). Although these devices have become increasingly sophisticated, many may need additional modification or customization to meet the specific needs of a person with an SCI.

AT may be categorized as being no-tech, low-tech, or high-tech. No-tech solutions typically involve changes in the ways that people do things to meet an individual's needs. For example, when a person with SCI enters a clothing store in a power wheelchair, he might be confronted with very narrow aisles that are not accessible. Store employees can provide a simple solution by bringing articles of clothing to the customer to examine. This requires no special technology and no major change in how business is conducted.

Generally, low-technology devices are simple in design, inexpensive, readily available, and require little, if any, training for effective use. For example, a flexible drinking straw may assist a person who has limited use of his hands or cannot hold a cup. Velcro fasteners on articles of clothing may enable a person to button his shirt or tie his shoes (Figure 12-1).

BOX 12-1 | Examples of Assistive Technologies Within Major Product Categories

Mobility: Assist individuals to maneuver in their environments of choice
- Walkers
- Canes
- Manual and power wheelchairs
- Scooters
- Portable ramps
- Adapted driving devices and customized vans

Sensory assistance: Assist individuals who have vision or hearing loss
- Tactile and auditory mobility aids
- Auditory signaling devices
- Print and computer screen magnification devices
- Audiotapes
- Vibrating pagers and alarm clocks

Communication: Assist individuals to send and receive messages in spoken and written form
- Adapted telephones
- Voice-controlled computer input
- Writing aids
- Speech output devices

Personal care: Enable independence in ADL such as grooming, bathing, dressing, eating
- Eating utensils with angled or built-up handles
- Razor holders
- Reachers
- Nonslip placemats under dinner plates
- Bath sponges
- Transfer boards
- Commode chairs

Recreation: Enable participation in social activities, team sports, and other forms of recreation
- Adapted games
- Gardening aids
- Sports wheelchairs

Data from Scherer MJ: *Assistive technology: matching device and consumer for successful rehabilitation*, Washington, DC, 2002, American Psychological Association Books.

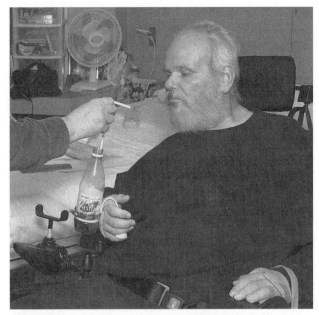

FIGURE 12-1 No-tech and low-tech AT devices are important to activities of daily living. This individual with SCI cannot grasp the bottle; however, he can use both a flexible straw and Velcro hand brace for independent drinking from the bottle of soda.

High-technology devices, on the other hand, tend to be more complex in design, expensive, harder to acquire, and requiring training and greater skill level to use effectively. For example, a person with a cervical SCI who has difficulty speaking might benefit from a commercially purchased augmentative and alternative communication (AAC) device that would pronounce words or phrases when he touches the buttons on a display panel.

AT devices may also be categorized by the specific type of assistance they provide[3,4]:

- Activities of daily living: devices that enable an individual in eating, dressing, grooming, and toileting
- AAC: devices that enable an individual to communicate more effectively
- Computer applications: hardware, software, and peripheral devices or attachments that help an individual to access the computer
- Environmental control systems: devices that assist an individual to do things in the environment, such as turning on lights, cooking, and controlling the television or VCR
- Home or work-site modifications: accessible ramps, lowered counter tops, and modified office work surfaces
- Prosthetics and orthotics: devices that replace or supplement loss of functioning in a body part, such as braces and splints
- Mobility aids: wheelchairs, scooters, and walkers
- Seating and positioning: skilled wheelchair fitting; cushions, molds, and inserts for the wheelchair that help to maintain an individual's proper body positioning
- Aids for vision or hearing: hearing aids, amplification and magnification devices
- Vehicle modifications: breath-controlled braking or steering mechanism; mechanized lifts

In each of these categories a wide range of devices is available. Table 12-1 lists Web sites where information about these devices can be found.

TABLE 12-1	**Web Site Resources for Assistive Technology**	
Site	URL	Content
ABLEDATA Database	http://www.abledata.com/	ABLEDATA is an electronic database of information with listings for AT and rehabilitation equipment available in the United States. It contains more than 22,000 products with detailed descriptions of the items, company contact information, and distributor listings. Fact sheets and consumer guides on various ATs and equipment are also available.
Accessible Environments	http://www.accessibleenvironments.net/homepage.htm	The largest supplier of accessibility products and equipment for creation of barrier-free environments in the home and workplace
Spinal Cord Injury Information Network	http://www.spinalcord.uab.edu/show.asp?durki=19679	Comprehensive listing of vendors by product category
National Spinal Cord Injury Association	http://www.spinalcord.org	Provides a wealth of information and resources, including hot links to sites related to AT and SCI
USA TechGuide to Assistive Technology Choices	http://www.usatech-guide.org	United Spinal Association Web guide to wheelchair and AT choices, related information and articles, wheelchair views and reviews. Promoting user involvement in the selection of appropriate AT. Empowerment by choice
Paralyzed Veterans of America	http://www.pva.org	Devoted to veterans of the armed forces who have SCI or dysfunction

Although AT devices offer individuals with SCI great potential to fully participate in society, AT services are sometimes more important. The term "assistive technology service" refers to any service that directly assists an individual with a disability in the selection, acquisition, or use of an AT device.[2] Often AT devices cannot be effectively identified, purchased, modified, customized, or implemented without the advice and skill of specific AT services. For example, it is necessary to evaluate the specific needs of an individual with SCI and include on-site visits to the environment where the person will potentially use AT devices. A team approach involving rehabilitation professionals from various disciplines who are familiar with the patient and have technological expertise in specific areas (e.g., occupational therapy, physical therapy, dietetics, physiatry) as well as the patient, family, and other caregivers will provide the best long-term results.[3,5]

During the evaluation process, it will be determined which AT device needs to be selected, designed, fitted, customized, adapted, applied, retained, repaired, or replaced. All these activities are important AT services that ensure appropriate AT device matches with the patient. AT services for purchasing, leasing, or obtaining AT devices are of particular importance to individuals with SCI, their families, and rehabilitation team members because they focus on ensuring that the device is delivered to the patient. In addition, it must be recognized that a variety of funding sources may be needed for these devices and services, depending on the age of the person with an SCI, the nature of his disability, the availability of resources, and the criteria for eligibility used by the various funders.[3,4]

Identifying and procuring a device is the first step in the process. Once obtained, the device needs to be implemented by using as many services as necessary to ensure that its potential to help the patient is fully realized.

Sometimes, AT devices are most effectively implemented in coordination with specific AT services:

- Therapies: physical, occupational, speech or language pathology
- Interventions: behavior modification, counseling
- Services associated with existing education and rehabilitation programs: transportation, vocational training

Other important AT services include the training and technical assistance provided directly to the patient, his family, caregivers, or colleagues who may be substantially involved in the technology's use and maintenance. Individuals with SCI and their rehabilitation team may access their state's Technology Assistance Project for information and support during the decision-making phase of the AT process. State projects for such assistance are funded under the Technology-Related Assistance for Individuals with Disabilities Act of 1994.[2]

IMPORTANCE OF THE ASSISTIVE TECHNOLOGY ASSESSMENT PROCESS

The process of selecting AT devices and services is central to both short- and long-term success of AT device use. Such a process, of necessity, considers the variety of personal characteristics that an individual with SCI brings to assessment and specific features of the device or service being considered. In addition to these characteristics and features, rehabilitation professionals need to consider a multiplicity of issues that potentially affect successful implementation of an AT device or service. These issues include cultural background of the patient and family, values and preferences of the user; and stigma associated with unwanted attention to the AT in public settings. When not considered, such sociocultural concerns may cause the patient and his family to abandon needed AT.[6,7]

Research has examined the impact of lifestyle and culture on the rehabilitation process and device usage.[8-11] A dynamic interaction has been documented between varying aspects in the life of an individual with disability that include differences in device acceptability from normative age-related physical and psychological traits, stage in the life cycle, and stage in the life of the family.[12,13] Such research clearly supports the importance of continuous communication between rehabilitation team members as they develop a comprehensive understanding of the patient from clinical and sociocultural perspectives and before making recommendations about AT devices or services.

The Matching Person and Technology (MPT) framework has been developed to enhance traditional models and has proven successful in ensuring the best choices of AT for individuals with a wide range of disabilities in various rehabilitation and service settings worldwide.[5,14]

MATCHING THE INDIVIDUAL AND TECHNOLOGY: A PROCESS FOR ENSURING ASSISTIVE TECHNOLOGY SUCCESS

To ensure that appropriate AT devices and services are identified and provided, rehabilitation team members must make sure that the patient is a participant in the process and also work closely with the family members or other caregivers.[15] The MPT process of selecting appropriate technological solutions includes consideration of three domains: (1) personal characteristics and preferences, (2) environment of use, and (3) characteristics of the technology or service.[11] These areas of influence form an interrelated foundation for decisions that will be made about AT devices and services (Figure 12-2).

Personal Characteristics and Preferences

The planning process begins with a careful exploration of the patient's skills, abilities, experiences, values, and preferences. Together the team and patient assess and define appropriate AT devices and services.[16,17] Personal characteristics and preferences include the patient's cognitive abilities, functional capabilities, cultural values, experience and expectations, and technology acculturation. Table 12-2 provides sample questions that team members may use to fully define the patient's capabilities.

Cognitive Ability

The patient's level of cognitive ability is a critical component in the AT assessment process because traumatic brain injury (TBI) and SCI often occur together.[18] Deficits in memory, concentration, executive functioning, and organizational skills may pose special challenges in planning solutions for care and independence with AT equipment.[19] Similarly, the ability to scan a visual field and plan specific sequences of motor activities becomes very important in considering the right match to specific AT devices and services. For example, a high-tech computerized communication system requires a user to visually scan a display panel containing many icons, words, or phrases and make selections by using planned motor responses (Figure 12-3). A low-tech alternative requires a user to simply nod his head in response to questions asked by a communication partner.

Life satisfaction for people with SCI is associated with the ability to communicate and participate socially with others.[20,21] Depending on the degree of injury sustained, varying linguistic skills may be present and pose unique possibilities related to AT devices and services. Typically, communication skills in individuals with

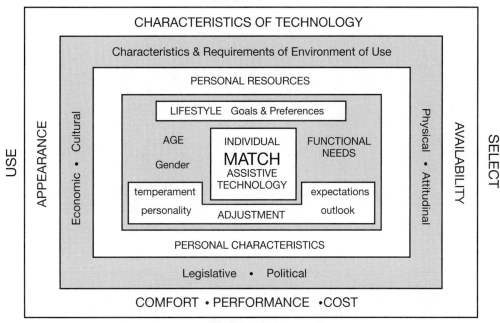

FIGURE 12-2 Influences on reaching an optimal AT and user match. (Courtesy Institute for Matching Person & Technology, Inc., © 2000. Used with permission.)

TABLE 12-2	**Considerations for Personal Characteristics and Preferences in Choosing Assistive Technology Devices and Services**
Consideration	Sample Team Questions
Cognitive abilities	Is traumatic brain injury present in addition to SCI? If so, what daily life activities have been affected? Can the individual profitably use complex, computerized devices? How well does the individual work with multiple steps? Sequencing?
Functional capabilities	Have the following capabilities been assessed for limitations and strengths (to use for limitations in other areas)? Eyesight, hearing, speech Understanding, remembering Physical strength, stamina Upper extremity control Grasping and use of fingers Lower extremity control Mobility
Personal experiences	How does this person handle stress? Failure? Challenges?
Personal expectations	What are this person's goals and dreams? What role will AT play in achieving those goals? Does he believe AT use will enhance his quality of lie?
Cultural values	What is the nature of this person's family support? Support from friends and coworkers? Will the individual feel self-conscious using this device around others?
Technology acculturation	What type of exposure has this person had with technology use? Have his experiences with technology been satisfying or frustrating?
Customary patterns	What is this person's typical routine and how will AT use affect his routine?

SCI focus on functional activities: writing, typing, reading, using the telephone, and selecting sequences of symbols that have meaning attached to them. Each of these activities can be facilitated with use of AT solutions.[17]

Functional Capabilities

Functional capabilities for individuals with SCI can include a wide range of activities (see Chapters 6 and 7). In this analysis, the focus is on sensory skills, physical abilities, and mobility capabilities. Sensory skills such as vision and hearing are key considerations because AT devices and services will require the ability to interact visually or auditorily with devices or people providing specific services.[17]

Physical abilities include consideration of the patient's strength, vitality, and fine and gross motor coordination. AT devices, and participation in AT services such as physical and occupational therapy, require varying degrees of physical skill. Matching the patient's physical ability and the technology is

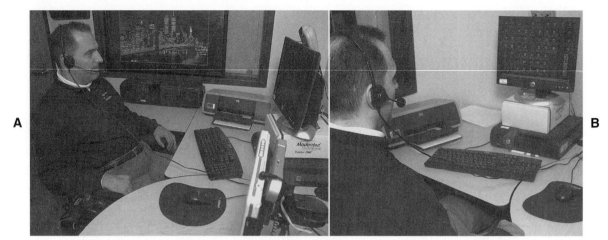

FIGURE 12-3 The ability to use computer equipment effectively requires an understanding of the interrelationships between types of hardware (**A**) as well as the cognitive skill to recognize, remember, and apply multiple sequences when working with software programs (**B**).

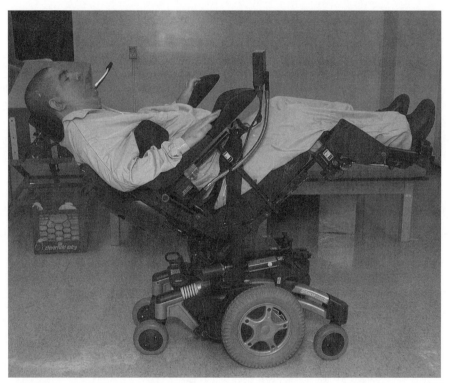

FIGURE 12-4 A power wheelchair operated by sip-n-puff technology is a sophisticated device dependent on the user's ability to control the chair's movement through respiratory breaths. Training and commitment combine to give this individual with a high-level cervical injury freedom of movement and a sense of accomplishment that increases his life satisfaction.

integral to successful use. Careful consideration also should be given to the muscle strength and work capacity indicated by the patient's current status and prognosis.[17]

Mobility and transportation capabilities refer to a person's ability to move freely in his immediate surroundings and are very important for individuals with SCI.[17,21] There are increasingly sophisticated low- and high-tech solutions to assist mobility and transportation (Figure 12-4). Matching a patient with the best seating technology and teaching him the highest level of wheelchair skills possible with his physical abilities are among the most important AT services for individuals with SCI (see Chapters 11 and 15).

Cultural Values

Cultural values are increasingly found to play an important role in AT decision-making processes.[17,22-24] Individuals with SCI from varying cultural backgrounds (e.g., Hispanic American, African American, Asian American, American Indian) will have value systems that are often quite different from those raised in cultures derived from Western Europe. When the backgrounds of health professionals and patients vary, there is a chance that the health care provider will be insensitive to the influence and importance of these differing value systems.[3,25-27] For example, individuals with SCI and their family members of various cultural groups may hold values that differ substantively from their health care providers with regard to preferred styles of communication, roles within the family unit, individual achievement (versus group participation and unity), and independence versus dependence.

Experience and Expectations

Personal life experiences can have a powerful influence on a person's desire to use AT devices or services.[11,13,28] Personal experience with technology typically results in a unique perspective developed over time, which affects evaluations and interventions provided as well as resulting experiences. Technology users evaluate and use devices and services on the basis of objective and subjective social, cultural, and lifetime contexts.[28] Today, many individuals with SCI and their families will have had previous experiences with AT devices and services, which provide a wealth of experience to enhance the decision-making process. They may have clearly perceived desires for specific types of devices and services on the basis of their past experiences. Conversely, individuals and their family members who do not have such experience may tend to rely more on the recommendations of technology professionals.

Personal expectations become important in the AT matching process when the patient or family members believe or hope that AT devices and services will do more than is possible in reality. In such instances the patient may abdicate personal responsibility for the appropriate use of recommended devices and services.[29,30] During AT assessment, such attitudes cannot be ignored because they may contribute to disappointment, frustration, and anger when AT devices and services fail to live up to expectations.[31] Consequently, it is critical that AT professionals clearly understand the expectations of the individual with SCI and provide meaningful information to him about device features and capabilities as well as anticipated involvement of family members, caregivers, and intervention personnel to ensure success of the device.

Goals and aspirations interrelate with an individual's experience and expectations. They become particularly significant in the face of the life changes and challenges that occur with SCI and are related to an individual's satisfaction with his current life situation.[32,33] Research shows that life satisfaction and subjective rating of well-being decrease as obstacles to social functioning increase.[33] Yet, in the face of equal challenges and obstacles, some individuals maintain high goals and expectations of themselves while others lower their personal aspirations considerably. In either instance, the AT devices and services considered will necessarily vary markedly.

Normative expectations refer to those societal-based norms that are typically age based. People hold changing expectations for individuals as they age. For example, the expectations for behavior and developmental functioning for a young child are different from those for an adolescent and different from those for an adult, which further vary as the adult ages.[17] Because of these normative expectations, research has suggested dynamic interaction factors between devices and user.[8,10,11,34] In addition, there appear to be differences among people across time in AT acceptability on the basis of the person's age-related normative psychological and physical capabilities, life cycle changes, and family life stage.[10,13]

TABLE 12-3	Environmental Considerations in Choosing Assistive Technology Devices and Services
Consideration	Sample Team Questions
Architectural environment	Will the AT device fit physically into all desired environments (car, living room, kitchen)? Are changes in the environment necessary to accommodate AT device use?
Psychosocial environment	Will the AT meet the person's needs in various situations and environments? Do technology service assistance and accommodations exist for successful use of this device?

Technology Acculturation

Technology acculturation is closely related to life experience because it is based on the extent that an individual has used technology in the past. Although everyone has had varying experiences with technology, it is acculturation that influences how an individual will view the ability of technology to make a meaningful difference in his life. It will also greatly affect the willingness of a person with SCI to use AT devices and services.[1]

Environmental Considerations

After the team has a comprehensive understanding of the patient with SCI, it turns its focus to the environment in which this individual will use AT devices and services.[3,17,35] Any environmental setting, whether it is a home, a workplace, or a community environment, will have differing demands and characteristics that may affect the success of an AT solution. These influences may be categorized as (1) physical, (2) cultural, (3) attitudinal, (4) economic, and (5) legislative and political.[3,36] Table 12-3 provides sample questions that team members may use to clarify the architectural and psychosocial environmental factors that influence choices of AT devices and services.

Physical Factors

Physical influences include architectural spaces of the environment in which the individual with SCI will live and work. Architectural barriers still exist, although their removal has long been mandated by federal legislation.[37-39] Under the Americans with Disabilities Act of 1990,[37] all new buildings are required to conform to rigorous design constraints to enable access by people with disabilities; however, many older buildings, and particularly physical facilities in places of public accommodation, still present barriers to full access and participation. Team members must give careful consideration to the physical spaces in which the individual with SCI will use the AT devices and services that are being considered and be mindful of potential barriers that could minimize the effectiveness of or present particular challenges to the use of AT solutions in those spaces.

Cultural Factors

Cultural factors, although unique to an individual, exert considerable influence over the environments that a person with SCI comes in contact with.[1] Although any individual with SCI brings his own unique cultural values to an assessment setting, the process of acculturation (i.e., the extent to which outside societal forces affect changes in behavior on the part of the individual) varies markedly from person to person. Acculturation involves giving up old ways and adopting new ways,[40] or the extent to which people from one cultural background participate in the values and practices of a dominant society.

People from other backgrounds may demonstrate any of four distinct acculturation patterns that affect the extent to which they approach or avoid interaction with a dominant culture and the degree to which they maintain or relinquish attributes of their native culture.[1] These patterns include assimilation, integration, separation, and marginalization.[41-43] Assimilation occurs to the extent that a person desires contact with the dominant culture while not necessarily maintaining an identity with his native culture. Integration occurs when a person who wants to maintain his cultural identity also desires a high level of interaction with the dominant culture. Separation occurs when a person has a little interaction with the dominant culture (and related microcultural groups) while desiring a close connection with and affirmation by his native culture. Marginalization occurs when a person chooses not to identify with either his native culture or the dominant culture, which can be demonstrated in cases of enforced cultural loss combined with enforced segregation.

Team members must be cognizant of these powerful cultural influences while also striving to understand their own cultural value systems and how their values may affect their perceptions of the person with SCI, their communication style, and their preferences for AT.

Attitudinal Factors

Attitudinal factors encompass specific community values and attitudes that may be held by individuals and groups with whom the person with SCI will live and work. If community attitudes reflect marginalization of people with disabilities or their devaluation as human beings, numerous barriers including discriminatory policies and procedures and insensitivity to the existence of physical barriers may exist. Such barriers can substantively affect the effectiveness of AT devices and solutions.[3] Team members are challenged to understand the value system and attitudes of communities within which the person with SCI will be using AT devices and solutions; failure to do so often can result in negative experiences on the part of the AT user.

Economic Factors

Economic factors include user, family, and community resources available in the AT decision-making process. The issue of financing AT devices and services is particularly important because it can often become the most significant service system barrier.[35,44,45] AT services include evaluations, purchasing, leasing, maintenance, repair, and training. Unfortunately, the realities of potentially limited funding for existing service systems (e.g., public schools, vocational rehabilitation) presents a major challenge to team members and underscores the importance of effective practices of identifying appropriate technologies for persons with SCI.[46-48] Multiple sources including state, federal, and private sources such as Medicaid, Vocational Rehabilitation, the Social Security Administration, CHAMPUS (Civilian Health and Medical Program of Uniformed Services), and private insurance often need to be accessed.[45,49] Sometimes inexpensive AT devices or those that can be modified, customized, or made by service system personnel at minimal cost are the only ones made available to some individuals.

Team members may consider leasing as an alternative to purchasing expensive devices, thus minimizing hidden expenses.[35,50] Leasing may be considered an AT service under existing federal legislation.[2]

Another economic issue related to expensive devices that are prescribed for individuals with SCI is protection from theft and damage, depending on where particular devices are to be used. Although a rehabilitation facility may have coverage for theft or damage as long as a device in on site, liability issues may need to be examined if the device leaves the facility.

Integrally linked to financing AT devices are personnel training needs.[51-55] Effective team members cannot ignore the necessity of training personnel, including staff, patients, family members, and other caregivers, in the correct and efficient use of AT devices.[44,51,54] Although many AT devices can easily be used without training, more sophisticated devices such as keyboard emulators, nondedicated speech devices, and environmental control systems may require considerable personnel training commitments. It is also important to give thought to attitudes held by the professionals who will require training in the use of AT devices. Some professionals and some family members of individuals with SCI will not want to learn to use technology that is being considered. Professional resistance to using devices, whether intentional or not, has been observed when devices are made inaccessible to children.[56]

Although the benefits of technology for a person (and family) with SCI, may occur after their delivery, the resources of the service delivery system, understanding and belief in technology, technological competence of the team professionals, the person himself, and the interest, resources, and persistence of the individual's families, all are related to positive outcomes.

Legislative and Political Factors

Legislative and political factors include forces that serve to make AT devices and services available and affordable. This includes legislation and its mandated activities and services. It also includes the policies and procedures adopted by such federal agencies as the Social Security Administration and the Department of Veterans Affairs. It is important that patients, clients, family members and friends, and health care providers understand the importance of continued communication with legislative representatives and government agencies to encourage support of legislation and policies that increase access to AT equipment and services as well as to the greater community environment.

TABLE 12-4 | Technological Considerations in Choosing Assistive Technology Devices and Services

Consideration	Sample Team Questions
Range of devices	Have all alternative AT devices been considered? Non-tech, low-tech, and high-tech?
Potential to enhance levels of performance	Does this AT product do everything desired? Does it require some skills or capabilities the individual does not have? Can these AT products or services be adapted to changing needs?
Cost	Does this AT product have extra features that make it more versatile? Are there extra features that will not be used? Are adaptations or additional parts necessary for this device? Are all fiscal aspects of the product or service accounted for so that there will be no hidden costs?
Ease of use	Are the parts of the AT product (e.g., knobs, switches, straps) accessible and easy to use?
Comfort	Does the AT device have essential stability for a variety of situations and environments? Is it comfortable to use?
Dependability	Does the AT device perform reliably? Are there human override capabilities? Can it be repaired locally?
Transportability	Is the AT device portable? Is its size and weight manageable for this person? Can it be moved by car or van?
Longevity and durability	Does the AT device have the durability needed in a variety of situations and environments? Are special features needed because of the weather conditions or physical features of the local area?

Characteristics of Technology

Specific features of AT devices and services are typically examined after the team has formulated a profile of the patient's needs and preferences and environmental parameters have been determined.[17,36] The potential for an AT device to enhance levels of performance must also be carefully considered. The team applies its understanding of the patient's performance levels by forming a plan that addresses the individual and family's priorities, concerns, and resources. Many AT devices are designed to perform specific functions in home, community, and other natural settings, whereas other devices may have multiple uses across tasks and settings. Table 12-4 provides sample questions that team members may use to ensure that the technological considerations of AT devices and services being considered will provide the best match to the patient's needs.

Availability

The range of AT devices available and their potential applications make this a time-intensive process. Vendor catalogs, databases, and representatives can help the team locate appropriate devices and provide demonstrations with hands-on opportunities to test the devices being considered. In addition, many state projects funded under the Technology-Related Assistance for Individuals with Disabilities Act have demonstration centers that afford people with SCI and their families or caregivers experience with a range of AT devices.[2]

Opportunity for hands-on experience and trial use has repeatedly been identified as a prerequisite to AT decision making by both people with disabilities and their family members.[57,58] Effective team members should ensure that the person with SCI has an opportunity to use an AT device before purchase.[16,17] Documentation for use is also important and needs to be provided either through product manuals or vendor demonstrations.

It is important to realize that advantages of AT devices and services that may seem obvious to team professionals at the time of assessment in a clinical setting may not be so apparent to the user or in settings outside the rehabilitation center or clinic. For example, computer applications that enable the person with SCI to access the Internet for information and other support services may be unavailable if there is limited access to telephone lines or electrical outlets in the home. Similarly, if the individual with SCI lives in an area with high unemployment, having AT devices and services that were targeted to facilitate getting and maintaining a job might not accomplish that goal.[22]

Cost

The cost of AT is often identified as a primary barrier to acquiring AT devices and services.[57,59] Of particular importance to the team is the real cost of the device, including costs associated with assembling, obtaining special parts and batteries, maintenance requirements, and additional devices that are required to operate the device being considered. For example, such additional devices could include alternate means of inputting data into a computer with a mouthstick, head pointer, or voice input software. When hidden expenses are encountered, they should be considered on the front end of the decision-making process so that specified providers and payors can be identified to fund the necessary services.

Comfort and Appearance

The comfort of AT devices has also been identified as a factor for consideration during the decision-making process.[3,35] The team should include careful assessment of the patient's physical abilities and the demands to operate or use any AT device and the level of physical, emotional, and social comfort experienced during its use in natural settings. Some devices may be used with great ease and comfort, whereas others can only be used for short periods before the person will become tired or uncomfortable. Although appearance may add a spark to AT appeal and user acceptance as exemplified by the souped-up, hot rod look of some wheelchairs, the functional capabilities of AT are more enduring. It should not be underestimated, however, that a large part of an individual's acceptance and life satisfaction is entwined with a positive self-image. The ability of wheelchair users to express masculinity or femininity through the appearance of their chair can be an important statement (Figure 12-5).

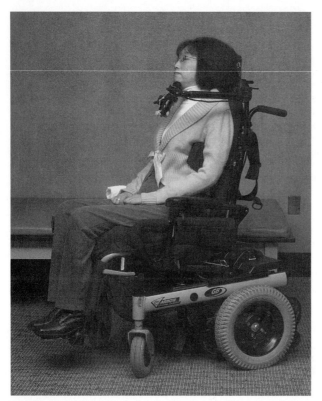

FIGURE 12-5 Comfort and appearance as well as function are important characteristics of AT devices. Individuals with SCI who use a wheelchair for mobility often want to reflect their personality through their chair as well as through the clothes they wear. This individual enjoys feeling like a "girly-girl" with her pink sweater and bow that match the trim on her chair.

Ease of use and simplicity of operation of an AT device are important considerations for the user and family members or other caregivers.[58] When complex devices are prescribed that require inordinate training commitments by service providers, family members, and the person with SCI, reluctance to those time investments may be seen.[56] In addition, if the cognitive or motor demands of the device exceed the person's performance levels, both the individual and his caregivers may be resistant to using it with the result of technology abandonment.[60]

Performance
Dependability of the device includes the extent to which its performance matches manufacturer claims and its ability to meet the needs of the user.[61] Team members will assess the ability of AT devices to provide performance or evaluation data necessary for the documentation of the patient's progress toward meeting his goals.

Repair and maintenance considerations should also be considered during decision-making processes because some AT devices require lengthy or frequent repairs.[17,61] Team members can request information from vendors about product testing, reliability, and repair records for devices. When independent information is not available, team members may contact other individuals who have used the device to obtain their perspectives on its dependability, reliability, and repair and maintenance issues. Team members should also ask vendors about backup or

loaner equipment provided by the manufacturer when a device needs repair and what kind of a warranty is available. If a warranty is not available, team members should identify local companies or individuals that can provide parts or repair damaged AT devices.[35]

Transportability of the device across and within naturalistic settings may also be an important factor for team members to consider.[62] Sometimes bulky or heavy devices are chosen for an individual with SCI who has limited strength and vitality, but they may end up being difficult to move around in the environment or to transport.[63] Conversely, smaller devices may be cumbersome for some people with SCI to transport, requiring a special case, satchel, or bag, or the help of a designated assistant. Team members need to ensure availability of the AT device for identified targeted tasks in their plan.

Longevity and durability become important considerations because some AT devices may need to be handled carefully with sensitivity to varying levels of abuse (e.g., spills, being dropped), whereas other devices are specifically designed to resist very rugged use. Product manuals should provide information about longevity and durability or direct contact with the manufacturer may be helpful.[35]

Adaptability in meeting the changing needs of an individual user over time must also be carefully considered because many AT devices are purchased for continuous use.[61] Devices that may be used across many settings may be preferable and more cost-effective compared with those that perform only one function or are meant for use in one location. Some AT devices, however, are designed to perform a specific function and cannot be adapted. Before an AT device is purchased, team members should identify potential modifications that may be needed over time so that such modifications can be weighed against available fiscal and human resources in the service system (e.g., rehabilitation personnel, community volunteers).

Compatibility with other devices, or the extent to which a device being considered can be used with other AT solutions or other supports, may become an important consideration as well. Team members also should consider the patient's current and future needs when examining the ability of the AT to be used with other devices.[35,56]

The user's sense of safety and security when using an AT device is important for effective and continued use. Safety features of all devices should be assessed during the decision-making process. Not all AT devices may prove safe for use across all environmental settings.[17] Some devices may require that one or more people be present to assist while the individual with SCI operates the device. Others may have sharp edges or features that could increase the likelihood of injury under certain circumstances. In addition, the team needs to ensure that any AT device will remain safe and usable when exposed to water, moisture, and extremes of temperature.

Emerging Research and Educational Modules
In keeping with the World Health Organizations International Classification of Functioning, Disability, and Health (ICF), this chapter advocates that assessment for AT devices and services be evaluated in the context of the whole person and his

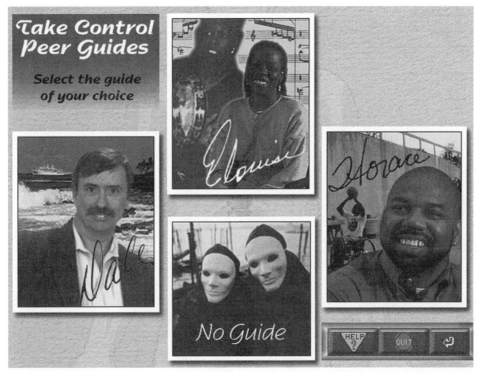

FIGURE 12-6 Peer-guided features incorporated into the "Take Control: Multimedia Guide to Spinal Cord Injury" program can provide the user with positive reinforcement for using AT devices and services and enrich his knowledge base. (Courtesy Alan G. VanBiervliet.)

environment.[64] The ICF holistically includes home, recreation, work, school, and community within the typology of health and functioning. The tool provides a standard language and framework to describe health and health-related states and is intended for use in classification and research on the effects of health conditions, health services, and health outcomes. ICF synthesizes a biopsychosocial model that integrates the biological, individual, and social perspectives of health and care (see Figure 5-2).

The model illustrates the interactions between health condition and its context (i.e., contextual factors including the environmental and personal factors) to produce a picture of "the person in his world."[64] The intent is to perpetuate an interactive and dynamic model.

Integrity of body structures and functions, activity, and participation can be facilitated by contextual factors, such as AT, that promote health and function. Conversely, impairment, limitation, and restriction denote problems in health and function. Contextual factors that have a negative impact on health and function are barriers so that:

- Lack of trained personnel to assist in choosing and obtaining AT devices or services constitutes a barrier
- Policies that set a low priority on resource allocation for AT devices or services constitute a barrier
- Personal history of perceived failure with AT that may hinder future use of AT devices or services constitute a barrier

The ICF emphasis on health and wellness helps identify barriers that were previously misunderstood. It also renders increased significance to outcomes-based research and health care results.

There is a growing recognition by the government of the United States that AT service delivery must be outcomes based.

Recent federal legislation, the Rehabilitation Act Amendments of 1998,[65] reflects interest by the federal government that recipients of specific types of grants submit information to measure project outcomes and performance. Federal initiatives, such as the Assistive Technology Outcomes (ATOMS)[66] and Consortium on Assistive Technology Outcomes Research (CATOR)[67] Projects, have been developed to examine AT service delivery practices nationally and to develop recommendations for the field regarding how AT outcomes should be measured. The MPT process is being used in these projects to elicit useful outcome data.

In recent years, the availability of high-quality health care–related training materials aimed at improving care and lifestyle for patients and clients with chronic conditions has incorporated the holistic ICF view of health and wellness in interactive educational modules. Programs specifically designed for individuals with SCI can provide a new AT service that supports the use of AT devices recommended by team members.

For example, "Take Control: Multimedia Guide to Spinal Cord Injury (SCI) Volumes 1-4" is a series of CD-ROM programs that combine photos, video clips, animation, illustrations, narration, personal experiences, and games into a rich, engaging environment for learning about SCI.[68,69] This innovative tool uses a peer guide concept in which the user selects a guide and then is lead through multiple learning paths (Figure 12-6).[30] Each guide has an accompanying biographical sketch with a brief digital movie in which the guide introduces himself in his own words.[26] The programs provide many options—tutorials, learning games, an encyclopedia on SCI—allowing the user to explore presented information in any order or at any depth.

CLINICAL CASE STUDY Assessment and Match for Effective Assistive Technology Case 1

Patient History

Mario Garbelli is a 48-year-old man with a C4 tetraplegia, ASIA A diagnosis. He was weaned from a ventilator during his acute rehabilitation. He has not had any significant medical complications during his rehabilitation. Mario is currently 16 weeks post injury and is attending outpatient rehabilitation. His tilt-in-space wheelchair has been ordered.

Mario is a partner in a large law firm that is located 10 miles from his home. He has a wife and two teenaged children. His wife currently does not work outside the home. He has excellent insurance and health care benefits.

Patient's Self-Assessment

Mario plans to return to work as soon as possible and his law firm is implementing an AT environment to facilitate his continued place in the firm.

Team Goals

Evaluate patient needs for AT in his home, workplace, and community that will provide efficient and effective means for the greatest independence with consideration of wheelchair use and his cognitive capacity to learn and implement technology. Evaluate patient's expected positioning in the tilt-in-space wheelchair to determine the AT needs during all upright activities.

Patient Goals

"I want to be able to return to my law practice and resume as full a schedule as possible."

Assessment and Match for Effective Assistive Technology Case 2

Patient History

Betsy Downing is a 20-year-old woman with a C6 tetraplegia, ASIA B diagnosis resulting from a motor vehicle accident. She was injured 13 weeks ago and is now attending outpatient therapy. Her acute-care hospital course was complicated by a urinary tract infection. During her acute rehabilitation stay she had a prolonged period of adjustment to upright tolerance with several incidences of syncope. She has been medically stable for the past 5 weeks.

Betsy is currently living at home with her parents, who are in the final stages of modifying their home for wheelchair accessibility. Betsy was injured during the summer between her sophomore and junior years in college. She is a chemical engineering major.

Patient's Self-Assessment

Betsy plans to return to college and reside in an accessible dorm. Her college is located approximately 100 miles from her parents'

home. Most of the college campus is already accessible and it has agreed to provide any other necessary accommodations to ensure Betsy's success.

Team Goals

Evaluate patient needs for AT in her home, school, and community that will provide efficient and effective means for the greatest independence with consideration of wheelchair use and cognitive capacity to learn and implement technology.

Patient Goals

"I want to be able to complete my college degree and do engineering research."

Assessment and Match for Effective Assistive Technology Case 3

Patient History

Larry Mullen is a 74-year-old man with a C5 tetraplegia, ASIA A diagnosis. He was injured 15 weeks ago as the result of a fall from a stepladder. His acute-care hospital stay was complicated with a deep venous thrombosis of his right lower limb and an episode of pneumonia. Larry is now medically stable and is in the process of his final wheelchair evaluation as an outpatient.

Larry is a retired plumber. He and his wife, Janice, live in a one-bedroom condominium located on the ground floor. His home has no mortgage. Larry and Janice have three married children and six grandchildren. All family members live nearby and are in good health. Larry was self-employed and has only Social Security benefits.

Patient's Self-Assessment

Larry wants to again be active in the condominium association and continue to meet his other retired pals at the local coffee shop.

Team Goals

Evaluate patient needs for AT in his home and community that will provide efficient and effective means for the greatest independence with consideration of wheelchair use and his cognitive ability to learn and implement technology given his role as a retired tradesman.

Patient Goals

"I want to enjoy my final years with my family and friends."

Critical Thinking Exercises

The three preceding case studies discuss patients who will require AT to fulfill their personal recovery goals. This chapter summarizes broad concepts that are essential to the patient assessment process before assistive services and technology can be determined. By using a team meeting context, describe the roles of the team members in considering the selection of the most efficient and cost-effective AT for each patient. Assume that all three of the patients will have fully accessible homes.

1. What are the three characteristics that must be considered when the team evaluates these patients with SCI for AT services and technology?
2. Describe the differences among no-tech, low-tech, and high-tech ATs. Give examples of each type of AT.
3. After the team identifies and procures an AT device for the patient, what are the next steps?
4. During a team meeting, on the basis of the patient information provided, what individual, environmental, and technological considerations will warrant team discussion?

SUMMARY

Achieving an optimal match between an individual with SCI and technology devices and services by focusing on the person who uses (or is expected to use) a particular AT device is the target of interventions by rehabilitation professionals in this chapter. The evolution of more enlightened AT policies will involve understanding the features and aims of person-focused programs. It is crucial that the individual's functioning is considered in the choice of device and instruction in its use. It is equally important, however, that an evaluation is made of the person's attitudes, knowledge, and comfort with respect to technology in general and the device in particular. An evaluation for person and technology matching also should include information about the person's environment (both physical and sociocultural) and preferred goals within the domains of activity and participation. To reduce the likelihood of technology abandonment, the AT evaluation should facilitate prediction of how the person will respond to a given technology, what methods of teaching will facilitate the person's acceptance of the technology, or what alternative devices or resources might be better accepted or more appropriate for other reasons.

The need exists to take into account cultural and attitudinal influences on resource selection and use as well as economic, physical, and legislative and political considerations. Individuals with disabilities vary in their desire for assistive technology versus personal assistance versus help from family members. Often, this choice reflects one's cultural mores and expectations. Family members may resent the use or presence of AT in the home. To use a truly idiographic, person-centered approach requires understanding such influences and pressures, the level of program and professional trust, and language differences (e.g., an immigrant may communicate well only in his native language). Therefore it is imperative that the consumer be involved in a dialog that identifies such needs and preferences. Consumer preferences and goals need to drive the AT matching process; obstacles to optimal AT use and the need for additional supports and resources must be identified and strategies for training in use implemented.

REFERENCES

1. Parette HP, Huer MB, Scherer M: Effects of acculturation on assistive technology service delivery, *J Special Educ Technol* 19:31-41, 2004.
2. Technology-Related Assistance for Individuals with Disabilities Act of 1994, P.L. 103-218, (March 9, 1994). 29 U.S.C. 2201 et seq: U.S. Statutes at Large, 108, 50–97.
3. Scherer MJ: *Living in the state of stuck: how technology impacts the lives of people with disabilities*, ed 3, Cambridge, MA, 2000, Brookline.
4. AbleData: *Informed consumer's guide to funding assistive technology*:http://www.abledata.com/text2/funding.htm. Accessed January 29, 2004.
5. Scherer MJ: Matching person and technology homepage: http://members.aol.com/IMPT97/MPT.html. Accessed January 25, 2004.
6. Cushman LA, Scherer MJ: Measuring the relationship of assistive technology use, functional status over time, and consumer-therapist perceptions of ATs, *Assist Technol* 8:103-109, 1996.
7. Scherer MJ, Galvin JC: An outcomes perspective of quality pathways to the most appropriate technology. In Galvin JC, Scherer MJ, editors: *Evaluating, selecting and using appropriate assistive technology*, Gaithersburg, MD, 1996, Aspen.
8. Becker G, Kaufman S: Old age, rehabilitation, and research: a review of the issues, *Gerontologist* 28:459-468, 1988.
9. Gitlin LN, Luborsky MR, Schemm RL: Emerging concerns of older stroke patients about assistive device use, *Gerontologist* 38:169-180, 1998.
10. Murphy RF, Scheer J, Murphy Y, et al: Physical disability and social liminality: a study in the rituals of adversity, *Soc Sci Med* 26:235-242, 1988.
11. Scheer J, Luborsky M: The cultural context of polio biographies, *Orthopedics* 14:1173-1181, 1991.
12. Murphy R: *The body silent*, New York, 1990, Norton.
13. Luborsky MR: Adaptive device appraisal by lifelong-users facing new losses: culture, identity, and life history factors. In Hafferty F, Hey SC, Kiger G, editors: *Translating disability: at the individual, institutional, and societal levels*, Salem, OR, 1991, Society for Disability Studies and Willamette University.
14. Scherer MJ: *The matching person and technology (MPT) model manual*, ed 3, Webster, NY, 1998, Institute for Matching Person & Technology.
15. National Spinal Cord Injury Association: *Factsheet 4a: choosing a spinal cord injury rehabilitation facility*: http://users.erols.com/nscia/resource/factshts/fact04a.html. Accessed January 28, 2004.
16. Gray DB, Quatrano LA, Lieberman ML: *Designing and using assistive technology: the human perspective*, Baltimore, MD, 1998, Brookes.
17. King TW: *Assistive technology: essential human factors*, Boston, MA, 1999, Allyn & Bacon.
18. Davidoff G, Morris J, Roth E, et al: Cognitive dysfunction and mild closed head injury in traumatic spinal cord injury, *Arch Phys Med Rehabil* 66:489-491, 1985.
19. Slater MJ, Vecchio S: *Traumatic brain injury: the overlooked diagnosis in spinal cord injuries*: http://www.slatervecchio.com/articles/Verdict_Sept_97.htm. Accessed January 28, 2004.
20. Chase BW, Cornille CA, English RW: Life satisfaction among persons with spinal cord injuries, *J Rehabil* 2000: http://www.findarticles.com/cf_dls/m0825/3_66/66032255/p1/article.jhtml?term=. Accessed January 29, 2004.
21. Cull JG, Hardy RE: *Physical medicine and rehabilitation approaches in spinal cord injury*, Springfield, IL, 1997, Charles C Thomas.
22. Dogbo N: *Success story: assistive technology and ethnic minorities*: http://www.atnet.org/CR4AT/PositionPapers/Minorities.html. Accessed January 29, 2004.
23. Hourcade JJ, Parette HP, Huer MB: Family and cultural alert! Considerations in assistive technology assessment, *Teach Except Child* 30:40-44, 1997.
24. Kemp C, Parette HP: Barriers to minority parent involvement in assistive technology (AT) decision-making processes, *Educ Train Mental Retard Develop Disabil* 35:384-392, 2000.
25. Lynch EW, Hanson MJ: *Developing cross-cultural competence: a guide for working with children and families*, ed 2, Baltimore, MD, 1997, Brookes.
26. Parette HP, Huer MB, VanBiervliet A: Cultural issues and assistive technology. In Edyburn DL, Higgins K, Boone R, editors: *The handbook of special education technology research and practice*, Whitefish Bay, WI, 2005, Knowledge by Design.
27. Roseberry-McKibbin C: *Multicultural students with special language needs*, ed 2, Oceanside, CA, 2002, Academic Communication Associates.

28. Luborsky M: The cultural context of polio biographies, *Orthopedics* 11:1173-1181, 1993.

29. Margalit M: *Effective technology integration for disabled children*, New York, 1990, Springer-Verlag.

30. VanBiervliet A, Parette HP: *Families, cultures and AAC* [CD-ROM], Little Rock, AR, 1999, Southeast Missouri State University and University of Arkansas for Medical Sciences.

31. Parette HP, Angelo DH: Augmentative and alternative communication impact on families: trends and future directions, *J Special Educ Technol* 30:77-98, 1996.

32. Decker SD, Schulz R: Correlates of life satisfaction in middle-aged and elderly spinal cord injured persons, *Am J Occup Ther* 39: 740-745, 1985.

33. Nosek MA, Fuhrer MJ, Potter C: Life satisfaction of people with physical disabilities: relationship to personal assistance, disability status, and handicap, *Rehabil Psych* 40:191-202, 1985.

34. Stein H: Rehabilitation and chronic illness in American culture, *Ethos* 7:153-176, 1979.

35. Parette HP: Effective and promising assistive technology practices for students with mental retardation and developmental disabilities. In Hilton A, Ringlaben R, editors: *Effective and promising practices in developmental disabilities*, Austin, TX, 1998, PRO-ED.

36. Scherer MJ: Connecting to learn: educational and assistive technologies for people with disabilities, Washington, DC, 2004, American Psychological Association Books.

37. Americans with Disabilities Act of 1990, P.L. 101-336, (July 26, 1990). 42 U.S.C.A. 122101 et seq: U.S. Statutes at Large, 104, 327-378.

38. Rehabilitation Act of 1973, P.L. 93-112, (1973). 500-504, 87 Stat. 355, 390-394 (current version at 29 U.S.C. 790-794d).

39. Telecommunications Act of 1996, P.L. 104-104, (1996). 110 Stat. 56.

40. Ruiz RA: Cultural and historical perspectives in counseling Hispanics. In Sue DW, editor: *Counseling the culturally different: theory and practice*, New York, 1981, Wiley & Sons.

41. Berry JW, Kim U, Power S, et al: Acculturation attitudes in plural societies, *Appl Psych* 38:185-206, 1989.

42. Berry JW, Poortinga YH, Segall MH, et al: *Cross-cultural psychology: research and application*, Cambridge, 1992, Cambridge University Press.

43. Berry JW, Sam DL: Acculturation and adaptation. In Berry JW, Segall MH, Kagitcibasi C, editors: *Handbook of cross-cultural psychology, vol. 3: social behavior and applications*, ed 2, Boston, 1997, Allyn & Bacon.

44. Church G, Glennen S: Assistive technology program development, In Church G, Glennen S, editors: *The handbook of assistive technology*, San Diego, CA, 1992, Singular.

45. Wallace JF: Creative financing of assistive technology. In Flippo KF, Inge KJ, Barcus JM, editors: *Assistive technology: a resource for school, work, and community*, Baltimore, 1995, Brookes.

46. Hager RM: *Funding of assistive technology: state vocational rehabilitation agencies and their obligation to maximize employment* (1999): http://www.nls.org/vrbooklt.htm. Accessed January 31, 2004.

47. Kemp CE, Hourcade JJ, Parette HP: Building an initial information base: assistive technology funding resources for school-aged students with disabilities, *J Special Educ Technol* 15:15-24, 2000.

48. Sheldon J: *Funding of assistive technology: work incentives for persons with disabilities under the social security and SSI programs—using the work incentives to fund AT and make work a reality* (2002): http://www.nls.org/wkboklet.htm. Accessed January 31, 2004.

49. Mann WC, Lane JP: *Assistive technology for persons with disabilities: the role of occupational therapy*, Rockville, MD, 1991, American Occupational Therapy Association.

50. Hofmann AC: *The many faces of funding*, Mill Valley, CA, 1994, Phonic Ear.

51. Bryant DP, Bryant BR: *Assistive technology for people with disabilities*, Boston, MA, 2003, Allyn & Bacon.

52. Culp DM, Ambrosi DM, Berniger T, et al: Augmentative and alternative communication aid use: a followup study, *Augment Altern Commun* 2:19-24, 1986.

53. Inge KJ, Flippo KF, Barcus JM: Staff development for assistive technology personnel. In Flippo KF, Inge KJ, Barcus JM, editors: *Assistive technology: a resource for school, work, and community*, Baltimore, 1995, Brookes.

54. Lindsey JD: *Technology & exceptional individuals*, ed 3, Austin, TX, 2000, Pro-Ed.

55. Todis B: Tools for the task? Perspectives on assistive technology in educational settings, *J Spec Educ Technol* 13:49-61, 1996.

56. Parette HP, Brotherson MJ, Hourcade JJ, et al: Family-centered assistive technology assessment, *Interv School Clinic* 32:104-112, 1996.

57. Hayward BJ, Elliott BG: *National evaluation of state grants for technology-related assistance for individuals with disabilities programs. Final report: perspectives of consumers: findings from focus groups,* vol. II, Research Triangle Park, 1992, Research Triangle Institute.

58. Parette HP, VanBiervliet A: *Assistive technology curriculum for Arkansans with disabilities* (ERIC Document Reproduction Service, ED 324 886), Little Rock, AR, 1990, University of Arkansas at Little Rock.

59. Uslan MM: Barriers to acquiring assistive technology: cost and lack of information, *J Vision Impair Blindness* 86:402-407, 1992.

60. Dillard D: *National study on abandonment of technology: 1989 annual report on the national rehabilitation hospital's rehabilitation engineering center's evaluation of assistive technology* (Cooperative Agreement No. H133E0016), Washington, DC, 1989, National Institute on Disability and Rehabilitation Research.

61. Galvin J, Scherer MJ: *Evaluating, selecting, and using appropriate assistive technology*, Gaithersburg, MD, 1996, Aspen.

62. Batavia AI, Hammer GS: Toward the development of consumer-based criteria for the evaluation of assistive devices, *J Rehabil Res Dev* 27:425-436, 1990.

63. Carey DM, Sale P: Practical considerations in the use of technology to facilitate the inclusion of students with severe disabilities, *Technol Disabil* 3:77-86, 1994.

64. World Health Organization: *International Classification of Functioning, Disability and Health (ICF)*: www3.who.int/icf/. Accessed September 21, 2007.

65. Rehabilitation Act Amendments of 1998, PL 105-220, 112 STAT 936.

66. Assistive Technology Outcomes: *Welcome*: http://www.uwm.edu/CHS/atoms/. Accessed February 1, 2004.

67. Consortium on Assistive Technology Outcomes Research: *Welcome*: http://www.atoutcomes.com/pages/highlights.html. Accessed February 1, 2004.

68. VanBiervliet A: Multimedia and SCI: educational strategies for the 21st century, *Top Spinal Cord Injury Rehabil* 5:33-49, 1999.

69. VanBiervliet A, McCluer S: *Take control: multimedia guide for spinal cord injury*, vol. I [CD-ROM], Little Rock, 1996, Arkansas Spinal Cord Commission and Program Development Associates.

SOLUTIONS TO CHAPTER 12 CLINICAL CASE STUDY

Assessment and Match for Effective Assistive Technology Cases 1 Through 3

1. The rehabilitation team must consider each patient on the basis of the following:

- Personal characteristics and preferences, including cognitive ability, functional capabilities, cultural values, experience and expectations, and technology acculturation
- Environmental considerations, including physical factors, cultural factors, attitudinal factors, economic factors, and legislative and political factors
- Characteristics of technology, including availability, cost, comfort and appearance, and performance

2. AT can be described as no-tech, solutions that involve changes in the way people do things to meet an individual's needs; low-tech, devices that are simple in design, inexpensive, readily available, and require little, if any, training for effective use; and high-tech, devices that are more complex in design, expensive, harder to acquire, and require training and a greater skill level to use effectively.

- No-tech options might include removing area rugs to facilitate wheelchair propulsion, arranging furniture so that a wheelchair can be maneuvered in each room, arranging furniture so that an individual using a wheelchair can be fully part of the group.
- Low-tech options might include drinking straws, nonskid material to hold plates or other objects on the table or desk, a book stand to prop up a book to make reading easier, an angled mirror in the bathroom for grooming, Velcro closures for clothing, large power switches that can be controlled with a tenodesis grip rather than fine motor control.
- High-tech options might include computer applications using hardware, software, and peripheral devices or attachments that help an individual to access the computer such as voice recognition systems; environmental control systems that assist an individual in turning on lights, cooking, and controlling the television or VCR.

3. After an AT device has been identified and procured, it needs to be implemented by as many services as necessary to ensure that its potential to help the patient is fully realized. In some instances a device is best implemented in coordination with specific AT services, such as therapies, interventions, or services associated with existing education and rehabilitation programs including transportation or vocational training. AT services can also include training and technical assistance provided directly to the patient, his family, caregivers, or those colleagues who may be substantially involved in the technology's use and maintenance.

4. During a team meeting, the needs of each patient will be discussed to ensure the best match for AT and services. Discussion should include their work, school, and home cultures for acceptance of AT devices.

- Mario Garbelli will require high-tech AT and services to return to his job because of his high level of tetraplegia and limited use of his upper limbs. Appropriate technology that promotes ease of telephone use and the ability to produce written communications will be needed in both his home and office. Voice recognition software should be explored for communication. Mario should be evaluated for a tilt-in-space wheelchair using the most efficient propulsion techniques: chin, head, or mouth control. His power wheelchair should include options for tilting for pressure relief and reclining for comfort. Transportation to and from work along with options to work part time from home should be discussed with Mario and colleagues from his law firm. Maintenance and repair will be critical in the selection of all equipment: Is the manufacturer reliable and timely with repairs? Warranty packages should be reviewed during the selection process of all AT devices. Dependability, durability, repair record, leasing versus purchase, and trial of all AT devices needs to be considered for this patient during the selection process. Team members should assess and discuss the patient's background with computer use and evaluate his need for instruction and continuing education. Mario's expectations and attitudes toward work, technology, and the sociocultural and attitudinal issues he will find in his law firm will all affect the establishment of team goals. Environmental considerations and barriers in the workplace should be addressed (the home is assumed to be fully accessible). Economic impact in the workplace and home as it relates to insurance coverage and future finances should be considered.
- Betsy Downing will require special assessment when considering wheelchair accommodation for her return to a college campus setting. Maintenance and repair ease will be critical in the selection of a wheelchair(s) as well as the purchase of other AT devices. Campus accessibility and accommodations for power wheelchair or push activation power assist wheelchair use will be critical. It is also important to evaluate Betsy's computer use background to facilitate her ability to handle her course load. The ease and efficiency with which she uses her computer will play a large role in her ability to take class notes (although lectures could also be audiotaped or copies of notes could be obtained from other classmates). Dependability, durability, record of repair, leasing versus purchase, and hands-on trials of all AT devices should be considered for Betsy during the selection process. Economic and insurance issues will affect all AT device purchases and are related to the auto insurance company settlement that will cover Betsy's care. Self-care for all ADL requirements will also need team discussion and input to choose the most appropriate AT devices and services, including a personal attendant. Advisement of scheduling of classes to allow for morning and evening personal care needs should be considered.
- Social and home access and ADL care will be the most important issues for Larry Mullen. The team will need to explore how to economically support a personal aide along with AT devices required for Larry's ADLs. Mobility devices will be very important for Larry's access at home and in the community. Wheelchairs should be explored for their ease of use at home and their portability, which will assist with transportation and independence when Larry visits his children's homes and is out in the greater community. Wheelchair selection will be critical for this patient for independence with propulsion and transfers. Maintenance and repair ease also will be important during selection and purchase of wheelchair(s) and AT devices, but given the patient's mechanical expertise he should understand the importance of maintenance. Dependability, durability, repair record, leasing versus purchase, and hands-on trials of all AT devices need to be considered for this patient. AT for personal care and ADL should be considered so not to burden his family.

CHAPTER THIRTEEN

Using Assistive Technology

Gabriella Stiefbold, OTR, ATP, and Terrence Carolan, PT, ATP, MS

I have used a headset-mounted computer mouse since 1990. I also use a chin-controlled joystick that is mounted to my motorized wheelchair. I have found it is much more convenient than asking people to push my chair around all day and to type for me on the computer. The equipment I use helps me to be independent at home as well as at school and work. Without assistive equipment a lot more disabled people would be home collecting disability benefits instead of out working productively, which is not only bad for a person's quality of life but also is an inefficient allocation of resources.

Karen (C3-4 SCI)

Assistive technology (AT) is an integral part of interventions for the individual with spinal cord injury (SCI). Regardless of the level of technological assistance—no technology, low technology, or high technology—AT allows people with SCI to access their environment in ways that may not be possible without such help. Although some individuals with SCI can require part-time or full-time attendant care, access to computers, telephones, home automation, and other mainstream technology can allow many individuals with SCI to return to their former roles at home, in the community, and at work.

AT has been defined "as any item, piece of equipment, or product system, whether acquired commercially, modified, or customized. Such equipment is used to increase, maintain, or improve functional capabilities of individuals with disabilities."[1] AT affects all aspects of an individual's daily life, including personal care, communication, interfaces throughout the home, mobility, education, work, and recreation. Each component may allow the user to do specific tasks or a range of tasks that allow him to be more independent or function more effectively. Some are sophisticated electronic technologies and others are as simple as a suction cup or clothes hook. Lange and Smith[2] have defined the high-technology electronic aids to daily living (EADLs) as a blend of robotics, computers, and other adaptive equipment that increase independence in self-care, mobility, communication, education, and vocation.

Data from the 2006 Model Systems Report indicates that 64% of individuals with SCI admitted to a model system for rehabilitation worked before their injuries. One year after injury, 32% of those with paraplegia and 24% of those with tetraplegia had returned to work.[3] Rigby et al.[4] compared functional abilities as a result of use of EADLs by using structured interviews with 32 individuals with tetraplegia where half were EADL users and the other half were nonusers. The authors used three scales that included the Functional Autonomy Measuring scale, Lincoln Outcome Measures for Environmental Controls scale, and Psychological Impact of Assistive Devices (PIAD) scale to assess the impact of EADLs in tetraplegia. The authors concluded that EADL users performed significantly better for instrumental daily activities in the majority of the 12 tasks tested. EADL users also had control over many more household devices, which not only optimized their independence but also had a positive psychosocial effect on their sense of competence, adaptability, and self-esteem. Those who did not use EADLs were more dependent on others for their daily living skills.[4]

THE CLIENT'S PERSPECTIVE   Assistive Technologies

Talking with other people who have SCI is often the best resource for adaptive equipment and AT.

Helpful Hints
- Shower chairs with suction cups
- Keep reachers near the pantry and every closet
- Reachers with suction cups work the best
- Slide boards are great for transfers of different heights
- Take a slide board along when traveling because hotel beds always are different heights

Sarah Everhart Skeels and Scott Chesney

To further emphasize the psychosocial impact of EADLs, Jutai et al.[5] examined the anticipated impact at two time points on users who were eligible but had not yet received any devices with actual users using the PIAD scale. The results indicated a positive benefit on autonomy, functional independence, and psychological well-being for both groups, thus supporting the application of EADLs as providing psychosocial benefit, even if the device had not yet been received.

This conclusion was further supported when Ripat and Strock[6] examined the participants who had not yet received their devices at late intervals of between 3 and 6 months. Interestingly, although the EADLs induced a positive sense of competence and confidence, 1 month after receiving the device there was a reduced psychosocial impact explained as an effect of the individual to balance his highly positive view of how the device would affect his life on the basis of experience versus reality. At 3 and 6 months after, his perception of benefit returned to its original level. The results from these studies demonstrate the need to include AT evaluation and instruction as part of the rehabilitation program to boost the number of individuals who return to work and decrease the assistance on others needed for daily living skills.

EVALUATION

A comprehensive evaluation will help to determine the best technology fit to the patient's overall needs. Rust and Smith[7] discuss the importance of documenting the use of AT devices and their impact on functional outcomes to provide evidence of clinical benefit to insurers as well as scientific evidence about outcome effectiveness. A therapist in an inpatient setting should incorporate frequent re-evaluations in the treatment program to allow for trialing multiple devices, assessing preferences, and documenting the effectiveness of each.

A thorough assessment of the individual with an SCI for appropriate AT is crucial for a successful outcome and to ensure that the individual will use the prescribed equipment. Initial medical and therapy assessments, including American Spinal Injury Association (ASIA) scores (see Chapters 1 and 6) and manual muscle testing (see Chapter 6), will enable an optimal AT match to the patient and his potential for functional success. Psychological readiness and cognitive ability also must be considered before introduction of AT (see Chapter 12). For example, an individual who is newly injured may be ready to trial devices that would allow him access to basic devices, such as the phone and television, but may need some time and exposure to technology before discussing devices for home automation.

Assessment should begin with an interview to determine the patient's interest level in AT and to obtain an inventory of devices the individual would like to control. This will vary with each individual, from those interested in controlling a single device such as a television remote to others who want to control a wide range of devices within their environment, such as computers, entertainment systems, and extensive home automation systems. This inventory will assist the clinicians in guiding the individual toward a discussion of both high- and low-technology options.

During the initial assessment, the clinician will determine the patient's prior level of technology use in his work, home, or school environments to ascertain his familiarity with technology. In addition, it also is important to discover what role he wants technology to play in his current life. The clinician can then provide a variety of options for the individual to consider and assist him in achieving his goals. A person who attended school full time and had an active lifestyle at home should be introduced to options that can enable him to complete all aspects of schoolwork, interact with friends and family, and participate in activities to maintain his active lifestyle. Someone who is retired and used to a sedentary lifestyle may simply want to be able to keep in touch with friends and be able to watch his favorite television programs. The student may have had extensive experience in the use of technology as a result of school demands, whereas the older adult may have had far less experience with technology. Both these individuals have technology goals but will require varied levels of AT interventions.

After the assessment of a patient's interest in and need for AT, it is necessary to determine the most consistent and reliable site of access for technology use. Initial evaluations can guide decisions about the best site for consistent upper limb, head movement, or ample voice output for a voice-activated system. The factors that determine site of access are important (Clinical Note: Factors in Determining Site of Access). Switch testers can be used during the assessment to determine an optimal site for access.

CLINICAL NOTE **Factors in Determining Site of Assistive Technology Access**

- Location of the device
- Time of day
- Frequency of use
- Consistent accuracy

Location of the device is essential to its proper use. For example, an individual who wishes to use a voice-activated computer system may need to work in an area where noise levels are fairly low to avoid sound interference. The possibility of the patient disturbing those around him while using a voice-activated system also should be considered when choosing a location. Individuals who want to access infrared devices outdoors may encounter interference from sunlight, which could hinder the reliability of the device. Time of day and frequency of device use also could dictate the ways in which an individual uses a device. For example, patients sometimes have changes in voice output in the evening or when supine in bed. In such cases, an alternative means may be recommended to allow access at all times of the day. It is imperative to ensure consistent accuracy for use of the prescribed device to ensure continued usage.

MEDIA OF TRANSMISSION

Throughout the world, information is communicated in a variety of ways. Electronic mail and data can be sent from one computer to another by dial-up modems, cable connections, digital subscriber lines, or wirelessly. Personal digital assistants (PDAs) can also communicate information wirelessly. Televisions can be controlled with an infrared remote control. Speech itself can be an effective way of transmitting information through voice recognition applications. These patterns also hold true in the world of AT. Data can be transmitted by standard house wiring, infrared control, ultrasound, radio frequency, and speech (Table 13-1). EADL systems frequently have hybrid capabilities that enable switching power to remote devices.

Standard House Wiring

Standard house wiring operates on 110-volt alternating current (AC) in North America and can be used to communicate basic information from a control center to appliances, such as lamps or appliances (Figure 13-1). One example of an EADL control system that relies on house wiring is produced by X10 (Irvine, Calif.). X10 technology is a language that allows compatible products to communicate with each other using the existing electrical wiring in the home; it grew out of the beginnings of the home automation industry in the 1970s to target able-bodied people with remote-controlled conveniences and was quickly adapted for disability-related products.[8] Easy installation starts with a transmitter that is plugged or wired into the home's standard wiring. It sends control signals to a receiver at another site, which allows an individual to turn appliances on or off. X10 appliances are plugged directly into an appliance module, which then is plugged directly into an electrical outlet. Because these installations are simple and rely on existing wiring, they are cost-effective as well.

In addition, new integrated modules can control a house full of lights and appliances (LiteTouch, Inc., Salt Lake City, Utah, and Elan Home Systems, LLC, Lexington, Ky., in collaboration with Elan VIA! Integrations Partner program marshaling the electronic industry's manufacturers for unprecedented support of integrated systems).[9] In a single family dwelling, the signals used to control X10 modules will not travel through the home power transformer so there is no risk of interfacing with the devices in nearby homes. One drawback, however, is the possibility of mixed signals in apartment complexes, where users could inadvertently

TABLE 13-1 | **Advantages and Disadvantages of Various Media of Transmission**

Media of Transmission	Advantages	Disadvantages
AC house wiring	Ease of setup Low cost	Possibility of commands being misinterpreted while being transmitted through the wiring Can only turn appliances on or off
Infrared	Ability to carry multiple signals that can be used in controlling an appliance with a variety of features Can travel across the distance of an average-size room	Cannot travel through solid objects
Ultrasound	Highly portable because easy to relocate receiver modules	Able to transmit only a small number of functions Does not have the versatility of infrared transmission Cannot travel through solid barriers
Radio frequency	Increased transmission distance Can transmit through walls or other solid objects Can carry both discrete commands and speech Ability to transmit a large number of commands	Interference from other radio frequencies can be an obstacle to use
Voice control	Voice recognition software continues to make strong advances	Can only be effectively used over the distance that speech can travel Quality of the transmission is dependent on variables including background noise, quality of speech, and volume

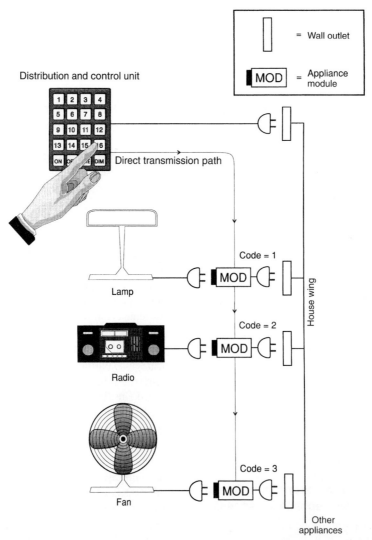

FIGURE 13-1 A direct-selection EADL. Each appliance has a numerical code, and the keypad is used to select the appropriate module. Control functions such as ON, OFF, and DIM are also activated by pressing the proper key on the keypad. This figure also illustrates the use of house wiring for distribution of the control signals to the appliance modules. (From Cook AM, Polgar JM: *Cook and Hussey's assistive technologies: principles and practice*, ed 3, St. Louis, 2008, Mosby Elsevier, Figure 14-8, p. 469.)

control each other's devices.[8] Other drawbacks include the possibility of commands being misinterpreted while being transmitted through the wiring or interference with other appliances that generate "noise" in the powerline, such as a hair dryer or vacuum. Noise filters are now available to overcome this problem.

When devices need to be controlled from two sources of power lines (e.g., 220-volt AC current used by some large appliances), a phase cross-over is available from integrated modules to solve this problem. Wall switches can be replaced with the integrated controller units in permanent installations because the modules do not prevent local control of the receptacles and switches. That allows others to use these switches in a standard manner so that a light switch can be controlled manually or by remote control.[8]

Infrared

Infrared is one of the most common means of data transmission. Whenever a person uses a remote control to turn on a television, he is likely using infrared technology to affect change. Similarly, when a person uses AT to control the features of a television, DVD player, or audio receiver, infrared technology is probably the media of transmission (Figure 13-2). Infrared signals work on a dispersed line of sight basis by mimicking signals of standard remote control devices.[8]

Infrared EADL control is programmed using standard sequences for commercially available products such as DVD players. The configured systems store the information codes that have been transferred from a conventional remote. This allows a number of codes to be stored for a variety of interactions within the home environment; however, significant setup time is required on the part of users or caregivers to program the device.[8,10]

Infrared light has the ability to carry multiple signals that can be used in controlling an appliance with a variety of features. It can travel across the distance of an average-size room but cannot travel through solid objects or around corners. A controller must be aimed at the device for the signals to be received, which means that an EADL cannot access a device in another room. X10 Powermid transmitter technology overcomes such restraints by converting infrared signals into radio frequencies that can pass through walls. Additional Powermid transmitters can enable a person with SCI to control any infrared device in a home from any room and are available internationally from numerous retailers including Crutchfield and Target.

In addition to programmable infrared EADL controllers, increasingly more sophisticated infrared universal remote control units can be used to access a variety of devices; however, control often requires a high level of dexterity. Home audio-video interoperability (HAVi) specifications have been designed to target this problem and encourage home electronics manufacturers to work toward the use of a single remote control unit. One advantage of HAVi is its ability to add new devices to its network. This industry standard has been jointly developed by major corporations including Hitachi, Panasonic Philips, Sharp, and Toshiba.[11] Another industry group, the Infrared Data Association, has focused on standards to allow personal computers, augmentative communication devices, and PDAs to control home electronics.[8]

Perhaps the most promising new technology standard is known as V2. It promotes the ability of EADLs to control settings on a

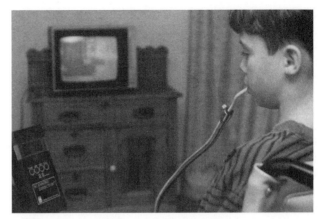

FIGURE 13-2 A trainable infrared EADL with scanning access. The EADL is shown mounted to a wheelchair. It is positioned so there is a line-of-sight link to the television for use of infrared control. (From Cook AM, Polgar JM: *Cook and Hussey's assistive technologies: principles and practice*, ed 3, St. Louis, 2008, Mosby Elsevier, Figure 14-12, p 474. Courtesy APT Technology, Inc., DU-IT CSG, Inc., Shreve, Ohio.)

thermostat in a hall or "press" a push button at a crosswalk.[12] This new standard enables fully functional remote operation of products through intermediate devices and intelligent agents. The method allows a person to execute a specific command without having to walk through a chain of menus and provides entirely visual, audio, or natural language interfaces. It also is bidirectional, which allows product status to be communicated to the user and to the remote when a selected temperature is reached or the laundry cycle complete.

Ultrasound

Ultrasound is a sound frequency that can be used to transmit only a small number of functions. It does not have the versatility of infrared transmission, nor can it travel through solid barriers.

Radio Frequency

Radio frequency transmissions have the ability to transmit over larger distances, transmit through walls or other solid objects, and carry both discrete commands and speech. Some X10 devices use radio frequency to communicate between the X10 modules and the controller (e.g., Powermid transmitters). Wireless networking and Bluetooth technology is based on the transmission of data or voice over a specific radio frequency. Advantages include increased transmission distance, the ability to carry human speech, and the ability to transmit a large number of commands. Interference from other radio frequencies can be an obstacle to using this as a transmission medium.

Voice Control

Not only is speech a way to communicate, but it is also a medium of transmission. Voice recognition software continues to make strong advances, and can be found in cars, PDAs, cellular telephones, voice recognition software for word processing, and environmental control applications. Voice control can only be effectively used over the distance that speech can travel, and the quality of the transmission is dependent on variables including background noise, quality of speech, and volume.

SWITCH ACCESS

A person with SCI is often unable to control electronic devices through traditional means. Switches are tools that allow alternative means to execute a command in an electronic device (Clinical Note: Various Switch Characteristics). Depending on the level of control desired, a user can choose single, dual, or multiple switches. These refer to the number of possible selections that a user can access with one switch. Switches can be either wired or wireless. They can be momentary, latched, or proportional. Momentary switches activate the product only as long as the input is continued. Latched switches stay on once the switch is activated and are turned off only with a second activation of the switch. Proportional switches translate movement into movement of the assistive technology; the response is directly proportional to the user's input.

CLINICAL NOTE **Various Switch Characteristics**

- Single, dual, or multiple
- Wired or wireless
- Momentary, latched, or proportional

Table 13-2 illustrates examples of different types of switches. Pneumatic switches are triggered by intraoral pressure generated by the user. They are typically used with a tube attachment that is placed in the user's mouth. They can function as a single or dual switch, using sip-n-puff as discrete functions. Motion-based switches such as a self-calibrating auditory tone infrared switch or a fiberoptic switch cast light over part of a user's body. When movement interrupts that beam of light, the switch is triggered. Manual switches are the most common type of switch. Examples include any switch triggered by manual pressure at any access point of the body. Sensitivity of these switches varies greatly and should correlate closely with the evaluation of the user's strength and motor control.

When a clinician uses a switch with a patient for the first time, a switch tester can be a powerful teaching tool. A switch can be plugged into a switch tester and when activated, the switch tester can give both visual and audio feedback to the patient. This biofeedback can confirm that the switch has been successfully activated. When the patient masters a switches use, he can begin training with the chosen AT that it controls.

TABLE 13-2 | Switch Types

Pneumatic	Motion Based	Manual

A. TASH pneumatic switch

B. TASH SCATIR switch

C. TASH plate switch; light touch

D. TASH buddy button switch; medium to heavy touch

E. TASH heavy duty cap switch; heavy to medium touch

F. TASH micro light switch; light touch

Figures A-F courtesy Tash, Inc., Richmond, VA.

USING ELECTRONIC AIDS TO DAILY LIVING

EADLs provide individuals with needed access to personal devices, power mobility, and the overall environment. Although once referred to as environmental control units, that term has been restricted to devices that control environmental conditions such as thermostats.[8,13,14] Categories of EADLs that are particularly important to individuals with SCI include telephones, computers, and home automation devices.

Telephone Access

Patients find that one of the most important areas of EADL access is telephone access. Most individuals with SCI use telephone access as the basis for resuming normal day-to-day social contacts with friends and family. Because access to these social bonds may have been limited since their injury, relearning facility becomes a particularly strong motivational tool.

Telephone access has evolved from landline only systems to those with wireless capabilities and finally to mobile cellular telephones. Adaptive telephone systems using traditional landline phones provide individuals with phone access while in the home. Such systems can stand alone or be part of a system that provides other environmental access and can be controlled through switch activation or voice control. Some systems are wireless with a limited range from the telephone base. These systems provide a person desired contact with friends and family and access to emergency numbers; however, they have limited portability and cannot be used outside the home.

Low-technology options for landline users include large-button phones that an individual with only gross upper limb function (C5 to C7) can access with a universal cuff and peg. Other low-technology options include phone holders, some of which use goosenecks to hold the handset of the phone and allow the phone to be positioned next to an individual's ear. Phone cuffs are also available and attach to a handset allowing a person with limited hand function to hold a phone headset to his ear (Figure 13-3). Individuals who have active head movement may be able to use a mouthstick for phone access and the addition of a headset or a system with speakerphone capabilities can allow for hands-free use of the phone.

Cellular telephones have significantly changed the landscape for phone access. Recommendations for individuals with SCI who want to access a telephone now include a variety of cellular products using creative positioning of the handset to enable a user with limited upper limb strength to access keys on the phone or flip the phone open or closed. Individuals with some upper limb function can use low-technology adaptive equipment such as finger or typing pegs to manage cell phone buttons.

Voice activation capabilities, available on many cellular phones, can allow a person with little or no upper limb use to access a cellular phone. Indeed, these options used in conjunction with a headset can allow for private telephone access in multiple environments. Clinicians evaluating for phone access should consider the patient's voice quality output at varied times of the day. Changes in voice output may limit voice recognition abilities. Also, some cellular telephones have limited access because a button must be pressed to open the phone line before voice control can be used and many patients lack the ability to use their upper limbs to push any cell phone button. Currently there are a limited number of cell phones that allow truly hands-free voice-controlled dialing; however, this feature is expected to increase in the short term.

The emergence of Bluetooth technologies has created new opportunities for individuals with SCI to use cell phones and other wireless applications. A Bluetooth headset allows a user to speak on a headset without having a physical connection to the phone set, as long as the headset stays within a set distance of the phone base (Figure 13-4, *A*). The headset also has buttons that allow the user to open a line and end a call (Figure 13-4, *B*). An individual with available gross upper limb movement can access the switch to open and close the phone line and then use voice dialing to make the call. Manufacturers vary the designs of their headset pieces and some have buttons that are large enough to allow for creative adaptations (e.g., building up the button piece to allow for ease of access). A switch mount positioned close to the headset can provide a surface for people who use cervical and head movement for their primary control to press against when activating the Bluetooth headset.

Other technologies include PDA access using voice recognition software. For individuals with SCI who are returning to school or work, access to mobile planners in addition to their workstation has improved quality of life and organization of work, home, and school functions. Systems that integrate phone, PDA functions, and Microsoft- based applications (e.g., Excel and PowerPoint) are available with voice recognition for phone access and other functions that require some upper limb control. Individuals with limited upper limb control (C6 to C7) should be able to access these integrated systems. Voice recognition options can be used to access the phone function while adaptations using a typing peg are used to access other applications, including e-mail and computer-based programs. Although these technologies do not address the needs of individuals with higher SCIs who have significant upper limb limitations, they do make a tremendous impact on the lives of many people with SCI who were previously without access to such sophisticated technology.

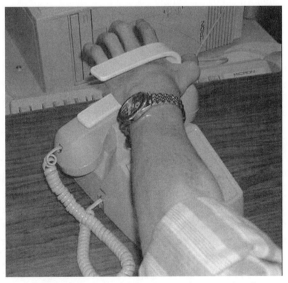

FIGURE 13-3 Accessible phone with universal cuff.

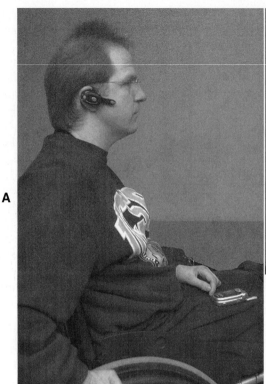

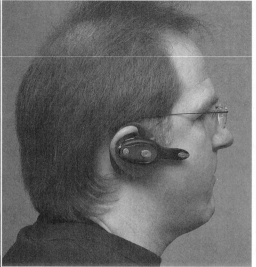

FIGURE 13-4 A, Client uses a cell phone with Bluetooth headset. **B,** Close-up of Bluetooth ear piece.

Computer Access

Computer access is a common area of interest for individuals after SCI. Initial evaluations should incorporate a needs assessment related to computer use. Discussion should include prior computer experience, the purpose of computer usage, and all applications that will be accessed for leisure, work, or school functions. Accommodations made to enable computer access for individuals with SCI can assist in return to a gainful work environment. For individuals with limited mobility, computer access can serve to bridge the gap to the world of technology, gain needed information through the Internet, keep in contact with friends and family, and lead to potential employment by telecommuting or job site modification.[15]

The initial evaluation also should provide information about the individual's available upper limb function. People with some gross upper limb function may benefit from low-technology adaptive equipment to access a computer. Others with a complete C6 SCI can use a simple typing peg adaptation, which relies on the remaining strength of the wrist extensors to push the pegs. Individuals with little or no upper limb function who have active head movement (C3 to C4) can use a mouthstick to access keyboard (Figure 13-5).

Page management is often a concern for those returning to school or work, and ways to accommodate these functions can be incorporated into the computer access evaluation. Low-technology options that facilitate page management include bookstands and simple book holders that allow easy positioning of books, magazines, and other literature so that an individual can turn pages with an adapted peg (see Figure 9-30).

It is helpful to begin training with low-technology options when introducing computer access and then proceed as needed

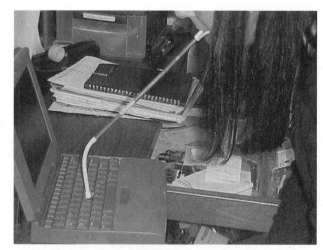

FIGURE 13-5 Patient uses mouthstick to type.

to more refined higher technology. Low-technology devices are then a familiar alternative if technical problems arise with more complex systems or funding difficulties are encountered and new equipment is delayed.

Integrated System Access

The Quartet Simplicity and PROXi (Quartet Technologies, Inc, Tyngsboro, Mass.) are system devices that allow a user with limited or no upper limb function to control a personal computer through EADL. Although the demands of computer control are much greater than those of an EADL, some computer-based systems are designed as combinations of specific input technologies and remote controls systems or specialized features such as a hospital bed.

The strength of these integrated systems is that the user needs to learn only one single control strategy to have access to all the electronic devices and information systems within the environment. Their weakness lies in the possibility of loosing control of the entire environment if the electronic component fails.[16]

Keyboard Access

Physical keyboards include devices or controls that provide individual switches for each operation that is produced and switch combinations that modify desired actions. Adapted keyboards may be classified according to scale, timing, and pattern. A conventional computer keyboard may be too large for a person with SCI to handle easily because of limited movement of his shoulders, elbows, or hands. Thus changing its scale may be indicated. Alternatives to conventional keyboards may include offering smaller keys, a smaller number of keys, less space between the keys, or any combination thereof. Some key size reductions can be accomplished by increasing the slope of the key sides, which maintains the same touch areas while allowing the overall key dimensions to be smaller. The Cherry keyboard (Cherry Corporation, Pleasant Prairie, Wis.) accomplishes this key reduction and also provides an option of 84 keys versus the typical 104 keys.

On the contrary, keypads on PDAs are usually so small that they may require fine motor control by individual digits and therefore are not optimal for a person with SCI. Compact keyboards can be adapted with universal wireless options that allow the addition of a larger more usable keyboard for use by a person with SCI and limited hand function.[16]

Changing the keyboard timing is another way to enhance its function. The autorepeat behavior of a keyboard may be adjusted for individuals with limited motor function. People who press keys with a mouthstick or finger splint to type may accidentally engage wrong keys. For this reason, the immediate response keyboards may not be desirable. Through the "slow key" feature, a small delay may be added before the key takes action and very brief key presses ignored. The disadvantage of this feature is that typing becomes slower and less automatic.[16]

People with SCI may also benefit from alternate keyboard patterns such as the Chubon keyboard, which provides an option for single digit typing.[17] Disadvantages include the limited portability because the adapted keyboard includes altered labels to the key caps making it difficult for other users. In addition, the keyboard layout is interpreted in the software of the computer, so the alternative layout must be programmed on each computer where it is used. One option is to use an adapted USB keyboard that can be carried between computers. Another is computer software that enables the keyboard configuration to be remapped to any new computer without installing itself on the host computer.[16]

Mouse Access

A trackball-type mouse offers an inexpensive option for data input into a computer (Figure 13-6, A). The mouse was initially created to address ergonomic issues and related hand position for individuals who typed frequently. The systems are easy for an individual with gross upper limb movements to use with or without adaptive devices to assist him. In addition, there is the switch-adapted mouse trackball (i.e., SAM-Trackball, RJ Cooper & Associates, Laguna Niguel, Calif.) that allows the separation of mouse movement from clicking without moving the mouse. There is also an after-market trackpad, similar to those found on laptops, that are USB based so they do not require any special drivers for operation. Low-technology adaptations include finger pegs on dolphin splints (Figure 13-6, B) and universal cuffs holding peg splints (Figure 13-6, C).

For individuals with higher cervical injuries, a head-pointing mouse can provide access to the computer. Users report a high-level of accuracy with HeadMaster (Prentke Romich Wooster, Ohio).[18] Such head-pointing devices use infrared light reflected from a small target worn by the user, in which the light source works in tandem with a camera placed on the computer monitor. When the user moves the target into the infrared camera's field of view, the movement is converted to mouse cursor movements. The advantages of this system are that the user is not tethered and does not need to wear unsightly hardware. Although infrared head-pointing devices provide minimally intrusive mouse movement, they do not provide a means of mouse clicking. A system known as dwell-clicking allows the user to hold the mouse cursor in one location for a period of time so that it can generate the desired click (SmartNav from NaturalPoint); however, it requires the user to access the software control to determine whether he wants single or double clicks. This means that the user must stop for a short period of time for each mouse action to occur, significantly slowing performance.

Voice Recognition Access

The most common high-technology option for computer access is voice recognition software. Voice recognition uses voice output to navigate a computer, perform word processing, and even use the Internet. The system requires the user to don a headset or have a microphone positioned at the desktop (Figure 13-7). Consideration should be given to an individual's voice output and any evident variations in voice strength during different times of the day because the software requires consistency of volume to work optimally.

Training an individual to be independent with voice recognition software can take as little as 15 minutes; however, decreased vocal output variations require additional training. It will take approximately 2 to 4 weeks of steady use before the program consistently recognizes an individual's voice. It is important that this time commitment is explained to a client beginning training so that he knows what to expect and can decide whether the system will be an appropriate match for his needs. Although PC-based voice recognition software has been the standard, Mac-based voice recognition software is available.

Emulation Access

Mouse emulators are systems that allow computer access by mouse movements controlled by external sources other than a standard mouse. These systems are typically used in conjunction with on-screen keyboard software. With this software, a keyboard is created on the computer screen and the individual types words and uses any of the standard keyboard functions by moving the mouse and clicking over the desired letter or number. Several types of mouse emulation systems are available.

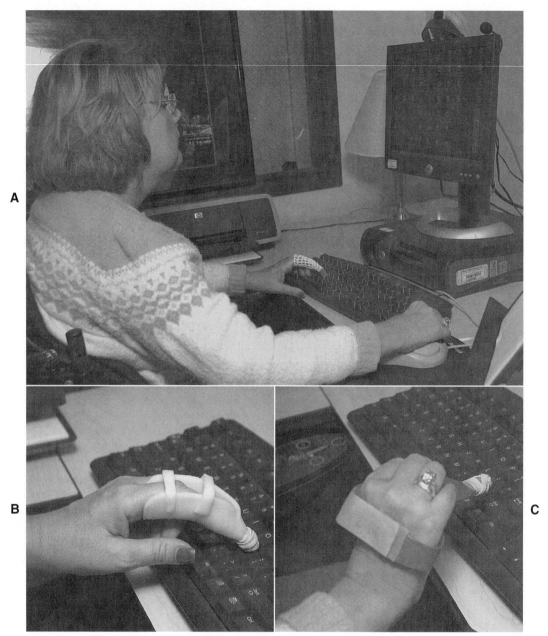

FIGURE 13-6 A, Client accesses the computer by using both a trackball mouse under the right palmar surface of her hand and a peg splint on her left index finger. **B,** Close-up of a client using a finger peg in a dolphin splint to type. **C,** Close-up of a client using a universal cuff with peg splint in place to type.

Simple plug-and-play systems plug into the existing mouse port. These systems allow for mouse stylus control with head or eye movement and click and drag functions controlled by sips and puffs. Other complex systems use infrared transmission or Web cameras to target consistent head movement, facial movement, or any other consistent movement of a body part to enable control of the mouse. Click, double click, and drag functions are performed with sips and puffs or by the amount of time an individual holds his gaze on a desired spot. One system uses movement of the pupil to control a mouse for computer access, allowing individuals with the highest level of injury (C1 to C2) who have no active head or neck movement to access a computer with the movement of their eyes.

Individuals who require higher technology options or those with limited head and neck function also may use electronic page-turning devices for switch-activated page turning. Such systems use any type of switch to turn pages, from a simple button switch to a pneumatic (e.g., sip-n-puff) driven system. Limitations include the size of books that can be used with the system as well as the potential for inaccuracy in the number of pages that are turned.

Alternative Access
Alternative access systems depend on a host computer system to which an AT device is attached. USB ports now allow AT devices and resident software to travel between computers, allowing users greater flexibility.

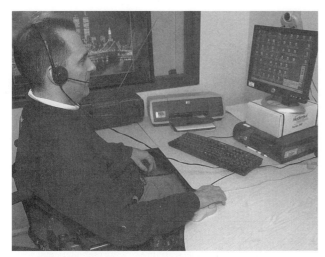

FIGURE 13-7 Client uses a voice-activated system for computer access. He also has some upper limb function to control a trackball mouse (see Figure 9-33 of a client using a voice activation system without a trackball mouse).

Individuals with SCI whose computer usage was minimal before their injury may find Internet use and e-mail to be their most important focus areas. For others who relied on a high level of computer usage or who have potential to be employed in an area requiring computer access, it is essential to determine the best fit for computer access. In both cases, it is important to keep in mind ease of use and time efficiency when determining appropriate computer access recommendations.

Environmental Access

When evaluating patients for environmental access, it is important to consider low-technology options first. Simple devices such as a touch lamp converter may be recommended that will allow a light to be turned on and off in response to gross touch. Other simple EADL direct-selection devices discussed previously include house-wired systems that use a single command center box with appliance modules for each appliance to be accessed (see Figure 13-1). These systems are used for simple on-and-off functions of many electrically powered devices and are relatively inexpensive and simple to use. An individual who wishes to control a limited number of items can do so with large-button remote controls, voice-activated systems, or higher end options with switch access. It is also possible for a person using a power switching EADL to control the room temperature through a small heater, which is useful when he spends part of each day alone. Electric hospital beds, however, may be more difficult to control because different beds use different input signals; therefore, it is vital to make sure that the client's EADL can control his model bed.[16]

A world of devices is available and they range from simple to more complex systems, such as infrared systems with integrated features that can control hundreds of commands (Figure 13-8). These systems allow a range of options from a few functions, such as the control of the TV and lights, to a fully integrated system that accesses a full entertainment system, automatic door opener, curtain controls, automatic water faucet, and many other electronic functions throughout the home. For example, special lighting modules can be used to dim or brighten a room's lighting in addition to switching power on and off, although they only work with incandescent lighting.

Mainstream home automation systems have bridged the gap between environmental access for individuals with a disability and home automation systems available to anyone who wants to control electrical function in their home. Many of these systems can integrate house wiring to be controlled by switch access or touch screens. Mainstream technology has also introduced an array of items such as miniature vacuums and lawnmowers that perform their tasks independently with limited setup from the user.

Simple systems to control home electronics can vary significantly in cost from hundreds to upwards of thousands of dollars for full home automation systems. It is therefore essential to carefully consider the client's needs and ensure that the individual will be able to use all the integrated technology. For some clients, such systems will be the difference between spending time independently and requiring an assistant at all times.

Environmental access facilitated through home automation provides tools that can improve a client's quality of life and decrease dependence on others.[13] When an individual is evaluated for AT integration, discharge placement must be considered as well as what areas of the home environment the individual would like to control. High-technology systems designed for carefully prioritized and individualized access options will provide the best service to the client.

POWER MOBILITY INTEGRATION

Power mobility systems have traditionally remained separate from other ATs. Manufacturers have opted to integrate existing high-end technology systems into the wheelchair electronics to control a device or devices within the environment through the driver controls of the wheelchair. This sometimes offers additional independence to power mobility users.

Systems that could integrate power mobility drive functions, however, are often underused or not ordered because of the additional cost and their inherent limitations.

Several power mobility manufacturers have addressed this by incorporating environmental control into the electronics of their power mobility system (Figure 13-9). This makes environmental control easier to obtain at a reasonable price because these power mobility systems are funded far more frequently by insurers than other forms of assistive technology (e.g., computer access devices and home automation). Bluetooth technologies are also being incorporated into power drive controls, giving the user Bluetooth control of power mobility functions. Obviously, AT should be designed to travel with the client whenever possible rather than remain resident on a specific device or in a specific environment.[16]

ERGONOMICS AND COMPUTER WORKSTATION SETUP

Ergonomics is a key area of concern across all population groups with the goal of preventing repetitive strain injuries, eyestrain, and compromised posture and positioning. For those who are disabled and certainly for individuals with SCI, this concern is even greater and must be adequately addressed. For a client with

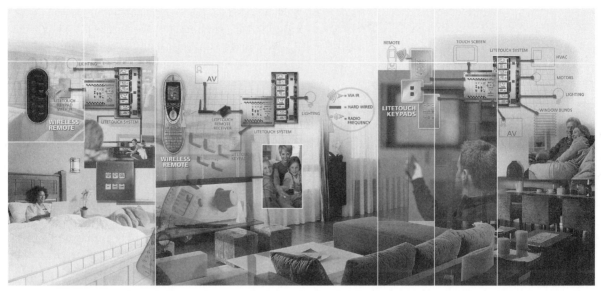

FIGURE 13-8 LiteTouch, Inc, lighting and AV control solutions for the whole home. (Courtesy LiteTouch, Inc., Salt Lake City, UT.)

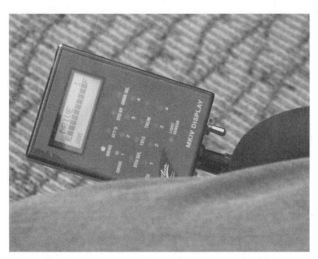

FIGURE 13-9 Integrated controls on a power wheelchair.

SCI, the issue of ergonomics and adequate workstation setup should be incorporated into discussions about home accessibility and functional access.[15]

Desk height is the primary factor for workstation setup and is determined by using both wheelchair seat to floor height and, more important, floor to top of knee height. These dimensions will vary for power mobility users and manual mobility users. Table height should allow for 3 to 4 inches of additional clearance above the knee of an individual in his wheelchair. Upper leg length must also be considered. A longer upper leg length will require a greater depth dimension for the desk or workstation to provide optimal access to the entire station (Figure 13-10). Simulation of a computer station setup is an important step because it will allow assessing the patient's upper limb excursion and will help in positioning frequently used items within the individual's reach.

The client should be seated appropriately in his wheelchair seating system, with optimal line of sight to the computer screen. The computer monitor should be positioned in front of the individual, rather than off to one side, to avoid prolonged positions of trunk or cervical rotation. Wheelchair options such as desk length arms and swing-away joysticks for power mobility users will allow for additional accessibility to the workstation. The clinician should discuss power tilt versus reclining chairs with clients who will need power seat functions for weight shifts. Power recline features will allow for pressure relief without leaving the desk area, whereas power tilt will require the individual to move out of the desk space for pressure relief. Individuals who require very specific positioning to control head or voice-controlled systems may find power recline to be a better option to avoid repeated moves in and out of the desk area (Figure 13-11). Accessories on the desk, such as a bookstand to hold paperwork and rotating file holders, can further promote ease of access at the computer station.

Ergonomic issues should be discussed with all clients with SCI who plan to use a computer workstation, including those with paraplegia who will need few physical adaptations to their workstation. All individuals should be instructed in correct ergonomics for their workstation including computer monitor placement in an effort to help prevent pain and overuse problems.

MAINSTREAM TECHNOLOGY

Mainstream technology has made a tremendous impact on the lives of individuals with SCI. Before mainstream technology became readily available, options for individuals with SCI were limited to low-technology or high-technology devices with expensive price tags. In 1997, Holme et al[19] reported that high cost and lack of third-party reimbursement were key factors deterring therapists from recommending environmental control units for home use. Mainstream technology has now introduced significantly less expensive options that in many cases

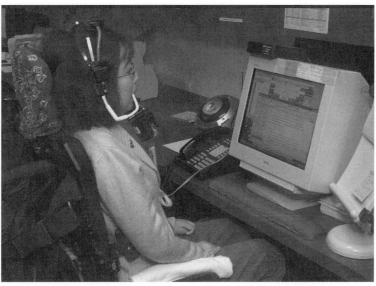

FIGURE 13-10 Client at computer workstation using pneumatic-controlled software and good ergonomics with adequate workstation setup providing optimal line of sight to computer monitor.

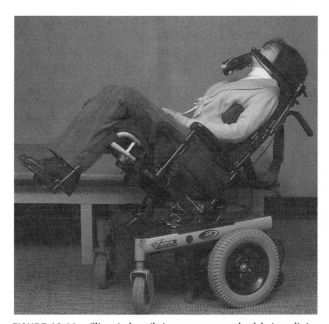

FIGURE 13-11 Client in her tilt-in-space power wheelchair reclining to perform pressure relief of the ischial tuberosities.

offer a greater variety of functions than previously existing technologies.

Broadband services through local Internet providers have provided additional opportunity for wireless Internet access to individuals with SCI. For laptop users, this feature can be an important addition to access in the community environment where wireless access has become increasingly available.

Other integrated technologies have also emerged that combine access to two important and common areas of interest: television and computer. Computer manufacturers have integrated computer technologies with television access, allowing for television viewing through the computer monitor. Therefore an individual who is able to access his computer by any mouse emulator or voice recognition system can now also access a television and DVD player, which can provide other functions such as listening to music. This exciting merging of technologies will increasingly allow for greater independence with multiple home-based devices.

New options for electronic page turning include true electronic readers created for the mainstream market with applications to the disabled community. Pages can be viewed digitally and mimic the look of text. Systems are compact and similar to the size of a small hardcover novel. Pages can be turned with the use of buttons on the system, which can be accessible by typing peg adaptations (Figure 13-12) or mouthstick use. The cost of this system is significantly lower than the cost of previous electronically driven page turners. They also provide an individual with a wide array of available text selections because e-books can be downloaded onto the system for reading and are often from the public library. Integration of switches such as pneumatic sip-n-puff systems or voice-activated systems would significantly improve access to this system for individuals with SCI.

New leisure devices are also a part of mainstream technologies. MP3 players and iPod devices have become a standard for access to music and videos. Many of these systems are inherently easy for individuals with limited or no hand function to use. The system may be accessed with gentle hand movements or by peg or mouthstick (Figure 13-13).

Emerging mainstream technologies have provided an explosion of devices that serve the able-bodied and disabled populations. Further refinement of these technologies will improve access to mainstream technology for individuals with SCI and limit the need to use high-technology systems that previously were the only options. It is essential for clinicians to keep abreast of emerging technologies to provide consumers with SCI the best options for their accessibility needs. Table 13-3 provides a summary of recommended devices for each level of cervical SCI.

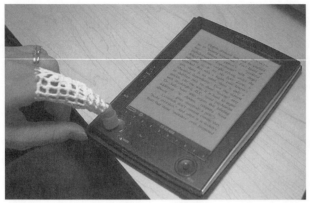

FIGURE 13-12 Client reading from a Sony reader using an adaptive peg to access the button that turns the pages.

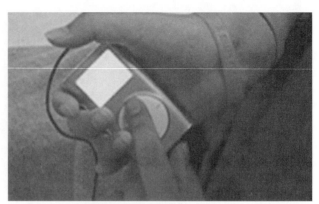

FIGURE 13-13 Patient using an iPod.

TABLE 13-3	**Summary of Recommended Devices for Each Level of Spinal Cord Injury**			
Injury Level	Key Muscles Innervated	Environmental Access	Telephone Access	Computer Access
C1-2 tetraplegia	Trace; head/neck flexion, rotation, extension; jaw motion, eye blink, eyebrow	Voice, pneumatic, or motion-triggered switch control	Landline use with pneumatic or voice control; cell phone access with voice dialing, computer telephone with computer access listed below	Voice recognition software; eye control mouse emulation; pneumatic mouse click control, mouthstick
C3 tetraplegia	Same as C1-2 with addition of improved neck stability, control, and active range of motion	Voice, pneumatic, head switch control, or motion-triggered switch	Landline use with pneumatic or voice control or head switch access; cell phone access with Bluetooth headset and voice dialing	Voice recognition software, eye and head-controlled mouse emulation with pneumatic mouse click control
C4 tetraplegia	Cervical flexion, extension, lateral flexion, rotation; scapular elevation and rotation; some shoulder abduction (10 to 15 degrees) with trapezius assist	Voice, pneumatic, head switch control, or motion-triggered switch	Landline use with pneumatic or voice control or head switch access; cell phone access with Bluetooth headset and voice dialing	Voice recognition software, head-controlled mouse emulation with pneumatic mouse click control
C5 tetraplegia	Partial shoulder abduction and flexion; active elbow flexion and some supination; generally, C5 motion is one of imbalance	Switch-controlled access point: hand or forearm or remote control; X10 control with universal cuff or peg; touch lamp	Traditional phone with modified phone holder, universal cuff with peg for dialing; headset phone use; cell phone with Bluetooth or peg for dialing or voice dialing	Voice recognition software; trackball mouse or head-controlled mouse emulation if weak; typing peg or universal cuff for typing
C6 tetraplegia	Include those available at C5 and scapular abduction, horizontal adduction, wrist extension, and pronation	Switch-controlled access point: hand or forearm or remote control; X10 control with universal cuff or peg; touch lamp	Traditional phone with modified phone holder; universal cuff with peg for dialing; headset phone use; cell phone with Bluetooth or peg for dialing or voice dialing	Voice recognition software; trackball mouse emulation if weak; typing peg or universal cuff for typing
C7-8 tetraplegia	Include those available at C6 and increased scapular motion and stability, triceps, wrist extension, and flexion, elbow extension; some finger extension, thumb abduction; C8 also has finger flexion and extension along with overall greater strength	Switch-controlled access point: hand or forearm or remote control; X10 control with universal cuff or peg; touch lamp	Traditional phone with modified phone holder, greater finger peg use for dialing, typing, and remote control access; headset phone use; cell phone with Bluetooth or peg for dialing or voice dialing	Voice recognition software; trackball mouse emulation if weak; typing peg or universal cuff for typing

ASSESSMENT IN REHABILITATION AND IN USER SATISFACTION

It is generally accepted that EADLs play an important role in providing a means of access and control for individuals with SCI. Despite how carefully clinicians evaluate and match a patient's needs with the appropriate technologies, it is important to know how AT affects rehabilitation outcomes and how satisfied the consumer is and remains once discharged to the home environment. Unfortunately, little research exists to support whether AT has an impact on rehabilitation outcomes or whether consumers are satisfied with their devices. In 2005, Rust and Smith[7] reviewed 100 instruments that measured rehabilitation of health outcomes. Each of the instruments was evaluated according to the degree the scale assessed AT, the content of the scale, and the scoring of the instrument. The authors found that 30% of the instruments ignored AT. When AT was included, there was a greater tendency to reduce the health outcome score as a result of using the AT than allowing the use of AT to attain the highest possible score. Further research is needed to standardize the use and scoring criteria for examining rehabilitation outcomes for patients using AT.

Regarding consumer satisfaction with AT, in 2002 Shone et al[20] interviewed 40 EADL users and nonusers about their views and experiences with EADLs using the Functional Independence Measure and the Quebec User Evaluation of Satisfaction with assistive Technology (QUEST). Overall, consumers were well satisfied with their EADLs even after a second assessment 6 months later, although some consumers expressed concern about the cost and associated services of the technologies. Although this study evaluated individuals with degenerative neuromuscular conditions rather than SCI, it reflects the importance of using a questionnaire that explores other dimensions such as the effect of the EADL on quality of life and other psychosocial factors. Outcome measures such as the QUEST[21] may help substantiate payment by insurance companies for sophisticated devices. Therefore, both assessing use of AT and documenting its impact on rehabilitation outcomes with consistent scoring criteria and the psychosocial value to consumers is necessary if AT is to become available to more people with SCI.

CLINICAL CASE STUDY **Using Assistive Technology**

Patient History

Gina Parsons is a 52-year-old woman with a C4 tetraplegia, ASIA A diagnosis. She had a spinal cord compression injury as the result of a motor vehicle accident. Gina had a urinary tract infection during her acute-care stay. Ten weeks after her injury, she is medically and orthopedically stable. She is currently still an inpatient in an acute rehabilitation hospital.

Gina is a law librarian at a university near her home. Her husband is overseeing the renovation of their home, where they are converting the downstairs study into a bedroom. There is a full bath on the first floor, which is being modified for full accessibility and is next to the new bedroom. Gina's 26-year-old daughter is married and lives approximately 10 miles away. Her 21-year-old son is a senior in college. Gina is currently trying out various wheelchairs in anticipation of ordering her own wheelchair.

Patient's Self-Assessment

Gina wants to return to her job, where most of her activities are accomplished on the computer. She also hopes to return to her volunteer work at the local soup kitchen.

Clinical Assessment
Patient Appearance
- Height 5 feet 1 inches, weight 102 pounds, body mass index 19.3

Cognitive Assessment
- Alert, oriented × 3

Cardiopulmonary Assessment
- Blood pressure 116/60 mm Hg, heart rate at rest 72 beats/min, respiratory rate 14 breaths/min, cough flows are ineffective, vital capacity significantly decreased

Musculoskeletal and Neuromuscular Assessment
- Motor assessment reveals C4 ASIA A, sensory C4
- Upper limb muscle strength consists of upper trapezius 4/5 bilaterally
- Deep tendon reflexes 3+ below the level of lesion

Integumentary and Sensory Assessment
- Skin is intact throughout and sensory intact to C4.

Range of Motion Assessment
- Passive range of motion is within normal limits at both upper limbs except for shoulder flexion, which is limited to 165 degrees bilaterally.
- Straight leg raise (SLR) is 95 degrees in both lower limbs and dorsiflexion is 5 degrees; all other motions in the lower limbs are within functional limits.

Mobility and ADL Assessment
- Dependent with bed mobility and transfers to all surfaces
- Dependent with pressure relief in manual wheelchair; verbal cues required for pressure relief in power tilt-in-space wheelchair with sip-n-puff control
- Independent in power wheelchair maneuvering on level surfaces with sip-n-puff control
- Dependent in all self-care activities of daily living

Evaluation of Clinical Assessment

Gina Parsons is a 52-year-old woman with a C4 tetraplegia, ASIA A diagnosis. Gina is evaluating power wheelchairs and AT resources for return to work.

Patient's Care Needs
1. Evaluation of power wheelchairs for optimal postural alignment and pressure relief for prescription
2. Evaluate wheelchair maneuverability capabilities.
3. Evaluation of durable medical equipment needs to ease activities of daily living
4. Evaluation for return to home and work AT needs
5. Evaluation for home and work transportation needs
6. Evaluation for family and attendant training

Diagnosis and Prognosis

Diagnosis is C4 complete tetraplegia, ASIA A. Prognosis is to return to work with optimal power wheelchair for independent pressure relief, transport to and from home and work, and maneuvering in each environment. Skilled interventions for assessment and training of AT to maximize ease of activities of daily living at home and work.

Continued

CLINICAL CASE STUDY Using Assistive Technology—cont'd

Preferred Practice Patterns*

Impaired Muscle Performance (4C), Impairments Nonprogressive Spinal Cord Disorders (5H), Primary Prevention/Risk Reduction for Cardiovascular/Pulmonary Disorders (6A), Primary Prevention/Risk Reduction for Integumentary Disorders (7A)

Team Goals

1. Team to evaluate optimal wheelchair positioning
2. Team to evaluate power wheelchairs for prescription
3. Team to design a pressure relief program to prevent integumentary disorders
4. Team to evaluate patient knowledge on range of motion maintenance
5. Team to evaluate AT for return to work and ease of activities of daily living
6. Team to assess van transportation needs

Patient Goals

"I want to be able to return to my job, attend my son's college graduation, and enjoy my husband and family."

Care Plan

Treatment Plan and Rationale

- Initiate wheelchair seating evaluation
- Initiate wheelchair maneuvering evaluation
- Initiate assistive technology evaluation
- Initiate physical therapy interventions for optimal pressure relief
- Initiation of home and work van lift and transport evaluation

Interventions

- Instruct patient in joint range of motion for prevention of contracture
- Instruct patient in proper pressure relief provided by family member and wheelchair tilting features
- Instruct patient in wheelchair maneuvering using sip-n-puff and chin control options on all surfaces
- Instruct patient in AT options to maximize independence in home and work functions and ease activities of daily living
- Instruct patient in use of van lift and transportation options
- Instruct patient how to educate family and personal assistants in everyday care

Documentation and Team Communication

- Team will complete wheelchair prescription.
- Team will order equipment for home activities of daily living and EADL.
- Team will order AT to meet home and work requirements.
- Team will document pressure relief schedule and train family members.
- Team will report selected transportation option.

Follow-Up Assessment

- Biweekly team conferences for timely attainment of goals
- Reassessment for consultation with other services

Critical Thinking Exercises

Consider factors that will influence patient education, therapy, and team care decisions unique to Gina's SCI when answering the following questions:

1. What AT can allow Gina to return to her former role at home?
2. What AT can allow Gina to return to her former role in the community?
3. What AT can allow Gina to return to her former role at work?

*Guide to physical therapist practice, rev. ed. 2, Alexandria, VA, 2003, American Physical Therapy Association.

SUMMARY

Access to technology has a significant impact on the lives of individuals with SCI. Quality-of-life issues are frequently mentioned in the literature regarding AT.[4] There is also the assumption that use of AT allows for better coping strategies for their disability because of the gain of control these individuals experience as they are actively using ATs to control the environment.[15] A needs assessment looking at prior usage and potential for future usage will help with decision making for access to technologies. If the goal is to allow for access to technology from wireless locations and while in a power mobility system, users should be introduced to integrated systems that can provide access by wheelchair drive controls. Mainstream technology should be considered whenever possible because it can offer lower pricing and greater variety for individuals with SCI.

REFERENCES

1. Technology-Related Assistance for Individuals with Disabilities Act of 1994, P. L. 103-218, (March 9, 1994). 29 U.S.C. 2201 et seq: U.S. Statutes at Large, 108, 50–97.
2. Lange ML, Smith R: Technology and occupation: contemporary viewpoints, *Am J Occup Ther* 56:107-109, 2002.
3. National Spinal Cord Injury Statistics Center: *Spinal cord injury facts and figures at a glance,* University of Alabama, Birmingham: http://www.spinalcord.uab.edu. Accessed June 2006.
4. Rigby P, Ryan S, Joos S et al: Impact of electronic aids to daily living on the lives of persons with cervical spinal cord injuries, *Assist Technol* 17:89-97, 2005.
5. Jutai J, Rigby P, Ryan S et al: Psychosocial impact of electronic aids to daily living, *Assist Technol* 12:123-131, 2000.

6. Ripat J, Strock A: Users' perceptions of the impact of electronic aids to daily living throughout the acquisition process, *Assist Technol* 16:63-72, 2004.

7. Rust KL, Smith RO: Assistive technology in the measurement of rehabilitation and health outcomes: a review and analysis of instruments, *Am J Phys Med Rehabil* 84:780-793, 2005.

8. Anson D: Assistive technology. In Pendleton HM, Schultz-Krohn W, editors: *Pedretti's occupational therapy: practice skills for physical dysfunction*, ed 6, St. Louis, 2006, Mosby Elsevier.

9. LiteTouch, Inc.: www.litetouch.com and Elan Home Systems: www.elanhomesystems.com. Accessed September 25, 2007.

10. Cook AM, Polgar JM: *Cook and Hussey's assistive technologies: principles and practice*, ed 3, St. Louis, 2008, Mosby Elsevier.

11. Teirikangas J: *HAVi white paper:* http://www.tml.tkk.fi/studies or jussi.teirikangas.hut.fi. Accessed July 5, 2007.

12. V2 standards whitepaper, V1.8, (revised February 2005): www.myurc.org/whitepaper.php. Accessed July 5, 2007.

13. Craig A, Tran Y, McIsaac P et al: The efficacy and benefits of environmental control systems for the severely disabled, *Med Sci Monit* 11:RA32-39, 2005.

14. MacNeil V: Electronic aids to daily living, *Team Rehabil Rep* 9:53-56, 1998.

15. McKinley W, Tewskbury MA, Sitter P et al: Assistive technology and computer adaptations for individuals with spinal cord injury, *Neurorehabilitation* 19:141-146, 2004.

16. Anson D: Computer and EADL access for individuals with spinal cord injury, *Top Spinal Cord Inj Rehabil* 11:42-60, 2006.

17. Chubon RA, Hester MR: An enhanced standard computer keyboard system for single-finger and typing-stick typing, *J Rehabil Res Dev* 25:17-24, 1988.

18. Kanny EM, Anson DK: A pilot study comparing mouse and mouse-emulating interface devices for graphic input, *Assist Technol* 3:50-58, 1991.

19. Holme SA, Kanny EM, Guthrie MR et al: The use of environmental control units by occupational therapists in spinal cord injury and disease services, *Am J Occup Ther* 51:42-48, 1997.

20. Shone SM, Ryan S, Rigby PJ et al: Toward a comprehensive evaluation of the impact of electronic aids to daily living: evaluation of consumer satisfaction, *Disabil Rehabil* 24:115-125, 2002.

21. Demers L, Weiss-Lambrou R, Ska B: Quebec user evaluation of satisfaction with assistive technology (QUEST): a new outcome measure. In Sprigle S, editor: *Let's tango: partnering people and technology. Proceedings of RESNA 1997 annual conference*, Arlington, VA, 1997, RESNA.

SOLUTIONS TO CHAPTER 13 CLINICAL CASE STUDY

Using Assistive Technology

1. Several assistive devices should be evaluated for home activities. After Gina's power wheelchair has been chosen and the home environment is made ready, arrangements for ATs to facilitate home entry and perform household functions from the wheelchair and bed can be made. For example, a wheelchair-mounted remote control can be programmed to turn on exterior lighting using integrated technology to enable safe entry into the home. Also from the wheelchair, the same integrated technology can be used to program the thermostat because individuals with tetraplegia have problems with their temperature control and the ability to control the thermostat is essential for comfort and safety in the home environment. Depending on what functions Gina will need to perform when her husband and adult children are not present, other assistive devices can be adopted. For example, Gina will want to be able to turn various electronic devices in her home on and off such as a TV, music system, and lights. She also will want to control these same functions when she is in bed by using an electronically programmed remote control that can manage multiple household functions, including elevation of the head of her bed. Most important, telephone access needs to be embedded within the wheelchair and bed systems to allow for outside and emergency communication. This high-technology assistive device controller will allow Gina to operate control switches on the telephone using sip-n-puff or chin controls. Practice in learning how to operate these devices will be essential in making and answering calls, using call waiting, and becoming independent in her home environment.

2. For Gina to return to her former role in the community, transportation services will need to be arranged. Her role as a soup kitchen volunteer will need to be modified from serving food to managing others who serve the food. Her access will require power-wheeled mobility that can maneuver in tight spaces. Gina will need to develop a high level of wheelchair mobility skills and the ability to perform wheelchair tilting features for pressure relief throughout the day. Again, a wheelchair mounted control box that can enable sip-n-puff or chin control to make telephone calls will be essential.

3. For Gina to return to work as a law librarian, many of the same features needed to return to her home and community will be necessary, such as sip-n-puff and chin control of the control box to make phone calls and manage pressure relief positions. In addition, computer use will be essential to accomplish her work responsibilities. This will require an ergonomic workstation in her work environment where Gina will be able to have the computer screen elevated on a desk so that she can view it without compromising neck posture. In addition, Gina will have to learn to type using sip-n-puff controls because a voice-activated system would not be realistic in a library. This will require training and practice to enable specialized features such as typing capital letters and other specialized notations. A wireless laptop mounted on her lap tray that can upload periodicals and other databases is another option to provide access within the library work environment. This will allow Gina to move away from the workstation to provide library support to patrons by searching the database mounted on a lap tray and operated with her sip-n-puff controller.

CHAPTER FOURTEEN

Accessible Home Modification and Durable Medical Equipment

Sean McCarthy, OTR/L, ATP, MS, and Cynthia Nead, Senior COTA

During the 25-plus years that I've lived with a disability, it has always been essential to lead my life as normally as possible. With that in mind, it was important to my wife and me that we make our house look like a home and not like a hospital or institution. Our accessible home design has not only increased my confidence and independence, it has allowed me to share special moments with the significant people in my life. Our newly remodeled kitchen is a joy to work in and looks sharp.

(Michael C5-6 SCI)

Since 1973, federally funded model spinal cord injury (SCI) care systems have been generating data from numerous research projects oriented toward the establishment of an effective, goal-oriented continuum of care for individuals with SCI. Advances in the medical management and rehabilitation of individuals with SCI have contributed to improved functional outcomes and a move toward independent living in progressively shorter periods of time. In the past, the majority of individuals with SCI were not expected to return to a level of functional independence comparable with their preinjury status. Today, the establishment of coordinated systems of SCI care and the passage of major disability legislation has contributed to more effective rehabilitation that is directed toward discharging patients to their homes.

According to the National Spinal Cord Injury Statistical Center (NSCISC) in Birmingham, Alabama, approximately 88% of all individuals who were discharged from a model SCI center since 1999 have been sent to a private residence that was most often their home before the onset of injury.[1] This positive trend toward successful discharge to the private home has been precipitated by numerous advances in the medical management of SCI in conjunction with changes in society's perception of disability. Federally mandated accessibility laws have made public accommodations and federally funded housing more accessible to millions of individuals with disabilities. Principles of universal design have slowly begun to change the way in which private residences are built so that each home is made more accessible to all people of varying levels of ability. Until universal design principles are fully integrated into the U.S. housing market, however, the majority of homes will require extensive modifications to ensure accessibility for individuals with SCIs. This chapter identifies the process of ensuring the successful discharge of individuals with SCI after inpatient rehabilitation. Particular emphasis is placed on discharge planning to the home environment; however, alternative discharge placements for individuals with SCI are also reviewed. Specifically, the home assessment process is outlined along with general wheelchair-accessible home modification suggestions. Essential accessibility legislation, housing design characteristics, and sources of home modification funding are also reviewed. In addition, information is provided about the durable medical equipment (DME) needs of individuals with SCI.

REHABILITATION CENTER ENVIRONMENT

The National Institute on Disability and Rehabilitation Research (NIDRR) was created by congress in 1978 under the U.S. Department of Education to assist with the coordination of research programs that would serve to promote independent living among individuals with disabilities. In addition to funding research that has supported the Americans with Disabilities Act (ADA) of 2004[2] and the integration of universal design principles into the built environment, NIDRR currently sponsors 14 model SCI care systems located throughout the United States.[3] Each model system is responsible for the collection of information relative to the continuity of SCI care starting with admission to the acute care setting, to inpatient rehabilitation, and, finally, after discharge from the model system. The NSCISC is responsible for assembling all information collected by each model system into the SCI database. This information has played an integral role in the way in which rehabilitation services are delivered and has ultimately assisted in improving the quality of life of individuals with SCI.

Each of these federally funded model systems are composed, in part, of acute rehabilitation centers that offer coordinated inpatient, outpatient, and community-based rehabilitative services oriented toward maximizing functional performance and community reintegration after SCI. Each model center relies on an interdisciplinary, patient-focused approach to rehabilitation to develop a plan of care that is tailored to individual needs. Highly trained medical and rehabilitative staff evaluate newly injured individuals admitted to a model rehabilitation center and initiate the discharge planning process immediately. Discharge planning is discussed by clinicians from all disciplines with a patient and his family on admission to ensure that all members of the rehabilitation team are working toward the same functional end in an appropriate and timely manner. If the patient is to be discharged to his home, inevitably some home modifications must be undertaken to ensure wheelchair accessibility. It is during the inpatient phase of the rehabilitation process that the patient and his family are given the tools and information needed to ensure a safe and successful discharge to the home.

INSTITUTIONAL AND GROUP CARE ENVIRONMENTS

Unfortunately, approximately 12% of individuals with SCI are unable to return to their homes after inpatient rehabilitation, with 5% being discharged to nursing homes.[1] The remaining 7% are discharged to other hospitals, group homes, assisted living centers, or other facilities on both a permanent and nonpermanent basis.[1] Individuals are often discharged to such alternative environments because of medical instability, inadequate funding, inability to complete home modifications, lack of family support, and any other internal or external factor that would make discharge to the home inappropriate or unsafe. It is important to have a general understanding of the overall structure and function of many of these alternative discharge environments to assist in the attainment of an optimal match between the individual and the given discharge location.

Nursing homes or long-term care facilities offer a variety of services ranging from rehabilitation to custodial care.[4] Custodial care is oriented toward serving the needs of individuals without rehabilitation goals, who require consistent nursing services. Long-term care facilities are often reserved for individuals who require consistent supervision, significant assistance with all activities of daily living (ADL), and lack an appropriate family support system. Individuals with remaining rehabilitation goals may be admitted to a facility that offers a subacute level of care. Subacute units are often part of long-term care facilities but may also be associated with acute-care hospitals and rehabilitation centers.[4]

Subacute programs offer less intense rehabilitation than acute-level programs do and often serve as transitional care centers for individuals who are waiting for the completion of home modifications but no longer require the intensive therapeutic services offered by the acute rehabilitation setting. Admission to subacute programs is highly dependent on insurance coverage, bed availability, and the presence of measurable and appropriate therapeutic goals. In contrast to facility-based subacute and long-term care discharge placements, some individuals with SCIs may be placed in community-based group homes that act as private residences equipped with 24-hour supervision. Group homes are typically operated by nonprofit societies and provide residents with peer support, counseling, and independent living skills training. Younger individuals who may be capable of more independent living and are seeking services such as vocational skills training often prefer the group home setting.

Ultimately, there are multiple factors that determine an appropriate discharge placement for each individual. However, the safety of the individual must always serve as a guide to making informed decisions regarding both temporary and long-term discharge plans.

ACCESSIBLE HOUSING
Housing Designs

Four types of housing design are considered by rehabilitation specialists when assessing the needs of an individual with SCI: accessible, adaptable, transgenerational, and universal. Each type of housing design has a primary objective that is interrelated to the formulation of a home designed to meet the needs of clients with SCI and their families.

Accessible design meets prescribed code requirements for individuals with specific disabilities.[5] For example, the 1990 ADA accessibility guidelines defined the minimum code requirements for wheelchair accessibility in public buildings.[6,7] These codes include the components of an accessible route through the house, turning space allowances, ramp slope allowances, and many other elements for building accessibility. Each of these accessibility guidelines is based on the minimum clear width of a standard

adult manual wheelchair, which is defined as 32 inches wide and 48 inches long. Power wheelchairs are larger and may require additional clearance space. The accessible guidelines established by the ADA commonly invoke a hospital-like or institutional look that is devoid of individuality and is often negatively received by individuals and the housing marketplace.[8]

Unfortunately, many inexperienced architects and builders rely heavily on broad-based accessibility standards to provide wheelchair-accessible housing to individuals after SCI. It is important to understand that considerable variability exists among both wheelchair users and the wheelchairs currently available in the marketplace. Accessibility guidelines do not take such variation into account and should never serve as a substitute for individualized home assessment based on the specific functional abilities and goals of the individual. These guidelines were developed to articulate the civic minimal requirements that must be implemented by places of employment, public accommodations, and commercial facilities. Minimum accessibility guidelines are often inappropriate for the creation of a truly wheelchair accessible private home and often do little more than provide access through the home's front door and bathroom.

Adaptable housing design refers to modifications made to an existing or standard design for the purpose of making a home usable by an individual.[9] Examples include the removal of cabinets from under the kitchen sink and the addition of insulation around the sink's plumbing to allow for safe wheelchair access to avoid leg burns from touching hot pipes with insensate skin. Clients with SCI who return to their homes after rehabilitation tend to prefer adaptable housing designs. The extent of adaptations required depends on the functional abilities of the client and on the current level of the home's accessibility. Extensive home adaptations are often costly and time-consuming ventures that must be considered early during inpatient rehabilitation to ensure readiness at discharge. The ability to adapt the design of the home to the specific needs of the individual wheelchair user is essential to ensuring a positive transition from inpatient rehabilitation to home.

Transgenerational housing describes a design that takes into account those changes that occur over an individual's life span.[9] It is important to consider this concept when making home modification recommendations for manual wheelchair users who potentially may change to a power wheelchair over time. Differences between manual and power wheelchairs include turning radius, weight, and overall dimensions; accommodation to these essential features will affect the home design. It also is important to identify potential functional changes that individuals with SCI may achieve over time to decrease the need for additional home adaptation in the future.

Universal design allows products and environments to be used by all people, to the greatest extent possible, without need for adaptation or specialized design.[10] Homes that are universally designed strive to be as accessible as possible to the widest range of individuals with varied abilities. Universal design includes all of the major design categories and is primarily found in new construction. The principles of universal design may be used as a guide for making informed decisions concerning the individual

BOX 14-1 | Principles of Universal Design

PRINCIPLE ONE: Equitable Use

The design is useful and marketable to people with diverse abilities.

- Provide the same means of use for all users: identical whenever possible; equivalent when not.
- Avoid segregating or stigmatizing any users.
- Provisions for privacy, security, and safety should be equally available to all users.
- Make the design appealing to all users.

PRINCIPLE TWO: Flexibility in Use

The design accommodates a wide range of individual preferences and abilities

- Provide choice in methods of use.
- Accommodate right- or left-handed access and use.
- Facilitate the user's accuracy and precision.
- Provide adaptability to the user's pace.

PRINCIPLE THREE: Simple and Intuitive Use

Use of the design is easy to understand, regardless of the user's experience, knowledge, language skills, or current concentration level.

- Eliminate unnecessary complexity.
- Be consistent with user expectations and intuition.
- Accommodate a wide range of literacy and language skills.
- Arrange information consistent with its importance.
- Provide effective prompting and feedback during and after task completion.

PRINCIPLE FOUR: Perceptible Information

The design communicates necessary information effectively to the user, regardless of ambient conditions or the user's sensory abilities.

- Use different modes (pictorial, verbal, tactile) for redundant presentation of essential information.
- Provide adequate contrast between essential information and its surroundings.
- Maximize "legibility" of essential information.
- Differentiate elements in ways that can be described (i.e., make it easy to give instructions or directions).
- Provide compatibility with a variety of techniques or devices used by people with sensory limitations.

PRINCIPLE FIVE: Tolerance for Error

The design minimizes hazards and the adverse consequences of accidental or unintended actions.

- Arrange elements to minimize hazards and errors: most used elements, most accessible; hazardous elements eliminated, isolated, or shielded.
- Provide warnings of hazards and errors.
- Provide fail-safe features.
- Discourage unconscious action in tasks that require vigilance.

PRINCIPLE SIX: Low Physical Effort

The design can be used efficiently and comfortably and with a minimum of fatigue

- Allow user to maintain a neutral body position.
- Use reasonable operating forces.
- Minimize repetitive actions.
- Minimize sustained physical effort.

PRINCIPLE SEVEN: Size and Space for Approach and Use

Appropriate size and space is provided for approach, reach, manipulation, and use regardless of user's body size, posture, or mobility.

- Provide a clear line of sight to important elements for any seated or standing user.
- Make reach to all components comfortable for any seated or standing user.
- Accommodate variations in hand and grip size.
- Provide adequate space for the use of assistive devices or personal assistance.

From Connell BR, Jones M, Mace R et al: *The principles of universal design*, version 2.0, Raleigh, NC, 1997, North Carolina State University.

home modification needs of a new wheelchair user and his family and their needs over the course of their life spans (Box 14-1).[10] Such homes consider changes that occur throughout the life span and allow individuals with disabilities and other family members to coexist without disruption or limitation in participation within the home.

Incorporation of universal design concepts into new housing construction will minimize the need for extensive home modifications that are often costly and aesthetically displeasing. In addition, the universally designed home may reduce the need for assistive technology devices and the use of special services. Unfortunately, the majority of homes are still built using standard design codes instead of the principles of universal design. When the principles of universal design are more readily accepted as a vital component in the construction of new housing, the process of providing wheelchair-accessible homes will become a less laborious and costly venture for patients who wish to return to their homes after discharge from rehabilitation. Responsible health care professionals may use the principles of universal design as

tools to guide the home assessment process, to respect the aesthetics of the home by minimizing the institutional look, and to aid in the successful integration of clients with SCI into their homes. Easter Seals Disability Services has developed supporting information for home accessibility through a partnership with Century 21 Realty, which provides brochures on the availability of easy-access housing.[11]

Public and Private Housing Legislation

The successful return home by individuals with SCI depends on many factors, including medical status, functional status, family structure, financial assets, and the availability of wheelchair-accessible housing.[12] The ability to locate wheelchair-accessible housing has and continues to be a fundamental problem in the United States. According to Steinfeld et al,[13] only 10% of the 100 million housing units available in the United States are accessible. Since the early 1960s, the federal government has slowly recognized the problem of limited wheelchair accessibility in the public sector and more recently in the context of the private home. In

1988, Congress passed the Fair Housing Amendments Act, which requires that all new multifamily dwellings consisting of four or more units, public and private, is accessible to individuals with disabilities.[8]

This act included accessibility provisions for rental housing, by clearly articulating a wheelchair user's right to make necessary home modifications to allow for accessibility.[13] It is important for the responsible members of the rehabilitation team to understand the legal rights of tenants and the obligations of landlords when attempting to make reasonable and necessary accessibility modifications to a rented home. The Fair Housing Amendments Act was the first to acknowledge that homes designed according to standard accessibility guidelines do not necessarily ensure access for all individuals with disabilities.[8]

In 1990, the ADA was enacted and established full civil rights protections to individuals with disabilities.[6,7] Overall, the ADA does not specifically address housing accessibility except for public facilities such as motels, hotels, and dormitories.[5] Title III of the ADA is of particular importance, however, because it established accessibility guidelines for all public buildings, businesses, and homes that are either partially or fully funded by the federal government.[6,7] Although the ADA served as a major victory for individuals with disabilities in the realm of public accommodations, it did little to change the accessibility status of private single-family homes.

THE CLIENT'S PERSPECTIVE   Accessibility Standards

It's important to understand that most environments don't meet accessibility standards. Many of the homes of our friends and family will not have accessible bathrooms, nor will hotels or other spaces we may encounter in our journeys. We have to develop our own list criteria for what we need to be comfortable within any environment, which needs to take into account the amount of time we will be spending in that location. We should know the width of our chairs, from wheel to wheel or push rim to push rim, so that we know how wide a doorway needs to be to wheel through it. That way, we can tell someone to measure the space before we get to the location so we'll know whether we can get in. Always being as prepared as possible makes our experiences more comfortable, and if we know we will not be comfortable, it can be appropriate to try and change the location or just decline the invitation.

Sarah Everhart Skeels

Currently, there are no state or federal accessibility laws that apply to the construction of single-family homes or other forms of private housing. Some states have introduced bills to create ordinances or guidelines on how new homes can be built with use of universal design features.[14] Numerous states and cities have established visitability ordinance initiatives, which pertain to the construction of publicly and privately funded homes. The concept of visitability refers to homes that are constructed with at least one no-step entrance and at least one half-bath (preferably a full bath) on the main floor and that provide for 32 inches of clear passage through all interior doors, including bathrooms.[15] By embracing the concept of visitability in the construction of individual homes, the choices in homes that individuals with

SCI can reside in or visit will be dramatically increased without the need for extensive adaptation. Many supporters of the visitability movement argue that universal design in construction is a right that should be afforded to all people.[14] For this right to someday be realized, education, training, and advocacy need to continue in both mainstream society and the housing industry. Increasing awareness about the benefits of universal design will facilitate positive changes in home access for everyone, including individuals with SCI.

Home Modification Funding Sources

Making a home accessible for individuals with SCI is essential to ensuring a positive transition from inpatient rehabilitation to life in the community. Rehabilitation professionals, patients, families, and medical insurers agree that home modifications are necessary for the majority of patients who wish to return to their residences. Major medical insurers, including Medicare and Medicaid, however, disagree with heath care providers and patients when it comes to funding necessary modifications. Although there is considerable variability between each person's health care benefits, there is little variability when it comes to covering home modifications. The majority of insurance benefits do not offer coverage for home modification costs, and insurers often require that a home assessment be carried out before the approval of other benefits, such as coverage of DME. Lack of funding from medical insurers places the burden of financing home modifications on the patient and his family.

There are instances in which home modification costs are covered by third-party insurers. Individuals who are injured while at work and are in receipt of Workers' Compensation benefits typically receive funding for necessary home modifications. In addition, some automobile insurance benefits may be used to fund home modifications, but automobile insurance policies typically have a preset funding limit that may also be used to cover medical bills. Therefore, it is important to identify what insurance coverage is designated as primary or secondary so that automobile insurance funds may potentially be held for home modification costs. It is also important to refer patients to their designated social service worker or case manager so that they fully understand and appropriately manage their insurance benefits.

In some instances, funding may be provided from designated federal legislation, such as Section 504 of the Rehabilitation Act of 1973. According to section 504, landlords who are in receipt of federal housing funds are required to pay for accessible home modifications.[13] For those individuals who do not reside in federally assisted housing, the U.S. Department of Housing and Urban Development (HUD) offers home improvement loan programs that make it easier to finance affordable home modifications. In addition, HUD provides contact information for local housing and community development offices that have the ability to access community block grants and other home improvement funds.

In addition, local charitable organizations, independent fund raisers, and community service groups offer another avenue to funding, labor, or necessary materials required to successfully modify the home for wheelchair access.[13] Ultimately, the burden of financing home modifications for the majority of individuals with SCI falls on the patient and his family. To enhance successful rehabilitation, the therapy team needs to provide as much information as possible about potential funding sources early in the inpatient rehabilitation process.

Preparing for Discharge: Home Accessibility Assessment

When a patient with SCI is admitted to an inpatient rehabilitation facility, members of the therapy team including the physiatrist, occupational therapist, physical therapist, nursing staff, social worker, and psychologist complete their initial evaluations and formulate a treatment plan in preparation for discharge. The ultimate discharge plan must be formulated and discussed with the patient and designated family members during weekly team conferences that are initiated on admission. Home accessibility and discharge placement plays an integral part in team discussions from the beginning so that the home will be ready at discharge.

After the initial evaluations and the formulation of long-term goals, the patient is issued a preliminary home evaluation form that is to be completed by friends or family members (Figure 14-1). This form can be used as a means to forecast the extent of needed home modifications. It will also provide preliminary information about the home that team members can use for more in-depth assessment when needed. The specific information shows the home's design (single story or two story) and overall layout with essential dimensions. It also allows areas of concern to indicate the home's ownership status (owned or rented) and number of inhabitants (family members or roommates). The rehabilitation team can use this home assessment when making a home visit.

Sometimes, the preliminary home assessment reveals that few modifications are necessary and a more formal assessment is not needed. In these cases, the patient and his family may be educated about basic reorganization of the home and given literature about ramping for an accessible entrance and exit to the home. Typically, however, a patient requires a more in-depth review of the home by trained members of the rehabilitation team to ensure appropriate accessibility. Several patient factors may influence the home evaluation (Clinical Note: Patient Status Influencing Home Evaluation).

In these cases, the preliminary home evaluation form identifies problem areas that may serve as significant obstacles to establishing appropriate wheelchair accessibility. Formal, on-site home evaluation is required to identify all potential accessibility problem areas and to provide viable home modification suggestions. The home evaluation is typically conducted by the therapy team's occupational therapist in conjunction with the patient's home caregivers. Before this evaluation, the occupational therapist needs to gather specific patient information from each member of the rehabilitation team. The home evaluation and modification recommendations must always start with the functional needs and goals of the patient to ensure that the home environment is safe, appealing, and accessible.

A detailed home evaluation that includes photographs and sample graphs of hallway and room spaces can be used to document additional measurements, comments, and problem areas associated with the home's design. An in-home evaluation allows

CLINICAL NOTE Patient Status Influencing Home Evaluation

- Patient's diagnosis including level of injury and American Spinal Injury Association classification
- Patient's medical status including prognosis for recovery
- Patient's functional status including ability to transfer and ambulate
- Type of mobility device(s) used: manual or power wheelchair
- DME: sleep support surfaces, transfer aids, bathroom equipment
- Patient's goals: What parts of the home are deemed most important by the patient? What activities of daily living does the patient wish to engage in within the home?

the evaluating therapist to systematically assess the primary features of the home to serve as a guide to ensure that all salient aspects of the home are evaluated for accessibility. The rehabilitation team will use both approaches to generate a final home accessibility report, which includes the current status and recommendations to ensure accessibility. The final report is reviewed with the patient and his home caregivers to make sure that everyone understands the recommendations and that all goals are considered.

The patient and his family are then referred to qualified building professionals who have experience with accessible architecture and construction. These professionals bring the expertise to evaluate the home's structural components and to ensure the feasibility of all home modification recommendations. The occupational therapist must work closely with the architect or contractor to make sure that the home modification process is oriented toward the creation of a safe, patient-focused, and accessible home environment.

HOME MODIFICATIONS

General guidelines for establishing a wheelchair-accessible residence are used as a starting point on which to base specific recommendations (Box 14-2). Accessible floor plans commonly used by individuals with SCI will be described subsequently. In all cases, consultation with a qualified architect or contractor is important to ensure that the necessary modifications are consistent with the appropriate building code. Often, however, building codes, safety codes, and ADA recommendations will conflict. In those cases it is necessary to use guidelines that apply the least restrictive recommendations.[16] For instance, if a fire code states that the exit door must be 30 inches wide but the ADA states it must be 32 inches wide, then the door must be 32 inches wide to allow wheelchair accommodation.

The patient and his home caregivers should become familiar with the architects and contractors in their geographical area. It is important to visit previously remodeled homes and talk with their occupants about workmanship and usage satisfaction. Discovering the advantages and disadvantages of their experiences helps to clarify decisions for the current modification

Family dynamics are important to the planning as well. Family includes anyone who is living within the residence where the

PRELIMINARY HOME EVALUATION FORM

In order to provide ease of patient transition from the inpatient setting to home, please complete this form and return it to the therapy department as soon as possible. This information will assist in identifying potential durable medical equipment needs and will serve as a starting point from which accessibility recommendations can be made.

If you have any questions, please contact:_____ Phone #:_____

PATIENT: _____ Room #: _____ Phone #: _____

HOME ADDRESS: _____

HOME & ENTRANCE EVALUATION

HOME	House ❑ Apartment ❑ Townhouse ❑ Other ❑ No. of Floors ___
APPROACH	Level ❑ Sloped ❑ Paved ❑ Stone ❑ Other ❑
PRIMARY ENTRANCE	Stairs ❑ Number ____ Stair height _____ Railings ❑ R❑ L❑ Both ❑ Landing ❑ Width & depth _____ Other ❑
ENTRANCE DOOR	Width (door to molding) _____ Width (molding to molding) _____ Opens In ❑ Opens Out ❑ Screen door ❑ Lever handle ❑
SECONDARY ENTRANCE	Stairs ❑ Number ____ Stair height _____ Railings ❑ R❑ L❑ Both ❑ Landing ❑ Width & depth _____ Other ❑
ENTRANCE DOOR	Width (door to molding) _____ Width (molding to molding) _____ Opens In ❑ Opens Out ❑ Screen door ❑ Lever handle ❑

INTERIOR ACCESS EVALUATION

HALLWAYS	Width _____ Carpeted ❑ Hardwood ❑ Tile ❑ Other ❑
INTERIOR STAIRS	Yes ❑ Number __ Width ___ Depth ___ Height ___ Railings ❑ R❑ L❑ Both ❑
INTERIOR DOORS	Width (door to molding) _____ Width (molding to molding) _____ Opens In ❑ Opens Out ❑ Lever handle ❑ Other ❑
OTHER AREAS OF CONCERN:	

COMMUNAL LIVING AREAS

LIVING ROOM	Dimensions:	Floor surface:	Clear path for wc access (32" min) ❑	Please provide room diagram.
DINING ROOM	Dimensions:	Floor surface:	Clear path for wc access (32" min) ❑	Table height (floor to base) _____
KITCHEN	Dimensions:	Floor surface:	Clear path for wc access (32" min) ❑	Counter height ___
KITCHEN APPLIANCES	Refrigerator: Side-by-side ❑ Top-bottom ❑	Sink: Lever faucet ❑ Clearance: _____	Stove/oven: Gas ❑ Electric ❑ Controls: Front ❑ Rear ❑	Kitchen table ❑ Height (floor to base): _____

FIGURE 14-1 Preliminary home evaluation form. *Continued*

patient with SCI will reside. Daily routines influence the home modifications needed; the more a person with an SCI is alone, the more modifications are required. For instance, if there is someone at home to help with meal preparation, then the kitchen modifications can be kept to a minimum; if not, counter height and cabinet and appliance access must be considered. Operating appliances, environmental temperature control, getting in and out of bed, bathing, toileting, dressing, and meal preparation are all areas for consideration to ensure that the person with SCI can perform these functions either independently or with caregiver assistance (see Chapter 9). Importantly, the person with an SCI must be able to vacate the home independently in the case of

OTHER AREAS OF CONCERN:				
PERSONAL LIVING AREAS				
BEDROOM	Dimensions:	Floor surface:	Location:	Please provide room diagram.
BED	Height:	Clearance: Under _____ Along right side _____ Left side _____ In front to nearest object or wall _____		
BATHROOM	Dimensions:	Floor surface:	Location:	Please provide room diagram.
SHOWER & TUB	Interior height: _____	Exterior height: _____	Width: _____	Curtain ❑ Glass door ❑
SHOWER STALL	Width: _____	Depth: _____	Other:	
SINK	Height (floor to base) _____	Lever faucet ❑	Describe area under sink:	
TOILET	Height _____	Distances: From right edge _____ Left edge _____ In front of toilet to the nearest object or wall _____		
OTHER AREAS OF CONCERN:				
RECOMMENDATIONS (Rehabilitation Team):				

FIGURE 14-1, cont'd Preliminary home evaluation form.

a fire or other emergency, regardless of whether a caregiver is present.

In addition, it is important to understand that people with SCI are extremely sensitive to extremes in temperature and they are unable to regulate their own body temperatures. Often the most obvious place to begin the home remodeling is a garage or basement area; however, one drawback to these two areas is that stringent temperature controls must be added along with high levels of insulation. Air conditioning is required in warm weather and heat in cold weather, both with independently operated thermostat controls. Because these two areas may be isolated from the rest of the home, their use may increase social isolation and present major access problems to other key areas of the home.

Home Exterior

Accessible parking in a covered area that provides protection from inclement weather needs to be positioned as close as possible to the nearest accessible entrance to the home. Wheelchair-accessible parking spaces for cars measure at least 8 feet wide and allow for at least 5 feet of space along side the car to facilitate transfers. If the patient will use a van equipped with a lift, at least 8 feet of space is required to accommodate a van lift that projects from the side of the vehicle (Figure 14-2). For vans that are equipped with a rear entry lift, at least 25 feet of length from the van door is necessary to accommodate the van's ramp.

The parking surface and accessible route to the front entrance should consist of a smooth, continuous, and level surface

BOX 14-2 | General Considerations for an Accessible Home

- Make all rooms of the house accessible.
- Ensure that primary living areas have complete wheelchair access, including doors to any room with a minimum clearance width of 32 inches if the doorway does not require a turn to access and a minimum clearance width of 36 inches if the doorway requires a 90-degree turn to access.
- Alter thresholds to be no greater than 1 inch, allowing the person in the wheelchair to maneuver.
- Install and maintain smoke detectors throughout the home.
- Use hardwood or uncarpeted floors for easiest wheelchair travel; a low pile, high-density type carpet is recommended if it is in place or desired.
- Remove or rearrange furniture that will impede wheelchair access.
- Notify police and fire departments that an individual with a disability resides in the home and provide them with the bedroom location.
- Install an intercom system between the bedroom and main living areas.

- Provide backup power if the individual is dependent on equipment for life support (e.g., ventilator).
- Make sure light switches are at a height of no more than 36 inches.
- Remove molding surrounded doorways if more space is needed to gain wheelchair accessibility.
- Place lazy Susans or circular rotating shelves in cabinets and the refrigerator to allow easy access.
- Consider installing power door openers using a remote or push plate on the wall to accommodate independent access by the wheelchair user.
- Use power window or drapery openers for individuals with SCI who are alone for long periods and may need to regulate temperature or light in a room.
- Eliminate throw rugs because they pose a hazard for ambulation, transfers, and wheelchair use.

Data from Eberhardt K: Home modifications for persons with spinal cord injury, *OT Pract* November:*24-27*, 1998; Stiens S, Kirshblum S, Groah S et al: Spinal cord injury medicine, 4: optimal participation in life after spinal cord injury: physical, psychological, and economic reintegration into the environment, *Arch Phys Med Rehabil* 83(1 Suppl):S72-S81, 2002; and Easter Seals: *Easter Seals disability services partnership with Century 21 on home accessibility*:: http://www.easterseals.com/site/PageServer?pagename=ntlc_easyaccesshousing_tips. Accessed May 2007.

THE CLIENT'S PERSPECTIVE   Transition from Rehab to Home

Remember that we are all individuals and our routines won't match everyone else's regardless of whether we have a disability or are able-bodied.
 Helpful Hints:
- Use everything you've learned in rehab and integrate most of it into your daily routine, but like everything else, some things will need to be adapted to fit comfort levels and time constraints
- Flexibility is always key
- Some days are completely smooth sailing; on others, everything seems to go wrong
- Maintain focus, even when rushing to get somewhere
- Make sure you get out of the house as much as possible, even if it's just to roll around the neighborhood or the mall; it will get you involved with what's going on outside of your life
- Keep a sense of humor
- Know that life is full of challenges and sometimes things just go wrong
- Adjust the schedule because it's going to take more time to do things in the beginning
- Learn to budget time because it helps minimize our stress and the stress of others who may be helping us
- Repetition leads to gradual ease, and down the road we'll need less time and energy to accomplish the same tasks
- We need to be patient with ourselves and those around us as we work through this adjustment period

Scott Chesney and Sarah Everhart Skeels

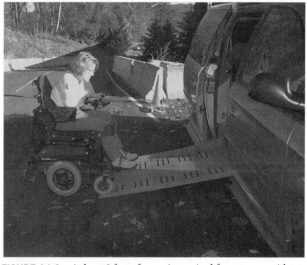

FIGURE 14-2 At least 8 feet of space is required for a person with tetraplegia using a power wheelchair to negotiate a side entry ramp to an accessible van.

Entrances

It is important that all entrance areas also are well lit and their surfaces consist of smooth, continuous, level, and skid-resistant materials that enhance traction and allow for proper drainage.[17] When steps are present, several options are available for remodeling the home's entry, including the addition of prefabricated or custom-built ramping, regrading the ground leading up to the entrance, or installation of mechanical lifts.

There are numerous prefabricated ramping systems available on the market today. The advantages of prefabricated ramps include portability, cost containment, and increased ease of

that does not exceed a slope greater than 20 inches of length for every 1 inch in height. These areas need to be well lit for increased safety and may be equipped with motion sensitive lighting to allow for hands-free illumination of the area.

installation. In general, ramps are constructed of fire retardant materials and built with a slope not exceeding 12 inches in length for every 1 inch in rise (Figure 14-3, *A, B,* and *D*).

A covered ramp offers protection from inclement weather. The required dimensions include a path 36 to 40 inches wide with a level platform at all landings, including at the doorway, of at least 5 feet by 5 feet (Figure 14-3, *A* and *C*). Adequate space at the doorway landing is critical for safe door management.

Safety requirements include curbs approximately 4 inches in height along with handrails positioned at a minimum of 2 feet 6 inches in height on both sides of the ramp. Ramps are divided into 10- to 12-foot sections with the number and size of expansion joints kept to a minimum. Whenever the ramp changes direction, a platform landing separates it (Figure 14-4). These landings also provide rest areas. The amount of space available, functional ability of the patient, and type of mobility device used all contribute to the final design of the ramp.

The most attractive option for adapting entrances with stairways is to regrade the home's front landscape so that it is level with the front entrance. Interestingly, regrading is often less expensive then installing a ramp but should adhere to the same slope and safety requirements.

Mechanical lifts are often necessary for homes with dramatic level changes and minimal space to accommodate the appropriate amount of ramping (Figure 14-5, *A* and *C*). In addition, safety devices such as ramp gates are important considerations (Figure 14-5, *B*). Unfortunately, mechanical lifts require maintenance and an external power source and may not be aesthetically pleasing. As with any custom device, mechanical lifts must be installed by qualified home modification professionals.

The entrance door landing must be level with the living space floor. The entrance door needs to swing inward away from the confined space of the porch landing and steps and is unencumbered by a storm door. The entryway must be at least 32 inches wide as measured from door to molding if no turn is involved in the landing space during door management. Lever-type door handles are easier to open for people with limited hand function. The use of offset door hinges allows the door to swing clear of the doorway.

Because individuals with restricted mobility are vulnerable to hazards, especially fire, two remotely located exits from any residence are recommended. An accessible secondary exit allows all occupants the opportunity to vacate the house in the event of an emergency.

General Considerations Within the Home

As mentioned previously, individuals with SCI have difficulty regulating their body temperatures below the level of injury in both hot and cold environments. Therefore, the ability to regulate the temperature of the home by heating and air conditioning is critical to the health and safety of the individual. Position temperature controls at a height to allow for independent access from the wheelchair.

A backup generator or external power source is often necessary to power life-sustaining medical equipment, such as a ventilator, during temporary losses of power. Equipping the home with an intercom system provides for daily communication within the house or during an emergency.

In multistory homes, floor-to-floor access is desirable and may be necessary. One option available for individuals with good transfer skills is a stair-glide. Stair-glides are seats that glide up and down a track that has been mounted to an existing staircase. Stair-glides are available from numerous manufacturers in a variety of configurations. Some models are manufactured to accommodate curved or even spiral staircases. Despite their ability to manage numerous types of staircases, some staircases may not be appropriate for safe use with individuals with SCI. A qualified contractor or product representative should always be consulted regarding the safe and appropriate installation of a stair-glide. In addition, it is critical to select a stair-glide that has the appropriate weight capacity, seating dimensions, and support needed for safe management on the staircase. It is also important to examine the dimensions of a given stair-glide relative to the overall dimensions of the staircase because there needs to be adequate room for a caregiver or other household member to access the staircase.

Stair-glides suitable for most individuals with SCI should be equipped with folding arms, an adjustable seat height, padded seating surfaces, accessible controls, and the ability to swivel the seat away from the staircase up to 90 degrees (Figure 14-6). These factors will allow for safe and appropriate transfers, positioning, stability, skin protection, and control of the device.

Overall, stair-glides are typically less expensive and easier to install than wheelchair lifts and elevators. However, stair-glides require additional transfers for floor-to-floor access and force the need for a secondary wheelchair. Unfortunately, a secondary wheelchair for the home is commonly not covered by most insurance companies and should be factored into the overall equipment cost.

When a stair-glide is not feasible because of construction or cost constraints, a wheelchair that can negotiate stairs, such as the Scalamobil, can be used. This portable, battery-powered device aids a person in a wheelchair to ascend and descend steps with the help of one person (Figure 14-7). The Scalamobil is not compatible with all manual wheelchairs and is not able to assist individuals seated in a power wheelchair. Those individuals who are appropriate for power wheelchair mobility may consider a wheelchair with stair-climbing capability, such as the iBOT 4000 (Independence Technology, Inc.). Appropriate users can ascend and descend properly constructed stairs equipped with one or two railings independently or by means of the assistance of a trained caregiver. Before considering the Scalamobil or the iBOT 4000, it is important to review wheelchair compatibility, stair compatibility, cost of the device versus the cost of modifying the home, and the need for a trained caregiver to operate either device safely.

Mechanical lifts or elevators can be installed to allow individuals who lack good postural control and transfer skills access to multiple floors. Careful attention to the overall dimensions and weight capacity of a residential lift or elevator will ensure that the wheelchair fits and has the necessary radius for entrance and exit maneuverability. Contact a lift manufacturer to determine how best to meet the patient's needs. Again a backup power source is required to operate stair-glides and lifts, thereby ensuring safe exit from the home in case of an emergency during an electrical power outage.

Doorways

All doorways need to be a minimum of 32 inches wide for a manual wheelchair and 34 inches wide for a power wheelchair. If the wheelchair user cannot access the doorway head on and a turn is required, the doorway must be 36 inches wide. Offset hinges

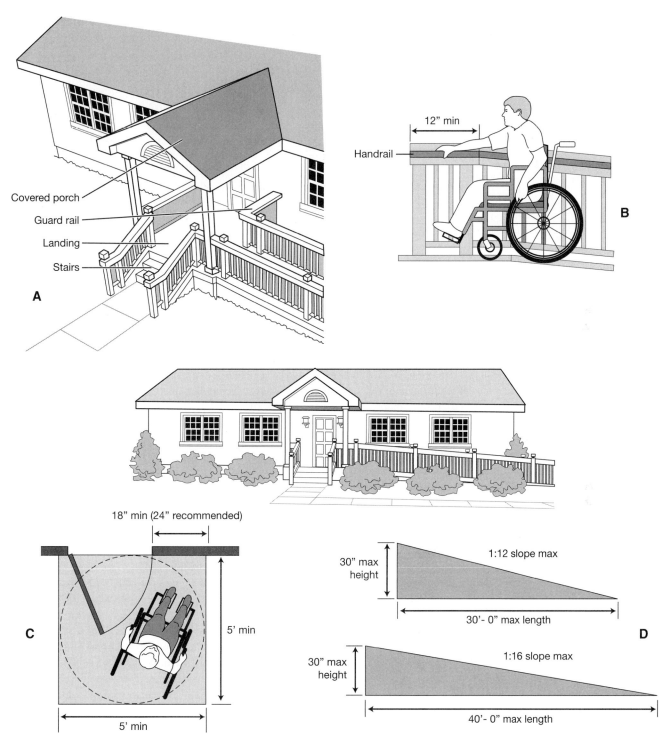

FIGURE 14-3 **A,** A covered landing protects against inclement weather and acts as a good transition between the stairs and ramp. **B,** Guardrails and balustrades should be 30 to 36 inches above the ramp floor with easy-to-grip round or oval handrails sections that are at least 12 inches long. **C,** The landing configuration at the front door entrance allows space for the door to open. It includes both the minimum 5 × 5 foot entry clearance opening and at least 18 inches of space on the latch side of the door. **D,** Two possible slope configurations: (1) a 1:12 slope (i.e., 12 inches of ramp for every inch of rise) resulting in a 30-foot length to achieve a 30 inch height and (2) a 1:16 slope resulting in a longer ramp of 40 feet in length over the same 30-inch height, which can be an easier rise for some individuals to push or walk up. (Adapted from Duncan R: *Wood ramp design: how to add a ramp that looks good and works too*, Raleigh, NC, 2004, Center for Universal Design, North Carolina State University.)

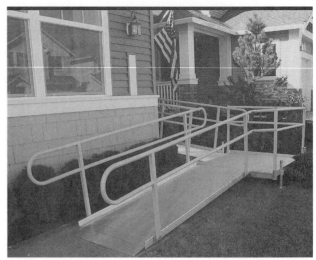

FIGURE 14-4 Exterior ramps can be configured in a number of ways to be compact and cost efficient. The L-shaped EZ-Access modular ramp has a platform that allows for safe maneuvering around the turn and an opportunity for resting. (Courtesy HomeCare Products, Inc., and Abby Lifts Inc., Toms River, NJ.)

increase overall door width up to 2 inches by allowing the door to swing flush with the door jamb when open. In addition, door threshold heights must be kept at 1 inch or less for smooth and unobstructed wheelchair access.

Lever style or U-shaped door handles are preferred over standard knobs, especially for individuals with tetraplegia who have impaired hand function. Lever-style door handles are easier to open because less torque is required to depress the handle. Patients who lack upper extremity function and rely on a power wheelchair equipped with specialty controls may need to use automatic or externally powered door openers. The existing wheelchair electronics and an electronic aid to daily living (EADL) can facilitate safe access through externally powered doors (see Chapter 13).

Hallways, Interior Doors, and Lighting

Hallways need to be a minimum of 36 inches in width when turning is not required. The minimum amount of space required to complete a 360-degree turn in the hallway is 5 feet by 5 feet for a manual wheelchair and 6 feet by 6 feet for a power wheelchair. The best floor surfaces are firm surfaces such as wood or smooth tile. Low pile carpeting is usually acceptable as well. All throw rugs and obstacles, however, must be removed so that wheelchair management is unimpeded.

Similarly to exterior doorways, all interior door widths need to measure a minimum of 32 inches for a manual wheelchair and 34 inches for a power wheelchair. If the wheelchair user is unable to access the doorway head on, thus requiring a turn, a doorway width of 36 inches may be necessary. Door threshold heights cannot exceed 1 inch to allow for smooth and unobstructed access.

In situations were limited space is available; a pocket door may be installed. Pocket doors can be mounted on the outside of the wall or built to slide inside the wall itself. Pocket doors are often used for bathroom access where inward swinging doors might obstruct access.

Light switches need to be located at all room and hallway entrances so that they are handy and can be illuminated for safe wheelchair access. Position all light switches at approximately 36 inches in height to allow for access from the wheelchair. A variety of light switch controls are available to accommodate the dexterity needs of the patient. Natural lighting should not be overlooked because primary windows may need to be positioned so that an unobstructed view of the outside is possible from a wheelchair-seated position. Windows may also be equipped with handles consistent with the patient's level of dexterity for opening and closing.

Bedrooms

Ideally, the wheelchair-accessible bedroom consists of adequate floor space along the bedside to allow for transfers and a full 360-degree turn. To accomplish this, remove all unnecessary furniture from the bedroom, leaving the bed, dresser, possibly a counter or desk space for vocational or computer activities, and medical equipment including a commode. Overall floor space of at least 10 feet by 14 feet with a minimum of 3 feet of floor space along side the bed is required; another passageway with a minimum of 4 feet is necessary at the end of the bed and again in front of the dressers and closet. The room should allow at least one 5 foot by 5 foot area clear of furniture for maneuvering the wheelchair.

The optimal bed height depends on the overall seat to floor height of the individual's wheelchair. Position the bed at a height that is level with the top of the wheelchair user's seat cushion. For individuals who are transferred from chair to bed by a mechanical lift, approximately 10 to 13 inches of clearance is necessary underneath the bed to accommodate the base for the free-standing lift (Figure 14-8, *A*). Lifts that are controlled by an overhead track system may be another alternative in the home environment (Figure 14-8, *B*).

An adequate number of electrical outlets should be available to accommodate the needs of individuals with high tetraplegia.

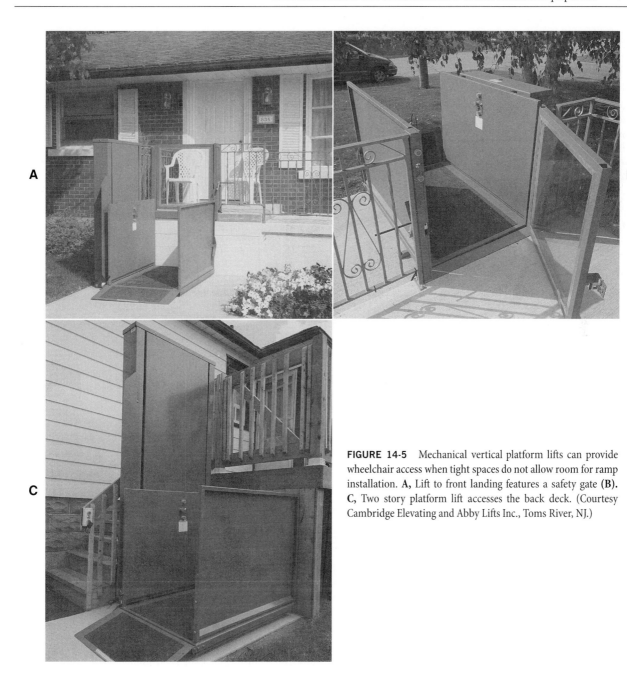

FIGURE 14-5 Mechanical vertical platform lifts can provide wheelchair access when tight spaces do not allow room for ramp installation. **A,** Lift to front landing features a safety gate **(B). C,** Two story platform lift accesses the back deck. (Courtesy Cambridge Elevating and Abby Lifts Inc., Toms River, NJ.)

Additional equipment, such as a hospital bed, respiratory equipment, and EADL devices that require electricity are often used. The layout of the room needs to consider essential appliances, including lighting and telephone, so that both can be readily available when the individual is in bed.

A roll-in closet equipped with lowered rods and shelving is ideal for the wheelchair user who possesses adequate arm and hand function to access his clothing. The closet door for a built-in closet needs a clearance width of 32 inches and a minimum 5 foot by 5 foot turning space. Folding, sliding, or pocket style doors may be a better alternative because standard doors often impede access and wheelchair maneuverability. Closet rods and shelving height are dependent on the wheelchair user's seated height and reach but are generally positioned between 36 and 48 inches in height and are no deeper than 16 inches.

Bathrooms

Depending on the person's level of injury, the bathroom is generally the room that needs the greatest modifications. First, the wheelchair accessible bathroom needs to be adjacent to the bedroom with a minimum of 8 feet by 10 feet of floor space. All electrical outlets, towel racks, and light switches should be positioned 36 inches to 40 inches from the floor. Mirrors and medicine cabinets should be positioned for viewing and access from the seated position. The bottom of the mirror or medicine cabinet is generally mounted at 40 inches from the floor.

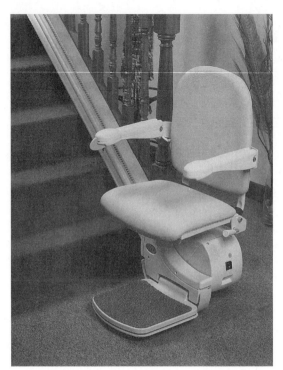

FIGURE 14-6 Stair lifts can provide access to a home's second story. The best configurations for individuals with SCI will have arms that flip up to allow transfer onto the chair and an extended footrest to support the feet without need for excessive knee bending. It also is important that the seat and footrest flip up to enable able-bodied individuals to still use the staircase. (Courtesy Sterling Stair Lifts, Inc. and Abby Lifts Inc., Toms River, NJ.)

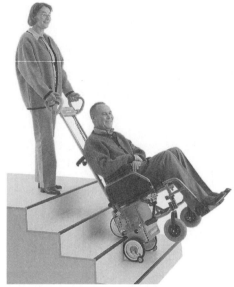

FIGURE 14-7 The Scalamobil is a lightweight, battery-operated portable stair climber that attaches to manual wheelchairs and allows a caregiver to ascend or descend stairs with an occupied wheelchair. The device will carry a maximum of 300 pounds on one battery charge. (Courtesy Frank Mobility Systems, Inc., Oakdale, PA.)

The swing of the bathroom door should be outward, into the bedroom, and away from the more confined space of the bathroom and provide at least the standard 32-inch-wide doorway clearance with a level threshold. Again the wheelchair turning radius needs to be an area 5 feet by 5 feet, clear of fixtures, for easy maneuvering. This turning space may overlap bathroom fixture floor clearance with at least 4 feet of clear space in front of all bathroom fixtures (Box 14-3).

Bathroom sinks need to be wall mounted either without a cabinet or with a large enough opening to accommodate a wheelchair easily (Figure 14-9). There are specific minimum dimensions for the position of the sink and other fixtures. For individuals with limited hand dexterity, lever-style handles on doors, sinks, and shower controls work better than do knob-type handles. Piping is contained within the wall or routed to the side of the sink to prevent burns or scraping the wheelchair user's lower extremities. If pipes must be exposed, they need to be insulated.

A standard shape and height (i.e., 14 inches) toilet is recommended for use with either a padded commode seat or a roll-in shower commode chair (Figure 14-10). Elevated or handicap designed toilets are generally inappropriate and are not compatible with recommended DME. Some toilet styles, such as those with an elongated toilet seat, also limit DME compatibility and are not recommended. Provide adequate space alongside the toilet to accommodate equipment dimensions, wheelchair maneuverability, and transfers.

Grab bars are often used alongside the toilet for stability during transfers, clothing management, and toileting (Figure 14-11, *A*). Attach all grab bars securely to wall studs with 1.5 inches of space between the wall and the bar to ensure adequate grip space. Grab bar positioning depends on the type of transfer and stability requirements of the individual. Transferring to the toilet requires that the wheelchair can be maneuvered next to the toilet (Figure 14-11, *B*).

Standard tubs or shower stalls may be used in conjunction with padded tub benches or shower seats if the functional level of the individual permits (see Figure 14-18, *A* and *B*). Replace glass shower doors with a shower curtain to accommodate a tub bench base that either hangs over or is positioned on top of the tub's wall. High-functioning patients who wish to limit the number of transfers necessary to complete their bathing, toileting, and personal hygiene routines often use a roll-in shower chair (Figure 14-12). A roll-in shower chair is required for individuals with higher injury levels who need additional positioning or stability while completing their personal hygiene with caregiver assistance.

A roll-in shower can be constructed by using nonslip surfaces with two or three tiled sides, a sloped floor for water drainage, and a ceiling-mounted tracked shower curtain for water containment (Figure 14-13, *A*). Keep the entrance to the shower stall free of any curb or threshold. A minimum of 5 feet by 5 feet of space is needed to accommodate most roll-in shower chairs (Figure 14-13, *B*). A hand-held shower head should be installed at an adjustable height. A heat lamp is an important addition to assist with temperature control because many patients require a significant amount of time to complete their bathroom routines. In addition, antiscald mechanisms should be installed and the water heater thermostat set no higher than 120° F for increased safety.

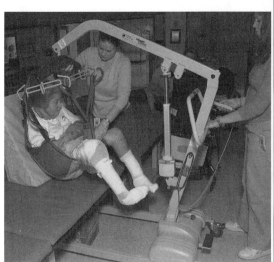
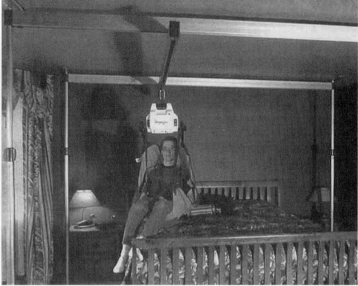

FIGURE 14-8 **A,** An individual is secured in a mechanical lift with the lift base positioned under a therapeutic mat demonstrating the need for under mat or bed space requirements when using this technology. **B,** An overhead track lift system provides another option for dependent bed transfers when space considerations do not allow for a free-standing mechanical lift. (**B,** Courtesy Easytrack Patient Lift System, Sunrise Medical, Carlsbad, CA.)

BOX 14-3 | Bathroom Fixture Placements

Sink and Mirror
- Wall-mount sink without cabinet or with large keyhole for knee clearance (27 inches high, 30 inches wide, 19 inches deep).
- Mount sink rim no higher than 34 inches from the floor and 27 inches deep.
- Choose sink with bowl depth that does not exceed 6.5 inches.
- Clear floor space in front of sink of 30 inches wide and 48 inches in length.
- Insulate sink pipes and drains to prevent scrapes and burns; pipes recessed, offset horizontally or located behind the wall are best.
- Allow countertop space adjacent to the sink that does not exceed a height of 34 inches.
- Hang mirror for viewing from both a seated and standing position with the lower edge mounted no more than 40 inches above the floor and the top edge mounted no less than 6 feet 2 inches.

Toilet
- Use a standard-height toilet (14-inch rim height) with a standard rolling shower-commode chair or over-the-toilet commode.
- Provide space on both sides of the toilet to accommodate an over-the-toilet commode.
- Provide a minimum of 18 inches clearance from midline of the toilet.
- Allow clear floor space 4 feet × 4 feet in front of the toilet to allow for over-the-toilet commode back-in access.

Roll-In Shower
- Construct a tiled, two- or three-sided, roll-in shower.
- Floor clearance needs to be a minimum of 5 × 5 feet.
- Use nonslip floor material, slightly sloped for water drainage without curb or threshold.
- Install shower spray unit that adapts for use in a fixed or hand-held spray position with adjustable height and extended (-6 foot) shower hose with an on-off lever on the handle.
- Install thermostatic antiscald controls to prevent sudden changes in water temperature.
- Use a ceiling-hung track shower curtain to contain water.
- Use a wall-mounted seat for added stability rather than a tub bench.
- Provide adequate cabinet space for storage of hygiene equipment and supplies.
- Provide heat light and ventilating unit for temperature control.

Kitchen and Dining Rooms

When individuals with SCI are able to engage in meal preparation, the kitchen area needs at least one accessible workspace (Figure 14-14, *A*). Optimal counter heights are between 30 inches to 35 inches above the floor with approximately 24 inches of depth and 27 inches to 30 inches in height under the counter for lower extremity clearance. Providing a pullout surface for workspace can easily accommodate these specifications (Figure 14-14, *B*). Pullouts can also help bridge the carrying gap between appliances and the counter.

Recessed toe space of approximately 6 inches in depth and 8 to 11 inches in height provides access for wheelchair front rigging, which allows the chair to be positioned closer to the counter (Figure 14-14, *C*). A minimum of 5 feet of clear floor space needs to be present between all accessible cabinets and kitchen walls. Adequate upper and lower storage cabinets should be installed within reach from the seated position; the minimum usable shelf height is 18 inches and maximum usable shelf height is 4 feet 6 inches. In addition, cabinets that are equipped with roll-out shelves or lazy Susan units allow

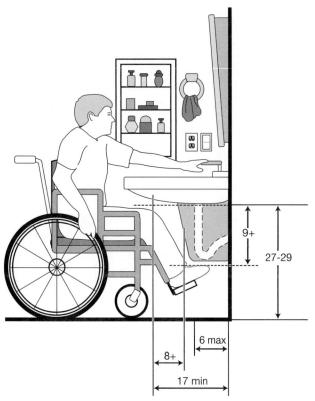

FIGURE 14-9 A lateral view of a bathroom sink layout illustrates wheelchair user access with knee space below sink and an insulated cover protecting insensate skin from hot water pipes. The mirror is mounted low and tilted downward to allow easier viewing. The wall adjacent to the basin accommodates electrical outlets, towel holder, and medicine cabinet—all within easy reach.

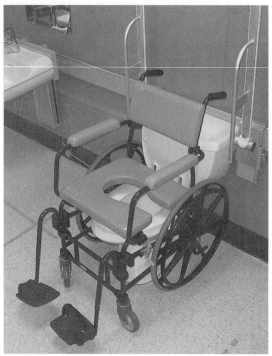

FIGURE 14-10 Commode chairs need to have padded seats, backs, and armrests because bowel routines may require long periods of sitting and it is important to protect the skin during this period. The seat opening allows access to the perineal region.

for unimpeded access to stored kitchen items (Figure 14-14, *D* and *E*).

Gas-style stove tops with front-mounted burners and front- or side-mounted controls are recommended as the best units to avoid burns (Figure 14-14, *F*). If the controls are mounted on the back of the stove, it is possible to purchase a switch package that can be mounted on the side.[18] Such adapter packages can be purchased from a company that specializes in products for people with visual impairments. A wall-mounted mirror may be positioned at an angle above the stove to allow for a clear view of pots positioned on the stove top.[18] Ovens should be wall mounted and positioned to allow for easy access to interior oven racks (Figure 14-14, *A* and *G*).

Microwave units are mounted at a height that allows the person with SCI to reach inside. Flat control panel buttons may be built up with small furniture bumpers to allow patients with limited hand dexterity access. Refrigerators with side-by-side mounted doors are best suited for independent freezer access. Roll-out shelving is ideal for access of items located at the rear of the refrigerator. The most frequently used items should be kept on the lower shelves. If the door is difficult to open, a loop can be attached to the door handle to ensure easier opening.

A kitchen sink with shallow depth is ideally positioned at 29 to 31 inches from the floor. A single-control, lever-style faucet

handle may be positioned at the side of the sink for increased ease of access (Figure 14-15, *A*). The cabinets can be removed from underneath the sink to allow the wheelchair and user access; pipes should be insulated or recessed to prevent burns (Figure 14-15, *B*).

The dining room should allow ample space to maneuver the wheelchair and be devoid of unnecessary furniture. The dining room table needs to have adequate underneath leg space to allow for unimpeded wheelchair access with a height consistent with the wheelchair user's seated height (i.e., generally positioned at 30 inches from the floor). It is important to consider knee depth clearance as well, taking care to measure the wheelchair from back to the front of the footrest.

In conjunction with the therapy team's recommendations, the family or other caregivers play a major role in deciding what modifications are necessary. When planning how to organize the remodeled space, using two dowels—one 32 inches long and the other 36 inches long—helps visualize where cabinets and appliances need to be located. In fact, if caregivers hold the dowel horizontally and walk throughout the home, they will see where potential problem places exist. Again, if the clearance involves a turn, the area needs to be 36 inches wide, and straight approach access needs 32 inches.

DURABLE MEDICAL EQUIPMENT

DME consists of a variety of devices and support surfaces that are designed to meet the self-care, mobility, pressure management, and positioning needs of individuals with disabilities. Someone with SCI often requires specialized DME that is designed to meet

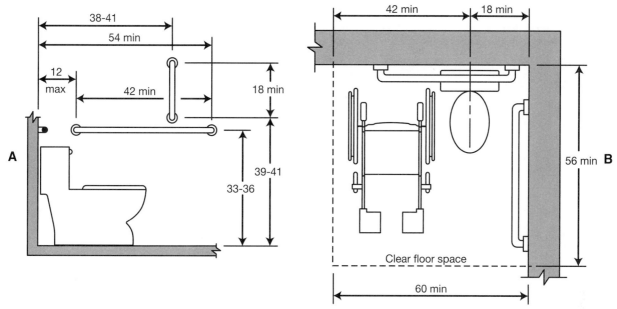

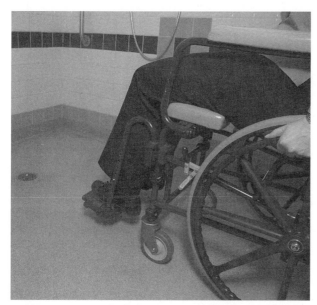

FIGURE 14-11 Consideration must be given to grab bar placement when configuring toilet placement. Locating the toilet an extra 3 inches from the wall (18 inches from wall to midline) allows space for the grab bar. **A,** Configuration for wall-mounted grab bars, **B,** View from above of wall-mounted grab bars.

FIGURE 14-12 An individual enters an accessible roll-in shower by using a shower-commode chair. Note that there is no ledge to roll over; the shower floor is angled toward the drain to avoid water flooding outside the shower area.

his unique needs. And these DME requirements are contingent on a number of factors, including level of injury, functional status, home accessibility, and personal goals.

Numerous equipment manufacturers make a variety of competing DME products, some with distinct advantages and others with disadvantages. It is commonly the responsibility of the occupational or physical therapist to identify appropriate equipment that is consistent with the patient's medical and functional status. It is important for the patient to try out all DME before a prescription is generated. During the trial process, the therapist will work with the equipment vendors to educate the patient about the pros and cons of a given product. This allows the patient to make an educated decision regarding recommended equipment options. It is important that the therapist responsible for equipment trials keep up to date on all new equipment and the requirements for its safe use.

Insurance coverage for DME varies considerably across various private insurance payers and state-run Medicaid programs. Coverage criteria under Medicare are typically more rigid than some other plans; in fact, it does not cover certain items, such as bathing equipment, under any circumstances. Many insurance companies will consider funding prescribed DME as long as medical necessity is established. The therapist also typically writes the letters of medical necessity that outline the need for the prescribed piece of equipment on the basis of the individual's medical status and functional level. It is important for the prescribing therapist to have first-hand knowledge of the patient's DME coverage so that the necessary documentation is included along with each prescription. Although insurance coverage should be considered early in the equipment trial process to prevent a delay on discharge, it should never dictate what equipment is recommended.

DME commonly used by individuals with SCI is based on equipment recommendations after individualized assessment by qualified therapists who consider the needs of the patient first. Products often prescribed include mobile arm supports (see Figure 9-4), sleep support surfaces, transfer aids, and bathroom equipment.

Sleep Support Surfaces

Individuals with SCI often require adjustable hospital beds that are designed to provide support and assistance with a variety of medical and functional tasks. Home care hospital beds are typically categorized by level of adjustability that can be operated manually, with semielectric controls, or with fully electric controls. Patients with tetraplegia generally rely on hospital beds

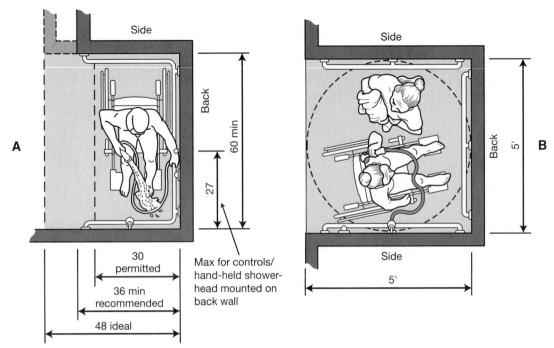

FIGURE 14-13 **A,** An illustration of an individual managing independent wheelchair access to a curbless shower viewed from above shows why a 48-inch width is ideal while a permitted 30-inch width would be unduly cramped. **B,** A 5 × 5 foot radius is required for a curbless shower in which caregiver access is needed to assist an individual with showering. (Adapted from Young LC, Pace RJ: *Curbless showers: an installation guide,* Raleigh, NC, 2003, Center for Universal Design, North Carolina State University.)

with at least semielectric controls to assist with positioning, postural drainage, bed mobility, transfers, and certain self-care tasks. Those with high tetraplegia may require a hospital bed with fully electric controls that is capable of multiple adjustments, including the ability to assume positions that assist in the management of respiratory secretions and edema control, such as the Trendelenburg (i.e., supine with head lower than the feet) and reverse Trendelenburg (i.e., supine with head higher than feet) positions (see Chapter 4). Individuals with paraplegia may also benefit from adjustable hospital beds with electric controls to provide assistance and support during self-catheterization, lower body dressing, and bed mobility.

People with SCI are at risk for the development of pressure ulcers as a result of insensate skin, incontinence, and immobility. Numerous specialty mattresses and mattress overlays are available in the market, designed to meet the pressure management needs of a variety of patients (see Figure 3-9, *A* and *B*). These mattresses and overlays are composed of a variety of materials used alone or in combination including foam, air, gel, viscous fluid, and ventilated honeycomb. In addition to the use of a variety of materials, each mattress or overlay uses different features that provide unique therapeutic functions for a given patient.[19,20]

The Centers for Medicare and Medicaid Services (CMS) categorizes all support surfaces into three groups (Clinical Note: Classification of Mattress Surfaces to Prevent Pressure). Reimbursement coverage for these support surfaces is often based on these guidelines. Overall, CMS coverage guidelines relate to specific criteria that include documentation about the patient's mobility, continence, sensory, circulatory, and nutritional status.[21] A history of pressure ulceration and a history of myocutaneous flap surgery are also included in the coverage criteria. In addition, the

---

CLINICAL NOTE **Classification of Mattress Surfaces to Prevent Pressure Ulcers**

- Group I surfaces are unpowered mattress overlays or mattresses that are used for pressure ulcer prevention (Maklebust, 2005).
- Group II surfaces include both powered and more advanced unpowered support surfaces (Brienza, 2005). Group II surfaces also consist of both mattress overlays and mattress systems.
- Group III surfaces are composed of air-fluidized beds that are high-air-loss systems (Brienza, 2005). These systems are made of ceramic silicone beads that are fluidized by warm air that is pressurized and forced through the beads (Brienza, 2005).

Data from Brienza DM, Geyer MJ: Using support surfaces to manage tissue integrity, *Adv Skin Wound Care* 18:151-157, 2005; Maklebust J: Choosing the right support surface, *Adv Skin Wound Care* 18:158-161, 2005; Centers for Medicare and Medicaid Services: http://www.cms.hhs.gov. Accessed June 2007; and Brienza DM: Measuring pressure, *Adv Provid Postacute Care* May/June:81-82, 2005.

presence of a pressure ulcer or multiple pressure ulcers, their severity, location, and documentation regarding a comprehensive ulcer treatment program are additional factors in meeting CMS's coverage criteria. Clinicians need to understand the importance of the specific requirements regarding the documentation necessary for coverage by a given insurance plan.

Individuals with high-level tetraplegia who are dependent for position changes are at great risk for skin breakdown and require maximal pressure relief. Low-air-loss mattresses are commonly recommended for such individuals because of their ideal pressure management qualities. Some low-air-loss mattresses may also be equipped with alternating pressure and or lateral rotation features. Alternating pressure is a feature that systematically

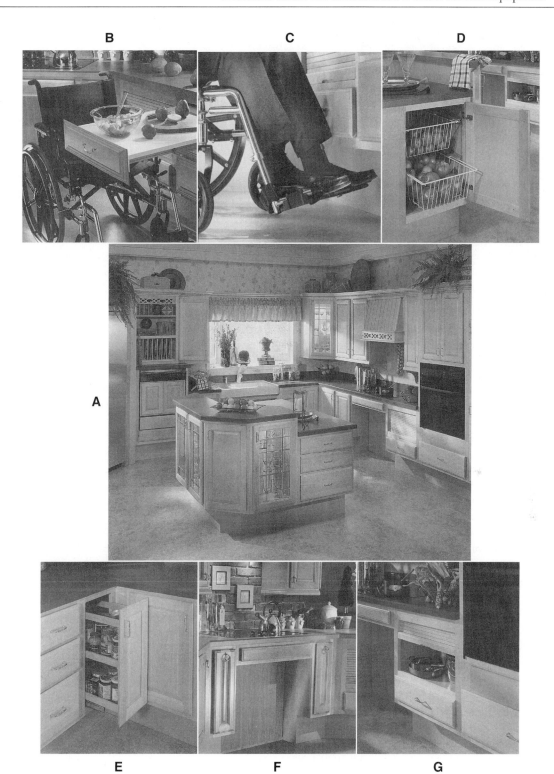

FIGURE 14-14 A wheelchair accessible kitchen (**A**) combines lower countertops, accessible shelves and drawers, and cabinet floor cutouts to allow space for wheelchair footrests, thereby increasing functional reach space. **B,** A wheelchair accessible pullout extends the counter workspace during kitchen preparation and can be pushed in to give the appearance of a kitchen drawer. **C,** Close-up of floor cutouts. **D,** Slide-out baskets and (**E**) shelves provides easy access to food and pots and pans. **F,** Cooktop with cutout for wheelchair accessibility also has controls mounted at the front to avoid the possibility of burns from making the user reach over hot burners. **G,** Wall oven placed at a height accessible for wheelchair users. (Courtesy Kraftmaid, Middlefield, OH.)

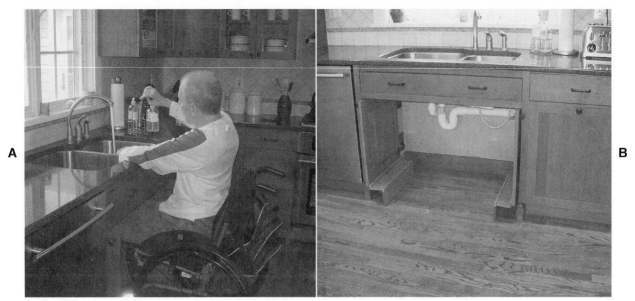

FIGURE 14-15 **A,** An individual with tetraplegia uses a kitchen sink with wheelchair accessible opening and single lever handle. **B,** The water pipes underneath the sink are configured to prevent contact with and possible scalding of insensate skin.

alters pressure distribution by periodically inflating and deflating air-filled compartments to shift a patient's body weight to varied points of contact.[19] Lateral rotation is a feature that automatically turns the patient up to 30 degrees from side to side at preset intervals. Air-based mattresses are ideal for pressure relief but must be inflated to the appropriate pressure and require an external power source.

Because low-air-loss mattresses shift with weight and are therefore less stable, transferring can be difficult. Individuals with lower-level tetraplegia who are less dependent for transfers and self-care may use foam-based mattresses or a combination of air and foam-based mattresses or gel and foam-based mattresses. These mattresses continue to provide needed pressure relief but also provide a firmer base of support that makes transfers, bed mobility, and self-care easier.

Individuals who are independent with bed mobility and do not have a history of skin breakdown often choose mattress overlays that are positioned on top of a standard mattress. Mattress overlays are considerably thinner than full mattresses, may not require an external power source, and are used by active individuals as a preventive measure. Many individuals with low-level paraplegia do not rely on any specialty sleep surface and are able to manage their skin care by positioning and routine turning schedules.

A prescription for a specialty mattress product is contingent on the presence and severity of a given pressure ulcer, history of pressure ulcer development, bed mobility status, continence status, and nutritional status. The rehabilitation team will consider each of these factors when making decisions about the type of support surfaces appropriate for a given patient.

Objective data regarding the pressure distribution qualities of a given surface can be obtained by using interface pressure mapping in which a flexible mat equipped with transducers measure the pressure between the body and the support surface (Figure 14-16). The data are electronically sent to a computer that displays a color-coded representation of load distribution

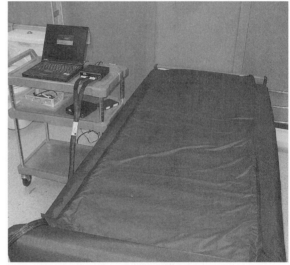

FIGURE 14-16 Pressure mapping in bed is used to quantify the areas of pressure from the support surface to the patient's body when in the supine, prone, or side-lying positions. Pressure mapping is used to assist in the elimination of inappropriate mattresses. Pressure mapping results are used in conjunction with other clinical information to identify an appropriate mattress that will prevent pressure ulcers during bed rest and sleep.

(Figure 14-17, *A* and *B*).[22] The rehabilitation team uses pressure mapping as an adjunct to clinical reasoning, support surface trials, visual inspection of the skin, functional transfer training, and ADL training on the recommended support surface. Because interface pressure is only one of many factors that contribute to pressure ulcer development, some clinicians recommend that pressure mapping be used to assist in excluding clinically inappropriate support surface options.[22] In addition, subjective feedback from the patient regarding comfort and positioning should be considered to assist in obtaining an appropriate match between the patient and the support surface.

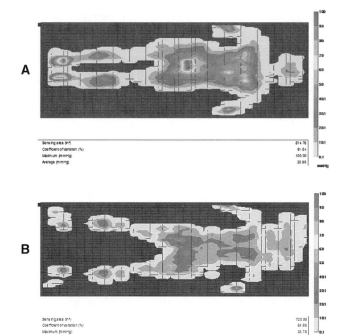

FIGURE 14-17 **A,** A three-dimensional pressure map of an individual lying on a bed with an inadequate mattress. Note the high peaks in the map indicating areas of excessive pressure around the shoulder blades, sacrum, and heels. **B,** A three-dimensional pressure map of the same individual using a mattress that significantly minimizes pressure, as indicated with reduced pressure peaks.

Transfer Aids

The ability to transfer into and out of the wheelchair depends on a number of factors, including the functional status of the patient's upper and lower limbs, sitting balance, the height of the transfer surface, and the type of surface to be transferred onto. Individuals with tetraplegia and some with high-level paraplegia need to use a transfer board to safely move into and out of their wheelchairs (see Chapters 7 and 8).

Transfer boards are available in a variety of shapes and sizes and are manufactured out of different materials ranging from wood to plastic (see Figure 8-10). Most standard-length transfer boards are approximately 24 inches in length, but transfer boards are also made in longer lengths to accommodate transfers to a surface that is positioned at a greater distance from the wheelchair. These types of transfer boards are at least 29 inches in length and may be used to transfer into and out of a vehicle. Many transfer boards are made with cutouts designed to provide assistance with board placement. These cutouts can be horizontally, vertically, or obliquely oriented and are of particular importance to patients with tetraplegia, who lack the significant hand function needed to successfully position a transfer board.

Individuals with higher-level tetraplegia who have decreased upper extremity function and poor sitting balance may require a caregiver-assisted transfer with specialty boards (see Figure 8-23) or lifts to safely complete functional transfers. There are two categories of patient lifts: floor based and ceiling based. Floor-based lifts are usually operated by a manual crank, hydraulic pump, or a powered actuator (see Figure 14-8, *A*). Power lifters are the simplest to use because the caregiver expends little manual effort

raising and lowering the patient and because they are equipped with rechargeable batteries. Each lift is available with a variety of slings that support the patient and with numerous configurations, sizes, and weight capacities to meet a wide range of body shapes, weights, and sizes. Lift slings are manufactured with or without a head support and are made of many materials ranging from polyester to nylon mesh. Nylon mesh slings are ideal for bathing applications because they are water permeable and dry relatively quickly.

Ceiling-mounted lifts can be installed as permanent or temporary applications in specific areas of the home such as the bedroom or bathroom to assist with functional transfers (see Figure 14-8, *B*). Advantages of ceiling-mounted lifts include increased ease of access to smaller spaces and increased ease of maneuverability regardless of flooring surface. Permanently mounted ceiling lifts often require expensive home modifications and installation costs to ensure their safe use; portable ceiling lifts do not require costly extensive modifications but cannot be installed where there is a suspended ceiling. Lifts mounted to the ceiling are also compatible with a variety of slings designed to meet the needs of individuals with varying positional requirements.

Bathroom Equipment

Bathroom equipment for individuals with SCI runs the gamut from standard off-the-shelf tub benches to custom configured roll-in shower-commode chairs. All DME used in bathrooms needs to have padded surfaces to protect insensate skin from breakdown. The ability to choose between custom equipment and standard DME is contingent on a review of the patient's functional status, medical status, and home evaluation report findings.

A patient whose home has a tub and who is more independent with transfers can rely on a padded tub bench for bathing. Tub benches are commonly constructed of stainless steel, anodized aluminum, or polyvinyl chloride piping. Some tub benches are configured so that two support legs are located outside the tub's wall (Figure 14-18, *A*). These tub benches often make water containment more difficult and may contribute to the development of an unsafe transferring environment. Other tub benches keep four legs contained within the tub and have a transfer surface positioned on top of the tub's wall (Figure 14-18, *B*). These benches are also often equipped with a groove along the top surface of the bench that is mounted above the tub's wall. This design helps keep water in the tub because the shower curtain can be tucked into the groove during bathing. Some tub benches are portable and may be collapsed and placed in a supplied storage bag for travel.

Patients who rely on a tub bench for bathing generally use a padded commode chair for toileting. Commode chairs are also produced in a variety of styles and configurations designed to meet the needs of a variety of individuals. People with SCI often require a U-shaped commode seat opening that can be oriented to the left, right, front, or back to allow for independent access to the perianal region during bowel program completion (see Figure 14-10). It is important to consider seat orientation because units that can only be positioned in a front or rearward make bowel management difficult for some patients. If stability during toileting is a concern, some commodes are equipped with a back support and armrests that can be dropped out of the way during transfers. It is also important that the chair is adjustable in height to allow a level transfer from the wheelchair.

Roll-in combination shower-commode chairs are often recommended for individuals with high-level tetraplegia or for those who wish to limit the number of transfers necessary to complete their bathing and toileting routines. Accessible bathroom facilities equipped with a standard toilet and a roll-in shower are necessary to accommodate a roll-in shower-commode chair. Shower-commode chairs equipped with manual tilt in space or recline capabilities are ideally suited for patients with tetraplegia who are dependent on a caregiver for transfers, bathing, and toileting.

These shower-commode chairs can also be equipped with arm troughs, seat-chest belts, lateral trunk supports, and headrests to provide maximal postural support and positioning. Those with higher functioning tetraplegia and paraplegia who are capable of independent transferring and self-propelling a wheelchair may use lower-profile roll-in chairs. Such chairs are equipped with 24-inch rear wheels, push rims, flip back armrests, and lower seat back heights to allow for increased ease of propulsion and independent transfers. Manufacturers of high-end bathroom equipment are often able to modify their shower-commode chairs to meet specific custom needs for stability, mobility, and functional requirements. Before such custom modification, consideration should be given to the altered chair dimensions and its effect on toilet and shower stall access.

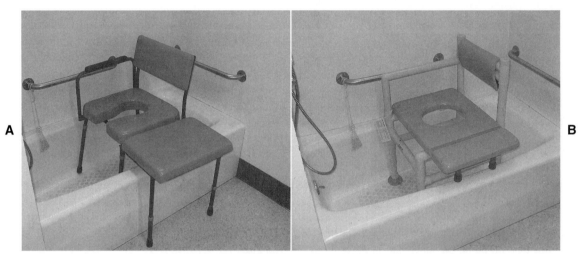

FIGURE 14-18 **A,** Tub bench with legs both inside and outside of tub. **B,** Polyvinyl chloride plastic tub bench with all four legs inside the tub.

CLINICAL CASE STUDY **Home Modifications Case 1**

Patient History
Robert Elvy is a 73-year-old man with a C7 tetraplegia, American Spinal Cord Association (ASIA) B diagnosis resulting from a fall. He is medically stable at 24 weeks after injury. His spinal surgery was followed by a sternal occipital mandibular immobilizer for 6 weeks and hard collar for 3. His initial acute care hospital stay was complicated by a deep vein thrombosis in his right lower limb, and his rehabilitation was interrupted by a return to acute care because of pneumonia. His total time in acute care and rehabilitation was 16 weeks.

Robert has a mild left thoracic right lumbar structural scoliosis. After his discharge from rehabilitation he and his wife went to Arizona to live with their daughter so that renovations for accessibility modification could be completed in their home. He has been an outpatient in Arizona for 8 weeks and is looking forward to returning home when his home's renovations are complete.

Robert is a retired high school math teacher. He uses a power reclining wheelchair with a manual wheelchair for back up. He lives in a one-story ranch home with his wife Ruth, age 68 years, who is a retired administrative assistant. Ruth is currently her husband's primary caretaker. Both Robert and his wife are collecting a pension, which supports their regular monthly expenses. They have two married children and four grandchildren. Their daughter lives in Atlanta and their son in Arizona. They already owned a van, and a power lift

and hand controls have been installed. Robert has passed his hand control driving exam.

Patient's Self-Assessment
Robert is focused on completing his rehabilitation therapy and returning to his adapted home. He wants to continue an active and high-quality retirement.

Clinical Assessment
Patient Appearance
• Height 6 feet 0 inches, weight 200 pounds, body mass index 27.1

Cognitive Assessment
• Alert, oriented × 3

Cardiopulmonary Assessment
• * Blood pressure 116/70 mm Hg, heart rate at rest 68 beats/min, respiratory rate 14 breaths/min, cough flows are ineffective (<360 L/min), vital capacity is reduced (between 1.5 and 2.5 L)

Musculoskeletal and Neuromuscular Assessment
• Motor assessment reveals C7 ASIA B, motor is intact to the C7 level
• Deep tendon reflexes 3+ below the level of lesion

CLINICAL CASE STUDY Home Modifications Case 1—cont'd

Integumentary and Sensory Assessment
- Skin is intact throughout, sensory intact throughout

Range of Motion Assessment
- Passive and active motion is within normal limits in both upper limbs.
- Straight leg raise is 85 degrees in both lower limbs and dorsiflexion is 0 degrees, all other motions in the lower limbs are within functional limits.

Mobility and Activities of Daily Living Assessment
- Independent with bed mobility
- Independent in transfers to level surfaces, requires minimal assistance for uneven transfers, and is dependent for floor to wheelchair to floor
- Independent with pressure relief
- Independent in power and manual wheelchair maneuvering on all surfaces
- Does not perform high level wheelchair skills such as wheelies
- Dependent in bowel and bladder care
- Independent in upper body dressing and requires moderate assistance in lower body dressing
- Independent in driving

Evaluation of Clinical Assessment
Robert Elvy is a 73-year-old man with a C7 tetraplegia, ASIA B diagnosis from a fall. He is medically stable at 24 weeks after injury. His home renovations are near completion.

Patient's Care Needs
1. Completion of home modifications

Diagnosis and Prognosis
Diagnosis is C7, ASIA B. Prognosis is for modified independence with adaptive equipment, after set-up from a caregiver, with routine activities of daily living in a modified home environment.

Preferred Practice Patterns*
Impaired Muscle Performance (4C), Impairments Non-progressive Spinal Cord Disorders (5H), Primary Prevention/Risk Reduction for Cardiovascular/Pulmonary Disorders (6A), Primary Prevention/Risk Reduction for Integumentary Disorders (7A)

Team Goals
1. Team to develop and follow up monitoring home modification recommendations

Patient Goals
"I want my home to be as comfortable as possible for me and my wife."

Care Plan
Treatment Plan and Rationale
- Home modification

Interventions
- Follow-up home evaluation was completed before Robert's inpatient discharge.
- Repeat home evaluation to determine needs for manual and power wheelchair use and the use of temporary modifications such as portable ramps until the final renovations are completed

Documentation and Team Communication
- Team drafted, updated, and reviewed home modification plan with the patient and his wife.
- Team consulted case worker regarding insurance allowances for home modifications for accessibility.

Follow-Up Assessment
- Consult with vendors about home modifications as needed.

Critical Thinking Exercises
Consider what home modifications and DME applications will influence Robert's ability to access his home, live actively and productively, and be important to his successful adaptation.
1. Describe home modifications to consider when completing the home evaluation for this patient.
2. Assuming that the home has an attached two-car garage with one step to enter a laundry area 6 feet by 5 feet and a front entrance with two steps to enter directly into the living room, what recommendations would you propose for home entrance?
3. Describe Robert's bedroom needs.
4. Describe the ideal bathroom for Robert including equipment.
5. What general recommendations would you give Robert and Ruth related to furniture layout in both the living room and dining room?

*Guide to physical therapist practice, rev. ed. 2, Alexandria, VA, 2003, American Physical Therapy Association.

CLINICAL CASE STUDY Home Modifications Case 2

Patient History
Mary Pressman is a 25-year-old woman with a T10 paraplegia, ASIA A diagnosis. She was injured in a motor vehicle accident. She also had a fractured left femur with an open reduction internal fixation but is now orthopedically stable. She is 40 weeks after injury and has completed her inpatient and outpatient rehabilitation.

Mary is a computer programmer and works for a large company. Her company provided a long-term disability option, which she has taken. She received full funding for her wheelchair. She is engaged and her fiancé works for the same company in the marketing division. Mary and her fiancé are in the process of looking for a home to purchase.

Mary has temporarily moved back home with her parents until the wedding. Her parents have a bedroom and bathroom on the first floor that she can access with her manual wheelchair. Her previous lifestyle was a very active one; she was an avid cyclist and swimmer.

Patient's Self-Assessment
Mary wants to return to her previous active lifestyle as soon as possible.

Continued

CLINICAL CASE STUDY Home Modifications Case 2—cont'd

Clinical Assessment
Patient Appearance
- Height 5 feet 2 inches, weight 105 pounds, body mass index 19.2

Cognitive Assessment
- Alert, oriented × 3

Cardiopulmonary Assessment
- Blood pressure 116/70 mm Hg, heart rate at rest 68 beats/min, respiratory rate 14 breaths/min, cough flows and vital capacity are within normal limits

Musculoskeletal and Neuromuscular Assessment
- Motor assessment reveals T10 paraplegia, ASIA A, sensory intact to T10
- Deep tendon reflexes 3+ below the level of lesion

Integumentary and Sensory Assessment
- Skin is intact throughout, sensory intact to T10

Range of Motion Assessment
- Passive and active motion is within normal limits in both upper limbs.
- Straight leg raise is 110 degrees in both lower limbs and dorsiflexion is 7 degrees; all other motions in the lower limbs are within functional limits.

Mobility and ADL Assessment
- Independent with bed mobility
- Independent in transfers to all surfaces
- Independent with pressure relief
- Independent in manual wheelchair maneuvering on all surfaces
- Independent in high-level wheelchair skills
- Independent in bowel and bladder care
- Independent in upper body dressing and lower body dressing
- Independent in driving

Evaluation of Clinical Assessment
Mary Pressman is a 25-year-old woman with a T10 paraplegia, ASIA A diagnosis. She was injured in a motor vehicle accident where she also had a fractured left femur. She underwent an open reduction internal fixation and is now orthopedically stable. She is 40 weeks after injury and has completed her inpatient and outpatient rehabilitation.

Patient's Care Needs
1. Completion of home modifications

Diagnosis and Prognosis
Diagnosis is T10 paraplegia, ASIA A. Prognosis is for full independence in all activities with modified home environment.

Preferred Practice Patterns*
Impaired Muscle Performance (4C), Impairments Nonprogressive Spinal Cord Disorders (5H), Primary Prevention/Risk Reduction for Cardiovascular/Pulmonary Disorders (6A), Primary Prevention/Risk Reduction for Integumentary Disorders (7A)

Team Goals
1. Team to develop recommendations for home modification as needed

Patient Goals
"I want a home that my fiancé and I find comfortable and one we can raise a family in."

Care Plan
Treatment Plan and Rationale
- Make recommendations for new home to be purchased for possible home modification
- Assess temporary home environment while living with parents

Interventions
- Conduct home evaluation consultation
- Consult with patient about potential vendors and general contractors who are familiar with making and adapting an accessible home

Documentation and Team Communication
- Team to compile home modification plan as requested by the patient
- Team to document needs to case worker for insurance authorization for specialized home equipment and modifications

Follow-Up Assessment
- Consult on home modification as needed

Critical Thinking Exercises
On the basis of Mary's injury level, job, and active lifestyle, consider what home modifications and DME applications that she will need to fulfill her goal of an accessible and livable home in which to begin her marriage and raise a family.
1. What recommendations would you make for an accessible kitchen to meet Mary's needs?
2. What recommendations would you make for Mary considering an accessible bedroom?
3. What advice would you offer Mary and her fiancé while they are shopping for a home if new construction is not available and construction modifications will be needed?

*Guide to physical therapist practice, rev. ed. 2, Alexandria, VA, 2003, American Physical Therapy Association.

SUMMARY

The home accessibility assessment and modification process is directly related to the DME considerations of the patient with SCI. A complete understanding of the individual's potential DME requirements must be obtained before the initiation of the formal home accessibility assessment. More specific knowledge of equipment dimensions and configurations is necessary before the initiation of specific home modifications. The ability to integrate product knowledge with accessible housing design is critical to the creation of an optimal patient-product match and for ensuring a successful discharge to the home. Although movement toward universal housing design will eventually make major home modifications easier, specific patient accommodation requirements will still need to be met.

REFERENCES

1. National Spinal Cord Injury Statistics Center: *Spinal cord injury facts and figures at a glance,* University of Alabama at Birmingham.: http://www.spinalcord.uab.edu. Accessed March 2007.

2. Americans with Disability Act: Standards for Accessible Design, 28 CFR Part 36, Washington, DC, Revised July 1, 2004, Department of Justice, pp 507-508.

3. National Institute on Disability and Rehabilitation Research: *http://www.ed.gov/about/offices/list/osers/nidrr/index.html.* Accessed May 2007.

4. Baigis J, Larson E, Haskey MY: Predictors of functional status in patients in a chronic-care facility, *Clin Perform Qual Health Care* 6:28-32, 1998.

5. Mace R: Universal design in housing, *Assist Technol* 10:21-28, 1998.

6. Eastern Paralyzed Veterans Association: *Barrier free design: selected federal laws and ADA accessibility guidelines,* New York, 1996, The Association.

7. Concrete Change: *Laws on disability access to housing: a summary:* http://www.concretechange.org/lawsoverview.htm. Accessed May 2007.

8. Peterson W: Public policy affecting universal design, *Assist Technol* 10:13-20, 1998.

9. Story M: Maximizing usability: the principles of universal design, *Assist Technol* 10:4-12, 1998.

10. Connell BR, Jones M, Mace R, et al: *The principals of universal design,* version 2.0, Raleigh, NC, 1997, North Carolina State University.

11. Easter Seals: *Easter Seals disability services partnership with Century 21 on home accessibility:* http://www.easterseals.com/site/PageServer?pagename=ntlc_easyaccesshousing_tips. Accessed May 2007.

12. Forrest G, Gombas G: Wheelchair accessible housing: its role in cost containment in spinal cord injury, *Arch Phys Med Rehabil* 76:450-452, 1995.

13. Steinfeld E, Levine D, Shea S: Home modifications and the fair housing law, *Technol Disabil* 8:15-35, 1998.

14. Jeserich M: Building better homes, *AT Journal* 60:1-5, 2002: http://www.atnet.org/news/nov02/110101.htm. Accessed March 2007.

15. National Organization on Disability: *Strategies for accessibility and visitability:* http://www.nod.org/content. Accessed 2007.

16. Eberhardt K: Home modifications for persons with spinal cord injury, *OT Pract* 3:24-27, 1998.

17. Karp G: *Life on wheels,* Sebastopol, CA, 1999, O'Reilly.

18. Hopkins HL, Smith HD: *Willard and Spackman's occupational therapy,* ed 8, Philadelphia, 1993, JB Lippincott.

19. Brienza DM, Geyer MJ: Using support surfaces to manage tissue integrity, *Adv Skin Wound Care* 18:151-157, 2005.

20. Maklebust J: Choosing the right support surface, *Adv Skin Wound Care* 18:158-161, 2005.

21. Centers for Medicare and Medicaid Services, http://www.cms.hhs.gov. Accessed June 2007.

22. Brienza DM: Measuring pressure, *Adv Provid Postacute Care* May/June:81-82, 2005.

SOLUTIONS TO CHAPTER 14 CLINICAL CASE STUDY

Home Modifications Case 1

1. The patient's front entrance and garage entrance to the home must be considered. Eight feet of space is required to accommodate a van lift that projects from the side of the vehicle; therefore, the attached garage must be assessed to determine whether it allows adequate space for the van's lift and the power wheelchair to exit and enter the home. Adequate lighting and protection related to inclement weather must also be considered when assessing entrances. The turning radius once inside the home at all junctions must be assessed to determine whether the power wheelchair can be accommodated. Evaluation for modifications of both hallway (36 inches) and doorway width (34 to 36 inches) throughout the home must also be assessed.

Special needs related to Robert's C7 tetraplegia, ASIA B diagnosis for bedroom and bathroom design and equipment must be carefully considered (see below). All modifications must take into account that this patient does not have hand function; therefore, controls for his environment must be at the level that he will be able to reach and doors should swing inward.

2. The entrance from the garage to the home would be preferred for this patient for vehicle access and entrance to the house during inclement weather. The modification of a ramp with a one-step entrance versus two steps at the front door would be easier to complete. A permanent ramp in the garage with a surface that consists of smooth, continuous, level, and skid-resistant materials that is well lit would be optimal. The required dimensions include a path 36 to 40 inches wide with a level platform at all landings including at least 5 × 5 feet at the doorway.

A portable prefabricated ramp for the front door or to bring when visiting friends and family would be recommended; ramp weight may be an important consideration because of Ruth's age. The width of the door at the garage entrance and the turning area to the kitchen from the laundry room must accommodate the power wheelchair. Consider the turning radius of the power wheelchair, which can vary on the basis of wheelchair size and location of drive mechanism (i.e., mid wheel drive versus front or rear wheel drive).

3. Robert's bedroom must provide adequate space for a 36-inch turning radius for the power wheelchair between the bed, furniture, and closet. Lever handles are recommended for all doors or a swing door. All lighting controls should be no higher than 36 inches and a control should be located outside the bedroom entrance as well as inside. Adequate bed height for the patient to perform a level transfer from the wheelchair should be considered as well as space for a mechanical lift if it is needed because Ruth should not be required to lift Robert given their ages.

A specialty mattress should be considered as well as the required electronic controls for the selected bed. A roll-in closet with appropriate equipment would be ideal. Robert lacks hand function and is 73 years old; therefore, his ability to perform independent lower body dressing and grooming is most likely unrealistic.

4. The ideal bathroom for Robert would include a roll-in shower with a sloped nonskid floor for water drainage, a ceiling-mounted tracked shower curtain for containment of water, a 5-foot turning radius, and a padded roll-in shower-commode chair that can be used for toileting as well. An antiscald mechanism should be installed or the water heater's thermostat set no higher than 120° F for increased safety.

Ideally, the sink should have lever fixtures and be wall mounted. All mirrors should be mounted no more than 40 inches from the floor. The door should swing out and accessible directly to the bedroom if this home's design can accommodate that. (See Box 14-3 for specific details.)

5. The furniture layout in the living and dining rooms should allow for power wheelchair maneuverability, and table heights should be adjusted to allow clearance of the wheelchair for optimal patient positioning when eating. EADLs and environmental controls should be considered to meet Robert and Ruth's needs and lifestyle.

SOLUTIONS TO CHAPTER 14 CLINICAL CASE STUDY

Home Modifications Case 2

1. The kitchen would require full accessibility from the manual wheelchair level. The counter height should be a minimum of 30 inches from the floor and 24 inches deep with 27 to 30 inches in height under the counter for lower limb clearance. A pullout surface for workspace could accommodate these specifications. Recessed toe space of approximately 6 inches in depth and 8 to 11 inches in height provides space for the wheelchair front rigging and allows it to be positioned closer to the counter.

Cabinets with roll out shelves or lazy Susan units are ideal. A minimum of 5 feet of clear floor space needs to be present between all accessible cabinets and kitchen walls. Gas-style stove tops with front-mounted burners and front- or side-mounted controls are recommended as the best units to avoid burns. A wall-mounted mirror may be positioned at an angle above the stove to allow for a clear view of pots positioned on the stove top. Ovens should be wall mounted and positioned to allow for easy access to interior oven racks. Other kitchen appliances should be mounted or placed at an adequate height that allows Mary to reach them, taking into consideration that she is a petite 5 feet 2inches.

A side-by-side refrigerator with mounted doors is best because it allows independent freezer access. Rollout shelving is ideal for access of items located at the rear of the refrigerator. The kitchen sink should be shallow and ideally positioned at 29 to 31 inches from the floor. A single control, lever-style, faucet handle may be positioned at the side of the sink for increased ease of access. There should not be cabinets underneath the sink and pipes should be configured so that they are out of the way and insulated. Cabinets should be within reach from the seated position. Mary should be interviewed about the evaluation so that she can have input into all recommendations.

2. Mary should have recommendations for adequate floor space alongside the bed to allow for transfers and a full 360-degree turn with the manual wheelchair. A minimum overall floor space of at least 10 feet by 14 feet with a minimum of 3 feet of floor space alongside the bed is required. Another passageway with a minimum of 4 feet is necessary at the end of the bed and again in front of the dressers and closet space. The room should allow at least one 5 × 5 foot area clear of furniture for wheelchair maneuvering. Bed height should be considered carefully for Mary in relationship to her wheelchair level to minimize the potential of shoulder injury during transfers.

An adequate number of electrical outlets need to be available to accommodate lifestyle needs, including the use of a computer in the bedroom. If a telephone is in the bedroom, it should be placed at an appropriate access height. A roll-in closet or built-in closet with folding or pocket door and equipped with lowered rods and shelving within Mary's reaching distance would be ideal.

3. Mary has undergone a major traumatic life change and is embarking on another major life change as she marries. The psychosocial considerations in this case scenario would most ideally be met by a string team approach that can address multiple needs. The team should work cohesively regarding advisement about the home purchase as well. A home that can be renovated to meet the needs addressed in the above solutions, in the most economical fashion, incorporating the principles of universal design as outlined in this chapter would be appropriate. Additional considerations related to vehicle access and access to and from the home as well as exterior home entrances should be considered.

Other home layout considerations include room sizes, doorway and hallway widths, as well as floor surfaces and transitions. Home size also must be considered when planning for a family. Proximity to work, family, and friends of the community in which Mary and her fiancé choose to live also is important. Access to adequate medical care is another consideration for this couple. In addition, a community that offers accessible recreational and leisure activities that are compatible with Mary's active lifestyle interests should be considered. Appropriate planning and counseling is critical as well as providing Mary with adequate resources to make the most ideal informed decisions for her future success.

CHAPTER FIFTEEN

Wheelchair Skills

Alicia Koontz, RET, ATP, PhD, and Mary Shea, OTR, ATP, MA

Learning things like how to do wheelies and get up and down curbs are skills that everyone should know. It's hard at first but with the techniques the therapists teach you and a little time it gets easier. You learn how to handle the bumps in the sidewalk and other obstacles you may come across. Your confidence gets stronger and that's key…being confident and believing in yourself. This makes you stronger in mind and body and gives you greater independence.

Derrick (T9 SCI)

A wheelchair is the primary means of mobility for most individuals with a spinal cord injury (SCI). This chapter focuses on the techniques that are necessary to appropriately fit users to wheelchairs and the components of manual and power wheelchairs that are essential for individuals with SCI to function as safely and independently as possible.

Wheelchair skills are not just about performing wheelies or for the benefit of a few young, active individuals; wheelchair skills are essential for all individuals who use a wheelchair for mobility and environmental access. Wheelchair skills include propulsion training: learning how to push the wheel to decrease the risk of upper limb overuse injuries, learning how to bump over a door saddle that separates one room from another, learning to open doors, and learning to direct others to help you (e.g., up or down steps). These skills form the necessary knowledge base for anyone who uses a wheelchair to get in and around his home or his friends' and families' homes, to exit a house in an emergency situation, and to negotiate the community.

In the United States, an average of 36,559 wheelchair-related accidents each year are serious enough to require the user to seek attention in an emergency department.[1] In addition, an average of 51 deaths are caused by wheelchair-related accidents each year.[2] Between 1973 and 1987, there were 770 wheelchair-related deaths reported to the U.S. Consumer Product Safety Commission (USCPSC), 68.5% of which were attributed to falls and tips.[2] Of the 2066 nonfatal accidents reported between 1986 and 1990 to the USCPSC, falls and tips were the cause 73.2% of the time [2] (see Chapter 20).

It is important that an individual who uses a wheelchair receive instruction and training on wheelchair propulsion techniques to minimize his risk of injury and secondary complications such as repetitive strain injuries. Research has shown that individuals with SCI who use manual wheelchairs are at an increased risk for development of pain and repetitive strain injuries at the shoulder and wrist.[3-5] The technique that an individual uses to propel a wheelchair has been associated with the development of carpal tunnel syndrome and rotator cuff conditions.[6,7] Emerging evidence suggests that propulsion technique, type of wheelchair, and the way the wheelchair is fitted to a person can reduce injurious forces and the risk of injury.[8] Selecting the most appropriate wheelchair, adjusting it properly, and training the client in safe and effective use of the wheelchair in a variety of settings are all important elements to minimize each individual's risk of upper limb pain and injury. Consequently, this chapter initially provides an introduction to wheelchair type and fit and focuses on specific wheelchair skills with manual and power wheelchairs.

MANUAL WHEELCHAIRS
Wheelchair Type and Fit

The type of wheelchair and its fit to the individual client will influence his ability to perform wheelchair skills. For the majority of individuals with SCI who use manual wheelchairs as their means of mobility, the most commonly seen wheelchairs in accordance with the Centers for Medicare and Medicaid Services (CMS) K-Code classification include depot (K0001), lightweight (K0004), and ultralight (K0005). The depot wheelchair is designed for short-term hospital or institutional use and weighs at least 35 pounds; it is not adjustable. The lightweight wheelchair weighs between 30 pounds and 35 pounds and is designed with a minimum of adjustment capabilities. Ultralight wheelchairs weigh less than 30 pounds and are adjustable. Titanium chairs weighing less than 20 pounds are now available; however, they are not typically covered for individuals with paraplegia. Although reimbursement for titanium chairs is possible under the K9 code, few vendors are willing to chance coverage because it is rare. Four primary reasons support the use of ultralight wheelchairs (Box 15-1). Manual wheelchair users with SCI who will be using a wheelchair as their primary means of mobility will benefit from using an ultralight, durable manual wheelchair, which can be fully customized to fit their individual needs.

Force Required for Propulsion

An ultralight chair requires less force for propulsion. Rolling resistance is related to body and wheelchair weight.[9] Therefore a lighter wheelchair will reduce the forces needed to propel the chair

---

BOX 15-1 | Reasons for Using Ultralight Weight Wheelchair

- Less force is required for more energy-efficient propulsion.
- Maximum adjustability to customize fit to meet individual client's needs
- Higher quality construction and more durable components
- Cost-effective

and thus the forces transmitted into the upper limb joints. One study directly compared ultralight and depot wheelchairs. It reported that, when using an ultralight wheelchair, individuals with SCI pushed at faster speeds, traveled further distances, and used less energy.[10] The reduction of force becomes most important for maximum safety and independence when ascending ramps and outdoor surfaces such as sloped sidewalks and streets.

Maximum Adjustability Is Important to Fit

Only ultralight weight wheelchairs have axle and seating components that can be set up to fit the user. If more weight is over the front casters, it is more difficult to push and maneuver the wheelchair. Research shows that rolling resistance is lower with larger-diameter wheels.[9] Therefore adjusting the frame so that more of the client's weight is centered over or slightly behind the rear wheels will reduce rolling resistance. Such adjustments should be performed with caution because they can also make the wheelchair tip back more easily.

Ultralight wheelchairs allow for customizability of rear axle position and other adjustments such as camber and seat angle. This setup is important to truly fit the wheelchair to an individual for good hand-to-wheel access for a positive impact on propulsion mechanics. Most of the ultralight weight wheelchairs have a good degree of axle and seat angle adjustability to maximize fit to an individual. This adjustability is important for individuals with new injuries because they initially need the wheelchair set up for more stability and safety and, as they gain wheelchair skill proficiency, the wheelchair components can be adjusted for maximum performance and improved shoulder biomechanics. It should be noted that, despite current advances in technology and research, the CMS has not modified or updated the manual wheelchair coding criteria and reimbursement schedules to reflect these advances. As a result, true ultralight wheelchairs are in a miscellaneous code at this time. These are wheelchairs that are either made of titanium or have almost no adjustability. The customizability of these wheelchairs to an individual is done when the wheelchair is specified and ordered. This type of wheelchair is essential to maximize "fit" for maximal upper limb joint protection to maximize independence and safety with functioning at a wheelchair level.

High-Quality Components

Ultralight wheelchairs are made out of stronger, higher-grade materials and better components than are other wheelchairs. This includes the materials used for the frame and the components such as bearings that can reduce rolling resistance. A more durable frame and better components result in fewer repairs and, consequently, less down time without the wheelchair. This is absolutely essential for individuals who use wheelchairs because their safety and mobility can be severely compromised when parts fail. When the chair is out of commission, an individual's ability to perform life roles and activities of daily living (ADL) are also compromised. This has far-reaching implications: an individual may not be able to supervise his children properly or meet school or work-related responsibilities.

Research shows that ultralight wheelchairs outperform both depot and lightweight-type wheelchairs when internationally accepted fatigue-testing standards are applied.[11,12] Titanium frame

wheelchairs have a further advantage in that the material titanium also assists to dampen vibration from the environment and thus minimize the damaging effects of vibration on an individual's spine and shoulders.[13]

Economic Impact

Ultralight wheelchairs have been shown to last 13.2 times longer than depot wheelchairs and therefore cost about 3.5 times less to operate.[11] In comparison with lightweight wheelchairs, ultralights lasted 4.8 times longer and were 2.3 times less expensive to operate than lightweight wheelchairs.[12] When tested to failure, ultralight wheelchairs had the longest survival rate and had fewer catastrophic failures than depot and lightweight wheelchairs[14] Premature failures of wheelchairs place the individuals at risk for injury and compromise their ability to perform their life roles and ADLs. Consequently, the initial higher cost of ultralight weight chairs is more than made up for in durability.

Wheelchair Setup

After a client is positioned in his wheelchair with optimal upright sitting posture and pressure distribution (see Chapter 11), his wheel access is assessed to ensure optimal contact for efficient wheelchair propulsion technique and safety with performance. For an individual with a new injury, the wheel axle is placed more posteriorly and incrementally shifted anteriorly as his proficiency with wheelchair mobility skills increases. Antitippers are also used to ensure maximum safety with functioning at a wheelchair level. Other wheelchair considerations that can affect a client's ability to perform wheelchair skills are camber (angle at which rear wheel is tilted or slanted), seat width, seat angle, and armrests.

Rear Wheel Axle

The most critical wheelchair adjustment affecting propulsion technique and skills is position of the rear wheel axle. An ultralight wheelchair allows for both fore-aft and vertical height setup of the axle. The axle is generally shifted upward to increase a client's access to the wheel. For some wheelchair models, the rear seat is brought lower, independent of the wheel position; this, in turn, usually shifts the client's rear seat to floor height. It is important to ensure each client has the hip range to tolerate this increased seat angle to ensure he is seated with the most upright posture possible. This is extremely important because posture affects the shoulder girdle position. If an individual is seated with a kyphotic posture (i.e., collapsed trunk) (see Figure 11-4), then his shoulder girdle is in an elevated and protracted position, which changes the normal alignment and places him at an increased risk for shoulder injuries.

Moving the axle forward places more of the user's weight over the large wheel and brings the rear wheels closer to the front of the body (Figure 15-1). This enables greater access to the push-rim for a longer stroke.[15] In addition, more weight is shifted over the larger wheels so rolling resistance is less[9] and it is easier to pop into a wheelie to ascend curbs. Such adjustments should be done with training and caution, however, because moving the axle forward can make the wheelchair more unstable and cause backward tipping. This can compromise wheelchair stability when an individual negotiates the wheelchair over uneven surfaces such as a ramp or sidewalk.

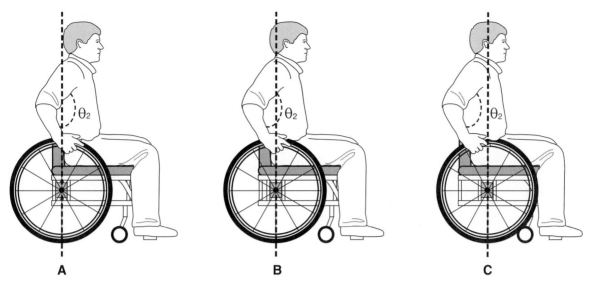

FIGURE 15-1 The position of the wheelchair axle can give the client increased access to the push rim for a more efficient stroke. **A,** The axle is mounted at the back of the seat, constricting the client's access to the push rim. **B,** The axle is mounted in line with the client's shoulder and hand when placed on the top of the rim; his elbow angle between 100 and 120 degrees is optimum for efficient propulsion. **C,** The axle is mounted forward, causing the wheelchair seat to shift rearward, bringing the rear wheels closer to the front of the body.

Wheelchair users often have difficulty maintaining a supported seated posture when subjected to external forces, which may include gravity when descending different terrain such as hills, ramps, and sidewalk slopes.[16] These external forces can be induced by ordinary obstacles that an individual encounters every day, thus increasing the risk of falling. Consequently, any wheelchair adjustments should be performed with caution on the basis of the client's trials over both level and uneven surfaces to ensure maximum safety with mobility.

Ideally, a more forward axle position is preferred because it has been associated with less muscle effort, smoother joint excursions, and lower stroke frequencies (number of times a client strikes the push rim).[17] In a study of 40 wheelchair users in their own manual wheelchairs, a more forward axle position was associated with lower peak forces, less rapid loading of the push rim, fewer strokes to go the same speed, and greater hand contact with the push rim.[18] Two of these parameters, stroke frequency and rate of loading the push rim, have been associated with damage to the median nerve.[7] A lower stroke frequency and rate of loading may help protect the median nerve from injury.

Because moving the rear axle forward has been proven to decrease rearward stability of the wheelchair, thus making the wheelchair more unstable in the backward direction,[19] wheelchairs are often delivered with the axle in the most rearward position possible. As a result, it is necessary for wheelchair vendors and clinicians to adjust the wheelchair setup. Considering the effect of such movement on chair stability, it is recommended that the axle be moved forward incrementally and training occurs to ensure the individual in the wheelchair has sufficient stability for safety.

When fitting an individual for his second or third wheelchair, the axle can be preset in a similar position to that of the existing wheelchair with antitippers in place (Figure 15-2, *A*). Antitippers should be used to minimize rearward falls (Figure 15-2, *B*), particularly with individuals who have more recent SCIs. Antitippers

should be positioned to allow the client to slightly tip the wheelchair and clear the front casters a minimum of 1 inch from the floor—a movement that is often necessary to negotiate door saddles. In other words, the antitippers with wheel components should not be so close to the floor that they prevent the client from using a slight wheelie to move across a door saddle. Extreme caution should be used to ensure that a client is safe until he has learned the necessary skills for maximum safety with functional mobility. If antitippers are set low, they might need to be removed, or rotated in an upward direction, to allow the client to negotiate a curb and pop a wheelie. Clinical judgment is essential to find the right antitipper height for each individual client.

In addition, it is important to explain to the client that adding weight to the chair can affect stability. Therefore, packages or backpacks should ideally be located underneath the seat of the chair[20] to ensure the weight distribution in the wheelchair is not changed. Finally, it is important for clinicians to remember that adjusting the axle position can affect wheel alignment and seat angle. Consequently, other adjustments, such as caster alignment, may be needed to keep the wheelchair in good alignment.

Rear axle height also affects wheelchair skills. Raising the axle lowers the seat, and lowering the axle raises the seat. In general, studies have shown that a lower seat position improves propulsion biomechanics. A lower seat position has been associated with greater upper limb motions,[15,21] greater hand contact with the push rim,[18,21] lower frequency, and higher mechanical efficiency.[21] These findings are obviously intuitive because lower seat heights give greater access to the push rim.

A lower seat height also increases stability of the wheelchair. Research agrees that the ideal seat height is the point at which the angle between the upper arm and forearm is between 100 and 120 degrees when the hand is resting on the top dead center of the push-rim (see Figure 11-22).[18,21] An alternative method that can be used to approximate the same ideal position is to have the client rest with

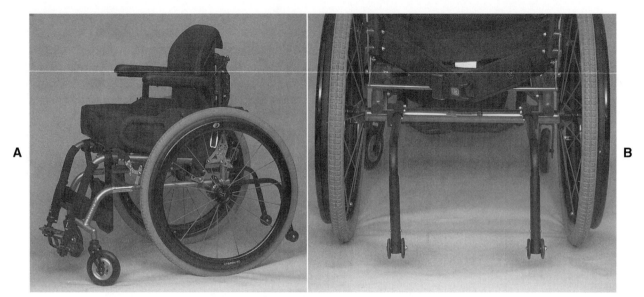

FIGURE 15-2   Antitippers shown from **A,** the lateral perspective, and **B,** the back of a wheelchair.

his arms hanging straight down at his side. His fingertips should be at the same level as the axle of the wheel. If the seat height is too high, less of the push rim can be accessed and a higher stroke frequency is used to go the desired speed. Adjusting seat height through vertical axle movement can affect alignment; thus other adjustments, such as caster alignment and height, may be needed to keep the wheelchair in good alignment.

Camber

As with any feature, adding camber to make the wheelchair's wheels angle outward at the bottom has both advantages and disadvantages (Table 15-1) (see Figure 11-31). Camber of the wheel allows for continuation of the normal biomechanical angle of the glenohumeral joint, can increase side-to-side stability, and greatly facilitates turning of the wheelchair. The main disadvantage to camber is that it can significantly increase the overall width of the wheelchair and consequently compromises environmental access (e.g., the ability to fit the chair through a 28-inch-wide standard doorway). Two, four, and six degrees of camber are commonly seen on everyday wheelchairs as long as the overall width is less than 28 inches.

Wheelchair Width and Depth

When the size of a client's wheelchair is determined, the width should be as narrow as possible without causing pressure on the bony hip prominences. If the seat width is too wide, a client will use greater shoulder abduction and access less of the push rim for wheelchair skills. This is a major concern because performing forceful motions (e.g., pushing a wheelchair) into a flexed, internally rotated, and abducted shoulder position predisposes individuals with SCI to shoulder impingement injury.

Optimizing seat depth is essential to ensure proper fit and pressure distribution. Adjustment to the seat back angle is necessary for optimal posture and balance and is paramount to preserving upper limb function. When seat depth is determined, the pelvis should be supported in as neutral a position as possible and measurements taken from the back of the pelvis to just shy of popliteal fossa (see Chapter 11).

Seat Slope or Angle

A posterior scat angle can be achieved by either raising the axle or, in a squeeze frame wheelchair, by lowering the rear seat to floor height. This effectively lowers and angles the seat back. This adjustment adds stability to the wheelchair user, increases hand-to-wheel access, and may make it easier to push and maneuver the wheelchair. Extreme care should, however, be taken with this adjustment because it increases weight posterior to the wheelchair axle, thus increasing the chance of tipping. In a squeeze frame wheelchair, it decreases the seat angle. Consequently, it is important to ensure that the client has sufficient hip range of motion to sit at this angle (see Chapter 11). Back angle adjustment often accompanies a seat angle adjustment because it changes a client's orientation in the wheelchair. Also, because of the lower rear seat height, transfers out of the wheelchair may be more difficult with a more posterior seat angle. The transfer change can often be resolved with additional transfer training.

Armrests

The type of armrest and its setup is extremely important to hand access of the push rim. A standard armrest with a pad in its standard position can provide individuals with an increased feeling of stability in the wheelchair. However, it compromises an individual's wheel access because he usually has to abduct his arms to clear the armpad and access the push rims. This is similar to having too wide a seat and can predispose individuals to shoulder impingement injury. Armrests, if needed, should be mounted in line with the seat frame. This can be accomplished by reversing the armpad on a standard, removable armrest or by using the padded, swing-away, tubular-style armrest.

Propulsion Technique

A number of ergonomic studies have strongly implicated frequency of task completion as a risk factor for repetitive strain injury or pain at the wrists[22-25] and shoulder.[26-28] Wheelchair

TABLE 15-1	Advantages and Disadvantages of Wheelchair Wheel Camber	
Advantages	**Disadvantages**
Brings top of wheels inward and closer to the body, enabling arms to access more of the push rim	Wider wheelchairs can be problematic in tight areas
Improved biomechanics: reduces shoulder abduction because the wheels are closer to the body	Diminished traction and uneven tire wear on a conventional tire
Increases wheelchair lateral stability	
Reduces rolling resistance because less of the tire contacts the ground	
Protects client's hands when pushing in tight areas because the wheels make contact first with walls and door frames	

propulsion, with a stroke occurring approximately once per second, exceeds what the majority of studies consider a frequent task. A study specifically involving wheelchair users with paraplegia found that median nerve injury was related to the frequency of propulsion.[7] The more often the individual with SCI pushed on the rim to go a constant speed, the more nerve damage he had. Median nerve injury is the basic process behind the development of carpal tunnel syndrome.

Studies in the ergonomic literature have demonstrated that higher forces are correlated with injuries or pain at the wrist [22,23,25] and shoulder.[27,28] The forces defined as high in these studies are almost always exceeded during wheelchair propulsion.[29] Two studies in the SCI literature have examined the effects of high forces during wheelchair propulsion. In one study that involved individuals with paraplegia, the rate of force loading to the push rim was correlated with median nerve damage.[7] A higher rate of loading, which is closely related to higher force, was associated with greater median nerve injury. When the same research subjects were followed up longitudinally, decrements in median nerve function over time were predicted by the forces exerted on the push rim at the start of the study.[30] These results strongly suggest that higher peak forces lead to injury.

Research findings from the ergonomic and SCI literature relate injury risk to repetitive force tasks and indicate that individuals who use wheelchairs should learn to use propulsion techniques that minimize forces and decrease the frequency of the propulsive stroke.[8] Propulsion patterns of persons with SCI have been examined in detail.[31-35] Although the path of the hand is constrained by the arc of the push rim during the delivery of propulsive forces, there is more freedom in upper limb motion when the hand is off the rim and preparing for the next stroke, which is referred to as the recovery part of the stroke.

Four distinct patterns of recovery have been identified: semicircular (A), arc (B), single-loop over (C), and double-loop over (D) (Figure 15-3). In one study, the single-loop over form of propulsion (Figure 15-3, C), which consists of having the hand above the push rim during recovery, was the most prevalent pattern in individuals with paraplegia.[32] Another study also consisting

of manual wheelchair users with paraplegia did not find any one pattern to be more prevalent on a level treadmill but found that as the treadmill incline increased, individuals were quick to switch to an arc form of propulsion.[35] This was an expected finding because when traversing a ramp, the wheelchair has a greater tendency to roll backwards during recovery, and quick strokes are necessary to keep the wheelchair moving forward. In the arc form of propulsion, the hands remain close to the handrim during recovery to enable for grabbing the pushrim more readily.

For propulsion over level surfaces, the semicircular pattern, in which the user's hand drops below the push rim during recovery, has been shown to have better biomechanics (Figure 15-3, A). The semicircular pattern has been associated with lower stroke frequency,[32] greater time spent in the push phase relative to the recovery phase,[32] and less angular joint velocity and acceleration.[31] The semicircular pattern is preferred because the hand follows an elliptical pattern with no abrupt changes in direction and no extra hand movements. By applying forces to the push rim in smooth, long strokes, the same amount of energy is imparted to the rim with less high-peak forces or a large rate of force loading. A long stroke, for example, as shown in Figure 15-3, A, as opposed to a short stroke (Figure 15-3, B) or interrupted stroke (Figure 15-3, D), is also likely to minimize the number of strokes needed to push at a desired speed.

The previous research findings suggest that individuals who use wheelchairs should be educated on propulsion technique to maximize their efficiency and minimize their risk for repetitive strain injuries.[8,31-34] Consequently, it is important to begin wheelchair skills training with educating clients about their potential for injury and a more efficient technique to propel their wheelchairs.

After a client is set up in the wheelchair with sufficient wheel access, he should be instructed to compare the wheel to the face of a clock. Training should emphasize trying to start contact with the wheel at about 10 o'clock and to release contact at about 2 to 3 o'clock with normal propulsion. This will result in a longer, more energy efficient stroke. For the recovery phase (discussed above), the SCI literature supports the semicircular recovery pattern in which the client releases the stroke around 2 to 3 o'clock and keeps his hand beneath the handrim as he brings his hand down below the push rim and directly back around until he is again at the 10 o'clock position on the handrim.

Wheelchair Parts Management and Basic Maintenance

All clients and their caregivers, as necessary, should be trained in full wheelchair seating system parts management and basic maintenance. Basic wheelchair parts management training can include wheel lock negotiation, footplate and legrest movement, flip up and down and/or swing away removal, removal and replacement of armrests, cushion, back support wheel, and antitipper. Because wheelchairs are carefully designed for durability and low maintenance, clients should expect their personal maintenance to be limited to inspection, tightening loose components, and cleaning activities (Table 15-2). Trained technicians should be sought when the wheelchair is not functioning properly and skilled maintenance is needed.

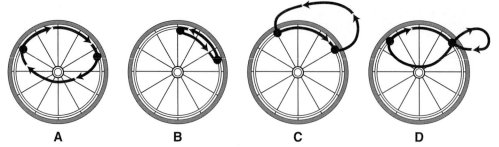

FIGURE 15-3 Four propulsion patterns used by individuals with paraplegia. The thick black line on the wheel is the path followed by the hand, and the arrows indicate the direction the hand moves. The circles indicate hand and push rim contact and hand release.

Evaluating Wheelchair Skills

Outcome measures are important to ensure quality of care in the rehabilitation process. For example, outcome tools such as the Functional Independence Measure (FIM) and Craig Handicap Assessment and Reporting Technique (CRAIG) document the client's overall function and performance and are used to aid in evaluating the effectiveness and efficiency of services and interventions provided. Preliminary tools for evaluating power wheelchair skills have been developed, but surprisingly few have been developed for manual wheelchair skills. The most comprehensive tool currently available is the Wheelchair Skills Test (WST). The WST is a systematic instrument intended to objectively, simply, and inexpensively evaluate and document a wide range of representative manual wheelchair skills (www.wheelchair-skillsprogram.ca/). The test is administered on a specific person in his wheelchair. Skills are evaluated in a standardized setting with specific equipment and materials (e.g., pylons, transfer bench, gravel) and environmental obstacles (e.g., curbs, incline, door, door threshold). Examples of the types of skills evaluated include apply/release brakes; move armrests and footrests away and restore; turn in place; turn while moving; stationary wheelie; wheelie turn; wheelie forward/backward; three-point turns; parallel parking; reaching to floor, in/out of knapsack, and for high object; and enter/exit through a door; curb and incline ascent/descent; transfer in/out of wheelchair; and fold/open wheelchair (if non-rigid frame). The clinician responsible for wheelchair training should report whether an individual skill is a goal by answering the question "Is it reasonable to expect this person to be able to perform this skill in this wheelchair at discharge from the rehabilitation program?" The clinician should take into consideration the client's aspirations, anticipated level of function, wheelchair equipment and postdischarge setting. The clinician should consider input available to that point from the client, his family, and other team members. For each skill, the client receives a score of pass, fail, or not applicable.

The WST has been found to be practical, safe, and well tolerated and to exhibit good to excellent reliability, excellent content validity, fair construct, and concurrent validity.[36] The WST may be used early in the course of a rehabilitation program as a diagnostic measure to determine which, if any, skills or wheelchair changes need to be addressed during the rehabilitation process or how much training will be necessary to ensure safe and effective wheelchair use. Repeating the test on completion of the rehabilitation program provides an outcome measure that reflects the effectiveness of the wheelchair skills training program and interventions.

The Wheelchair Circuit is another tool that can be used to assess progress with wheelchair skills.[37] This test includes nine standardized tasks related to ADLs, not only wheelchair skills. The tasks in this circuit are figure-8 shape using the wheelchair, crossing a doorstep in a wheelchair, mounting a platform in a wheelchair, a wheelchair sprint of 15 meters, walking 15 meters, wheelchair driving on a treadmill for 5 minutes at a speed of 0.83 meter/second, wheelchair driving on a treadmill at a 3% slope at 0.56 meter/second, wheelchair driving on a treadmill at a 6% slope at 0.56 meter/second, and transfer. Interrater and intrarater reliability have been established for the tasks except for crossing a doorstep and mounting a platform, and therefore the authors do not recommend these tasks for assessment of mobility. Overall further validation of the wheelchair circuit is needed to test validation of scoring the test.[37] Clinicians are advised to apply the use of this circuit using those tasks applicable to the client because not all of the tasks may be performed by all individuals with SCI.

Training in Advanced Wheelchair Skills

Advanced wheelchair skills are essential for all individuals who use their wheelchair outdoors in the community. It is therefore imperative that individuals with SCI learn to safely negotiate common obstacles within the community at a wheelchair level. This includes the ability to instruct or perform techniques to ascend and descend curbs, ramps, and stairs, to negotiate doorways and uneven surfaces, and perform floor transfers. These advanced skills should be initiated after the client has become proficient in basic skills, including wheelchair propulsion on level surfaces, weight shifts, transfers, mat and bed mobility, and basic ADLs. Individuals should use a wheelchair that is optimally fitted to them to ensure appropriate body mechanics for efficient propulsion technique and to facilitate advanced-level wheelchair mobility skills. A pelvic belt is strongly recommended to maximize contact and stability between the client and the wheelchair. It is necessary to obtain clearance from the client's physician before performing advanced wheelchair skills training to ensure that spinal stability and skin integrity will not be compromised. As a client is learning these techniques, his caregiver should be trained to assist with advanced skills to ensure maximum safety. Also, if a client presents with decreased cognition or safety concerns, his caregiver should be trained in advanced-level skills to ensure maximum safety with mobility indoors and in the community.

Individuals in wheelchairs and caregivers should be educated on caster position and the importance of a forward facing caster for maximum safety and stability with forward reach, picking

TABLE 15-2 | Checklist for Basic Wheelchair Maintenance

Inspection	On Receipt	Weekly	Monthly	Periodically
General				
Wheelchair opens and folds easily	✓			✓
Wheelchair rolls straight with no excess drag or pull	✓	✓		
Footrests flop up and down easily	✓			✓
Legrests swing away and latch easily	✓			✓
Backrest folds and latches easily	✓			✓
Armrests easy to move and latch	✓			✓
All nuts and bolts are snug	✓			✓
Wheels				
Axle threads in easily or slides in and latches properly	✓			✓
No squeaking, binding, or excessive side motion while turning	✓	✓		
All spokes and nipples are tight and not bent or nicked	✓			✓
Tire pressure is correct and equal on both sides	✓	✓		
No cracks, looseness, bulges in tires	✓		✓	
Casters				
No cracks, looseness, or bulges in caster tires	✓		✓	
No wobbling of caster wheel	✓	✓		
No excessive play in the caster spindle	✓	✓		
Caster housing is aligned vertically	✓	✓		
Wheel Locks				
Do not interfere with tire when rolling	✓		✓	
Easily activated and released by operator	✓	✓		
Hold tires firmly in place while activated	✓	✓		
Electrical System				
Wires show no cracks, splits, or breaks	✓			✓
Indicators and horn work properly	✓	✓		
Controls work smoothly and continually	✓	✓	✓	
Battery cases are clean and free from fluids	✓			✓
Motor runs smoothly and quietly	✓			
Upholstery				
No tears, rips, burn marks, or excessive fraying	✓			✓
No excessive stretching (e.g., hammocking)	✓		✓	
Upholstery is clean	✓	✓		

Adapted from Cooper RA: *Wheelchair selection and configuration*, New York. 1998, Demos Medical Publishing, Inc., Figure 14-18, p 389.

items up from the floor, and transfer to and from the wheelchair (Figure 15-4). Slightly reversing the wheelchair will facilitate caster change from the normal training position to a forward facing position (Figure 15-4). This is essential to increase the wheel base for increased stability with forward maneuvers and function. It is especially important for wheelchair to floor transfers.

Protective Response with Falls

Despite all efforts to minimize the risk of a fall, there is always the possibility that an individual in a wheelchair will fall backward in his wheelchair, especially if it is set up for performance over stability. It is therefore imperative that individuals in wheelchairs learn to protect themselves when falling. Even after learning these techniques to minimize the impact of the fall, a client should always be encouraged to follow up with his physician in the event of a fall at home or in the community.

Learning to fall safely should always be practiced on a padded surface to avoid injury to the client and unnecessary

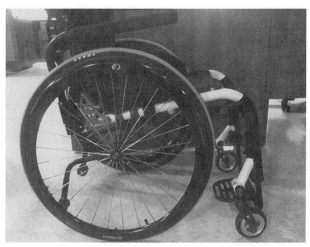

FIGURE 15-4 A forward-facing caster is essential for maximum safety with reaching activities, transfers, and picking up items from the floor.

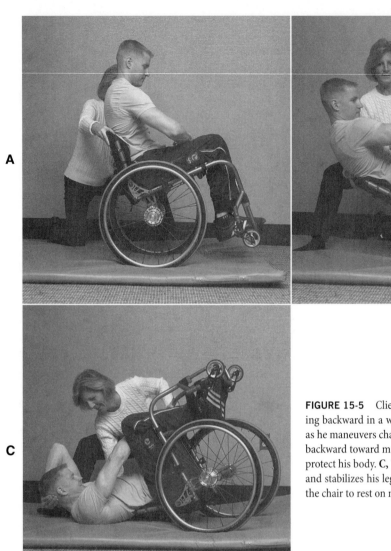

FIGURE 15-5 Client demonstrates protective responses to falling backward in a wheelchair. **A,** The therapist guards the client as he maneuvers chair into wheelie. **B,** The therapist guides chair backward toward mat as the client begins to position his arms to protect his body. **C,** The client protects his head with his one arm and stabilizes his legs with his other arm as the therapist guides the chair to rest on mat.

damage to the chair. The therapist should initiate the training for this response by dependently tilting the wheelchair back (Figure 15-5, *A*), and slowly lowering it to the floor while the client performs the proper protective response (Figure 15-5, *B*). The most important protective response when the wheelchair has tipped backward beyond a position of recovery is to protect the head. The client should be instructed to tuck his chin to his chest, cover the back of his head with one arm, and block his knees with the other arm to ensure that his knees do not fall forward and hit him in the face (Figure 15-5, *C*). The therapist can facilitate proficiency with this task by gradually increasing the speed of the dependent tilt back and eventually the client is allowed to fall backward from a wheelie in a controlled manner with therapist assistance.

Wheelies

Although wheelies may appear to be a way of showing off, they are actually the foundation of many advanced wheelchair skills and are essential for independence and safety with indoor and outdoor mobility. When moving in a wheelchair across uneven surfaces (e.g., grass or gravel), the casters may get caught and result in a fall or significant strain with propulsion. If wheelies have been mastered, one can move across uneven surfaces using only the large rear wheels to decrease this strain. In addition, wheelies are a vital component in advanced wheelchair skills such as ascending and descending a curb.

When wheelie training is initiated, it is often easier to begin with maintaining a wheelie rather than attaining a wheelie. The therapist can instruct the client in this skill by tilting his chair backward to his balance point and then have him negotiate the wheels forward and backward through a very small range to allow him to become aware of the boundaries of his balance point. This will give him a good understanding and feel for his balance point so that he is aware of what he is attempting to achieve. Verbal clues should be kept to a minimum so that the client can feel the wheel. The client should be encouraged to keep only a light pressure on the wheel rims and to allow the wheel to move. In addition, a client who is able, should be instructed to lean his trunk and forehead slightly forward when balancing to keep his center of gravity over the wheelchair's base of support (Figure 15-6). It is important to note that individuals with some hand function (i.e., C7 level of injury) have the potential to be independent in achieving their balance point and popping wheelies.

When a client becomes comfortable with balancing in a wheelie, he can progress to popping or attaining a wheelie. To assume a wheelie from a static position have the client either perform a short backward stroke and then propel forward with a quick, strong stroke to lift the casters off the floor or push the wheels forward with a quick strong stroke as the client leans backward to lift the casters off the floor. The objective is for the client to pop into a wheelie, immediately find his balance point, and then maintain that balanced position. The therapist should guard the client from behind the wheelchair with both hands lightly on or near the wheelchair. It is important for the therapist to avoid transmitting any pressure through her hands and to allow the chair to move so the client can get a feel for his balance point. The therapist should be prepared to prevent the wheelchair from falling backward or landing forcefully on the casters. When initiating wheelies, the therapist should also provide verbal feedback to help the client remain relaxed and to instruct him in the proper balance correction techniques. Verbalization of the technique is used to complement what the client is experiencing at a particular time. For example, in the wheelie, if the wheelchair is tipping backward, the client should bring the wheels backward to bring the wheelchair more forward; conversely, if falling forward, the client should bring the wheels forward in an attempt to regain his balance point. After a client understands what is happening with the wheel and his balance point, it is again helpful to keep verbal cues to a minimum and allow him to experience the balance point and maintaining a wheelie.

When a client begins to attain and maintain a wheelie independently, he is ready to progress to propulsion in a wheelie. This is an opportunity to have the client practice propelling forward and backward and turning in a wheelie position to really get a feel for his balance point. As the client masters this, have him negotiate the wheelchair up and down a ramp in the wheelie to really get a firm sense of his balance point. Concise verbal communication between the therapist and client will help allow the therapist to safely guard the client without providing excessive hands-on assistance. Also, using a strap on the back rigidizer bar can allow the therapist to adequately guard the client for an extended period of time without straining her back muscles. The proper protective responses described previously should be reinforced during the wheelie training.

A more advanced wheelchair skill for clients who are independent in dynamic wheelies may be to descend an incline in a wheelie. The client will coast toward the ramp in a wheelie and allow the wheel rims to smoothly glide through his grasp. As the client is learning proficiency with this skill, the therapist should follow behind the wheelchair with both hands, providing contact guard to the wheelchair to prevent posterior tipping or slamming down forward.

Door Management
The first step in negotiating most doors is developing the ability to manipulate keys and door knobs. For individuals without full grasp, wrist extension may be used to hook the level handle.

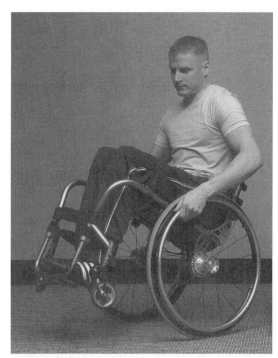

FIGURE 15-6 The client performs a wheelie with his trunk leaning slightly forward to keep his center of gravity over the wheelchair base of support. The carpet resistance is helpful to master control of the wheelie.

Different techniques can be used to maneuver a wheelchair through a doorway, depending on how it opens and whether the hinge is spring loaded.

Pushing a Door Open
An individual in a wheelchair should approach the door in a forward direction and position himself directly in front of the door to maximize physical access to manipulate the doorknob and the door. If a doorknob is present, it should be released. Then the client should use his arm closest to the hinged side to push the door open. His contralateral upper limb should stabilize the wheelchair by holding its handrim. The client can use the front or side of the wheelchair or intermittently push with his hand closest to the hinge to stabilize a spring-loaded door in the open position while he propels through the doorway using his other hand on the wheelchair handrim (Figure 15-7). Once a door is open, the client can use both hands on the handrims to negotiate the threshold. If the door is spring loaded, when able to reach the door frame, the client can let go of the wheel rim and pull the wheelchair through using the frame. To prevent injury, clients should be instructed to avoid using their footplates or feet to push or hold a spring loaded door open.

Pulling a Door Open
To pull a door open, a client should approach the door from the unhinged side, keeping the wheelchair behind the opening arc of the door. The chair should be slightly angled toward the door. This will allow the client to reach the handle with the upper limb closest to the door. The client can use his arm farthest from the door to push on the wall next to the door and stabilize his body and the wheelchair. After the client opens the door, he can propel the wheelchair through with both hands.

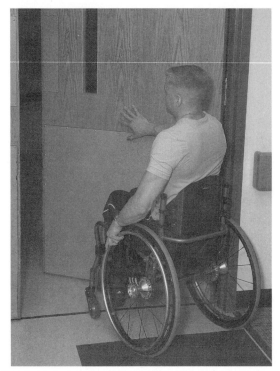

FIGURE 15-7   The client in manual wheelchair pushes door open.

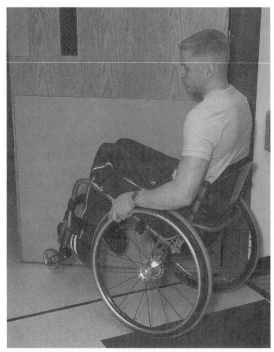

FIGURE 15-8   The client in manual wheelchair clears the threshold and moves through the doorway.

If the doorway has a door saddle, the client should perform a slight wheelie to negotiate it. In Figure 15-8, the client demonstrates how to pop the casters to clear the threshold while almost in wheelie position. After the casters have cleared, the client should grasp both handrims and propel the rear wheels over the threshold.

Ramps
Ascending a Ramp

Client Techniques. Initially, to ascend a ramp or incline the client should first check the antitippers to ensure that they are locked in the down position. In addition, to prevent the wheelchair from tipping backward, the client should lean forward as far as possible (respecting any precautions he may have) and maintain this position while propelling up the ramp (Figure 15-9). The wheelchair is propelled up the ramp by use of short, quick strokes, toward the front of the wheel, keeping the chair in constant forward motion. This will enable the client's momentum to assist with the elevation. If the wheelchair comes to a complete stop, it is much more difficult for the client to resume the ascension.

If a client has high-mounted wheel locks on his wheelchair, care should be taken to avoid getting his thumbs caught in the locks. Some clients may choose to get low-mounted wheel locks for this reason. The therapist or caregiver should guard the client from behind to assist the client if necessary and to ensure that he does not tip backward. Grade Aids are a wheelchair accessory that is available for clients who may have difficulty propelling up an incline. It is a device that is placed near the wheel locks to prevent the wheelchair from rolling backward between strokes.

As a client becomes more proficient with wheelchair mobility skills, he will most likely remove the antitippers. The therapist or caregiver should guard the client as he initially begins using the

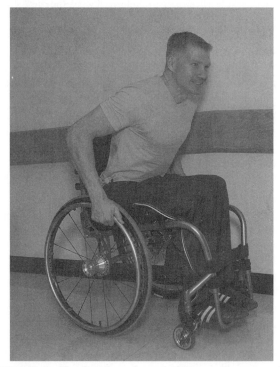

FIGURE 15-9   The client leans forward while ascending a ramp in a manual wheelchair.

wheelchair with the antitippers in the up position to ensure that the body's forward lean is 100% stable for negotiation of the different grades of inclines.

Caregiver Techniques. When pushing an individual in a wheelchair up a ramp, the caregiver should first make sure that the antitippers are in place. The caregiver should begin with her elbows flexed and lean forward into the wheelchair to attain a low center of gravity. As the caregiver pushes the client up the ramp, her elbows can move into an extended locked position and she should use her lower limb strength to negotiate the wheelchair up the ramp and onto a flat, level surface. The caregiver should be reminded to keep her head up and torso aligned throughout the maneuver to reinforce proper body mechanics. Proper body mechanics are essential to minimize the risk of injury for the caregiver. For steeper incline grades, the antitippers may need to be adjusted to clear the ramp, and the caregiver should use caution and make sure she has the strength to perform the task safely.

Descending a Ramp

Client Techniques. To descend a ramp, the client should approach the ramp forward, lean as far back as possible, and allow the wheelchair rims to smoothly glide through his grasp. The speed of the descent is controlled by the amount of friction applied to the wheel rims by the client. If a client does not have hand function, this is done by the heels of the hands squeezing in against the outside of the wheel rims. It is strongly recommended that clients wear push gloves when propelling down a ramp to avoid skin breakdown or friction burns. The posterior lean of the trunk while a client is descending the ramp is essential for maximum control over his body and subsequently the wheelchair. The therapist can guard the client from behind with one hand on the wheelchair and the other hand in front of the client's trunk to prevent forward flexion until he can hold himself back sufficiently to ensure trunk stability (Figure 15-10). The client is independent with descending a ramp when complete control is consistently maintained throughout descent and the client can stop or turn on command. If a ramp is particularly steep, a client may choose to zigzag down the ramp to ensure greater control over the wheelchair rather than going straight down the incline.

Caregiver Techniques. For clients who do not have sufficient control to negotiate the wheelchair down a ramp, the easiest and safest technique is for the caregiver to bring the client down the ramp backward. In this position, the caregiver is between the client and the bottom of the incline and there is minimal chance that the caregiver will lose her grip and the client descend the incline uncontrolled. There are two ways the caregiver may position herself to accomplish this. In the first, the caregiver is on the ramp with the wheelchair backed to the edge of the decline. The caregiver may then lean into the wheelchair facing up the incline keeping both elbows extended and head up (as when pushing a client up a ramp). The second position is to stand sideways with her hip against the wheelchair (Figure 15-11). With either position, the caregiver should slowly negotiate the wheelchair down the ramp by using the muscles in her lower limbs. It is important for the caregiver to periodically check behind for people or obstacles. A caregiver can also assist a client down a ramp with the wheelchair facing forward. The caregiver handling is pictured in Figure 15-10.

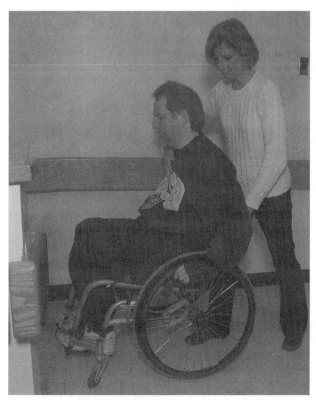

FIGURE 15-10 The therapist guards a client as he descends a ramp in a manual wheelchair.

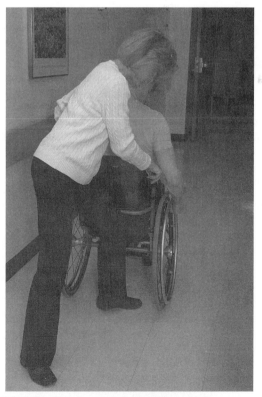

FIGURE 15-11 The client is dependently brought down a ramp by a therapist coming down the ramp backward. The therapist stands sideways with her hip against the wheelchair backrest to avoid inadvertent loss of control down the ramp by the patient. The therapist or caregiver should strive to keep her elbows slightly flexed and use her leg muscles to protect her back.

Curbs

Although many public areas are now equipped with curb cuts, they are not always conveniently located and at times they are 2 to 3 inches above the surface of the street. In addition to being used on curbs, the following techniques are also useful for negotiating elevated thresholds, single steps, or uneven sidewalks.

Dynamic Wheelies: Rolling and Popping

This is a prerequisite to curb negotiation. The client, who previously learned to pop a wheelie from a static position, must now learn to pop a wheelie while the chair is moving forward. This roll-and-pop skill can be initiated by having the client propel down a hallway and every 15 feet add a quick, strong forward stroke while shifting trunk weight posteriorly to lift the casters off the ground and pop into a wheelie. After a client masters this skill, he will need to work on timing his pop so that when he approaches a curb the casters land up on the curb.

Ascending a Curb

Client Techniques. The easiest approach to teaching curb negotiation is to separate the task into its component parts and then combine them to optimize the use of momentum. Start with a small curb, approximately 2 inches, and progress to increased heights as appropriate to the client's skill level. The antitipper should be shifted upward or removed to perform this activity, and the therapist should be directly behind the wheelchair ready to guard the client as necessary.

The client should approach the curb in a forward direction, pop into a wheelie, and land the casters on the curb. After the casters are on the curb, the client must immediately lean forward (Figure 15-12, *A*) and propel the rear wheels up the curb (Figure 15-12, *B*). A client may ascend a low curb even if he hesitates when approaching and popping onto the curb. As higher curbs (e.g., 4 to 6 inches) are attempted, however, the momentum of the forward movement is crucial for the individual in the wheelchair

to successfully ascend the curb. If an individual hesitates, he will lose momentum and will not be able to ascend higher curbs.

The client should be guarded from behind to ensure that he does not fall backward and, if necessary, to provide assistance to clear the casters and propel the rear wheels up the curb. Verbal cueing is helpful for teaching the client to time his pop and optimize his forward momentum.

Caregiver Techniques. If a caregiver is going to be trained to negotiate the wheelchair up a curb, she should be instructed in the proper technique to minimize her risk for injury. To dependently lift a wheelchair up a curb, threshold, or single step, start approximately 2 feet from the elevation to avoid bumping the client's feet or the wheelchair footplates against the curb. The caregiver should begin by rotating the antitippers into the up position. The caregiver should use her foot on the lower rear frame of the wheelchair (next to the antitipper) to bring the wheelchair into a wheelie position with the casters high enough to clear the elevation. In the wheelie, she rolls the wheelchair forward until both rear wheels are against the curb; then she slowly lowers the casters onto the elevated area (e.g., step or sidewalk). The caregiver should then position herself sideways with one hip against the wheelchair and the other leg out in a backward direction, giving her a wide base of support (Figure 15-13, *A*). She should bend her legs to use her lower limb strength and body weight to lift and roll the rear wheels up the elevation (Figure 15-13, *B*). As the rear wheels ascend the curb, the caregiver's body momentum will help move the wheelchair forward and onto the elevation (Figure 15-13, *C*). It is important to make sure that both rear wheels remain in contact with the curb at all times. If the rear wheels do not remain in contact with the curb, increased weight will be transferred to the casters, which may swivel and make this task more difficult. To avoid injury, it is important to reinforce proper body mechanics when instructing this procedure. After maneuvering over the curb, it is imperative to remember to reposition the antitippers in the downward-facing position.

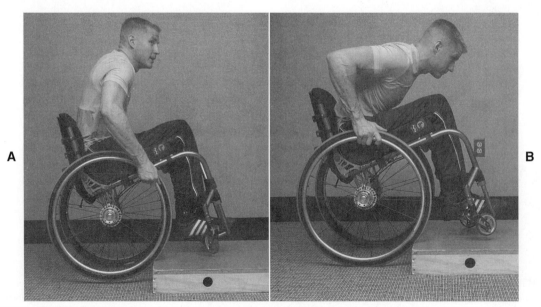

FIGURE 15-12 The client ascends a curb. **A,** The casters are up on curb, and **B,** the client leans forward to propel rear wheels up curb.

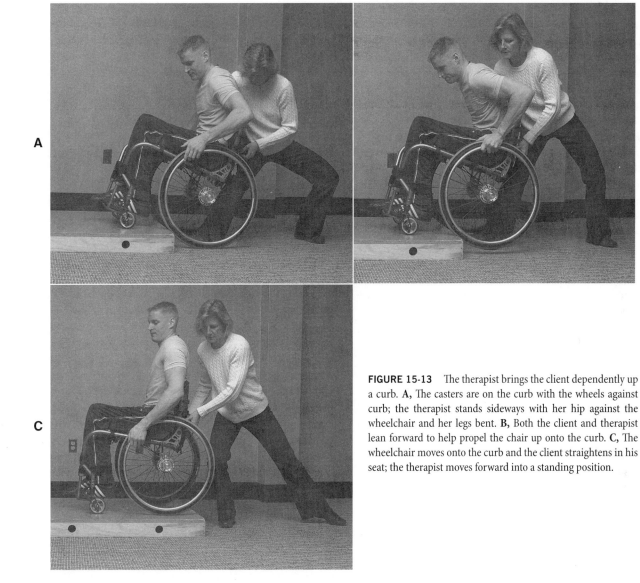

FIGURE 15-13 The therapist brings the client dependently up a curb. **A,** The casters are on the curb with the wheels against curb; the therapist stands sideways with her hip against the wheelchair and her legs bent. **B,** Both the client and therapist lean forward to help propel the chair up onto the curb. **C,** The wheelchair moves onto the curb and the client straightens in his seat; the therapist moves forward into a standing position.

Descending a Curb

Client Techniques. The safest and easiest way to descend a curb is backward. The client should back the wheelchair up to the edge of the curb and make sure that the wheelchair is completely square with the curb (i.e., both rear wheels are an even distance from the curb). While leaning forward, the client then controls the rear wheel descent from the curb by allowing the handrims to slowly slide through his grasp. When both rear wheels are on the bottom surface, the client should then back away slightly (about 4 inches) and perform a sharp turn by holding one wheel steady and propelling forward on the other to rotate the wheelchair and remove the casters from the curb without banging against it. The caregiver guards from the rear, as in ascending curbs, to minimize the risk of tipping backward and to ensure a controlled descent from the curb.

As a client progresses with his wheelchair mobility skills, he can learn to descend a curb forward in a wheelie. This is a much faster technique and allows the client to smoothly continue forward in the direction he is going. To accomplish this technique, the client coasts in a wheelie at a steady speed with the wheelchair square to the curb. He allows the handrims to slide freely through a light grasp as he descends the curb. The client can then continue on without slowing or stopping. The caregiver guards from behind the client to prevent him from tipping backward. It is extremely important that the client is independent in dynamic wheelies and protective falls before attempting this maneuver.

Caregiver Techniques. The safest way for a caregiver to move an individual in a wheelchair down a curb is to bring the wheelchair down backward. The caregiver should first turn the antitippers of the wheelchair facing upward and position the wheelchair with the rear wheels square at the edge of the curb. She then positions herself on the street sideways with a wide base of support and one hip against the back of the wheelchair and the other leg out into the street. This is the same biomechanics as in Figure 15-13. The direction is just reversed. The rear wheels are guided to roll down the curb as the caregiver shifts her weight and bends with her hips and knees. When the rear wheels are on the street surface, the wheelchair is tipped back into a wheelie. While remaining in a wheelie (i.e., balance point), the chair is rolled away from the curb. After the casters are clear, the caregiver shifts one foot to the lower rear frame of the wheelchair to assist with slowly lowering the casters to the floor. The antitippers must then be shifted into the down position. It is very important that the caregiver perform this descent with proper biomechanics to minimize her risk of injury.

Floor Transfers

Many clients will tell you that they do not need to learn floor transfers because they have no intention of performing any activities on the floor. There is always the possibility, however, of falling out of a wheelchair, and if a client has children it is important to be able to play with them on the floor. Therefore it is important to review floor transfers with all clients with SCI.

If a client has fallen backward in his wheelchair and remained in the wheelchair, he may choose to simply right the wheelchair from this tilted-back position. If the client is out of the wheelchair on the floor, he may choose to position the wheelchair upright and then transfer from the floor into the wheelchair in its upright position. Keep in mind that for an individual with a high-level injury independence may mean directing others to assist him back into the wheelchair. As always, good judgment is of paramount importance. The individual with SCI should be aware of the abilities of his friends, family, and caregivers. If necessary, the best solution may be to call 911 and have the police or first aid squad come to lift the individual into his wheelchair rather than having friends or family members attempt it.

Righting a Wheelchair from a Tilted-Back Position

The tilted-back position is often the position an individual will land in when he falls backward in his wheelchair. Starting with the wheelchair resting on the floor in a tilted-back position, the client must first appropriately reposition himself in the wheelchair. His buttocks should be firmly back in the seat, his knees hooked over the front edge of the seat with the feet on or behind the footplates, the seatbelt snugly tightened, and the wheel locks in the locked position. The client should then be trained to reach across to the front corner of the seat and grasp the wheelchair frame. This position will allow him to prop up onto his opposite elbow on the floor. By pulling on the wheelchair with one arm and pushing off the opposite elbow the client can work up onto an extended arm. Then by shifting his weight through his upper body away from his extended arm, he should shift his extended arm on the floor around the side of the wheelchair while pulling up on the locked wheel with the other arm until the wheelchair frame resumes its upright position. It is not uncommon for an individual to have a long torso; consequently, his arms cannot reach sufficiently to perform this maneuver. This individual may be successful by using a forceful extension/flexion thrust to attain an upright position or, depending on his level of injury, he may need assistance from another person to attain an upright position.

During the initial training in this activity, two people should guard the client. One person should be positioned behind the wheelchair to assist the client in properly positioning himself and to protect his head in case he falls backward. The second person should be positioned in front of the wheelchair and holding onto the frame of the chair. Using this technique, they can help to right the chair and ensure that the client's feet do not get caught under the chair as it is brought into an upright position. As the client becomes more proficient with this activity one person may guard him from either the front or back position, depending on the client's needs.

A slight modification of this technique can also be used for caregivers to perform a dependent floor-to-wheelchair or wheelchair-to-floor transfer. In a wheelchair-to-floor transfer, the caregiver should be positioned behind the wheelchair and lower it by using the same techniques and safety precautions (i.e., pelvic/seat belt) described previously. For a floor-to-wheelchair transfer, the client should be positioned supine on the floor with his knees to his chest. The wheelchair can be placed under his buttocks (Figure 15-14).

The client is positioned in the wheelchair as previously described. If able, the client can assist by hooking his upper limbs onto the armrests or frame and pulling himself as far forward as possible. Last, by using proper biomechanics, the caregiver should position herself behind the wheelchair and lift it to an upright position (Figure 15-15, *A*). If a second assistant is available, she may assist in front as previously described (Figure 15-15, *B*).

Wheelchair-Floor Transfers

Anterior floor transfers not only require strong upper limbs but also good balance during high-level position changes. This maneuver should always be practiced on a soft surface, or the client should wear kneepads to avoid skin breakdown. The wheelchair should be positioned for maximum front stability with the caster in the forward facing direction (see Figure 15-4).

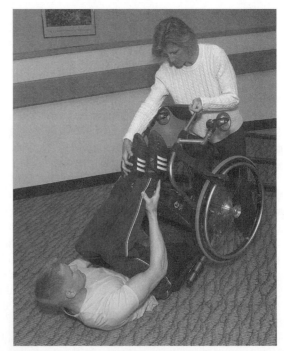

FIGURE 15-14 The therapist positions the wheelchair under the client for a dependent floor-to-wheelchair transfer. The client is on the floor with knees to chest and the wheelchair is placed under his buttocks.

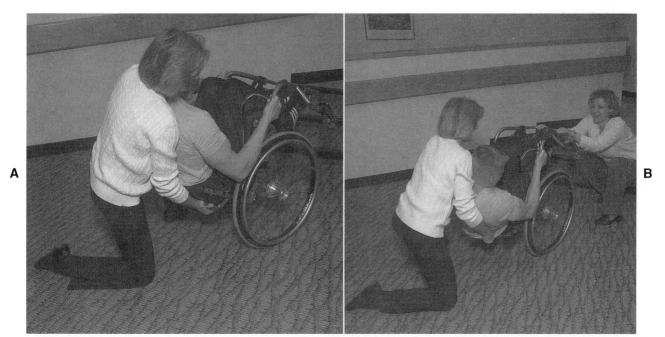

FIGURE 15-15 Dependent righting of tilted-back wheelchair. **A,** The client leans forward and hooks frame with upper limbs; the therapist is behind the chair and shifts her weight from right leg kneeling on floor to half-kneeling left leg to help pivot wheelchair upward. **B,** Two caregivers working together at opposite ends of the wheelchair easily pivot the chair into upright position.

If the wheelchair has swing-away legrests or flip-up footplates, they should be moved out of the way and the client's feet tucked slightly to one side of the wheelchair. If the wheelchair has a rigid front and a fixed footplate, the client can position his feet in front of the footplate or with his feet slightly off to one side of it. The client then shifts his buttocks to the front half of the seat, leans forward, and places one hand on the floor as far forward as possible (Figure 15-16, *A*). The client shifts so that his knees are next to his extended arm on the floor to control his knees coming to the floor. The therapist guards his pelvis to prevent him from landing on the floor with excessive force (Figure 15-16, *B*).

Floor-Wheelchair Transfers: Anterior Approach
To transfer up into the wheelchair from the floor, the client starts in a side-sit position in front of the wheelchair (Figure 5-17, *A*). With the arm farthest from the wheelchair, he should reach for the front corner of the opposite seat frame. With his elbow immediately next to the wheelchair seat, he should place his elbow on the front corner of the seat. Then, he pushes down into the wheelchair frame as he levers his body up into a tall kneel position (Figure 15-17, *B*). At this point, the client's knees should be midline and slightly in front of the footplate and his body facing the wheelchair. The client or therapist, depending on the client's level of independence, may need to readjust his knees to obtain this position. He can do this by lifting his body weight with his arms on the front sides of the wheelchair seat.

The client then reaches across to the back corner of the seat with one hand so that both hands are on the same side of the chair, one on the front and one on the back corner of the seat (Figure 15-18, *A*). As the client pushes down, he shifts his weight over his hands. This will lift his knees off the floor, and the angle

of his upper body will help to twist his body to allow his hip to rest on the corner of the seat (Figure 15-18, *B*). The therapist should guard throughout this activity and can facilitate the twist at the pelvis, as needed. The client can then push up on the armrests or the wheels to adjust himself and assume an upright, symmetrical sitting position. This is an extremely difficult activity that requires significant upper body strength. As an individual is learning this technique, he may have trouble lifting himself high enough and may get caught on the wheelchair cushion when performing the transfer. If this is the case, the activity can be graded and made easier by removing the cushion before the transfer. After the client is back in the wheelchair, he can then transfer onto a level surface, replace the cushion, and return to the wheelchair or he can have a caregiver replace the cushion as he lifts his buttocks off of the seat sling. It is recommended that when a client is being introduced to this transfer, a second person be available to steady the wheelchair or provide additional assistance to the client.

Floor-Wheelchair Transfers: Lateral Approach
Clients with extremely strong and flexible upper limbs may be able to perform a lateral transfer to and from the floor with the lateral transfer technique described in Chapter 8 (Figure 15-19). It is a very advanced technique to lift the buttocks high enough to clear the seat of the wheelchair. A client needs to be proficient in uneven lateral transfers before considering this technique. A strategy to grade this transfer is to position a stool next to the wheelchair. A patient can first perform a lateral transfer to the stool and then from the stool to the wheelchair. This intermediary step will make the transfer easier to perform. A gel pad can be placed on the stool to minimize buttock pressure concerns.

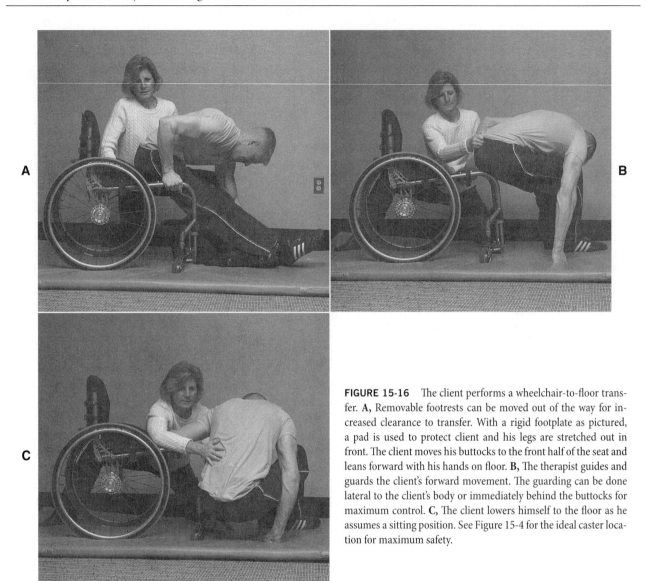

FIGURE 15-16 The client performs a wheelchair-to-floor transfer. **A,** Removable footrests can be moved out of the way for increased clearance to transfer. With a rigid footplate as pictured, a pad is used to protect client and his legs are stretched out in front. The client moves his buttocks to the front half of the seat and leans forward with his hands on floor. **B,** The therapist guides and guards the client's forward movement. The guarding can be done lateral to the client's body or immediately behind the buttocks for maximum control. **C,** The client lowers himself to the floor as he assumes a sitting position. See Figure 15-4 for the ideal caster location for maximum safety.

Stair Negotiation

Stair negotiation requires exceptional upper limb strength and is considered by many to be the most difficult of all advanced wheelchair skills. Although it is possible for an individual to perform this independently, it requires a significant amount of upper limb strength and energy. It is not recommended as an everyday activity because individuals with SCI need to protect their upper limb joints from unnecessary use or overuse.

Ascending Stairs in a Wheelchair

First and foremost, before attempting to negotiate steps with an individual in a wheelchair, it is important to check the condition of the set of stairs. The stairs should be a sturdy set of steps to handle the combined size and weight of the client, the assistant, and the wheelchair. The steps themselves should be in good condition (no worn carpeting coming up), dry, and clear of debris. It is also important to assess the sturdiness of the handrim if the client is going to assist. Ascending stairs in a wheelchair can be performed by either a one-person assist technique or a two-person

assist technique. Both of these techniques are reviewed below, along with several safety considerations.

For the one-person assist technique, the client has to have full upper limb innervation and strength. The client should start with his wheelchair backed up against the first step and the seatbelt firmly fastened across his hips. The client then turns toward the railing and grasps the railing with both hands, one arm more posterior than the other. Using the railing, he can pull himself into a wheelie (Figure 15-20). The client can then proceed to lift the wheelchair up one stair at a time by maintaining a wheelie and pulling up on the railing. The client will readjust his hand position once he stabilizes himself on a step. The therapist assists from behind with one or both hands on the wheelchair frame rigidizer bar or push handles of a folding wheelchair.

It is important to note that wheelchair manufacturers do not recommend lifting a client up or down the stairs or curbs using push handles that are mounted onto the rigidizer bar of a rigid wheelchair. When a client reaches the top of the stairs, the hand reaching across the body releases the railing and grasps its

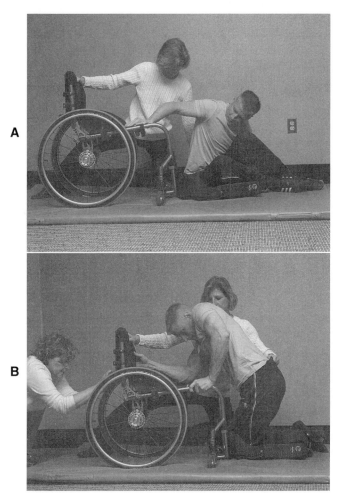

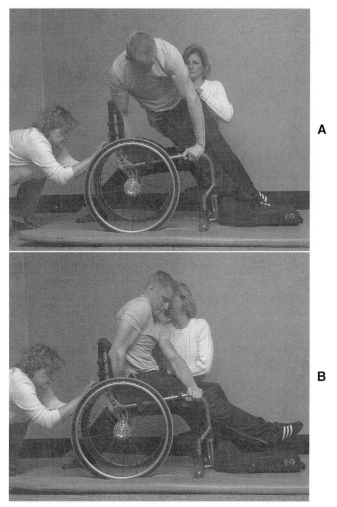

FIGURE 15-17 The client assumes a tall kneel in front of the wheelchair in preparation for floor-to-wheelchair transfer using the anterior approach. **A,** The client assumes a modified longsit position in front of wheelchair slightly off to the side. **B,** The client pulls himself up to tall kneel in front of the wheelchair.

FIGURE 15-18 The client twists into seat in floor-to-wheelchair transfer. **A,** This is a client with good upper body strength, both arms on one side of seat with one arm on the front and one arm on the back of the seating surface. This is essential to raise his body up above chair seat and twist it into position. **B,** The client lowers into an upright position in the chair seat.

corresponding wheel rim while the other hand remains on the railing to adequately stabilize the wheelchair. The client then propels the wheelchair backward with the hand on the rim until the wheelchair is in its upright position and clear of the stairs.

Because of the significant amount of upper body strength and strain this technique entails, most clients opt to use a two-person technique for maximum safety and joint protection. To perform the two-person assisted technique, the client positions his chair facing away from the stairs with his rear wheels against the bottom step. The antitippers should be removed from the chair. The stronger assistant will lead the lift and is positioned at the client's head with both hands securely on the frame of the wheelchair or on the integrated push handles (taking into consideration the previously reported risks). A second assistant is positioned at the client's feet, and grasps the front of the wheelchair frame.

Removable components (e.g., legrests, armrests, backrests) of the chair must never be used to lift the chair because these parts are not stable and can easily come out of position during the lift. If a client's wheelchair has swing away legrests, they may be removed to allow the second assistant to gain a better grasp on

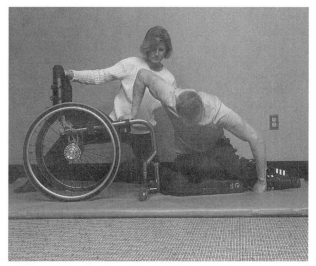

FIGURE 15-19 The client performs a floor-to-wheelchair lateral transfer.

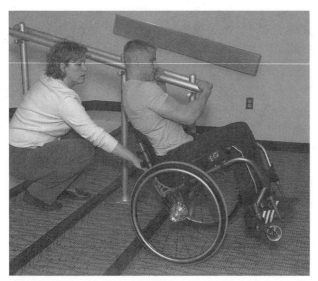

FIGURE 15-20 The client ascends the stairs in a wheelchair assisted by therapist using a rear-facing technique.

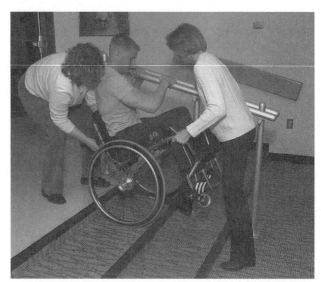

FIGURE 15-21 Two therapists lift a client in his wheelchair down stairs; the top caregiver steadies the chair while the bottom caregiver places one foot on the step that the wheelchair is moving toward and moves her other foot down a step as the chair descends.

the frame. In this situation it is important to take care to protect the client's legs from injury. As standard protocol, caregivers should be instructed to use proper body mechanics to minimize their risk of injury. A helpful hint is to instruct the assistants to maintain good communication and good eye contact with each other during the lift. This will facilitate safety and good mechanics with head up, back straight, and knees bent.

After the assistants are in position, the client is tipped into a wheelie, and the lead caregiver positions one foot on the step the wheelchair will be lifted to and the other foot one step above. The assistants roll the wheels of the wheelchair up one step on the lead assistant's command. Both rear wheels should remain in contact with the stairs throughout this activity. The lead assistant will be lifting the majority of the client's weight. The second assistant will help with the lifting and is responsible for stabilizing the wheelchair by applying a horizontal force and keeping the rear wheels in contact with the next step (Figure 15-21). This is done to ensure that the wheelchair does not roll back down the step and will allow the lead assistant to reposition his feet for the lift to the next step. The assistants repeat this procedure, ascending one step at a time until reaching the top. When the client is secure on the next level and away from the stairs, the rear antitippers and any other parts removed from the chair should be replaced.

Descending Stairs in a Wheelchair

Clients with full hand function may descend stairs backward with the assistance of one person. The client should back the wheelchair to the edge of the top step, place one or both hands on the railing if he has adequate upper body strength to assist in a hand-over-hand technique. Another option is to place an arm on the handrail and the other hand on the corresponding wheel handrim. He then leans forward (when guiding his chair by the handrim) to enable his trunk to rest on his thighs. The assistant is behind the client on the lower part of the flight of stairs to help control the descent of the wheelchair. The client slowly lowers the back wheels down one step at a time (Figure 15-22).

As the chair descends, the casters and footplates can forcefully hit each step. Clients should be warned that this will happen so that they do not become frightened by the loud noise it will make. When the back wheels are on the floor, the client then spins the casters off the bottom step using the technique described for descending a curb. This descending stairs technique is a quick and fairly easy way to descend stairs with the assistance of only one person. It can, however, cause damage to the wheelchair and should therefore only be used when absolutely necessary.

If a client is unable to actively assist in descending the stairs, two assistants are necessary for maximum safety. The technique is similar to ascending the stairs with two assistants. The antitippers are removed and this time the wheelchair is positioned facing the stairs. The lead assistant is behind the wheelchair and the second assistant is in front of the wheelchair, approximately two to three steps below the chair. The lead assistant should tip the wheelchair into a wheelie and roll the rear wheels to the edge of the top step. On the lead assistant's command, the wheelchair is lowered one step at a time. The second assistant will provide a backward horizontal force to stabilize the chair and ensure that it is lowered in a controlled manner one step at a time. After descending the stairs, the antitippers are replaced.

Bumping

Another option to ascend or descend stairs is to bump, which involves going up or down the stairs on the buttocks. Before initiating this activity, the client must demonstrate sufficient unsupported sitting stability and should be proficient in floor transfers and lateral transfers between uneven surfaces. This technique can pose a threat to skin integrity; therefore it is vital that clients have good safety awareness and are vigilant with skin inspection. The Jay Protector by Sunrise Medical, Inc. (www.sunrisemedical.com/index.jsp) is an example of a protective covering for the buttocks that should be worn to decrease the risk of skin breakdown during bumping. It is strongly recommended that it be worn during training and be ordered for any client who will be required to bump up and down stairs on a semi-regular basis.

A client can be trained in the basic technique by bumping up and down a padded curb-type surface placed on the therapy mat before bumping up and down an actual staircase. The curb can be the usual therapy curb for wheelchair mobility skills and is used to simulate a step. A two-inch curb should be used initially with progression to higher curbs based on the client's success and skill level. Bumping is usually initiated with the client in a long sit position, with his back to the front of the curb on a slight angle. Most clients will find it easiest if the hand closer to the curb is placed up on the curb and the other hand placed on the mat next to their hip. The client then positions his knees in flexion so that his feet will not drag along the mat and limit his ability to bump up and down the curb. The client should extend his elbows and depress his shoulders to lift his buttocks from the mat. Simultaneously, the client uses the head-hips relationship described in Chapter 8. He should tuck his head and maneuver his upper body forward to allow his hips to be levered up and back and gently lowered onto the curb. If the client has pain in the glenohumeral joint, the activity should be discontinued.

To descend the curb, the client should lift his buttocks, as when ascending the curb, and simultaneously swing his head and upper body backward to facilitate the hips moving forward to clear the edge of the curb. When descending the curb, the client must be careful to avoid sliding off the curb. Therapist position: the therapist takes a position in front of him to provide assistance at the hips and ensure that adequate clearance is obtained and sitting stability is not lost when the client is practicing this technique on the mat.

Ascending Stairs on Buttocks

To position oneself for bumping up stairs, the client may either perform a transfer to the floor in front of the stairs or perform a lateral transfer directly to the second step. The client then places both feet one to two steps below the buttocks and will reposition them in this manner as each step is ascended to avoid getting his ankles caught on the edge of the step (Figure 15-23). The client then ascends the steps by using the same technique discussed above. When he reaches the top of the stairs, the client will perform a floor-to-wheelchair transfer.

A client may also be instructed in bringing his wheelchair with him as he ascends the stairs. This is a very difficult activity requiring extraordinary strength and balance and will be successfully achieved by few clients and only on four- to six-step staircases. The technique for this is initiated when the client is sitting on the second step. He should position the wheelchair in a tilted back position with its push handles resting on the step beside his buttocks. If the staircase is narrow and the client has a folding wheelchair, he may remove the cushion, throw it to the top of the stairs and fold the chair. When ascending a step the hand that would normally be on the step next to the client's hip will now be positioned on the push handle resting on the step. After each step is ascended, the wheelchair is pulled up the step stabilized by resting it on the push handle and wheel, and the procedure is repeated until the top of the stairs is reached.

A variation to this technique, especially useful for those chairs without push handles, is to use a strap hooked to the chair to pull it up the steps. When a therapist is guarding a client during training of this technique, a second person may be required. This may be necessary because it is vital to provide assistance at the client's hips to ensure that adequate clearance is obtained and balance is not lost. The second assistant is necessary to ensure that the wheelchair does not fall down the stairs and get damaged.

Descending Stairs on Buttocks

To position himself for bumping down stairs, the client will perform a wheelchair-to-floor transfer and scoot to the top of the stairs. The client places both feet two steps below his

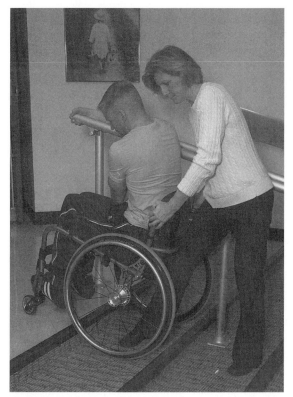

FIGURE 15-22 The client descends stairs in his wheelchair with the therapist assisting.

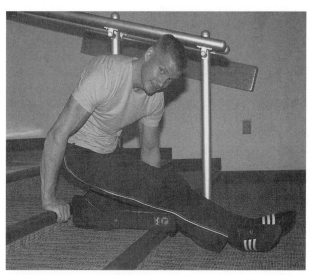

FIGURE 15-23 The client bumps up steps using his chair cushion in an emergency situation because his Jay Protector was at home.

buttocks and will reposition them in this manner as each step is descended. The client then descends the stairs as described above for descending the curb. Once the client reaches the second-to-last step, he may perform a lateral transfer into his wheelchair or he may descend to the bottom of the stairs and then perform a floor-to-wheelchair transfer. Clients with exceptional balance and upper body strength may bring their wheelchair with them as they descend the stairs by reversing the technique described above with ascending stairs.

Elevator Negotiation

When entering an elevator, it is important that the client considers the gap between the elevator and the floor. This gap is supposed to be within ½ inch; however, that is often not the case. If the gap is between ½ inch and 2 inches, a client should negotiate it the same way he negotiates a curb or a door threshold. If the gap is greater than 2 inches, he should wait for another elevator or get appropriate assistance because a large gap can present an unsafe situation.

As often as possible individuals in a wheelchair should ride in the elevator facing forward. This will increase an individual's safety with exiting in an emergency situation and when others enter the elevator. Being in a forward position will allow a client physical access to elevator buttons, visual access to others who are entering and exiting, visual access to the floor the elevator is on, and visual access of the gap between the door and the floor for safe techniques when exiting. In addition, this allows an individual in a wheelchair to observe the same elevator etiquette that everyone else observes.

When entering an elevator, the client should check to see whether the elevator is crowded. If the elevator is not crowded, it may be easier to enter facing forward and then turn around in the elevator to ride facing forward. If there is insufficient room in the elevator to turn around or the client is accompanied by a caregiver or colleague who can hold the elevator door, he should reverse into the elevator so that exiting is more efficient.

That being said, if the elevator is crowded, at times it may be easier to enter in a forward position to avoid hitting others and to remain in that position. In this case, an individual should be cautious when exiting the elevator and note the floor-to-elevator gap and the location of other riders.

Escalators

Negotiating escalators is a very advanced and complex wheelchair skill. If there is a ramp or elevator in the same building, it is recommended that the ramp or elevator be used over the escalator. Using the escalator requires a significant amount of wheelchair skill to avoid injury to the client or to the personal assistant. It is important to note that some public places may not permit wheelchairs on escalators, especially if they have an elevator or ramp. The majority of individuals who use escalators out of necessity usually have an assistant with them for maximum safety. There are many variables that need to be considered with escalators because they are constantly moving and cannot easily be stopped (Box 15-2).

Ascending Escalators in a Wheelchair

When an individual negotiates an upward-moving escalator with assistance, there are several steps that are recommended for successful completion of this challenging task. First, the client

---

| BOX 15-2 | Factors to Consider When Negotiating Escalators |

- Steepness of the steps
- Speed of the handrail
- Handrail speed relative to step speed
- Ability to lean forward in the wheelchair
- Ability to push the wheelchair forward and backward
- Sufficient hand strength to grasp the escalator rails

---

and assistant should observe the escalator before approaching to see whether the steps are wide enough to accommodate the chair wheels. A pelvic belt should be secured to maintain good wheelchair and individual contact. According to Axelson et al,[36] a series of steps should follow next. After positioning the wheelchair on the escalator platform, the client and assistant should visualize the goal to position the front wheels and back wheels to be staggered across an upper step and a lower step. The client should pull his body forward to pull the wheelchair onto the escalator with the footrest positioned on one step and the rear wheels on the third step down. Depending on the escalator and an individual's wheelchair setup, the front casters will either rest on or dangle above the middle step.

Immediately, the client should grab the escalator handrail with one hand and his own wheelchair push rim with the other hand. Next, as the escalator starts to incline, the client should lean forward to avoid backward tipping. The rail may be perceived to be moving faster than the steps, so the client should let the rail gently slip through his hand to "keep pace" with the step speed. Conversely, if the handrails move more slowly than the steps, pressure should be applied to the push rim to avoid slipping backward; forward movement of the handrail hand will be necessary to keep up with the wheels. As the escalator steps level out at the top, the client should gradually sit more upright to maintain balance. When all four of the wheels are at the same level, a push off the handrails to move off the escalator is needed. Care should be taken to avoid catching the wheelchair casters where the steps move below the floor.

There are several important considerations for the assistant as well. An assistant should always follow an individual in a wheelchair onto the escalator with one foot one step below the wheelchair and her other foot used as a brace two steps below the wheelchair. The assistant should be facing upward with hands resting lightly on the push handles or the back posts to prevent them from falling backward. The assistant should not put pressure on the wheelchair unless the wheelchair begins to tip or slide backward down the escalator. If these steps are followed by both the client and assistant, risk of injury from use of the escalator should be minimal.

Descending Escalators in a Wheelchair: Reverse Technique

When an individual using a wheelchair negotiates a downward-moving escalator with assistance, Axelson et al[38] suggest that the following steps be followed for successful and safe completion of the task. First, the assistant should step onto the escalator before the client and stand facing upward. Until the client is ready and has rolled on the escalator platform, the assistant may have to walk up against the downward-moving escalator. When the assistant is on the escalator, the client will roll the wheelchair backward onto the escalator until his rear wheels are one step lower than the front casters. At this time, the assistant should stand one step below the rear wheels. Again, the client should then immediately lean forward and grasp one handrail as high as possible while simultaneously applying pressure to the push rim with the other hand to avoid slipping backward. The client should push the wheelchair forward so that the rear wheels are secure on a step. The assistant should keep her hands on the push handles or rigidizer bar times to be sure that the client does not roll or tip over backward. This guarding should be maintained until the client reaches the bottom of the escalator and all four of the wheels are on level ground. When the escalator bottom platform is reached, the client should push off from the handrails and propel the wheelchair backward off the track. The assistant should also back up as the client reaches the escalator platform to allow the client to reverse off the escalator.

POWER WHEELCHAIRS

There are several general rules of thumb that should be kept in mind when instructing clients in power mobility (Box 15-3). There are also several common misconceptions about power wheelchairs (Clinical Note: Common Misconceptions About Power Wheelchairs). To truly appreciate what is involved in driving a power wheelchair, it is recommended, if possible, to get in a power wheelchair and perform 3 hours of normal indoor and outdoor daily routine (e.g., go to a local store, deli, or neighbor). This will provide a better understanding of the challenges that come up in the course of performing everyday activities. Many of us have had formal training when learning how to drive a car. It certainly did not come naturally, and it was not common sense. It only became that way after learning the rules of the road and an extended amount of time and practice.

CLINICAL NOTE **Common Misconceptions About Power Wheelchairs**

- The only individual who needs training to drive a power wheelchair is one who uses alternative access methods such as a pneumatic controller or a head array.
- Driving a power wheelchair is something that comes naturally.
- Driving a power wheelchair is simply common sense.

Power Wheelchair Base Styles

When initially teaching an individual to drive a power wheelchair, it is important to consider the base style he is using. As mentioned in Chapter 11, there are three different power wheelchair drive bases: rear wheel drive (RWD), mid wheel drive (MWD), and front wheel drive (FWD) (see Figure 11-39). The drive wheel placement determines the drive base style. Consequently, the RWD wheelchair is a base with the drive wheel in the rear and the FWD base is a base with the drive wheel in the front, near the individual's feet. Depending on the type of power wheelchair base being used, wheelchair maneuverability varies

and there are different guidelines on what direction to approach a curb.

For all the drive base styles, the surface that is being negotiated affects how the wheelchair will perform. Therefore, for a first-time user it is important to begin on open, flat, smooth, level indoor surfaces and progress to uneven surfaces and tighter areas. The following sequence of skills discussed is a loose framework that describes a hierarchy of power wheelchair mobility skills because each skill is loosely based on preceding skills.

Training in Power Wheelchair Mobility Skills
Level, Open Surfaces

For level, open surfaces, it is important for an individual to feel comfortable with negotiating the wheelchair in a straight path on the right side of the hallway or sidewalk. This is important to maximize success with maneuvering traffic flow in open areas. When an individual demonstrates good success with maneuvering the wheelchair in open areas, he is ready to progress to negotiating turns.

Turning to Negotiate Open Doorways

For full accessibility, it is important for an individual to master the way a wheelchair turns. The feel of the turn is different in each of the different drive wheel styles and accommodation should be made to allow for adequate clearance. For example, in an FWD power base, more of the turn happens behind the driver. With an FWD base and with standard tight doorways, it is important to maneuver the wheelchair close to the doorway and to initiate the turn when the footrests are two thirds of the way into the doorway. This technique will allow for adequate clearance of the back end. In contrast, in an RWD base, the turn happens in front of the driver. In an RWD power base, it is important to make a wider turn by initiating the turn sooner when the wheelchair is further from the doorway (e.g., middle of hallway). With practice, each individual will develop a feel for how his wheelchair maneuvers and this will become a more intuitive skill. As with maneuvering in open areas, it is important to maneuver the wheelchair toward the right side of the doorway to maximize traffic flow.

Another major component of negotiating doorways is the ability to proportionally use the joystick or alternative controller to slow down the chair to safely negotiate the turn. Doorway negotiation activities can reinforce the concept of driving a wheelchair proportionally for maximum control.

Threshold Negotiation

Before maneuvering uneven surfaces, it is important to ensure that the driver is aware of the threshold and slows down as he approaches it. The individual should then gently guide the wheelchair over it. This is similar to negotiating a speed bump with a car. It is important to slow down to allow each set of wheels to smoothly transition over the surface.

Ramps

When negotiating ramps in a power wheelchair, it is important to use good judgment and make sure that the ramp is stable, free of debris, and not so steep that it will jeopardize the stability of the wheelchair. The ramp should be approached in the forward direction for maximum visual access and to negotiate the ramp safely. When ascending

BOX 15-3 | General Rules of Thumb for Power Mobility Training

- Pay particular attention to each client's style of mobility.
- Remember that there are drivers and nondrivers. Wheelchair electronics can be modified to support both ends of this continuum to ensure that each individual is as safe and independent as possible with mobility in his power wheelchair.
- Emphasize to clients and caregivers that joysticks operate as both steering wheel and gas pedal combined in one unit. They can be used to negotiate the wheelchair through 360 degrees of movement and the harder they are pushed the faster the wheelchair will move.
- For individuals with dexterity issues, place a larger handle or U-shaped device on the stem of the joystick to increase the lever arm. The joystick then requires less effort from the client to negotiate the wheelchair and move at a more rapid pace.
- Make sure that there is sufficient foot support (footrest) clearance to negotiate uneven indoor surfaces (e.g., door thresholds and ramps) and outdoor surfaces.
- Make sure the antitippers on a rear wheel drive power wheelchair have sufficient clearance to negotiate uneven surfaces outdoors so that the wheelchair does not get hung up with insufficient drive wheel contact with the ground.

- Make sure incline entrances and curbs to be negotiated are within guidelines for a mid wheel drive power wheelchair so that the chair drive wheel does not get hung up with insufficient drive wheel contact with the ground.
- Stress use of a pelvic belt as a minimal precaution when clients drive a power wheelchair; it is just as important as using a seat belt when driving a car. Pelvic belt use also maximizes pelvic alignment and stability so that a client is able to stay seated upright in his wheelchair without sliding forward. The pelvic belt strap should be positioned between a 60- to 90-degree angle relative to the seat pan.
- Suggest a chest strap to provide anterior chest support for clients with trunk instability as a helpful addition to the pelvic belt. If more aggressive anterior support is required for stability in the wheelchair, there are several harness models available that stabilize the upper torso and maximize distribution of external forces.
- Recommend back supports with lateral contours or separate lateral supports to provide a client with lateral torso stability in the wheelchair for maximum safety on uneven surfaces.
- Consult the owner's manual for each specific wheelchair model to ensure that manufacturer guidelines are followed when teaching a client skills for his wheelchair.

a ramp, because of the angle of the wheelchair with the front up and the back trailing behind, gravity forces the torso back, increasing the trunk forces against the backrest of the wheelchair. It should be noted that when negotiating a steeper grade ramp with the RWD wheelchair, an individual may need to lean forward to maximize the wheelchair's stability. To do this, the client with a low cervical injury may use a chest strap that is maintained in a slightly loosened position. The loosened strap provides a space into which the trunk is allowed to forwardly lean without complete loss of balance forward.

When descending a ramp, the back end of the wheelchair is higher than the front end. This can result in a client's loss of balance in the anterior direction. He can counteract this by using power recline or power tilt. This will shift the seating system backward slightly for improved stability. A chest strap or harness can also be used for more aggressive support. Some individuals also hook an arm over the push handle on top of the back support for increased stability with descending inclines. Care should be taken with hooking to ensure that it does not exacerbate pain or anterior instability in the glenohumeral joint. Initially, it is important for individuals to descend an unfamiliar ramp slowly to maximize traction and control. As an individual becomes familiar with a particular ramp, he may increase his speed to a more normal pace. In addition, when a ramp is quite steep an individual may choose to zigzag up or down it rather than going straight up or down.

Curb Cuts

The concepts for negotiating curb cuts are the same as for negotiating ramps. Three additional challenges may be a terrain change (a rougher or smoother surface), sloping off to one side or the other, or the curb interface with the street. Good visual scanning with advanced planning and good judgment are essential skills for maximum safety and success when negotiating curb cuts in the community. The techniques for ascending and descending curbs described subsequently may need to be used when negotiating curb cuts that are not level with the street.

For curb cuts that are sloped off to one side or the other, it is helpful to have a client shift his head toward the higher side of the slope to maximize torso stability when negotiating a more aggressively side-sloped curb cut. The lateral contours of a back support and lateral supports are helpful to provide an individual with adequate torso stability for maximum safety when negotiating the wheelchair up or down aggressively sloped curb cuts.

Unfortunately, curb cuts are often not fabricated to the guidelines set by the Americans With Disabilities Act (ADA). Consequently, as an individual attempts to negotiate an unfamiliar curb cut, he may get caught in the transition. For individuals with all types of wheelchairs, the footrests may get stuck. If an individual has a power tilt, power-elevating legrests, or power-elevating seat feature, these can be used to obtain adequate footplate clearance. The best situation would be to reverse the same way he approached this curb cut and find an alternative route. For individuals with an MWD power wheelchair, negotiating this transition may result in the wheelchair high centering. This means that the front and rear wheels make contact with the uneven surfaces, but the middle drive wheel gets suspended and is an unable to make sufficient contact to mobilize the wheelchair. For an FWD power wheelchair with front antitipper wheels may have a problem with negotiating curb cuts. Similar to the MWD model, the front tipper wheel and rear casters may be making contact with the uneven surfaces of the curb cut and street. This could result in the front drive wheel being suspended and unable to make sufficient contact with the ground to mobilize the wheelchair.

Curb and Step Negotiation

To negotiate a curb in a power wheelchair, the client should approach the curb as symmetrically as possible with both sides of his wheelchair. The technique for descending a curb differs depending on the power wheelchair base being used. In an MWD and an FWD power wheelchair base, an individual should approach a curb forward to ascend and descend it. This maximizes an individual's visual field and consequently his safety when heading into the street with a power wheelchair. For curbs taller than 1 inch, in an RWD power wheelchair the client should approach a curb forward to ascend it but in reverse to descend it. This increases torso stability against the back support for maximum safety with descending the wheelchair into the street.

Ascending a Curb

One major advantage to an RWD power base is its ability to negotiate curbs and its ability to be lifted up a 5- to 7-inch step. An RWD power base can be maneuvered up a 4-inch curb with ease by negotiating a wheelie so that the rear drive wheels absorb most of the impact from the curb. Modification to the wheelchair's electronic parameters, including higher acceleration with forward speed, will help the client to perform this maneuver. By using his head, neck, and upper body, the individual in the wheelchair can shift his weight in a posterior direction in the wheelchair seating to increase weight behind the drive wheel while simultaneously pushing forward on the joystick. This will lighten the front end of the wheelchair for increased clearance of the curb by the caster. However, similarly to negotiating a curb in a manual wheelchair, timing is crucial to allow the caster to clear the curb. An individual can also use power recline or tilt to assist with the posterior weight shift as long as it does not compromise his visual field of the curb and the area in front of the wheelchair. It is important to practice this technique initially on a level, open surface before progressing to 2-, 3-, and 4-inch-high curbs.

The therapist should also be aware of the following challenges: the slope of the street down toward the curb and the timing of the weight shift for adequate caster clearance of the curb. When the slope of the street goes downhill toward the curb, as is common for water drainage, it makes it more difficult for the individual in the wheelchair to shift his weight posterior of the drive wheel, which is essential to lighten the weight on the casters to facilitate curb negotiation.

To ascend a 1- to 3-inch curb in an MWD or an FWD power wheelchair, it is important to approach the curb as symmetrically as possible. When the client has set up his approach in a straight, symmetrical manner, approximately 2 to 3 feet in front of the curb, he should gently accelerate the joystick to climb the curb. The wheelchair movement should be at an even, smooth pace without stops and starts. This will provide the wheelchair with the momentum to move over the curb as smoothly as possible (Figure 15-24). It is important that the wheelchair negotiates the curb in a symmetrical manner for maximum stability. If the wheelchair negotiates the curb on a diagonal, it has the potential to tip off to the side.

Ascending One Step

With assistance from a trained caregiver, an RWD power base can be maneuvered up and over a 5- to 7-inch curb or step. This is a very advanced skill and is not encouraged just for the sake of doing this. Unfortunately, it is often a necessary skill for everyday life for individuals who live in city environments where entrances to favorite restaurants or stores may be configured with such steps. The preferred method for negotiating this step is to use a portable ramp. If a portable ramp is not available or practical, a caregiver and client

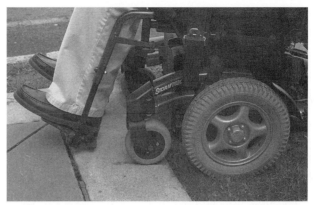

FIGURE 15-24 The client ascends a 1-inch curb in a wheelchair with a mid wheel drive power base.

can be trained in a safe two-person technique to negotiate the step. The technique is similar to negotiating a wheelchair up a 4-inch curb with a caregiver's weight on the back of the wheelchair to maximize the posterior weight shift for adequate caster clearance over the step. After the casters are up on the step, the caregiver should then position his body sideways to use the push handles and her hip and knee muscles to propel the rear wheels up and forward as the individual in the wheelchair gently pushes the joystick in a forward direction. Again, for maximum user and caregiver safety, this skill is not recommended as a first choice to negotiate a 5- to 7-inch step entrance. A portable ramp is strongly recommended to negotiate a 5- to 7-inch step.

FWD and MWD power wheelchairs cannot be maneuvered up a step in the manner described previously. A portable ramp is essential for an individual with the FWD or MWD wheelchair to negotiate a 4- to 7-inch curb or step.

Descending a Curb

To descend a 1- to 4-inch curb in the RWD power wheelchair, the wheelchair should be reversed down the curb for maximum stability and safety. Initially, the individual using the wheelchair should maneuver it up to the curb in a forward approach to visually inspect the curb for a stable, intact, nonslippery surface and the street so that there is minimal traffic activity. He should then turn the wheelchair so that the back of the wheelchair is at a 90-degree angle to the curb. At this point, he can gently reverse the wheelchair down the curb so that both drive wheels transition down the curb at the same time. After the drive wheels are on the street, the wheelchair should be maneuvered backward to allow for about 4 inches of drive wheel clearance of the curb. He should then move the joystick in a sharp left or right direction so that the wheelchair spins, the casters come off the curb, and stop when the wheelchair is facing forward in the street. This technique is important to maximize the individual's visual field of what is happening in the street so that he can safely continue on his way.

To descend a 1- to 3-inch curb in FWD and MWD power wheelchairs, it is important to visually inspect the curb for stable, intact, nonslippery surface. When the curb is visually acceptable to the driver, he should approach the curb in a forward direction, again at a symmetrical, 90-degree angle to the curb. He should gently move the joystick in a smooth, consistent manner to maneuver the wheelchair down the curb (Figure 15-25). For maximum control and safety, care should be taken to proceed at a normal pace and not too fast when negotiating down the curb.

Tighter Normal Environments and Crowded Areas

Most everyday environments, with the exception of some department stores and supermarkets, do not have sufficient room to maneuver a power wheelchair with ease. Consequently, it is important to ensure that the electronics are adjusted and the client well trained to ensure that he has good control with maneuvering in tight normal areas. This is especially important when negotiating semicrowded and crowded areas so that the individual in the wheelchair can respond as a defensive wheelchair driver. When an individual is familiar with the basic operation of the wheelchair, he should be instructed to watch the more dynamic elements of the environment, especially other people. It is important to interpret and predict the actions of others so that he can plan his movement accordingly and minimize the risk of hitting and injuring others with the wheelchair. Unfortunately, it is not unusual for an individual in a wheelchair to be moving smoothly down the sidewalk behind a person who suddenly stops in the middle of the sidewalk to answer a cell phone or look across the street. It is clear who is at fault here but there are no written rules, no brake lights, no hazard or turn signals with mobility on sidewalks. It is important for the individual in the wheelchair to be prepared for these situations so that he can be successful in avoiding them as often as possible.

Elevator Negotiation

The ADA states that elevator doors should be at least 36 inches wide and remain open for at least 5 seconds. If that is not the case with a particular elevator you are working with, it is important to discuss this issue with building management to see whether the elevator can be reprogrammed to maximize safety and access.

After an individual is comfortable negotiating the wheelchair in the reverse direction, it is helpful to practice maneuvering the wheelchair backward through a standard door as a prerequisite skill for elevator negotiation. When an individual can move the chair backward through a standard door within a reasonable time frame, actual elevators can be used for training.

Entering an Elevator

As often as possible, the client should position himself in the elevator facing forward. This is an important safety issue so that he has a clear visual field of everyone who enters and exits the elevator after him, has visual access to the floor the elevator is on, has easy access for evacuation out the door in an emergency situation, has visual access of the gap between the door and the floor, and has ease and maximum safety during normal exiting of the elevator.

Before advancing into an elevator, it is important to get a good visual understanding of the interface between the floor and the actual elevator to be aware of rises or drops to the elevator floor. If the rise or fall to the elevator floor is within 2 inches, negotiate this as you would a curb. If the difference between the surfaces is greater than 2 inches, it is better to err on the side of safety and wait for the next elevator to see if it aligns better with the floor.

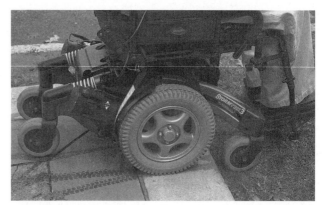

FIGURE 15-25 The client descends a 1-inch curb in a wheelchair with a mid wheel drive power base.

If the elevator is empty and there is sufficient room to turn around in the elevator, it is easier to enter in the forward position and then turn around. If the elevator has a few people in it, as a general rule of thumb, it is better to reverse into the elevator so that the wheelchair remains in a forward-facing position. If the elevator is crowded, it may be better to wait for the next elevator or to enter the elevator in a forward position and be prepared to reverse out to allow others to exit.

When reversing into the elevator, it is important to know whether the elevator door is wide enough to accommodate the wheelchair. If it is, the individual in the wheelchair can align himself with one side of the door and use that as a guide to reverse through the door. This is especially helpful for individuals with limited neck movement and those who use alternative controllers, such as a pneumatic controller or a head array (see Figure 11-43).

Exiting an Elevator

In the forward-facing position in the elevator, it is easy to exit the elevator by driving straight out the door. If the individual in the wheelchair had to enter the elevator forward and could not turn around, he should position himself so that he can see one side of the door and use that as a visual guide to reverse out through the doorway. It is important to ask and make sure that there is no one positioned behind the wheelchair or waiting in the elevator entrance to maximize safety when exiting in reverse.

The rise or drop between the actual floor and the elevator should also be addressed. It is difficult for the individual in the wheelchair to see when he is in a crowded elevator with the exit behind the wheelchair. It is important that the individual in the wheelchair ask for help to better understand this transition and safely exit the elevator.

Door Management

Doorway management is an advanced wheelchair mobility skill because it requires an individual to maneuver within a constricted space to physically access the door. It also can necessitate opening a door with a doorknob or door handle, releasing a latch, stabilizing the door in an open position, and negotiating the wheelchair up and over a threshold. Consequently, these tasks should be performed at a slow, controlled speed to maximize safety and success.

As often as possible, it is helpful to ask for and accept assistance when negotiating doors with a power wheelchair. This is

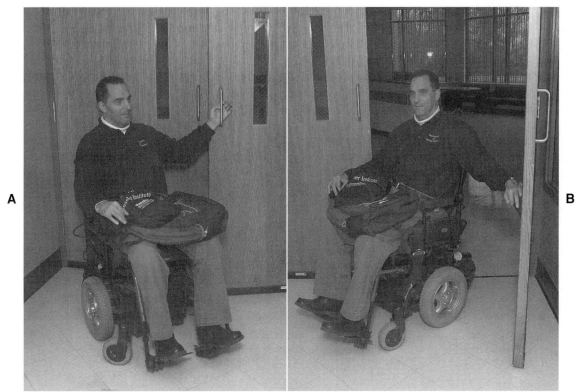

FIGURE 15-26 The client turns his power wheelchair to negotiate through a doorway. **A,** Opening the door and **B,** turning into a doorway in a mid wheel drive power wheelchair requires initiating the turn sooner before the wheelchair enters the doorway. This individual finds it easier to reverse through the doorway as he stabilizes it with his left upper extremity.

important to maximize safety and minimize upper limb joint stress on the individual in the power wheelchair. That being said, door management is an important skill to learn for maximum safety in an emergency situation and for times when the individual in the wheelchair is alone and needs to be able to negotiate a door to enter or exit a particular area.

Pushing a Door Open

Pushing a door open is not difficult as long as the person in the wheelchair can manipulate the door handle. The individual in the wheelchair should approach the door in a forward or forward and slightly lateral direction to maximize physical reach and access to the door handle. As much as space will allow, the wheelchair footrests should be within the door space so that once the door latch is released, the individual in the wheelchair can use his footrests to gently push the door forward. This contact should be as close to the door handle side as possible to maximize leverage and success. The individual in the wheelchair can use his arm on the side of the door hinge to assist with holding the door open as the wheelchair clears the doorway.

The door may need to be closed after the individual is on the other side. This can easily be accomplished by turning the wheelchair around. The individual can then initiate the movement by reaching with his arm and then gently pushing the door completely closed with the wheelchair footrests.

If the door is spring-loaded the same technique described above is used. However, the technique requires a greater amount of arm strength and more agile maneuvering of the wheelchair.

Pulling a Door Open

Negotiating a door that opens towards the wheelchair is an even more advanced mobility skill that requires the individual in the wheelchair to make contact with the handle and pull it toward him while reversing the wheelchair with the other arm (Figure 15-26, *A*). He then maneuvers around the door to hold it open and move into the entrance.

An ideal situation would be to have sufficient space for the wheelchair on the side of the door near the handle. If the wheelchair can be positioned on the side of the door to allow the individual to open it without having to reverse the wheelchair, that is preferable to minimize the maneuvering. After the individual releases the latch and initiates the movement to open the door, he can maneuver the wheelchair so that the side of the wheelchair and footrests can hold the door. This will allow him to reposition his arm on the other side of the door to push it open wider for sufficient access to enable the wheelchair to clear the doorway. To close the door after the individual negotiates the threshold is similar to the starting technique. It requires that he turn around, face the door, position the wheelchair close to the door handle, and slowly reverse the wheelchair as he holds the door handle with his free arm. This will allow him to pull the door closed.

Again, if the door is spring loaded, the same technique described previously is used to open it. However, this is a significant challenge because it takes a greater amount of arm strength and more agile maneuvering of the wheelchair. Refer to the techniques described in the manual wheelchair section for additional strategies to maximize success.

CLINICAL CASE STUDY Development of Wheelchair Skills

Patient History

John McCoy is a 26-year-old man with a T12 paraplegia, American Spinal Injury Association (ASIA) A diagnosis resulting from a fracture dislocation sustained in a motor vehicle accident. His fracture was stabilized 1 day after injury by surgical decompression laminectomy and fusion of spinal levels T9 to L2. He wore a thoracic lumbar spinal orthosis for 4 weeks after surgery. John's acute-care course was complicated by a grade 2 pressure ulcer on his sacrum, which required 2 weeks of bed rest to heal. After discharge from the acute-care hospital, John completed 4 weeks of inpatient rehabilitation where he gained independence in all ADLs.

John has been discharged and is now attending outpatient therapy for his wheelchair prescription and training in advanced wheelchair skills. He is currently using a rental wheelchair.

John lives with his girlfriend in a wheelchair-accessible apartment. He is a computer engineer and works as a computer programmer and troubleshooter, which requires him to be on the road traveling locally in his car from location to location. He has found that loading and unloading his wheelchair from the car is very fatiguing and is looking forward to a lighter-weight permanent wheelchair that can meet his needs for high maneuverability on a variety of terrain.

Patient's Self-Assessment

John wants to improve his mobility skills to facilitate access in the community and at work.

Clinical Assessment
Patient Appearance

- Height 5 feet 10 inches, weight 150 pounds, body mass index 21.5
- Posture: John's posture in the wheelchair is with a collapsed, symmetrical trunk.

Cognitive Assessment

- Alert, oriented × 3

Cardiopulmonary Assessment

- Blood pressure 112/65 mm Hg, heart rate at rest 76 beats/min, respiratory rate 12 breaths/min, vital capacity is within normal limits

Musculoskeletal and Neuromuscular Assessment

- Upper limb muscle strength is 5/5 trunk is 4/5 and lower limbs 0/5.
- Deep tendon reflexes are 2+ in the upper limbs and 0 in the lower limbs.

Integumentary and Sensory Assessment

- Skin is intact throughout, history of grade 2 sacral pressure ulcer.
- Sensation is absent below T12.

Range of Motion Assessment

- Supine mat assessment revealed passive range of motion is within normal limits throughout his extremities. Excellent hip flexion to 105 degrees and hamstring range within normal limit.

Mobility and ADL Assessment

- Independent in all self-care activities including dressing, grooming, hygiene, bowel and bladder management, basic wheelchair management and propulsion, and driving maximum assistance with high-level wheelchair skills.
- Nonambulatory

Equipment

- Tub bench, rental manual wheelchair, 2-door sedan adapted with hand controls

Evaluation of Clinical Assessment

John McCoy is a 26-year-old man with a T12 paraplegia, ASIA A diagnosis from a motor vehicle accident. He is 12 weeks post injury and is being admitted for outpatient physical therapy for wheelchair prescription and training in advanced manual wheelchair skills. His 2-week delay in starting therapy was caused by a waiting list.

Patient's Care Needs

1. Functional training for advanced wheelchair skills for independence in the home, work, and community
2. Education in wheelchair maintenance and management of wheelchair components

Diagnosis and Prognosis

Diagnosis is T12 paraplegia, ASIA A. Prognosis is for full mobility independence with manual wheelchair skills for home, work, and community.

Preferred Practice Pattern*

Impaired Muscle Performance (4C), Joint Mobility, Motor Function, Muscle Performance, and Range of Motion Associated With Fracture (4G), Impairments Nonprogressive Spinal Cord Disorders (5H), Prevention/Risk Reduction for Integumentary Disorders (7A)

Team Goals

1. Patient to demonstrate good understanding of pros and cons of wheelchair options to actively participate in decision making.
2. Patient to be independent with loading and unloading wheelchair from car incorporating good body mechanics.
3. Patient to be independent with all community mobility in wheelchair including three to four steps.
4. Patient to be independent with wheelchairs parts, management, care, and maintenance.

Patient Goals

"I want to be fitted for and receive a lightweight wheelchair and to get around in it independently."

Care Plan
Treatment Plan and Rationale

- Complete a wheelchair mobility training needs assessment.
- Initiate a trial and evaluation program so that John can assess several wheelchairs for optimal posture, propulsion, and ease of maneuverability in his home, work, and the community.
- Schedule advanced wheelchair skills training for independent function in the home, work, and community.
- Schedule John to attend a wheelchair seating clinic for prescription of his manual wheelchair.
- Plan to educate and train patient in wheelchair maintenance and wheelchair component management.

Interventions

- Training with propulsion and advanced wheelchair skills with a variety of seating simulations to promote independence on all terrain.
- Specify wheelchair seating system order with team, including vendor.
- Training via education and demonstration with wheelchair maintenance and taking wheelchair apart and putting it back together.
- Educate patient in body mechanics and ergonomics and train patient in car transfers incorporating these techniques.

CLINICAL CASE STUDY Development of Wheelchair Skills—cont'd

Documentation and Team Communication

- Team will specify the wheelchair prescription together.
- Team will discuss progress on learning the safe execution of advanced wheelchair skills.
- Team will review consistency in wheelchair maintenance and management.
- Team will document level of independence in all wheelchair skills and car transfers.
- Letter of medical necessity to be completed and all supporting documentation for wheelchair.

Follow-Up Assessment

- "Fit" and delivery of wheelchair and seating system.
- Follow up on use of wheelchair at home, work, and community to determine needs for additional practice of advanced wheelchair skills in unique environments and terrain.

Critical Thinking Exercises

Consider factors, especially of lifestyle and work demands, that will influence John's independence and safety regarding independent mobility. On the basis of the preceding case study summary and outlined care plan, answer the following questions:

1. What type of wheelchair would you recommend for John? What is the optimal propulsion technique?
2. When initially instructing John in wheelies, what skills should have preceded this instruction? How should the instruction progress?
3. Describe how you would have John negotiate stairs if an elevator was out of order with one person assisting.
4. How would you instruct John to descend an 8-inch or higher curb?
5. What is the optimal method for John to transfer from the floor back into his wheelchair?

*Guide to physical therapist practice, rev. ed. 2, Alexandria, VA, 2003, American Physical Therapy Association.

SUMMARY

The community is filled with obstacles such as steps and uneven surfaces. Consequently, for individuals who use a wheelchair as their primary means of mobility, proficiency with advanced wheelchair skills is essential for maximum safety and independence. Each client will find that independence includes being aware of his abilities and being able to independently instruct others to assist him when necessary. Overuse injuries resulting from the repetitive strain of wheelchair use can be devastating, resulting in loss of independence and a reduced quality of life. Rehabilitation and continuing training that includes the provision of evidence-based clinical practices in wheelchair skills, appropriate wheelchair setup, and instruction in propulsion techniques can protect upper limb function in individuals with SCI who depend on wheelchairs for mobility. The therapeutic techniques and progression of advanced wheelchair techniques described in this chapter are consistent with current practice. As with any therapeutic technique, therapeutic judgment should override these techniques and all can and should be modified as necessary to meet individual client abilities.

REFERENCES

1. Ummat S, Kirby RL: Nonfatal wheelchair-related accidents reported to the National Electronic Injury Surveillance System, *Am J Phys Med Rehabil* 73:163-167, 1994.
2. Calder CJ, Kirby RL: Fatal wheelchair-related accidents in the United States, *Am J Phys Med Rehabil* 69:184-190, 1990.
3. Sie IH, Waters RL, Adkins RH et al: Upper extremity pain in the postrehabilitation spinal cord injured client, *Arch Phys Med Rehabil* 73:44-48, 1992.
4. Gellman H, Sie I, Waters RL: Late complications of the weight-bearing upper extremity in the paraplegic client, *Clin Orthop* 233:132-135, 1988.
5. Nichols PJ, Norman PA, Ennis JR: Wheelchair user's shoulder? Shoulder pain in clients with spinal cord lesions, *Scand J Rehabil Med* 11:29-32, 1979.
6. Boninger ML, Dicianno BE, Cooper RA et al: Shoulder magnetic resonance imaging abnormalities, wheelchair propulsion, and gender, *Arch Phys Med Rehabil* 84:1615-1620, 2002.
7. Boninger ML, Cooper RA, Baldwin MA et al: Wheelchair pushrim kinetics: body weight and median nerve function, *Arch Phys Med Rehabil* 80:910-915, 1999.
8. Koontz AM, Boninger ML: Proper propulsion: understanding how wheelchair users propel themselves can lead to prevention of repetitive strain injury, *Rehab Management* 4:18-21, 2003.
9. Brubaker CE: Wheelchair prescription: an analysis of factors that affect mobility and performance, *J Rehabil Res Dev* 23:19-26, 1986.
10. Beekman CE, Miller-Porter L, Schoneberger M: Energy cost of propulsion in standard and ultralight wheelchairs in people with spinal cord injuries, *Phys Ther* 79:146-158, 1999.
11. Cooper RA, Robertson RN, Lawrence B et al: Life-cycle analysis of depot versus rehabilitation manual wheelchairs, *J Rehabil Res Dev* 33:45-55, 1996.
12. Cooper RA, Gonzalez J, Lawrence B et al: Performance of selected lightweight wheelchairs on ANSI/RESNA tests: American National Standards Institute-Rehabilitation Engineering and Assistive Technology Society of North America, *Arch Phys Med Rehabil* 78:1138-1144, 1997.
13. Kwarciak AM: *Performance analysis of suspension manual wheelchairs* [thesis], Pittsburgh, PA, 2003, University of Pittsburgh, Department of Bioengineering.
14. Fitzgerald SG, Cooper RA, Boninger ML et al: Comparison of fatigue life for 3 types of manual wheelchairs, *Arch Phys Med Rehabil* 82:1484-1488, 2001.
15. Hughes CJ, Weimar WH, Sheth PN et al: Biomechanics of wheelchair propulsion as a function of seat position and user-to-chair interface, *Arch Phys Med Rehabil* 73:263-269, 1992.

16. Cooper RA, Dvorznak MJ, O'Connor TJ et al: Braking electric-powered wheelchairs: effect of braking method, seatbelt, and legrests, *Arch Phys Med Rehabil* 79:1244-1249, 1998.

17. Masse LC, Lamontagne M, O'Riain MD: Biomechanical analysis of wheelchair propulsion for various seating positions, *J Rehabil Res Dev* 29:12-28, 1992.

18. Boninger ML, Baldwin MA, Cooper RA, et al: Manual wheelchair pushrim biomechanics and axle position, *Arch Phys Med Rehabil* 81:608-613, 2000.

19. Majaess GG, Kirby RL, Ackroyd-Stolarz SA et al: Influence of seat position on the static and dynamic forward and rear stability of occupied wheelchairs, *Arch Phys Med Rehabil* 74:977-982, 1993.

20. Kirby RL, Ashton BD, Ackroyd-Stolarz SA et al: Adding loads to occupied wheelchairs: effect on static rear and forward stability, *Arch Phys Med Rehabil* 77:183-186, 1996.

21. van der Woude LHV, Veeger DJ, Rozendal RH et al: Seat height in handrim wheelchair propulsion, *J Rehabil Res Dev* 26:31-50, 1989.

22. Werner RA, Franzblau A, Albers JW et al: Median mononeuropathy among active workers—are there differences between symptomatic and asymptomatic workers, *Am J Ind Med* 33:374-378, 1998.

23. Silverstein BA, Fine LJ, Armstrong TJ: Occupational factors and carpal tunnel syndrome, *Am J Ind Med* 11:343-358, 1987.

24. Loslever P, Ranaivosoa A: Biomechanical and epidemiological investigation of carpal tunnel syndrome at workplaces with high risk factors, *Ergonomics* 36:537-555, 1993.

25. Roquelaure Y, Mechali S, Dano C et al: Occupational and personal risk factors for carpal tunnel syndrome in industrial workers, *Scand J Work Environ Health* 23:364-369, 1997.

26. Cohen RB, Williams GR: Impingement syndrome and rotator cuff disease as repetitive motion disorders, *Clin Orthop* 351:95-101, 1998.

27. Frost P, Bonde JP, Mikkelsen S et al: Risk of shoulder tendinitis in relation to shoulder loads in monotonous repetitive work, *Am J Ind Med* 41:11-18, 2002.

28. Andersen JH, Kaergaard A, Frost P et al: Physical, psychosocial, and individual risk factors for neck/shoulder pain with pressure tenderness in the muscles among workers performing monotonous, repetitive work, *Spine* 27:660-667, 2002.

29. Boninger ML, Cooper RA, Robertson RN et al: 3-D pushrim forces during two speeds of wheelchair propulsion, *Am J Phys Med Rehabil* 76:420-426, 1997.

30. Boninger ML, Koontz AM, Sisto SA et al: Pushrim biomechanics and injury prevention in spinal cord injury: recommendations based on CULP-SCI Investigations, *J Rehabil Res Dev* 42:9-19, 2005.

31. Shimada SD, Robertson RN, Bonninger ML et al: Kinematic characterization of wheelchair propulsion, *J Rehabil Res Dev* 35:210-218, 1998.

32. Boninger ML, Souza AL, Cooper RA, et al: Propulsion patterns and pushrim biomechanics in manual wheelchair propulsion, *Arch Phys Med Rehabil* 83:718-723, 2002.

33. Sanderson DJ, Sommer HJ: Kinematic features of wheelchair propulsion, *J Biomech* 18:423-429, 1985.

34. Veeger HEJ, van der Woude LHV, Rozendal RH: Wheelchair propulsion technique at different speeds, *Scand J Rehabil Med* 21:197-203, 1989.

35. Richter WM, Rodriguez R, Woods KR et al: Stroke pattern and handrim biomechanics for level and uphill wheelchair propulsion at self-selected speeds, *Arch Phys Med Rehabil* 88:81-87, 2007.

36. Kirby RL, Swuste J, Dupuis DJ et al: The Wheelchair Skills Test: a pilot study of a new outcome measure, *Arch Phys Med Rehabil* 83:10-18, 2002.

37. Kilkens OJ, Post MW, van der Woude LH et al: The wheelchair circuit: reliability of a test to assess mobility in persons with spinal cord injuries, *Arch Phys Med Rehabil* 83:1783-1788, 2002.

38. Axelson P, Yamada Chesney D, Minkel J et al: Escalators, In Wong AK, Pasternak M, editors: *The manual wheelchair training guide*, Santa Cruz, CA, 1998, Pax Press, Division of Beneficial Designs.

SOLUTIONS TO CHAPTER 15 CLINICAL CASE STUDY

Development of Wheelchair Skills

1. The lightest weight wheelchair should be recommended for John McCoy. Although this technology is more expensive at the outset, it is less expensive to operate and will last longer because it is made of titanium. The customization of "fit" will maximize hand to wheel access and posture. The weight of the wheelchair will allow ease of propulsion and decreased joint strain with loading and unloading the wheelchair from the car and will therefore serve as a prevention of potential shoulder injury. In addition, stroke frequency and rate of loading the push rim will be less compared with a conventional wheelchair, which will help to minimize median nerve damage over time. The semicircular technique for wheelchair propulsion is the optimal method for propulsion. Because of the long-term effects of wheelchair propulsion and possibilities of upper limb injuries, instruction in propulsion technique is extremely important.

2. Protective response to falling should be taught before progressing to the wheelies. The therapist should guide John through a series of backward falls at various rates with the client practicing head protection by tucking his head and protecting his face with upper limb by holding his lower limbs down so that they do not fall backward, hitting John in the face with the impact of the fall. After John has become proficient with protective responses, the progression to wheelies begins with the therapist guarding from behind beginning with stationary control of balance in the wheelie position. A surface with higher rolling resistance (e.g., carpet) should be used. To assume a wheelie from a static position, John will perform a backward stroke and then propel forward with a quick, strong stroke to lift the casters off the floor and immediately find his balance point. The therapist always guards from behind. John will then progress to assuming wheelie position from a level position and then moving forward and backward in a wheelie, turning in a wheelie, and climbing curbs. Climbing curbs should begin with a 2-inch curb and progress to higher levels, depending on John's mobility needs within the community.

3. John may be able to ascend stairs with assistance from one person if the elevator is not working. He will back up to the steps and grasp one railing with both hands, assume a wheelie by pulling on the railing, and lift the wheelchair up one stair at a time by pulling hand over hand on the railing. The therapist or person assisting John lifts from behind with both hands on the wheelchair frame or in a folding chair, the push handles. After John reaches the top of the stairs, he releases one arm and grasps its corresponding wheel rim while the other hand remains on the railing to stabilize the chair. John can then propel backward with his hand on the rim until the wheelchair is upright.

SOLUTIONS TO CHAPTER 15 CLINICAL CASE STUDY

Development of Wheelchair Skills—cont'd

4. The safest method to descend an 8-inch curb is in a backward position. John can perform this maneuver by dropping his chair's rear wheels slowly and evenly off the curb while allowing the handrims to slowly slide through his grasp. It is extremely important that John leans forward as he lowers the wheelchair. When both rear wheels are on the bottom surface, he will back up about 5 inches and make a sharp turn by holding one wheel steady while propelling backward on the other so that the casters move from the curb without banging against the curb. If an assistant is present, she should guard from behind.

5. John should use an anterior approach starting from a sidelong sit position and then pull into a tall kneel position with both hands on the front corners of the wheelchair frame and his knees positioned midline. He can now reach across to the back corner of the seat with one hand so that both hands are on the same side of the chair on the front and back corners. Next he shifts his weight over his hands and pushes down into the seat lifting his knees off the floor. While he lifts, he also twists his trunk to allow his hip to rest on the seat. John then performs a push-up to reposition his hips for equal weight-bearing distribution.

CHAPTER SIXTEEN

Ambulation

Andrea Behrman, PT, PhD, Erica Druin, MPT, Mark Bowden, PT, MS, and Susan Harkema, PhD

I could not wait to try and stand again. With the help of long leg braces I did. Once I stood I wanted to take steps. It was very hard to maintain my balance relying on the muscles that I had left. It took hard work and self confidence to become independent with crutches. The psychological benefit of standing up and seeing things the way they once were is a tremendous feeling. I am so happy that I am able to stand once again.

Nick (T10 SCI)

Asked to try walking without his rolling walker, BJ pondered a moment and then responded to the question: Yes, I'll try, but you know that I was taught to walk again with six legs, not two.

BJ (C7 ASIA C SCI)

Spinal cord injury (SCI) is one of the most disabling health problems facing adults today. Paralysis of lower limb muscles resulting in the loss of the ability to walk, impaired walking, and disability are major consequences of SCI. Any clinician who works with individuals who have SCI will undoubtedly be asked at some point in her career, "Will I ever walk again?" The answer, of course, depends on many variables, which will be discussed in more detail later in this chapter. There are physiological and economic costs to be considered, and successful outcomes depend very heavily on an intense physical and psychological commitment on the part of the trainee. Training paradigms will range from those that are purely compensatory, such as bracing and electrical stimulation, which allow even those with complete injuries the capacity for limited stepping, to recovery-based paradigms based on animal and human models of the neurobiological control of locomotion. The comments from Nick and BJ at the beginning of this chapter provide insight not only about the desire to walk but also exemplify compensation strategies for sensorimotor deficits as the mainstay of rehabilitation for upright mobility. This chapter introduces an impending paradigm shift from compensation-based to activity-based therapies capitalizing on neuroplasticity within the central nervous system as the basis for walking recovery programs.[1] As the science of rehabilitation emerges, the only thing that can be said with any degree of certainty is that clinicians should never answer the above question negatively, and more important, physical therapists should never be the limiting factor in an individual's desire to walk again.

WHAT IS WALKING?

For clear goals to be set and attained, the clinician, patient, family, and all those involved must be clear as to what the definition of walking may be. Is it merely the ability to cross an indoor, level terrain to get from point A to point B, or does walking imply symmetrical, coordinated movements that resemble those of the patient before he was injured? Is walking an outcome for exercise, limited or full household ambulation, or some degree of community ambulation? Does walking allow for physical assistance, the use of an assistance device, or the use of some sort of orthosis, and does it contain a definable requirement for endurance?

All the above questions need to be answered and mutually agreed on by all those involved when engaging in gait rehabilitation in those with SCI.

Clinical treatment paradigms are often based on the World Health Organization's International Classification of Functioning, Disability, and Health Model of Functioning and Disability (see Figure 5-2). In terms of SCI ambulation, interventions are often based on the level of "body functions and structures" by promoting maximum capacity muscle strength, range, and endurance in muscles that can be voluntarily activated above and below the lesion.[2] Activity level interventions aim to compensate for nonremediable deficits of paralysis and weakness by using braces and assistive devices and by teaching new behavioral strategies or skills for ambulation and mobility.[2-4] As mentioned previously, however, interventions must also take into account personal and environmental factors and additionally focus on an individual's ability to participate in community activities that require or are assisted by ambulatory function.

Of particular importance is the clinicians' definition of independence. The Functional Independence Measure (FIM), which is the gold standard for inpatient rehabilitation outcomes, defines independent ambulation as being able to walk 150 feet without any physical assistance; modified independence allows for the use of an assistive device.[5] Independence cannot be ascertained, however, unless ambulation skills meet the needs of an individual's environment. For example, is the individual independent going up and down steps, ramps, and on uneven terrain? Given that research has posited normal velocity at 1.0 m/s to 1.67 m/s,[6] that 0.8 m/s can predict community ambulation in poststroke populations,[7] and that an excess of 1.2 m/s is required to cross some urban streets,[8] is an individual's gait speed fast enough to truly predict independence? Last, because it has been well documented that community independence requires an individual to traverse approximately 1000 feet at a time,[8,9] can community independence be accurately predicted on the basis of a FIM measure of 6 or 7 with the criterion of 150 feet? The purpose here is not to criticize FIM but rather imply that it alone is not sufficient to define independent gait and should be used in concert with other outcome measures.

PROGNOSIS FOR WALKING

The large majority of individuals with complete spinal cord injuries as defined by the American Spinal Injury Association (ASIA) Impairment Scale (see Figure 6-12) will need to rely on purely compensatory techniques to achieve even minimal levels of ambulation. Injuries in 89% of those classified as ASIA A during the first week of injury will remain complete, and only 3% to 6% of those whose injuries convert to motor incomplete will gain enough strength to assist with ambulation.[3] Approximately 50% of individuals with an ASIA B diagnosis will become ambulatory and most of them will have preserved sacral sensation for pain and temperature.[3] This observation implies that sparing in the spinothalamic tracts is a good prognostic indicator for the adjacent lateral corticospinal tracts. Without spinothalamic tract sparing, the likelihood of ambulation decreases to approximately 10% to 33%.[3] The majority of people diagnosed within the first week of injury as motor incomplete eventually ambulate for their primary means of locomotion, although the prognosis decreases significantly with age.[10] Typically, the prognosis for ambulatory potential is directly proportional to the amount of motor activity seen on evaluation, and most, if not all, individuals initially diagnosed with ASIA D within the first 3 days after injury move on to full-time ambulation.[10] It should be noted that different researchers use varying definitions of independent walking; thus results from prognostication research should not be evaluated individually.

BENEFITS AND COSTS

Physiologically and psychologically, there are many benefits to regaining ambulatory function after SCI. Although it is debatable, there is some evidence that weight bearing helps prevent the osteopenia that often accompanies acute SCI.[11] There is believed to be a decrease in spasticity and the incidence of pressure ulcer formation.[12,13] In addition, many believe that standing and walking have positive impacts on bowel and bladder regulation and can decrease the incidence of urinary tract infections[12,13] (Clinical Note: Benefits of Ambulation After Spinal Cord Injury).

CLINICAL NOTE   **Benefits of Ambulation After Spinal Cord Injury**

- Helps prevent osteopenia
- Decrease in spasticity
- Decreased incidence of pressure ulcer formation
- Positive impact on bowel and bladder regulation
- Decreased incidence of urinary tract infections
- Psychological benefits and motivation
- Reported improvements in quality of life

Psychologically, many, if not all, will at some point in their rehabilitation after SCI list ambulation as one of their primary goals. Even the limited ability to stand provides the opportunity to interact with the world from the same viewpoint as before the injury and can provide some psychological benefit and motivation. Those with SCI who have been able to undergo a long-term standing program not only report several health-related benefits such as improved circulation, skin integrity, spasticity control, and bowel and bladder function, but also improvements in sleep,

pain, fatigue, and general well-being.[12] These improvements in quality of life are felt even if programs are initiated years after injury.[13]

Because of the sensory impairments associated with SCI, clinicians must take special precautions in gait training, particularly if the therapy involves extensive bracing. Fabrication of the orthosis should include careful evaluation of fit and materials to avoid any undue pressure points. Any movable joints in the orthoses should be aligned with anatomical joint lines to decrease the potential effects of shear. Skin integrity should be maintained through careful evaluation and inspection of the fit of the orthosis and the monitoring of any reddened areas after doffing, and all individuals should be educated on independent skin inspection to be done after each wear (Clinical Note: Costs of Ambulation After Spinal Cord Injury).

CLINICAL NOTE   **Costs of Ambulation After Spinal Cord Injury**

- Possible skin issues from bracing
- Risk of hyperflexibility
- Long-term shoulder conditions
- Increased likelihood of falls
- Increased energy requirements

In addition to potential skin issues, there is a risk of causing hyperflexibility, not only at the joints proximal to bracing but also potentially in the vertebrae at or near the original fracture sites. The introduction of bracing and the possible side effects may also increase the incidence of autonomic dysreflexia and an action plan should be developed to quickly deal with any possible occurrences. Heavy use of the upper limbs during ambulation places a significant, repetitive strain on the shoulder complex, which it was not designed to handle, and long-term conditions are often seen in this population. In addition, by retraining the ability to walk, the clinician is also increasing the client's risk-taking behavior and likelihood of falls, and proper safety education should be a part of any gait training program. Last, and perhaps most significantly, walking after SCI is an incredibly intense undertaking physiologically, and the energy requirements are much higher than normal ambulation and even self-propelling a manual wheelchair.[14] Because of this energy expenditure, many find that compensatory approaches to walking do not lead to community ambulation but rather are best used for limited household use, and sadly, many forego the benefits of walking because of the excessiveness of the energy requirements.

Because the upper limbs are doing all of the work previously done by the lower limbs and often must compensate for trunk weakness as well, oxygen consumption may be as much as 160% greater than normal.[14] Oxygen consumption depends on the individual's strength level, and it is negatively correlated with the lower limb motor score.[14] Energy expenditure is also linked to the level of orthotic management that is required to achieve ambulation. For example, those who require bilateral knee-ankle-foot orthoses (KAFO) use 226% of the oxygen of normal walkers, walk only at 0.32 m/s, and load 79% of their body weight through the upper limbs.[14] By comparison, those who walk with only the need of one ankle foot orthosis (AFO) increase oxygen expenditure by 81%, walk at 0.8 m/s, and load 13.9% of their body weight through the upper limbs. For those who persist with brace walking, however, the speed more than doubles and the energy costs are cut in half.[15]

As a result of the physiological costs, very few individuals who use bilateral KAFOs are able to ambulate full time in the community. Hussey and Stauffer[16] suggested in 1973 that those who were able to walk in the community had intact pelvic control, bilateral 3/5 hip flexor strength, and at least a 3/5 in one of the knee extensors, allowing the individual to ambulate with a maximum of one KAFO and use a reciprocal gait pattern. This predictive categorization has held true for over 30 years and has only recently been challenged with the relatively recent advances in locomotion research.

CONSIDERATIONS FOR CONVENTIONAL GAIT TRAINING

Numerous factors should be considered before initiation of conventional gait training in patients with SCI, including the individual's motor control, range of motion (ROM), muscle tone, sensation, functional abilities, posture, skin integrity, and autonomic function.

Motor Control

The amount of spared lower limb strength is perhaps the best predictor of an individual's walking ability. The Lower Extremity Motor Score, which is the sum of the 10 key lower limb muscles (e.g., left and right hip flexors, knee extensors, ankle dorsiflexors, long toe extensors, and ankle plantar flexors) is a predictor for locomotor function, with higher LEMS predicting improved capacity.[10, 17-19] In addition to ambulatory capacity, lower limb motor control is predictive of gait speed and 6-minute walk distance.[20] Intact trunk control, especially pelvic control, greatly enhances the person's ability to independently ambulate and reduces necessary energy expenditure. Last, if the person is to ambulate by using compensatory techniques, upper limb strength, especially in the elbow extensors, is prerequisite.

Range of Motion

A patient's ROM is important to consider for conventional gait training. To best maintain standing in bilateral long leg braces, a patient assumes the "parastance" position (Figure 16-1, A). The parastance position refers to a posture where the weight line falls posterior to the hips and anterior to the knees and ankles. To obtain this position, the patient needs hip extension and dorsiflexion beyond neutral and full knee extension. This will optimize the patient's ability to be biomechanically stable in stance with orthoses without lower limb muscle strength. If a patient does not have this ROM available, he will experience increased demands on the upper limbs for weight bearing and may be at greater risk for falling (Figure 16-1, B).

Muscle Tone

The effects of hypertonicity are varied and debatable. It is important to determine whether an individual is hypertonic, in what joints, and what exacerbates or ameliorates the spasticity.

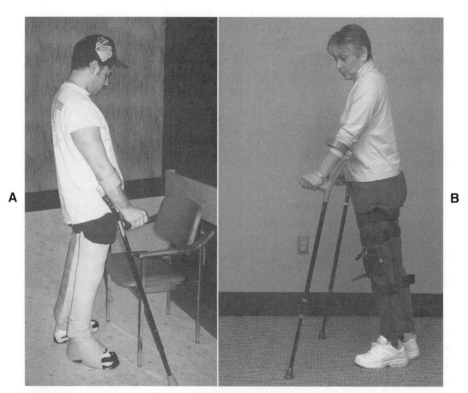

FIGURE 16-1 **A,** A patient wearing long leg splints stands in the parastance position in which his weight line falls posterior to his hips and anterior to his knees and ankles. This position allows him to achieve optimum stability in stance without lower limb strength. **B,** A patient with tight hip flexors is unable to obtain hip extension beyond neutral and as a result cannot achieve full parastance position. She consequently needs to bear more weight through her upper limbs and may be at greater risk for falling.

The predominant pattern (i.e., flexor or extensor) can help guide early treatment goals and orthotic needs.

Sensation

As mentioned previously, intact pain and temperature sensation is a good prognostic indicator for subsequent motor recovery, and proprioception is also correlated with ambulatory capacity. In addition to its prognostic function, it is important to evaluate whether paresthesias limit function or would cause problems when donning prostheses.

Functional Abilities

A patient's function must be addressed to be able to coordinate an expansive and thorough rehabilitation program. Gait training should not be done in lieu of wheelchair level functional training unless it is believed with some certainty that mobility gained with gait training carries over to functional capacity. This is of particular importance in inpatient rehabilitation, where discharging someone with as much independence as possible is the primary goal versus the individual's desire to work solely on walking.

Posture

A person's ability to assume and maintain an adequate posture must be assessed before initiation of gait training. A person's ability to extend his hips beyond a neutral position will assist in the maintenance of static balance during stance. Likewise, the absence of trunk control may necessitate the use of platform attachments on a walker. In fact, the Consortium for Spinal Cord Medicine Clinical Practice Guidelines consider any complete injury above T10 as nonfunctional because of the importance of postural control.[3]

Skin Integrity

Skin integrity is of vital importance for those who will undergo training with braces, and treatment plans must be organized in concert with the sensation findings from above. A complete history of previous pressure ulcers and type of management (e.g., conservative versus surgical) must be obtained to create a wearing schedule for orthoses.

Autonomic Function

A history of any autonomic dysreflexia should be noted in the evaluation and the therapist should document any part of the intervention that may cause an event (e.g., poorly fitting orthoses, straps that are applied too tightly, kinked catheter tubing). The treatment team should have a clearly defined procedure in place should a patient complain of dysreflexia-type symptoms.

OUTCOMES

As mentioned previously, it is very important to quantify as many important elements of walking as possible and not rely on one measure to be the definitive outcome. In addition to summary index scores, it is important to gather information on speed of walking, endurance, balance, and quality of movements. When the information provided is viewed as a whole, the various types of outcome measures act together in concert (Clinical Note: Outcome Measures Used to Assess Ambulation).

CLINICAL NOTE Outcome Measures Used to Assess Ambulation

- FIM
- Ten Meter Walking Test for Speed
- Dynamic Gait Index
- Berg Balance Test
- Six-Minute Walking Test for Endurance
- Walking Index for SCI
- SCI Functional Ambulation Inventory
- Community Walking Activity

Measures of Functional Independence

The FIM defines mobility on a seven-point scale ranging from being totally dependent on others for the activity (0) to being independent (7) (see Figure 6-15). Independence is defined as being able to walk 150 feet on a level walkway without any external physical assistance or an assistive device.[5] A modified independent score (6) may be given if the individual does not require external assistance but can only complete the activity with an assistive device.

Speed—The 10-Meter Walk Test

Gait speed is a fast, easy, inexpensive, and reliable method of quantifying gait ability. Timing of gait performance enhances objectivity and provides greater ability to identify differences in ability than do many qualitative assessments.[21-23] More specifically, gait speed is a strong discriminator between household and community ambulators in individuals after a stroke. Excellent (interclass correlation coefficients [(ICCs] >0.97) interrater and intrarater reliability estimates for self-paced timed forward walking using a stopwatch have been reported.[2] Individuals should be given a 3-meter warm-up distance before the 10-meter distance and 3 meters beyond the 10 meters to continue walking so that the effects of acceleration and deceleration are not scored. The time that it takes to traverse the 10 meters at the subject's usual pace should be recorded. Automated walkway systems such as the GaitRite and the GaitMat II can be used to quantify gait speed over a shorter distance and eliminate the need for stopwatches and calculations. The GaitMat II has been proven valid and reliable in the poststroke population,[24] and the GaitRite is valid and reliable in healthy subjects[25] and with individuals with Parkinson's disease,[26] but not with SCI.

Dynamic Balance During Gait

The ability to adapt to the environment reactively or proactively during walking has been identified as a critical feature of community ambulation.[27] The Dynamic Gait Index (DGI) evaluates the ability to adapt to changes in task demands. The DGI rates performance from 0 (poor) to 3 (excellent) on eight different gait tasks, including gait on even surfaces, gait when changing speeds, gait and head turns in a vertical or horizontal direction, stepping over or around obstacles, and gait with pivot turns and steps. The DGI incorporates items identified as key components necessary for community ambulation, including forward walking velocity,[6] stopping suddenly,[8] moving the head,[28] and obstacle negotiation.[29] Excellent interrater (ICCs, 0.97) and intrarater reliability (ICCs, 0.96) has been reported for the DGI.[22]

Berg Balance Test

The Berg Blance Test (BBT) is a 14-item test that requires an individual to perform everyday tasks of increasing difficulty, including postures and movements associated with daily tasks such as sitting, moving from one chair to another, standing up, turning around, picking up an item from the floor, and the performance of more challenging tasks such as standing on one foot. Evaluators rate each item on a five-point ordinal scale according to whether the task is successfully performed, the distance reached, and the amount of (1) time to maintain a position, (2) physical assistance or supervision required for safety, and (3) time to complete the task. Content validity, interrater reliability (ICC = 0.98), concurrent validity, intrarater reliability (ICC = 0.98), and criterion validity have been established for the BBT in evaluating older adults and community-dwelling frail older adults.[30,31] A score of less than 45 (out of a total possible 56 points) has been established as a threshold for balance impairment, predictor of falls, and strongly associated with decrements in effective and safe ambulation in the community.[30]

Endurance

The 6-minute walk test is a submaximal test of aerobic capacity and has been shown to be a valid and reliable measure of endurance in older adults.[32,33] The trainee is simply asked to walk at a comfortable speed for 6 minutes while someone monitors the distance traveled.

Walking Index for Spinal Cord Injury

The Walking Index for Spinal Cord Injury, Version II (WISCI II) was selected as an instrument to categorize the level of physical assistance and use of assistive devices or braces required for walking (Figure 16-2). The WISCI II, a valid and reliable instrument,[34] consists of a 20-item scale with a score of 1 as the most dependent and 20 as the most independent.

Observational Gait Analysis

The Spinal Cord Injury Functional Ambulation Inventory (SCI-PAI) was developed as a way to quantify observational gait analysis specific for the SCI population. The SCI-PAI is a valid and reliable measure of walking ability for those with SCI and is sensitive to changes resulting from a gait-training intervention.[35]

Community Walking Activity

If possible, it is very valuable to collect information on the amount of walking a patient is able to perform outside the clinical setting. This can be accomplished with simple measures such as diaries or questionnaires or with more technologically advanced methods such as accelerometers or the Step Activity Monitor (Figure 16-3), which not only counts the number of steps taken in the day, but also counts strides and observes activity during predetermined time spans (e.g., per minute or hour), providing more information than basic accelerometers.[36]

CONVENTIONAL GAIT TRAINING

Conventional rehabilitation after SCI emphasizes promoting functional gains through strengthening and endurance training of the muscles under voluntary control and compensation for nonremediable deficits of paralysis and weakness by using braces and assistive devices for support.[2,37] Successful mobility is often dependent on learning a new behavior, often requiring bracing with assistive devices. Using this compensatory approach, the probability of achieving ambulation increases as voluntary muscle strength surpasses targeted thresholds of lower limb motor scores.[38-40] Learning new behaviors and techniques are often in the form of learning new gait patterns, having the appropriate braces prescribed and fitted, and learning novel mobility skills incorporating the newly acquired bracing and assistive devices. Because many of the compensatory issues relate to complete injuries, except where otherwise specified, the following guidelines are relevant to those with complete SCI using bilateral KAFOs.

When initiating gait training it can be quite cumbersome and expensive to try to provide and fit patients with KAFOs for training. Rather, the use of long leg splints is simple and less expensive (see Figure 16-1, A). Splints can be made from narrow padded wooden boards held in place with ace wraps. The board should extend from just below the ischial tuberosity to just above the Achilles tendon. The ace wraps are used in a figure-eight pattern to completely enclose the board on the leg to prevent slippage. In addition, the ankle should be ace wrapped into a dorsiflexed position, being careful to avoid ankle inversion.

Training typically begins in the parallel bars. It should be noted that the patient will have a tendency to pull on the bars to assume stance and to help maintain his balance. If he is allowed to rely on this method of support when working in the parallel bars, it will become a habit that is very difficult to break when progressing to other assistive devices. The therapist should constantly remind him to maintain pressure on the bars in a downward direction only (Figure 16-4, A). Instructing the patient to keep his hands open, rather than wrapping his fingers tightly around the bars, can reinforce this training.

A patient should work toward maintaining static standing balance in the parastance position with unilateral upper limb support. Few patients will be able to maintain their balance for more than several seconds without any upper limb support. If a patient allows his weight line to move anterior to his hips, unrestricted hip flexion will occur and the patient will jackknife and fall backward. When guarding a patient, the therapist must prevent jackknifing by placing one hand at the pelvis ready to provide an anterior force and the other hand at the upper trunk ready to provide a posterior force (Figure 16-5). In addition, the therapist can help stabilize a patient who is losing balance by grabbing his guarding belt. These interventions allow the therapist to help a patient regain his parastance position.

After a patient has gained a feel for where his balance point is located in the parastance position and has learned to regain this position when displaced, he may begin to work on lifting his body and then lowering himself directly into the parastance position (see Figure 16-4, A and B). When he has mastered this skill, he will be ready to begin work on ambulation within the parallel bars. Eventually the patient may master the four-point gait, which is dependent on his upper body strength, body balance, and control. In addition to stabilizing his balance and maintaining the parastance position, the patient will learn how to turn within the bars. This maneuver requires the patient to change his hand placement and trunk orientation so that he can face the right bar (Figure 16-6, A);

WISCI II Levels

Level	Devices	Braces	Assistance	Distance
0				Unable
1	Parallel bars	Braces	2 people	Less than 10 meters
2	Parallel bars	Braces	2 people	10 meters
3	Parallel bars	Braces	1 person	10 meters
4	Parallel bars	No braces	1 person	10 meters
5	Parallel bars	Braces	No assistance	10 meters
6	Walker	Braces	1 person	10 meters
7	Two crutches	Braces	1 person	10 meters
8	Walker	No braces	1 person	10 meters
9	Walker	Braces	No assistance	10 meters
10	One cane/crutch	Braces	1 person	10 meters
11	Two crutches	No braces	1 person	10 meters
12	Two crutches	Braces	No assistance	10 meters
13	Walker	No braces	No assistance	10 meters
14	One cane/crutch	No braces	1 person	10 meters
15	One cane/crutch	Braces	No assistance	10 meters
16	Two crutches	No braces	No assistance	10 meters
17	No devices	No braces	1 person	10 meters
18	No devices	Braces	No assistance	10 meters
19	One cane/crutch	No braces	No assistance	10 meters
20	No devices	No braces	No assistance	10 meters

SCORING SHEET (WISCI II)

Patient Name _____ Date _____

Check descriptors that apply to current walking performance, then assign the highest level of walking performance. (In scoring a level, choose the level at which the patient is safe as judged by the therapist, with patient's comfort level described. If devices other than stated in the standard definitions are used, they should be documented as descriptors. If there is a discrepancy between two observers, the higher level should be chosen.)

Descriptors

Gait: Reciprocal _____; swing through _____

Devices		Braces		Assistance		Patient reported comfort level	
// bars < 10 meters		Long leg braces: Uses 2 Uses 1		Max assist x 2 people		Very comfortable	
// bars 10 meters		Short leg braces: Uses 2 Uses 1		Min/Mod assist x 2 people		Slightly comfortable	
Walker: Standard Rolling Platform		Locked at knee _____ Unlocked at knee _____		Min/Mod assist x 1 person		Neither comfortable nor uncomfortable	
Crutches: Uses 2 Uses 1		Other:				Slightly uncomfortable	
Canes: Quad Uses 2 Uses 1						Very uncomfortable	
No devices		No braces		No assistance			

Level assigned: _____

FIGURE 16-2 The Walking Index for SCI, Version II (WISCI II). (From Dittuno PL, Dittuno Jr JF Jr: Walking index for spinal cord injury (WISCI II): scale revision, *Spinal Cord* 39:654-656, 2001.)

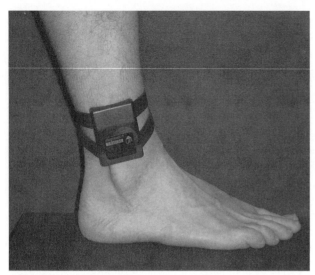

FIGURE 16-3 A step activity monitor is positioned on the outside of the ankle to collect valuable information about the amount of walking a patient is able to perform.

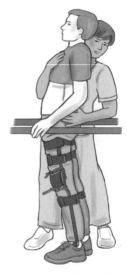

FIGURE 16-5 To prevent a patient from jackknifing when he is using bilateral KAFOs, the therapist should keep one hand at his pelvis while gripping a guarding belt to provide an anterior force and the other at his upper trunk to provide a posterior force.

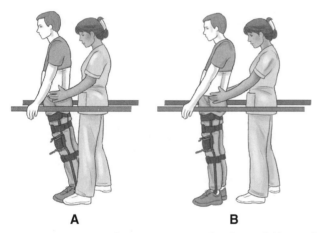

A   **B**

FIGURE 16-4 Patients begin gait training within the parallel bars and are taught to assume and maintain the parastance position with the weight line behind their hips. They lean on the anterior hip structures while making attempts to lift their hands and hold static balance. **A,** The patient then leans forward, placing a downward force on the parallel bars, lifts the legs, and **B,** returns to the parastance position.

next he moves both hands to the bar he is facing and assumes the parastance position (Figure 16-6, *B*). He can now move his right hand to the opposite bar and twist his trunk to produce the momentum to complete the turn (Figure 16-6, *C*).

Gait Patterns

There are various types of gait patterns that an individual with bilateral KAFOs may use. A reciprocal gait pattern is best used by individuals with active hip flexion. Those without active hip flexion may also use this pattern if they are able to compensate by hiking their hips and performing a posterior pelvic tilt to advance one leg at a time. Another option is a swing-through gait pattern, which involves lifting the body (Figure 16-7, *A* to *C*) and allowing the lower limbs to swing forward, landing in front of the hands

(Figure 16-7, *D*). As soon as the patient's feet land, he must immediately regain the parastance position (Figure 16-7, *E*). After he is stable, his hands are advanced so that he can swing his lower limbs in front of his hands again (Figure 16-7, *F*). When guarding a patient performing a swing-through gait pattern, the therapist must remember that preventing the patient from jackknifing is of primary importance (Figure 16-8).

A swing-to gait is similar to the swing-through gait; rather than having the feet land in front of the hands, the feet now land slightly behind the hands. This allows the patient to more easily maintain his balance. For patients who do not have the upper body strength to clear their feet for a swing-through or swing-to gait, a drag-to gait may be used. This is essentially the same as the swing-to gait pattern without the patient lifting his body up for foot clearance, which makes it a slower and less functional gait pattern.

Although ambulation begins within the parallel bars, patients should be advanced to free-standing assistive devices quickly so they do not begin to rely exclusively on the security of the bars. When assistive devices are advanced, enough time should be taken to allow the patient to gain a sense of his balance point with the new device before ambulation is initiated. The transition to forearm crutches may be smoother if the patient first works with one parallel bar and one forearm crutch before progressing to bilateral forearm crutches. Patients who use a reciprocal or swing-through gait should ultimately use forearm crutches; those using a swing-to or drag-to gait may use forearm crutches but will more likely use a walker.

Braces

A wide variety of braces are available to compensate for motor deficits associated with SCI (Figure 16-9, *A* and *B*). Because most orthotic devices are custom made, in a clinic it is impossible to stock a full range of braces that will exactly or even closely fit the individual. In addition, keeping a large variety of assistive options in the clinic is likely cost-prohibitive. Long-leg splints described

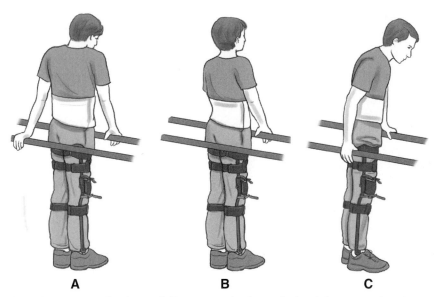

A **B** **C**

FIGURE 16-6 A patient learns how to turn within the parallel bars. **A,** First he changes his hand placement and trunk orientation so that he faces the right bar. **B,** While maintaining the parastance position, he moves his other hand to the facing bar. **C,** Then he moves his right hand to the opposite bar, twisting his trunk to complete a full turn.

previously or adjustable KAFOs that can be reconfigured for a variety of patients permit evaluation and preliminary training. Adjustable KAFOs that offer the ability to unlock the knee and provide adjustable angles at the ankle will allow for a fairly thorough evaluation. This will also give the patient the opportunity to understand the intense physiological cost involved in walking with braces. The clinician will increase the likelihood of follow-through by identifying patients who can overcome the significant limitations of this type of locomotion. Table 16-1 lists examples with descriptions of various types of orthoses used for SCI rehabilitation.

Training for Patients with Incomplete Spinal Cord Injury

Conventional training for those with incomplete SCI (iSCI) often mirrors other types of gait training by incorporating traditional and specialized techniques such as neurodevelopmental treatment (NDT) and proprioceptive neuromuscular facilitation (PNF). These patients, however, deserve special consideration because of the transient nature of the neurological recovery inherent within their diagnosis. Specifically, the widely recognized use of bracing and orthotic devices requires caution in clinical application.

- Do not block recovering motion. Patients with iSCI often have neurological recovery for at least 1 year after injury and sometimes for even longer. As a result, it is imperative that rigid braces not be used because they may prevent activity within the recovering motor units and potentially slow down or halt the recovery process.
- Do not brace a functioning joint to assist proximal or distal joints. Common problems with patients with SCI include instability at the knee and genu recurvatum. Setting a rigid ankle AFO in slight plantarflexion or dorsiflexion, respectively, may reduce these problems. This should only be done if there is a problem at the ankle for which the proposed solution is appropriate. Otherwise, joint conditions requiring orthotic management should be handled at the area of the problem.

- Understand the impact of bracing on mechanics. Bracing, especially rigid bracing of a joint, often causes undesirable effects in the biomechanics of motion. For example, a rigid ankle is not able to dorsiflex, which prevents the tibia from translating forward on a stationary foot. This in turn prevents the limb from moving into terminal stance in a normal fashion. Such changes in the mechanics of gait must be compensated for through a short stride length, circumduction, or hip-hike (elevation of the pelvis to clear the foot for hip flexion). This is only one example in what could be myriad complications. Bracing may be necessary, but the unintended secondary results need to be considered beforehand.
- Recognize upper motor neuron (UMN) versus lower motor neuron injuries (LMN). LMN injuries are a possibility when the injury is below the T10 level and demonstrate more flaccid paralysis than UMN injuries. Physiological return is often slower in this population, and they may require more aggressive bracing earlier in the delivery of care.

Functional Activities
Donning and Doffing Orthoses

A person may not be considered truly independent unless he is also independent in the application and removal of the braces that are required for ambulation. The most common technique is to don the KAFOs from a long-sitting position, either on a bed or mat table, if available. The individual rests the KAFO beside the straightened lower limb, lifts the leg with one hand while sliding the orthosis under with the other hand. This technique requires a great deal of hamstring flexibility (usually approximately 110 degrees, but it may vary depending on arm length and body type) because the process includes manipulation of stabilization straps and shoes distally. Sit-to-stand may happen from the bed or mat or the individual may transfer into the wheelchair before standing.

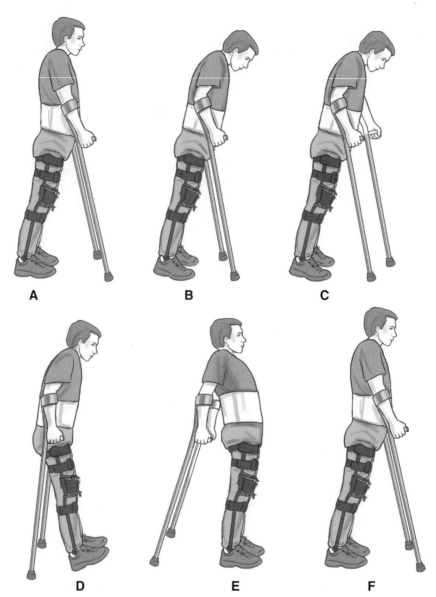

FIGURE 16-7 When a patient practices the swing-through gait patten using bilateral KAFOs and forearm crutches, he begins in the parastance position (see Figure 16-1, *A*). He leans forward onto the forearm crutches **(A)** and applies a downward force on the crutches **(B),** lifting his lower body off the floor surface **(C).** With the help of this momentum, his legs swing through, relying on the control of his shoulder and trunk muscles **(D),** and his legs land in unison in front of the crutches **(E),** which helps to push his hips forward off the crutches behind and toward the parastance position. He then swings his crutches forward to prepare for the next step **(F).**

Sit-to-Stand

Performing sit-to-stand while wearing bilateral KAFOs or long-leg splints and using an assistive device can be very challenging. Sit-to-stand may be performed by using a pop-up method or a turn-around method. The pop-up method involves placing both hands on the walker or forearm crutches (Lofstrand crutches), bending forward at the hips, and pushing straight down with the upper limbs to lift the body into a standing position (Figure 16-10, *A*). When he is lifting into upright, a patient may pull his lower limbs back underneath so he ends up in stance with his legs in line with or slightly behind their upper limbs. Sometimes a patient who is using forearm crutches will leave his feet out in front (Figure 16-10, *B*), so he ends up with his feet in front of the crutches (the same as the end position of a swing-through gait) (Figure 16-10, *C*) and will then need to adjust the position of his forearm crutches.

It should be noted that the shoulders are in a compromised position when the pop-up technique is used during sit-to-stand. During this technique the patient is lifting his body weight with his shoulders in abduction and internal rotation. This is a biomechanically weak position and a prime one to cause impingement of the shoulder. An alternate technique that is less strenuous to the shoulders is the turn-around method. To perform this technique, the patient crosses one leg over the other (Figure 16-11, *A*), turns toward the bottom leg until facing the chair (Figure 16-11, *B*), and then pushes up to stance (Figure 16-11, *C*). He then reaches for his assistive device, which should have been positioned within reach next to the chair, and assumes the parastance position (Figure 16-11, *D*). Although this technique requires less upper limb strength, many patients do not like it because of how it looks and because it takes longer to perform than the pop-up method.

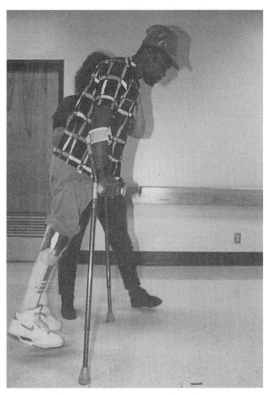

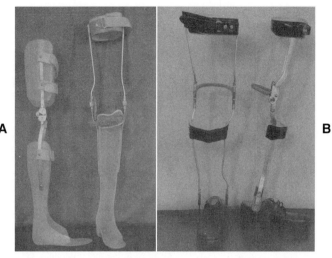

FIGURE 16-9 **A,** Combination plastic and metal KAFOs. **B,** The Scott-Craig KAFO is a special design for SCI. The orthosis consists of double uprights, offset knee joints with locks and ball control, one posterior thigh band, a hinged anterior tibial band, an ankle joint with anterior and posterior adjustable pin stops, a cushion heel, and specially designed foot plates made of steel. (From Umphred DA: *Neurological rehabilitation*, ed 4, St. Louis, 2001, Mosby.)

FIGURE 16-8 The patient initiates a swing-through gait pattern using bilateral plastic molded KAFOs and forearm crutches. Notice that the therapist guards the patient to prevent him from jackknifing by placing one hand at his pelvis ready to provide an anterior force and her other hand at the upper trunk ready to provide a posterior force if his balance is compromised.

Maneuvering Curbs

After successful ambulation on level surfaces has been achieved, the patient may initiate higher levels of functional activity. When ascending a curb, the patient places his assistive device up on the curb, leans forward over his upper limbs, lifts his body weight, and simultaneously places both feet up on the curb. He must quickly assume the parastance position to avoid jackknifing. When descending a curb, the patient may place his assistive device down first, or if he is using forearm crutches, he may choose to lower his feet first and then bring his forearm crutches down. If moving his assistive device first, he should place it far enough out in front of the curb to allow the hips to remain forward and decrease his chance of jackknifing. The patient then simultaneously brings both feet down off the curb. If moving his legs down first, he must have sufficient range of motion in his shoulders and the ability to quickly attain the parastance position. Then nearly simultaneously, he must lift his crutches down from the curb behind him. It cannot be stated often enough that a patient must learn to immediately regain the parastance position when his feet land in going up or down a curb so that he remains balanced.

Ascending and Descending Stairs

Ascending stairs may be performed the same way as ascending a curb. If a rail is available, it should be used; otherwise, bilateral forearm crutches may be used. Ascending stairs with one rail and one forearm crutch is much easier than using two forearm crutches because of the stability provided by the rail. Depending on the patient's upper body strength and balance, the patient will carry the second crutch by holding it along the rail or allowing it to hang off the forearm (Figure 16-12, *A*). Some patients prefer to hold the second crutch in their forearm crutch hand. The patient begins by placing his forearm crutch (on the side of his body away from the rail) on the first step. He then lifts his body weight using one forearm crutch and the hand rail and lowering his feet onto the first step (Figure 16-12, *B*); he follows through by edging his feet forward on the step and assuming the parastance position (Figure 16-12, *C*).

Patients who have active hip flexion on at least one side have the option of using a different technique for ascending stairs. The patient stands sideways holding the rail with both hands with his stronger leg closer to the stairs. He then lifts the stronger leg and places it on the first step. Using momentum, he swings the other leg onto the step, placing it behind the first leg.

Patients who ascend sideways also may descend in the same manner. The weaker leg should be lowered first, placing it back far enough to leave room for the other leg to be lifted off the step and then placed in front (Figure 16-13). Patients who do not have the hip strength to descend sideways may find going backward the easier method. In this case, the patient lifts his body weight using bilateral forearm crutches placed on the same step his feet are on or uses one hand rail and one forearm crutch (Figure 16-14, *A*). After he lifts himself up, he gently lowers his feet down a step, making sure to land in the parastance position (Figure 16-14, *B*).

Ascending and Descending a Ramp

When ascending and descending a ramp, patients may use a reciprocal gait pattern or a swing-to or drag-to gait pattern. Patients would find it very difficult to maintain balance using a swing-through gait pattern on a ramp. Another option is to ascend and

TABLE 16-1 | Options for Mechanical Orthosis

Orthoses	Description	Outcomes
Swivel walker	Rigid body structure with fixation at hips, knees, and ankles provided by a leather chest pad, polypropylene sacral band, hinged knee bar assembly, and footclamp assembly Swiveling footplates mounted beneath body frame	Ambulation achieved by rocking side-to-side using head and upper trunk movements Clearing one footplate from the ground causes the frame to automatically swivel forward on the other footplate Used without assistive devices Slow and restricted to level surfaces only
Parawalker (hip guidance orthosis [HGO])	KAFOs attached to rigid body brace, which helps maintain the hips in minimal abduction Support provided at the chest by a leather strap and at the buttocks by a polypropylene band attached directly to the hip joint housing Low friction hip joint with flexion-extension stops Shoe plates incorporate a rocker sole and are fastened to the metal uprights, positioning the ankles in dorsiflexion	Patient leans forward, placing hips in full extension and shifts weight toward the stance side, allowing the opposite leg to swing forward under the influence of gravity Used with assistive devices (e.g., forearm crutches)
Reciprocating gait orthosis (RGO)	Includes thoracic support up to the xiphoid process, a cable coupling system, a custom-molded pelvic assembly, and bilateral plastic molded KAFOs Cable system provides hip joint stability by preventing simultaneous flexion of hips and allowing unilateral hip flexion-extension in a reciprocal manner when a step is taken Ratchet knee joint prevents the knee from flexing even if not fully extended Hip joint has two locking positions: full hip extension and 20 degrees of flexion, thus allowing for normal upright posture and a forward center of gravity to better accommodate ambulation up an incline	Because of the cable system, as the patient shifts his weight onto the forward stance leg (creating hip extension on the stance side), flexion is transmitted to the contralateral leg to aid it in the swing-through phase
Advanced reciprocating gait orthoses (ARGO)	Version of RGO with the following modifications: Single encased cable used to reduce friction Hip and knee joint are connected by a knee lock actuating cable so that the hip mechanism releases the knee lock Compressed gas strut provides a knee extension movement to augment coming up to standing and controlling hip flexion when sitting down	Mechanism of use same as with RGO
Walkabout orthosis	Bilateral plastic molded KAFOs joined by a single-axis hip joint unit located between the thighs under the perineum Thoracolumbar or lumbar soft corset is incorporated into the system to stabilize the trunk and has cross-straps to the hip joints that help the legs to swing	Patient performs reciprocal gait with a short cadence because of the height gap between the positions of the orthotic hip joint and physiological hip joint
Craig-Scott orthosis	Double metal upright KAFOs Supporting bands eliminated except for rigid posterior thigh band and anterior tibial band Offset knee joint with bail locks Cushioned heel and extended shoe plate Solid ankle set in 5-10 degrees of dorsiflexion	Designed for use with swing-through or swing-to gait pattern
Plastic molded KAFOs	Uses same biomechanical principles as Craig-Scott orthosis but typically uses drop locks as opposed to bail locks at knee joints	Follows same principles as Craig-Scott orthosis for swing-through or swing-to gait but may also be used for reciprocal gait pattern Lighter weight and more cosmetic than Craig-Scott orthosis Precautions should be taken regarding risk of skin problems

TABLE 16-1 | Options for Mechanical Orthosis—cont'd

Orthoses	Description	Outcomes
Vannini-Rizzoli stabilizing limb orthosis (V-RLSO)	Polypropylene orthosis encloses the lower leg from 2 cm below the distal pole of the patella to the toes Orthosis is inserted into a specially designed leather boot (different varieties are available for different weather) Insole of the orthosis is angled to achieve 10 to 15 degrees of plantarflexion, thus shifting the center of gravity of the user forward and anterior to the ankle joint	Angle of plantarflexion in which the foot is maintained stabilizes the knee in standing Static equilibrium is controlled by maintaining an upper body position in which the head is held high, with hips and knees in an extended position Ambulation achieved with help of assistive device by shifting center of mass slightly to the side and forward then bringing unweighted foot forward in a pendulum fashion

Data from Nene AV, Hermens HJ, Zilvold G: Paraplegic locomotion: a review, *Spinal Cord* 34:507-524, 1996; Seymour RJ, Knapp CF, Anderson TR et al: Paraplegic use of the Orlau swivel walker: case report, *Arch Phys Med Rehabil* 63:490-494, 1982; Farmer IR, Poiner R, Rose GK et al: The adult Orlau swivel walker—ambulation for paraplegic and tetraplegic patients, *Paraplegia* 20:248-254, 1982; Butler PB, Poiner R, Farmer IR et al: Use of the Orlau swivel walker for the severely handicapped patient, *Physiotherapy* 68:324-326, 1982; Butler PB, Major RE, Patrick H: The technique of reciprocal walking using the hip guidance orthosis (hgo) with crutches. *Prosthet Orthot Int* 8:33-38, 1984; Major RE, Stallard J, Rose GK: The dynamics of walking using the hip guidance orthosis (hgo) with crutches, *Prosthet Orthot Int* 5:19-22, 1981; Saitoh E, Suzuki T, Sonoda S et al: Clinical experience with a new hip-knee-ankle-foot orthotic system using a medial single hipjoint for paraplegic standing and walking. *Am J Phys Med Rehabil,* 75:198-203, 1996; Lehmann JF, Warren CG, Hertling D et al: Craig-Scott orthosis: a biomechanical and functional evaluation, *Arch Phys Med Rehabil* 57:438-442, 1976; Lyles M, Munday J: Report on the evaluation of the Vannini-Rizzoli stabilizing limb orthosis, *J Rehabil Res Dev* 29:77-104, 1992.

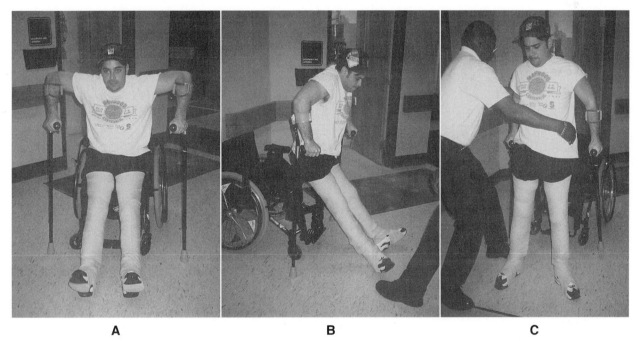

A **B** **C**

FIGURE 16-10 The patient performs the pop-up method of sit-to-stand using bilateral long leg splints and forearm crutches. **A,** The patient bends forward at the hips at the same time that he pushes straight down with his upper limbs on the forearm crutches to lift his body. **B,** Because he has kept his feet out in front as he popped-up to stance; he will need **C,** to adjust the position of his forearm crutches to achieve parastance.

descend the ramp sideways. To do this, a patient should elevate the pelvis to perform relative hip abduction and adduction to move one leg at a time up or down the ramp. Patients may also choose to zigzag up or down the incline if it is particularly steep.

Falling

When a patient walks there is always the risk he will fall. Patients with SCI walking with bilateral KAFOs should, therefore, be instructed in how to reduce the risk of injury if they fall and how to then resume a standing position. If a patient with bilateral KAFOs feels as though he cannot prevent himself from falling, he should do everything possible to ensure the fall is forward. If he jackknifes and falls backward, he will not be able to protect himself. When

falling forward he can throw his assistive device out of the way to keep from landing on it and put his hands out to break the fall.

If possible, he should bend at the hips as he falls forward and allow his elbows to bend as his hands hit the ground to decrease the force transmitted through his arms (Figure 16-15). When he is on the ground, the patient should retrieve his walker or forearm crutches. The patient then positions the assistive device so that it will be reachable when he is again in an upright position. He can place the forearm crutches with the handles pointing inward at about the level of his knees and the tips of the crutches near his head. Then he should assume a prone position with his hips in full external rotation. The patient pushes up, walking his hands back toward his feet (Figure 16-16, *A*). He picks up one forearm

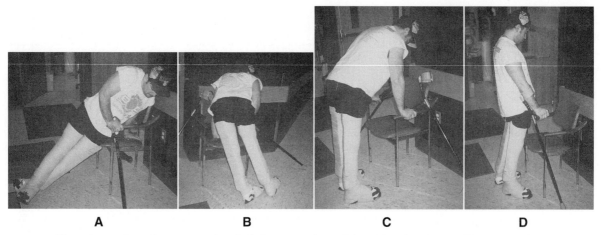

FIGURE 16-11 The patient performs the turn-around method of sit-to-stand using bilateral long leg splints and forearm crutches. **A,** With his forearm crutches positioned next to his chair, the patient crosses one leg over the other. **B,** He then turns his body towards his lower leg until he is facing the chair. **C,** After pushing himself into a stance position, he reaches **D,** for his forearm crutches and assumes the parastance position.

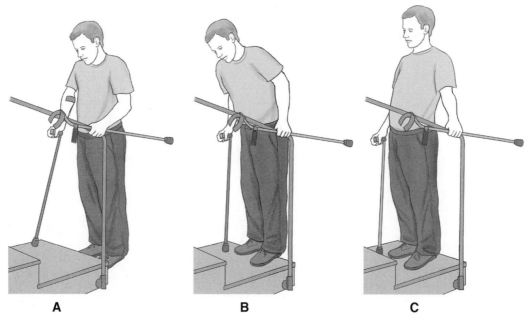

FIGURE 16-12 **A,** A patient ascends a railed stairway by holding his unused crutch in his rail hand oriented horizontally and placing the other crutch on the step above. Although this requires good hand size and grip, it also allows for a strong grip onto the forearm crutch. Another option might be to hold the unused crutch in the crutch hand to allow for a stronger grip on the railing. **B,** He then pushes down on the crutch and railing to elevate his feet to the step above. Care should be taken to clear the lip of the step when present by proper placement of the crutch on the step above before elevating the body. **C,** The patient lands on the step above ultimately with his entire feet fully placed on the stair tread and assumes the parastance position until ready to ascend the next step.

crutch (Figure 16-16, *B*), maintains his balance, and picks up the second forearm crutch (Figure 16-16, *C*). Then he works his forearm crutches in closer and as soon as possible drops his pelvis forward to assume the parastance position. Patients using a walker will have the walker placed over their hips. As the patient walks his hands back toward his feet, he comes up underneath the walker and places one hand at a time onto the lower side rungs of the walker. The patient then moves his hands up onto the walker handles and as soon as possible allows his pelvis to drop forward to assume the parastance position.

Progression of Conventional Gait Training

Ambulation skills progress and the patient gains independence by using the following steps:

- Decrease support on the upper limbs by moving out of the parallel bars and progressively advancing to less-supportive assistive devices.
- Reduce the amount of physical assistance during a treatment session.
- Start with level terrain and progress onto uneven terrain, ramps, curbs, and stairs.

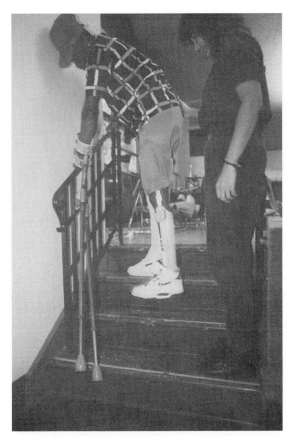

FIGURE 16-13 The patient descends the stairs sideways using one KAFO and one long-leg splint. Facing and holding on to one rail with both hands, he lowers his first leg and places it far enough back to leave room for the other leg to be lifted off the step and placed in front of the first. Notice that the patient is carrying his forearm crutches along by allowing them to dangle from his forearm.

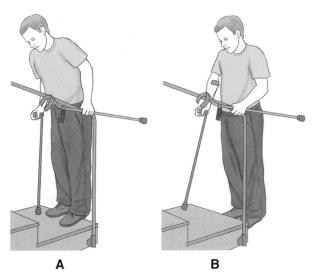

A **B**

FIGURE 16-14 **A,** A patient uses the forearm crutch in his right hand as he descends the final stair to the floor level in the backward direction while holding the rail with his left hand along with his unused crutch held horizontally. **B,** He lowers himself to the floor level and assumes the parastance position. Depending on the patient's upper body strength and balance, he could also carry the unused forearm crutch in his right hand.

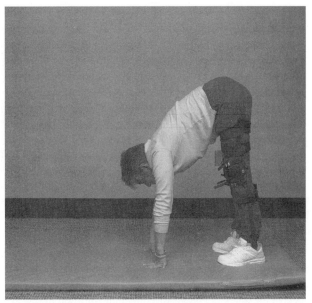

FIGURE 16-15 A patient's hamstring flexibility allows her to bend at the hips when she falls forward, resulting in the transmission of decreased force through her arms when her hands hit the ground.

- Evaluate the need for bracing continually and provide the least restrictive option. For example, unlock the knee joint in a KAFO for the patient with returning knee extensor strength to determine whether an AFO would be sufficient.
- Progress the gait pattern from drag-to to swing-to or swing-through or progress from four-point to two-point gait patterns.
- Improve endurance by progressively challenging the patient during gait activities and by providing adjunctive cardiovascular therapies.
- Increase the speed of walking during training to more closely approximate normal speeds and to meet the demands of the community.

ADJUNCTIVE THERAPIES

Depending on the individual's goals and needs, one or a variety of adjunctive therapies may assist in progression of independence. For those with complete injuries, functional electrical stimulation (FES) may help maintain muscle bulk and reduce spasticity, although it is not shown to increase any voluntary strength or increase motor unit activation. Parastep, a program of synchronized FES, has been shown to help those with complete injuries walk without bracing (see Figure 17-9) but does not have any functional carryover once the stimulation is removed[41] and it carries a high physiological and metabolic cost.[42] For those with incomplete injuries, cardiovascular and endurance training may assist in tolerating some of the physiological costs of walking. Rhythmical, symmetrical activities such as pedaling a stationary bicycle have face validity as adjunctive therapies and are often used in the clinic, although the exact physiological impact and mechanism of training is unclear at this time. Last, aquatic therapy is often used in conjunction with or as a precursor to overground treatment. The buoyancy of the water reduces the body weight of the individual, making it easier to maintain postural control and take independent steps when not possible

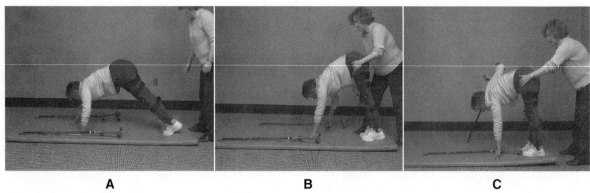

FIGURE 16-16 A patient comes to stances from a prone position on the floor by using forearm crutches. **A,** The patient pushes up and walks her hands back toward her feet. **B,** She picks up the first forearm crutch, stabilizes her balance, and **C,** reaches for the other forearm crutch. After she has both crutches in place, she will work them in closer to her body, and as soon as possible will drop her pelvis forward to assume the parastance position.

overground. Walking in a pool may be progressed by having the patient ambulate in more shallow water, reducing the buoyancy effect of the water and progressively loading the lower limbs.

EMERGING APPROACHES TO REHABILITATION OF WALKING

In the last 25 years, advances in the rehabilitation of ambulation after SCI have focused predominantly on achieving ambulation for people with complete SCI. Advances that have emerged include the use of FES (Parastep),[43,44] bracing (i.e., Louisiana State University–Reciprocating Gait Orthosis [LSU-RGO]),[45] and implanted electrical stimulation.[46] Each strategy compensates for the lack of voluntary muscle control to achieve walking, standing, or sit to stand. Though promising, these technological advances have remained primarily experimental and outside the realm of usual care.

During this same period, basic scientists were investigating the role of the spinal cord in the control of walking. They found that with intense, repetitive training midthoracic spinalized cats can respond to, interpret, and integrate peripheral input associated with walking to generate a coordinated stepping response.[47] Spinalized cats were trained on a treadmill while partially suspended with trunk support and manual assistance for stepping.[47-49] Specificity of training was further confirmed by Edgerton et al[50] observing that stand-trained cats could then stand, step-trained cats could then step, but that neither of the trained cats could perform the opposite, untrained task. Barbeau et al[51-53] translated this paradigm to humans for retraining walking after SCI and stroke, applying similar training principles and experience-dependent training by using an overhead lift for body weight support (BWS) with a treadmill and therapists to assist the legs.

Because of the high visibility of the body weight support system and the treadmill (BWST), many clinicians and manufacturers name the therapy that uses this modality as body weight–supported treadmill training, supported treadmill training, partial weight-supported treadmill training, or other derivations. Such terminology emphasizes the modality yet fails to identify the specific goal of the training: locomotor rehabilitation. Within the goal of locomotor training, subgoals of endurance, balance, and posture may also be relevant. Furthermore, a singular focus on the modality infers that the modality is the sole, critical component of the training. The BWST provides a safe, convenient, and permissive environment. The training, however, is better defined by its theoretical

basis in providing the sensory experience of walking, task specificity, and activity-dependent plasticity. The experience may be promoted in any training environment, including the home, community, or overground, or while stepping with a BWST. The clinician would be better served understanding the training guidelines that direct locomotor training, how to progress the patient, and the basis for clinical decision making regardless of the modality.

Wernig et al[54] has termed these guidelines the "rules of spinal locomotion," whereas Behrman and Harkema[39] refer to the training as locomotor training that encompasses defined principles or guidelines subserving the overall locomotor therapeutic program. "Train like you walk" provides a concise overview of the training. The BWS and treadmill provide a controlled environment for providing the specific afferent input associated with the task of walking and yet a permissive environment in generating a stepping response. For the purposes of this chapter, the therapeutic approach will be referred to as locomotor training (LT), an activity-based therapy.

The training guidelines[39,55] were derived from basic and applied science findings and include (1) maximize weight bearing through the legs and minimize or eliminate weight bearing through the arms,[56-62] (2) provide sensory input consistent with the motor task; specifically standing or walking,[63-66] (3) promote postural control and optimize the trunk, limb, and pelvic kinematics for walking and associated motor tasks,[62,67 68] and (4) maximize the recovery and use of normal movement patterns and minimize the use of compensatory movement strategies.[62] Furthermore, advocated strategies should be applied uniformly across training components or environments to optimize the locomotor outcome of the training (Table 16-2).

LT focuses on the goal of achieving independent community walking at normal walking speeds without an assistive device, bracing, or use of compensatory movements. Although in reality not all people will achieve this goal, aiming for this goal directs therapists to ask what is limiting the individual from achieving this outcome. These limiting factors then become the stepwise goals for training. As described by Forssberg,[69] then Barbeau et al,[27] walking for successful community ambulation is a complex task. To walk requires control to produce (1) a reciprocal stepping pattern, (2) maintenance of upright posture,[70] and (3) adaptation of walking to the behavioral goals of the person and the constraints imposed by the environment[27] (Figure 16-17).

TABLE 16-2 | Locomotor Training Goals and Progression

Goal	Retraining Occurs in Body Weight Support and Treadmill Environment	Overground Assessment	Community Environment
Independent community walking with maximized weight bearing (load) through the lower limbs and sustained appropriate trunk posture, limb kinematics, and coordinated stepping	• Maximize loading of lower limbs • Eliminate or minimize loading of arms • Use BWS necessary to achieve upright posture and coordinated stepping • Use increased load during rests between stepping trials to practice upright trunk control and postural alignment without loading the arms • Gradually increase load during stepping to foster coordinated stepping	• Use horizontal poles for balance as opposed to upper limb weight-bearing support	• Use arms for balance and minimal weight bearing if an assistive device is used • Emphasize loading primarily through the lower limbs • Stress maximizing lower limb loading and decreasing arm loading on assistive devices
Overground walking at normal (or preinjury) speed	• Train at normal walking speeds: most easily achieved during step training in the BWST where trainers can control speed • Approximate normal walking speeds in early training with manual assistance • Diminish manual assistance at the same speed as patient progresses • Challenge patient to maintain independent stepping at varying speeds later in training	• Use horizontal poles for minimal balance, promote arms wing, and provide verbal cues to facilitate speed of walking • Begin stepping overground from a diagonal stance position to promote forward progression at the initial stride	• Encourage speed with safe ambulation • Introduce assistive devices that promote a fluid, forward advancing gait pattern to approximate normal speed (e.g., rolling walker, bilateral crutches, or canes that may afford a normal walking speed) • Use of a two-point gait pattern versus a four-point pattern may also promote speed
Achieve corequisite dynamic postural control for community walking and locomotor specific kinematics (e.g., upright trunk, reciprocal stepping pattern, interlimb coordination)	• Achieve upright posture during standing and walking either independently or with manual assist, bungees, or BWS • Primary initial goal is to achieve upright posture and trunk/pelvic control • Achieve weight shift or load transfer from one limb to another consistent with forward progression • Achieve alternating loading and unloading with interlimb temporal-spatial symmetry within the participant's ability or with manual assistance • Refine kinematics for flexion and extension associated with swing and stance phases • Progress to postural and kinematic control of stepping using BWST (e.g., degree of BWS required, use of lateral bungees attached horizontally between the pelvic band and BWS platform to maintain lateral or anterior-posterior stability, assist from a manual trainer at the pelvis or trunk, ability to maintain head and trunk alignment) • Achieve hip extension on a loaded and extended lower limb critical for advancement of swing phase	• Progress to postural control using horizontal poles for support for arm loading and balance or manual assist as required • Sustain upright trunk • Use speed to promote appropriate and normal limb kinematics • Use postural control and limb kinematics to progress from weight shifting in stride position to stepping overground with upright posture, weight shift, and stepping pattern • Promote achieving hip extension	• Practice body alignment until patient can independently align his shoulders over hips in standing and walking • Promote maintenance of posture and kinematics during community walking based on type of gait pattern used (two-point versus four-point), type of assistive device, need for guarding • Use the least restrictive device to promote upright trunk and good stepping kinematics

Continued

TABLE 16-2 | Locomotor Training Goals and Progression—cont'd

Goal	Retraining Occurs in Body Weight Support and Treadmill Environment	Overground Assessment	Community Environment
Achieve necessary endurance to sustain walking in the community	• Measure endurance and progress by the continuous duration of a single bout of stepping (or standing) or by the total time spent stepping (or standing) • Demonstrate improved endurance when a patient can walk four 5-minute bouts of training compared with ten 2-minute bouts • Achieve 20-30 minutes of total stepping time (even if multiple training bouts are needed) • Increase duration of stepping bouts • Provide intermittent manual assistance initially to increase the total duration and length of the training bouts • Step independently for 30 minutes on the treadmill	• Do not promote endurance for overground stepping	• Use distance walked during a 2- or 6-minute timed session to assess endurance • Progress endurance by increasing total duration or frequency of standing or walking at home with proper trunk and limb kinematics • Provide instruction and safe devices to accomplish endurance progression and continued improvement in translation from formal sessions to home and community use • Encourage patient to self-select amount of time spent standing and walking outside training sessions and be cognizant of goal for independent walking
Achieve independence in community ambulation as highest level of ability and ultimate outcome	• Achieve independence from manual assistance by trainers at the trunk, pelvis, or legs • Achieve independence from body weight support • Achieve independence from bungees attached between the BWS frame and pelvis for trunk and pelvic stability • Gain upright posture with head up and looking forward and head aligned over the shoulders, pelvis, and feet • Perform weight shift with loading at foot contact or heel strike • Maintain ability as BWS is decreased and in conjunction with a coordinated stepping pattern • Adjust speed and load often to identify best conditions for stepping	• Maintain upright posture, limb kinematics for stepping and loading • Initiate walking and achieve normal walking speeds without manual assistance or guarding	• Achieve independent control of upright posture and kinematics at home and in community • Progress to no use of braces • Use least restrictive device and progress to no assistive device • Progress to no need for guarding during community walking
Achieve adaptability to meet patient's behavioral goals and negotiate the environment	• Emphasize consistent, coordinated stepping pattern in early training rather than adaptability • Initiating adaptability through stepping as treadmill speed increases and stops • Challenge adaptability in later training after stepping pattern has stabilized and independent trunk control is attained • Increase adaptability by using abrupt starts and stops of the treadmill, varying speeds, carrying items while walking, walking up and down inclines, or stepping over obstacles • Achieve adaptability late in training by practicing independent stepping at a speed approximating normal or allowing coordinated stepping with as little BWS as possible	• Establish independent and coordinated gait • Introduce varying behavioral goals (e.g., speed, terrain) • Provide experience to afford check for adaptability without assistive devices • Identify ongoing challenges to accomplishing independent community ambulation	• Negotiate obstacles and uneven terrain, vary speed demands for walking, and add attentional demands during the tasks of walking to practice adaptability • Reinforce practice with experience at home and in community • Encourage patient to accomplish his own goals at home, work, or in community whether pushing a grocery cart for the first time, climbing stairs, or feeding the cattle • Encourage patient to use consistent application of the locomotor training principles (e.g., standing upright while pushing the grocery cart as opposed to leaning on it for support)

Data from Visintin M, Barbeau H: The effects of parallel bars, body weight support and speed on the modulation of the locomotor pattern of spastic paretic gait: a preliminary communication, *Paraplegia* 32:540-553, 1994; Dobkin BH, Harkema S, Requejo P et al: Modulation of locomotor-like EMG activity in subjects with complete and incomplete spinal cord injury, *J Neurol Rehabil* 9:183-190, 1995; Sullivan KJ, Knowlton BJ , Dobkin BH: Step training with body weight support: effect of treadmill speed and practice paradigms on poststroke locomotor recovery, *Arch Phys Med Rehabil* 83:683-91, 2002; Beres-Jones JA, Harkema SJ: The human spinal cord interprets velocity-dependent afferent input during stepping, *Brain* 127(pt 10):2232-2246. Epub 2004 Aug 2; Craik RL, Dutterer L: Spatial and temporal characteristics of foot fall patterns. In Craik RL, Oatis CA, editors: *Gait analysis: theory and application*, 1995, St Louis, MO, Mosby-Year Book, pp. 143-158; Macpherson JM, Fung JA, Jacobs R: Postural orientation, equilibrium, and the spinal cord, *Adv Neurol* 72:227-232, 1997 (review); Butland RJ, Pang J, Gross ER et al: Two-, six-, and 12-minute walking tests in respiratory disease, *BMJ* 284:1607-1608, 1982.

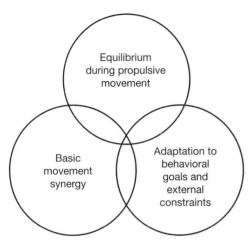

FIGURE 16-17 The nervous system's requirements for functional walking control. (From Barbeau H, Ladouceur M, Norman KE et al: Walking after spinal cord injury: evaluation, treatment, and functional recovery, *Arch Phys Med Rehabil* 80:225-235, 1999.)

Because the effects of SCI compromise each of the neural control requirements for walking, a successful intervention program should address rehabilitation of each requirement.

Locomotor Training Aims and Components

The specific aims for LT differ across three components of training yet provide an integrated continuum translating the capacity developed in the BWST to overground assessment to use in the home and community.

In the step training component, training is designed to develop the capacity to step well. Intense practice emphasizes facilitating coordinated stepping with normal walking kinematics approximating normal gait speeds. Use of the BWST and manual trainers affords a highly constrained environment for optimally providing the ensemble of sensory information specific to walking and thus promoting a coordinated stepping response. Coordinated stepping reflects a reciprocal stepping synergy characterized by the spatial and temporal pattern of walking; trunk, lower limb, and upper limb kinematics; and speed. Repetition provided by the treadmill increases the opportunity for greater stepping practice (Figure 16-18). Step training continues only as good steps are demonstrated. Thus, early training bouts may be abbreviated; however, their length increases as the number of coordinated steps increases.

Overground assessment immediately follows step training on the treadmill and consists of evaluating the patient's ability to stand and walk on level surfaces. The intent is to assess what factors are limiting this individual from walking independently in the community at normal walking speeds without an assistive device, brace, or compensatory movements. The individual is asked to stand independently; if he is unable to do so, then manual assistance is provided to achieve the task-specific kinematics for standing. The assessment overground occurs with minimal manual support for balance or kinematics according to the training guidelines. For example, horizontal poles may be used for balance or to coordinate arm swing, but they are not used for upper limb weight bearing (Figure 16-19).

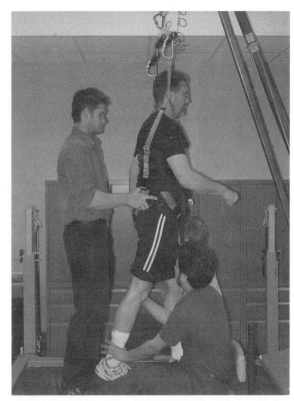

FIGURE 16-18 A patient performs step training on a treadmill with body weight support.

Overground evaluation thus provides a quick assessment of the patient's ability to transfer skills acquired while step training on the BWST to overground. The trainers use this assessment to direct the training goals for the next day in step training with the BWST and to identify goals for community gait training. Skills that are lacking for independent overground walking, the presence of gait deviations, or visible compensatory strategies are identified and targeted as goals for the next day's step training.

For each training session, community ambulation training immediately follows overground assessment. The aim of community ambulation training is to afford the participant the knowledge and tools to apply the training guidelines beyond the daily, clinic-based treatment session to his everyday life and to prepare him for independent home and community walking. Thus, the participant is empowered to apply knowledge of walking from the training experience into everyday activities involving standing and walking. Safety in performing such tasks is a primary consideration. If the individual cannot stand or walk independently, then activities are identified that may reinforce the guidelines at home. For instance, the patient can practice weight bearing through the legs when doing transfers, sitting upright in the chair, or performing a stand-pivot transfer with assistance. As abilities improve, time standing may be increased or the frequency of walking at home increased. Proper posture may be practiced. Whatever the activity, how it is to be performed is established by its consistency with the guidelines. If the individual can stand or walk but requires assistance, assistive devices (e.g., forearm crutches, cane, walker) may be introduced (Figure 16-20).

The use of devices, however, is adapted for consistency with the training guidelines. Selection of a device may be based on safety,

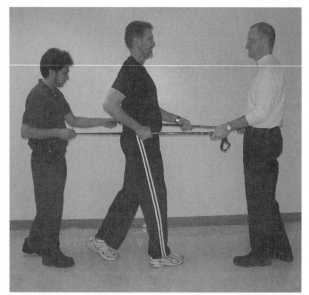

FIGURE 16-19 A patient performs overground step training by using horizontal poles for balance or to coordinate arm swing.

allowing increased time for standing and walking at home or in the community, and its use consistent with a pattern of walking that follows the "train like you walk" premise. For instance, a rolling walker may promote speed, whereas bilateral forearm crutches may promote reciprocal arms coordinated with the legs in a two-point pattern. Both devices, however, encourage weight bearing through the arms unless the individual is instructed how to minimize load bearing on the arms and to emphasize load bearing on the legs with an upright posture. This posture is likely experienced and practiced while training on the BWST and is now transferred to his everyday standing and walking activities.

Progression of Locomotor Training

Progression of skills advances across each of the three training components in every LT session. Goals are established for load, speed, postural control and kinematics, endurance, independence, and adaptability (Clinical Note: Domains for Progression During Locomotor Training). Progression often occurs at different rates across these domains. Progression in one domain may require temporary regression in another because of an interactive effect. For instance, progressing toward an independent walking goal while on the treadmill may require a decrease in the treadmill speed for several bouts of training while altering the BWS to maintain a coordinated stepping pattern. LT across time may emphasize different domains for progression, providing a framework for decision making and advancement. A training priority may shift

---

CLINICAL NOTE **Domains for Progression During Locomotor Training**

- Load
- Speed
- Postural control and kinematics
- Endurance
- Independence
- Adaptability

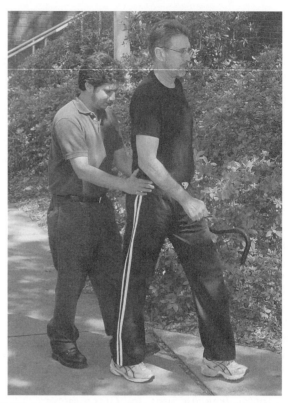

FIGURE 16-20 A patient performs community ambulation training with an assistive device. While practicing, the patient is instructed how to minimize load bearing on the arms and emphasize load bearing on the legs with an upright posture.

from an early emphasis on achieving an upright posture and stepping endurance of a total of 30 minutes to increasing body weight load and speed to mid training goals for independent trunk control with continued load progression, to late training foci of continued independence and adaptability.

Therapeutic Process

Interactions between the training team and the individual emphasize the trainer as an educator providing knowledge of the training guidelines and their use in training at home or the community. Education begins the first day emphasizing why an upright stance is critical to attaining hip extension and its relationship to activating hip flexion. Working toward independent control of upright posture then becomes a goal not only for daily training in the clinic but also a responsibility for an individual at home or his community. The training team also identifies with the individual the factors limiting successful walking full time, independently, in the home and community at a normal walking speed without using assistive device, braces, or compensatory movements. These factors become goals for the following training sessions. For instance, if lack of endurance is preventing full-time ambulation, then it becomes an emphasis for training using the BWST and for the community. Goals are then set to increase the duration of training bouts to ultimately achieve 30 minutes of continuous stepping.

LT is in its infancy as a therapeutic strategy for retraining walking after SCI. Research is promising, but much needs to be defined to provide the evidence-based practice for the recovery of walking after SCI. Reviewing the literature in which a body

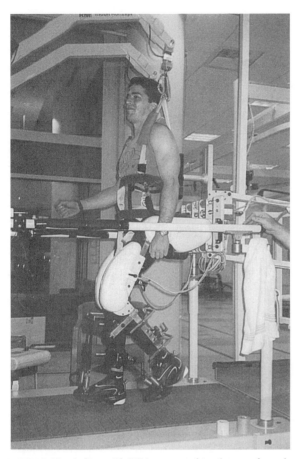

FIGURE 16-21 A client with SCI is supported in a harness from above while he uses the Lokomat robotic-assisted gait training device, which integrates computer control of the hip and knee joints that are synchronized with the a treadmill speed.

weight support and treadmill modalities are applied indicates variability in the training parameters and progression guidelines (e.g., speed, BWS, manual assistance, intensity, duration, frequency), population studied (e.g., acute and chronic, ASIA impairment classification), inclusion of overground training or other conventional therapies, and outcomes measured. Over the last 13 years, seven research reports detail training that used a BWST modality in people with chronic SCI.[39,54,71-75] The number of subjects in this research examining chronic SCI (i.e., those who have completed inpatient rehabilitation) range from one to 44: n = 1-8[39,71-74] to n = 44[74] to research examining people soon after SCI (n = 1,[39] n = 45,[74] and n = 200). For instance, only three

reports applied guidelines for training in a continuum from the treadmill to overground,[39,71,74,75] whereas others combined BWS with conventional therapies.[54] Gait speed and distance walked are the most frequent outcome measures, indicating improvements in excess of 150%[39,71] in overground gait speed and 200 meters in distance walked.[74] Improvement, though, may vary in clinical meaningfulness (e.g., 0.118 to 0.318 m/s or 0.09 to 0.33 m/s) or distance walked (e.g., 0 to 200 meters). Outcome measures that further examine actual amount of activity, increased participation, or impact on quality of life will be advantageous in examining the effectiveness of LT and consumer satisfaction. Research combining use of the BWS and treadmill with electrical stimulation also report improved coordination during walking and increases in gait speed.[76,77] Other combinations of therapies have yet to be tested, such as strength training and LT.

We are at a crossroads with advances in technology and measurement instrumentation, so we can advance our understanding of such interventions, their effect, and the mechanisms accounting for behavioral improvements. Conventional gait training with an emphasis on a compensation strategy for deficits after SCI has been compared with the emerging LT approach as the foundation for treatment and a paradigm shift towards recovery of walking as a goal (Table 16-3). Our rush to provide this therapy must be tempered in the necessity and opportunity to provide clinicians with answers to who, what, when, where, and how to guide clinical practice, the evidence for clinical decision making. As the manufacturing of BWS systems has proliferated, parallel efforts are under way by engineers to design robotic devices to replace manual trainers or augment manual training with BWS and treadmill.[78-80] Roles for such devices are far from being established and clinical practice guidelines need to be developed to place robotics within an entire locomotor retraining program. The Lokomat (Hocoma, Inc.) encases the patient's legs in a robotic-assisted gait training device while his weight is supported by a padded body harness, thereby making it easier to move thorough various gait patterns (Figure 16-21). Force transducers at the hips and knee joints can measure the interaction between the patient and the Lokomat. Software modules are available to change the passive guidance characteristics and to provide biofeedback in real time to enhance performance. Benefits of such therapy may reduce metabolic expenditures and improve training. Although questions of who, what, when, and how still need to be answered, early clinical results show promise.[81,82] Will robotics allow earlier intervention, assist in maintaining health post-SCI, or provide greater intensity to training?

TABLE 16-3 | **Comparison of Conventional Gait Training and Locomotor Training**

Strategy	Conventional Gait Training	Locomotor Training
Overall training goals and approach	• Achieve upright standing and walking mobility by: • Maximizing voluntary motor control and strength • Compensating for weakness or paralysis with bracing or assistive devices • Teaching new behavioral strategies for ambulation that incorporate use of braces, crutches, or compensatory movements • Retraining postural and motor control by facilitation techniques (PNF, NDT, muscle strengthening, aquatic therapy) and in-task and out-of-task training	• Promote recovery of walking by providing locomotor-specific sensory input through intense practice and using the intrinsic mechanisms of the nervous system to generate stepping response • Achieve independent community ambulation at normal walking speeds, without the use of braces or assistive devices and without the use of compensatory movements • Use training principles: load, sensory cues, kinematics, maximize recovery by use of normal movements, minimize use of compensatory movements
Patient evaluation and prediction of walking potential	• Evaluate voluntary motor control through manual muscle testing and ASIA evaluation • Evaluate sensation, posture, upper limb strength, range of motion • Predict walking potential based on degree of voluntary motor control, ASIA classification, ASIA lower limb motor scores, age, and preservation of sensation	• Evaluate the patient's ability to generate a stepping response and maintain upright posture when placed on a treadmill at or close to normal walking speed with body weight support and manual assistance, as needed to generate an optimal stepping pattern and posture • Understand indications of walking potential are related to activation of coordinated stepping and upright posture in this environment
Training location	• Use overground surfaces within parallel bars or with assistive devices and guarding of patient by therapists, physical therapy assistants, or aides	• Use step training with body weight support, treadmill to retrain capacity to step • Use overground environment to assess translation of skills from treadmill to overground and any gait deviations to be addressed in step training • Use community ambulation training to translate abilities and principles to home and community use • Use manual trainers as required for training in all environments
Training emphasis	• Use top-down approach in which patient is taught a new strategy for ambulation and often a new gait pattern that incorporates new equipment for weight support (assistive devices) and limb control (bracing) (i.e., similar to learning a new or novel skill) • Include cognitive demands apparent in learning a new skill	• Use bottom-up approach in which aim is to provide sensory experience of walking most consistent with actual walking guided by limb kinematics, posture, loading, and speed of walking with aim of taking advantage of nervous system's capacity to generate steps • Includes cognitive demands of learning and applying the locomotor principles
Use of assistive devices	• Introduce assistive devices immediately with the initiation of gait training or in conjunction with use of parallel bars • Use upper limbs for weight bearing immediately with parallel bars or assistive devices • Select devices that compensate for leg, arm, and trunk weakness or impaired balance; provide independence and safety • Understand that typical posture with a device promotes forward trunk lean and emphasis on weight bearing on the arms • Select gait pattern from swing-through, swing-to, four-point, to two-point • Progress devices on the basis of developing better control; device selected may be the terminal device	• Introduce assistive device only during community ambulation training, thus minimizing or eliminating upper limb weight bearing capacity training for stepping • Select the least restrictive device or one most consistent with the locomotor (LT) principles • Select device-based ability to allow consistent practice in the home or community, independence, and safety • Choose gait pattern so that device or device height is adapted for more consistency with the LT principles (e.g., landing foot first versus crutch first, raising height of walker to promote upright posture vs. leaning forward on walker) • Use more than one assistive device type during training (e.g., one device may afford endurance to be used in the community; another may challenge balance or afford arm swing to be used at home) • Encourage progression to regain upright posture, balance, limb kinematics, and gait speed from step training and translation to community ambulation • Encourage bilateral devices over single device use (e.g., crutch or cane) to promote greater step symmetry and coordination; use to practice walking • Encourage upright posture and diminished arm weight bearing by using walking or exercise poles

TABLE 16-3 | Comparison of Conventional Gait Training and Locomotor Training—cont'd

Strategy	Conventional Gait Training	Locomotor Training
Progression	• Load arms immediately in parallel bars or with assistive device use • Brace early as needed to maintain extension and upright standing • Speed of walking is slow at first • Provide therapists/physical therapy assistants/aides for guarding and manual assistance for controlling device, limb movements, and posture • Gain strength or control in new mobility task • Gain independence on level terrain and progress to independence in negotiating obstacles and uneven terrain • Gain endurance • Change bracing or assistive device use • Diminish stability of device with progression • Change gait pattern: four-point to two-point or step-to to step-through	• Depends on early, mid, and late phase training: Load legs as much as possible in BWS treadmill • Do not use braces in BWS treadmill • Do not weight bear on the arms • Approximate normal walking speed during first and early to intermediate sessions • Provide assistance with manual trainers for trunk posture and pelvic or limb kinematics • Advance development of trunk and pelvic control as a first priority • Progress by diminishing BWS first, then manual assistance in step training • Provide opportunity for individual to practice task independently in a safe environment on treadmill with BWS, adjust speed first to allow a permissive environment for practice, then increase BWS if needed for independent practice • Practice may occur at an individual body segment and/or as a whole • Continue to transfer skill acquired on the treadmill to overground and community application

Adapted from Behrman AL, Bowden MG, Nair P: Neuroplasticity after spinal cord injury and locomotor training: a paradigm shift in the foundation for rehabilitation and recovery, *Phys Ther* 86:1406-1425, 2006.

CLINICAL CASE STUDY | Ambulation Conventional Gait Training

Patient History
Michael Price is a 27-year-old man referred to physical therapy with a C8 tetraplegia, ASIA D diagnosis. Surgical posterior spinal fusion was performed, followed by halo traction for 16 weeks. After the halo orthosis was removed, Michael was in a Philadelphia collar for 1 week and a soft collar for 2 weeks. He is now 25 weeks post injury and is an outpatient in physical therapy for ambulation training.

Michael is a dentist and recently also completed a residency in orthodontics. He works in a practice with two other dentists. Michael is engaged to be married. He and his fiancée live in a wheelchair-accessible apartment building with elevator access to their one-bedroom unit on the twelfth floor. His fiancée works as an accountant. They have postponed the wedding because of his injury but hope to be married within the next year.

Patient's Self-Assessment
Michael wants to return to his dental practice within the next 8 weeks. During the past several weeks Michael has regained a significant amount of strength in his legs. He hopes to eliminate his wheelchair and, most important to him right now, walk down the aisle on his wedding day.

Clinical Assessment
Patient Appearance
• Height 5 feet 11 inches, weight 156 pounds, body mass index 21.8

Cognitive Assessment
• Alert, oriented × 3

Cardiopulmonary Assessment
• Blood pressure 118/68 mm Hg, heart rate at rest 68 beats/min, respiratory rate 12 breaths/min, cough flows are ineffective (<360 L/min), vital capacity is reduced (between 1.5 and 2.5 L)

Musculoskeletal and Neuromuscular Assessment

Muscle Groups	Left	Right
Elbow flexors (C5)	5	5
Wrist extensors (C6)	5	5
Elbow extensors (C7)	5	5
Finger flexors (C8)	4	5
Finger abductors (T1)	4	4
Hip flexors (L2)	3	4
Knee extensors (L3)	3	4
Ankle dorsiflexors (L4)	2	3
Long toe extensors (L5)	0	0
Ankle plantar flexors (S1)	0	0

• Motor assessment reveals C8 incomplete ASIA D.
• Knee flexion and hip extension is 2 out of 5 bilaterally; sensation in all modalities is preserved throughout.
• Deep tendon reflexes 3+ below the level of lesion

Integumentary and Sensory Assessment
• Skin is intact throughout, sensory intact throughout.

Range of Motion Assessment
• Passive and active motion is within normal limits in both upper limbs.
• Straight leg raise is 104 degrees in both lower limbs and dorsiflexion is 7 degrees; all other motions in the lower limbs are within functional limits.

Mobility and ADL Assessment
• Independent with bed mobility
• Independent in transfers to all surfaces including floor to wheelchair
• Independent with pressure relief
• Independent in manual wheelchair maneuvering on all surfaces
• Independent in high-level wheelchair skills except ascending and descending stairs, which requires minimal assistance of one person for eight stairs

Continued

CLINICAL CASE STUDY — Ambulation Conventional Gait Training—cont'd

- Independent in bowel and bladder care
- Independent in upper and lower body dressing
- Independent in driving

Evaluation of Clinical Assessment

Michael Price is a 27-year-old man with a C8 incomplete tetraplegia, ASIA D diagnosis who has had a recent return of strength in his lower limbs. He is attending an outpatient physical therapy program for ambulation evaluation and training with appropriate orthoses and assistive devices.

Patient's Care Needs

1. Evaluation for physical therapy to gain more independence in standing and walking
2. Consultation for orthotics clinic as needed
3. Evaluation and instruction for home exercise regimen or activities to promote independent walking at work.

Diagnosis and Prognosis

Diagnosis of C8 incomplete tetraplegia, ASIA D. Prognosis is for return to community ambulation with appropriate orthoses and assistive devices

Preferred Practice Patterns*

Impaired Muscle Performance (4C), Impairments Nonprogressive Spinal Cord Disorders (5H), Primary Prevention/Risk Reduction for Cardiovascular/Pulmonary Disorders (6A), Primary Prevention/Risk Reduction for Integumentary Disorders (7A)

Team Goals

1. Team to evaluate ambulation
2. Team to instruct with appropriate orthoses and assistive devices for independence in community ambulation
3. Team to assess independence on elevations with appropriate orthoses and assistive devices
4. Team to establish an education plan for patient in home and work environments
5. Team to instruct patient in home exercise regimen

Team Goals

- Independent ambulation with or without assistive or orthotic support to return to work as a dentist

Patient Goals

"I want to walk down the aisle at my wedding."

Care Plan

Treatment Plan and Rationale

- Completion of a physical therapy evaluation for achieving independent ambulation with or without orthoses and assistive devices
- Evaluate the level of independence without assistive or orthotic devices.
- Review and update home and work exercise program for enhancing recovery of locomotion.

Interventions

- Implement intense repetitive practice of ambulation on a treadmill and overground.
- Practice performing home exercises to be sure that the therapeutic goals are understood.

Documentation and Team Communication

- Team will document physical therapy evaluation and referral to orthotics clinic as needed.
- Team will discuss need for prescription of orthotic devices or assistive devices when nearing discharge.

Follow-Up Assessment

- Reassessment of independence in ambulation status in 4 weeks with further training as needed

Critical Thinking Exercises

Consider factors that will influence Michael's treatment and instruction for community ambulation when answering the following questions:

1. Would you expect Michael to be a full-time ambulator?
2. Would bracing be recommended for Michael? If so, what kind?
3. What type of assistive device would you use at the beginning of Michael's training and what might he progress to?
4. What gait pattern would you recommend for Michael? Why?
5. How would you train Michael to negotiate elevations, both ascending and descending?
6. If Michael had not experienced significant return of strength in his lower limbs and was ultimately going to require KAFOs, how would you instruct him on falling and resuming stance?
7. Would BWS with a treadmill be an option for Michael? Why or why not?

*Guide to physical therapist practice, rev. ed. 2, Alexandria, VA, 2003, American Physical Therapy Association.

CLINICAL CASE STUDY — An Activity-Based, Locomotor-Training Perspective

Patient History (using previous case history)
Mobility and ADL Assessment

- Locomotor capacity
  - Stepping, standing, and weight shift (lateral in stance and diagonal in stride position) is assessed in the BWS and treadmill environment with manual trainers.
  - Stepping including the capacity to load the leg (transition to weight-bearing), support weight during the stance phase, transition to swing, and swing are examined by optimizing the afferent, task-specific experience of walking.
  - Balance is assessed as the amount of BWS required and manual assistance required for proper pelvic motion and upright posture during stepping.
  - Independence in stepping, balance, standing, and weight shift are then assessed in the BWS and treadmill environment.

- For stepping, the treadmill speed is reduced and the speed is identified at which independence in limb and trunk control is achieved.
- This is limb and trunk control representing recovery of preinjury function and not compensatory behaviors.
- Adaptability to environmental obstacles and personal goals for walking may also be assessed by altering treadmill speed, providing abrupt stop/starts, inclines, and stepping over obstacles.
- The combination of BWS, speed (nearing normal), and manual assistance that affords an optimal stepping pattern approximating normal is assessed and recorded.
- These parameters will become the starting point for training and progression of locomotor skill.
- The same strategy of assessment is applied to the task of standing and weight shift.

CLINICAL CASE STUDY | **An Activity-Based, Locomotor-Training Perspective—cont'd**

- Overground walking
  - The capacity to transfer the skills demonstrated in the treadmill environment is assessed overground using minimal manual assistance and no assistive devices and braces and includes the ability to sit, come from sit to standing, stand, and step overground.
  - Stepping, balance, and adaptability are assessed as to what are limiting factors for achieving independent ambulation.
- Community ambulation
  - Standing in the home, safely, with minimal UE support and appropriate posture.
  - Weight shift in standing and stride position.
  - Use of an assistive device may be introduced to promote standing and walking, though the specific device and gait pattern will be selected to provide the least restrictive device in approximating the kinematics and spatial-temporal characteristics of walking minimizing UE load-bearing for continued training of the skill of walking.
  - The guidelines for LT remain the focus for selection of activities in the home and community.

Standardized assessments at the impairment level (e.g., strength, ROM, sensation) complement the stepping evaluation in the treadmill environment.

Evaluation of Clinical Assessment

Michael Price is a 27-year-old man with a C8 incomplete tetraplegia, ASIA D diagnosis who has had a recent return of strength in his lower limbs. He is attending an outpatient physical therapy program for ambulation evaluation and training using locomotor training principles

Patient's Care Needs

With Michael's prioritization of goals, the ability to walk down the aisle will be addressed within the broader scope of achieving independent, full-time ambulation via recovery of function. Distance, speed, obstacles (carpet), and independence necessary will be identified and used as short-term goals for walking skill development and training. The long-term goals for wheelchair elimination and return to practice also require identification of the specific demands of his home and work environment.

Diagnosis and Prognosis

Diagnosis of C8 incomplete tetraplegia, ASIA D. Prognosis is for return to community ambulation without minimal to no orthotic and minimal use of assistive devices

Team Goals

1. Team to evaluate ambulation
2. Team to instruct with appropriate locomotor training and progression for independence in community ambulation
3. Team to assess independence on elevations
4. Team to establish an education plan for patient in home and work exercise
5. Team to instruct patient in home exercise regimen

Patient Goals

1. To walk down the aisle at his wedding.
2. To eliminate use of his wheelchair.
3. To return to his practice as a dentist.

Care Plan

Treatment Plan and Rationale

- Complete work/home-based evaluation for specific requirements for standing and walking.
- Establish home and community-based activities daily to support transfer of skills from treadmill environment to home.
- Reassess achievement of goal: walking down aisle, then progress to long-term goals.

Interventions

- Implement intense, repetitive practice of stepping and co-requisite balance daily on a treadmill with BWS and manual trainers. Progress daily.
- Assess independence in BWS/treadmill environment and capacity overground.
- Continue to transfer skills to home.

Critical Thinking Exercises

Consider factors that will influence Michael's treatment and instruction for community ambulation when answering the following questions:

1. Would you expect Michael to be ambulatory full-time in the community?
2. What gait pattern would you recommend for Michael? Why?
3. Would locomotor training be an option for Michael? If yes, how would it be progressed?
4. If locomotor training were applied, what practice environments would be selected?

SUMMARY

This chapter examines the spectrum of rehabilitation and training for ambulation after SCI, spanning approaches that provide total compensation to training that aims to enhance the recovery of walking. Interestingly, although certain tools and equipment are common to both conventional and the emerging LT approaches, the means and rationale for their use differ substantially when considering how they are introduced and used in the process. A paradigm shift may occur influencing the provision of physical rehabilitation of walking. Assistive devices and modalities will likely emerge that promote a therapy consistent with LT guidelines; however, the guidelines may be implemented in any environment. Continued partnership with basic scientists[83,84] and applied researchers working with individuals with SCI is critical to establishing the science for our clinical practice and enhancing walking outcomes.

REFERENCES

1. Behrman AL, Bowden MG, Nair P: Neuroplasticity after spinal cord injury and locomotor training: a paradigm shift in the foundation for rehabilitation and recovery, *Phys Ther* 86:1406-1425, 2006.
2. Somers MF: *Spinal cord injury: functional rehabilitation,* ed 2, Upper Saddle River, NJ, 2001, Prentice-Hall.
3. Consortium for Spinal Cord Medicine: *Outcomes following traumatic spinal cord injury: clinical practice guidelines for health-care professionals,* Washington, DC, 1999, Paralyzed Veterans of America.
4. Atrice M, Gonter M, Griffin D et al: Traumatic spinal cord injury. In Umphred DA, editor, *Neurological rehabilitation,* ed 3, St. Louis, 1995, Mosby.
5. Uniform Data System for Medical Rehabilitation: *FIM instrument,* Buffalo, NY, 1997, State University of New York at Buffalo.
6. Waters RL, Lunsford BR, Perry J et al: Energy-speed relationship of walking: standard tables, *J Orthop Res* 6:215-222, 1988.
7. Perry J, Garrett M, Gronley JK et al: Classification of walking handicap in the stroke population, *Stroke* 26:982-989, 1995.

8. Lerner-Frankiel MB, Varcas S, Brown MB et al: Functional community ambulation: what are your criteria? *Clin Manag Phys Ther* 6:12-15, 1986.

9. Lapointe R, Lajoie Y, Serresse O et al: Functional community ambulation requirements in incomplete spinal cord injured subjects, *Spinal Cord* 39:327-335, 2001.

10. Burns SP, Golding DG, Rolle WA Jr et al: Recovery of ambulation in motor-incomplete tetraplegia, *Arch Phys Med Rehabil* 78:1169-1172, 1997.

11. de Bruin ED F-RP, Herzog RE, Dietz V et al: Changes of tibia bone properties after spinal cord injury: effects of early intervention, *Arch Phys Med Rehabil* 80:214-220, 1999.

12. Eng JJ, Levins SM, Townson AF et al: Use of prolonged standing for individuals with spinal cord injuries, *Phys Ther* 81:1392-1399, 2001.

13. Walter JS, Sola PG, Sacks J et al: Indications for a home standing program for individuals with spinal cord injury, *J Spinal Cord Med* 22:152-158, 1999.

14. Waters RL, Mulroy S: The energy expenditure of normal and pathologic gait, *Gait Posture* 9:207-231, 1999.

15. Chantraine A, Crielaard JM, Onkelinx A et al: Energy expenditure of ambulation in paraplegics: effects of long term use of bracing, *Paraplegia* 22:173-181, 1984.

16. Hussey RW, Stauffer ES: Spinal cord injury: requirements for ambulation, *Arch Phys Med Rehabil* 54:544-547, 1973.

17. Waters RL, Adkins R, Yakura J et al: Prediction of ambulatory performance based on motor scores derived from standards of the American Spinal Injury Association, *Arch Phys Med Rehabil* 75:756-760, 1994.

18. Waters RL, Adkins RH, Yakura JS et al: Motor and sensory recovery following incomplete tetraplegia, *Arch Phys Med Rehabil* 75:306-311, 1994.

19. Waters RL, Adkins RH, Yakura JS et al: Motor and sensory recovery following incomplete paraplegia, *Arch Phys Med Rehabil* 75:67-72, 1994.

20. Kim CM, Eng JJ, Whittaker MW: Level walking and ambulatory capacity in persons with incomplete spinal cord injury: relationship with muscle strength, *Spinal Cord* 42:156-162, 2004.

21. Creel GL, Light KE, Thigpen MT: Concurrent and construct validity of scores on the timed movement battery, *Phys Ther* 81:789-798, 2001.

22. Shumway-Cook A, Baldwin M, Polissar NL et al: Predicting the probability for falls in community-dwelling older adults, *Phys Ther* 77:812-819, 1997.

23. Williams ME, Gaylord SA, Gerritty MS: The timed manual performance test as a predictor of hospitalization and death in community-based elderly population, *J Am Geriatar Soc* 42:21-27, 1994.

24. Pomeroy VM, Chambers SH, Giakas G et al: Reliability of measurement of tempo-spatial parameters of gait after stroke using GaitMat II, *Clin Rehabil* 18:222-227, 2004.

25. Bilney B, Morris M, Webster K: Concurrent related validity of the GAITRite walkway system for quantification of the spatial and temporal parameters of gait, *Gait Posture* 17:68-74, 2003.

26. Nelson AJ, Zwick D, Brody S et al: The validity of the GaitRite and the Functional Ambulation Performance scoring system in the analysis of Parkinson gait, *NeuroRehabilitation* 17:255-262, 2002.

27. Barbeau H, Ladouceur M, Norman KE et al: Walking after spinal cord injury: evaluation, treatment, and functional recovery, *Arch Phys Med Rehabil* 80:225-235, 1999.

28. Richards C.L., Malouin F., Dean C.M.: Gait in stroke: assessment and rehabilitation, *Clin Geriatr Med* 17:833-855, 1999.

29. Dean CM, Richards CL, Malouin F: Task-related circuit training improves performance of locomotor tasks in chronic stroke: a randomized, controlled pilot trial, *Arch Phys Med Rehabil* 81:409-417, 2000.

30. Berg KO, Maki BE, Williams JI et al: Clinical and laboratory measures of postural balance in an elderly population, *Arch Phys Med Rehabil* 73:1073-1080, 1992.

31. Berg KO, Wood-Dauphinee SL Williams JI et al: Measuring balance in the elderly: validation of an instrument, *Can J Public Health* 83 (2 Suppl):S7-S11, 1992.

32. Steffen TM, Hacker TA, Mollinger L: Age- and gender-related test performance in community-dwelling elderly people: Six-Minute Walk Test, Berg Balance Scale, Timed Up & Go Test, and gait speeds, *Phys Ther* 82:128-137, 2002.

33. Troosters T, Gosselink R, Decramer M: Six-minute walk test: a valuable test, when properly standardized [letter], *Phys Ther* 82:826-827; author reply 827-828, 2002.

34. Dittuno PL, Dittuno Jr JF Jr: Walking index for spinal cord injury (WISCI II): scale revision, *Spinal Cord* 39:654-656, 2001.

35. Field-Fote EC, Fluet GG, Schafer SD, et al: The Spinal Cord Injury Functional Ambulation Inventory (SCI-FAI), *J Rehabil Med* 33:177-181, 2001.

36. Coleman KL, Smith DG, Boone DA et al: Step activity monitor: long-term, continuous recording of ambulatory function, *J Rehabil Res Dev* 36:8-18, 1999.

37. Behrman AL, Tomlinson SS: "I want to walk": an approach to physical therapy management of the individual with an incomplete spinal cord injury, *Neurol Rep* 17:7-12, 1993.

38. Trimble MH, Kukulka CG, Behrman AL: The effect of treadmill gait training on low-frequency depression of the soleus H-reflex: comparison of a spinal cord injured man to normal subjects, *Neurosci Lett* 246:186-188, 1998.

39. Behrman AL, Harkema SJ: Locomotor training after human spinal cord injury: a series of case studies, *Phys Ther* 80:688-700, 2000.

40. Basso D, Behrman AL, Harkema SJ: Recovery of walking after central nervous system insult: basic research in the controlled locomotion as a foundation for developing rehabilitation strategies, *Neurol Rep* 24:47-54, 2000.

41. Chaplin E: Functional neuromuscular stimulation for mobility in people with spinal cord injuries: the Parastep I System, *J Spinal Cord Med* 19:99-105, 1996.

42. Winchester P, Carollo JJ, Habasevich R: Physiologic costs of reciprocal gait in FES assisted walking, *Paraplegia* 32:680-686, 1994.

43. Wieler M, Stein RB, Ladouceur M et al: Multicenter evaluation of electrical stimulation systems for walking, *Arch Phys Med Rehabil* 80:495-500, 1999.

44. Brissot R, Gallien P, Le Bot MP et al: Clinical experience with functional electrical stimulation-assisted gait with Parastep in spinal cord–injured patients, *Spine* 25:501-508, 2000.

45. Dall PM, Muller B, Stallard I et al: The functional use of the reciprocal hip mechanism during gait for paraplegic patients walking in the Louisiana State University reciprocating gait orthosis, *Prosthet Orthot Int* 23:152-162, 1999.

46. Stein RB, Bélanger M, Wheeler G et al: Electrical systems for improving locomotion after incomplete spinal cord injury: an assessment, *Arch Phys Med Rehabil* 74:954-959, 1993.

47. Barbeau H: Locomotor training in neurorehabilitation: emerging rehabilitation concepts, *Neurorehabil Neural Repair* 17:3-11, 2003.

48. Edgerton VR dLR, Tillakaratne N, Recktenwald MR et al: Use-dependent plasticity in spinal stepping and standing, *Adv Neurol* 72:233-247, 1997.

49. Rossignol IS, Barbeau H: New approaches to locomotor rehabilitation in spinal cord injury, *Ann Neurol* 37:555-556, 1995.

50. Edgerton VR, de Leon RD, Tillakaratne N et al: Use-dependent plasticity in spinal stepping and standing, *Adv Neurol* 72:233-247, 1997.

51. Finch L, Barbeau H, Arsenault B: Influence of body weight support on normal human gait: development of a gait retraining strategy, *Phys Ther* 71:842-856, 1991.

52. Barbeau H, Wainberg M, Finch L: Description and application of a system for locomotor rehabilitation, *Med Biol Eng Comput* 25:341-344, 1987.

53. Barbeau H, Danakas M, Arsenault B: The effects of locomotor training in spinal cord injured subjects: a preliminary study, *Restor Neurol Neurosci* 5:81-84, 1993.

54. Wernig A, Muller S, Nanassy A et al: Laufband therapy based on 'rules of spinal locomotion' is effective in spinal cord injured persons, *Eur J Neurosci* 7:823-829, 1995.

55. Behrman AL, Lawless AR, Davis SB et al: Locomotor training progression and outcomes after incomplete spinal cord injury, *Phys Ther* 85:1356-1371, 2005.

56. Barbeau H, Rossignol S: Enhancement of locomotor recovery following spinal cord injury, *Curr Opin Neurol* 7:517-524, 1994.

57. Dietz V, Gollhofer A, Kleiber M, Trippel M: Regulation of bipedal stance: dependency on "load" receptors, *Exp Brain Res* 89:229-231, 1992.

58. Duysens J, Pearson KG: Inhibition of flexor burst generation by loading ankle extensor muscles in walking cats, *Brain Res* 187:321-332, 1980.

59. Prochazka A, Bennett DJ, Stephens MJ et al: Measurement of rigidity in Parkinson's disease, *Move Disord* 12:24-32, 1997.

60. Dietz V: Locomotor training in paraplegic patients [letter; comment], *Ann Neurol* 38:965, 1995.

61. Harkema SJ, Hurley SL, Patel UK et al: Human lumbosacral spinal cord interprets loading during stepping, *J Neurophysiol* 77:797-811, 1997.

62. Visintin M, Barbeau H: The effects of body weight support on the locomotor pattern of spastic paretic patients, *Can J Neurol Sci* 16: 315-325, 1989.

63. Grillner S, Rossignol S: On the initiation of the swing phase of locomotion in chronic spinal cats, *Brain Res* 146:269-277, 1978.

64. Pearson KG, Rossignol S: Fictive motor patterns in chronic spinal cats, *J Neurophysiol* 66:1874-1887, 1991.

65. Lam T, Pearson KG: Proprioceptive modulation of hip flexor activity during the swing phase of locomotion in decerebrate cats, *J Neurophysiol* 86:1321-1332, 2001.

66. Dietz V, Muller R, Colombo G: Locomotor activity in spinal man: significance of afferent input from joint and load receptors, *Brain* 125:2626-2634, 2002.

67. Dietz V: Human neuronal control of automatic functional movements: interaction between central programs and afferent input, *Physiol Rev* 72:33-69, 1992.

68. Field-Fote EC, Tepavac D: Improved intralimb coordination in people with incomplete spinal cord injury following training with body weight support and electrical stimulation, *Phys Ther* 82:707-715, 2002.

69. Forssberg H: Stumbling corrective reaction: a phase-dependent compensatory reaction during locomotion, *J Neurophysiol* 42:936-953, 1979.

70. Horak FB, Macpherson JM, Peterson BW: Postural orientation and equilibrium. In Rowell LB, Shepherd JT, editors: *Exercise: regulation and integration of multiple systems*, New York, 1996, American Physiological Society.

71. Protas EJ, Holmes SA, Qureshy H et al: Supported treadmill ambulation training after spinal cord injury: a pilot study, *Arch Phys Med Rehabil* 82:825-831, 2001.

72. Gardner MB, Holden MK, Leikauskas JM et al: Partial body weight support with treadmill locomotion to improve gait after incomplete spinal cord injury: a single-subject experimental design, *Phys Ther* 78:361-374, 1998.

73. Trimble MH, Behrman AL, Flynn SM et al: Acute effects of locomotor training on overground walking speed and H-reflex modulation in individuals with incomplete spinal cord injury, *J Spinal Cord Med* 24:74-80, 2001.

74. Wernig A, Muller S: Laufband locomotion with body weight support improved walking in persons with severe spinal cord injuries, *Paraplegia* 30:229-238, 1992.

75. Dobkin BH, Apple D, Barbeau H et al: Methods for a randomized trail of weight supported treadmill training versus conventional training for walking during inpatient rehabilitation after incomplete spinal cord injury, *Neurorehabil Neural Repair* 17:153-167, 2003.

76. Field-Fote E: Spinal cord stimulation facilitates functional walking in a chronic, incomplete spinal cord injured subject, *Spinal Cord* 40:428, 2002.

77. Field-Fote EC: Combined use of body weight support, functional electric stimulation, and treadmill training to improve walking ability in individuals with chronic incomplete spinal cord injury, *Arch Phys Med Rehabil* 82:818-824, 2001.

78. Hornby TG, Zemon DH, Campbell D: Robotic-assisted, body-weight–supported treadmill training in individuals following motor incomplete spinal cord injury, *Phys Ther* 85:52-66, 2005.

79. Colombo G, Joerg M, Schreier R et al: Treadmill training of paraplegic patients using a robotic orthosis, *J Rehabil Res Dev* 37:693-700, 2000.

80. Colombo G, Wirz M, Dietz V: Driven gait orthosis for improvement of locomotor training in paraplegic patients, *Spinal Cord* 39:252-255, 2001.

81. Hidler JM, Wall AE: Alterations in muscle activation patterns during robotic-assisted walking, *Clin Biomech (Bristol, Avon)* 20:184-193, 2005.

82. Lunenburger L, Colombo F, Riener R: Biofeedback for robotic gait rehabilitation, *J Neuroengineering Rehabil* 4:1, 2007. Published online January 23, 2007.

83. Kleim JA, Jones TA: Principles of experience-dependent neural plasticity: implications for rehabilitation after brain damage, *American Journal of Speech Hearing and Language Research* (in press).

84. Adkins DL, Boychuk J, Remple MS et al: Motor training indices experience specific patterns of plasticity in the motor cortex and spinal cord, *J Appl Physiol* 101:1776-1782, 2006.

SOLUTIONS TO CHAPTER 16 CLINICAL CASE STUDY

Ambulation

1. Typically in an individual with an ASIA D injury, the prognosis for ambulatory potential is directly proportional to the amount of motor activity seen on evaluation, and most, if not all, individuals will be able to ambulate full time. In this case, Michael is not symmetrical in his muscle recovery and the posterior musculature of his lower limbs is weak. This imbalance must be considered in the training and progression of ambulation and may ultimately influence his ambulation outcome.

2. Because of the imbalance in strength between Michael's right and left lower limbs and the weakness of the posterior lower limb muscles bilaterally, control at each joint during ambulation will be compromised. Evaluation in the parallel bars with and without orthoses should be performed. Trunk control will play a large part in this process while Michael learns his balance point during both swing and stance phases of training and it will vary for each limb. Stabilization from muscle imbalances may or may not ultimately be needed at his ankle(s) and knee(s).

3. Michael's training progression with an assistive device will begin within the parallel bars and progress to a walker and ultimately to forearm crutches. He will need to rely on the assistive device for balance during swing phase and to regain an upright posture and balance during stance.

4. Michael should be instructed in a variety of gait patterns, including swing-to, swing-through, four-point, and two-point. Because of the muscle imbalance in his lower limbs and trunk weakness, different gait patterns may be more efficient in a variety of environmental situations. It would appear that a four- or two-point gait would be the objective for training, but ultimately the decisions about which pattern to use in different situations will rest with Michael. The more options he has available to him, the greater his ability will be to solve problems as he faces them in his environment. The clinician should keep in mind that Michael's overall imbalance of muscle control will affect his gait pattern, which will be slower than normal and may not

Continued

Ambulation

appear normal. Slower velocity may ultimately affect his endurance for long distance ambulation because his gait will be less efficient.

5. Elevation training may be initiated in the parallel bars using a small curb of 2 inches; progressing to 4- and 6-inch curbs. Trunk control and upper body strength will influence the technique performed in both cases. Ascending a curb may be taught by placing the assistive device up on the curb, leaning forward over the upper limbs, lifting the body weight, and simultaneously placing both feet up on the curb ensuring that the toes clear the rim of the curb. Descending the curb, the assistive device is placed down first and then both feet are simultaneously brought down off the curb, ensuring that the majority of his body weight is forward over the assistive devices to avoid jackknifing. Because of his motor recovery, Michael may also be evaluated for single-limb curb ascent and descent in the parallel bars to see if this is ultimately a safer and more efficient approach.

Another option would be to ascend or descend stairs sideways with the stronger leg closer to the stairs, holding the rail with both hands (see Figure 16-13). Michael would lift the stronger right leg and place it on the first step. He would then bring the left leg onto the step placing it next to or behind the right leg depending on the depth of the step. He would lower the weaker leg first, placing it back far enough to leave room for the other leg to be lifted off the step and then placed in front. However, because of the return of strength in his lower limbs, forward-facing variations should be attempted with the stairs as they were with curbs. He may even be able to progress to step over step. During training, Michael should work on using two rails, one rail, and no rail because all of these situations may arise in different environments. When presented with no railing, a method such as used with the curb may be needed. It should be noted that extra caution must be taken with stair descent because the forces of gravity can make eccentric control of the quadriceps and upper limbs challenging.

6. If a patient in bilateral KAFOs feels that he is going to fall, he should do whatever he can to fall forward so that he can protect himself from injury. He should throw his assistive device out of the way so that he does not land on it and put his hands out for protection. If possible, he should bend at the hips and allow his elbows to bend as his hands hit the ground to decrease the force transmitted through his arms. After he is on the ground, he can place his forearm crutches with the handles pointing inward at about his knee level with the tips of the crutches located near his head. He should assume the prone position with his hips in full external rotation. He then pushes up, walking his hands back toward his feet. He picks up one forearm crutch, maintains his balance in a tripod, picks up the second crutch, works both crutches in closer, and as soon as possible drops his pelvis forward to assume the parastance position. If he is using a walker, it should be placed over his hips. As he walks his hands back toward his feet, he will come up underneath the walker and place one hand at a time onto its lower side rungs. He will then move his hands up onto the handles of the walker and as soon as possible allow his pelvis to drop forward to assume the parastance position.

7. Locomotor training provides a safe, convenient, and permissive environment for a patient to relearn progressive ambulation. Should the time, finances, and staffing be available for BWST this may be a very helpful means for motor relearning because of Michael's regained strength and progression in learning how to use his available musculature. The safety that is provided with a gradual increase of his body weight would be a positive effect of using this method. In addition, this approach may have a positive effect on relearning a reciprocal gait pattern, which would be a reasonable goal for this patient. However, because of the staffing and time commitment required this method might not be feasible or available.

An Activity-Based, Locomotor Training Perspective

In the first case study example, the primary basis for ambulation prognosis is based on an evaluation of the capacity to demonstrate voluntary LE muscle activation and strength via manual muscle tests. Assistive devices and orthotics are listed as a primary tool for solving the problem of walking disability and for achieving community ambulation. The emphasis is consistent with a compensation-based approach to strength deficits to achieve ambulation.

In comparison, an activity-based approach, via the same case study, but from a locomotor training perspective emphasizes activation of the nervous system below the level of the lesion during an evaluation and subsequent training. The nervous system's capacity is

assessed during the task of locomotion in a permissive environment using a treadmill with a body weight support system, overhead safety to catch the person should he stumble or fall, and the assistance of manual trainers at the pelvis/trunk and each leg.

Transfer of such capacity to overground is assessed in an environment that affords a means to observe such function. From these two assessments, the factors limiting successful walking are identified relative to stepping, balance, and adaptability. Refer to Table 16-3 for a detailed, step-by-step comparison of conventional gait training and locomotor training from evaluation and goal setting through training.

CHAPTER SEVENTEEN

Functional Electrical Stimulation

Pouran D. Faghri, MD, FACSM, MS, Susan V. Garstang, MD, and Sue Kida, PT, MHA

There are a lot of physical benefits to using FES. I think the increased blood flow and muscle mass is really important for improved skin integrity. I've had my injury over 9 years and I have yet to develop any pressure sores. I also really like the ERGYS—it gives the rider a tremendous high. There's no better feeling than coming off that bike; your head is clear and your energy is up, and you feel ready to take on the world!

Sarah (T4 SCI)

HISTORY

Electrical stimulation uses electrical current to stimulate intact motor or sensory nerves, thereby producing a neurological response. It has been used in the medical arena for a variety of maladies since 400 BCE. Krueger was the first to use electrical stimulation on paralyzed limbs in 1744, when static electricity was used to treat paralysis.[1] Throughout the 1800s, electrical stimulation was applied as a treatment for a variety of complaints, which marked the latter half of the nineteenth century as the Golden Age of Medical Electricity because of rapid discoveries and changes that occurred in the field. The first significant application of electrical stimulation to improve muscle function dates back to 1950, with the invention of the cardiac pacemaker. Next phrenic nerve pacemakers were introduced in the 1960s to assist respiration (see Chapter 4).

The first real effort to apply electrical stimulation for therapeutic use came in 1961 when Liberson et al[2] used a portable stimulator and placed electrodes above the peroneal nerve of the fossa poplitea. The stimulator was placed in the shoe of a hemiplegic patient's affected foot to counteract footdrop. As the patient lifted his heel, the stimulator was triggered, thus causing dorsiflexion of the foot. After this application, the term functional electrotherapy was used for the first time as a rehabilitative aid, evolving into modern-day functional electrical stimulation (FES).

During the same decade, Kantrowitz was beginning to apply FES to patients with spinal cord injury (SCI). His team stimulated the quadriceps and glutei to aid in static standing.[3] Surface electrodes were placed over the medial quadriceps and medial glutei in both legs. On stimulation, the patient was able to rise from his wheelchair and remain standing. A formal report of this research does not exist, which renders many details such as standing time, stimulation type, and electrode characteristics unknown.

In 1963, Long[4] created an electrically activated flexor-hinge orthosis, used to cause finger extension and hand opening in a patient with tetraplegia. The next year, a cybernetic model that explained the mechanism behind conscious movement was developed at Case Institute of Technology in Cleveland, and this model, when presented in schematic form by Vodovnik et al,[5] introduced the concept of neural bypass theory. Their findings set precedence for control of paralyzed limbs by FES. Vodovnik et al[5] introduced the first stimulator controlled through electromyography. Voltage signals detected by the left trapezius muscle during movement were used as a visual feedback. From the behavior of

the signal, the stimulation current was adjusted accordingly and applied to the extensor digitorum. The use of electromyogram in conjunction with FES is still widely used.[6]

Mooney[7] introduced the first implantable stimulator in 1969. His design was later modified by Shuck in 1973 to stimulate the peroneal nerve during the swing phase of gait analysis.[6] During this period, rehabilitation engineering centers were created by the U.S. Department of Health, Education, and Welfare.[8] Rancho Los Amigos Hospital in California was among the first five of these centers. In 1970, Ranchos researchers attempted the implantations of a multichannel stimulator in man—the first of its kind—an application that included gait correction in a hemiplegic patient as well as fixation of the knee and hip in a paraplegic patient.[6]

FES was studied only in adult patients until 1971. Applications in children determined that use of FES at younger ages could aid in psychomotor and behavioral development and increase "communicativeness" of the child patients. These experiments were also not fully documented, leaving many questions unanswered as to the number of children tested, indications, and the success rate.[6] From the 1970s to the present day, FES applications have undergone many modifications in an attempt to improve comfort, efficiency, and results.

USES OF FUNCTIONAL ELECTRICAL STIMULATION IN SPINAL CORD INJURY

FES can be used for many applications in those with SCI. These include maintaining or increasing range of motion (ROM), correction of contractures, muscle strengthening, facilitation of voluntary motor function, inhibition of spasticity, orthotic substitution, prevention of circulatory hypotension and orthostatic hypotension, and exercise (Box 17-1).[3,9] Most activities performed with FES combine these basic applications to enhance the functions of standing, gait, or grasp. Electrical stimulation has also been used to assist in respiration, and in the treatment of scoliosis, pain alleviation, spasticity reduction, and bladder and bowel function.

FES applications include FES-cycle ergometry for lower limb conditioning and training, which was developed during the 1970s and approved by the U.S. Food and Drug Administration (FDA) in 1984. The FineTech-Brindley stimulator, known as VOCARE in the United States, aids in bladder control and was introduced in Europe in 1984 and obtained FDA approval in 1998.[10] The first

---

BOX 17-1 | **Applications of Functional Electrical Stimulation in Spinal Cord Injury**

- Strengthening and endurance
- Cardiovascular reconditioning
- Enhancement of upper limb function
- Standing and gait
- Augmentation of bladder function
- Phrenic nerve stimulation
- Wound healing
- Prevention of DVT
- Reduction of osteoporosis
- Management of ejaculatory failure
- FES-enhanced cough
- ROM
- Facilitation of voluntary responses
- Orthotic substitution

---

report of the use of FES to achieve walking for a patient with complete paraplegia appeared in 1983.[11] The Parastep system, used to aid walking in patients with SCI, was introduced in 1989 and gained FDA approval in 1994. The neuroprosthetic Freehand system developed to augment upper limb function was first implanted in 1986 and received FDA approval in 1997.[9,12] Originally developed and approved by the FDA as the Handmaster wrist-hand orthosis, the NESS H200 is an FES device that assists individuals with neurological disorders perform functional activities of the forearm and hand.[13,14]

CONTRAINDICATIONS AND PRECAUTIONS

There are several absolute contraindications to electrical stimulation that are applicable to every device that is discussed in this chapter.[1,3] Electrical stimulation must not be used in the following cases:

- With patients who have a demand cardiac pacemaker or phrenic pacemaker because it may interfere with the sensing or pacing functions of those applications
- Over the carotid sinus to avoid stimulation of the baroreceptors causing vasodilation and bradycardia
- Over malignant tumors because it has been shown in animal models to cause tumor spread and metastasis

Relative contraindications include pregnancy because the safety and effect on fetus are not known; severe osteoporosis because of the risk of fracture with strong muscle contraction; seizure disorder because of theoretical concern about triggering seizures; or in patients with history of cardiac conduction disturbances in whom electrocardiogram monitoring should be used during the first few sessions to assess the effect on the heart during stimulation.

There are also general precautions for the use of FES. Patients must have intact peripheral nerves; electrical stimulation is challenging in lower motor neuron injuries (e.g., cauda equina syndrome). Individuals with higher SCIs can also have components of peripheral nerve injury in addition to the central nervous system injury, thus making electrical stimulation difficult for the muscles innervated at those levels. Electrical current should not be applied directly to skin because it may result in tissue damage. Proper skin preparation is discussed later. Rapid muscle fatigue or pain is possible if proper

stimulation parameter selection is not made. To prevent such damages, the therapist must consider both the amplitude and pulse duration of the current intensity. In addition, electrical heating produced by a current source has been found to cause toxic compound accumulation and temperature increases in tissue.[15]

If the patient has insensate skin, there is an increased risk of burns or irritation. In those with diabetes, the skin must be monitored closely, again because of decreased sensation and increased risk of skin irritation. Patients who are sensate may find it difficult to tolerate the necessary stimulus intensity; indeed, in some patients, FES may worsen neurogenic pain. When a patient is prone to spasticity, the stimulation may exacerbate the spastic response both at the time the stimulus is delivered and over the long term (weeks). Patients who have SCI above T6 may also be at risk for autonomic dysreflexia (AD). One study demonstrated that FES of the lower limbs with frequencies of 50 Hz provoked AD in 8 of 10 patients with SCI above T6[16]; however, using frequencies of 30 to 35 Hz was not tied to significant episodes of AD. Before using FES in a patient with SCI, it is wise to obtain medical clearance for performing active exercise with the muscles that will be stimulated and to monitor blood pressure throughout. Other contraindications and precautions specific to particular applications of FES are discussed when each use is described. Absolute and relative contraindications, general precautions, and limitations are listed in the Clinical Note: Contraindications and Precautions for Functional Electrical Stimulation.

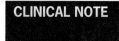 **CLINICAL NOTE** | **Contraindications and Precautions for Functional Electrical Stimulation**

Absolute Contraindications
- Should not be used if the patient has a demand cardiac pacemaker or phrenic pacemaker
- Not to be used over the carotid sinus
- Must not be used over malignant tumors

Relative Contraindications
- Pregnancy
- Osteoporosis
- Seizure disorder
- History of cardiac conduction disturbances
- Severe respiratory disease
- Spinal instability
- Pathological or unhealed fractures
- Joint disarticulation
- Fixed contractures in the lower limbs

General Precautions
- Risk of burns or irritation if patient has insensate skin
- Risk of intolerance for sensate patient
- Risk of worsening neurogenic pain
- Risk of worsening spasticity
- Risk for AD in patients with lesions above T6
- Risk of orthopedic instability in the area of electrode placement
- Risk to open wounds or incision sites
- Risk of heterotopic ossification impeding ROM in lower limbs

- Risk to metal hardware in the femur
- Risk of hypertension
- Risk of hypotension
- Risk of venous thrombosis

Limiting Factors
- Ineffective in lower motor neuron injuries
- Severe obesity
- Severe spasticity or flaccidity
- Limited ROM in the knees or hips
- Motivation
- Realism
- Frequent UTI or other infections

PHYSIOLOGY OF FUNCTIONAL ELECTRICAL STIMULATION

FES works by using electrical current to stimulate intact peripheral nerves, thereby eliciting a muscle contraction. If peripheral nerves are damaged, which occurs with a lower motor neuron injury, the muscle needs to be stimulated directly to elicit a response. Stimulating denervated muscles requires a more potent stimulus level consisting of higher amplitudes and longer pulse durations and is technically a more difficult endeavor.[17]

In general, a single pulse of stimulation provokes a single action potential in a number of individual nerve fibers near the stimulating electrode. These action potentials are propagated toward the neuromuscular junction, and a single muscle twitch results.[17] A train of individual stimulus pulses at a constant frequency summates the muscle twitches and forms a smooth contraction.

In normal human physiology, small diameter motor neurons innervate type I muscle fibers; these are the first recruited motor units during a muscle contraction.[1] Type I fibers are slow-twitch oxidative fibers, which are resistant to fatigue and contract during periods of low levels of exertion. Later in the time course of the muscle contraction, larger diameter neurons, which innervate type II muscle fibers, are recruited to produce a maximal muscle contraction. Type II muscle fibers are fast twitch, glycolytic, and fatigue more quickly.

In contrast to normal physiology, electrical stimulation provides selective activation of the larger motor neurons because they are easier to stimulate because of their lower threshold of excitation.[1,17] The muscle fibers that are innervated by the larger axons (i.e., type II fibers) tend to fatigue more quickly, which is why muscles stimulated by FES fatigue sooner than those subject to a volitional motor response. This phenomenon is caused by the reversal of the normal recruitment order of skeletal muscle fibers, as described above.

In addition, in normal physiology, there is asynchronous activation of multiple geographically diffuse motor units that produces the total muscle response of a smooth contraction distributed evenly across the muscle.[1] This allows for a maintained, slowly fatiguing contraction with a steady force response. In contrast to normal physiology, when FES is used to stimulate motor neurons and units, they are excited synchronously with preferential activation of motor units in the proximity of the stimulation. Thus, fewer motor units are activated further away from the source of stimulation. This again leads to rapid fatigue and the need for a higher stimulation output to maintain a strong muscle contraction.

The reversal of the normal recruitment order and the asynchronous activation of motor units results in FES being less efficient and less selective than normal physiology.[1,18] Again, the end result of these differences is faster muscle fatigue. Fatigue can be minimized by using lower frequencies, alternating on periods with off (i.e., rest periods), changing the duty cycle (ratio of stimulus on vs. off), cyclically stimulating multiple heads of a muscle group, or periodically changing postures to provide muscle groups with periods of rest. Therefore, once a patient with SCI can volitionally contract his muscle by using normal physiological responses, electrical stimulation support should be reduced or eliminated.

FUNCTIONAL ELECTRICAL STIMULATION SYSTEMS

Several factors affect the muscular response to FES (Clinical Note: Factors That Affect Muscular Response to Functional Electrical Stimulation). The settings of the stimulation parameters such as amplitude, pulse width, frequency, and type of waveform will affect the response to electrical stimulation. In addition, the impedance, or resistance to current flow inherent in different tissues, will affect the response to electrical stimulation. Impedance is the sum of resistive, capacitive, and inductive tissue components that limit the flow of current. The lower the impedance of the tissue, the greater the flow of current will be through the tissue. More current is needed to pass through higher impedance tissues (e.g., subcutaneous fat) than through muscle itself. Finally, electrode size and orientation and types of electrode systems used will affect the results obtained with FES.

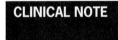 **CLINICAL NOTE** **Factors That Affect Muscular Response to Functional Electrical Stimulation**

Stimulation parameters
- Amplitude
- Pulse width
- Frequency
- Type of waveform

Impedance
Electrode size and orientation
Types of electrode systems used

Parameters

All FES systems have multiple parameters that optimize the response to electrical stimulation.[19] The results of the applied electrical stimulation and the patient's tolerance of this stimulation will depend on how these parameters, including waveform, amplitude, current duration, frequency, ramping, and the duty cycle, are adjusted. Figure 17-1 illustrates the stimulation components that can be manipulated when FES is modulated.

Waveform

A waveform is a stimulus pulse consisting of a phase that may be positive or negative, a shape (e.g., sine or rectangular), and an amplitude. There are many types of waveforms available that elicit neural excitation and lead to a muscular contraction. The

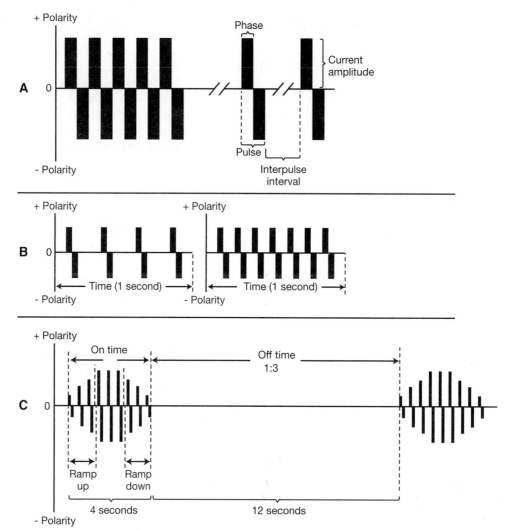

FIGURE 17-1   Waveforms that represent the current used in FES can be manipulated in a number of ways. **A,** Using a symmetrical biphasic current in which there is an equal electrode pulse in both positive and negative directions reduces skin irritation and chemical reactions and is therefore best tolerated by the patient. **B,** The frequency or pulse rate of individual electrical pulses affects the quality of the muscle response and the rate of muscle fatigue; it should be adjusted to prompt the best outcomes. **C,** Rise and fall of the current allows the patient to accommodate to the current's stimulation and is integral to on time; the duty cycle is the ratio of on time to off time.

FES unit's effectiveness depends on a type of waveform that affects both the excitability and the fatigability of the muscle. This waveform also influences the amount of sensory disturbance with stimulation.

On the basis of their investigation of constant current stimulation with small electrodes, Poletto and Van Doren[15] reported that monophasic stimulation is more appropriate for limited-time laboratory use and biphasic stimulation is better suited for longer-term applications. McNeal and Baker[20] focused on regions of excitability and techniques of stimulation applicable to quadriceps and hamstring muscles positioned at different knee angles. On the basis of a scale of perceived comfort, they concluded that subjects preferred biphasic waveforms in comparison with monophasic waveforms. Previous work conducted by Bowman and Baker had also supported these preferences.[20]

It should be noted that direct current is not adequate to produce a tetanic muscle contraction and may cause increased skin irritation and discomfort from unwanted stimulation. Therefore, pulsatile current should be used. Pulsatile current is some

variation of a rectangular pulse, which is effective at producing muscle contraction and can be further broken down into monophasic, asymmetrical biphasic, or symmetrical biphasic waveforms.

Monophasic pulsatile current is unidirectional and causes electrode polarization and equal ion flow in tissues. It can cause electrode deterioration and skin irritation. Asymmetrical biphasic current activates an electrode pulse that is greater in one direction but balanced by other aspects of the waveform so that the average current flow is zero. The acting phase positive current goes through the positive electrode into the skin or tissue, during the passive or balancing phase the current returns out the negative electrode, and the amplitude of the current returns to zero. The possibility of chemical reactions and skin irritation still exist with this waveform.

In symmetrical biphasic current, there is an equal ion electrode pulse in both the positive and negative directions and depolarization occurs under both electrodes; therefore, both electrodes are active. This reduces skin irritation and chemical reactions, making symmetrical biphasic current the most comfortable and least noxious waveform (Figure 17-1, *A*).

Amplitude

Amplitude refers to the magnitude of current applied during the pulse cycle. It determines both the sensory and motor response. Increasing the intensity recruits more motor units. A training period, however, may be necessary if a patient cannot tolerate the electrical stimulation high enough to achieve the desired response.

Research has shown a correlation between amplitude and frequency as perceived by patients. Frequency refers to the number of pulses generated per second. Both parameters show discrepancies between the produced and perceived values. In work by Van Doren,[21] perceived amplitude and frequency were compared for a 10 charge-balanced, constant current, biphasic pulse with an actual frequency or 1000 Hz. The mathematical correlation between the two factors was represented as follows:

$$A = m\log(F) + b$$

in which A = amplitude (expressed in dB units), F = stimulus frequency (Hz), and b = the calculated slope (dB/octave).

By use of this expression, contours for perceived amplitude and frequency were measured at predetermined reference values. Reference amplitudes were 3, 6, 9, and 12 dB with a 16-Hz reference stimulus. Reference frequencies were 8, 16, and 32 Hz with a sweep for matching amplitude from 3 dB to 12 dB at 1-dB increments. The result of this research showed amplitude to have no effect on perceived frequency. Frequency was found, however, to have a small but significant effect on amplitude perception that varied with the amplitude of the reference stimulus frequency.[21]

Current Duration

Current duration (e.g., pulse width or pulse duration) is the amount of time that the electrical current is delivered. In other words, it is the time that it takes to begin and end all phases and interphase intervals within one pulse. The current duration affects the intensity required to generate a motor response, thus affecting the comfort of the stimulation. Because current duration affects the amount of current (or intensity) required to generate a motor response, the interaction of these settings alters the effectiveness and comfort of the FES. When the current duration is decreased, increased intensity is required to elicit a motor response. Conversely, when the current duration is increased, less intensity is required to elicit a motor response. When using FES to elicit a motor response, it is important to remember this relationship so that these parameters may be adjusted together to provide the best and most comfortable response.

Frequency

Frequency (i.e., pulse rate) is the rate of individual electrical pulses, delivered in trains of pulses at a specified frequency (Figure 17-1, *B*). The frequency affects the quality of the muscle response and the rate of muscle fatigue. Depending on the muscle mass, a fused contraction (tetanization) can occur with 15 pulses per second

(pps) to 50 pps. An average pulse rate is about 25 to 30 pps but this depends on the muscle and its innervation. Higher frequencies above those required to achieve tetanus should be avoided because they can fatigue the muscle faster.

Ramping

The rate of rise and fall of current is called ramping. Rise time allows for sensory accommodation to the stimulation and thus affects the comfort of stimulation. In the presence of severe spasticity, a rapid rise time can evoke abnormal reflexes; therefore, when patients with severe spasticity are stimulated, the rise time may need to be increased significantly to allow for sufficient time to achieve the desired response without triggering spasticity. Keep in mind that when lengthening the rise time for accommodation, the on time also needs to be adjusted to allow sufficient time to produce a tetanic contraction. Fall time is less significant because the muscle will stop contracting as the stimulus decreases during fall time. The ramp time must be added onto the total stimulation time because the ramp time is not included in the total muscle stimulation time.

Duty Cycle

The duty cycle is the ratio of on time to the total cycle of stimulation, characterized by the relationship between the time the unit is on and the time the unit is off (Figure 17-1, *C*). This is also referred to as on:off time. This ratio is important because a muscle needs adequate rest to avoid fatigue. A duty cycle of 1:1 may cause muscles to fatigue quickly, whereas 1:5 is best to prevent fatigue, and 1:3 is functionally the most practical. Initially, a 4-second on and 12-second off cycle is recommended, in which the rise time and fall time are included in the total on-time.

Adjustment of these various stimulation parameters will affect the quality of the muscle contraction.[17] The amplitude and the pulse width need to be adequate to meet or exceed the threshold of excitability of the stimulated tissue. Increasing amplitude can result in the excitation of additional nerve fibers, but it is only effective if there are still motor units left to recruit. Increasing pulse width can also increase excitation of additional nerve fibers, resulting in an increased muscle contraction. In electrical stimulation, pulse amplitude and width are used to increase recruitment, whereas pulse frequency alters temporal summation and affects the rate at which the muscle fatigues (Clinical Note: Understanding Pulse Amplitude, Pulse Width, and Pulse Frequency).

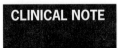

CLINICAL NOTE | **Understanding Pulse Amplitude, Pulse Width, and Pulse Frequency**

In electrical stimulation, pulse amplitude and width are used to increase recruitment, whereas pulse frequency alters temporal summation and affects the rate at which the muscle fatigues.

- Pulse amplitude: magnitude of current applied during the pulse cycle that will determine both the sensory and motor responses
- Pulse width: current duration in the amount of time that the electrical current is delivered; the time to begin and end all phases and interphase intervals within one pulse
- Pulse frequency: number of pulses generated per second

In summary, although the combination of stimulation parameters is specific to each application, there are some general parametric values. In a topical review of FES as compiled by Rushton,[22] the recorded range of frequencies used for neuromuscular stimulation spanned from 10 to 100 Hz. Stimulation involving the lower limbs uses frequency values of 30 Hz. The most common pulse train used is a rectangular stimulating current pulse. Pulse durations range from 5 to 500 microseconds. Monophasic or biphasic waveforms are often used, incorporating either a constant voltage or current source. The objective of selecting an appropriate parameter combination is to maximize muscle activation by using as little stimulation as possible; however, not all parameters may be minimized at once. Efforts to minimize any particular parameter will result in a complete change to the existing parametric combination.[22] Rushton also emphasized the importance of pulse type. Response characteristics and the likelihood for electrolytic nerve damage may potentially be affected through improper selection of pulse type. For such reasons, it is suggested that stimulation pulses be charge balanced or that biphasic stimulation pulses be used.[23]

The most advanced applications of stimulators involve implantable hardware for chronic disease. Stimulation incorporating constant current sources, programmable waveforms, and electrically isolated bipolar sources are required in these instances. Future research may include optimization and modification of these systems.

Components of Functional Electrical Stimulation Systems

All FES systems have some or all of the following components: control switch, stimulator, sensors, electrodes, and power source.

Control Switch

A control switch activates and regulates the current that will cause excitation of the muscles. This is typically an on-off switch, but can also be proportional so that it is controlled by body position.

Stimulator

A stimulator or control unit interprets signals from the control switch and then delivers the appropriate preprogrammed electrical signals to the target nerves through the electrodes.

Sensors

Sensors fulfill two major roles: (1) they detect patient commands or volition to inform the stimulator which action is desired and (2) they measure the state of the muscle being stimulated or the state of the body. Sensors can detect position, force, and acceleration and can be either external or implanted. Sensors can also be event detectors or provide continuous measurement of a physical quantity to a certain resolution (i.e., force).

Electrodes

Electrodes deliver electrical stimulation to the nerves at the motor point. The types of electrodes used with FES include surface electrodes, percutaneous electrodes, or implanted systems.[17]

Electrodes play a major role in the effectiveness and success of a stimulation program. Varying the type of electrode will alter the amount of conductivity and ease of use. Placement is also important to the muscle response and may require some searching of motor points and repetition to be effective. Electrode size and orientation influence current density, which is the amount of current flow per unit area and is maximal at the interface between the tissue and the electrode, decreasing with distance from the electrodes. Closely spaced electrodes allow for more superficial stimulation, whereas electrodes spaced further apart allow for deeper tissue stimulation (Figure 17-2). In addition, larger electrodes stimulate more superficially as the current is spread out, and smaller electrodes stimulate deeper tissue. Muscles should always be stimulated with the electrodes placed longitudinally, if possible, because a muscle will contract four times better when stimulated in the longitudinal direction as opposed to the transverse direction.[24]

Surface electrodes are applied directly to the skin surface over the motor point (Figure 17-3, A). They are the most commonly used type of electrode for FES and are easily applied and removed. Disadvantages include variation in electrode recruitment characteristics, lack of selectivity in obtaining a discrete response from a given muscle, inability to stimulate deep muscles, especially the hip extensors, external wire connections, skin reactions, and prolonged donning and doffing times. Surface electrodes also concomitantly deliver sensory stimulation that can provoke unwanted reflex responses or spasticity. Comfort may be an issue for patients with intact or partial sensation although the waveform settings can be altered to alleviate discomfort. In addition, skin burns or irritation can develop, especially when sensation is diminished or absent.

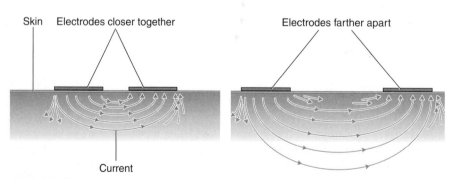

FIGURE 17-2   Electrode spacing affects current movement through tissue. When the electrodes are closer together, the current travels more superficially. When the electrodes are farther apart, the current goes deeper. (From Cameron MH: *Physical agents in rehabilitation: from research to practice,* ed 2, St. Louis, 2003, WB Saunders.)

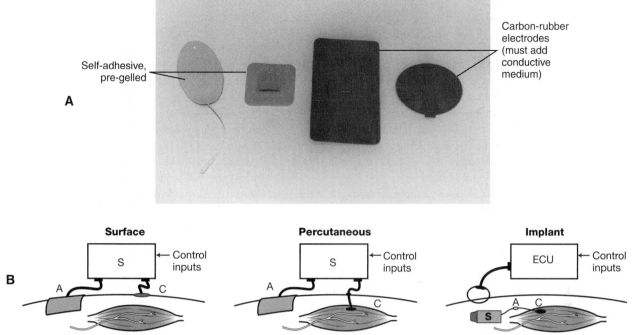

FIGURE 17-3 **A,** Examples of different types of surface electrodes used in FES. **B,** Schematic showing neuroprosthetic system configurations in which single-channel monopolar stimulation of one muscle near its motor point is shown for a surface, percutaneous, and implanted system. *S,* Stimulator; *A,* anode (reference electrode); *C,* cathode (active electrode); *ECU,* external control unit. (**A,** from Cameron MH: *Physical agents in rehabilitation: from research to practice,* ed 2, St. Louis, 2003, WB Saunders; **B,** from Peckham PH, Knutson JS: Functional electrical stimulation for neuromuscular applications, *Annu Rev Biomed Eng* 7:327-360, 2005.)

Percutaneous intramuscular electrodes are implanted in the muscle close to the anatomic motor point and exit through the skin. The stimulator and controls are outside the body. The electrodes need to be periodically replaced, and the electrode entry site needs to be maintained. Surgically implanted electrodes are entirely implanted inside the body and connected to a stimulator outside the body that supplies stimulus waveforms. The internal receiver gets information from an external control unit by radio waves. Electrodes can be attached to the epineurium, sewn on the muscle sheath in the vicinity of the motor point, or placed with a cuff around the nerve (e.g., perineural electrodes). Intraneural electrodes, consisting of a very fine wire inserted into the nerve fascicle, are in the early stages of development. Implanted electrode systems are more convenient, and the muscle recruitment characteristics remain constant. Mechanical attachment or nerve stimulation can cause nerve damage, however, and the electrode attachment sites can become infected. Figure 17-3, *B,* presents a schematic comparison of surface, percutaneous, and surgically implanted electrodes.

Power Source
The power source is typically supplied by one or several batteries. Prolonged use of the system raises the issues of weight and cosmesis and the frequent need for new batteries.

Means of Regulation
Open-Loop Control
Open-loop control is characterized by the patient sending out a command that delivers a certain amount of stimulation, regardless of the actual response of the muscle. Only visual or auditory feedback is available to direct the patient to alter the command.

This type of system is useful when exact precision is unnecessary. An open-loop control system does not modify its signal regardless of a patient's movement or consequences thereof. The pattern of stimulation is predetermined in this case.[23] The muscles in question will receive the same amount of current per stimulation. There are three types of open-loop controls: user control, cyclical control, and triggered cycle control.[22]

A user-controlled open-loop system is the most basic type of control available. It allows the patient to stimulate muscles or movement upon command. An example of this type of application is the sacral anterior root stimulator implant, which is primarily used in bladder control. If the patient wishes to empty his bladder, he can activate a hand switch. This controller also allows the patient to adjust the strength of the stimulus.

A cyclical open-loop system is characterized as a set of stimulation settings that are run continuously at a set cycle length. These settings and frequency remain constant until adjustments are made to the system. This type of open-loop system is used in phrenic pacers (see Chapter 4).

Phrenic pacers may also incorporate a triggered cycle open-loop control systems. As mentioned previously, the cycle is predetermined but only initiates when an inspiratory effort is made. Such inspiratory efforts can be the R wave of the myocardium in cardiac assist stimulators, a foot-drop, or a toe-lift in gait applications.[22] Currently open-loop control systems are considered standard for standing and walking applications.[23] These loops are simplistic in nature because they do not incorporate the use of any sensors. This also makes them a more economical choice of stimulation control. The lack of constant stimulation adjustment, however, has made them secondary to closed-loop controls.

Closed-Loop Control

Closed-loop control is characterized by the electrical stimulation being initiated through the user's command and then modified on the basis of some feedback measurement such as force or position. Some systems are programmed to modify the stimulus without the user's awareness, on the basis of input from sensors, whereas other systems use visual or auditory feedback from the user to modify the command. With closed-loop control, the delivery of electric stimulation is continuously modulated to control the quality being measured by the sensors.

Because a closed-loop control system is so sensitive to patient performance, there has been a constant increase in the number of applications associated with FES research. Applications for a closed-loop system include exercises such as leg lifts, bicycling, and walking,[23] as well as complex systems involving sphincter activation regulation and motion control in several types of gait analysis. Crago et al[25] reported about a closed-loop system applied in prostheses intended for urinary bladder control. Because relative pressure changes within the bladder itself are impossible to obtain, pressure changes across the urethral sphincter were measured. These values were closely approximated to absolute pressure changes in the bladder. Changes in transurethral pressure exceeding threshold would activate a closed-loop feedback control designed to regulate sphincter stimulation. Stimulation duration would last for several seconds or until baseline pressures were met, although because of physical differences between patients, threshold pressure values for this system would vary accordingly.

Closed-loop systems have also proven to be beneficial in stance and gait performance; when controlling stance in patients with paraplegia, closed-loop systems provide resistance to internal and external disturbances. These controllers compensate for muscle fatigue and upper limb motions. In turn, the patient has a sense of confidence that his legs will not buckle while performing activities in the standing state. In some cases, patients were able to remain standing for as long as 75 minutes.[25]

A hybrid system combines closed-loop controllers with orthotics. The objective of this combination is to minimize disadvantages associated with both methods and maximize their advantages. Andrews et al[26] described closed-loop control implementation in conjunction with a floor-reaction, ankle-foot orthosis to stimulate quadriceps. A force sensor placed within the orthotic component helped regulate the amount of stimulation required to keep the knee extended. Incorporation of both the controller and orthotic components reduced the amount of quadriceps stimulation needed and minimized the amount of muscle fatigue and hyperextension in the knee.

EFFECTS OF FUNCTIONAL ELECTRICAL STIMULATION
Changes in Muscle Morphological Features

After SCI, there are decreases in type I muscle fibers, the oxidative enzyme succinate dehydrogenase activity, and the capillary-to-fiber ratio in comparison to that of healthy control muscles.[1,27] These factors result in muscles that fatigue more readily with exertion. In addition, after SCI there is a loss of muscle bulk, a reduction in the amount of force that the muscles are capable of

producing, and a decrease in overall lean body mass with an increase in fat mass.

The use of FES has been shown to produce changes in the muscle at the level of the muscle fiber and even at the intracellular level.[28] Continuous low-frequency electrical stimulation of skeletal muscles results in transformation of the muscle fiber from type II fibers to fibers with type I characteristics.[27] This means that the fast-twitch fibers are converted to slow-twitch fibers and thus become more resistant to fatigue. Continuous electrical stimulation at 20 Hz of the tibialis anterior in patients with SCI has been shown to result in an increase in the proportion of type I fibers from 14% to 25%.[27] FES has also been shown to enhance the oxidative capacity of the muscle, as demonstrated by an increase in the activity of succinate dehydrogenase, which also makes the muscle less likely to fatigue.[27]

General Strengthening and Endurance

FES has been used after SCI for muscle strengthening and endurance training. Electrical stimulation to lower limb muscles after SCI causes an increased thigh circumference, improved muscle strength and endurance, increased quadriceps muscle area, and increased quadriceps muscle protein synthesis rates.[29] Daily FES in individuals with SCI increases endurance of the muscle to levels found in able-bodied control subjects with decreased fatigability.[30] Using FES-cycle ergometry causes gains in total lean body mass (LBM) of almost 8% with a decrease in percentage of body fat of 12%. These gains in lean body mass are primarily attributed to gains in the lower limb LBM, with increases of nearly 10% over baseline.

FES can be used with individuals with incomplete or complete SCIs. In those with complete injuries, FES can be used in the lower limbs to retard atrophy and promote muscular endurance and improve cardiovascular fitness, discussed subsequently. FES can also be used to augment function and strengthen partially innervated muscles. This applies both to incompletely innervated muscles in the zone of partial preservation (see Chapter 1) of those with complete injuries and to the partially innervated muscles of those with incomplete SCI.

Strengthening Incompletely Innervated Muscles

The advent of better prehospital emergency care and the consistent use of steroids immediately after injury have resulted in an increase of incomplete injuries. The use of FES with incomplete injuries can assist the patient with initiating volitional control over muscles that are receiving neural input, strengthening atrophied muscles, and maximizing functional capacity.

When FES is used to initiate volitional control or for strengthening, it is desirable to incorporate function into the activity. The muscles most typically stimulated for function in the upper limbs are the biceps for feeding activities and manual wheelchair propulsion, the triceps for carryover to transfer activities, and the wrist extensors to improve the strength of the tenodesis grasp. It should be noted that stimulation of the triceps area tends to produce a strong sensory response and is not as comfortable as other muscle groups. When the wrist extensors are stimulated, it is important to block finger extension to avoid overstretching the finger flexors so that the patient's tenodesis grasp is preserved.

In addition, both flexor and abductor shoulder muscles are commonly strengthened to allow for increased functional use of the arm. With significant shoulder atrophy, subluxation may be a problem. Stimulation of the supraspinatus and posterior deltoid muscles is often used to provide support to the joint and decrease pain. Faghri et al[31] found that electrical stimulation of supraspinatus and posterior deltoid muscles during the acute stage of recovery after stroke caused significant reduction in the pain and shudder sublimation in a group of hemiplegic stroke patients.

The muscles most typically stimulated for functional use in the lower limbs are the quadriceps to allow for stance, the ankle dorsiflexors for step response, and the hip abductors and extensors for stability in stance. In addition to strengthening the ankle dorsiflexors by stimulation of the peroneal nerve, a mass flexion withdrawal response can be elicited that not only lifts the foot up but also flexes the knee and hip to allow for stepping (Figure 17-4). Stimulation of the hip muscles may be difficult because of their size and location and may need to be done in the gravity-eliminated position to start, before incorporation into functional activities.

FES should be incorporated into traditional treatment programs as one of a group of effective tools in the treatment of patients with SCI. In addition to being used to initiate volitional motor control and to strengthen atrophied muscles, soft tissue contractures in patients with an incomplete SCI can be managed

in conjunction with serial casting, splinting, and stretching. In the clinical setting, FES has also been shown as a successful substitute for traditional types of orthoses in functional ambulation programs, stimulating enhanced stance stability or facilitating limb swing through during ambulation. Patients with an incomplete SCI benefit from using FES orthotics by initiating some functional carryover of volitional movement.

When FES is used with patients who have incomplete injuries, many of the stimulation parameters need to be adjusted carefully to allow for the best motor response within the patient's pain tolerance threshold. Current amplitude needs to be adjusted slowly to allow the patient to accommodate to the sensory discomfort. For most patients, FES requires some getting used to, so care should be taken not to exceed the patient's sensory tolerance. Even if the level of stimulation is not high enough to elicit a contraction at first, the patient should continue to be stimulated at the low level to allow for sensory adaptation and eventual tolerance to higher settings. Within 1 week, the patient should be able to adapt to appropriate stimulation levels to elicit a muscle response if stimulated at least one time per day. The length of the treatment session depends on the patient's goals and the muscle response. Sessions may range from 15 minutes up to several hours per day for strengthening.

When trying to elicit a muscular response in the patient with an incomplete SCI, the following factors may affect success:

- Excess adipose tissue impedes FES and is a poor conductor.
- Lower motor neuron involvement or severe muscle atrophy may cause lack of contraction response.
- Neural damage such as a nerve root or plexus injury coexisting with the SCI may cause lack of muscle response.
- Pain tolerance or hypersensitivity to stimulation may make treatment at the low levels of stimulation tolerated ineffective.
- Skin irritation and burns related to hypersensitivity from the polar effects of the stimulation when a symmetrical waveform is not selected

Contraindications to FES, in addition to the general contraindications for all types of FES reviewed previously, include orthopedic instability in the area of electrode placement, inappropriate stimulation in an area of muscle surgical transfer, and stimulation over open wounds or incision sites.

Goals and expectations of FES must be clearly understood before treatment is initiated. The patient needs to be voluntarily interested in participating and realistic about the treatment applications or the treatment will not be as effective. It is important that the patient understands that FES will not repair or regenerate nerves but rather may strengthen existing already innervated muscles and assist in improving function.

CARDIOVASCULAR RECONDITIONING

As the population with SCI ages and older adult patients survive their injuries, cardiovascular disease has become one of the main causes of morbidity and mortality in individuals with SCI.[15] Within the first 3 months of an SCI, a significant decline occurs in aerobic capacity, with declines in maximal oxygen consumption of more than 40%. In people with tetraplegia, data show a decrease in maximum heart rate, stroke volume, cardiac output,

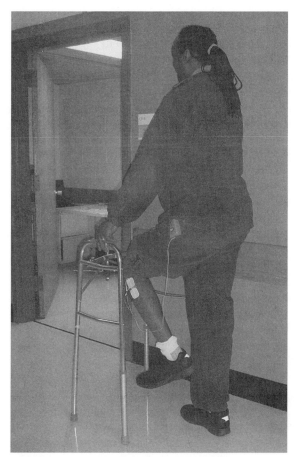

FIGURE 17-4 FES of the dorsiflexors through the peroneal nerve achieves mass lower limb flexor withdrawal, which not only lifts the foot up but also flexes the knee and hip to allow for stepping.

and the development of left ventricular atrophy.[32] Research on maximal oxygen consumption (VO_2) in individuals with chronic SCI reveal an inverse relationship to the level of SCI. In addition, people with SCI report decreases in lean body mass and increases in fat mass after injury (see Chapter 18).

To slow the decline of the cardiovascular system, it was obvious that most patients with SCI would benefit from some form of aerobic activity to prevent cardiac deconditioning but that they are unable to perform such activity at the required intensity level. A device to allow patients with SCI to perform aerobic activity using their larger leg muscles to help to prevent cardiac decline was needed; once developed it became known as a functional electrical stimulation leg cycle ergometry (FES-LCE) system. The prototype for this FES bicycle was developed in the late 1970s by Jerrold Petrofsky, an electrical engineer at Wright State University, and received FDA approval in 1984. Commercially available under the brand name of REGYS, it was followed less than 2 years later by the ERGYS, which is a home unit that allows individuals the option to exercise outside the clinic environment (Figure 17-5).

The REGYS and ERGYS are computerized closed-loop FES systems, which consist of a lower limb cycle ergometer in combination with a surface electrode system. The ergometer measures the work performed by the muscles. Both systems use two electrodes (i.e., active and ground) per muscle with a total of 12 electrodes dispersed over the quadriceps, glutei, and hamstring muscles. These electrodes are hooked up to color-coded wires to ensure stimulation of the correct muscle at the appropriate time. Muscle stimulation is activated sequentially to produce a smooth pedaling motion through the ergometer, with the feet placed into an open boot that is attached to the pedals. During the process, closed-loop feedback is provided by measuring the cycling rate, the impedance needed to deliver the stimulus, and the current being used. The microprocessor regulates the delivery of electrical stimulation to the patient to allow cycling rates between 35 and 50 revolutions/min (rpm). The system will automatically shut off if the impedance exceeds 16,000 ohms, if the current exceeds 220 volts, or if the cycling rate drops below 35 rpm.

If muscle response is poor when an individual begins an FES cycle ergometry program, assisted cycling is used to facilitate the desired response and build muscle contractility. The goal is for the patient to be able to cycle for an amount of time to produce an aerobic effect (i.e., at least 20 minutes 3 days a week). An added load or resistance on the flywheel is also available to continually increase the workload.

Unit parameters for the REGYS and ERGYS include various waveforms, pulse widths, pulse frequencies, and amplitudes. The current systems have the capacity for up to 16 different waveforms. Changing the waveform can allow for better performance in delivery of the stimulation depending on the individual patient's response to the stimulus and the factors that affect that response (e.g., atrophy, sensation, impedance). Currently, the units have pulse widths ranging from 300 to 500 microseconds. This range allows greater variability for individuals who are not as easily stimulated. Lengthening the pulse width allows for an increased response to electrical stimulation, but also increases the chance of polar effects beneath that electrode and the possibility of skin irritation or burns. Both systems have four options available for pulse frequency (30, 40, 50, and 60 pps). This variability allows for more options when stimulating the sensate patient. The amplitude can range from 0 to 140 mA. The variability in intensity again allows for more options when trying to get the desired muscle response.

Candidates

Candidates for FES-LCE include individuals with complete SCI above T12. FES cycle ergometry has been used with appropriate monitoring in individuals who are ventilator dependent, allowing them an effective exercise option. People with incomplete SCI above T12 and individuals with spina bifida who can tolerate

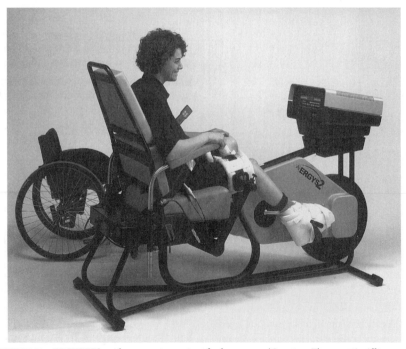

FIGURE 17-5 ERGYS FES-cycle ergometry system for home use. (Courtesy Therapeutic Alliances Inc.)

sufficient stimulation levels to obtain the desired results are also candidates. FES cycle ergometry may benefit individuals with incomplete injuries by helping to strengthen weak but intact muscles as well as providing aerobic exercise. FES is ineffective in stimulating lower motor neuron injuries below T12.

Contraindications

In addition to the contraindications listed previously for all types of FES, specific contraindications for FES-LCE include severe respiratory disease, spinal instability, pathological or unhealed fractures, joint disarticulation, and fixed contractures in the lower limbs.

General Precautions

Specific precautions for FES cycling include heterotopic ossification limiting ROM in the lower limbs, metal hardware in the femur, hypertension, hypotension, and venous thrombosis.

Limiting Factors

Limiting factors may include severe obesity, severe spasticity or flaccidity, limited ROM in the knees or hips, motivation, realism, and frequent urinary tract infections (UTI), or other infections. Clinical anecdotes indicate that individuals with frequent UTIs or those taking antibiotics do not cycle as well as when not compromised by these infections.

Risk Factors

Potential risk factors involved with FES include the following:

- Risk of cardiac insult or severe blood pressure fluctuations in patients with unstable cardiovascular systems
- Potential for joint disarticulation or fracture
- Potential to increase neurogenic pain
- Risk of increasing spasticity in susceptible patients
- Potential for skin irritation and burns during strong or prolonged levels of electrical stimulation
- Risk of outgrowing clothing, braces, or even wheelchairs as a result of increased muscle bulk

Benefits

Reported benefits of FES-LCE include improved cardiovascular status, increased respiratory capacity, increased muscle bulk, increased circulation and skin integrity, improved psychological well-being, temporarily decreased spasticity, and increased bone density (Clinical Note: Benefits of Functional Electrical Stimulation Cycle Ergometry). Research has supported many of these claims by analyzing the physiological responses and gains made with FES-LCE system use.[32-34]

CLINICAL NOTE **Benefits of Functional Electrical Stimulation Cycle Ergometry**

- Improved cardiovascular status
- Increased respiratory capacity
- Increased muscle bulk
- Increased circulation and skin integrity
- Improved psychological well-being
- Decreased spasticity (temporary)
- Increased bone density.

During FES-LCE, an increase occurs in aerobic capacity, as measured by an increase in peak oxygen consumption, pulmonary ventilation, heart rate, blood pressure, and cardiac output (i.e., enhanced venous return and improved left ventricular end-diastolic volume), with greater increases noted in subjects with paraplegia versus tetraplegia.[29,32,34] These increases are linear with the metabolic demand on the muscle. FES-LCE also results in increased blood flow in the lower limbs and reduced venous pooling during FES-LCE, which is associated with a reduced rate-pressure product and increased endurance.[35] In patients with tetraplegia, FES-LCE can result in an improvement in left ventricular mass.[35]

Physiological response to participating in a 12-week FES-LCE training program is similar to that of able-bodied athletes undergoing an exercise program. During submaximal exercise using FES-LCE, the heart rate and blood pressure response to any certain level of exercise decreases, indicating a training effect.[36] In addition, the endurance for ergometer pedaling increases because more work is done at a similar heart rate and systolic blood pressure and as muscle bulk is increased.[29] Individuals with paraplegia who regularly use FES-LCE have been shown to have decreases in their resting blood pressure (systolic and diastolic) after a 12-week FES-LCE program compared with values before initiation of the FES-LCE program.[36] Interestingly, after the same 12-week program, individuals with tetraplegia had an increase in resting systolic blood pressure and heart rate, with values normalizing from low pre-exercise levels.

Most FES cycling units now interface with either pregelled self-adhering electrodes or custom-measured garments for ease of application (Figure 17-6). Self-adhering electrodes tend to provide better contact with the skin than garments, although garments may be easier for a patient or caregiver to apply versus placement of electrodes. Garments do need to be cared for carefully and they last for approximately 1 year.

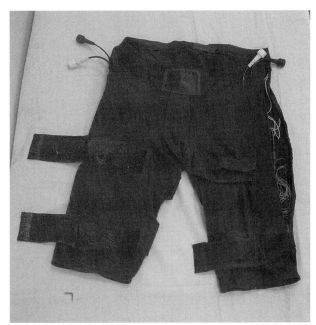

FIGURE 17-6 Pregelled, self-adhering electrodes embedded in garments for use with FES cycle.

Other devices continue to be developed that offer different stimulation parameters and ergonomics, but all work on essentially the same premise and with similar components. Another cycle ergometer, the RT300, is a stand-alone device that does not require the patient to transfer but rather allows access from his wheelchair (Figure 17-7). The patient secures his feet in the pedals, supports his legs with the leg guides, and uses surface electrodes to and from his leg muscle groups to interface with the computerized controls. Built-in safety features include spasm and fatigue detection and automatic speed control and a cut-off switch. The RT300 also incorporates Bluetooth technology to allow data collection from each session that monitors patient performance and progress. Such parameters as session duration, cycling velocity (rpm), fatigue resistance, and level of resistance can be monitored and recorded. Depending on a patient's individual needs and responses to stimulation, clinical performance may be better on one system versus the other.

Future Advances

Although there is sufficient evidence that FES-LCE exercise reduces the risk for development of secondary impairments in people with upper motor neuron lesions,[37,38] there is little understanding about how best to combine cycling with FES to maximize exercise performance. In terms of leg cycling exercise, performance can be evaluated on the basis of an individual's pedaling efficiency (i.e., mechanical efficiency), which is defined as the ratio between power output (PO) and power input (PI). During leg cycling, PI can be measured as the amount of force muscles contribute at an instantaneous cycling cadence, whereas PO is a measure of the product of cycling cadence and flywheel break resistance.

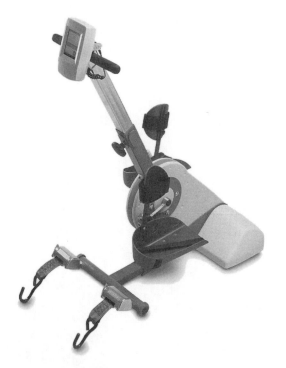

FIGURE 17-7 The RT300 is a portable, compact, and adjustable FES cycle that can be used from a wheelchair. The touch sensitive and color-coded graphical interface allows the user to control the therapy session. (Courtesy Restorative Therapies Inc.)

Research has found that most subjects who participate in FES-induced leg cycling have early muscle fatigue at very low PO levels. Low PO is generated by the stimulated muscles that elicit relatively high oxygen consumption (VO_2). Pollack et al[34] reported that the average untrained SCI subject could only briefly maintain cycling with marginal overall gains in cycling time and PO during 4 to 8 weeks of exercise. Moreover, others have reported that gross efficiency (i.e., mechanical efficiency/metabolic efficiency) during FES-induced leg cycling to be only 3% to 4% as opposed to 25% to 30% obtained by able-bodied individuals during standard upright leg cycling.[38] The energy lost during FES equates to more than 95% of the total energy that was invested in pedaling. The most important questions that should be answered are (1) how to improve the performance of FES-LCE by changing either the timing of stimulation or sequencing of stimulation and (2) how to develop strategies that reduce the strength requirements by either increasing the number of the muscles stimulated or individualizing the pattern of muscle activation to increase the number of people capable of using FES-ILC as a means of exercise. Researchers are trying to answer these questions by developing appropriate musculoskeletal models for FES-LCE and optimizing the cycling performance for these individuals.[39,40]

As technology continues to advance, it is anticipated that various options for FES cycling will become available in the marketplace that suit the needs of more consumers at affordable prices. The RT300 FES bike is an example of a product that may be an affordable alternative for clinic and home use.

RESTORATION OF UPPER LIMB FUNCTION

There are more than 54,000 individuals with C5 to C6 tetraplegia in the United States today and approximately 2000 new injuries each year.[41] These patients lack the ability to grasp and release objects without assistance. Neuroprostheses for the upper limb were initially developed by using surface electrodes in the 1960s.[12] Building on that pioneering work, several FES systems have been developed to restore controlled movement to the paralyzed hand. This involves substituting for palmar and lateral grasp and providing a means to change from one type of grasp to the other while also providing the ability to release objects.

The Freehand system is an implantable neuroprosthetic process that restores hand grasp function to selected SCI individuals and has been demonstrated to assist individuals with C5 to C6 tetraplegia in upper limb activities of daily living (ADL) skills. It is typically combined with tendon transfer surgery for optimal results (see Chapter 10). The first system was implanted in 1986 and the Freehand system received FDA approval in 1997. Offered at 22 facilities worldwide, the Freehand system became clinically successful and well accepted by patients; however, its manufacturer withdrew from the SCI market in 2001. At that time a second-generation Freehand system had been developed with the ability to provide greater upper limb function and research was continuing.[12]

Components of the original system include an implanted electrode system to eight selected forearm and hand muscles.[42] Some of the muscles stimulated include the extensor pollicis longus, flexor pollicis longus, extensor digitorum communis, flexor digitorum profundus, abductor pollicis brevis, and adductor pollicis brevis.[43] The electrode leads are then tunneled subcutaneously to an internal stimulator located in the upper chest. An electrical signal is generated by an external microprocessor and transmitted through an external transmitting coil placed over the implanted stimulator. A small positional joystick, which senses changes in shoulder position, is placed on the chest with a telescoping rod attached across the shoulder joint opposite the limb with the implanted electrodes. The joystick allows the user to proportionally regulate grasp force and hand opening with changes in shoulder position on the contralateral side. Shoulder retraction produces hand opening and protraction closes the hand. The system is controlled by a portable microprocessor. There is a subcutaneous electrode that gives sensory feedback, typically placed under the skin near the clavicle. The Freehand system uses a biphasic waveform with four amplitude settings varying from 2 to 20 MA.

Other upper limb FES systems have shown promise, including the Bionic Glove and FESMate. The Handmaster developed by NESS in Israel is commercially available worldwide as the NESS H200, a surface system FES technology that is FDA approved (Figure 17-8, A).[13,14] The H200 is a noninvasive device that is worn on the forearm and hand, which enables a patient to perform ADLs by helping the hand to open and close and increasing ROM and strength, in addition to improving circulation (Figure 17-8, B).[14] Although it is primarily marketed for patients with stroke, traumatic brain injury, multiple sclerosis, and cerebral palsy, Alon and McBride[14] have reported on the functional gains achieved in individuals with C5 to C6 SCI.

Candidates

SCI candidates for upper limb Freehand neuroprostheses implantation have C5 or C6 (motor level) tetraplegia, with intact lower motor neuron innervation of the forearm and hand muscles.[44] Patients must have functional ROM of the upper limb, adequate strength in the proximal muscles of the shoulder to perform functional tasks with the implanted device, intact vision, and be medically stable and skeletally mature. Implantation is possible and has been performed in those who have not reached skeletal maturity, but it is difficult because provisions for growth of the limb must be made.

Contraindications

In addition to general contraindications for FES described previously, additional contraindications for the Freehand system and the NESS H200 include uncontrolled upper limb spasticity, a history of active or recurrent sepsis, or an implanted cardiac or phrenic pacemaker.

Implantation of the Freehand System

Preparation for surgery over a 4- to 12-week period includes conditioning of involuntary muscles with a surface electrical stimulation program, strengthening of voluntary muscles, ROM of the arm and hand, and patient education as to unit use and function. The surgical procedure involves implantation of electrodes to excitable muscles, contracture release as needed, and commonly, tendon transfers to optimize function and substitute for function of denervated muscles. Surgery is normally performed on the dominant hand.

A postsurgical management of up to 12 weeks includes casted immobilization of 2 to 4 weeks. If the implant surgery is done in combination with tendon transfers, immobilization could be for a total of 6 to 8 weeks. It is very important that the patient understands the time frame to avoid frustration and to arrange for appropriate care needs. The rehabilitation phase consists of 4 to 6 weeks of stretching, strengthening, reconditioning, and retraining muscles including ADL functions. Patient education on unit use and function is also a vital component of this phase.

Continuing precautions that a patient with the Freehand system must follow are significant and include the following:
- Patients cannot have magnetic resonance imaging (MRI) of any part of the body (x-rays and computed tomography are fine).
- Patients cannot have therapeutic ultrasound over the area of the implanted system.
- Patients cannot have diathermy regardless of the site.

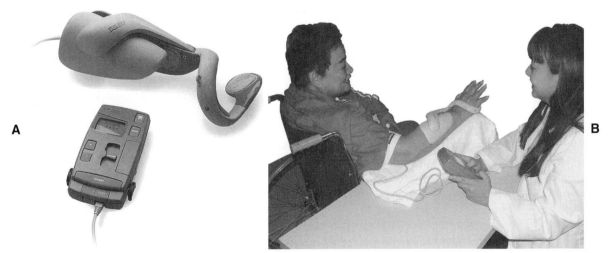

FIGURE 17-8   A, The NESS H200 is a noninvasive FES device that is worn on the forearm and hand and enables patients with neurological disorders to perform everyday activities that would not be possible without it. **B,** A therapist instructs the client in the various stimulation patterns that support tasks and are used for therapy. (Courtesy Bioness Inc.)

- Patients should avoid surface stimulation to the instrumented arm (including transcutaneous electrical nerve stimulation or electrodiagnostic studies).
- External parts of the system should not get wet.
- Patients need antibiotic prophylaxis before dental procedures.
- Patients should not have any procedures (blood pressure, intravenous injections, blood draws) on the instrumented arm.

As with the other previously stated FES precautions, at this time this device's effects are unknown on pregnancy, AD, or seizures, so precautions should be taken when dealing with these conditions. In addition, implantation of this system may result in blockage of x-rays and mammograms in areas of device placement. It has also been noted that stimulation with this unit leads to increased serum creatine phosphokinase (CPK) levels, which could mask cardiac symptoms of elevated CPK levels. Further testing would be necessary to identify a cardiac problem. Use of muscle relaxants may also affect the way the stimulated muscles react, so these medications may alter or prohibit functional outcome. It is recommended that this system be used with caution at all times because of the possibility of malfunction. Higher-risk activities of daily living (e.g., driving, carrying hot objects) may not be advisable. It is also imperative that skin checks are done daily to ensure that there are no signs of burns or device extrusion.

Benefits

Benefits of the Freehand system include increased level of activity performed, decreased assistance required, decreased time and effort required to perform ADLs, increased ROM, increased grasp force, improved grasp-release test, decreased reliance on orthoses, and excellent user satisfaction with increased self-esteem, confidence, independence, enhanced appearance, and potential cost savings.[24,45,46]

Benefits of the NESS H200 are a safe and noninvasive neuroprosthesis that allows ADL activities of grasp, lifting (e.g., utensils, video cassette, telephone), and release as well as improved grip strength and FES-induced finger motion.[12,13] The H200 provides a self-adjusting and superior fit enhanced by custom-fitted electrodes and multiple stimulation patterns that ensure reproducible contact during functional and therapeutic activities. In addition, it is noninvasive, versatile to many settings, cost efficient, and easy to use.

STANDING AND GAIT

The goals of lower limb FES for gait in individuals with SCI are to provide a system for ambulation that is safe, reliable, easy to use, functional for community distances, energy efficient, inexpensive, and cosmetically acceptable.[19,47] It has been estimated that approximately 11% of all patients with SCI in the United States are potential users of a lower limb FES system for gait.[48]

Ambulation systems currently are classified as (1) ambulation with orthoses, (2) hybrid systems using FES in combination with orthoses, and (3) FES systems using surface or implanted electrodes typically in conjunction with ankle-foot orthoses (AFO) to provide ankle stability. Hybrid systems seek to improve mobility

restoration by combining two technologies. Examples of hybrid systems include using a knee-ankle-foot orthosis with electrical stimulation to the quadriceps, or applying FES to gluteal muscles and quadriceps in combination with an orthotic system such as the ParaWalker.

As discussed in Chapter 16, energy expenditure during ambulation in patients with SCI is typically high. The goal of using FES with orthoses is to decrease the energy expended during gait to a level that is practical. The lowest energy expenditure during gait occurs with the use of a reciprocal gait orthosis (RGO) in combination with FES to the thigh muscles (hybrid system). The addition of FES to the thigh muscles with the RGO decreases energy expenditure by 16% and doubles the speed of ambulation (from 1.2 km/hr with the RGO alone to 2.4 km/hr with the hybrid system).[49] However, using the RGO involves a significant amount of bracing because the brace provides the bulk of the antigravity support. The practical implication is that these systems often take 30 to 45 minutes to don, after which the patient can walk for 800 meters and stand up and sit down four to six times before fatigue requires him to stop.

Other hybrid systems are under development. In one model, the patient wears a custom-made garment enhanced by surface electrodes in conjunction with the lightweight titanium graphite hip-knee-ankle-foot orthoses (HKAFO). The entire system weighs approximately 3 pounds and is undergoing FDA trials.

Another, the ParaWalker electrical stimulation hybrid orthosis, is an HKAFO that incorporates a rigid body brace.[50] Energy consumption with the ParaWalker is about 3.5 times greater than the patient's resting level. Electrical stimulation of the stance-side gluteal muscles reduces the energy cost of locomotion by approximately 6% to 8% compared with ambulation with the ParaWalker alone.

Research in implanted FES for ambulation has been in progress for 20 years and remains at trial phase without FDA approval. Implanted FES systems for gait were initially designed to use up to 50 active electrodes allowing for 25 muscle stimulation points in each leg without orthoses. As in upper limb implantable systems, the electrodes target specific muscles for stimulation to obtain precise responses to ambulation commands. A large number of channels were thought to be needed for the functional ambulation capacity that was desired. More recently, as implants have undergone modifications, the number of electrodes needed has been reduced. Implanted systems allow for ambulation on level surfaces and stairs. The stimulator includes a menu similar to that of a word processor with commands of walk, sit, stand, step up, and step down. Patients generally use walkers with hand control switches as the interface. Ideally, such systems should be totally implanted with closed-loop feedback. Potential complications associated with implanted electrode systems include infections in the area of electrode placement, fractures, and device extrusion.

Ambulation with systems that are primarily based on FES has been found to require more energy than using an RGO with FES, or long-leg braces, depending on the speed of ambulation. Marsolais et al[47,51] studied patients with SCI who had implanted intramuscular electrodes in nine muscles in the lower limbs and walked using FES and a rolling walker with a reciprocal gait. This group was then compared with another group using long-leg brace ambulation. During FES walking, energy consumption was 59% to 75% of maximal aerobic power. However, as the speed of FES walking increased, there was no increase in energy costs; energy efficiency equaled that of long-leg brace ambulation. At speeds between 0.4 and 0.6 m/s, FES walking energy costs were similar to those of long-leg brace ambulation.

There are several different approaches to lower limb surface FES for ambulation. The motor points of different muscles can be directly stimulated in a sequential fashion to provide movements. Alternately, nerves can be stimulated along their course before they enter the muscle. This is typically the technique used with the peroneal nerve to the ankle dorsiflexors. The stimulation provokes a reflex withdrawal of the foot (i.e., triple flexion withdrawal), which can then be used for gait. Another approach to augmenting gait is to maintain constant stimulation to a muscle such as the quadriceps and use a swing-to gait with crutches or a walker.

One of the primary systems used for standing and gait is the Parastep, which was introduced in 1989 and FDA approved in 1994 (Figure 17-9). It is an open-loop system, powered by 8 AA batteries that provide 2.5 hours of continual use under normal conditions. This system is primarily an FES system, with surface self-adhesive electrodes placed over the quadriceps, glutei or paraspinals, and peroneal nerves. The six channels can be used with a pulse rate of 24 pps, pulse duration of 120 to 150 microseconds, and intensity up to 300 mA. The system includes a front-wheeled walker connected by a cable to a microprocessor that is worn by the patient and typically is used with bilateral AFOs to provide ankle stability.

Candidates

Various factors should be considered when determining whether a patient should use FES for standing and gait (Clinical Note: Factors to Consider in Candidates for Functional Electrical Stimulation Standing and Gait). Candidates for FES-assisted standing and gait are typically patients with an SCI from T4 to T12, although such systems can be used with any individual who has an incomplete cervical SCI.[48] Stimulating patients with injuries above T6 may be problematic because of potential AD and decreased strength in the upper limbs, back, and chest muscles, which makes use of the upper limbs for weight bearing difficult and challenges upper body balance. Patients must have intact lower motor neuron innervation, and electrical stimulation of the muscles must provide contraction that is powerful enough to maintain locked knees in standing. In addition, patients need to demonstrate the cognitive ability to use the system and the motivation to participate in the training program and continued use of the system outside the clinic setting. Finally, patients need to be independent in transfers, have the upper body strength to lift their bodies out of the wheelchair into a standing position with a walker, be able to demonstrate standing balance for greater than 3 minutes without orthostasis, and have the ability to maintain standing posture with less than 20% of the body weight borne by the upper limbs. They should also exhibit the absence of joint disease in the lower limbs, full ROM at the ankles, functional ROM at the hips and knees (i.e., less than 10 degrees hip or knee contracture), and the absence of spasticity that might preclude standing.

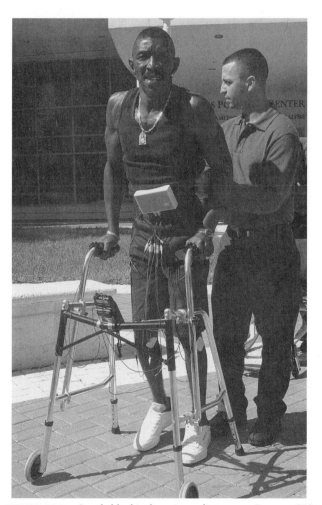

FIGURE 17-9 Guarded by his therapist, a client uses a Parastep FES system to enable ambulation. (Courtesy Dr. Mark S. Nash, The Miami Project to Cure Paralysis.)

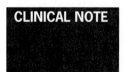

CLINICAL NOTE	Factors to Consider in Candidates for Functional Electrical Stimulation Standing and Gait

- Patient with lesions from T4 to T12
- Patient with intact lower motor neuron innervation
- Patient who demonstrates cognitive ability required for system use
- Patient who is motivated to participate in the training program and continue using system
- Patient who is independent in transfers
- Patient who has upper body strength to lift his body out of the wheelchair and into a standing position with a walker
- Patient who demonstrates standing balance for greater than 3 minutes without orthostasis
- Patient who is able to maintain standing posture with less than 20% of the body weight borne by the upper limbs
- Patient who has full ROM at ankles and functional ROM at hips and knees
- Patient without joint disease in the lower limbs
- Patient without spasticity that might limit standing

Contraindications

Contraindications to FES-assisted standing and gait include the general contraindications and precautions previously listed. In addition, patients should not use lower limb FES if they have a history of long bone fractures from osteoporosis or if their bone density is less than 55% on x-ray scan. Other contraindications include lower limb joint disease (e.g., arthritis or severe heterotopic ossification), decreased lower limb ROM with contractures, or severe lower limb spasticity that precludes standing.

Training

Before using an FES system for standing and gait, patients must undergo a training program. Training for the Parastep system focuses on several aspects:

- Increasing strength and endurance of the quadriceps in response to electrical stimulation
- Ability to reproduce the triple flexion response
- Cardiovascular endurance
- Maintenance of upright posture

In addition, standing and balance with the system should be practiced before the patient begins taking steps with FES stimulation. Finally, if use of the system is successful, training with the unit for use in the home setting is initiated.

Limitations

Limitations of FES-assisted ambulation systems include electrode failure, FES-induced muscle fatigue, excessive energy expenditure, FES-induced AD or spasticity, and cumbersome electrical hardware with an inefficient user-machine interface.[47] Reasons that patients discontinue using these systems include the time required to don and doff the apparatus, difficulties with operation, and problems incorporating use of the system into the home environment and living situation.[19] As practical applications, these systems may not be as functional as wheelchair mobility because the speed of ambulation with lower limb FES systems is slow, typically in the range of 0.1 to 0.4 m/sec. In addition, the average comfortable walking distance with these devices varies from 20 m to 200 m because of the rapid onset of muscle fatigue.

A follow-up study of the Parastep system revealed that none of the participants with an injury level above T4 reached independence with the system.[48] Thirty-one patients completed the training program. All patients could stand with the Parastep system; 92% could stand and take steps and 34% could eventually ambulate using the system without the assistance of another person. The average distance ambulated was 99 m without rest, and a total distance ambulated during a training session was 445 m. The review showed that 82% of the participants continued to use the system regularly at 6-month follow-up.

Benefits

The use of FES-assisted ambulation or hybrid systems increased strength of lower limbs, increased bulk of muscles, increased muscular and cardiovascular endurance, independent standing and ambulation, improved self-esteem, and a perception of enhanced well-being (Clinical Note: Benefits of Functional Electrical Stimulation–Assisted Ambulation or Hybrid Systems).[18,48,52]

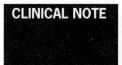

CLINICAL NOTE Benefits of Functional Electrical Stimulation–Assisted Ambulation or Hybrid Systems

- Increased strength of lower limbs
- Increased bulk of muscles
- Increased muscular and cardiovascular endurance
- Independent standing and ambulation
- Improved self-esteem
- Enhanced well-being

AUGMENTATION OF BLADDER FUNCTION

FES can also augment or restore bladder function in individuals with SCI. More than 2000 patients worldwide have been implanted with some type of electrical bladder stimulator over the last 40 years.[10] Bladder stimulation can enhance voiding capability, decrease infections, and achieve continence.

Candidates

Candidates for FES bladder augmentation systems generally have not responded to traditional techniques of bladder management, have frequent or chronic UTIs, show intolerance to catheterization, have frequent AD from bowel or bladder sources, or have uncontrolled incontinence (Clinical Note: Factors to Consider in Candidates for Functional Electrical Stimulation Bladder Systems). The patient must have intact reflex bladder contractions with a complete or incomplete suprasacral SCI with upper motor neuron preservation.

CLINICAL NOTE Factors to Consider in Candidates for Functional Electrical Stimulation Bladder Systems

- Patient who does not responded to traditional bladder management techniques
- Patient who has frequent or chronic UTIs
- Patient who has an intolerance to catheterization
- Patient who has frequent AD from bowel or bladder sources
- Patient who has uncontrolled incontinence
- Patient who has intact reflex bladder contractions with a complete or incomplete suprasacral SCI

Contraindications

Contraindications to FES bladder augmentation systems include severe bladder fibrosis with inadequate bladder compliance and capacity or reflex erections that are adequate for satisfactory intercourse.[42]

Application of Functional Electrical Stimulation Bladder Augmentation Systems

Electrical stimulation of the urinary system can be applied at a variety of sites: direct stimulation of the bladder wall, pelvic nerve stimulation, spinal cord stimulation, and sacral root stimulation (e.g., intradurally at the ventral roots or extradurally).[53,54] Direct stimulation of the bladder wall is accomplished by using multiple electrodes to the detrusor. This technique is compatible with lower motor neuron injuries. The spread of stimulation, however, can cause pain, defecation, erection, sphincter contraction, and contraction of pelvic and leg musculature. Success with the technique has been limited by problems with the interface between the electrodes and the bladder wall. Pelvic nerve stimulation is also limited because it is technically difficult to implant the electrodes and stimulation can cause reflexive external sphincter activity.

Direct spinal cord stimulation theoretically enables selective detrusor contraction; unfortunately, results vary greatly depending on the location of the electrode tip. The electrode tip needs to be implanted in the intermediolateral region of the sacral cord, and the parasympathetic motor neuron pool may be damaged in the process.

Sacral root stimulation is the technically optimal site for electrode attachment; this technique is most commonly used in patients with SCI.[55] Electrical stimulation is typically limited to the ventral part of the sacral roots. When the dorsal roots have been severed, an areflexic bladder, accompanied by increased capacity and no reflex contractions, results. Stimulation of the ventral part of the sacral root results in contraction of both the bladder and the sphincter.[55] Because the sphincter is striated muscle, it contracts and relaxes quickly. The smooth muscle of the detrusor contracts and relaxes slowly, which results in a poststimulus voiding pattern. This is characterized by bursts of voiding between pulse trains. This technique has been shown to result in complete bladder emptying.

Ventral root stimulation was introduced in 1984 in Europe. The original system is the FineTech-Brindley stimulator. At 6-month follow-up, complete continence during daytime was achieved in 73% of patients, and 86% of patients were continent at night. Long-term follow-up revealed that 85% of users could effectively void with the stimulator alone and had low residual urine volumes.[42] Significant increases in bladder capacity and compliance were achieved in all patients, and 95% of users had less than 60 ml of residual urine.[10] This FineTech stimulator is FDA approved and was marketed in the United States as VOCARE Bladder System by NeuroControl; however, it was not covered by Medicare and is currently available directly from FineTech-Brindley in England.

The system consists of a surgically implanted stimulator and receiver, which are connected to electrodes that are attached to the anterior sacral roots (i.e., S2 to S4). A posterior rhizotomy is performed at the time of implantation. Because the rhizotomy is permanent, it is important that the client understand the implications of this procedure. The system is controlled by an external microprocessor, and a transmitter is used to transmit signals through the skin to the receiver that is implanted subcutaneously. The system can be used starting 3 to 4 days after surgery. The control unit has three settings with different electrical parameters for augmentation of bowel, bladder, and erectile function, although currently there are no long-term data on the effects on bowel and erectile function.

Another system manufactured by Medtronic, Inc., called the InterStim neurostimulator, has been FDA approved for use in the United States since 1997. Although not developed for individuals with SCI, the device has been shown to greatly reduce or eliminate urinary urgency, resulting in incontinence for those individuals who have nonobstructive bladder dysfunction,[56] and therefore has similar indications as the FineTech system, which may make it an option of choice when conservative treatments are no longer effective. An additional advantage is that the system is completely reversible and can be removed at any time without damage to the nerves. The implantable neurostimulator is the device that generates the electrical impulses that are sent to the sacral nerve. The neurostimulator contains a battery and electronics to create these impulses. The device is most frequently placed under the skin of the buttock, although it may be placed in the abdomen. The hand-held patient programmer allows the client to turn the neurostimulator on and off and to adjust the stimulation within the safe settings programmed by the physician. Contraindications include the use of diathermy, ultrasound, MRI, radiation, pregnancy, multiple sclerosis, or under the age of 16 years.

In 2007, a Canadian expert panel identified research priorities for the development and testing of sacral stimulator protocols for the control of micturition in SCI without rhizotomy.[57]

OTHER USES OF FUNCTIONAL ELECTRICAL STIMULATION

Research has shown mixed results in using electrical stimulation to promote wound healing.[1] It may increase blood flow, the number and function of fibroblasts in tissue, and collagen, protein, and deoxyribonucleic acid synthesis. It causes changes in expression of cellular receptors for growth factors and enhances neurite growth and extension. Pulsed electrical stimulation with alternating polarities may be the most effective for wound healing. The FDA has not approved the use of FES in wound healing.

Significant osteoporosis can develop in patients with SCI, a process that begins immediately after injury. Several studies have looked at the issue of osteopenia reversal with FES. Immobilization as a result of SCI is associated with a marked increase in osteoclastic bone resorption and pronounced decrease in osteoblastic bone formation. This imbalance between bone resorption and bone formation has been associated with the level of immobility after SCI.[58,59,60] Individuals with incomplete SCI or who are mobilized early after injury have shown less bone loss.[61] Therefore, balancing bone formation activities and avoidance of bone resorption appear to be important in preventing osteoporosis after SCI. Bloomfield et al[62] and Mohr et al[63] have reported that the used FES-induced cycling resulted in an increase in distal femur bone density at higher loads. Of further interest, after 6 months of training it was determined that serum osteocalcin, which indicates bone formation, was increased in all subjects by an average of 78%, and urinary calcium and hydroxyproline, which indicate bone resorption, did not change in the same period.[62,63] In addition, Mohr et al found that the bone mineral density of the proximal tibia increased 10% after 12 months of FES-LCE training at a frequency of three times per week.[63] Long-term use of FES-LCE can produce small increments in bone mass, localized to the skeletal regions receiving the greatest mechanical strain. It has also been shown to increase bone mineral density of the lumbar spine and increase bone turnover without concomitant resorptive activity.[1]

Moreover, FES has been studied for the prevention of deep venous thrombosis (DVT) after SCI.[1] Faghri et al[64] evaluated the effects of FES of lower limb muscles (e.g., tibialis anterior, gastrocnemius, quadriceps, and hamstring muscle groups) during 30 minutes of upright standing on the central and peripheral hemodynamic response in persons with SCI. Fourteen individuals with SCI were tested during 30 minutes of standing. Central hemodynamic responses of stroke volume, cardiac output, heart rate, arterial blood pressure, total peripheral resistance, and rate-pressure product were evaluated with impedance cardiography. They conclude that FES of the lower limb could be used as an adjunct during standing to prevent orthostatic hypotension and circulatory hypokinesis. This effect may be more beneficial to those with tetraplegia who have a compromised autonomic nervous system and may not be able to adjust their hemodynamics to the change in position. Long-term intervention is necessary to further evaluate these effects. In other research, FES to the tibialis anterior and gastrocnemius-soleus muscle groups for 23 hours per day over a 28-day period in combination with low-dose heparin in patients with acute SCI showed a significant decrease in the incidence of DVT in comparison with a group receiving low-dose heparin alone.[1] This effect is thought due in part to the effects of FES in increasing plasma fibrinolytic activity, although this use is not clinically practical because it impedes mobilization and is poorly tolerated if any sensation is present.

The use of FES for the management of spasticity has produced mixed results according to Mysiw and Jackson.[1] One protocol that included 20 minutes of stimulation showed a significant improvement in the pendulum drop test, but this improvement did not persist past 24 hours. A protocol of 8 weeks of 20 minutes of electrical stimulation two times per day, 6 days a week, demonstrated a tendency toward increasing spasticity with long-term surface electrical stimulation.

In other work, the dorsiflexor muscles of four SCI participants were activated by means of surface electrical stimulation and the isometric ankle moment was measured.[65] Short bursts of constant stimulation frequency at seven different frequencies between 8 to 50 Hz triggered spastic reactions in all participants. The onset times of spastic activity during an electrically elicited contraction shortened with increased stimulation frequency. One stimulation burst may also have a spasticity reduction effect on a subsequent burst, indicating potential short-term benefit of stimulation on spasticity in isometric conditions.

FES may be used to improve ROM. This does not require active patient participation but is poorly tolerated in the sensate patient and may interfere with other types of therapy. In addition, significant improvements in the bulk and muscle strength have been reported after 7- to 12-week sessions of FES-induced knee extension exercise.[66] FES systems are under development to stimulate lower motor neuron injuries effectively to allow patients with those lesions the same benefits of FES exercise.

Research involving FES-induced standing transfers provides stimulation to selected muscles in the lower limbs controlled by a stand-to-sit switch.[67] This technology could enable patients with tetraplegia to transfer with less assistance or possibly even independently.

CLINICAL CASE STUDY Functional Electrical Stimulation Case 1

Patient History
Carl Greenspan is a 25-year-old man with a C5 tetraplegia, American Spinal Injury Association (ASIA) C diagnosis. He had a spinal cord compression injury from a motorcycle accident. Nine weeks after his injury, he is medically and orthopedically stable. He began regaining both motor function and sensory sensation at 3 weeks after injury and is still recovering strength throughout his body. He is currently attending outpatient physical and occupational therapy as well as behind-the-wheel driver's training. He is experiencing pain in his left shoulder: 0 at rest, 2 out of 10 with wheelchair propulsion, and 6 out of 10 when lifting weights greater than 5 pounds.

Carl is a recent college graduate with a master's degree in physical education. He is currently living with his parents. They have converted the downstairs study into a bedroom for him and there is a full bath on the first floor of the home. He has a rental manual wheelchair. Before his injury, Carl had been living in an apartment with two of his friends from college and was hunting for a job. He had worked in construction between college graduation and graduate school.

Patient's Self-Assessment
Carl hopes to teach physical education at the high school level and coach track and field.

Clinical Assessment
Patient Appearance
- Height 6 feet 1 inches, weight 170 pounds, body mass index 22.4

Cognitive Assessment
- Alert, oriented × 3

Cardiopulmonary Assessment
- Blood pressure 116/60 mm Hg, heart rate at rest 72 beats/min, respiratory rate 14 breaths/min, cough flows and vital capacity are reduced

Musculoskeletal and Neuromuscular Assessment

Muscle Groups	Left	Right
Elbow flexors (C5)	5	5
Wrist extensors (C6)	2	5
Elbow extensors (C7)	2	2
Finger flexors (C8)	2	2
Finger abductors (T1)	2	2
Hip flexors (L2)	2	4
Knee extensors (L3)	4	4
Ankle dorsiflexors (L4)	2	2
Long toe extensors (L5)	2	2
Ankle plantar flexors (S1)	2	2

- Motor assessment reveals C5 ASIA C, sensory assessment of light touch and pinprick is intact to C5 and impaired in all dermatomes from C6 to S4-S5.
- Deep tendon reflexes 3+ below the level of lesion

Integumentary and Sensory Assessment
- Skin is intact throughout and sensory intact to C5 with impairment in all dermatomes to light touch and pinprick from C6 to S4-S5.

Range of Motion Assessment
- Passive and active ROM is within normal limits at both upper limbs.

CLINICAL CASE STUDY Functional Electrical Stimulation Case 1—cont'd

- Straight leg raise is 90 degrees in both lower limbs and dorsiflexion is 2 degrees; all other motions in the lower limbs are within functional limits.

Mobility and ADL Assessment

- Independent with bed mobility and transfers to all surfaces
- Independent with pressure relief
- Independent in manual wheelchair maneuvering on all surfaces
- Independent in all self-care ADLs
- Currently unable to drive

Evaluation of Clinical Assessment

Carl Greenspan is a 25-year-old man with a C5 tetraplegia, ASIA C diagnosis. He is being seen for outpatient physical therapy, occupational therapy, and driver's training.

Patient's Care Needs

1. Evaluation of ambulation potential including assessment of orthotics and assistive devices needs and potential to benefit from FES
2. Evaluation of shoulder pain during functional tasks and responses to a shoulder physical examination
3. Evaluation for return to work needs
4. Evaluation for wheelchair for optimal postural alignment
5. Evaluation for driving

Diagnosis and Prognosis

Diagnosis is C5 incomplete tetraplegia, ASIA C with a prognosis of full recovery of left shoulder function with skilled interventions for restoration of maximal functional independence.

Preferred Practice Patterns*

Impaired Muscle Performance (4C), Impairments Nonprogressive Spinal Cord Disorders (5H), Primary Prevention/Risk Reduction for Cardiovascular/Pulmonary Disorders (6A), Primary Prevention/Risk Reduction for Integumentary Disorders (7A)

Team Goals

1. Team to decrease patient's left shoulder pain during functional activities, including weight-bearing activities with assistive devices during gait
2. Team to educate patient on prevention of future shoulder injuries
3. Team to evaluate the use of FES for the reduction of pain and facilitation of muscle recruitment
4. Team to evaluate ambulation, including FES to lower limb muscles
5. Team to discuss wheelchair design, postural alignment, and potential needs for wheelchair purchase
6. Team to discuss capacity to return to work or modified work
7. Patient to complete driver training instruction and pass the driver's examination

Patient Goals

"I want to be able to walk, teach physical education, and live on my own. I want to go back to sports without pain in my left shoulder."

Care Plan
Treatment Plan and Rationale

- Initiate physical therapy interventions for the reduction of pain in patient's left shoulder and restoration of pain-free function.
- Instruct patient about strategies for prevention of future shoulder injuries.
- Initiate driver's training instruction.
- Initiate ambulation training on all surfaces.

Interventions

- Instruct patient in joint protection to prevent upper limb injury.
- Initiate FES protocols applicable for restoration of upper limb function.
- Gait training with appropriate devices to maximize ambulation independence
- Initiate FES protocols applicable for restoration of lower limb function.
- Examine wheelchair propulsion in various wheelchairs to optimize alignment and minimize shoulder injury.

Documentation and Team Communication

- Team will complete The Wheelchair Users Shoulder Pain Index (WUSPI) biweekly.
- Team will refer patient to orthotics clinic for evaluation of lower limb orthotics related to FES impact on gait performance.
- Team will refer patient to wheelchair seating clinic for evaluation of wheelchair setup (alignment) to remove potential causes of shoulder pain resulting from poor wheelchair seating.
- Team will refer patient to driver's training and discuss potential vehicle modifications.
- Team will document patient's potential to return to work given functional independence.

Follow-Up Assessment

- Biweekly team conferences for timely attainment of goals
- Reassessment for consultation with other services

Critical Thinking Exercises

Consider factors that will influence patient education, therapy, and team care decisions unique to Carl's SCI when answering the following questions:

1. What potential FES interventions will facilitate muscle activation in the left upper limb and reduce pain?
2. What precautions should be considered when using FES with Carl?
3. What waveform is appropriate with the least amount of skin irritation?
4. What is the recommended stimulus frequency range for FES? What can happen as the frequency increases?
5. What considerations should the therapist make regarding electrode size and placement?
6. Describe FES use for Carl's lower limbs.

*Guide to physical therapist practice, rev. ed. 2, Alexandria, VA, 2003, American Physical Therapy Association.

CLINICAL CASE STUDY Functional Electrical Stimulation Case 2

Patient History

Jamie Blanchart is a 50-year-old woman with a T6 paraplegia, ASIA A diagnosis from a skiing injury. She is 3 years post injury. She completed both inpatient and outpatient therapy. Jamie has no medical complications at present but has a history of UTIs and two episodes of DVT.

Jamie is an accountant who works part time. She is married with two children, ages 18 and 20 years. She uses a lightweight manual wheelchair and drives an adapted van. Her home is fully accessible and includes a small workout room off her bedroom.

Patient's Self-Assessment

Jamie wants to perform exercise conditioning in her home to keep herself in optimal physical condition.

Clinical Assessment
Patient Appearance

- Height 5 feet 4 inches, weight 112 pounds, body mass index 19.2

Cognitive Assessment

- Alert, oriented × 3

Cardiopulmonary Assessment

- Blood pressure 110/70 mm Hg, heart rate at rest 76 beats/min, respiratory rate 14 breaths/min, cough flows are minimally ineffective, vital capacity is minimally reduced (2.5 L).

Musculoskeletal and Neuromuscular Assessment

- Motor assessment reveals T6 ASIA A, sensory T6.
- Deep tendon reflexes 3+ below the level of lesion

Integumentary and Sensory Assessment

- Skin is intact, sensory intact to T6.

Range of Motion Assessment

- Passive and active ROM is within normal limits at both upper limbs.
- Straight leg raise is 110 degrees in both lower limbs and dorsiflexion is 10 degrees; all other motions in the lower limbs are within functional limits.

Mobility and ADL Assessment

- Independent with bed mobility and transfers to all surfaces
- Independent with pressure relief
- Independent in manual wheelchair maneuvering on all surfaces including high-level wheelchair skills
- Independent in all self-care ADLs

Evaluation of Clinical Assessment

Jamie Blanchart is a 50-year-old woman with a T6 paraplegia, ASIA A diagnosis from a skiing injury. She is 3 years post injury and seeks instruction to keep herself in optimal physical condition.

Patient's Care Needs

1. Evaluation of exercise fitness equipment for home purchase and use
2. Education regarding exercise fitness equipment
3. Education regarding prevention of deconditioning with SCI

Diagnosis and Prognosis

Diagnosis is T6 complete paraplegia, ASIA A. Jamie's prognosis is excellent for effective management of fitness to reduce the risk of impaired muscle performance and cardiovascular-pulmonary disorders resulting from an acquired SCI.

Preferred Practice Patterns*

Impaired Muscle Performance (4C), Impairments Nonprogressive Spinal Cord Disorders (5H), Primary Prevention/Risk Reduction for Cardiovascular/Pulmonary Disorders (6A), Primary Prevention/Risk Reduction for Integumentary Disorders (7A)

Team Goals

1. Team to consult and assist patient with purchase of exercise equipment for use in her home
2. Team to instruct patient on prevention of secondary complications of SCI and the effects of exercise for prevention of physical decline
3. Team to discuss use of FES, including indications and contraindications

Patient Goals

"I want to be able to workout whenever it is convenient and I want to at home."

Care Plan
Treatment Plan & Rationale

- Evaluate and consult with patient and assist with purchase of exercise equipment for home.
- Educate patient about strategies for prevention of complications resulting from fitness decline in individuals with SCI.
- Instruct patient about potential uses of FES.

Interventions

- Initiate outpatient exercise and FES consultation.

Documentation and Team Communication

- Team consultation for patient purchase of exercise and FES equipment for home

Follow-Up Assessment

- Reassessment of consultation after 1 month

Critical Thinking Exercises

Consider factors that will influence patient education, therapy, and team care decisions unique to Jamie's SCI when answering the following questions:

1. What type of equipment for FES and conditioning should be recommended for Jamie to use at home? Why?
2. What are the benefits that Jamie might achieve?
3. What contraindications for Jamie need to be ruled out? What precautions should be considered?

---

*Guide to physical therapist practice, rev. ed. 2, Alexandria, VA, 2003, American Physical Therapy Association.

SUMMARY

FES technology affects a variety of areas in SCI rehabilitation and can be used to augment function in many situations. The technology has progressed significantly over the last 20 years with the development of numerous FDA-approved devices. It is important to understand the application of FES parameters to obtain the optimal contraction with the least sensory or skin disturbance and the lowest degree of muscle fatigue. FES produces different muscle recruitment patterns than those that occur during normal physiological contractions. Therefore, whenever volitional contraction is available, it is preferable and should be the goal. FES can improve muscle strength, endurance, and size. In addition, FES cycling produces cardiovascular conditioning. Other uses of FES include restoration of upper limb function, augmentation of bladder function, spasticity modulation, and standing for functional transfers. Widespread use of FES is limited by a variety of factors including an inefficient user-machine interface, high cost, FES-induced fatigue, user time requirements, and a limited number of appropriate candidates. Continuing research focuses on designing smaller components and better sensors for improved feedback and control of system functions. In addition, FES systems need to be developed that are individualized, more effective, easier to use, and more cost-effective.

REFERENCES

1. Mysiw W, Jackson R: Electrical stimulation. In Braddom RL, Buschbacher RM, editors: *Physical medicine and rehabilitation*, Philadelphia, 1996, WB Saunders.

2. Liberson WT, Holmquist HJ, Scot D et al: Functional electrotherapy: stimulation of the peroneal nerve synchronized with the swing phase of the gait of hemiplegic patients, *Arch Phys Med Rehabil* 42:101-105, 1960.

3. Sipski M, Delisa J: Functional electrical stimulation in spinal cord injury rehabilitation: a review of the literature, *Neurorehabilitation* 1:46-57, 1991.

4. Long C II: An electrophysiologic splint for the hand, *Arch Phys Med Rehabil* 44:499-503, 1963.

5. Vodovnik L, Long C II, Reswick JB et al: Myo-electric control of paralyzed muscles, *IEEE Trans Biomed Eng* 12:169-172, 1965.

6. Vodovnik L, Bajd T, Kralj A et al: Functional electrical stimulation for control of locomotor systems, *CRC Crit Rev Bioeng* 6:63-131, 1981.

7. Mooney V: A rationale for rehabilitation procedures based on the peripheral motor system, *Clin Orthop Relat Res* 63:7-13, 1969.

8. Reswick JB: How and when did the rehabilitation engineering center program come into being? *J Rehabil Res Dev* 39(6 Suppl): 11-16, 2002.

9. Peckham PH: Functional electrical stimulation: current status and future prospects of applications to the neuromuscular system in spinal cord injury, *Paraplegia* 25:279-288, 1987.

10. Van Kerrebroeck EV, van der Aa HE, Bosch JL et al: Sacral rhizotomies and electrical bladder stimulation in spinal cord injury, part I: clinical and urodynamic analysis, Dutch Study Group on Sacral Anterior Root Stimulation, *Eur Urol* 31:263-271, 1997.

11. Kralj A, Bajd T, Turk R: Gait restoration in paraplegic patients: a feasibility demonstration using multichannel surface electrode, *J Rehabil Res Devel* 20:3-20, 1983.

12. Peckham PH, Knutson JS: Functional electrical stimulation for neuromuscular applications, *Annu Rev Biomed Eng* 7:327-360, 2005.

13. Snoek GJ, Ilzerman MJ, in't Groen FA et al: Use of the NESS handmaster to restore handfunction in tetraplegia: clinical experience in ten patients, *Spinal Cord* 38:244-249, 2000.

14. Alon G, McBride K: Persons with C5 to C6 tetraplegia achieve selective functional gains using neuroprosthesis, *Arch Phys Med Rehabil* 84:119-124, 2003.

15. Poletto CJ, Van Doren CL: A high voltage, constant current stimulator for electrocutaneous stimulation through small electrodes, *IEEE Trans Biomed Eng* 46:929-936, 1999.

16. Ashley EA, Laskin JJ, Olenik LM et al: Evidence of autonomic dysreflexia during functional electrical stimulation in individuals with spinal cord injuries, *Paraplegia* 31:593-660, 1993.

17. Jaeger RJ: Principles underlying functional electrical stimulation techniques, *J Spinal Cord Med* 19:93-96, 1996.

18. Jacobs PL, Nash MS, Klose KJ et al: Evaluation of a training program for persons with SCI paraplegia using the Parastep 1 ambulation system, part 2: effects on physiological responses to peak arm ergometry, *Arch Phys Med Rehabil* 78:794-798, 1997.

19. Kralj A, Bajd T, Turk R: Enhancement of gait restoration in spinal injured patients by functional electrical stimulation, *Clin Orthop Relat Res* 233:34-43, 1988.

20. McNeal DR, Baker LL: Effects of joint angle, electrodes and waveform on electrical stimulation of the quadriceps and hamstrings, *Ann Biomed Eng* 16:299-310, 1988.

21. Van Doren CL: Contours of equal perceived amplitude and equal perceived frequency for electrocutaneous stimuli, *Percept Psychophys* 59:613-622, 1997.

22. Rushton DN: Functional electrical stimulation, *Physiol Meas* 18:241-275, 1997.

23. Jaeger RJ: Lower extremity applications of functional neuromuscular stimulation, *Assist Technol* 4:19-30, 1992.

24. Mulcahey MJ, Betz RR, Smith BT et al: Implanted functional electrical stimulation hand system in adolescents with spinal injuries: an evaluation, *Arch Phys Med Rehabil* 78:597-607, 1997.

25. Crago PE, Chizeck HJ, Neuman MR et al: Sensors for use with functional neuromuscular stimulation, *IEEE Trans Biomed Eng* 33:256-268, 1986.

26. Andrews BJ, Baxendale RH, Barnett R et al: Hybrid FES orthosis incorporating closed loop control and sensory feedback, *J Biomed Eng* 10:189-195, 1988.

27. Martin TP, Stein RB, Hoeppner PH et al: Influence of electrical stimulation on the morphological and metabolic properties of paralyzed muscle, *J Appl Physiol* 72:1401-1406, 1992.

28. Edwards BG, Marsolais EB: Metabolic responses to arm ergometry and functional neuromuscular stimulation, *J Rehabil Res Dev* 27:107-114, 1990.

29. Ragnarsson KT: Physiologic effects of functional electrical stimulation-induced exercises in spinal cord-injured individuals, *Clin Orthop Relat Res* 233:53-63, 1988.

30. Stein RB, Gordon T, Jefferson J et al: Optimal stimulation of paralyzed muscle after human spinal cord injury, *J Appl Physiol* 72:1393-1400, 1992.

31. Faghri PD, Rodgers MM, Glaser RM et al: The effects of functional electrical stimulation on shoulder subluxation, arm function recovery, and shoulder pain in hemiplegic stroke patients, *Arch Phys Med Rehabil* 75:73-79, 1994.

32. Nash MS, Bilsker MS, Kearney HM et al: Effects of electrically-stimulated exercise and passive motion on echocardiographically-derived wall motion and cardiodynamic function in tetraplegic persons, *Paraplegia* 33:80-89, 1995.

33. Hooker SP, Figoni SF, Glaser RM et al: Physiologic responses to prolonged electrically stimulated leg-cycle exercise in the spinal cord injured, *Arch Phys Med Rehabil* 71:863-869, 1990.

34. Pollack A, Axem K, Spielholz N et al: Aerobic training effects of electrically induced lower extremity exercises in spinal cord injured people, *Arch Phys Med Rehabil* 70:214-219, 1989.

35. Petrofsky J: Bicycle ergometer for paralyzed muscles, *J Clin Eng* 9:13-19, 1984.

36. Faghri P, Glaser R, Figoni S: Functional electrical stimulation cycle ergometer exercise: training effects on cardiorespiratory responses of spinal cord injured subjects at rest and during submaximal exercise, *Arch Phys Med Rehabil* 73:1085-1093, 1992.

37. Glaser R: Exercise and locomotion for the spinal cord injured. In Terjung R, editor: *Exercise and sports science reviews,* vol. 13, New York, 1985, Macmillan.

38. Petrofsky JS, Stacy R: The effect of training on endurance and the cardiovascular responses of individuals with paraplegia during dynamic exercise induced by functional electrical stimulation, *Eur J Appl Physiol Occup Physiol* 64487-492, 1992.

39. Schutte L, Rodgers M, Zajac F et al: *Improving the efficacy of electrical-stimulation induced leg cycle ergometry* [PhD dissertation], Palo Alto, CA, 1993, Stanford University.

40. Trumbower R, Faghri P: Improving pedal power during semireclined leg cycling, *IEEE Eng Med Biol Mag* 23:62-71, 2004.

41. Go B, DeVivo M, Richards J: The epidemiology of spinal cord injury. In Stover SL, DeLisa JA, Whiteneck GG, editors: *Spinal cord injury: clinical outcomes from the model systems,* Gaithersburg, MD, 1995, Aspen Publishers.

42. Smith B: Functional electrical stimulation, *Top Spinal Cord Inj Rehabil* 3:56-69, 1997.

43. Keith MW, Peckham PH, Thrope GB et al: Functional neuromuscular stimulation neuroprostheses for the tetraplegic hand, *Clin Orthop Relat Res* 233:25-33, 1988.

44. Keith MW, Peckham PH, Thrope GB et al: Implantable functional neuromuscular stimulation in the tetraplegic hand, *J Hand Surg [Am]* 14:524-530, 1989.

45. Stroh Wuolle K, Van Doren CL, Bryden AM et al: Satisfaction with and usage of a hand neuroprosthesis, *Arch Phys Med Rehabil* 80:206-213, 1999.

46. Wijman CA, Stroh KC, Van Doren CL et al: Functional evaluation of quadriplegic patients using a hand neuroprosthesis, *Arch Phys Med Rehabil* 71:1053-1057, 1990.

47. Marsolais EB, Kobetic R: Development of a practical electrical stimulation system for restoring gait in the paralyzed patient, *Clin Orthop Relat Res* 233:64-74, 1988.

48. Chaplin E: Functional neuromuscular stimulation for mobility in people with spinal cord injuries: the Parastep I system, *J Spinal Cord Med* 19:99-105, 1996.

49. Isakov E, Douglas R, Berns P: Ambulation using the reciprocating gait orthosis and functional electrical stimulation, *Paraplegia* 30:239-245, 1992.

50. Nene AV, Patrick JH: Energy cost of paraplegic locomotion using the ParaWalker—electrical stimulation "hybrid" orthosis, *Arch Phys Med Rehabil* 71:116-120, 1990.

51. Marsolais EB, Edwards BG: Energy costs of walking and standing with functional neuromuscular stimulation and long leg braces, *Arch Phys Med Rehabil* 69:243-249, 1988.

52. Guest RS, Klose KJ, Needham-Shropshire BM et al: Evaluation of a training program for persons with SCI paraplegia using the Parastep 1 ambulation system, part 4: effect on physical self-concept and depression, *Arch Phys Med Rehabil* 78:804-807, 1997.

53. DeVivo M, Stover SL: Long-term survival and causes of death. In Stover SL, DeLisa JA, Whiteneck GG, editors: *Spinal cord injury: clinical outcomes from the model systems,* Gaithersburg, MD, 1995, Aspen Publishers.

54. Rijkhoff NJ, Wijkstra H, van Kerrebroeck PE et al: Urinary bladder control by electrical stimulation: review of electrical stimulation techniques in spinal cord injury, *Neurourol Urodyn* 16:39-53, 1997.

55. Rijkhoff NJ, Wijkstra H, van Kerrebroeck PE et al: Selective detrusor activation by electrical sacral nerve root stimulation in spinal cord injury, *J Urol* 157:1504-1508, 1997.

56. Siegel SW, Catanzaro F, Dijkema HE et al: Long-term results of a multicenter study on sacral nerve stimulation for treatment of urinary urge incontinence, urgency-frequency, and retention, *Urology* 56(6 Suppl 1):87-91, 2000.

57. Hayes KC, Bassett-Spiers K, Das R et al: Research priorities for urological care following spinal cord injury: recommendations of an expert panel. The Ontario Neurotrauma Foundation International Expert Panel, Ontario, Canada, *Can J Urol* 14:3416-3423, 2007.

58. Garland JM: Regulation of apoptosis by cell metabolism, cytochrome c and the cytoskeleton, *Symp Soc Exp Biol* 52:81-118, 2000.

59. Marcus R: Role of exercise in preventing and treating osteoporosis, *Rheum Dis Clin North Am* 27:131-141, vi, 2001.

60. Minaire P: Immobilization osteoporosis: a review, *Clin Rheumatol* 8(2 Suppl):95-103, 1989.

61. Tsuzuku S, Ikegami Y, Yabe K: Bone mineral density differences between paraplegic and quadriplegic patients: a cross-sectional study, *Spinal Cord* 37:358-361, 1999.

62. Bloomfield SA, Mysiw WJ, Jackson RD: Bone mass and endocrine adaptations to training in spinal cord injured individuals, *Bone* 19:61-68, 1996.

63. Mohr T, Podenphant J, Biering-Sorensen F et al: Increased bone mineral density after prolonged electrically induced cycle training of paralyzed limbs in spinal cord injured man, *Calcif Tissue Int* 61:22-25, 1997.

64. Faghri PD, Yount JP, Pesce WJ et al: Circulatory hypokinesis and functional electric stimulation during standing in persons with spinal cord injury, *Arch Phys Med Rehabil* 82:1587-1595, 2001.

65. Mela P, Veltuj PH, Huijing PA: Excessive reflexes in spinal cord injury triggered by electrical stimulation, *Arch Physiol Biochem* 109:309-315, 2001.

66. Faghri P, Glaser R: Feasibility of using two FES exercise modes for spinal cord injured patients, *Clin Kinesiol* 44:62-68, 1989.

67. Triolo RJ, Bieri C, Uhlir J et al: Implanted functional neuromuscular stimulation systems for individuals with cervical spinal cord injuries: clinical case reports, *Arch Phys Med Rehabil* 77:1119-1128, 1996.

SOLUTIONS TO CHAPTER 17 CLINICAL CASE STUDY

Functional Electrical Stimulation Case 1

1. Stimulation to the posterior deltoid and supraspinatus muscles is the optimal FES intervention to avoid subluxation and reduce pain. Although it might be difficult to isolate the supraspinatus, extending and rotating the head to the opposite side will relax the trapezius (upper and middle fibers completely cover the supraspinatus) and allow palpation of the muscle. If the middle trapezius is not innervated, it may be possible to stimulate the supraspinatus, but this is unlikely because the trapezius is innervated by C2, C3, and C4. In addition, Carl has an incomplete injury, making partial innervation of the shoulder muscles possible. In this case just stimulating the posterior deltoid will be sufficient.

2. The therapist must take care to avoid skin irritation from the electrodes or potential skin burning over insensate areas. Tolerance of the stimulation over areas where Carl's sensation is intact also will need to be considered. Carl's lesion is above T6; therefore, AD could occur and the frequency of stimulation could influence this because it has been demonstrated at 50 Hz. Neurogenic pain or spasticity, if present, could be exacerbated.

3. A symmetrical biphasic current is optimal to avoid skin irritation.

4. A frequency of 10 to 100 Hz is recommended; however, muscle tetany will cause muscle fatigue.

5. Carl's body type and the muscles that will be stimulated must be considered because larger electrodes stimulate more superficially and smaller electrodes stimulate deeply. The posterior deltoid and supraspinatus are relatively superficial but they are not large muscles. This indicates that a smaller electrode could be the better choice; however, stimulation tolerance and muscle fatigue must be assessed. Another option if the stimulation intensity is not tolerated would be to keep the active reference electrodes relatively close together, thereby focusing stimulation superficially.

6. FES may be used on a variety of muscles for evaluation purposes. In Carl's case, FES must be closely monitored because he may gain even more motor recovery. His strongest muscle group in the left lower limb is the quadriceps (4 out of 5); he has right lower limb strength (4 out of 5) in both the hip flexors and quadriceps. Carl is lacking hip extension in the bilateral lower limbs and may not be able to tolerate the amount of stimulation necessary if his sensation is intact throughout the gluteal region.

Currently, Carl is not able to use an assistive device to support ambulation because of weakness although his emerging recovery allows for assessment of such supportive devices. If his motor recovery continues, an appropriate assistive device for his upper limbs should be evaluated along with orthoses for his lower limbs. FES could be used to facilitate or strengthen dorsiflexion. The optimal walking system for this patient is not known because recovery is still occurring. Reevaluation and a variety of FES augmentative treatments may be possible because Carl has an incomplete lesion.

SOLUTIONS TO CHAPTER 17 CLINICAL CASE STUDY

Functional Electrical Stimulation Case 2

1. FES cycle ergometry can be evaluated for Jamie with possible rental or purchase of an Ergys unit for her home. Jamie is a 50-year-old woman with a T6 paraplegia, ASIA A diagnosis; her injury level along with her T6 level of sensation would make this system a plausible fitness solution because absent sensation might allow a higher-intensity stimulation to generate a muscle contraction.

2. FES through cycling could enhance muscle strength and endurance, muscle circumference, and muscle protein synthesis rates. It may also improve Jamie's cardiovascular fitness. Other reported benefits include increased respiratory capacity, increased bone density, increased circulation and skin integrity, and improved psychological well-being.

3. Contraindications include severe respiratory disease, spinal instability, pathological or unhealed fractures, joint disarticulation, and fixed contractures in the lower limbs. Precautions include hypertension, hypotension, venous thrombosis, metal hardware in the femur, DVT, and heterotopic ossification in the lower limbs limiting ROM.

CHAPTER EIGHTEEN

Exercise and Fitness with Spinal Cord Injury

David R. Gater, Jr., MD, PhD

The best thing that ever happened to me since my injury 34 years ago was the rehabilitation hospital that taught me to be independent, despite my resistance. I have gotten back to a pretty normal life. Exercise is such a big part of my life in controlling my weight and making my arms strong. It also really helped my physical appearance. I really didn't like to exercise in the beginning but I quickly realized how much it helped me to do activities in every day life. I am very interested in working out at the gym. I pushed my insurance company to help support me in participating in an exercise program.

Trish (T 9-10 SCI)

Exercise is an important component in the gaining and maintaining of physical fitness. This chapter provides an overview of exercise considerations for the individual with a spinal cord injury (SCI). Specifically, work and anaerobic and aerobic capacity are discussed. Physiological adaptation resulting from an SCI should be considered when exercise programs and parameters are designed and implemented, which requires an understanding of body systems, including the autonomic nervous system (ANS), cardiovascular and pulmonary systems, and the endocrine system. The effect of problems with thermoregulation on individuals with SCI as it relates to exercise tolerance is reviewed, as well as metabolic alterations as a result of SCI to lipid profiles, glucose metabolism, body composition, and osteopenia. Guidelines for exercise screening described here can assist patients and clinicians to individualize exercise prescriptions. Finally, some barriers to exercise implementation are discussed.

DEFINITIONS OF FITNESS, EXERCISE, AND BENEFITS

It is important that the reader understands several key terms used in application to exercise with individuals who have spinal cord injuries. Physical fitness is a set of attributes that people have or can achieve that contribute to their ability to perform physical activity. For people with SCI, the level and completeness of their injury must first be considered because these components provide the framework and inherent limitations for physical fitness within this special population. Although discussed in earlier chapters (see Chapters 1 and 6), level and completeness of injury by American Spinal Injury Association (ASIA) classification (classes A-E) bear repeating because they influence not only total available working muscle mass but also neurologically and hormonally mediated energy responses and fitness capacity.

Level of injury (LOI) has an inverse relationship with voluntarily activated muscle mass, so that higher levels of SCI allow motor activation of fewer muscle groups. Although most muscles receive innervation from multiple nerve roots, only the major root contribution to each major muscle group is identified by the ASIA classification system to simplify and facilitate communication between clinicians. Complete SCI above the C3 nerve roots allows no voluntary motor function below the neck, although C3 weakly contributes to diaphragmatic contraction. C4 nerve roots provide voluntary control over the sternocleidomastoid and trapezius muscles, allowing head turning and shoulder shrugs; C4 also contributes to diaphragmatic excursion. C5 innervates scapular stabilizers, rotator cuff, and other shoulder musculature and elbow flexors; C5 also contributes to contraction of the diaphragm. The major additional function of C6 innervation is to the wrist extensors, which can also facilitate weak, passive finger grasp because of tenodesis (i.e., finger flexion from tightening of the finger flexor tendons associated with active wrist extension). C7 innervates the potentially largest muscle group of the upper extremity, the elbow extensors, and the wrist flexors and finger extensors. C8 innervates the finger flexors, whereas T1 additionally innervates the hand intrinsic musculature, notably the finger abductors.

Descending levels of thoracic nerve roots gain increasing motor function of the intercostal, abdominal, and paraspinal musculature, contributing to improved respiration, hemodynamic stability and truncal stability, which directly affect exercise options. The thoracolumbar spinal cord is also the origin of the sympathetic nervous system so that higher levels of SCI (e.g., cervical or upper thoracic) have either severely blunted or complete absence of ability to invoke or modulate sympathetic responses. Hence, in addition to limitations imposed by reduced functional musculature in SCI, exercise responses are further impaired by sympathetic, hormonal, and hemodynamic insufficiency.

Lumbosacral nerve roots contribute to voluntary control of lower extremity musculature and are therefore essential for normal gait and ambulation. L2 contributes primarily to hip flexors, whereas L3 plays the major role in contraction of knee extensors and hip adductors. L4 roots are essential for ankle dorsiflexion; L5 further contributes toe extensors and hip abductors, and S1 is necessary for ankle plantar flexion and hip extension. Sacral roots S2 to S5 are necessary for voluntary control of urinary and anal sphincters.

As indicated in Chapter 1, completeness of SCI plays a major factor in determining residual motor function. Motor complete SCI is classified as either ASIA A (no motor or sensory spared below the LOI) or ASIA B (sacral sensory sparing, but no voluntary motor function below the LOI). ASIA C indicates sacral sensory sparing, with less than antigravity motor function in the majority of muscle groups below the LOI. ASIA D includes sacral sensory sparing with at least antigravity (i.e., functional) motor strength in the majority of muscle groups below the LOI. ASIA E indicates full recovery of motor and sensory function below the LOI but may still yield abnormal gait and movement as a result of increased spasticity. There appears to be variability in ANS responses associated with incomplete SCI, lending increased importance to the functional graded exercise test in this population.

Spasticity is velocity-dependent muscle hypertonia and reflects disinhibition of reflex modulating pathways from the central nervous system (CNS), resulting in hyperreflexia, spasms, and increased resistance to passive stretch that often impair functional mobility (see Chapters 2 and 6). Spasticity may, however, facilitate transfers, exercise, and locomotion when appropriately used. Spasticity only occurs in upper motor neuron injuries and is therefore seldom present in conus and cauda equina injuries because of disruption of the final common pathway in motor control (i.e., afferent and efferent fibers conveyed in the peripheral nervous system). Although spasticity and hyperreflexia may contribute to increased whole body energy expenditure in upper motor neuron injuries, the flaccid paralysis of lower motor neuron injuries contributes almost nothing to basal metabolism. These points are of paramount importance when considering physical activity or exercise for improved fitness or weight loss in persons with SCI.

Physical activity has been defined as "any bodily movement produced by skeletal muscles which results in energy expenditure" and should be clearly distinguished from exercise, which is characterized as "a subset of physical activity that is planned, structured, and repetitive and has as a final or an intermediate objective the improvement or maintenance of physical fitness."[1] The distinction is an important one because a person may participate in physical activities that do not significantly improve physical fitness, although in sufficient quantities those activities may contribute to weight loss through increased caloric expenditure.

In a very broad sense, there are two types of exercise: anaerobic (which can be performed in short bursts without oxygen) and aerobic (which requires oxygen to sustain rhythmical movement), although at any given time during exercise training both are being used to a variable extent. Anaerobic exercise such as resistance training and sprinting can significantly improve measurable quantities of peak strength and power, whereas aerobic exercise is primarily used to improve endurance (time to exhaustion) and total work capacity, as measured by peak oxygen consumption or caloric expenditure. Central and peripheral mechanisms are involved in the adaptation to both types of exercise. Central mechanisms of adaptation include disinhibition of the CNS and ANS and hormonal alterations, which affect whole body metabolism, immune function, and cardiopulmonary dynamics. Peripheral mechanisms of exercise adaptation include enzymatic (affecting substrate storage and use) and structural (fiber cross-sectional area and capillary density) changes within skeletal muscle and sweat gland density within the skin. The two main principles of exercise training involve adaptation according to the specific type (specificity) and quantity (overload) of exercise used.[2] In addition, the principle of reversibility (use it or lose it) indicates that, when no longer subject to habitual stimulation, the body will revert its lowest level of function required to sustain life.

EFFECT OF EXERCISE ON FITNESS PARAMETERS
Work Capacity

Work capacity can be described as the maximal contribution of anaerobic and aerobic energy systems to administer force over a given distance in a specified time. Anaerobic capacity is most

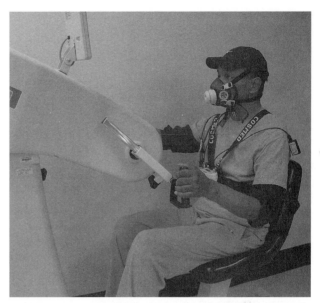

FIGURE 18-1   An individual with SCI performs a cycle ergometer–arm crank exercise test. Note the mask used to measure his levels of VO$_2$ during the test.

commonly reported in terms of peak power output, whereas aerobic capacity is usually expressed in terms of peak oxygen consumption.

Anaerobic Capacity

Anaerobic power in individuals with SCI is assessed by use of a Wingate Anaerobic Test (WAnT). The WAnT was developed in the 1970s at the Wingate Institute in Israel and is the most popular cycle ergometry test and in SCI must be performed on a cycle ergometer modified for arm cranking or a commercially available upper body ergometer (Figure 18-1). Although anaerobic power can also be assessed on a wheelchair ergometer, the results are more variable and less accurate because of the discontinuous application of force during wheelchair propulsion and the markedly reduced mechanical efficiency attributed to wheelchair propulsion compared with arm crank ergometry (ACE).

The most commonly used test length is 30 seconds, which is the time period for maximal effort where the major fuel source is anaerobic. A maximal effort or arm cranking is required during this 30-second period against a resistance based on body weight, but, as in the case of testing persons with SCI, it should be based on adjusted body mass (BM). As would be expected, people with higher levels of cervical injury have lower power outputs, primarily because of reduced muscle mass and stability but also because of presumed blunting of central drive. LOI must be taken into account when selecting the resistance load for the WAnT. The ranges of body mass (BM) to use for the determination of resistance using the WAnT for tetraplegia and paraplegia are listed in Clinical Note: Percent of Body Mass Used for Resistance During Wingate Anaerobic Test.

Peak power output for persons with tetraplegia sustained for 5 seconds peak power has been reported to range between 83

CLINICAL NOTE Percent Body Mass Used for Resistance During Wingate Anaerobic Test

- C5 tetraplegia = 1.5% body mass
- C6 tetraplegia = 2% body mass
- C7 tetraplegia = 3% body mass
- Paraplegia = 3.5% body mass

and 225 W for persons with tetraplagia and 300 W for persons with paraplegia. Clinical Note: Peak Power Output During Wingate Anaerobic Test Sustained for 5 Seconds summarizes the average workloads for C5 to C7 tetraplegia reported by Jacobs et al[3] and also includes the average workloads for people with paraplegia reported in other research by Jacobs et al.[4]

CLINICAL NOTE Peak Power Output During Wingate Anaerobic Test Sustained for 5 Seconds

- C5 tetraplegia = 83.2 ± 57.2 W
- C6 tetraplegia = 171.3 ± 47.5 W
- C7 tetraplegia = 224.5 ± 56.8 W
- Paraplegia = >300 W

Data from Jacobs PL, Mahoney ET, Johnson B: Reliability of arm Wingate anaerobic testing in persons with complete paraplegia, *J Spinal Cord Med* 26:141-144, 2003; Jacobs PL, Johnson BM, Mahoney ET et al: Effect of variable loading in the determination of upper-limb anaerobic power in persons with tetraplegia, *J Rehabil Res Develop* 41:9-14, 2004.

Anaerobic work capacity can also be reported as strength and weight lifting performance. In strict competition, men with paraplegia have been documented to lift more than 600 pounds in the traditional bench press, whereas women with SCI have bench pressed close to 300 pounds. There is a surprising lack of data about the impact of resistance training on strength and power application in persons with SCI. Hicks et al[5] recently demonstrated 19% to 34% increases in upper limb strength for persons with C4 to L1 SCI (complete and incomplete) after a 9-month, twice-weekly general exercise training program including both aerobic exercise and strength training.

Some may presume that exercise responses to resistance training would be similar to those seen in the able-bodied population, but no data have been presented to prove or refute such a hypothesis. The author intuits that blunted sympathetic and anabolic responses anticipated with higher levels of injury, combined with an overall reduced exercise volume, would result in diminished body composition, muscle hypertrophy, and strength changes compared with those observed in the able-bodied population. Greater frequency of resistance exercise may therefore be possible in this population, provided anabolic and catabolic hormonal ratios allowed sufficient recovery between sessions; it is unclear whether appropriate resistance training contributes to, or prevents, overuse, as is discussed later. A recent

cross-sectional study demonstrated a strong relationship between LOI and shoulder external rotator strength, with lower levels of injury associated with higher torques; no such relationship was demonstrated when assessing shoulder internal rotators, although truncal stability was more difficult to control for in the latter comparison.[6]

Aerobic Capacity

Peak aerobic capacity (VO_{2Peak}) represents a person's ability to maximally use oxygen in the performance of physical work, and it is dependent on CNS drive as well as peripheral influences on cardiovascular, pulmonary, endocrine, and musculoskeletal physiology. In a very simple sense, VO_2 (rate of oxygen consumption) reflects oxygen delivery and extraction (use) at the tissue level. VO_{2Peak} may be expressed mathematically in terms of cardiac output (CO) and the difference between arterial and venous oxygen concentrations: $VO_{2Peak} = CO \times (a - VO_2)$. CO reflects Heart rate (HR) × Left ventricular end-diastolic stroke volume (SV) ($CO = HR \times SV$), and it is also influenced by the vascular system's peripheral resistance (simply expressed as afterload [i.e., mean arterial blood pressure]). Oxygen concentration in the arterial blood depends on total blood volume and hemoglobin content and oxygen kinetics between the alveoli and pulmonary vascular system. Oxygen concentration in the venous blood reflects how much oxygen was extracted from arterial blood to be used by the peripheral tissues and during exercise reflects primarily the metabolic machinery available at the muscle level. The physical therapist must have at least a minimal grasp of how these organ systems are influenced by SCI to fully understand exercise testing results and how to optimally prescribe exercise for this special population.

PHYSIOLOGICAL SYSTEMS CONSIDERATIONS AND ADAPTATIONS WITH SPINAL CORD INJURY
Autonomic Nervous System

The ANS coordinates automatic life-sustaining processes and organizes visceral responses to somatic reactions (see Chapters 1, 2, and 3). It is composed of sympathetic and parasympathetic divisions, which regulate the action of smooth muscle and glands. During exercise, the CNS plays a key role in modifying autonomic responses over HR, SV, blood pressure (BP), blood flow, ventilation, thermoregulation, and metabolism by withdrawing parasympathetic influence and facilitating sympathetic responses; collectively this phenomenon is referred to as central drive.

The sympathetic nervous system is composed of preganglionic fibers derived from the thoracolumbar (T1 to L5) spinal cord that synapse on postganglionic fibers near the spinal cord in the sympathetic chain ganglia. The postganglionic fibers innervate smooth muscle, organs, and glands to facilitate the classic fight-or-flight response to sympathetic stimulation (e.g., increased HR, SV, ventilation, and sweating) with vasoconstriction of splanchnic vasculature and vasodilation of skeletal muscle vasculature. Most autonomic reflexes can be stimulated at the level of the spinal cord but are largely modulated by the supraspinal structures of the CNS, namely, the medulla, pons, and hypothalamus. In tetraplegia (cervical SCI), cortical and subcortical messages relayed along the spinal cord to the thoracic and lumbar sympathetic outflow tracts are interrupted, essentially blocking CNS-modulating influences. In addition, although sensory information from regions below the SCI is conveyed through the ANS, supraspinal modulation of reflex sympathetic responses below that level is blocked.

The parasympathetic nervous system, derived from the craniosacral portions of the CNS, promotes anabolic activity and energy conservation by reducing HR, SV, and ventilation and by increasing digestion. The cranial portion of the parasympathetic nervous system is not influenced by SCI; its effects on cardiac, pulmonary, and upper digestive structures are mediated primarily through the vagus nerve (cranial nerve X), which exits the CNS at the level of the medulla, above the spinal cord. Conversely, the sacral components of the parasympathetic nervous system arise from the lowest segments of the spinal cord and are no longer subject to modulating influences from the CNS after SCI, although sacral reflex parasympathetic pathways remain intact.

Cardiovascular Adaptation to Spinal Cord Injury

In response to acute cervical and upper thoracic SCI, cardiovascular adaptations after SCI occur. Bradycardia often ensues because of the disruption of cortical and subcortical influences on the sympathetic nervous system and the preservation of parasympathetic control on cardiac structures.[7-10] The bradycardia usually resolves in 2 to 6 weeks, likely as a result of withdrawal of parasympathetic tone over time and adaptive myocardial atrophy in the face of reduced left ventricular end-diastolic volumes and reduced afterload.[11-13] The cardiovascular system is further compromised by reduced sympathetic influence on peripheral and splanchnic vascular beds, resulting in reduced peripheral vascular resistance (diminished afterload), venous pooling (diminished venous tone and impaired muscle pump), and orthostatic hypotension. Venous pooling is also increased because of somatic impairment of ventilatory musculature, which subsequently reduces the negative transthoracic pressures responsible for end-diastolic ventricular filling associated with inspiration.

Pulmonary Adaptation to Spinal Cord Injury

Ventilation is significantly impaired in most individuals with SCI (see Chapter 4) because of paralysis of rib cage and abdominal musculature, reduced pulmonary compliance, and reduced diaphragmatic excursion.[14,15] The intercostal and abdominal muscles serve as expiratory muscles innervated by thoracic nerve roots from the spinal cord and are therefore no longer subject to voluntary control in tetraplegia and high paraplegia. The diaphragm is primarily responsible for inspiration and is innervated by the phrenic nerve, originating from cervical roots C3, C4, and C5. Complete spinal cord lesions above this level separate the breathing centers in the medulla from diaphragmatic control; these patients are ventilator dependent or require phrenic nerve pacing to the diaphragm to stimulate inspiration.[16,17] SCI involving the C3, C4, or C5 segments will have impaired ability to stimulate diaphragmatic excursion because of disruption of the phrenic nerve and assisted ventilation may be required.

Tetraplegia below C5 typically spares voluntary control of the diaphragm, although inspiration remains impaired from paralyzed abdominal muscles that allow abdominal contents, and subsequently the diaphragm, to descend. The diaphragm is left at a mechanical disadvantage, allowing diminished excursion during contraction and subsequent increased work during breathing. This effect is partially compensated for with the use of an abdominal binder, which returns the diaphragm to a higher, more functional position.[18] Hopman et al[19] demonstrated individuals with tetraplegia to have maximal inspiratory pressures of about 70%, maximal expiratory pressures of 46%, and inspiratory endurance only 40% of values obtained in able-bodied controls, with the ratio of inspiratory endurance to maximal inspiratory pressure 0.49 in those with tetraplegia compared with 0.82 in the able-bodied control subjects. Further, pulmonary function in complete tetraplegia is inversely related to the level of SCI[20,21] and length of disability[21] but may be improved with aggressive incentive spirometry and exercise training.[22-24]

Thermoregulation

The interruption of autonomic pathways in tetraplegia results in partially poikilothermic responses to thermal stress, providing these individuals much less ability to adapt to environmental and internally generated heat.[25] In complete tetraplegia afferent impulses relaying temperature information from the body are blocked at the spinal cord level, and although volume and osmoreceptors in the hypothalamus remain functional, efferent neural responses mediated through spinal cord pathways are obstructed, severely limiting sweat responses below the SCI. Although some investigators demonstrate no significant thermoregulatory activity in complete SCI,[26,27] others have reported at least partial, albeit significantly blunted, sweating responses below the level of SCI during thermal stress, suggesting the presence of thermoregulatory spinal reflexes.[28] The majority of sweat responses in tetraplegia, however, are relegated to regions above the level of SCI. In a practical sense, total plasma volume in SCI is reduced, and sweat excreted above the LOI is relatively concentrated, rather than the dilute sweat associated with exercise training.

Endocrine

Autonomic dysfunction and somatic paralysis in SCI may significantly affect metabolic and hormonal parameters in this population. Sympathomedullary responses are blunted in tetraplegia at rest,[29] and the adrenocortical-pituitary axis appears to be disrupted in SCI, with flattened circadian rhythms and poorly regulated corticosteroid responses.[30,31] As will be discussed, glucose intolerance occurs frequently in persons with SCI and is often accompanied by a state of hyperinsulinemia.[32,33] Although thyroid function may be altered in SCI for the short term, thyroid function tests are generally normal in healthy adults with SCI.[34] Conversely, testosterone and free testosterone levels in men with SCI are often reduced,[35] whereas growth hormone release is blunted[36] and depressed in the long term, as evidenced by reduced levels of insulin-like growth factor-1, a convenient indicator of chronic growth hormone secretion.[36,37] After the acute phase of SCI, ovulatory menstrual cycles are fairly well preserved, providing at least some cardioprotective and bone-sparing function in women.[38]

Autonomic Dysreflexia

For individuals with SCI above T6, an uncontrolled outflow of sympathetic activity in response to noxious stimuli below the SCI may occur, which is termed autonomic dysreflexia (see Chapters 2, 3, and 6), potentially resulting in life-threatening paroxysmal hypertension.[39] Information about noxious stimuli (e.g., distended bowel or bladder, lacerations, fractures, pressure sores, sunburn) from regions below the SCI is conveyed along afferent fibers of the ANS, which synapse with preganglionic efferent fibers in the spinal cord, stimulating reflex sympathetic responses below that level. Marked hypertension, mediated primarily by norepinephrine, can result in SCI lesions above T6 because of inability to autoregulate sympathetic outflow to the trunk, lower limbs and, most important, the greater splanchnic nerve, which arises at T7-T8 and provides innervation to the majority of the splanchnic vasculature bed.[40] Pressure receptors in the carotid bodies and aortic arch respond to the abrupt hypertension by stimulating medullary parasympathetic responses, resulting in bradycardia and vasodilation above the SCI, manifested as flushing, headache, hyperhidrosis, piloerection, pupillary dilation, and blurred vision. Such symptoms herald autonomic crisis, which can lead to intracerebral hemorrhages, seizures, arrhythmias, and death if not immediately and appropriately treated.

Despite these physiological limitations, both cross-sectional and longitudinal data have been demonstrated to support aerobic exercise training on VO_{2Peak} in SCI. For the sake of comparison, study results have been categorized into tables of high-, mid- and low-tetraplegia, as well as paraplegia, with ASIA classification or indications of when the individuals studied had complete or incomplete lesions, is also provided when available. To illustrate these studies of training effects in SCI, Tables 18-1, 18-2, and 18-3 summarize research with individuals with tetraplegia only. Results summarizing the training effects in paraplegia are outlined later in the chapter. The reader will note that, although many studies exist demonstrating VO_{2Peak} in SCI, relatively few demonstrate actual training interventions, and those training studies often mix groups without regard to level or completeness of injury. In general, however, it appears that peak exercise responses depend on the number and size of intact myotomes present and the degree to which the ANS is spared, particularly the sympathetic portion derived from the upper thoracic spinal cord. Persons with complete tetraplegia are especially limited in their aerobic capacity because of the combination of reduced working muscle mass, blunted sympathetic responses, and restrictive lung disease from intercostal and abdominal muscle paralysis; peak heart rates rarely exceed 120 beats/min.

Lipid Profiles

Lipid profiles should be considered when determining the risk for coronary artery disease (CAD). Although there are many different types of lipids, only a few are traditionally used to establish CAD risk. High-density lipoprotein (HDL-c) cholesterol is considered beneficial because it scavenges free fatty acids (FFA) and triglycerides (TG) from the blood and returns them to the liver where they can be packaged and removed. HDL-c levels greater than 60 mg/dl convey protection against CAD, whereas levels

below 40 mg/dl increase CAD risk. Low-density lipoproteins (LDL-c) are responsible for delivery of FFA and TG to the vascular endothelium, precipitating atherosclerosis. Total cholesterol levels reflect both HDL-c and LDL-c, with levels greater than 200 mg/dl associated with increased risk for CAD.

Individuals with SCI have similar total cholesterol levels but significantly lower HDL-c levels compared with able-bodied controls (42 ± 7.9 vs. 47 ± 6.7), particularly noticeable in the male population (39 ± 8.3 vs. 45 ± 7.0).[41] As seen in the able-bodied population, there appears to be a direct relationship between physical activity and HDL cholesterol (HDL-c) in persons with SCI.[42-44] Maki et al[45] noted that reduced HDL-c was significantly correlated with abdominal adiposity in 46 men with SCI, although activity levels were not described. Few training interventions have actually been examined for changes in cholesterol profiles in the population with SCI, however. A few studies have demonstrated no significant improvement in lipid profiles after 10 to 16 weeks of aerobic upper limb exercise in persons with SCI.[46,47] However, Hooker and Wells[48] demonstrated improved cholesterol profiles (total cholesterol/HDL-c from 5.0 to 4.0 mg/dl, HDL from 39 to 47 mg/dl) in patients with SCI who had completed 8 weeks of moderate upper limb exercise training. Although these data imply reduced CAD risk for those individuals with SCI who exercise regularly, longitudinal studies are lacking to substantiate this contention.

Body Composition

Body mass index (BMI) is calculated as a person's weight relative to squared height (Weight (kg)/Height (m^2)) and is the most commonly used indicator of obesity in our society. BMI ≥ 25 is considered overweight, whereas BMI ≥ 30 is considered obese and places the person at significantly higher risk for CAD, diabetes mellitus, osteoarthritis, and certain types of cancer. Obesity is more likely to occur in SCI because of the relative loss of metabolically active muscle tissue (sarcopenia), particularly in the lower limbs, resulting in 12% to 54% lower basal energy expenditure, depending on the level and completeness of SCI.[49-51] Bauman et al[52] have demonstrated significantly reduced muscle mass and viscera in SCI versus monozygotic able-bodied twins by using whole body potassium counts (2534 ± 911 mEq vs. 3515 ± 916 mEq); resting energy expenditures were similarly reduced in SCI versus able-bodied twins (1634 ± 290 vs. 1735 ± 295 kcal/d). Previously, Spungen et al[53] had reported that the monozygotic twins with acquired paraplegia had significantly more total body fat mass and percent fat per unit BMI than did their able-bodied twins. Similarly, a Canadian group has recently reported markedly lower fat-free body mass (FFM) in SCI versus able-bodied controls (69.2 ± 8.7 vs. 77.2 ± 7.2 kg), with higher fat mass (30.8 ± 8.7 vs. 22.8 ± 7.2 kg) despite similar BMIs.[54] Most recently, Spungen et al[55] have demonstrated that 133 men with SCI were 13.1% fatter per unit of BMI compared with age-, height-, and ethnicity-matched able-bodied control subjects. Thus the most typical measure for determining obesity (BMI) appears to grossly underestimate obesity in persons with SCI and would therefore also likely underestimate risk for obesity-related comorbidities. No studies to date have reported upper limb exercise to have significant changes in body composition for persons with SCI.

TABLE 18-1 | Maximal Exercise Performance Outcomes for Individuals With Tetraplegia at C6 or Above

Study	Mode	Sex	Status	n	Levels of SCI	Age (yr)	Mass (kg)	VO$_{2Peak}$ (ml · kg^{-1} · min^{-1})	HR (beats/min)	PO$_{Peak}$ (W)
Coutts et al, 1983[120]	WCE	M	UT	2	C6	27.0 ± 4.2	70.2 ± 9.0	15.3 ± 3.7	100 ± 17	30 ± 9
Dicarlo, 1982[121]	ACE	M	T	1	C6	24	74	17.0	120	48
Lasko-McCarthy & Davis, 1991[122]	WCE	M	UT	12	C5-C6	29.1 ± 3.4	73.3 ± 9.6	9.4 ± 3.2	112	NA
Lassau-Wray et al, 2000[123]	ACE	M	UT	5	C4-C5	32.4 ± 3.2	63.1 ± 4.0	11.5 ± 1.1	122 ± 7	NA
Ready, 1984[23]	ACE	F	T	1	C6	19.0	50.8	15.6	113	37.5
Simard et al, 1993[124]	WCE ACE	M/F	UT	25	C5-C6	34.4 ± 8.9	71.8 ± 11.5	WC 10.4 ± 3.7AC 10.8 ± 3.6	NA	10 ± 13 19 ± 15
Wicks, 1983	WCE/ACE	MF	T	81	C5-6	28.8 ± 4.021	67.9 ± 14.7 43.6	WC 14.7 ± 5.2/ACE 13.7 ± 4.1WC 17.2/ACE 14.8	146/143 136/150	NA

Mode, Form of exercise; *C*, complete injury; *I*, incomplete injury; *M*, male; *F*, female; *T*, trained; *UT*, untrained; *NA*, not available.

TABLE 18-2 | Maximal Exercise Performance Outcomes for Individuals With C7 Tetraplegia

Study	Mode	Sex	Status	n	Level of SCI	Lesion Extent	Age (yr)	Mass (kg)	VO$_{2Peak}$ (ml · kg^{-1} · min^{-1})	HR (beats/min)	PO$_{Peak}$ (W)
Burkett, 1990[126]	WCE	M/F	UT	4	C4-7	1C/3I	26.5 ± 2.8	60.2 ± 7.4	8.9 ± 2.2	134 ± 26	NA
Coutts et al, 1983[120]	WCE	M	UT	3	C7	NA	27.0 ± 2.5	75.2 ± 19.3	11.3 ± 1.2	111 ± 25	22 ± 8
Coutts & Stogryn, 1987[127]	WCE	M	T	2	C6-C7	NA	25 ± 1.0	59.4 ± 0.2	17.1 ± 0.2	102 ± 1.0	29 ± 10
Dicarlo et al, 1983[128]	ACE	M	T	2	C5-C7	NA	26.5 ± 2.5	52.6 ± 2.6	20.2 ± 0.1	NA	66 ± 7
Gass & Camp, 1979[129]	WCE	M	T	1	C6-C7	NA	N/A	54.6	19.4	120	NA
Schmid et al, 1998[130]	WCE	M	UT	20	C5-C7	NA	33.8 ± 6.7	74.8 ± 14.5	13.7 ± 3.2	110 ± 17	33 ± 9
Simard et al, 1993[124]	WCE ACE	M/F	UT	22	C7	NA	33.5 ± 9.5	61.7 ± 10.3	WC 13.9 ± 5.3 AC 15.2 ± 4.7	NA	21 ± 19 28 ± 16
Whiting et al, 1983[131]	WCE	M	T	2	C5-C7	NA	27 ± 2.5	86.4 ± 4.6	12.8 ± 1.3	131 ± 1.3	50 ± 0
Wicks, 1983[125]	WCE/ACE	MF	T	51	C7	NA	28.8 ± 4.035	63.3 ± 9.770.5	WC 14.9 ± 4.6/ACE 13.1 ± 2.2WC 13.8/ACE 11.7	123/130 125/117	NA

Mode, Form of exercise; *Lesion extent*, degree of completeness of injury or ASIA levels; *C*, complete injury; *I*, incomplete injury; *M*, male; *F*, female; *T*, trained; *UT*, untrained; *NA*, not available.

TABLE 18-3 | **Maximal Exercise Performance Outcomes for Individuals With C8 Tetraplegia**

Study	Mode	Sex	Status	n	Levels of SCI	Lesion Extent	Age (yr)	Mass (kg)	VO_{2Peak} (ml • kg^{-1} • min^{-1})	HR (beats/min)	PO_{Peak} (W)
Bhambhani et al, 1995[132]	WCE	M	T	8	C5-C8	NA	31.8±6.2	72.1±6.4	19.8±4.0	NA	NA
Coutts et al, 1983[120]	WCE	M	UT	3	C8	NA	33.0±5.5	64.2±10	16.2±2.9	117±11	22±4
Erikkson et al, 1988[133]	WCE	M	UT/T	12/8	C5-C8	NA	29±5/32±11	63.6±11/62.1±11	13.9±1.9/17.4±5.1	119±18/118±24	NA
Gass et al, 1980[134]	WCE	M	T	7	C5-T4	NA	34.6±9.5	83.3±13.8	12.7±5.9	129±19	NA
Hjeltues/Janssen, 1990[135]	ACE	M	UT	10/10/3	C5-C8	C/I/I	36/47/41	NA	14±4.6/23±11/20±5.3	NA	NA
Hopman et al, 1996[136]	WCE	M/F	UT	7	C4-C8	NA	26.6±6.9	77.6±23.4	8.1±3.1	NA	21±15
Hopman et al, 1996[136]	WCE	M	T	8	C4-C8	NA	32.7±13	73.6±17.2	14.0±5.7	NA	50±29
Janssen et al., 1993[137]	WCE	M	UT	9	C5-C8	5C/4I	32.9±9.4	81.2±14.9	13.6±3.1	NA	NA
Janssen, 1997[138]	WCE	M	UT	8	C5-C8	NA	37.3±10	83.1±15.1	14.3±4.4	NA	NA
Lasko-McCarthy & Davis, 1991)[122]	WCE	M	UT	10	C7-C8	NA	28.9±6.3	70.3±7.7	15.1±4.0	127	NA
Lassau-Wray et al, 2000[124]	ACE	M	UT	5	C6-C8	NA	29.6±1.3	61.8±2.9	18.8±1.5	170±1	NA
McLean & Skinner, 1995[113]	ACE	M	T	7	C5-T1	NA	33.3	66.3±17.7	12.4	122	35.6
Noreau & Shephard, 1995[132]	WCE	M	UT	8	C5-C8	NA	31±15	NA	7.5±1.8	110±12	10±7
Ready, 1984[23]	ACE	M	T	5	C6-C8	NA	25.5±1.5	71.7±7.6	15.0±4.1	122±13	43±13
Simard et al., 1993[124]	WCE ACE	M/F	UT	3	C8	NA	35±17.0	56.0±7.0	WC 14.2±2.3 AC 14.4 (4.5)	NA	NA / 23±15
Van Loan et al, 1987[140]	ACE	M/F	UT	13	C5-C8	NA	29.6±2.5	62.2±3.4	12.0±3.3	109±17	23±3

Mode, Form of exercise; Lesion extent, degree of completeness of injury or ASIA levels; *C,* complete injury; *I,* incomplete injury; *M,* male; *F,* female; *T,* trained; *UT,* untrained; *NA,* not available.

Glucose Metabolism

Impaired glucose tolerance has been reported in a large percentage (up to 70%) of patients with SCI; it is characterized by hyperinsulinemia in response to a glucose challenge for this population.[56] Petry et al[57] found that glycosylated hemoglobin (HbA1c) levels above 6.0 g/dl in patients with SCI significantly correlated with impaired glucose tolerance or frank diabetes; they recommended routine HbA1c screening for patients with SCI. Aksnes et al[32] noted an association between whole-body insulin-mediated glucose uptake and skeletal muscle mass in those with tetraplegia, suggesting loss of muscle mass as the primary reason for insulin insensitivity. The hyperinsulinemia in these patients may therefore be related to body composition changes, as has been reported in the general population.[58] Bauman and Spungen[59] reported that only 44% of veterans with SCI had normal 2-hour oral glucose tolerance test results by the existing World Health Organization standards at the time. Of note, 62% of those with tetraplegia and 50% with paraplegia with a mean duration of injury of 17 years had abnormal glucose tolerance test results compared with only 18% of age-matched control subjects with similar BMI; fully 22% with SCI were found to be frankly diabetic.[59] No studies to date have demonstrated upper limb exercise training to have significant changes in glucose tolerance for persons with SCI.

Osteopenia

Neurogenic osteopenia in complete SCI results from the withdrawal of stress and strain on bone as modeled by Wolff's law.[60] Paralysis of skeletal musculature below the level of SCI prevents the usual application of external forces (muscle contraction and gravitational loading) required to prevent bone resorption. As a result, urinary excretion of calcium, hydroxyproline, magnesium, and phosphorus are significantly increased, particularly within the first 3 months but remaining so for up to 18 months after acute tetraplegia, indicating an overall trend of bone resorption.[61-63] In addition, plasma parathormone and 1,25-(OH)2 vitamin D (calcitriol) levels are reduced both short and long term, whereas calcitonin levels initially increase and remain elevated above control levels and to a greater extent in subjects with chronic tetraplegia than in subjects with paraplegia.[64] Bone mineral loss as determined by dual-energy x-ray absorptiometry (DEXA) is rapid and linear within the first 4 months of SCI, occurring to a greater extent in the pelvis and lower limbs in individuals with tetraplegia and paraplegia.[65] Interestingly, significant bone mineral loss also occurs in the upper limbs, even in those with paraplegia, without return to baseline. Homeostasis at 67% of original bone mass is achieved at about 16 months after injury, barely above fracture threshold.[65] Even in patients with complete neurological recovery after SCI, bone mineral content remains below preinjury levels 1 year later.[66]

EFFECTS OF EXERCISE ON UPPER LIMB REPETITIVE STRAIN

Upper limb overuse injuries in individuals who are wheelchair reliant are reported by 51% to 81% of respondents surveyed, most frequently at the shoulder.[67-70] One study reported that 55% of patients with tetraplegia had upper limb pain, 45% of which was attributed to shoulder conditions, whereas an additional 33%

were cervical in origin.[69] Magnetic resonance imaging (MRI) in one study detected rotator cuff tears in 73% of symptomatic individuals with paraplegia compared with 59% of symptomatic able-bodied subjects; 54% of all individuals with paraplegia tested (including 11 whom were asymptomatic) were found to have rotator cuff tears, the majority of which were full thickness.[71] It appears that these injuries may be age related because a younger group of individuals with more recent SCI had few rotator cuff injuries by MRI, but a relationship between BMI and shoulder degenerative arthritis was demonstrated even in this relatively young population.[72]

Besides rotator cuff tears, shoulder conditions in SCI frequently include capsular contracture or capsulitis, anterior instability, rotator cuff impingement, osteoarthritis, and osteonecrosis.[73] Those with tetraplegia are especially at risk for shoulder conditions because of rotator cuff limitations, pectoral and latissimus dorsi weakness, truncal instability, and increased functional demand.[74] Additional upper limb overuse syndromes in SCI include bicipital tendinitis, lateral epicondylitis, ulnar neuropathy at the elbow, DeQuervain's tenosynovitis, and carpal tunnel syndrome.[75] These problems can be markedly debilitating in the person with SCI who relies heavily on residual function in the upper limbs for activities of daily living (ADLs) and mobility. Although strengthening scapular stabilizers and rotator cuff muscles would appear to reduce rotator cuff tears and preserve shoulder joint integrity, only two studies have been reported to use such a prophylactic program in SCI. Curtis et al[76] demonstrated significantly reduced shoulder pain in patients with tetraplegia or paraplegia who had completed 6 months of daily anterior shoulder stretching and posterior shoulder strengthening with Thera-Band exercises (one set) three times weekly compared with nonexercising control subjects (see Figure 8-5). Hicks et al[5] demonstrated significant reductions in pain, improved upper limb strength, and improved perceived quality of life in persons with SCI after 9 months of twice-weekly combined aerobic and strengthening exercises. Resistance exercises included muscle groups from forearm/wrist, elbow flexors, elbow extensors, shoulder, back, abdominals, and legs (appropriate subjects) performed as two sets of up to 15 repetitions (70% to 80% 1 repetition maximum [RM]) each.

EXERCISE SCREENING

The American College of Sports Medicine (ACSM) has established guidelines for medical screening and exercise testing in the able-bodied population.[77] Absolute contraindications for graded exercise testing (GXT) for both able-bodied and individuals with SCI is listed in Table 18-4.

Individuals with SCI reported in Model Systems data have standardized mortality ratios of 1.2 and 6.4 (compared with 1.0 in the able-bodied population) for ischemic heart disease and nonischemic heart disease, respectively,[78] suggesting that stricter guidelines for screening should be used for this population. Conservatively, it is therefore recommended that, for the purposes of risk stratification, men ≥40 years of age and women ≥50 years of age who have SCI be considered as having at least moderate risk for untoward events during exercise, independent of the CAD risk factor thresholds for use with ACSM risk stratification. It is further recommended that individuals with SCI obtain medical

TABLE 18-4	**Absolute Contraindications to Graded Exercise Testing in the Able-Bodied and in Individuals with Spinal Cord Injury**	
Contraindications		Additional Contraindications with SCI
Acute change in resting ECG		Uncontrolled autonomic dysreflexia
Unstable angina		Orthostatic hypotension
Uncontrolled symptomatic arrhythmias or hemodynamic compromise		Recent deep vein thrombosis or pulmonary emboli
Severe symptomatic aortic stenosis		Grade 3-4 pressure ulcers
Uncontrolled symptomatic congestive heart failure		
Acute pulmonary embolism or infarction		
Acute myocarditis or pericarditis		
Suspected or known dissecting aneurysm		
Acute infections		

TABLE 18-5	**Relative Contraindications to Graded Exercise Testing in the Able-Bodied and in Individuals with Spinal Cord Injury**	
Contraindications		Additional Contraindications with SCI
Left main coronary stenosis		Active tendonitis
Moderate stenotic valvular heart disease		Chronic heterotopic ossification
Electrolyte abnormalities		Peripheral neuropathy
Severe arterial hypertension (systolic BP >200 torr; diastolic BP 110 torr)		Grade 1-2 pressure ulcers
Tachyarrhythmias or bradyarrhythmias		Spasticity
Hypertrophic cardiomyopathy or other outflow tract obstruction		
Neuromuscular, musculoskeletal, or rheumatoid disorders that are exacerbated by exercise		
High-degree atrioventricular block		
Ventricular aneurysm		
Uncontrolled metabolic disease		
Chronic infectious disease		

clearance from a physician knowledgeable in SCI care, including a 12-lead electrocardiogram (ECG) and risk profile assessment, before participation in a strenuous exercise program. Relative contraindications for exercise testing for the able-bodied and individuals with SCI are defined in Table 18-5.

Should an exercise test be indicated or desired, the next step is to determine the most appropriate testing mode and protocol. The relative advantages and disadvantages of the three most common modes of exercise stress testing (field testing, ACE, and wheelchair ergometry [WCE]) for the population with SCI were well described by Davis in 1993.[79] Field testing is perhaps the easiest, least expensive, and mobility-specific method, and it has been demonstrated to provide a fair estimate of VO_{2Peak} in selected wheelchair users,[80,81] although recent data have failed to significantly correlate field testing with actual VO_{2Peak}.[82] Significant variability can occur with differences in terrain, wind speed, temperature, and humidity. ACE is the most established and widely validated upper limb test used for SCI, but it lacks mobility specificity; nonetheless, it remains the method of choice for VO_{2Peak} assessment in this population when clinical trials are performed.[79] Conversely, WCE is mobility specific to those who perform community mobility with a manual wheelchair, but it lacks availability, interinstitutional reliability/validity data, and typically requires greater maintenance. Several systems have been developed and tested, including wheelchairs mounted on a motorized treadmill,[83] low friction rollers,

and specialized devices to simulate overground propulsion.[84,85] Compared with ACE, WCE has been found to induce lower,[86] similar,[87] or greater[88] VO_{2Peak} responses, but with lower peak power output,[89] indicating reduced mechanical efficiency.

Recently, devices have been developed to assess all-extremity oxygen consumption, which may be appropriate for persons with incomplete SCI and for monitoring aerobic fitness in persons with SCI by using combined upper limb and functional electrical stimulation (FES) of the lower limbs for exercise training. Typically, these hybrid devices incorporate both ACE and leg cycle ergometry (LCE) for determination of total-body VO_{2Peak}. Advantages include improved venous return to the heart with subsequent increased SV and CO, as well as increased total muscle mass contributing to greater VO_{2Peak}.[90,91] VO_{2Peak} described when using these devices is not strongly correlated, however, with an individual's upper limb VO_{2Peak} or ability to perform community mobility and ADLs.[90]

Protocols for people with SCI may use continuous incremental graded protocols or discontinuous multilevel protocols for use with ACE or WCE.[85,92] Continuous protocols have well-defined submaximal or maximal end-point criteria and are progressive with increasing levels of exercise intensity. The primary disadvantage to the standard continuous protocol is that it requires too much time for practical completion, with the subject fatiguing at less than maximal capacity.

Many exercise physiologists prefer discontinuous, submaximal protocols for stress testing wheelchair users because the protocols are comfortable, safe, and relatively easy to administer. Unfortunately, prediction of VO_{2Peak} from these submaximal protocols is not as reliable as would be expected, and ischemia from coronary insufficiency at higher workloads may be missed altogether. A typical WCE protocol would use a constant speed (3 km/hr^{-1}) with a metronome-guided crank rate of 50 revolutions per minute and an initial resistance of 5 W. Each stage would last 4 to 6 minutes with 5-minute rest intervals and progressive 5- to 10-W increments used with each new stage to a predetermined power output (PO) of 30 W. A submaximal ACE protocol would use similar stages but with twice the PO levels. The equation most commonly used to predict VO_{2Peak} from submaximal HR in these protocols is that provided by Glaser et al,[93] which was developed by using (n = 30) able-bodied women and therefore is likely inappropriate for subjects with SCI. Regression equations developed by Hooker et al[94] for individuals with high- and low-lesion paraplegia failed to indicate the completeness of the injuries, although HR/VO_2 relationships appeared fairly strong for the two separate groups.[94]

To measure VO_{2Peak} and peak power output (PO_{Peak}), a continuous, shortened protocol can be used, allowing an initial intensity level of 50% of the predicted maximal PO (determined from submaximal testing), shortening each stage of testing to 2 minutes and allowing no rest between stages. A similar protocol has been described by Langbein et al[85] by using the Veterans Administration–developed Wheelchair Aerobic Fitness Trainer (WAFT), a wheelchair ergometer that can accommodate the user's own wheelchair. They use a continuous protocol with a fixed speed of 2 miles/hr^{-1}, initial intensity of 6 W, and 5- to 7-W increments between 3-minute stages; 20 seconds of rest between stages allows for BP determination. In addition to oxygen consumption and PO, BP, ECG, and perceived exertion should be monitored at the end of each exercise stage. Unfortunately, ECG monitoring during ACE or WCE is frequently impaired because of movement artifact and should therefore be continued during the first 10 seconds of the resting periods between stages to improve sensitivity for ischemic changes.

The correlation between GXT and CAD has not been clearly established in the population with SCI, although Bauman et al[95] demonstrated GXT ECG abnormalities in only 5 of 13 subjects found to have abnormalities on exercise thallium single-photon emission computerized tomography studies. The multistage ACE protocol provided 3-minute stages of 12-W increments starting with an initial workload of 36 W, allowing 30- to 45-second interruptions between stages for ECG and BP acquisition and using end points of 85% maximal predicted heart rate (MPHR = 220 – Age) or until symptoms limited continuation. Using an end point of 85% MPHR possibly precluded ischemic findings that may have occurred at higher heart rates.

For individuals undergoing testing to rule out ischemic heart disease, postexercise echocardiography[96] or nuclear imaging studies[97] may significantly improve the sensitivity and specificity of the exercise stress test. Termination of the test should be consistent with ACSM guidelines (Boxes 18-1 and 18-2).[98]

Special considerations should be made to accommodate varying levels of impairment found with SCI during the GXT. The arm crank or wheelchair ergometer should be adjusted appropriately to allow optimal efficiency and to reduce musculoskeletal injuries at the shoulder, elbow, and wrist, and straps should be applied to the torso to prevent truncal instability. For those individuals lacking significant triceps function, arm ergometers that allow pulling rather than pushing cyclical movements are preferred to optimize elbow flexor involvement. Wheelchair gloves or flexion mitts with Velcro straps are important to prevent blisters, lacerations, and abrasions, especially for those with tetraplegia whose hands and fingers are insensate or unable to sufficiently grasp. Velcro straps and cuffed weights are commonly used for resistance training equipment modifications, and abdominal binders and leg wraps may be used to facilitate improved pulmonary dynamics and greater venous return, reducing the risk for circulatory hypokinesis during maximal exercise.

Body composition analysis is another parameter commonly used in the fitness assessment of the person with SCI but it is not without limitations. Although recently touted as the gold standard for determining body composition in SCI,[99,100] even DEXA introduces significant error because it cannot account for hydration status and fails to measure a relatively large portion of upper limb tissue. Compared with the able-bodied population, persons with SCI are known to have reduced FFM density,[101,102] total body water,[103] and bone density.[104,105] Failure to account for

---

BOX 18-1 | Absolute Indications for Graded Exercise Test Discontinuation in Able-Bodied Populations

- Systolic BP ↓ of 10 torr from baseline despite ↑ workload, when accompanied by other evidence of ischemia
- Moderate to severe angina
- Increasing nervous system symptoms (e.g., ataxia, dizziness)
- Signs of poor perfusion (e.g., cyanosis or pallor)
- Technical difficulties (e.g., ECG or BP monitoring)
- Sustained ventricular tachycardia (1 mm ST in leads without diagnostic Q-waves, other than ECG leads V1 or a VR)
- Subject's desire to stop

BOX 18-2 | Relative Indications for Graded Exercise Test Discontinuation in Able-Bodied Populations

- Systolic BP ↓ of 10 torr from baseline despite ↑ workload, when accompanied by other evidence of ischemia
- ST or QRS changes such as excessive ST depression (>2 mm horizontal or downsloping ST ↓ or marked axis shift)
- Arrhythmias other than sustained ventricular tachycardia, including multifocal premature ventricular contractions (PVCs), triplets of PVCs, supraventricular tachycardia, heart block, or bradyarrhythmias
- Fatigue, dyspnea, wheezing, leg cramps, or claudication
- Bundle branch block development or intraventricular conduction delay that cannot be distinguished from ventricular tachycardia
- * Increasing chest pain
- * Hypertensive responses (e.g., SBP>250t or DBP>115t in absence of definitive evidence)

these differences when using standardized equations has lead to significant error in reporting percent body fat (% BF) by skinfold analysis, bioelectrical impedance, hydrostatic weighing, and even DEXA in the population with SCI.[106]

Further, fluid shifts are position dependent in individuals with SCI and subsequently require that timing and positioning during body composition assessment be standardized. Because of the known differences in FFM density, total body water, and bone density compared with able-bodied populations, four-compartment body composition modeling[107] should be used to determine % BF in persons with SCI until regression-based equations specific to SCI have been generated. A review of body composition analyses in SCI was completed by Kocina,[108] which indicated that body fat for men and women with SCI ranged between 25% to 32%. Unfortunately, the review also indicated the significant limitations associated with body composition analyses result from the differences in fat-free body density, bone mineral density, and total body water peculiar to this population. As noted previously, four-compartment body composition modeling is strongly recommended for individuals with SCI until regression-based equations specific to SCI have been generated.

Additional fitness testing appropriate for the person with SCI could include pulmonary function tests (see Chapter 4), quantified strength and flexibility measures (see Chapter 6), DEXA scan to determine bone mineral density, radiographs of paralyzed limbs to exclude asymptomatic fractures, lipid profiles, and HbA1c to rule out glucose intolerance or diabetes.

Anticipated Responses to Exercise Testing in Spinal Cord Injury

The peak responses to exercise testing in SCI have been fairly well documented over the past three decades. Further delineation of these studies for paraplegia is outlined in Tables 18-6, 18-7, and 18-8. Unfortunately, the level and completeness of SCI in this literature was often discounted when the protocols used were designed, leading to a fairly large range of responses. In general, however, it appears that peak exercise responses depend on the number and size of intact myotomes present and the degree to which the autonomic nervous system is spared, particularly the sympathetic portion derived from the upper thoracic spinal cord. Individuals with tetraplegia and high paraplegia are especially limited in their aerobic capacity because of the combination of reduced working muscle mass, blunted sympathetic responses, and restrictive lung disease from intercostal and abdominal muscle paralysis. Peak HRs rarely exceed 120 beats/min in T1 to T3 paraplegia, and although variable responses occur in T4 to T6 paraplegia, most persons with SCI below T7 have the capacity for similar peak HR responses as their age-matched able-bodied cohorts. Similar trends have been reported for BP responses to graded exercise in persons with SCI, although circulatory hypokinesis typically limits the peak BP responses to significantly less than those seen in able-bodied individuals.

When screening for CAD, it is recommended that ECG recordings be performed during the final seconds of each exercise stage and 10 seconds into each rest period to allow adequate tracings for ECG interpretation because upper limb work usually precipitates significant movement artifact during ECG monitoring.

As the person with SCI approaches peak exercise capacity, it is likely he will become relatively hypotensive despite leg wraps and abdominal binders. Individuals with tetraplegia often have resting BPs somewhere around 90/60 mm Hg and should be closely monitored for symptoms of hypotension and presyncope during strenuous exercise. Should symptomatic hypotension (systolic pressure drop >20 torr) occur, exercise testing should be halted and the person tilted back in his wheelchair to elevate the lower limbs above the level of the heart, promoting venous return. Ideally, this position would also be used at the end of an exercise stress test to maximally invoke the Frank-Starling mechanism for myocardial contractility, increasing the likelihood of creating ischemia in the presence of CAD. In the rare event that cardiopulmonary resuscitation (CPR) becomes necessary, it is safest and easiest to tilt the wheelchair back until the cradled head is safely resting on the padded floor, lifting the person's legs until the chair can be removed from beneath the torso, with CPR and Advanced Cardiac Life Support administered as per American Heart Association guidelines.[109]

EXERCISE PRESCRIPTION

As indicated previously, it is important to establish the level of neurological injury and the completeness of the lesion because this has tremendous implications in exercise prescription. Individuals with complete lesions at or above C4 will be relegated to FES-LCE or Hybrid exercise equipment (see Chapter 17). The person with C5 tetraplegia will require exercises that do not use active wrist extension, elbow extension, or grasp, whereas those with C6 lesions have active wrist extension but little or no elbow extension or grasp. C7 tetraplegia allows voluntary elbow extension, but without grasp, whereas individuals with C8 lesions have all function of the upper limbs except finger abduction and adduction. The prescription must be modified to allow accommodation of these differences. Furthermore, a complete lesion precludes automatic control of sympathetic responses below that level, whereas incomplete SCI may allow varying degrees of sympathetic response. In addition, a person with an incomplete SCI who has relative sparing of sensation in the lower limbs may not be able to tolerate FES-LCE or Hybrid exercise modes because of pain.

Succinct, precise, and quantifiable goals will optimize chances of a successful outcome, with several short-term and intermediate goals provided to allow continued feedback and motivation. Most individuals with SCI will have aerobic fitness levels well below that of the sedentary able-bodied population, whose VO_{2Peak} may be <28 ml/kg/min, and although peak exercise capacity is most easily quantified by determining VO_{2Peak} and PO on a maximal graded exercise test, this may not be practical for all individuals. Of note, peak HRs for persons with SCI performing a GTX do not necessarily correlate with peak capacity. Other measurable components of fitness include muscle strength and endurance, flexibility, pulmonary function, and body composition. Assessment of CAD risk stratification and fitness level is essential to safely and appropriately prescribe the initial level of intensity and exercise duration and should be performed, as previously indicated. In addition, the contraindications previously listed should be closely observed and

TABLE 18-6 | Maximal Exercise Performance Outcomes for Individuals with High Paraplegia

Study	Mode	Sex	Status	n	Levels of SCI	Lesion Extent	Age (yr)	Mass (kg)	VO_{2Peak} (ml/kg⁻¹/min⁻¹)	HR (beats/min)	PO_{Peak} (W)
Coutts et al, 1983[120]	WCE	M	UT	3	T1-T5	NA	29±4.2	80.7±19.0	22.3±7.5	167±26	48±13
Gass et al., 1995[141]	WCE ACE	M	UT	9	T2-T4	C	30.8±2.4	70.2±3.4	23.8±2.0 / 24.8±1.7	177±3 / 177±4	NA
Hjeltues & Janssen, 1990[135]	ACE	M	UT	6	T1-T6	C	33	NA	17±6.5	NA	NA
Hooker et al, 1993[94]	ACE	M	UT	13	T1-T6	NA	25.6±6.9	65.4±8.6	17.9±4.1	167±28	71±15
Janssen et al, 1993[137]	WCE	M	UT	6	T1-T5	C/I	38.8±9.0	82.8±10.6	17.6±4.0	NA	NA
Lassau-Wray et al, 2000[123]	ACE	M	UT	5	T1-T6	NA	33.4±3.6	68.8±3.9	27.0±0.8	170±1	NA
Lin et al, 1993[142]	ACE	M	UT	9	T1-T5	NA	32.9±2.4	54.9±2.5	17.4±1.0	167±8	33±4
Schmid et al, 1998[143]	WCE	M	UT	10	T1-T5	NA	35.6±12	72.3±10.2	25.1±5.7	172±13	67±27
Wicks, 1983[125]	WCE ACE	M	T	11	T1-T5	NA	30.2±8.0	70.5±13.6	WCE 22.0±5.2 / ACE 23.0±5.9	172±14 / 174±18	34±8 / 98±26
Wicks, 1983[125]	WCE ACE	F	T	1	T1-T5	NA	22	47.7	WCE 24.5 / ACE 29.1	176 176	34 82

Mode, Form of exercise; *Lesion extent*, degree of completeness of injury or ASIA levels; *C*, complete injury; *I*, incomplete injury; *M*, male; *F*, female; *T*, trained; *UT*, untrained; *NA*, not available.

TABLE 18-7 | Maximal Exercise Performance Outcomes for Individuals with Mid Paraplegia

Study	Mode	Sex	Status	n	Levels of SCI	Lesion Extent	Age (yr)	Mass (kg)	VO_{2Peak} (ml/kg⁻¹/min⁻¹)	HR (beats/min)	PO_{Peak} (W)
Bernard et al, 2000[144]	WCE	M	T	6	T4-8	C	31.6±2.9	62.8±7.2	28.4±2.2	183±5.4	NA
Coutts et al., 1983[120]	WCE	M/F	UT	3	T6-T10	NA	29±4.0	70.7±12.9	21.3±9.2	185±5	46±21
Coutts & Stogryn 1987[127]	WCE	F	T	1	T10-T11	NA	22	49.15	29.9	192	50
Hjeltues & Janssen, 1990[135]	ACE	M	UT	14	T7-T11	C	38	NA	26±8.5	NA	NA
Hjeltues & Janssen, 1990[135]	ACE	F	UT	2	T7-T11	C	26	NA	23±1.0	NA	NA
Hooker et al, 1993[94]	ACE	M	UT	14	T7-T12	NA	25.0±5.6	67.2±11.7	20.6±4.6	175±18	81±14
Hooker & Wells, 1992[145]	ACE	M	T	6	T4-T12	NA	35.3±6.6	63.2±4.3	43.1±7.4	180±10	142±9
Hooker & Wells, 1992[145]	ACE	F	T	1	T10	NA	33	52.4	38.0	167	102
Janssen et al, 1993[137]	WCE	M	UT	15	T6-T10	C/I	33.4±12	78.6±16.0	21.2±6.6	NA	NA
Janssen, 1997[138]	WCE	M	UT	10	T6-T10	NA	31.6±6.6	79.7±15.1	24.3±6.1	NA	84±23
Lin et al, 1993[142]	ACE	M	UT	11	T6-T10	NA	25.6±1.9	59.7±3.5	17.7±0.9	181±7	47±2
Schmid et al, 1998[143]	WCE	M	UT	10	T5-T10	NA	36.5±6.5	73.5±11.9	29.6±7.2	182±19	79±20
Scheider et al, 1999[146]	ACE	M	T	6	T10-T12	NA	32.0±4	70.8±7.9	29.6±2.2	185±4	120±5
Wicks, 1983[125]	WCE ACE	M	T	10	T6-T10	NA	27.5±7.4	70.3±16.9	WCE 27.8±6.4 / ACE 28.0±6.2	178±15 / 174±18	41±7 / 113±16
Wicks, 1983[125]	WCE ACE	F	T	4	T6-T10	NA	28.2±7.9	61.5±16.9	WCE 17.5±8.3 / ACE 21.7±8.3	170±12 / 175±16	28±5 / 65±13

Mode, Form of exercise; *Lesion extent*, degree of completeness of injury or ASIA levels; *C*, complete injury; *I*, incomplete injury; *M*, male; *F*, female; *T*, trained; *UT*, untrained; *NA*, not available.

TABLE 18-8 | Maximal Exercise Performance Outcomes for Individuals with Low Paraplegia

Study	Mode	Sex	Status	n	Levels of SCI	Lesion Extent	Age (yr)	Mass (kg)	VO_{2Peak} (ml/kg⁻¹/min⁻¹)	HR (beats/min)	PO_{Peak} (W)
Barstow et al, 2000[147]	ACE	M	UT	8	T4-L1	C	34.3±6.7	73.1±11.8	19.7±4.8	167±16.4	58±12
Bernard et al, 2000[144]	WCE	M	T	6	T11-L3	4C:2I	28.3±2.7	68.5±9.4	34.2±3.8	168±7.6	NA
Burkett, 1990[126]	WCE	M	UT	7	T5-L1	I	30.8±3.9	64.6±3.3	24.7±2.8	182±20	NA
Burkett, 1990[126]	WCE	M	T	4	T5-L3	3C:1I	32.8±2.9	75.2±9.0	28.1±2.2	163±16	NA
Burkett, 1990[126]	WCE	F	UT	5	T3-L2	3C:2I	29.0±5.6	55.6±5.0	15.9±2.2	166±21	NA
Cooper et al, 1992[148]	WCE	M	T	11	T3-L2	NA	30.9±5.8	65.9±6.1	38.1±4.3	NA	NA
Coutts et al, 1983[120]	WCE	M	UT	4/3	T11-L3/ L4-S2	NA	29±5.0/ 28±2.5	72.6±17.8/ 66.6±14.9	37.6±11.0/ 33.7±12.1	190±8/ 188±10	89±23/ 68±15
Coutts & Stogryn 1987[127]	WCE	M	T	2	T9-L2	NA	27.5±3.5	76.6±9.1	44.0±6.8	183±5.5	117±4
Erikkson et al, 1988[133]	WCE	M	UT/T	10/T	T1-S2	NA	33±11/31±4	79.3±19.8/ 65.1±10.6	22.0±6.7/ 33.6±6.7	186±9/ 183±13	NA
Hjeltues & Janssen, 1990[135]	ACE	M	UT	8/11	T12-L3/ L4-S2	C	37/53	NA	28±6.8/24±7.1	NA	NA
Hjeltues & Janssen, 1990[135]	ACE	F	UT	2	T12-L3/ L4-S2	C	27/35	NA	23±1.5/40	NA	NA
Janssen et al, 1993[137]	WCE	M	UT	12/2	T11-L3/ L4-S2	C/I	33.0±15/39.5	78.9±21.9/ 68.4	25.7±7.8/31.3	NA	NA
Janssen, 1997[138]	WCE	M	UT	14	T11-L3	NA	40.6±16	85.6±21.4	25.6±8.3	NA	84±23
Lassau-Wray et al, 2000[123]	ACE	M	UT	5	T7-T12	NA	28.2±3.3	62.6±6.0	27.6±2.1	174±1	NA
Lin et al, 1993[142]	ACE	M	UT	19	T11-L3	NA	30.9±2.0	58.5±1.6	21.3±0.9	182±4	51±3
Schmid et al, 1998[147]	WCE	M	UT	10	T11-S2	NA	33.0±9.1	74.6±11.2	30.1±9.5	176±19	72±32
Van Loan et al, 1987[140]	ACE	M/F	UT	8	T4-L3	NA	25.2±2.9	60.2±2.8	25.3±7.4	160±32	85±13
Wicks, 1983[125]	WCE ACE	M	T	17/7	T11-L3/ L4-S2	NA	26.1±6.5/ 36.0±4.7	64.8±14./ 159.9±7.5	WCE 31.2±7.6 ACE 31.0±6.6 WCE 36.1±4.7 ACE 37.7±4.5	177±15 174±18 178±15 174±18	42±7 116±19 40±7 121±9
Wicks, 1983[125]	WCE ACE	F	T	2	T11-L3/ L4-S2	NA	21.5±3.5 30.0±0.0	44.1±2.0 50.6±4.2	WCE 30.2±0.2 ACE 32.7±4.1 WCE 16.4±11 ACE 22.0±4.8	178±14 175±2 169±2 180±8	34±7 90±12 26±12 65±7

Mode, Form of exercise; Lesion extent, degree of completeness of injury or ASIA levels; C, complete injury; I, incomplete injury; M, male; F, female; T, trained; UT, untrained; NA, not available.

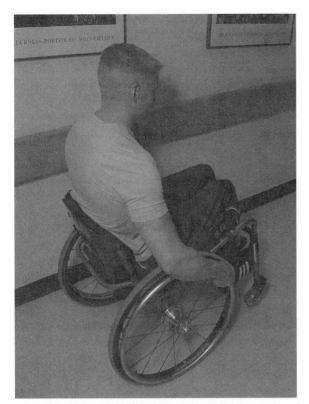

FIGURE 18-2 An individual with paraplegia includes exercise in his daily routine by propulsion of his manual wheelchair. He is seen here negotiating an interior incline. His upper body strength benefits from practicing on challenging surfaces such as steep inclines.

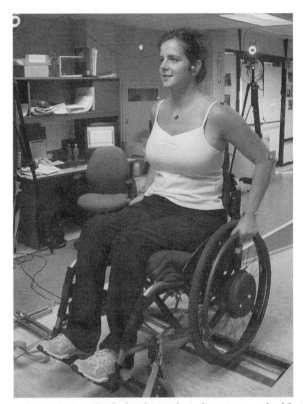

FIGURE 18-3 An individual with paraplegia demonstrates wheelchair ergometer exercise.

physician clearance provided before continuing with the exercise prescription.

The informed choice of exercise mode should be made by the patient because this will dictate, to a large degree, patient compliance. The person prescribing the exercise should be aware of the available options including manual wheelchair propulsion (Figure 18-2), ACE, WCE (Figure 18-3), FES-LCE (see Figure 17-5), ACE plus FES-LCE (Hybrid), and resistance training equipment, as well as the advantages and disadvantages applicable to each.

A consensus statement recently generated by the Centers for Disease Control and Prevention and the ACSM has recommended that "every US adult should accumulate 30 minutes or more of moderate-intensity physical activity on most, preferably all, days of the week."[110] Moderate activity was defined by the panel as activity performed at 3 to 6 metabolic equivalents (METS) (i.e., 10.5-21 ml/kg^{-1}/min^{-1}),[77] which is near VO_{2Peak} for some individuals with SCI but still a helpful guideline when appropriately modified for this population. The most appropriate way to monitor and prescribe intensity of aerobic exercise for the individual with SCI remains somewhat at controversy.[111] Recommended guidelines for the able-bodied population suggest that exercise intensity should be within 60% to 90% of maximal HR or 50% to 85% of maximal VO_2 to significantly improve cardiovascular fitness parameters.[112] HR responses in tetraplegia and high paraplegia, however, are subject to parasympathetic

withdrawal more than sympathetic stimulation, resulting in significantly lower maximal heart rates (130 vs. 180-200 beats/min seen in able-bodied subjects) and contributing to the great deal of variability noted between VO_{2Peak} and HR in this population.[113] Janssen et al[114] developed regression equations predicting heart rate reserve values of 30% to 80% corresponding to 50% to 85% VO_{2Peak} in those with high paraplegia and tetraplegia, but again, variability seemed large. Although improvements have been demonstrated while using exercise intensity of 60% to 85% HR_{max} in the population with SCI, it is not clear that heart rate is the best way to monitor intensity. McLean and Skinner[113] recommended prescribing intensity as a percentage of PO_{Peak}, but this would require constant reevaluation to maintain optimal training intensity because PO_{Peak} would be expected to increase linearly with training. Rate of perceived exertion (RPE) may be the most appropriate scale on which to base prescribed exercise intensity for individuals with tetraplegia and high paraplegia because it has been used with good success in cardiac transplant patients who have denervated hearts,[115] although this too has limitations.[116]

If the prescription is preceded by a graded exercise test, one may use the RPE values corresponding to 50% to 85% VO_{2Peak} to assign an exercise range; this should correspond to about 12 to 13 (somewhat hard) on the Borg RPE scale (Box 18-3).[117] Alternatively, 60% to 90% of HR_{max} may be assigned as the target heart rate zone if a person has a heart rate monitor, recognizing the limits of this technique; tetraplegia often precludes self-monitoring of the pulse. Without exercise testing, the ability to accurately

BOX 18-3	Borg Scale Rate of Perceived Exertion Scale, the 15-Grade Scale for Ratings of Perceived Exertion

6	No exertion at all
7 }	Extremely light
8 }	
9	Very light
10	
11	Light
12	
13	Somewhat hard
14	
15	Hard (heavy)
16	
17	Very hard
18	
19	Extremely hard
20	Maximal Exertion

Instructions to the Borg-RPE-Scale

During the work, we want you to rate your perception of exertion (i.e., how heavy and strenuous the exercise feels to you and how tired you are). The perception of exertion is mainly felt as strain and fatigue in your muscles and as breathlessness or aches in the chest.

Use this scale from 6 to 20, where **6** means "No exertion at all" and **20** means "Maximal exertion."

9	Very light. As for a healthy person taking a short walk at his or her own pace.
13	Somewhat hard. It still feels OK to continue.
15	It is hard and tiring, but continuing is not terribly difficult.
17	Very hard. It is very strenuous. You can still go on, but you really have to push yourself and you are very tired.
19	An extremely strenuous level. For most people this is the most strenuous exercise they have ever experienced.

Try to appraise your feeling of exertion and fatigue as spontaneously and as honestly as possible, without thinking about what the actual physical load is. Try not to underestimate nor to overestimate. It is your own feeling of effort and exertion that is important, not how it compares with other people's feelings. Look at the scale and the expressions and then give a number. You can equally well use even as odd numbers. Any questions?

From Brog G: *Borg's perceived exertion and pain scales*, Champaign, IL, 1998, Human Kinetics, p. 31.

assign exercise intensity will be markedly impaired. A final consideration would be to have an individual use the three- to five-word sentence rule; if he is able to speak in three- to five-word sentences during exercise, he should be within an appropriate intensity range.

When using the FES-LCE or Hybrid exercise systems, it should be recognized that a detailed protocol needs to be used to avoid complications such as autonomic dysreflexia or lower limb fractures. Commercial systems will have manufacturer's recommendations for initial settings, duration, frequency, and precautions that should be closely followed. Initial intensity levels will necessarily be less than those used in upper limb protocols.

The duration of a single aerobic exercise bout will vary depending on fitness levels but should be preceded and followed by a 10-minute warmup and extend between 20 and 60 minutes in length.[110] Prolonged exercise tolerance in persons with SCI has received little attention in the literature, and it is therefore recommended that progression of exercise duration be monitored closely and that individuals replenish with small amounts of fluids frequently while exercising. If prolonged exercise (>2 hours) is anticipated, intermittent catheterization should be performed on a scheduled basis or, alternatively, an indwelling catheter is recommended to reduce the likelihood that, with fluid replenishment, bladder distention would induce autonomic dysreflexia in those at risk.

Aerobic exercise should be performed no fewer than 3 days a week to maintain fitness but may occur up to 5 days a week for optimal gains in cardiopulmonary fitness without negative consequences, particularly when performed at relatively low intensity levels.[97] Individuals with SCI may require increased exercise frequency to optimize caloric expenditure but should be judiciously monitored to reduce the incidence of upper limb overuse syndromes. A person with SCI who has a VO_{2Peak} <15.5 mg/kg^{-1}/min-1 (<3 METS) may require multiple bouts of exercise daily, each lasting 5 to 15 minutes, until he is able to tolerate 20- to 30-minute sessions.

The initial stages of an aerobic exercise program should focus more on developing the habit of exercise rather than the intensity and duration of exercise because exercise adherence may decrease if the program is too rigorously initiated. The duration of the early exercise bouts may be limited by the individual's muscular endurance; as is often the case with upper limb work. As earlier indicated, short sessions of 5 to 15 minutes two to four times daily may be appropriate early in the course of an exercise training program. Individuals should be told to expect delayed-onset muscle soreness, which may persist during the first 2 weeks of the exercise program, but which should subside after that, despite increasing intensity or duration. This conditioning stage should last 6 to 8 weeks.

The improvement stage is marked by rapid improvement and progression of intensity and frequency of exercise. After duration of exercise is extended to 30 minutes, intensity may be increased if the individual feels time constraints become a limiting factor. As duration and intensity of exercise are increased, however, frequency should be decreased to prevent overtraining. Maintenance of exercise conditioning is required once an individual has achieved his goals, or by the reversibility principle, benefits will be lost. The most important factor in extended exercise compliance is that the activity be enjoyable and usable.

Little research has been done in the area of resistance training for neurologically intact muscle in SCI; it is unclear whether individuals with SCI have different responses to resistance training than do able-bodied people.[111] As earlier indicated, testosterone, free testosterone, and growth hormone levels are significantly reduced in individuals with SCI, and their responses to exercise appear blunted, perhaps a reflection of reduced overall muscle mass used during exercise bouts. Although muscle groups that remain neurologically intact and under voluntary control should respond to an imposed stress, hormonal responses may not be

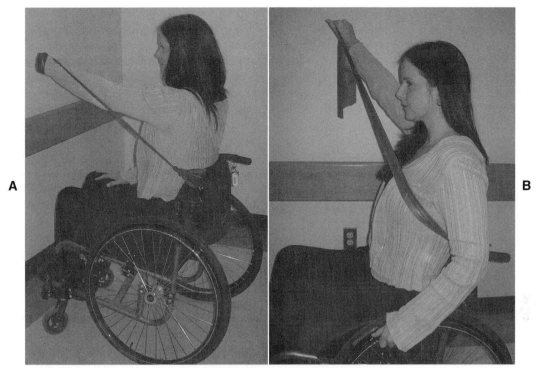

FIGURE 18-4 A person with paraplegia uses Thera-Band to strengthen her upper limbs. **A,** Thera-Band is attached to the wheelchair push handle to allow her to do strengthening exercises in any environment without needing to transfer out of the chair. Movements can be performed in the forward direction to work on elbow, shoulder, and scapula muscles. **B,** She can also perform movements in the diagonal direction to mimic the proprioceptive neuromuscular facilitation approach to strengthening. Handles (not shown) that can be attached to these elastic bands are available and useful for individuals who do not have adequate hand grip.

adequate to stimulate hypertrophy to the extent seen in the able-bodied population.

Minimally, scapular stabilization and rotator cuff resistance exercises should be used in all individuals with SCI capable of voluntary control of these muscles. Initial intervention should include two sets of 10 repetitions, with 6-second isometric contractions for shoulder protractors, retractors, elevators and depressors, and for internal and external shoulder rotators, progressing to dynamic Thera-Band exercises as static strength plateaus (Figure 18-4). Strength and hypertrophy gains will typically plateau with Thera-Band exercises as well, and additional gains will require increased resistance and volume of exercise (Figure 18-5). Although dumbbells and free weights may be used under close supervision, paralyzed lower limbs and truncal musculature significantly reduce a person's ability to balance even small objects when lying supine or when seated without significant truncal support. Whether free weights are used, or isotonic/isokinetic machines, wheelchair brakes should be set before lifting, and care should be taken not to exceed the wheelchair's weight and stress limitations as provided by the manufacturer. As per the ACSM guidelines for muscular strength and endurance, a prescription of one set to exhaustion of 8 to 12 repetitions for each of the major muscle groups that remain neurologically intact, two to three times a week, is recommended.[112] Circuit resistance training combining resistance exercise with arm cranking has demonstrated positive effects on both strength and fitness in individuals with paraplegia.[111] Progression and maintenance should be individualized according to the person's need and goals.

BARRIERS TO IMPLEMENTATION

To successfully participate in an exercise program, the person with tetraplegia must have access to a mildly temperate climate or thermally controlled environment (to avoid the risk of hypothermia and hyperthermia), appropriate seating and positioning (to reduce the risk of pressure sores, autonomic dysreflexia, spasticity, and musculoskeletal trauma), and adapted equipment for resistance or aerobic training. Unfortunately, few commercial fitness centers are cognizant of these needs, and many fail to even provide appropriate access to wheelchair users. A recent survey of physical fitness facilities in a major metropolitan city demonstrated that none of the 34 facilities reviewed met all of the 1990 Americans With Disabilities Act requirements for accessibility as mandated by Title III, with lowest compliance reported in the areas of restrooms, locker rooms, drinking fountains, and space around exercise equipment.[118] More recently, Rimmer et al[119] have developed and validated an instrument to determine accessibility of fitness and recreational environments, which can be used by the physical therapist to assist clients in finding appropriate facilities.

Because of the significant risks associated with exercise in this population, the initial stages of exercise training should be performed under the supervision of an exercise physiologist or physical therapist well versed in SCI exercise responses

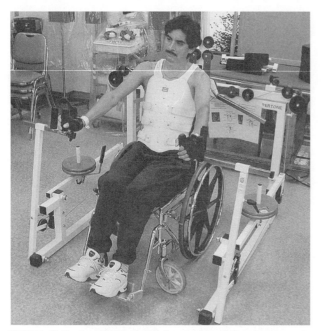

FIGURE 18-5 An individual with impaired hand function can use a rickshaw-type strength training gym equipment if he uses a Velcro mitt to facilitate his grip on the machine handle. (From Pendleton HH, Schulz-Krohn W: *Pedretti's occupational therapy*, ed. 6, St. Louis, 2006, Mosby.)

(Figures 18-6 and 18-7). HR and BP responses should be monitored during these initial stages to assess for possible episodes of exercise-induced autonomic dysreflexia or hypotension. For upper limb aerobic exercise, the arm crank or wheelchair ergometer should be adjusted appropriately to allow optimal efficiency and to reduce musculoskeletal injuries at the shoulder, elbow, and wrist, and straps should be applied to the torso to prevent truncal instability. Wheelchair gloves or flexion mitts are important to prevent blisters, lacerations, and abrasions, especially for those with tetraplegia whose hands and fingers are insensate. Upper arm bands or Co-Ban tape may be used to prevent abrasions at the medial upper arm with wheelchair propulsion. Velcro straps and cuffed weights are commonly used for resistance training equipment modifications. Abdominal binders and leg wraps may be used to facilitate improved pulmonary dynamics and greater venous return, allowing improved CO by the Frank-Starling mechanism. FES-LCE and Hybrid systems are now commercially available but remain fairly expensive to purchase and maintain relative to ACE. The individual's time constraints, transportation availability, required assistance, and financial constraints should also be discussed because these factors will significantly affect compliance with the exercise program. Recognizing these considerations, rehabilitation professionals often may incorporate exercise and strength training into task-specific activities that are functional in origin (Figure 18-8).

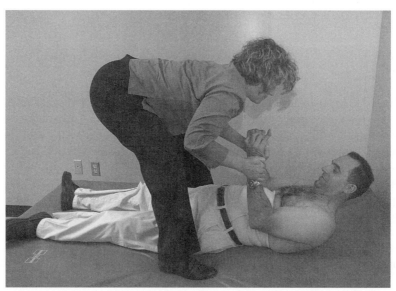

FIGURE 18-6 The therapist may use a pull-up method for strengthening concentric and eccentric biceps so that the patient learns how to lift his own body weight or how to use an overhead bed trapeze. It is essential for the therapist to maintain good body mechanics during exercise sessions.

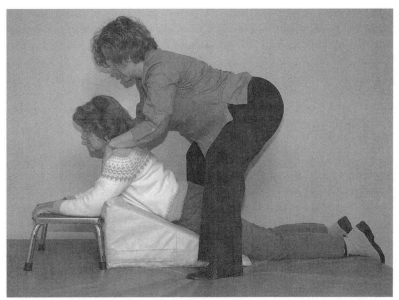

FIGURE 18-7 Upper body strengthening may be accomplished by using weight bearing through the patient's elbows to promote contraction around the shoulder muscles, which are needed for body stabilization. When the therapist resists shoulder motion in all directions, these shoulder stabilizers are strengthened and the patient learns the importance of stability before functional position changes can be accomplished. The therapist needs to maintain good body position during intervention maneuvers.

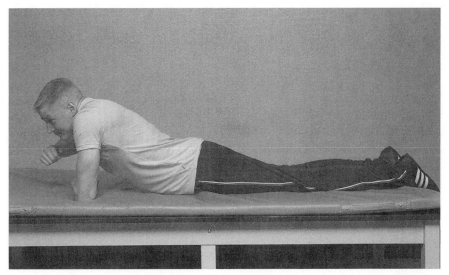

FIGURE 18-8 Strength training can be incorporated in to task-specific activities that are functional in origin. This individual needs to perform a prone "army crawl" maneuver to move around in his bed. The task becomes an upper body therapeutic strengthening technique as well.

CLINICAL CASE STUDY Exercise and Fitness for Individuals with a Spinal Cord Injury Case 1

Patient History

Jake Boyd is a 23-year-old man with a C7 tetraplegia, ASIA A diagnosis resulting from a football injury. He is 1 year post injury and medically stable. His acute care and rehabilitation were completed without medical complications.

Jake is currently in his senior year in college and is a computer science major. He uses a power wheelchair to get around campus but relies on his manual wheelchair at home. He lives at home with his parents and two brothers, ages 15 and 17 years. The family room is on the first floor and has been converted to an accessible bedroom with a bathroom.

Patient's Self-Assessment

Jake's lifestyle has always been very active. He was a football player and wrestler in high school and on the tennis team earlier in his college career. He wants to be able to resume exercise and fitness activities and participation in team sports.

Clinical Assessment
Patient Appearance

- Height 5 feet 10 inches, weight 160 pounds, body mass index 23
- Atrophy in the forearm and hand, limiting grip capacity for using arm crank ergometry

Cognitive Assessment

- Alert, oriented × 3

Cardiopulmonary Assessment

- BP 112/60 mm Hg, HR at rest 66 beats/min, respiratory rate 13 breaths/min, cough flows are ineffective (<360 L/min), vital capacity is reduced (between 1.5 and 2.5 L)

Musculoskeletal and Neuromuscular Assessment

- Motor assessment reveals C7 ASIA A, motor is intact to the C7 level; sensory intact to T4
- * Deep tendon reflexes 3+ below the level of lesion

Integumentary and Sensory Assessment

- Skin is intact throughout with light touch sensation intact to T4.

Range of Motion Assessment

- Passive and active range of motion is within normal limits in both upper limbs
- Straight leg raise is 102 degrees in both lower limbs and dorsiflexion is 3 degrees; all other motions in the lower limbs are within functional limits.

Mobility and ADL Assessment

- Independent with bed mobility
- Independent in transfers to all surfaces, except floor to wheelchair to floor requires moderate assistance
- Independent with pressure relief
- Independent in manual wheelchair maneuvering on all surfaces
- Independent in high-level wheelchair skills except ascending and descending stairs, which requires the assistance of two people
- Dependent in bowel and bladder care
- Independent in upper body dressing and requires minimal assistance for lower body dressing
- Independent in driving

Evaluation of Clinical Assessment

Jake Boyd is a 23-year-old man with a C7 tetraplegia, ASIA A diagnosis resulting from a football injury. He is 1 year post injury and medically stable. His acute care and rehabilitation were completed without medical complications. He is being seen for GXT with ACE to develop a wellness and exercise fitness program.

Patient's Care Needs

1. Prescription for GXT with ACE
2. Consultation for wellness program in the wellness department
3. Education regarding fitness and wellness for safety and prevention of secondary conditions after spinal cord injury such as cardiovascular disease

Diagnosis and Prognosis

Diagnosis is C7 complete tetraplegia, ASIA A. Prognosis is good for Jake to gain improved fitness through adherence to the prescribed exercise program that emphasizes prevention of secondary complications.

Preferred Practice Patterns*

Impaired Muscle Performance (4C), Impairments Nonprogressive Spinal Cord Disorders (5H), Primary Prevention/Risk Reduction for Cardiovascular/Pulmonary Disorders (6A), Primary Prevention/Risk Reduction for Integumentary Disorders (7A)

Team Goals

1. Team to complete a graded exercise test
2. Team to design and evaluate an exercise fitness and wellness program
3. Team to educate Jake regarding fitness and wellness for safety and prevention of secondary conditions after SCI

Patient Goals

"I want to be able to exercise again and feel that exercise high I used to get."

Care Plan
Treatment Plan and Rationale:

- Complete GXT with ACE as basis for design of a fitness exercise and wellness program for Jake to enable primary prevention of secondary complications after SCI
- Design individualized exercise fitness and wellness program for Jake

Interventions

- Strengthening and cardiopulmonary fitness exercises
- Outpatient wellness department evaluation and consultation

Documentation and Team Communication

- Aerobic capacity and fitness exercise prescription
- Wellness team evaluation and team meeting

Follow-Up Assessment

- Reassessment of the exercise prescription every 4 weeks for 4 months

Critical Thinking Exercises

Consider factors including lifestyle and exercise needs and restrictions that are important to Jake's evaluation and exercise prescription when answering the following questions:

1. What issues are inherent in Jake's case relating to parasympathetic and sympathetic exercise restrictions?
2. What are some considerations for stabilizing Jake when performing crank testing?
3. What BP considerations are required for exercise testing?
4. What are some considerations for strength training with Jake?

*Guide to physical therapist practice, rev. ed.2, Alexandria, VA, 2003, American Physical Therapy Association.

CLINICAL CASE STUDY Exercise and Fitness for Individuals with a Spinal Cord Injury Case 2

Patient History

Sally Jones is a 56-year-old woman with a T11 ASIA A paraplegia diagnosis. She was injured 10 years ago in a motor vehicle accident. She has maintained a healthy lifestyle since her injury without hospitalizations.

Sally is a high school math teacher. She is married with two grown children. She has been active intermittently in wheelchair racing. She owns a manual wheelchair and a racing wheelchair.

Patient's Self-Assessment

Sally would like to take part in a consistent exercise program because she has recently noted fatigue at the end of her workday. She has been inconsistent about exercising over the past year.

Clinical Assessment
Patient Appearance
- Height 5 feet 1 inches, weight 109 pounds, body mass index 20.6

Cognitive Assessment
- Alert, oriented × 3

Cardiopulmonary Assessment
- BP 116/60 mm Hg, HR at rest 78 beats/min, respiratory rate 14 breaths/min, cough flows are effective and vital capacity is functional

Musculoskeletal and Neuromuscular Assessment
- Motor assessment reveals T11 ASIA A, sensory intact to T11
- Deep tendon reflexes 1+ below the level of lesion

Integumentary and Sensory Assessment
- Skin is intact throughout, sensory intact to T11

Range of Motion Assessment
- Passive and active motion is within normal limits in both upper limbs.
- Straight leg raise is 110 degrees in both lower limbs and dorsiflexion is 7 degrees; all other motions in the lower limbs are within functional limits.

Mobility and ADL Assessment
- Independent with bed mobility
- Independent in transfers to all surfaces
- Independent with pressure relief
- Independent in manual wheelchair maneuvering on all surfaces
- Independent in high-level wheelchair skills
- Independent in bowel and bladder care
- Independent in upper and lower body dressing
- Independent in driving

Evaluation of Clinical Assessment

Sally Jones is a 56-year-old woman with a T11 ASIA A paraplegia diagnosis. She was injured 10 years ago in a motor vehicle accident. She has maintained a healthy lifestyle since her injury without hospitalizations. She is seeking a wellness exercise fitness test and exercise program.

Patient's Care Needs
1. Prescription for GXT with ACE
2. Consultation for wellness program in the wellness department
3. Education regarding fitness and wellness for safety and prevention of secondary conditions after SCI

Diagnosis and Prognosis

Diagnosis is T11 complete paraplegia ASIA A. Prognosis is excellent for Sally to gain improved fitness with adherence to the prescribed exercise program that emphasizes prevention of secondary conditions after SCI.

Preferred Practice Patterns*

Impaired Muscle Performance (4C), Impairments Nonprogressive Spinal Cord Disorders (5H), Primary Prevention/Risk Reduction for Cardiovascular/Pulmonary Disorders (6A), Primary Prevention/Risk Reduction for Integumentary Disorders (7A)

Team Goals
1. Team to complete a GXT with ACE
2. Team to design and evaluate an exercise fitness and wellness program
3. Team to educate Sally regarding fitness and wellness for safety and prevention of secondary conditions after SCI

Patient Goals

"I want to be consistent with my exercise program and doing exercise regularly."

Care Plan
Treatment Plan & Rationale
- Complete GXT with ACE as a basis for design of a fitness exercise and wellness program for Sally to enable primary prevention of secondary conditions after SCI
- Design individualized wellness exercise fitness program for Sally

Interventions
- Outpatient wellness department consultation for evaluation of results from exercise testing and exercise prescription

Documentation & Team Communication
- Wellness team evaluation and team meeting
- Exercise prescription and methods for progressing workloads

Follow-Up Assessment
- Reassessment of the exercise prescription every 4 weeks for 4 months

Critical Thinking Exercises

Consider factors including lifestyle and exercise needs and restrictions that are important to Sally's evaluation and exercise prescription when answering the following questions:
1. What pre-exercise medical testing would you recommend for Sally?
2. Given Sally's injury level, what procedure(s) should be used to measure VO_{2peak} and peak PO?
3. What are some considerations in prescribing and selecting Sally's aerobic training program?
4. Once an aerobic program has been selected, how should that program progress?

*Guide to physical therapist practice, rev. ed 2, Alexandria, VA, 2003, American Physical Therapy Association.

SUMMARY

Exercise is an important component toward gaining and maintaining physical fitness in SCI. Physiological adaptation resultant from SCI should be considered when designing and implementing exercise programs and parameters. Systems such as the ANS, the cardiovascular and pulmonary systems, and the endocrine system play an important role in the outcomes of exercise performance and tolerance. Metabolic alterations as a result of SCI are affected, and parameters such as lipid profiles, glucose metabolism, body composition, and osteopenia should be considered when testing and training individuals with SCI. Following the guidelines for exercise screening enables patients and clinicians to design and individualize safe and effective exercise programs. Finally, every effort to remove barriers to exercise implementation should be made to enhance the potential for exercise compliance.

REFERENCES

1. Casperson CJ, Powell KE, Christenson GM: Physical activity, exercise, and physical fitness: definitions and distinctions for health-related research, *Public Health Rep* 100:126-131, 1985.
2. Skinner JS: General principles of exercise prescription. In Skinner JS, editor: *Exercise testing and exercise prescription for special cases: theoretical basis and clinical application*, Philadelphia, 1993, Lea & Febiger.
3. Jacobs PL, Johnson BM, Mahoney ET et al: Effect of variable loading in the determination of upper-limb anaerobic power in persons with tetraplegia, *J Rehabil Res Dev* 41:9-14, 2004.
4. Jacobs PL, Mahoney ET, Johnson B: Reliability of arm Wingate anaerobic testing in persons with complete paraplegia, *J Spinal Cord Med* 26:141-144, 2003.
5. Hicks AL, Martin KA, Ditor DS et al: Long-term exercise training in persons with spinal cord injury: effects on strength, arm ergometry performance and psychological well-being, *Spinal Cord* 41:34-43, 2003.
6. Bernard PL, Codine P, Minier J: Isokinetic shoulder rotator muscles in wheelchair athletes, *Spinal Cord.* 42:222-229, 2004.
7. Gilgoff IS, Davidson SL, Hohn AR: Cardiac pacemaker in high spinal cord injury, *Arch Phys Med Rehabil* 72:603, 1991.
8. Kawamoto M, Sakimura S, Takasaki M: Transient increase of parasympathetic tone in patients with cervical spinal cord trauma, *Anaesth Intensive Care* 21:218-221, 1993.
9. Lehman K, Lane J Piepmeir J et al: Cardiovascular abnormalities accompanying acute spinal cord injury in humans: incidence, time course and severity, *J Am Coll Cardiol* 10:46-52, 1987.
10. Winslow E, Lesch M, Talano J et al: Spinal cord injuries associated with cardiopulmonary complications, *Spine* 11:809-812, 1986.
11. Dixit S: Bradycardia associated with high cervical spinal cord injury, *Surg Neurol* 43:514, 1995.
12. Kessler KM, Pina I, Green B et al: Cardiovascular findings in quadriplegic and paraplegic patients and in normal subjects, *J Cardiol* 58:525-530, 1986.
13. Nash MS, Bilsker M, Marcillo AE et al: Reversal of adaptive left ventricular atrophy following electrically-stimulated exercise training in human tetraplegics, *Paraplegia* 29:590-599, 1991.
14. DeTroyer A, Heilporn A: Respiratory mechanics in quadriplegia. The respiratory function of the intercostal muscles, *Am Rev Respir Dis* 122:591-600, 1980.
15. Haas F, Axen K, Pineda H et al: Temporal pulmonary function changes in cervical cord injury, *Arch Phys Med Rehabil* 66:139-144, 1985.
16. Creasey G, Elefteriades J, DiMarco A et al: Electrical stimulation to restore respiration, *J Rehabil Res Devel* 33:123-132, 1996.
17. Miller JI, Farmer JA, Stuart W et al: Phrenic nerve pacing of the quadriplegic patient, *Thorac Cardiovasc Surg* 99:35-40, 1990.
18. Maloney F: Pulmonary function in quadriplegia: effects of a corset, *Arch Phys Med Rehabil* 60:261-265, 1979.
19. Hopman MT, Van der Woude LH, Dallmeijer AJ et al: Respiratory muscle strength and endurance in individuals with tetraplegia, *Spinal Cord* 35:104-108, 1997.
20. Almenoff PL, Spungen AM, Lesser M et al: Pulmonary function survey in spinal cord injury: influences of smoking and level and completeness of injury, *Lung* 173:297-306, 1995.
21. Cooper RA, Baldini FD, Langbein WE et al: Prediction of pulmonary function in wheelchair users, *Paraplegia* 31:560-570, 1993.
22. Crane L, Klerk K, Ruhl A et al: The effect of exercise on pulmonary function in persons with quadriplegia, *Paraplegia* 32:435-441, 1994.
23. Ready AE: Response of quadriplegic athletes to maximal and submaximal exercise, *Physiother Can* 36:124-128, 1984.
24. Walker J, Cooney M, Norton S: Improved pulmonary function in chronic quadriplegics after pulmonary therapy and arm ergometry, *Paraplegia* 27:278-283, 1989.
25. Schmidt KD, Chan CW: Thermoregulation and fever in normal persons and in those with spinal cord injuries, *Mayo Clin Proc* 67:469-475, 1992.
26. Downey JA, Huckaba CE, Kelley PS et al: Sweating responses to central and peripheral heating in spinal man, *J Appl Physiol* 40:701-706, 1976.
27. Wallin BG, Stjernberg L: Sympathetic activity in man after spinal cord injury: outflow to skin below the lesion, *Brain* 107:183-198, 1984.
28. Huckaba CE, Frewin DB, Downey JA et al: Sweating responses of normal, paraplegic and anhidrotic subjects, *Arch Phys Med Rehabil* 57:268-274, 1976.
29. Krum H, Brown DJ, Rowe PR et al: Steady state plasma 3H-noradrenaline kinetics in quadriplegic chronic spinal cord injury patients, *J Autonomic Pharmacol* 10:221-226, 1990.
30. Claus-Walker JC, Halstead LS: Metabolic and endocrine changes in spinal cord injury, II: partial decentralization of the autonomic nervous system, *Arch Phys Med Rehabil* 63:576-580, 1982.
31. Wang LC, Huang YC, Lee EJ, Chen HH: Acute paraplegia in a patient with spinal tophi: a case report, *J Formos Med Assoc* 100:205-208, 2001.
32. Aksnes AK, Hjeltnes N, Wahlstrom EO et al: Intact glucose transport in morphologically altered denervated skeletal muscle from quadriplegic patients, *Am J Physiol Endocrinol Metabol* 34:E593-E600, 1996.
33. Zhong YG, Levy E, Bauman WA: The relationships among serum uric-acid, plasma-insulin, and serum-lipoprotein levels in subjects with spinal-cord injury, *Horm Metab Res* 27:283-286, 1995.
34. Bauman WA, Spungen AM: Metabolic changes in persons after spinal cord injury, *Phys Med Rehabil Clin North Am* 11:109-140, 2000.
35. Tsitouras PD, Zhong YG, Spungen AM et al: Serum testosterone and growth-hormone insulin-like growth-factor-I in adults with spinal-cord injury, *Horm Metab Res* 27:287-292, 1995.
36. Bauman WA, Spungen AM, Flanagan S et al: Blunted growth-hormone response to intravenous arginine in subjects with a spinal-cord injury, *Horm Metab Res* 26:152-156, 1994.
37. Shetty KR, Sutton CH, Mattson DE et al: Hyposomatomedinemia in quadriplegic men, *Am J Med Sci* 305:95-100, 1993.
38. Reame NE: A prospective study of the menstrual cycle and spinal cord injury, *Am J Phys Med Rehabil* 71:15-21, 1992.

39. Braddom RL, Rocco JF: Autonomic dysreflexia: a survey of current treatment, *Am J Phys Med Rehabil* 70:234-241, 1991.

40. Curt A, Nitsche B, Rodic B et al: Assessment of autonomic dysreflexia in patients with spinal cord injury, *J Neurol Neurosurg Psych* 62:473-477, 1997.

41. Bauman WA, Spungen AM, Adkins RH et al: Metabolic and endocrine changes in persons aging with spinal cord injury, *Assist Technol* 11:88-96, 1999.

42. Bostom AG, Toner MM, McArdle WD, et al: Lipid and lipoprotein profiles related to peak aerobic power in spinal cord injured males, *Med Sci Sport Exerc* 23:409-414, 1991.

43. Brenes G, Dearwater S, Shapera R et al: High density lipoprotein cholesterol concentrations in physically active and sedentary spinal cord injured patients, *Arch Phys Med Rehabil* 67:445-450, 1986.

44. Dallmeijer AJ, Hopman MT, Van der Woude LH: Lipid, lipoprotein, and apolipoprotein profiles in active and sedentary men with tetraplegia, *Arch Phys Med Rehabil* 78:1173-1176, 1997.

45. Maki KC, Briones ER, Langbein WE et al: Associations between serum lipids and indicators of adiposity in men with spinal cord injury, *Paraplegia* 33:102-109, 1995.

46. Duran FS, Lugo L, Ramirez L et al: Effects of an exercise program on the rehabilitation of patients with spinal cord injury, *Arch Phys Med Rehabil* 82:1349-1354, 2001.

47. Midha M, Schmitt JK, Sclater M: Exercise effect with the wheelchair aerobic fitness trainer on conditioning and metabolic function in disabled persons: a pilot study, *Arch Phys Med Rehabil* 80:258-261, 1999.

48. Hooker SP, Wells CL: Effects of low and moderate-intensity training in spinal cord injured persons, *Med Sci Sport Exerc* 21:18-22, 1989.

49. Mollinger LA, Sparr GB, El Ghatet AZ: Daily energy expenditure and basal metabolic rates of patients with spinal cord injury, *Arch Phys Med Rehabil* 66:420-426, 1999.

50. Monroe MB, Tataranni PA, Pratley R et al: Lower daily energy expenditure as measured by a respiratory chamber in subjects with spinal cord injury compared with control subjects, *Am J Clin Nutr* 68:1223-1227, 1998.

51. Sedlock DA, Laventure SJ: Body-composition and resting energy-expenditure in long-term spinal-cord injury, *Paraplegia* 28:448-454, 1990.

52. Bauman WA, Spungen AM, Wang J et al: The relationship between energy expenditure and lean tissue in monozygotic twins discordant for spinal cord injury, *J Rehabil Res Dev* 41:1-8, 2004.

53. Spungen AM, Wang J, Pierson RN et al: Soft tissue body composition differences in monozygotic twins discordant for spinal cord injury, *J Appl Physiol* 88:1310-1315, 2000.

54. Buchholz AC, McGillivray CF, Pencharz PB: Differences in resting metabolic rate between paraplegic and able-bodied subjects are explained by differences in body composition, *Am J Clin Nutr* 77:371-378, 2003.

55. Spungen AM, Adkins RH, Stewart CA et al: Factors influencing body composition in persons with spinal cord injury: a cross-sectional study, *J Appl Physiol* 95:2398-2407, 2003.

56. Duckworth WC, Jallepalli P, Solomon SS: Glucose-intolerance in spinal-cord injury, *Arch Phys Med Rehabil* 64:107-110, 1983.

57. Petry C, Rothstein JL, Bauman WA: Hemoglobin A1c as a predictor of glucose intolerance in spinal cord injury, *J Am Paraplegia Soc* 16:56, 1993.

58. Ykijarvinen H, Koivisto VA: Effects of body-composition on insulin sensitivity, *Diabetes* 32:965-969, 1983.

59. Bauman WA, Spungen AM: Disorders of carbohydrate and lipid-metabolism in veterans with paraplegia or quadriplegia: a model of premature aging, *Metabol Clin Exp* 43:749-756, 1994.

60. Wolff J: *Das Gesetz der Transformation der Knochen*, Berlin, 1892, Ahirshwald.

61. Claus-Walker JC, Campos RJ, Carter RE et al: Calcium excretion in quadriplegia, *Arch Phys Med Rehabil* 53:14-20, 1972.

62. Claus-Walker JC, Spencer WA, Carter RE et al: Bone metabolism in quadriplegia: dissociation between calciuria and hydroxyprolinuria, *Arch Phys Med Rehabil* 56:327-332, 1975.

63. Naftchi NE, Viau AT, Sell GH et al: Mineral metabolism in spinal cord injury, *Arch Phys Med Rehabil* 61:139-142, 1980.

64. Vaziri ND, Pandian MR, Segal JL et al: Vitamin D, parathormone, and calcitonin profiles in persons with long-standing spinal cord injury, *Arch Phys Med Rehabil* 75:766-769, 1994.

65. Garland DE, Stewart CA, Adkins RH et al: Osteoporosis after spinal cord injury, *J Orthop Res* 10:371-378, 1992.

66. Wilmet E, Ismail AA, Heilporn A et al: Longitudinal study of the bone mineral content and of soft tissue composition after spinal cord section, *Paraplegia* 33:674-677, 1995.

67. Curtis KA, Drysdale GA, Lanza D et al: Shoulder pain in wheelchair users with tetraplegia and paraplegia, *Arch Phys Med Rehabil* 80:453-457, 1999.

68. Gironda RJ, Clark ME, Neugaard B et al: Upper limb pain in a national sample of veterans with paraplegia, *J Spinal Cord Med* 27:120-127, 2004.

69. Sie IH, Waters RL, Adkins RH et al: Upper extremity pain in the postrehabilitation spinal-cord injured patient, *Arch Phys Med Rehabil* 73:44-48, 1992.

70. Dalyan M, Cardenas DD, Gerard B: Upper extremity pain after spinal cord injury, *Spinal Cord* 37:191-195, 1999.

71. Escobedo EM, Hunter JC, Hollister MC et al: MR imaging of rotator cuff tears in individuals with paraplegia, *AJR Am J Roentgenol* 168:919-923, 1997.

72. Boninger ML, Towers JD, Cooper RA et al: Shoulder imaging abnormalities in individuals with paraplegia, *J Rehabil Res Dev* 38:401-408, 2001.

73. Campbell CC, Koris MJ: Etiologies of shoulder pain in cervical spinal cord injury, *Clin Orthop Rel Res* 322:140-145, 1996.

74. Nyland J, Quigley P, Huang C et al: Preserving transfer independence among individuals with spinal cord injury, *Spinal Cord* 38:649-657, 2000.

75. Boninger ML, Impink BG, Cooper RA et al: Relation between median and ulnar nerve function and wrist kinematics during wheelchair propulsion, *Arch Phys Med Rehabil* 85:1141-1145, 2004.

76. Curtis KA, Tyner TM, Zachary L et al: Effect of a standard exercise protocol on shoulder pain in long-term wheelchair users, *Spinal Cord* 37:421-429, 1999.

77. ACSM: The recommended quantity and quality of exercise for developing and maintaining cardiorespiratory and muscular fitness in healthy adults, *Med Sci Sport Exerc* 22:265-274, 1990.

78. DeVivo MJ, Stover SL: Long-term survival and causes of death. In Stover SL, DeLisa JA, Whiteneck GS, editors: *Spinal cord injury*, Gaithersburg, MD, 1995, Aspen.

79. Davis GM: Exercise capacity of individuals with paraplegia, *Med Sci Sport Exerc* 25:423-432, 1993.

80. Franklin BA, Swnated KI, Grais SL et al: Field test estimation of maximal oxygen consumption in wheelchair users, *Arch Phys Med Rehabil* 71:574-578, 1990.

81. Rhodes EC, McKenzie DC, Coutts KD et al: A field test for the prediction of aerobic capacity in male paraplegics and quadraplegics, *Can J Appl Sport Sci* 6:182-186, 1981.

82. Vinet A, Bernard PL, Poulain M et al: Validation of an incremental field test for the direct assessment of peak oxygen uptake in wheelchair-dependent athletes, *Spinal Cord* 34:288-293, 1996.

83. van der Woude LHV, Veeger HE, Rozendal RH et al: Wheelchair racing: effects of rim diameter and speed on physiology and technique, *Med Sci Sport Exerc* 20:492-500, 1988.

84. Cooper RA: A force energy optimization model for wheelchair athletics, *IEEE Trans Syst Man Cybernetic* 20:444-449, 1990.

85. Langbein WE, Maki KC, Edwards LC et al: Initial clinical evaluation of a wheelchair ergometer for diagnostic exercise testing: a technical note, *J Rehabil Res Dev* 31:317-325, 1994.

86. Dallmeijer AJ, Zentgraaff IDB, Zijp NI et al: Submaximal physical strain and peak performance in handcycling versus handrim wheelchair propulsion, *Spinal Cord* 42:91-98, 2004.

87. Pitetti KH, Snoek G, Stray-Gundersen J: Maximal response wheelchair-confined subjects to four types of arm exercise, *Arch Phys Med Rehabil* 68:10-13, 1987.

88. Gass GC, Camp EM: The maximum physiological responses during incremental wheelchair and arm cranking exercise in male paraplegics, *Med Sci Sport Exerc* 16:355-359, 1984.

89. Glaser RM, Sawka MN, Brune MF et al: Physiological responses to maximal effort wheelchair ergometry and arm crank ergometry, *J Appl Physiol* 48:1060-1064, 1980.

90. Mutton DL, Scremin AM, Barstow TJ et al: Physiologic responses during functional electrical stimulation leg cycling and hybrid exercise in spinal cord injured subjects, *Arch Phys Med Rehabil* 78:712-718, 1997.

91. Phillips W, Burkett LN: Arm crank exercise with static leg FNS in persons with spinal cord injury, *Med Sci Sport Exerc* 27:530-535, 1995.

92. Apple DF: *Physical fitness: a guide for individuals with spinal cord injury*, Washington, DC, 1996, Department of Veteran Affairs, Veterans Health Administration, Rehabilitation Research and Development Service, Scientific and Technical Publication Section.

93. Glaser RM, Foley DM, Laubach LL et al: An exercise test to evaluate fitness for wheelchair activity, *Paraplegia* 16:341-349, 1979.

94. Hooker SP, Greenwood JD, Hatae DT et al: Oxygen uptake and heart rate relationship in persons with spinal cord injury, *Med Sci Sports Exerc* 25:1115-1119, 1993.

95. Bauman WA, Raza M, Spungen AM et al: Cardiac stress testing with thallium-201 imaging reveals silent ischemia in individuals with paraplegia, *Arch Phys Med Rehabil* 75:946-950, 1994.

96. Langbein WE, Edwards SC, Louie EK et al: Wheelchair exercise and digital echocardiography for the detection of heart disease, *Rehabil Res Dev Rep* 34:324-325, 1996.

97. Balady G, Weaver D, Rose L et al: Arm exercise-thallium imaging testing for the detection of coronary artery disease, *J Am Coll Cardiol* 9:84-88, 1987.

98. Franklin BE: *American College of Sports Medicine guidelines for exercise testing and prescription*, ed 6, Baltimore, 2000, Williams & Wilkins.

99. Jones LM, Goulding A, Gerrard DF: DEXA: a practical and accurate tool to demonstrate total and regional bone loss, lean tissue loss and fat mass gain in paraplegia, *Spinal Cord* 36:637-640, 1998.

100. Spungen AM, Bauman WA, Wang J et al: Measurement of body-fat in individuals with tetraplegia: a comparison of 8 clinical methods, *Paraplegia* 33:402-408, 1995.

101. Cardus D, McTaggart WG: Body composition in spinal cord injury, *Arch Phys Med Rehabil* 66:257-259, 1985.

102. Spungen AM, Bauman WA, Wang J et al: Reduced quality of fat free mass in paraplegia, *Clin Res* 40:280A-280A, 1992.

103. Rasmann Nuhliced DN, Spurr GB, Barboriak JJ: Body composition of patients with spinal cord injury, *Eur J Clin Nutr* 42:765-773, 1988.

104. Biering-Sorenssen F, Bohr H, Schaadt A: Bone mineral content of the lumbar spine and lower extremities years after spinal cord lesion, *Paraplegia* 26:293-301, 1988.

105. Finsen V, Indredavik B, Fougner KJ: Bone mineral and hormone status in paraplegics, *Paraplegia* 30:343-347, 1992.

106. Clasey JL, Kanaley JA, Wideman L et al: Validity of methods of body composition assessment in young and older men and women, *J Appl Physiol* 86:1728-1738, 1999.

107. Heymsfield SB, Lichtman S, Baumgartner RN et al: Body-composition of humans: comparison of 2 improved 4-compartment models that differ in expense, technical complexity, and radiation exposure, *Am J Clin Nutr* 52:52-58, 1990.

108. Kocina P: Body composition of spinal cord injured adults, *Sports Med* 23:48-60, 1997.

109. American Heart Association: *CPR and ECC guidelines*: www.americanheart.org. Accessed November 5, 2007.

110. Pate RR: Physical activity and health: dose-response issues, *Res Q Exerc Sport* 66:313-317, 1995.

111. Nash MS: Exercise as a health-promoting activity following spinal cord injury, *JNPT* 29:87-106, 2005.

112. Pollock ML, Evans WJ: Resistance training for health and disease: introduction, *Med Sci Sport Exerc* 31:10-11, 1999.

113. McLean KP, Skinner JS: Effect of body training position on outcomes of an aerobic training study on individuals with quadriplegia, *Arch Phys Med Rehabil* 76:139-150, 1995.

114. Janssen TW, van Oers CA, Veeger HE et al: Relationship between physical strain during standardised ADL tasks and physical capacity in men with spinal cord injuries, *Paraplegia* 32:844-59, 1994.

115. Kavanaugh T: Physical training in heart transplant recipients, *J Cardiovasc Risk* 3:154-59, 1996.

116. Shephard RJ, Kavanagh T, Mertens DJ et al: The place of perceived exertion ratings in exercise prescription for cardiac transplant patients before and after training, *Br J Sports Med* 30:116-21, 1996.

117. Borg G: *Borg's perceived exertion and pain scales*, Champaign, IL, 1998, Human Kinetics.

118. Figoni FS, Bell AA: Accessibility of physical fitness facilities in the Kansas City metropolitan area, *Top Spinal Cord Injury Rehabil* 3:66-78, 1998.

119. Rimmer JH, Riley B, Wang E et al: Development and validation of AIMFREE: accessibility instruments measuring fitness and recreation environments, *Disabil Rehabil* 26:1087-1095, 2004.

120. Coutts KD, Rhodes EC, McKenzie DC: Maximal exercise responses of tetraplegics and paraplegics, *J Appl Physiol* 55:479-482, 1983.

121. DiCarlo SE: Improved cardiopulmonary status after a two-month program of graded arm exercise in a patient with C6 quadriplegia, *Phys Ther* 62:456-459, 1982.

122. Lasko-McCarthey P, Davis JA: Effect of work rate increment on peak oxygen uptake during wheelchair ergometry in men with quadriplegia, *Eur J App Physiol* 63:349-353, 1991.

123. Lassau-Wray ER, Ward GR: Varying physiological response to arm-crank exercise in specific spinal injuries, *J Physiol Anthropol Appl Human Sci* 19:5-12, 2000.

124. Simard C, Noreau L, Pare G et al: [Maximal physiological response during exertion in quadriplegic subjects], *Can J Appl Physiol* 18:163-174, 1993 (French).

125. Wicks JR, Oldridge NB, Cameron BJ et al. Arm cranking a wheelchair ergometry in elite spinal cord-injured athletes, *Med Sci Sports Exerc* 15:224-231, 1983.

126. Burkett LN, Chisum J, Stone W et al: Exercise capacity of untrained spinal cord injured individuals and the relationship of peak oxygen uptake to level of injury, *Paraplegia* 28:512-521, 1990.

127. Coutts KD, Stogryn JL: Aerobic and anaerobic power of Canadian wheelchair track athletes, *Med Sci Sports Exerc* 19:62-65, 1987.

128. DiCarlo SE, Supp MD, Taylor HC: Effect of arm ergometry training on physical work capacity of individuals with spinal cord injuries, *Phys Ther* 63:1104-1107, 1983

129. Gass GC, Camp EM: Physiological characteristics of trained Australian paraplegic and tetraplegic subjects, *Med Sci Sports Exerc* 11:256-259, 1979

130. Schmid A, Huonker M, Stober P et al: Physical performance and cardiovascular and metabolic adaptation of elite female wheelchair basketball players in wheelchair ergometry and in competition, *Am J Phys Med Rehabil* 77:527-533, 1998.

131. Whiting RB, Dreisinger TE, Dalton RB et al: Improved physical fitness and work capacity in quadriplegics by wheelchair exercise, *Journal of Cardiac Rehabilitation* 3:251-255, 1983

132. Bhambhani YN, Burnham R, Wheeler GD et al: Physiological correlates of simulated wheelchair racing in trained quadriplegics, *Can J Appl Physiol* 20:65-77, 1995

133. Eriksson P, Lofstrom L, Ekblom B: Aerobic power during maximal exercise in untrained and well-trained persons with quadriplegia and paraplegia, *Scand J Rehabil Med* 20:141-147, 1988

134. Gass GC, Watson J, Camp EM et al: The effects of physical training on high level spinal lesion patients, *Scand J Rehabil Med* 12:61-65, 1980.

135. Hjeltnes N, Jansen T: Physical endurance capacity, functional status and medical complications in spinal cord injured subjects with long-standing lesions, *Paraplegia* 28:428-432, 1990.

136. Hopman MT, Dallmeijer AJ, Snoek G et al: The effect of training on cardiovascular responses to arm exercise in individuals with tetraplegia, *Eur J Appl Physiol Occup Physiol* 74:172-179, 1996.

137. Janssen TW, van Oers CA, Hollander AP et al: Isometric strength, sprint power, and aerobic power in individuals with a spinal cord injury, *Med Sci Sports Exerc* 25:863-870, 1993.

138. Janssen TW, van Oers CA, van Kamp GJ et al: Coronary heart disease risk indicators, aerobic power, and physical activity in men with spinal cord injuries, *Arch Phys Med Rehabil* 78:697-705, 1997.

139. Noreau L, Shephard RJ: Spinal cord injury, exercise and quality of life, *Sports Med* 20:226-250, 1995.

140. Van Loan M, McCluer S, Loftin JM et al: Comparisons of physiological responses to maximal arm exercise among able-bodied, paraplegics, and quadriplegics, *Paraplegia* 25:397-405, 1987.

141. Gass EM, Harvey LA, Gass GC: Maximal physiological responses during arm cranking and treadmill wheelchair propulsion in T4-T6 paraplegic men, *Paraplegia* 33:267-270, 1995.

142. Lin KH, Lai JS, Kao MJ et al: Anaerobic threshold and maximal oxygen-consumption during arm cranking exercise in paraplegia, *Arch Phys Med Rehabil* 74:515-520, 1993.

143. Schmid A, Huonker M, Barturen JM et al: Catecholamines, heart rate, and oxygen uptake during exercise in persons with spinal cord injury, *J Appl Physiol* 85:635-641, 1998.

144. Bernard PL, Mercier J, Varray A et al: Influence of lesion level on the cardioventilatory adaptations in paraplegic wheelchair athletes during muscular exercise, *Spinal Cord* 38:16-25, 2000

145. Hooker SP, Wells CL: Aerobic power of competitive paraplegic road racers, *Paraplegia* 30:428-436, 1992.

146. Schneider DA, Sedlock DA, Gass E et al: VO2peak and the gas-exchange anaerobic threshold during incremental arm cranking in able-bodied and paraplegic men, *Eur J Appl Physiol Occup Physiol* 80:292-297, 1999

147. Barstow TJ, Scremin AM, Mutton DL et al: Peak and kinetic cardiorespiratory responses during arm and leg exercise in patients with spinal cord injury, *Spinal Cord* 38:340-345, 2000.

148. Cooper RA, Horvath SM, Bedi JF et al: Maximal exercise response of paraplegic wheelchair road racers, *Paraplegia* 30:573-581, 1992.

SOLUTIONS TO CHAPTER 18 CLINICAL CASE STUDY

Exercise and Fitness for Individuals with a Spinal Cord Injury Case 1

1. Individuals with complete tetraplegia are limited in their aerobic capacity because of the combination of reduced working muscle mass, blunted sympathetic responses, and restrictive lung function from intercostal and abdominal muscle paralysis, which are needed for optimal respiration, hemodynamic stability, and truncal stability, affecting exercise options. Peak HRs rarely exceed 120 beats/min in complete tetraplegia. HR responses in tetraplegia are subject to parasympathetic withdrawal more than sympathetic stimulation, resulting in significantly lower maximal HRs (130 versus 180 to 200 beats/min seen in able-bodied persons) and contributing to the great deal of variability noted between VO_{2Peak} and HR in this population. The CNS is responsible for the controlling "central drive" during exercise, inhibiting parasympathetic activity, and allowing for sympathetic activity to increase the HR as needed.

The problem is that the parasympathetic withdrawal by the vagus nerve decreases output, but the counter of the sympathetic to increase HR and SV is reflexively lost. RPE may be the most appropriate scale on which to base prescribed exercise intensity for individuals with tetraplegia because it has been used with good success in cardiac transplant patients who have denervated hearts, although this too has limitations.[115, 116]

2. Special considerations should be made to accommodate Jake's C7 level of impairment during the GXT. The ACE or WCE should be adjusted appropriately to allow optimal efficiency and to reduce musculoskeletal injuries at the shoulder, elbow, and wrist. Straps should also be applied to the torso to prevent truncal instability. Because Jake has triceps function, the arm ergometer should allow both pushing and pulling. Wheelchair gloves or flexion mitts with Velcro straps should be used to position the hand onto the crank for stabilization and to prevent blisters, lacerations, and abrasions.

The GXT should be performed in the presence of a physician to monitor the ECG and manage a possible cardiovascular adverse event. ACSM guidelines for termination of a GXT should be strictly adhered to and may require a more conservative approach because of reduced cardiac acceleration in SCI. These termination points include criteria such as, but are not limited to, acute myocardial infarction or moderate to severe angina, serious arrhythmias, pallor or cyanosis, shortness of breath, CNS symptoms such as confusion, ECG changes such as ST segment depression, supraventricular tachycardia, and a bundle branch block. As a person with SCI approaches peak exercise capacity, it is likely he will become relatively hypotensive despite leg wraps and abdominal binders. Individuals with tetraplegia often have resting BPs of around 90/60 mm Hg and should be regularly monitored for symptoms of hypotension and presyncope during strenuous exercise. Should symptomatic hypotension (systolic pressure drop >20 mm Hg) occur, exercise testing should be halted and the person should be tilted back in his wheelchair to elevate the lower limbs above the level of the heart, promoting venous return. This position would also be used at the end of an exercise stress test that can be performed to detect whether specified exercise intensity evokes abnormalities in cardiac function, possibly signifying CAD. Leg elevation can be used at the end of this stress test to maximally invoke the Frank-Starling mechanism for myocardial contractility, increasing the likelihood of detecting ischemia in the presence of CAD.

Continued

SOLUTIONS TO CHAPTER 18 CLINICAL CASE STUDY

Exercise and Fitness for Individuals with a Spinal Cord Injury Case 1—cont'd

4. Research is needed in the area of resistance training for neurologically intact muscle in the presence of SCI. It is unclear whether individuals with SCI have responses to resistance training different from those of able-bodied people. It is known that testosterone, free testosterone, and growth hormone levels are significantly reduced in persons with SCI and that these hormone responses to exercise appear to be blunted, which perhaps is a reflection of reduced overall muscle mass used during exercise bouts. Although muscle groups that remain neurologically intact and under voluntary control should respond to imposed stress, hormonal responses may not be adequate to stimulate hypertrophy to the extent seen in the able-bodied population.

It is recommended that Jake be taught the scapular stabilization and rotator cuff resistance exercises. Initial interventions should include two sets of 10 repetitions, with 6-second isometric contractions for shoulder protractors, retractors, elevators, and depressors and for shoulder internal and external rotators, progressing to dynamic elastic exercise band (Thera-Band exercises as static strength plateaus. Strength and hypertrophy gains will typically plateau as well with Thera-Band exercises. Further gains will require increased resistance and volume or total time of exercise. Although dumbbells and free weights may be used under close supervision, paralyzed lower limbs and truncal musculature significantly reduce a person's ability to balance even small objects when lying supine or when seated without significant truncal support. When using free weights, isotonic or isokinetic machines, wheelchair brakes should be set prior to lifting. The ACSM guidelines for muscular strength and endurance prescribe one set with resistance so as to reach exhaustion performing 8 to 12 repetitions for each of the major muscle groups that remain neurologically intact at intervals of two to three times a week.

SOLUTIONS TO CHAPTER 18 CLINICAL CASE STUDY

Exercise and Fitness for Individuals with a Spinal Cord Injury Case 2

1. Conservatively, it is recommended that, for the purposes of risk stratification, women ≥50 years of age are considered as having at least moderate risk for untoward events during exercise, independent of the CAD risk factor thresholds for use with ACSM risk stratification. Medical supervision should be obtained from a physician knowledgeable in SCI care, including a 12-lead ECG and risk profile assessment, before participation in a GXT or a strenuous exercise program. Additional considerations in planning a strenuous exercise program or a GXT are this client's age, pulmonary function tests, strength and flexibility measures, a DEXA scan to determine bone mineral density, radiographs of paralyzed limbs to exclude asymptomatic fractures, blood assays including lipid profiles, and HbA1c to rule out glucose intolerance or diabetes.

2. Many exercise physiologists prefer discontinuous, submaximal protocols for maximal exercise or stress testing in wheelchair users, because they are comfortable, safe, and relatively easy to administer. A typical WCE protocol would use a constant speed (3 km/hr^{-1}) with a metronome-guided crank rate of 50 revolutions per minute and an initial resistance of 5 W. Each stage should last 4 to 6 minutes with 5-minute rest intervals and progressive 5- to 10-W increments should be used with each new stage to a predetermined PO of 30 W. A submaximal ACE protocol would use similar stages but with twice the PO levels. To measure VO$_{2Peak}$ and PO$_{Peak}$, a continuous, shortened protocol can be used, allowing an initial intensity level of 50% of the predicted maximal PO (determined from submaximal testing), shortening each stage of testing to 2 minutes and allowing no rest between stages. A similar protocol uses the Veterans Affairs–developed WAFT, a wheelchair ergometer that can accommodate the user's own wheelchair. These use a continuous protocol with a fixed speed of 2 miles/hr^{-1}, initial intensity of 6 W, and 5- to 7-W increments between 3-minute stages; 20 seconds of rest between stages allows for BP determination. In addition to oxygen consumption and PO, BP, ECG, and perceived exertion should be monitored at the end of each exercise stage. Unfortunately, ECG monitoring during ACE or WCE is frequently impaired because of movement artifact and should therefore be continued during the first 10 seconds of the resting periods between stages to improve sensitivity for detecting ischemic changes.

3. Sally should be informed of various exercise modes and choose the type she prefers because this will facilitate her compliance. The therapist prescribing the exercise will educate Sally about available options including manual wheelchair propulsion, ACE, WCE, FES-LCE, ACE plus FES-LCE (Hybrid), and resistance training equipment, as well as the advantages and disadvantages of each. A helpful guideline, when appropriately modified for this population, is that moderate activity is defined as activity performed at 3 to 6 METS (i.e., 10.5 to 21 ml/kg^{-1}/min^{-1}). The most appropriate way to monitor and prescribe intensity of aerobic exercise for the individual with SCI however, remains somewhat controversial. If the prescription is preceded by a GXT, the Borg RPE values corresponding to 50% to 85% VO$_{2Peak}$ may be used to assign an exercise range; this should correspond to about 12 to 13 (i.e., somewhat hard) on the Borg RPE scale.

4. The duration of a single aerobic exercise bout will vary depending on fitness level determined, in this case, by the exercise tests discussed previously. A 10-minute warm-up is recommended followed by 20 to 60 minutes at the recommended RPE. The progression of exercise duration should be monitored closely with small amounts of fluids given frequently during exercise. Aerobic exercise should be performed at least 3 days a week to maintain fitness, but it may occur up to 5 days a week for optimal gains in cardiopulmonary fitness without negative consequences, particularly when performed at relatively low intensity levels. Short and multiple bouts of exercise daily may be required initially, each lasting 5 to 15 minutes, until Sally is able to tolerate 20- to 30-minute sessions. Overuse syndromes of the upper limbs, however, must be monitored carefully. The initial stages of an aerobic exercise program should focus more on developing exercise as a habit. Sally should be instructed on delayed onset of muscle soreness that may last for the first 2 weeks of exercising. Conditioning should occur in 6 to 8 weeks. The intensity of exercise may increase after 30-minute duration of an exercise has been achieved. Once the desired exercise goals have been met, maintenance of the conditioning is required. The most important factor in extended exercise compliance is that Sally finds the activity to be enjoyable.

CHAPTER NINETEEN

Sports and Recreation for People with Spinal Cord Injuries

Ian Rice, OTR/L, MS, Rory A. Cooper, PhD, Rosemarie Cooper, ATP, MPT, Annmarie Kelleher, OTR/L, MS, and Amy Boyles, BA

Before I became paralyzed at the age of 15, I had dreams and aspirations of either playing basketball at the University of North Carolina in Chapel Hill or running the wishbone offense as quarterback for the University of Oklahoma Sooners' football team. One way or another, I was determined to get there…What I found, over time, is that I've made wonderful friends [of the folks] I've met over the years. Each has played a vital role in helping me become the man I am today, including the many friends I've made through wheelchair sports.

Scott (T8 SCI)

Sports and recreation are an important modality in the rehabilitation of individuals with a spinal cord injury (SCI).[1-3] Because the length of stay for inpatient rehabilitation has become so short, there is little time for people who have recently been spinal cord injured to gain much experience with sports and recreation. This makes it critical to expose people to sports and recreation opportunities through community-based sports organizations or outpatient recreational therapy services. Adjusting to SCI and the changes in lifestyle associated with it can be mitigated by exposing the individual to healthy activities that build strength, stamina, self-confidence, and a sense of belonging.[4] There are many appropriate activities for individuals with wide-ranging interests and abilities. As with any recreational activity, it will take time and commitment to attempt and become proficient in and find those sports that most interest and meet the needs of each individual, but it is worth the journey.

The recreational interests and abilities of each individual vary because of multiple factors. It is important to recognize that maintenance of a healthy lifestyle and regular participation in exercise and recreational activities have been shown to reduce the detrimental effects of SCI.[5] Some people have an innate talent or natural drive to participate in sports and to pursue competitive activities. For those interested, sporting competitions are available on regional to international levels. Indeed, athletes with SCI must dedicate considerable time when desirous of being competitive at the national and international levels. The Paralympics are the pinnacle of many competitive sports with a long and rich history of affiliation with the Olympic Games.[6] This chapter discusses training techniques for both recreational and organized sports, a variety of sports activities, the structure of sports organizations for people with SCI, and research related to wheelchair sports. The intent is to provide resources for individuals with SCI and their clinicians to expand participation in and enjoyment from sporting activities that range from croquet to rock climbing (Box 19-1). Whether spending time with friends, conquering a personal goal, or setting a world record, sports and recreation can play a vital role in life.

TRAINING TECHNIQUES

A carefully designed training program can help athletes reach their full potential. Training programs specific to wheelchair athletics are not unlike the training regimens performed by able-bodied athletes. For wheelchair athletes competing in individualized competition such as racing, attaining peak performance at the appropriate time is crucial. Maintaining peak conditioning during an entire competitive season is unrealistic: it is difficult for a racer to go into competitive situations earlier in the season with enough fitness to handle all of the elements of a race course. Therefore, athletes tend to construct their training and competition schedule to peak for a particular event. Often wheelchair racers will use smaller competitions to prepare for the more important races, and preliminary races may also serve to qualify athletes through to events requiring time or place standards such as the Boston Marathon or World Championships and Paralympics.

During any given racing season, handcyclists and wheelchair racers will work at different levels of exertion at different times. During early season workouts, handcyclists commonly train in the small chain ring or gear to maintain a high cadence of 90 to 100 revolutions per minute at relatively slow speeds. If an athlete trained this way all year long, his fitness would be incomplete. He would be unable to meet the demands of actual events, which generally are diverse topographically. To truly peak and be prepared for a major race, an athlete must be able to handle large gears with frequent accelerations of pace, including sprinting, surging, hill climbing, drafting, and coasting. As a result, training must gradually take on more intense and diverse aspects, incorporating as many racing scenarios as possible.

Team sports such as rugby or basketball require a slightly different training approach because every game is important to the ultimate success of the team. Given the logistics of team sports, it is necessary for athletes to peak before the season while maintaining high levels of performance throughout the season.

Periodization

Athletes involved in team sports can achieve these types of results through a training technique called periodization. This technique divides the year into training intervals. Defining the term simply, it uses a process of training that varies the timing and intensity of workouts to achieve specific results. Periodization also allows for changes in the intensity (e.g., heavy, moderate, and light resistance) and changes in the volume of exercise (e.g., sets × repetitions), which theoretically keeps the exercise stimulus effective.[7] For example, the year can be divided into a preseason, in-season, main-season, and end-season. Teams use similar divisions when training for a specific event: precompetition, initial competition, main competition, and postcompetition (macrocycle).

The five training regimens that an athlete should implement into his periodization program include endurance, speed, skill, strength, and flexibility. Realizing that each athlete and sport has different needs, time allocated to each regimen will differ; however, implementing all five can help facilitate peak performance.

BOX 19-1 | Resources for Athletes with Spinal Cord Injury

Adaptive Sports Association
P.O. Box 1884, Durango, CO 81302
Winter sports 970-385-2163
Summer sports 970-259-0374
Administration 970-259-0374
http://www.asadurango.com/site_map.html

Disabled Sports USA
451 Hungerford Dr., Suite 100 Rockville, MD 20850
Telephone: 301-217-0960
Fax: 301-217-0968
http://www.dsusa.org/

National Alliance for Accessible Golf
2805 E. 10th St., Bloomington, IN 47408
Telephone: 812-856-4422
TTY: 812-856-4421
Fax: 812-856-4480
http://www.accessgolf.org/

National Spinal Cord Injury Association
6701 Democracy Blvd., Suite 300-9, Bethesda, MD 20817
Telephone: 800-962-9629 or 301-214-4006
Fax: 301-881-9817
http://www.spinalcord.org/

National Veterans Wheelchair Games
http://www1.va.gov/vetevent/nvwg/2007/default.cfm

National Wheelchair Basketball Association
http://www.nwba.org/index.php

North American Riding for the Handicapped Association, Inc.
P.O. Box 33150, Denver, CO 80233
Telephone: 800-369-RIDE (7433)
Fax: 303- 252-4610
narha@narha.org

Paralyzed Veterans of America
801 18th St., NW, Washington, DC 20006
Telephone: 202- 872-1300 or 800-424-8200
http://www.pva.org

United States Handcycling Federation
P.O. Box 2245, Evergreen, CO 80437
Telephone: 303-679-2770
http://www.ushf.org/

United States Quad Rugby Association
5861 White Cypress Dr., Lake Worth, FL 33467-6230
Telephone: 561-964-1712
Fax: 561-642-4444
http://www.quadrugby.com/toc.htm

U.S. Paralympics
One Olympic Plaza, Colorado Springs, CO 80909
Telephone: 719-866-2030
Fax: 719-866-2029
http://www.usparalympics.com/

Wheelchair Sports, USA
10 Lake Circle Suite G19, Colorado Springs, CO 80906
Telephone: (719) 574-1150
http://www.wsusa.org/

Common Errors

When designing an appropriate training program, some of the common errors made by athletes should be considered. Harre[8] summarized typical errors made by athletes while designing a training program, and more recently other authors have expanded his work.[9,10] Common errors in training may neglect recovery and include excessive demands on speed, loads, and volume (Box 19-2).

The underlying theme reflected by these errors is one of imbalance between intensity and adequate recovery, which, with an inappropriate lifestyle or social environment, can lead to a situation of overtraining. Workout strategies that avoid overtraining have been summarized by several authors; Box 19-3 summarizes steps described by Pyne.[9]

Endurance Training

Endurance training typically focuses on training for a particular event because it involves elevating the heart rate over a prolonged period of time. A wheelchair road racer preparing for a 5K or 10K event, for example, would train that particular distance at least 3 days a week. This approach may vary among athletes; some may train more frequently and others less, depending on their capabilities and levels of ambition. Some will find that training for a 12K event is a good way to prepare for an actual 10K event. The extra 2000 meters prepares the athlete for every weather condition and terrain while also creating a mind set wherein the athlete, knowing he can easily complete a 10K, will push even harder during the competition.

On days when athletes do not do endurance training they should do interval training. This type of training stresses the cardiovascular and neuromuscular systems and thus prepares the body for competition (Box 19-4). In addition, athletes who compete in endurance events should also train in speed, skill, strength, and flexibility to reach the highest possible physical condition.

Speed Training

Speed training is part of a well-thought-out periodization program. Athletes who participate in sports such as basketball, rugby, track and field events, swimming, and weight training will benefit from speed training. Speed training can increase reaction time, which can be a vital component related to performance and ultimately success in competition.

BOX 19-2 | Common Errors in Training

- Recovery is often neglected with mistakes in the microcycle and macrocycle sequence. The macrocycle is the division of a year into phases of training periods where the emphasis is different in each phase. A microcycle is one week of specialized training within a macrocycle. There is inadequate use of general exercise sessions for recovery purposes.
- Demands on an athlete are made too quickly relative to capacity, compromising the adaptive process.
- After a break in training for illness or injury, the training load is increased too rapidly.
- High volume of both maximal and submaximal intensity training
- The overall volume of intense training is too high when the athlete is primarily engaged in an endurance sport.
- Excessive attention and time are spent in complex technical or mental aspects without adequate recovery or down time.
- Excessive number of competitions with maximum physical and psychological demands combined with frequent disturbance of the daily routine and insufficient training
- Bias of training method with insufficient balance
- The athlete lacks trust in the coach as a result of high expectations or goal setting, which has led to frequent performance failure.

BOX 19-3 | Workout Strategies to Avoid Overtraining

- Formulate a long-term performance goal for the season as the basis on which the training program is designed.
- Use a progressive and cyclical increase in training load.
- Use a logical sequence to the order of the training phases.
- Use a training process supported by scientific monitoring.
- Use intensive recovery techniques throughout the training program.
- Emphasize skill development and refinement throughout the training program.
- Use an underlying component for the improvement and maintenance of general athletic abilities.

Data from Pyne D: Designing an endurance training program. In *Proceedings of the National Coaching and Officiating Conference* (1996 Nov 30–Dec 3), Brisbane, 1996, Australian Coaching Council Inc.

Sprint training, in which the athlete performs short sprinting intervals, is the best method to train for speed. For example, when an athlete is competing in 100-meter events, a single training session would be separated into four different distances. A typical training day for a 100-meter athlete is shown in Box 19-5. The last set of repetitions is 10% longer than the event itself. Because the athlete has have trained to sprint for 110 meters, he will be able to drive through the entire 100 meters during competition. An athlete's performance often fades or slows during the last portion of a workout, so this method can ensure quality production and performance through an entire workout.

Plyometrics

Another aspect of speed training is a technique called plyometrics. Plyometric exercise integrates strength and power into a single training session, resulting in explosiveness. Plyometrics relies on an external force to store energy within the musculature. The stored energy is immediately followed by an equal and opposite

BOX 19-4 | Components of Interval Training for 400-Meter Sprinter

- Sprint a given distance: sprint 200 meters, coast or lightly propel for 100 meters, perform interval over again 5 to 10 times.
- Dramatically reduce speed for a shorter distance.
- Perform the interval over again.
- Approaching competition: increase the sprinting intervals and decrease the rest intervals.

BOX 19-5 | Typical Training Day for a 100-Meter Athlete

Distance (m)	Repetitions
80	3
90	3
100	3
110	3

reaction, using the natural elastic tendencies of the muscles to produce energy. Wheelchair sprinters can use a medicine ball or plyoball to perform upper body plyometrics. The athlete performs plyometrics by quickly catching and explosively passing the ball to a partner for multiple repetitions. The goal of plyometric exercises is to minimize the time the body has to recover from the external force (e.g., the thrown ball), thereby increasing the amount of energy stored within the muscle for optimal performance.[11]

Skill Training

Skill training is also applicable to sports. Skill training in the context of this chapter essentially is equivalent to specificity training, which many athletes overlook because they think it encompasses only the competitive event itself. Athletes, however, should regularly examine and break down the mechanics of their movements. For example, wheelchair sprinters should dissect stroking techniques into distinct phases—preparatory, propulsion, and recovery phase—and examine each phase for proper form and execution. Movements used by throwers in field events are also extremely technical. Consequently, athletes can benefit from analyzing the component parts of these movements. For example, research by Chow and Mindock[12] relates success in the discus throw to the inclination and angular speed of the upper arm at release, the ranges of motion of the shoulder girdle, upper arm, and forearm during the forward swing, and the average angular speed of the shoulder girdle during the forward swing. Knowledge of proper form in executing these types of movements undoubtedly can help an athlete to increase his performance. Usually, the athlete needs advice from a physical or occupational therapist or an individual who understands movement biomechanics to improve performance and efficiency.

Strength Training

Strength training techniques typically refer to resistance training, which can be accomplished through the use of free or machine weights, surgical tubing, body weight exercises, manual resistance, or any other form of activity that follows basic strength

TABLE 19-1	Advantages and Disadvantages of Free Weights Versus Machines	
	Advantages	Disadvantages
Free weights	Permit small increments of weight	Requires a spotter at all times
	Teach coordination and balance	
	Allow creation of specific exercises for specific sports	
Machines	Controls the direction of movement	Coordination and balance are minimized
	Does not allow extraneous movements that can contribute to injury	Cannot be modified to become sport specific because they are usually created to perform one basic exercise

BOX 19-6 | Principles of Specific Adaptations to Imposed Demands

- Progression
- Overload
- Volume
- Frequency
- Intensity
- Documentation
- Motivation
- Specificity

training principles. The wheelchair athlete can apply exercise principles that are similar to those unimpaired athletes use, but the wheelchair athlete does have some unique characteristics. The wheelchair athlete with SCI depends on relatively smaller muscle groups of the upper body than does the unimpaired athlete who relies on his legs to produce movement. Seiler[13] has commented on the physique of elite, able-bodied marathon runners compared with elite wheelchair marathon racers. He explained that, although both athletes were endurance and cardiovascular athletes, the wheelchair racers were extremely bulky compared with the runners. Wheelchair marathoners have a much smaller total volume of muscle to do the work of the marathon race. It is possible that wheelchair athletes may posses the ability to have greater hypertrophy response to endurance training, independent of supplemental strength training in a weight room.[13]

Free Weights Versus Machines

Strength training can be accomplished by using free weights or machines (e.g., Universal, Cybex, Nautilus). Resistance training should not focus solely on free weights or machines: it is best to use both methods to provide a comprehensive workout. Table 19-1 compares the advantages and disadvantages of free weights versus machines.

Although both machines and free weights produce strength gains, to a large extent the magnitude of gains in maximum strength as a result of resistance training depends on the similarity between the strength tests and the training exercise. This aspect of movement specificity has been noted in longitudinal studies and in reviews of the literature.[14-16] In addition, there is evidence that resistance exercise machines can improve sports performance. For example, hip sled exercises produced improvements in both vertical jump distance and leg power. Training on machines has also improved the 40-yard dash, softball and baseball throw, shot put, and vertical jump. Circuit training both with and without machines has been widely used in athletic training programs supervised by professional coaches in sports such as swimming, track and field, and baseball.[16]

Sets and Repetitions

The number of sets and repetitions per exercise depends on the purpose of the training program. Generally, sets should remain between two to five per exercise, with 6 to 15 repetitions per set. Conditioning programs often entail three sets per exercise with 10 to 12 repetitions. The weight allocated to each set should be moderate.

For more intense strength training, the repetitions should be reduced to six per set. The repetitions are reduced so higher weights can be used. Sets should typically be on the higher side (five) to properly overload the muscle. Endurance athletes should focus on lighter weights with higher repetitions (13 to 16), with the number of sets remaining around three to four. It is important to remember that these recommendations have been generalized. Each athlete must determine the optimal number of sets and repetitions on the basis of his personal experience. It is best to begin a weight-training program by implementing a general conditioning program, moving to a more strenuous program only after general conditioning is completed. Most important, athletes should implement weight-training programs that complement their athletic events.[11]

Popular Training Regimens

The principles of specific adaptation to imposed demands (SAID) include progression, overload, volume, frequency, intensity, documentation, motivation, and specificity (Box 19-6). These principles, which are often used with able-bodied people, can be applied similarly in disabled people.[17] The SAID principles describe the adaptation that occurs within muscle tissue when it is progressively stressed or overloaded.[17] If an individual physically stresses a muscle or muscle group to the point at which fatigue occurs while performing the exercise movement, he can adapt to that stress in the sense that the body will respond to the exercise more favorably the next time. If this physical stress is repeated and increased, the body will continue to increase strength by adapting neurological pathways,[18-22] increasing muscle size,[23,24] and increasing the mineral content of bone.[25] Opinions differ, however, regarding optimal weight-training regimens.

There is no one program that will suit every athlete. Athletes must consider their age, sex, weight, position, and particular sport when conditioning for the upcoming season. It is best initially to change training routines every few weeks to get an idea of what training program works best for an individual's particular needs.

BOX 19-7 | Common Training Routines

- Training the entire body in 1 day
- Dividing the body into upper and lower portions
- Exercising only one body part per day
- Three primary training days (push-pull workout)

This should be done in the early preseason so that the athlete's training program will be established before the preseason is well underway, allowing him to train hard for the greater part of the preseason.

Athletes tend to use four common training routines (Box 19-7). The first consists of training the entire body in 1 day in which the athlete performs fundamental exercises that train every major muscle of the body. A comprehensive weight-training program can include exercises such as the bench press, overhead/military press, seated rows, lat-pulls, squats, and standing calf raises. To prevent overtraining, at least 1 day should be spaced between each of these comprehensive workouts, allowing the athlete to devote off days to training regimens for skill, flexibility, endurance, or speed.

The second training routine consists of dividing the body into upper and lower portions. The individual dedicates one day to an upper body workout and focuses on the lower body on the second day. Although this training program focuses on the fundamental exercises previously mentioned, it uses a more intense workout because only one half of the body is exercised per workout. The higher intensity occurs by use of heavier weights or by performing more sets or repetitions. The training regimen should include at least one off day to allow the body to recover from a more intense workout.

The third (and least commonly used) weight training routine consists of exercising only one body part per day. This type of program allows the athlete to focus his training on a single body part. A sample chest workout would include exercises such as bench press, incline press, decline press, or close-grip chest press, thus overloading the chest musculature to facilitate strengthening. The remaining days should be dedicated to the back, arm, shoulder, and leg musculature. Although this type of workout is very taxing to the body, it allows each body part to rest for at least 3 or 4 days, ensuring proper recuperation of the muscles. This routine is useful not only for novice weightlifters but also, because of its taxing nature, well-conditioned athletes should use it when they are concentrating on building their strength.

The last (and very popular) routine is commonly referred to as the push-pull workout. The push-pull workout divides the training program into three primary training days. The first day focuses on the chest and triceps area (the push day). The second day focuses on the back and biceps musculature (the pull day). The last day exercises the leg and shoulder musculature. This program permits very intense workouts because each body part has at least 3 days to recuperate. Yet even with 3 days of muscle recuperation, individuals should dedicate at least one day to other training regimens after the last day of the entire push-pull routine.[11]

Flexibility Training

Flexibility training should be an integral part of every athlete's daily workout. Everyone should stretch before and after every workout, with static stretches held for at least 30 seconds. In addition, everyone should avoid ballistic stretching, which can injure muscles.

Before each training session begins, an athlete should complete a warmup session. This can consist of lightly pushing around the track a few times or performing high-repetition and low-weight sets in a weight room. After the warmup session, the athlete should perform a number of upper and lower limb stretches, especially those specific to the competitive activity.

After every training session, athletes should cool down and stretch. Cool downs can be similar to the exercises used to warm up and can help alleviate muscle tightness and prepare the body for stretching. Stretching sessions after a workout should be comprehensive: both the upper and lower body requires stretching after workouts. To ensure that all muscles are properly stretched, a postexercise stretching session should last at least 20 minutes.[11]

RECREATIONAL AND COMPETITIVE SPORTS

Any number of recreational and competitive sports may be of interest to individuals with SCI. Although this chapter cannot cover every sport, a variety are discussed. Athletes should review relevant literature and consult coaches for training in specific activities.

Archery

Archery was included as a sporting event in the first Paralympic Games in Rome, Italy, in 1960. The first international wheelchair archery competition, however, was held in 1948 in Stoke Mandeville, England, because of the efforts of Sir. Ludwig Guttman.[26] Paralympic archery consists of an Olympic round only, which measures 70 meters in both the qualification and finals. Both men and women compete with the option of either standing or sitting in a wheelchair. Depending on the severity of the disability, archers may use a body support to stand, an authorized strapping system, a mechanical release aid, an approved compound bow, elbow or wrist splint, and an assistant to load arrows into the bow if they are unable to so themselves independently. All devices must be approved for use on the basis of the individual's disability.[27] The sport allows for competition in singles and team events, with the scoring procedures identical to those used by athletes competing in the Olympic games.[27] Adaptive archery equipment can be found through organizations, including Adaptive Shooting, American Wheelchair Archers, National Wheelchair Shooting Federation, and Outdoor Buddies Hunting Program. In addition, local and national tournaments exist and are available regularly to recreational and competitive athletes seeking competition.

Athletics

Athletics includes track and field events, pentathlons, and marathons. The field throwing events allow competitors to use specially designed throwing chairs attached to a holding device, offering

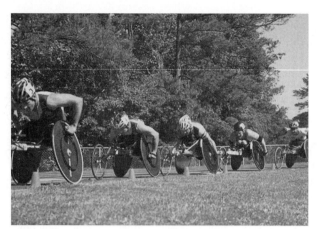

FIGURE 19-1 Elite paraplegic and amputee racers drafting in track competition.

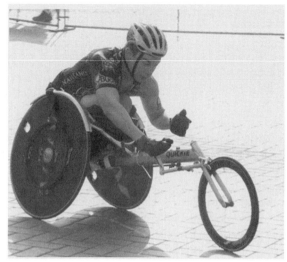

FIGURE 19-2 Individual with C7 tetraplegia using the kneeling position in his racing chair.

stability and support beyond what an individual's personal wheelchair could provide. Throwing chairs are much higher and do not have large wheels that could potentially interfere with the dynamic upper body movements required in throwing events. According to competition rules, the seat of an athlete's chair (including the cushion) for field events must not exceed 75 cm in height.[28] For wheelchair athletes, the chair design is important because it can significantly enhance performance depending on how well it matches the thrower's body and functional abilities. Consequently, athletes use chairs with different seat heights and configurations within the allowed parameters, to optimize support, positioning, and ultimately throwing execution.

Competitors in wheelchair athletics are classified on the basis of the neurological level of injury and the athlete's ability to effectively carry out movements necessary to complete a throwing task.[28] For the field events, there are nine different functional classes: F1 to F9. An F1 class equates to a neurological level of injury at roughly the C6 level. In contrast, the F9 class would have an extremely low level SCI in the sacral region or an incomplete cord lesion resulting in the ability to partially weight bear.[28] In addition, not all functional classes compete in the same events. For example, the javelin throw is not held for the F1 class because of the absence of sufficient hand function to control a javelin safely. F8 to F9 athletes are allowed to throw from a standing position and use an 800-g javelin. Wheelchair athletes in the other classes use a 600-g javelin and perform throws from throwing frames.[29] Therefore wheelchair athletes completing throws from throwing frames must rely entirely on the upper body and the support of the throwing frame to successfully execute throws. Any variations in throwing techniques used by wheelchair athletes are not specifically defined but are likely attributed to the differences in disability, chair design, and sitting position.[29]

Athletes with diminished hand function tend to use resin or adhesive-like substances to improve their grip. In addition, throwing implements such as the club and the shot vary in weight depending on the functional classification and sex of the athlete. The athletes having the highest neurological level of injury, roughly C6, compete in club throwing rather then the javelin.[28]

Track racers can compete in distances from 1000 meters through the marathon (Figure 19-1). The racing wheelchairs used by the athletes are customized and designed to fit the body of each user. This equipment, used in combination with correct propulsion biomechanics, can result in an extremely efficient means of movement.[30-33]

The design of a racing wheelchair optimizes the abilities of each user, incorporating features such as three-wheeled design, use of high pressure tubular tires, lightweight rims, precision hubs, carbon disc/spokes wheels, compensator steering, small push rings, ridged frame construction, and 2 to 15 degrees of wheel camber. The camber in a racing chair makes the chair more stable and allows the athlete to reach the bottom of the push rims without hitting the top of the wheels or push rim (see Figure 11-31). The fit of the racing chair to one's body and abilities is critical to overall performance as well. Most racing chair manufacturers require a number of anatomical measurements when a chair is ordered.[34] Typical body measurements include hip width, chest width, thigh length, arm length, trunk length, height, and weight. Wheelchair racers tend to sit in a position that promotes biomechanical efficiency and aerodynamics (Figure 19-2). Racers position themselves in a way in which the weaker portions of the body are brought close to those under voluntary control, which helps increase stability for wheelchair control and propulsion.[35]

The frame and seat cage of a racing chair are made to fit each individual, including different disability etiologies and levels as well. Both experience and etiology determine the location of rear axles with respect to the seat cage. Although experienced athletes with paraplegia prefer 15 to 25 cm from the seat back to the rear axles inserts, those with tetraplegia prefer 5 to 20 cm. Novice athletes generally choose more stable configurations. The seat cage upholstery adjustment and rear axle positions are fitted to allow athletes to position their shoulders over the front edge of the push rims, also creating room to reach the bottom of the push rims with both arms. Individuals with upper-level SCI tend to pull their knees up higher toward the chest (Figure 19-3) than do lower-level-injured athletes to further enhance stability, balance, and breathing.

Athletes with paraplegia, tetraplegia, or amputated limbs have different positioning preferences and each person has unique abilities and body structure. Generally speaking, there are three basic racing body positions available to racers: kneeling bucket, kneeling cage, and upright cage. The kneeling positions tend to be the lightest setup and the most aerodynamic and have allowed paraplegic and tetraplegic athletes to make tremendous performance gains over the years. Athletes inexperienced with the kneeling position may benefit from a kneeling cage, which affords them the flexibility of sitting upright or kneeling and permits more adjustment of body position. Upright cage seats work well for athletes with lower limb amputations and for athletes

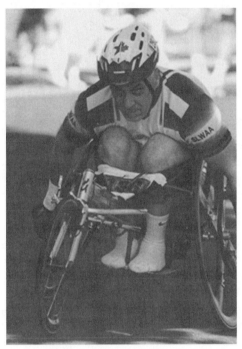

FIGURE 19-3 Individual with C6 tetraplegia using the cage position with foot plate on racing chair.

with low levels of paraplegia (i.e., those who have the trunk control to adjust body position while racing).[34]

A properly fitted racing chair can allow the user to make minor steering adjustments by swinging the upper body or hips. Racers often refer to this maneuver as "hipping" the chair. A racing chair's primary steering, however, is controlled by the upper body's interaction with the front wheel, where pressure can be applied to handle bars, which turn the front wheel left to right. When racing on a track an athlete should not rely on primary steering: an additional steering component called a compensator can be engaged with one hand while taking the chair around the curve of a track and then disengaged to accommodate the strait section of the track. Wheelchair racers can maintain chair control at high rates of speed for long distances not only because of the precision equipment and its fit but also because athletes use highly specialized propulsion strokes (Figure 19-4). The racing stroke is in part dependent on the athletes using special gloves available commercially or constructed independently by each racer. These gloves are often built using a combination of leather, foam, rubber, and self-molding plastics. Racing gloves promote solid contact between the glove surface and the push ring, which generally has a rubber-coated surface. This setup allows skilled athletes to keep up with the wheel at very high speeds and to deliver more force per stroke to the wheel, minimizing slips and other contact and release related inefficiencies. The motion of a propulsion stroke can best be described as a punching motion and it can take years to master.[31] Furthermore, aerodynamic positioning, as mentioned before, has initiated a propulsion technique where extensive shoulder extension and abduction during the back swing lead to increased hand speed at the impact energy transfer phase.[36,37]

Given the multitude physical and mechanical elements relevant to racing in combination with the reality that the propulsion technique can take substantial time to develop, new racers often find racing daunting. Novice racers typically enter the sport using previously owned equipment. Used equipment generally is loose fitting but can be adjusted with foam pads and additional

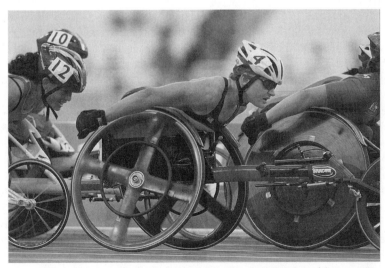

FIGURE 19-4 Wheelchair racers can maintain chair control at high rates of speed not only because of their precision equipment and its fit but also because they use highly specialized propulsion strokes. (Courtesy PVA Publications, Phoenix, Ariz.)

upholstery to accommodate the new occupant. It is important that athletes, particularly beginners, be able to reach brakes from a comfortable position, and the brake levers must be long enough and at the proper angle so that the athlete can apply sufficient leverage to stop the racing chair.[34] In addition, new racers are often relieved to know that racing competition separates athletes by functional class and sex to keep the playing field level. Most major road running races across the world have wheelchair divisions separated into tetraplegic and paraplegic events and tend to pay the top finishers in each class. Because racing can be profitable to the top athletes, many racers take training very seriously.

Marty Morse and Adam Bleakney[37] from the University of Illinois have collaborated to write a series of exercise training articles for wheelchair athletes for the magazine *Sports 'n Spokes*. One article in particular describes training methods for the wheelchair marathon. They describe wheelchair marathons as a series of sprints run off a steady pace. Successful training is therefore built around speed development. It presents drills for five areas of training for improved marathon performance. Each is based on the goals of developing maximal speed, acceleration, and the ability to sustain a high percentage of maximal speed for an extended period of time.

Basketball

Wheelchair basketball began in the 1940s because of interest among veterans to pursue sports and recreational activities.[38] Qualification tournaments are held before the Paralympic Games. Wheelchair users comprise the basketball team and have various diagnoses, including paraplegia, cerebral palsy, amputations, postpolio syndrome, or a disabling injury. Participants in wheelchair basketball are not required to use a wheelchair as their primary means of mobility or in their activities of daily living. Athletes compete on a court for 40 minutes with the same dimension and hoop height as specified by the International Basketball Federation.[39]

The player classification system used in wheelchair basketball covers each player and is based on his observed trunk movement during performance of basketball skills such as pushing the wheelchair, dribbling, passing, receiving, shooting, and rebounding. Point classes are 1.0, 1.5, 2.0, 2.5, 3.0, 3.5, 4.0, and 4.5 with each player assuming a point value equal to his classification. A 1.0 player is on the lowest end of relative function and is equivalent to that of a mid to upper thoracic SCI. A 4.5 point value would indicate a great degree of relative function (e.g., a sacral-level SCI or single leg amputee). The point values of the five participating players are combined to yield a team total. For International Wheelchair Basketball Federation world championships, Paralympic competitions, zonal championships, and the qualifying events leading up to these competitions, this team total may not exceed 14 points. The starting team and all subsequent player combinations by substitutions may not exceed this 14-point total. Each player is issued a player classification card that must be used during team play. The card indicates both the player's classification and describes any modifications to sitting position, the player's use of straps, and orthotic and prosthetic devices.

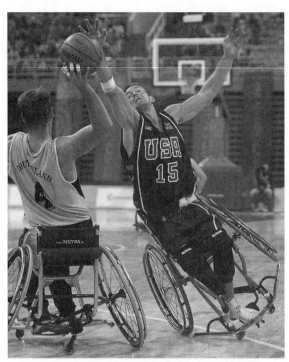

FIGURE 19-5 Basketball wheelchairs are designed to provide optimal speed, acceleration, and quick braking, as well as protect the player and chair from contact injuries. (Courtesy PVA Publications, Phoenix, Ariz.)

The varying degrees of disability among players require that they follow a basic rule of remaining firmly seated in the wheelchair at all times and not using a functional leg or leg stump for physical advantage over an opponent—a rule that is strictly enforced. An infraction of this rule during rebound or jump ball constitutes a physical advantage foul and is recorded in the official score book. Three such fouls disqualify a player from the game. Two free throws are awarded and the ball is given to the opposing team out of bounds. Additional rules of the game include (1) a player in possession of the ball may not push more than twice in succession with one or both hands in either direction without tapping the ball to the floor and (2) taking more than two consecutive pushes constitutes a traveling violation.

A player may, however, wheel the chair and dribble the ball simultaneously just as an able-bodied player runs and dribbles the ball simultaneously. There is no double dribble violation in wheelchair basketball. Furthermore, a player may remain within the opponents' restricted area (key) for no longer than 3 seconds. Staying in the area for a longer time will result in a 3-second violation. This restriction does not apply while the ball is in the air during a shot, during a rebound, or while the ball is dead.[40]

The type of wheelchair used in basketball is similar to an individual's personal wheelchair but incorporates other features that enhance its maneuverability.[4,41] Basketball wheelchairs are designed to be lightweight to allow for speed, acceleration, and quick braking (Figure 19-5). Although basketball is not a contact sport, some incidental contact is inevitable. Consequently, basketball wheelchairs use spoke guards to cover the rear wheel spokes to prevent wheel damage and illegal ramming and picking from the opposition. Made of high-impact plastic, spoke guards provide several additional benefits: they make it easier for players to pick up the ball from the floor by pushing it against the spoke guard and rolling it onto the lap; they protect hands and fingers from aggressive play when reaching for the ball; and they provide space to identify team affiliations and sponsor names.

The wheelchair must have four wheels, two large rear wheels and two front casters for front steering. The front casters tend to be made from extremely hard plastics, similar to in-line skate wheels, with precision roller bearings and are 5 cm in diameter. The rear wheels can be no large than 66 cm in diameter, and there must be a hand rim on each wheel. The seat height is limited to 53 cm from the floor, and the footrest should be no higher than 11 cm when the front wheels are in their forward movement position. In addition, players use high-pressure tires (i.e., 120 to 200 psi) with minimal or very low profile tread to maximize speed and maneuverability. High-pressure tires make it easier to push the wheelchair and help to make it faster on the court.

The footrest must also be designed to avoid damage to the playing surface. A cushion may be used, if it is made of flexible material and is no more than 10 cm thick, unless the player is classified as a 3.5-, 4.0-, or 4.5-point player, in which case it must be no thicker than 5 cm. The cushion must be the same size as the seat of the wheelchair. No black tires, gears, breaks, or steering devices are allowed on the chair. Camber is an important feature of basketball wheelchairs as well. Camber makes a wheelchair more responsive during turns and protects players' hands when two wheelchairs collide from the sides by limiting the collision to the bottom of the wheels and leaving a space at the top to protect the hands.[4]

Basketball wheelchair seats typically have a drop or seat bucketing of 5 to 15 degrees. Because basketball rules limit the maximum height of any portion of the seat, athletes usually try to make their seats as high as possible. Guards are an exception because lower seat heights and greater seat angles can make chairs faster and more maneuverable for ball handling. Referees check the players' wheelchairs before each game to ensure they meet the these requirements.

Cycling

Adaptive cycling allows an individual living with SCI to enjoy a form of exercise and recreational activity that has traditionally been a popular form of leisure as well. It is one of the fastest growing recreational activities for people with disabilities. The adaptive equipment consists of a handcycle that allows individuals with limited use of their lower limbs to use the strength of their upper limbs.[42,43] Relatively minimal modifications can be implemented to accommodate individuals with lower-level tetraplegia. Some of these modifications include hand cuffs that can be mounted to the arm crank handles and elastic abdominal binders that can be fitted around the user and the handcycle seat to increase trunk stability. A handcycle typically consists of a three-wheel setup to achieve the balance that a two-wheeled bicycle requires to function. Two-wheeled handcycles do exist but require a great deal of skill and balance. In addition, handcycle design allows the user to propel, steer, break, and change gears, all with the upper limbs and trunk.

Two types of handcycle designs are typical: upright and recumbent models. In an upright handcycle, the rider is in an upright position similar to a wheelchair. Upright handcycles use a pivot steer where only the front wheel turns while the cycle remains in an upright position. Transferring and balancing tend to be easier in the upright cycle. In a recumbent handcycle, the rider's torso may be reclined with legs positioned forward. These cycles may be lean-to-steer handcycles, where the rider leans to turn, causing the cycle to pivot at hinge points. Leaning to turn can be challenging if the rider lacks trunk stability, in which case it is better to use a pivot steering recumbent handcycle. Recumbent handcycles are lighter and faster, making them the choice for handcycle racing.

Fencing

Wheelchair users participate in fencing with their wheelchair secured to the floor to allow for safe, free movement of the upper body.[44] The sport consists of male and female athletes, with male athletes competing in the epee, foil, and saber, whereas women athletes participate in the epee and foil only. The foil has a flexible rectangular blade, approximately 35 inches in length, weighing less than 1 pound. The epee is similar in length to the foil, but is heavier, weighing approximately 27 ounces, with a larger guard and a much stiffer blade. The saber is the modern version of the slashing cavalry sword and is similar in length and weight to the foil.

Individuals participating in fencing are arranged into five functional classes that range from C5 to C6 level to sacral level. Individuals with high-level SCI may use bandages to fix the weapon to the hand if they lack sufficient grip strength. In terms of equipment, fencers compete from their wheelchairs, fixed into a fencing that is firmly attached to the ground. The frame positions athletes opposite one another at an angle 110 ± 2 degrees to a central axis bar connecting opponents. The inside front caster wheel of each athlete must be touching the central axis bar in the forward direction, and the wheelchairs are secured to ensure they do not move. The wheelchair back must be set at a 90-degree angle and the back height must be a minimum of 15 cm from the seat or seat cushion, which must have even thickness rather than be wedge-shaped. Fencers may use an armrest that is a minimum of 10 cm from the seat height, but only on the nonfencing arm side.

Protective clothing is mandatory and specific to the weapon being used. Protective gear includes protective plastrons, metallic jackets, lame apron, and hand protection (Figure 19-6). Fencers score points by hitting their target, which includes the whole of the upper body for the epee and saber. The saber also includes a lower target area, which includes any part of the body above a horizontal line drawn between the top of the folds formed by the thighs and the trunk of the fencer. Any portion of the chair or cushion above this line is also included in the target area.

The main objective of wheelchair fencing is for the first fencer to score 15 points (direct elimination) or 5 points (preliminary pool play) against the opponent. A point is awarded each time a fencer touches the opponent in the target area and direct elimination matches consist of three 3-minute periods.[44] Team events are composed of both male and female athletes who compete in the epee and foil. In addition, athletes are restricted to a maximum

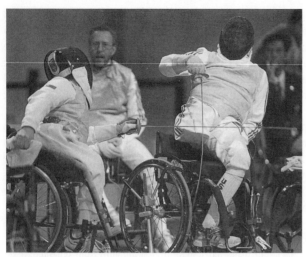

FIGURE 19-6 In fencing, protective clothing is mandatory and specific to the weapon being used. (Courtesy PVA Publications, Phoenix, Ariz.)

of two different weapons per event in the individual and team competitions.

Fishing

Fishing is an activity that can be adapted to meet the needs of a wide range of SCI levels. Many individuals prefer to transfer and fish from a boat while others may choose to fish from their wheelchairs. Fishing equipment can be hand-held or mounted to power and manual wheelchairs. In addition, there are numerous companies that sell adapted equipment designed to compensate for hand and upper limb weakness. Some of these devices include one-handed reel designs, knot ties, and rod holders.[45]

Football

Wheelchair football is played with manual chairs, power chairs, or scooters and typically requires five to fourteen players to hold a game. Players can use a standard football and may elect to wear protective equipment including bicycle helmets, eyewear, and gloves. Because of the equipment requirements, wheelchair football is played on a hard surface such as a gymnasium or parking lot. The game is considered touch football, but the players can decide on the level of contact before the game begins. This sport, like most team sports, uses a functional player classification system.[46]

Golf

Golf has become a popular sport for many active individuals living with an SCI. Consequently there are many assistive devices on the market that enable golfers with disabilities to play the game. These include golf clubs designed specifically to be swung from a seated position, mobility devices, gripping aids, practice facility equipment such as automated ball teeing devices, and ball retrieval aids. In addition, the Americans with Disabilities Act has allowed individuals with disabilities greater access to a wide range of recreational opportunities including golf courses. A number of golf associations also exist in the United States and internationally with the sole purpose of support for and to provide information to golfers playing with disabilities. Some of these

organizations include the United States Golf Association, the Resource Center for Individuals with Disabilities, and the National Alliance for Accessible Golf.

Horseback Riding

Depending on the rider's ambition, horseback riding offers many opportunities as both a recreational sport and a therapeutic activity. As a sport, it provides the rider with the opportunity to master skills necessary to confidently maneuver a horse through various outdoor courses and terrain. Adaptive riding equipment is available in the form of modified saddles and positioning devices, designed to provide additional support and stability of the rider when on the horse. Mechanical lifts are also available to assist individuals with physical disabilities to safely mount the horse.

Therapeutic riding involves teaching a rider the necessary skills and techniques to ride a horse as independently as possible and facilitates confidence and positive self-esteem through acquisition of these skills. Hippotherapy, a division of therapeutic riding, uses the rhythmical and repetitive movement of the horse (similar to human movement patterns of the pelvis when walking) and the body's natural tendency to adjust to this movement to focus on developing balance, body awareness, posture, coordination, and muscle tone in the rider. The North American Riding for the Handicapped Association (NARHA) is a nonprofit organization that promotes safe therapeutic riding for individuals with disabilities. The organization provides accreditation to therapeutic horseback riding centers in the United States to ensure that standards are established and maintained. Currently, the NARHA has more than 600 centers across the United States and more than 30,000 people with disabilities participate in their programs.

Off-Road Downhill

A variety of outdoor adventure activities exist for individuals with SCI. Ultimately, any individual interested in hiking, camping, or off-road navigation can do so with adaptations to the basic everyday manual and power wheelchairs. Mountain bike tires and other related off-road technologies allow for increased traction on soft, wet, or rough terrain. In addition, front casters have become larger to decrease rolling resistance, which reduces the likelihood of getting caught on obstacles.

In recent years additional highly specialized off-road wheelchairs have been developed by enthusiasts and engineers in the field (see Figure 11-40). Some of these wheelchair designs have independent wheel suspension and configurations that allow athletes to compete side by side with mountain bikers in dual slalom and downhill events, reaching speeds in excess of 50 miles per hour.[47]

Paddle Sports

Kayaking, canoeing, and rowing are sports that individuals with mobility impairments can participate in along with unimpaired individuals. Family and friends can benefit from this challenging exercise because it is safe and affordable and can be accessed in many different places. There are several ways for an individual with SCI to participate in paddling. Kayaks and canoes can accommodate a wide range of SCI levels using common adaptations for balance, kayak exit and entry, grip options for paddles, and overall kayak stability with use of outriggers. For individuals requiring more assistance, tandem kayaks are available. A paddling partner or instructor seated in the stern of tandem kayaks can help with steering and paddling when necessary. This type of kayak benefits beginners, individuals with limited paddling strength, and those with a variety of other impairments.

Power Lifting

Athletes competing in power lifting, which include the bench press and power lift, are classified by weight rather than by disability; hence, it is considered a cross-disability sport.[48] Athletes, however, must have at least 10% loss of function of their lower limbs to be eligible. All competitors lift against athletes in their weight class, which may include individuals with paralysis, lower limb amputations, or cerebral palsy. Regardless of the disability, athletes are required to have a maximum loss of 20 degrees of full extension in either elbow.[48] People with limitations of extension of joints require special approval from the classification officials to compete.

A lifter may be strapped to the bench with an official belt that is 10 cm wide. A competitor may wear a leather belt not exceeding 120 mm at its widest part with a thickness not exceeding 13 mm. The belt may not have any additional padding, bracing, or supports, leather or metal, either interior or exterior. The belt may be laminated, however, providing that each section of the leather is of the same width and extends the full length of the belt and it must be worn over the athlete's lifting costume.

Lifts are carried out on a square area measuring four meters on each side. If the lower part of the bench is too narrow for the lifter's legs, because of anatomical deformities, the referees may use a piece of wood to increase the width of the lower part of the bench, but only with agreement from an official jury. Any additional strapping used for support is allowed only on the legs, around the ankles, or just above the knees. For the bench press, the bar is lowered horizontally until it is 2.5 cm above the lifter's chest. The measurement must be made with a measuring stick 2.5 cm wide and 30 cm long. For the power lift, the lifter must lower the bar to his chest. Once the bar is motionless on the lifter's chest, the lifter presses upward to straight-arm length and holds the bar motionless until signaled a fair lift by the referee.[48]

Power Soccer

Indoor wheelchair soccer is a fast-paced game that can be played by individuals using primarily power wheelchairs. The sport is usually played inside in a gymnasium on a regulation basketball court although occasionally there are outdoor parking lot competitions (Figure 19-7). Many of the same skills required for wheelchair basketball are used in wheelchair soccer, such as quick movement, passing, dribbling, and shooting. In wheelchair soccer, a player may use hands, feet, or the wheelchair to move the ball. Team makeup is dependent on factors such as age, functional ability, and years of experience. Power soccer is a team sport played by individuals with various disabilities. It is unisex by design, and male and female participants are often on the same team.

The game's objective is to outscore the opponents by driving an oversized soccer ball (diameter 50 cm, pressure equal to 0.6 to 1.1 atmosphere) across the opposing team's goal line. A goal is scored when the ball passes over the goal line between the goal panels. If

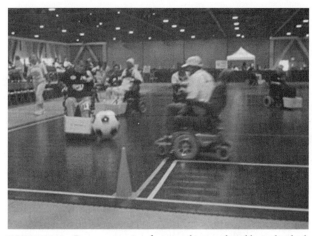

FIGURE 19-7 Power soccer is a fast-paced game played by individuals primarily using power wheelchairs on a smooth interior court.

the ball crosses the line as a direct result of a drop ball or a kick-in, however, it is not considered a goal. Foot guards are temporarily attached to chairs to help in controlling the ball and to prevent damage to wheelchairs. There are restrictions on the number and speed of electric wheelchairs (EW) used by the players: a maximum 2 EWs with a top speed of 6 km/h or a maximum 4 EWs with a top speed of 4.5 km/h. A team may use a combination of EWs during a match.

The game is similar to the nonstop action seen in a typical indoor soccer game. The match is played by two teams, with no more than four players on the court at any time. There is no goalkeeper. The match consists of two halves of 20 minutes each, with a 10-minute half-time break. If the scores are equal at the game's completion, the match is decided by extra time and eventually a penalty shootout if the scores are still drawn. A successful team uses court position, blocking, picking, and keeping the ball in the opponents' half.[49]

Rock Climbing

Rock climbing is an adventure sport that has attracted a significant number of individuals with SCI. Climbers can enjoy indoor rock climbing gyms as well as large-scale mountain expeditions. Climbing harnesses and other equipment have been designed to maximize upper limb efficiency while climbing; ascending gear tends to be extremely supportive and keeps a climber's body upright. Notable climbers with disabilities have successfully completed climbs at Mt. Rainier and Mt. McKinley, among other challenging heights.

Rugby

Quad rugby was originally called murder ball because of the aggressive nature of the game. Brad Mikkelsen teamed up with University of North Dakota's Disabled Student Services to create the first team, called the Wallbangers, and ultimately introduced rugby to the United States in 1981. In 1988, the United States Quad Rugby Association was formed to regulate and promote the sport on both national and international levels. Since its introduction, rugby has grown to become an international sport, with teams from around the world. Currently there are more than 45 organized teams in the United States with many new teams surfacing each year. Rugby first joined the Paralympics in 1996 as a demonstration event and then officially as a full medal sport at the 2000 Sydney Paralympic Games.

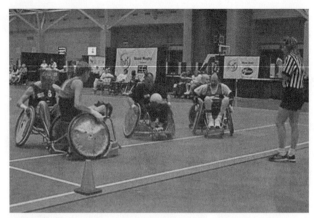

FIGURE 19-8 Quad rugby is a fast, rigorous game played indoors with two teams consisting of four players each.

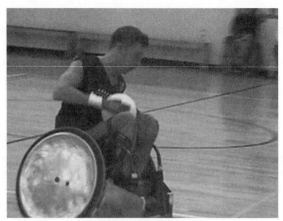

FIGURE 19-9 A rugby player maneuvers his fast, offensive-style chair especially built for scoring.

Players must have a combination of upper and lower limb impairment to be considered eligible to participate. Most of the players have sustained cervical-level spinal injuries and have some degree of tetraplegia as a result. Players are given a classification number, similar to basketball, based on a system that contains seven distinct classifications ranging from 0.5 to 3.5. A 0.5 player has the greatest impairment and is comparable to someone with C5 tetraplegia. Of those eligible to participate, the 3.5 player has the least impairment (i.e., C7 to C8 incomplete tetraplegia). Both men and women are encouraged to play and, because of the classification process, sex advantages are minimal. In addition, a team may have players with no more than a combined eight points out on a floor at any one time.

Played indoors, the game consists of two teams composed of four players—male or female (Figure 19-8). The objective of wheelchair rugby is for the players to cross the opponent's goal line (i.e., two wheels must cross the goal) while the player has possession of the ball. At the same time that the team on offense is trying to advance the ball, the defense tries to halt their progress by creating turnovers. When a player is in possession of the ball, he must bounce the ball every 10 seconds and a team must get the ball across midline in 15 seconds or less. In addition, certain restrictions apply in the key area. Three defensive players are allowed in the key, and if a fourth enters, a penalty can be assessed or a goal awarded. An offensive player can only stay in the key area for 10 seconds or a turnover is awarded.[50]

Players tend to use extreme wheelchair configurations, elastic binders, foams, and special tacky gloves to improve performance. Similar to basketball, players often become extremely proficient in adapting their equipment to promote balance and speed, so much so that they often appear to possess significantly more functional capacity then their neurological injury level would indicate. The styles of wheelchairs used in rugby are strictly regulated to ensure fairness, but the chairs vary considerably depending on each player's preference, functional level, and team role. Players with the most extreme upper body deficits tend to take on more defensive blocking and picking roles and use chairs that have additional length and hardware that enables them to grab other players' chairs.

Players with more functional ability usually take on the role of ball handler and use offensive chairs built more for scoring, which requires speed and quick maneuverability (Figure 19-9). In addition, many ball handlers' chairs are designed to deflect or slide off other chairs to minimize the likelihood of getting caught up or stopped in a tangle of chairs. Regardless of functional abilities and classification, all rugby chairs have extreme amounts of camber, 16 to 20 degrees, significant bucketing, and antitip bars. The camber provides lateral stability, hand protection, and ease in turning. The bucketing (i.e., knees are high relative to rear end) helps with trunk balance and protection of the ball.

Sailing

Sailing consists of two classes: single-handed and crew boat (i.e., Sonar boats). The single-handed class consists of the sailor facing forward in the boat, with all controls accessible within an arm's reach. Sailors competing in crew are assigned a point classification based on their disability. Three individual sailors, with varying levels of disabilities, comprise the Sonar crew. The team must be composed of individuals not exceeding a total set point value similar to that of rugby and basketball. Sailors with disabilities are able to add adaptive seating or assistive arrangements to the boat provided they are temporary fixtures and are approved before the event. Furthermore, the large cockpit and balanced inboard rudder add stability to the boat, making the sport ideal for individuals with a variety of disabilities.[51]

Paralympic sailing is offered for athletes with physical disabilities and for those with vision loss. The International Paralympic Committee (IPC) follows the classification procedures developed by the International Foundation of Disabled Sailing, which are posted on the IPC website at www.paralympic.org. Classification tests for sailors with physical disabilities are designed to test the athlete's ability to compensate for the movement of the boat (stability), operate the control lines and tiller (hand function), move about in the boat (mobility), and see while racing (vision). Athletes who use prostheses or supportive devices while sailing must be classified under those conditions. During functional anatomical testing, performed in a room equipped with an examination table, athletes are judged on strength, movement, and coordination. During functional dock tests, performed on a Sonar boat at dockside, athletes are tested on tiller, sheeting, cleating, transferring, and hiking. The same tests also are performed during functional sailing tests in competition.[52]

There are seven classifications, with class 1 representing the least sailing ability and class 7, the most sailing ability. Sailors are assigned to different classes on the basis of their point scores in the classification tests. Each crew is allowed a maximum of 14 rating points. No sailing advantage is given to a crew with a total of less than 14 points. When sailors present themselves for classification, they are required to bring all their personal assistive devices, adaptations, prostheses, and orthotics that they intend to use during racing. Additional devices could include seating support, harnesses, and any other essential adaptations. Seats allow the sailors to position themselves so they can control the tiller and sheet without fear of falling. Seats can be as basic as a lawn chair modified to fit a cockpit or as complex as a translating seat, which allows a sailor to switch sides of the boat. Sailors often use transfer benches as well which allow them to switch sides when tacking or jibbing; these seats can be anything from a sturdy cooler in the middle of the cockpit (i.e., custom cockpit filler) to platforms that fill in the cockpit area. Boat modifications may not include any requiring drilling holes or installation of permanent fixtures. Any modifications to the sail may not raise more than 20 cm above the existing seat, increase the sailor's performance beyond that of an able-bodied person, be power assisted, or be judged unsafe. Boats must be equipped with radios for boat-to-boat and boat-to-shore communication. In addition, athletes must wear personal flotation devices. Support and rescue boats are required during all events and at least one boat must have a scuba (self-contained underwater breathing apparatus) diver available to assist with rescues.[52]

The Paralympics includes both the crew boat discipline with one skipper and two crew members and the single-handed discipline. The racing rules, including course specifications, are posted on the International Sailing Federation (ISAF) Web site at www.sailing.org. Boats used in the crew boat discipline include the American 210, Sonar, Squib, Surprise, or UFO. The boat used in the single-handed discipline is the International 2.4mR. Modifications to ISAF rules competition consists of a four-race series with points awarded for place finish in each race. Points are accumulated across races, with the low score winning the regatta.

SCUBA

Many individuals with a range of SCI levels participate in underwater activities. The Handicapped Scuba Association certifies individuals with disabilities and has established specific regulations indicating the level of support a disabled diver will need to dive. The extent of support a diver requires is largely a function of injury level and diving experience. Most individuals diving with disabilities, however, enjoy great freedom from the reduced effects of gravity when under water. Many disabled divers increase their abilities using equipment like webbed diving gloves for extra push and a special buoyancy compensator for a more comfortable dive.[53]

Shooting Sports

Shooting events are comprised of free and supported rifle and free pistol, both air and .22 caliber, shooting at distances from 10 to 50 m. Competition occurs in the form of individual men and women as well as mixed and team events; however, team competitions are not included in the Paralympic Games. Competitors are permitted to use assistive devices in an attempt to create equal competition among the athletes with different functional abilities. Depending on an individual's level of SCI, athletes may use various forms of approved assistance. Some of these supports include a specially prescribed stand used to support the weight of a rifle, a shooting table, or a person who assists the competitor to cock and load the gun and exchange shooting targets where necessary. Competitors with tetraplegia or paraplegia may not strap themselves to the chair to increase trunk stability for shooting. They may strap their knees together only if they have sought and received approval during their classification. The height of the wheelchair or chair back and push handles must be at least 30 mm below the armpits when the shoulders are in the resting position. The scapula, arms, or armpits cannot derive horizontal support from or rest on any part of the wheelchair. The use of wheelchair armrests or chair sides is not permitted during competition unless specifically authorized by the classification team. No part of the chair or competitor that touches the floor may be in front of the firing line.[54]

Skiing

Skiing is both a recreational and competitive sport. There are several options for snow skiers to choose from: alpine, downhill skiing, Nordic, cross-country, and sit-skiing with monoski or bi-ski configurations. Assistive devices such as adaptive seating, backrests, cushions, tethering ropes, roll bars, and outriggers allow skiers with disabilities to maintain a similar pace to that of unimpaired athletes. When an athlete is learning to ski, a guide can be used to assist new skiers down the slopes for direction and safety. Various types of sit-skis in combination with outriggers exist, offering a skier with a disability more or less support and stability when needed. Monoskis and bi-skis have become quite advanced and offer shock absorption systems, frames molded to body shape, and quick-release safety options. The outriggers that skiers use are an adapted version of a forearm crutch and a shortened ski. Outriggers provide extra balance and steering maneuverability not available from a typical ski pole.[55] In addition, many sit-skis, whether monoskis or bi-skis, have loading mechanisms, usually hydraulic, that enable an athlete to jack himself up into a high position for loading onto a ski lift. Many athletes can load onto lifts independently, whereas others may require assistance, depending on experience and level of SCI.

The monoski is typically the ski of choice for individuals wanting high-end performance, maneuverability, and speed. When using a monoski, the individual sits relatively high over the snow on one ski and can translate upper body, arm, and head movement into the ski more efficiently than with the bi-ski system. The monoski's sensitivity can make it more challenging to learn, particularly for individuals with less trunk control, upper thoracic and above injuries, and for novices hitting the slopes occasionally. Because of the dynamic nature and sensitivity of the monoski, there are some inherent risks. While athletes are moving at high speeds and balancing over the single ski, serious falls can occur. When falls happen, the mass of the equipment and body can translate through the shoulders, head, or neck, causing severe injury.[56] Experienced monoskiers can match the speeds and handle technical terrain with the same facility that experienced able-bodied downhill skiers demonstrate; however, sit-skiing biomechanics put different strains on the body. Research has found that the stress on the monoskiers' upper bodies occurring from normal skiing was three times that of stress occurring in the upper bodies of downhill skiers who stand.[56] Sit-skiing involves an elevated isometric muscle contraction component because the upper limbs must balance the entire body with outriggers.[56] Furthermore, other disabled skiing research has compared the incidence of injuries occurring in monoskiing with the incidences of injury occurring in other sports. Laskowski and Paul[57] compared the incidence of emergency department visits over a 4-year period and found that injury rates were not significantly different. Fractures and sprain incidence were nearly identical; the only category of injury found to be more frequent in sit-skiing was noticed in the bruise category, showing 18% of disabled compared with 11% of nondisabled skiers, respectively.[57]

For skiing novices or individuals with less trunk stability seeking the freedom and excitement of skiing, bi-skis can serve as an appropriate alternative. Bi-skis are similar to monoskis but the user balances on two skis that can angulate and shift to put the skis on edge. Bi-skis are much easier to control because they have a wider base of support and can be mastered more quickly with fewer falls.

Cross-country skiing, also called Nordic skiing, uses sit-ski technology as well. The Nordic sit-ski is composed of a seat balanced over a frame with two cross-country skis approximately 12 inches apart. Because cross-country skiing requires great strength and cardiovascular fitness, many wheelchair athletes find it to be a great cross-training application for sports such as racing and handcycling.

Sledge Hockey

Sledge hockey derives its name from the Norwegian word *sledge*, which means sled, and is referred to as sled hockey in some parts of Canada and the United States. Ice sled hockey was invented at a Stockholm, Sweden, rehabilitation center in the early 1960s by a group who, despite their physical impairments, wanted to continue playing hockey.[58] The ice surface, goal net, and pucks are all the same, and all U.S. hockey rules apply with some necessary adaptations resulting from the nature of the game and its participants.

The equipment used in the game consists of the sledge—a metal-framed oval sled with two blades and a small runner, a seat with a backrest, leg straps, and optional push handles The traditional hockey stick is shortened and modified with two picks attached to the end (i.e., metal pieces with a minimum of three teeth measuring a maximum of 4 mm).[59] The picks are used to provide traction while the player moves down the ice and also give leverage for the player to shoot the puck with the blade end of the stick. A player may secure his hands to the stick if his grip is not solid. Two-blade sledges that allow the puck to pass underneath replace skates, and the players use sticks with a spike-end and a blade-end. The chair backrest cannot protrude laterally beyond the armpits of the player when properly seated on the sledge, although it may be padded and should have rounded edges and corners with no hard or sharp obtrusions to the sides.

With a quick flip of the wrist, players are able to propel themselves using the spikes and then play the puck using the blade-end of the sticks. A player may use two sticks with blades to facilitate stick handling and ambidextrous shooting. Sticks are made of wood or other material approved by the International Ice Hockey Federation, such as aluminum or plastic. The stick must not have any projections and all edges must be beveled. The dimensions of the stick are as follows: maximum length 100 cm measured in a straight line from the toe to the pick end, maximum width 3 cm, maximum thickness 2.5 cm. The shaft must be straight and the blade's maximum length only 32 cm from the heel to the toe and have a width of between 5 to 7.5 cm at the toe (i.e., front of the blade). A goalkeeper's stick may be equipped with a larger blade that must not exceed 35 cm in length and 9 cm in height.

Sledge hockey games consist of three 15-minute stop-time periods. Protective gear must be worn at all times and includes a helmet with cage or shield, shin guards, shoulder pads, gloves, elbow pads, neck guard, and hockey pants. In addition, straps are used to secure a player's feet, ankles, knees, and hips to the sledge. Repeated loss of straps or adjustments on ice causing delay of game is penalized accordingly. There are six players on the ice at a time for each team: one goalie, three forwards, and two defense players. Sledge hockey is unique because it does not have a classification system; its only requirement states that a player must have a disability that would prevent him from playing able-bodied hockey.

Snowmobiling

Snowmobiles can be accessible to wheelchair users with use of hand controls rather than foot pedals to operate the vehicle. A rider should have good upper body strength and dependable hand control. Equipment modifications can include seat adjustments, other equipment relevant to the person's disability, and the attachment of looped rubber tubing to the foot platform to maintain the lower limbs in correct positions. Warm, layered clothing for individuals with poor or limited circulation in the lower limbs is advised. Snowmobiling is an easy way of being out in the outdoors and crisp winter air. The general features of snowmobiles are similar to wheelchairs: seat height, hand controls, no foot pedals or foot-activated controls. Selection of equipment is based on an individual's specific disability.

Softball

Wheelchair softball was designed to allow individuals with a physical disability to play a game similar to traditional softball and abides by the Amateur Softball Association of America's (ASAA) official rules for 16-inch slow pitch. Ten individuals play per team and, as in rugby and basketball, players are classified on the basis of functional abilities and only a specified quantity can legally be active on the playing field at one time. The playing field is a hard surface allowing for easier maneuverability of the wheelchairs to preserve the pace of the game. Individuals with tetraplegia can also be integrated into play because of the point classification system. Players with upper limb impairments are allowed more freedom for bat, grip, and glove alterations.

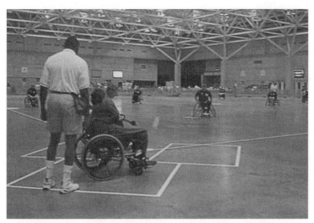

FIGURE 19-10 Wheelchair softball uses the official Amateur Softball Association of America's rules as its guide for indoor play with a diamond that has 50 feet between bases.

The official rules of the National Wheelchair Softball Association[59] do allow for some exceptions to the ASAA rules geared toward the wheelchair user. All participants must use manual wheelchairs with footplates, and the playing field must be a level smooth surface of blacktop or similar materials with 150 feet on the foul lines and 180 to 220 feet to straight center. The official diamond has 50 feet between all bases and 70 feet, 8.5 inches from home to second base (Figure 19-10). The base runner must be seated in his wheelchair and may tag or make contact with the base with either one or more wheels or his hand. If a runner is knocked out of his chair, he may proceed to the previous or next base by any means other than hopping, walking, or running and make contact with the base with any part of his body. A base runner may not place a lower limb on the ground or someone else's chair to stop his chair and if he does, the play is dead, resulting in a delay-dead ball situation.

All teams are required to have an individual with tetraplegia on their team in active play. Players with tetraplegia may alter the bat to improve the grip; however, alterations must be approved by the head umpire. If a team does not have someone with tetraplegia playing, the team is required to play with one less person on the field (i.e., nine rather then ten players). When a player is at bat there are rules set in place to prevent individuals with some lower limb movement from having unfair advantage. For example, a hitter cannot have a lower limb in contact with the ground when hitting. This action could help the batter unfairly stabilize himself. If this does occur, the batter is declared automatically out. A player's classification ranges from 1 to 3 points on the basis of his functional level. Someone with tetraplegia would receive a 1-point class and someone who has high functioning paraplegia (e.g., a low-level injury) would receive a 3-point class. A team of ten players may not exceed a total of 22 points.[59]

Swimming

The swimming events that take place at the Paralympic level include freestyle (50 to 1500 meter), backstroke (50 to 200 meter), breaststroke (50 to 200 meter), butterfly (50 to 200 meter), individual medley (150 and 400 meter), and relay events (4×50 meter free, 4×200 meter free, 4×50 meter medley,

4×100 meter medley). Athletes are classified and compete against others on the basis of how they move in the water with their hands, arms, trunk, and legs, which ultimately affects how starts and turns are performed. The level of an individual's SCI directly affects the types of strokes that he can perform. Stroke adaptations are permitted and specified within each stroke category and applied to swimmers' functional abilities, which are in turn indicated by swimmers' classifications. For example, in breast stroke competition swimmers may start in the water, off the side, or off the blocks. After the signal to start is given, one asymmetrical stroke is permitted to allow the swimmer to attain the breast position. Swimmers in specified classes may roll over on their backs to breathe but no attempts at forward propulsion are allowed. As an adaptation, swimmers who have completed their laps in relay races who are unable to immediately leave the water may stay in the water in an unused lane as long as they do not interfere with the other competitors or with timing equipment.[60]

Table Tennis

Table tennis can be played effectively with a power chair, a scooter, or a manual wheelchair. Standard four-wheel manual chairs are permitted; however, they are not as mobile as the three-wheeled chairs designed for tennis (i.e., with a minimum of two large wheels and one small wheel). In competition, men and woman can play individually and in teams. In addition, a wheelchair user is not permitted to strap any part of the body to the wheelchair unless medically necessary. For wheelchair play, the playing area may be reduced but should not be less than 8 meters long and 7 meters wide.

Disabled table tennis players are divided into 10 classes according to a functional classification system. Classes 1 to 5 compete in wheelchairs and classes 6 to 10 play standing. Activity mitts and Velcro straps can be used to secure the racket to the hand for participants with reduced hand function. When the ball is in play, the player may use the playing surface to restore his balance only after a shot has been played. In addition, when playing in a wheelchair, his feet are not permitted to touch the floor at any time during play. Players or teams score a point if the footrest or foot of an opponent touches the floor during play.[61] The game's objective is to use a hand-held paddle to pass the ball over a net onto the opponent's side of the table in a manner that prohibits the ball from being returned by the opponent. The game is played to 21 points, and a player must win by 2 points. A match is considered the best three of five games.

Tennis

Men and women who compete in singles and doubles tennis are required to use a wheelchair that is based on their having a diagnosis of a permanent mobility-related physical disability. Tennis is played on a court of the same size and net height as traditional tennis. Unlike traditional tennis, however, the ball is permitted two bounces on the court before it is returned. The same rules that apply to the athlete also apply equally to the wheelchair as a part of the body. Brakes are not permissible as stabilizers, and the athlete must keep one buttock in contact with the seat while hitting the ball (Figure 19-11).

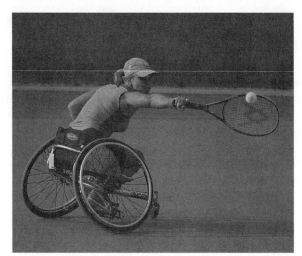

FIGURE 19-11 Wheelchair tennis is played on a court of the same size and net height as traditional tennis. Even though the ball is permitted two bounces, players must be agile and fast. (Courtesy PVA Publications, Phoenix, Ariz.)

Tennis players typically use a three-wheeled chair with a large amount of camber to maximize mobility around the court. Players with high-level SCI can play tennis by using a power wheelchair and longer rackets to compensate for length taken up for strapping the racket to the hand. Because players must cover the entire court with speed and agility, the tennis wheelchair is designed to meet these needs. The rear wheels of a tennis wheelchair are typically large at 61- to 66-cm diameter; they use high-pressure tires (i.e., 120 to 200 psi) to lower the chair's rolling resistance on the court and to increase speed; a single front caster is 5 cm in diameter, which makes the chair light and more maneuverable. The rear wheels are cambered to increase lateral stability during lateral shots and to make the chair turn faster. Tennis players, like rugby players, use a steep seat angle or dump, which helps keep them against the seat backs and gives them greater control over the wheelchair while also providing greater balance. Their knees tend to be flexed, with the feet on the footrest behind the knees (Figure 19-12). With the body in a relatively compact position, the combined inertia of rider and wheelchair is reduced (e.g., figure skaters bringing their arms in to spin faster) and makes the chair more maneuverable.[34,62]

Many players use chairs that have handles incorporated into the front of the seat, which can assist the player while leaning for a shot. The handles can also help keep players' knees in place when quick directional changes are necessary. In addition, straps can be used around the waist, knees, and ankles, depending on the player's balance. Wheelchair skills important to success in tennis include hand speed, an explosive first push to get to top speed as quickly as possible, quick stopping, and overall wheelchair control to deal with difficult bounces. Some general workout strategies used to develop many of these wheelchair skills include pushing up hills, drills where a player tows another wheelchair user holding on to the back of their chair, court sprints, backward pushing, and traversing cones. For more detailed information regarding wheelchair tennis, the International Wheelchair Tennis Federation has an excellent Web site at www.itfwheelchairtennis.com that provided detailed information and resources on the topic.

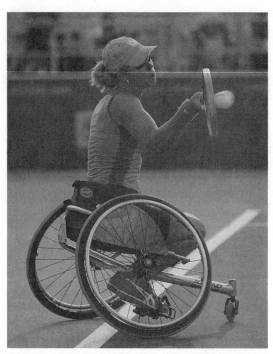

FIGURE 19-12 A tennis player keeps her knees flexed and her feet on the footrest, which is placed behind the knees. Her chair is considered a part of her body and the rules apply to it as well. (Courtesy PVA Publications, Phoenix, Ariz.)

Water Skiing

Water skiing is a popular water sport for individuals with SCI. Sit-ski design can incorporate a variety of adaptive features to suit a wide range of user levels. Ski modifications can compensate for trunk instability and hand weakness. Furthermore, some skis can be adjusted vertically, horizontally, and diagonally at the fin, allowing the user to fine-tune his equipment to meet individual skiing styles, user body weights, and varying boat velocities. At the competitive level skiing includes men and women's slalom, tricks, and jumping events.

ORGANIZATIONAL STRUCTURE OF SPORTS FOR PEOPLE WITH SPINAL CORD INJURY

Four major organizations coordinate sports competition for elite athletes active in the U.S. Paralympic movement. These groups are the IPC, the International Olympic Committee (IOC), the U.S. Olympic Committee (USOC), and United States Paralympics.

International Paralympic Committee

The IPC is an international nonprofit organization representing athletes of all sports and disabilities, run by individuals from nearly 160 national Paralympic committees worldwide. The IPC conducts the quadrennial summer and winter Paralympic Games and world and regional championships. The IPC sports committees create the rules of conduct applied to each sport, which include athlete classification rules and regulations, classifier coaching and officials training, and promotion of Paralympic sport worldwide.[63,64]

1. Identify Paralympic sports organizations for each of the Paralympic sports. Organizations to be considered for this status include the USOC-member national governing bodies and disability sport organizations and other organizations that can demonstrate the capability to direct a sports program for elite athletes with disabilities.
2. Develop a funding philosophy and secure financial support for Paralympic sports. Unlike the USOC, which is essentially restricted to seeking corporate support, private donations, and grant funding, U.S. Paralympics also has the flexibility to seek financial support from governmental agencies.
3. Facilitate the development of performance plans for each of the Paralympic sports. Performance plans typically include performance goals and plans for athlete identification and development, coach education, sports science support, and policy development.

Data from the U.S. Paralympics Web site: www.usparalympics.org.

International Olympic Committee

A relationship between the IPC and the IOC is essential because the Paralympic games have occurred in the same city and have used the same sporting venues and facilities as the Olympics since 1988.[6,64] In addition, the sports rules for able-bodied sports established by the international sports federations often serve as the framework for guidelines applied to Paralympic sports. Furthermore, participation and competition for some Paralympic sports often require athletes to be members of particular sports federations.[63,64]

Role of the U.S. Olympic Committee

The USOC serves as the National Paralympic Committee in the United States and is responsible for a variety of functions. Some of these include coaching, administrator and classifiers training, doping control, athlete development programs, and delegation representation in Paralympic Games and other major international IPC-sanctioned competitions.[63,64]

Role of U.S. Paralympics

U.S. Paralympics, a division of the USOC, was created in May 2001 to focus efforts on enhancing programs, funding, and the opportunities for individuals with physical disabilities to participate in Paralympic sports.[65] U.S. Paralympics has developed comprehensive and sustainable programs for elite athletes that are integrated into Olympic National Governing Bodies and has functioned as a platform to promote excellence in the lives of people with disabilities. Some of the specific goals of U.S. Paralympics goals promote the enhancement, development, and funding of elite sports competitions for disabled competitors (Box 19-8).

Because it takes talent, time, and support for any athlete to attain elite level status, National Disabled Sports Organizations (DSOs), a part of the USOC, has been developed to help promote the development of athletes with disabilities. These DSOs offer grass-roots programs for athletes. In the United States six DSOs are involved in the Paralympic movement (Box 19-9). Although the existing DSOs differ in the services they provide to athletes, typical features of these sports programs include athlete development camps, competition,

- National Disability Sports Alliance (NDSA)
- U.S. Association of Blind Athletes (USABA)
- Special Olympics International (SOI)
- Wheelchair Sports USA (WSUSA)
- Disabled Sports USA (DSUSA)
- Dwarf Athletic Association of America (DAAA)

and organization of networks of local clubs offering opportunities for athlete and official education and services.[63]

Paralympic Competition

Athletes who participate in the Paralympics have the privilege of representing their countries on a worldwide stage. Training for this level of competition takes years and countless hours of dedication. Participating athletes demonstrate athletic feats and a commitment of heart to the competition, which in turn inspires respect and admiration from their audiences and supporters. Sports have shown that SCI does not diminish the human spirit. The Paralympic movement has had a tremendously positive impact on the perceptions of society at large toward people with disabilities.

Athlete Classification Systems

Classification of athletes with disabilities helps to ensure fair competition among those with similar degrees of disability. The idea is to level the playing field for competitors and to allow individuals with similar physical attributes to compete against each other. Therefore it is important that the SCI classification system strives to achieve the following criteria:

- Be fair, with no individual having an edge solely on the basis of classification
- Enhance competition
- Enable individuals at different injury levels to compete on the same field
- Be easy to understand and apply

Because there is no ideal classification system that meets all the above criteria, there is consequently no uniformly accepted system. For example, athletes with SCI competing at the National Veterans Wheelchair Games are classified into seven classes on the basis of each individual's SCI level. Those with tetraplegia are classified into three classes: 1A (C4 to C6), 1B (C7), and 1C (C8); those with paraplegia are classified into four classes: II (T1 to T5), III (T6 to T10), and IV (T11 to L2), V (L3 to S5). The shortcomings of this system are related to their basis on a medical diagnosis confirmed or verified by the athlete's performance during a medical examination. The system fails to account for functional and performance capabilities of athletes with SCI in certain events using specialized sports equipment.

In the Paralympics, the largest sports competition for individuals with a variety of disabilities, several different classification schemes govern competition. Classifications evolved from simply assigning an athlete on the basis of type of disability such as blindness, SCI, amputation, and other orthopedic conditions to increasingly complex classification schemes resulting in a greater number of events that, unfortunately, decreased competition by reducing the number of competitors.[66]

The Paralympics have moved toward a functional classification system based on the athlete's ability to perform in a certain event. Wheelchair basketball is a leader in this movement because the wheelchair acts as an equalizer during the game, and skills in the wheelchair determine competition level.[67] Now classifiers observe a player's functions on the court during competitions and assign classifications on the basis of their observations. Observed trunk movement and stability during actual basketball participation, rather than the player's medical diagnosis or muscle function on an examining table, form the basis for his classification. On the basis of their classification, players are assigned a point value. With teams allowed only a predetermined maximum number on the court, the sum of the point value of all players cannot exceed this predetermined number.

Functional classification has made it harder for individuals with tetraplegia to compete, a situation that led, in part, to the development of wheelchair rugby. There are concerns that functional classification cannot work for all sports and many sports still use complex medical examinations to determine class. As seen in wheelchair basketball, many believe that the use of prosthetics or adaptive equipment may make it easier to combine individuals with different disabilities. Classification schemes currently used by the IPC are too complex for the purposes of this chapter. A full description is available on the IPC Web site: www. paralympic.org.

The Paralympic Games have become more inclusive and more successful over the years despite controversy over its classification system. They include exhibit events that are open and require no classification. Classification systems are anticipated to continue to evolve with time, approaching a more ideal solution.

RESEARCH RELATED TO WHEELCHAIR SPORTS

Research with physically impaired populations in relation to wheelchair sports is sparse. In general, a review of the literature relevant to wheelchair athletes with SCI reveals an emphasis on the biomechanics of wheelchair propulsion specific to wheelchair sports, exercise testing, training techniques, the physiological response to upper body activity, the thermoregulatory response to exercise, the occurrence of upper limb pain, and repetitive strain injury associated with wheelchair propulsion.[4,29,41,68-76] Studies specific to wheelchair sports have included wheelchair racing, basketball, field throwing events, handcycling, upper arm ergometry, and sit-skiing.[12,77-79] Research examining physiological variables tend to include measures of oxygen consumption, ventilation, heart rate, muscle contraction, electromyelography, and pain.[31,68,70, 80-85]

Physiological Research

Some specific and notable physiological findings include the work of Janssen et al,[80] who examined the physical capacity of male handcycle users and demonstrated that peak power output, maximal rate of oxygen consumption, and gross mechanical efficiency were associated with 10K race performance. In addition, multiple researchers have studied the kinematics of racing wheelchair propulsion and its relationship to efficiency. Cooper

and Bedi[83] reported that racing wheelchair propulsion has a gross mechanical efficiency over 30%, whereas Cooper[77] later reported that 10K wheelchair racers have a maximum gross efficiency of 35%. These findings indicate elite wheelchair racers are far more efficient than individuals propelling everyday chairs and able-bodied walkers, and above or comparable to runners and bicyclers.[83] Furthermore, research has shown that regular aerobic exercise in combination with strength training is important for all sports at the elite level.[4]

Several studies have measured cardiorespiratory function in wheelchair athletes as well. Van der Woude et al[71] investigated a wide range of athletes with SCI, testing them with a wheelchair ergometric sprint protocol, and reported oxygen consumption levels and heart rate. Their findings have indicated that performance in propulsion is highly variable across wheelchair athletes and is influenced by level of injury and training hours. Other research has tested road racers and handcyclists and reported that these activities require a high enough energy expenditure to maintain fitness and to potentially help to prevent cardiovascular diseases even at moderate intensity levels.[84]

In addition to these studies, which have been geared more toward sports-specific applications in elite wheelchair athletes, other findings in the physiological research arena point to the overall health benefits of active lifestyle. Studies have indicated that health benefits associated with exercise in wheelchair athletes does not necessarily put them at increased risk for injury.[85] In fact, a study by Fullerton et al[72] in 2003 found that the odds of having shoulder pain were twice as high among nonwheelchair athletes as they were among athletes. Curtis et al,[86] comparing two groups of individuals with SCI, found that wheelchair athletes had fewer physician visits and a trend toward fewer medical complications and fewer rehospitalizations compared with nonathletes. Sports participation did not lead to increased risk of medical complications and did not limit available time for vocational pursuits. These types of findings are of increased importance to individuals living with SCI because cardiovascular disease has been reported the number one cause of death in individuals surviving more than 30 years after SCI.[87] Research has also shown that sedentary individuals with SCI are far less fit than either their physically active counterparts or the sedentary unimpaired population.[11,88] Other resources available provide extensive detail on these subjects including work by Cooper et al,[88] who included chapters in their textbooks describing recreation technology and summarizing the benefits of exercise for people with disabilities. Frontera et al[89] have emphasized the importance of exercise physiology for successful rehabilitation, a healthy life after rehabilitation, and social reintegration.

Biomechanical Research

With the exception of wheelchair racing and wheelchair basketball, biomechanical studies related to wheelchair sports are not readily available. The research evaluated wheelchair propulsion during racing and primarily focused on improving physical performance and preventing secondary injury and extensively examined the biomechanics of this activity, especially such measures as segment angular and linear displacements, velocities, and accelerations.[90,91] More specifically, they studied the kinematics of the upper limbs during wheelchair propulsion to identify the most effective arm stroke pattern. O'Connor et al[92] showed that increased efficiency was related to minimizing head motion, a lower trunk angle, a larger push angle, and higher peak elbow height during recovery. Cooper et al[93] found that there was a maximal economy (i.e., steady-state oxygen consumption) for wheelchair athletes, which was associated with efficient biomechanics and level of fitness.

Generally speaking, literature has shown that the propulsion characteristics of experienced wheelchair athletes are different than those of inexperienced wheelchair users or control subjects. The differences are apparent and have been reported by many researchers. Experienced wheelchair users and athletes tend to push with significantly higher net mechanical efficiency. This efficiency has been quantified and reported by many researchers in a number of ways. Some of these optimal propulsion characteristics influencing efficiency are said to be a function of an individual having greater shoulder and elbow extension angles at initial hand-to-rim contact, maximal time spent in propulsion versus recovery, and lower

peak forces reached later in the propulsion cycle maintained for longer periods of time at elevated velocities. Experienced wheelchair users adapt their propulsion technique not by changing their style but by increasing the amplitude of their movements.[93-97]

In addition to training and experience, the functional potential or the athlete's level of SCI may affect propulsion characteristics and may explain contrasting results in the literature. Stroke pattern changes may be the result of the interaction of many factors including joint injury, muscle imbalance, fatigue, seating and positioning, weight distribution, balancing of the trunk, level of SCI, and the training attained after injury.[98] For example, a study by Dallmeijer et al[99] found that the level of injury of the wheelchair user can affect the orientation of the push angle on the hand rim. Individuals with tetraplegia were found to position their hands more backward relative to top-dead-center of the wheelchair push rim compared with individuals with paraplegia. Consequently, these elements need to be taken into consideration when biomechanical comparisons are made across heterogeneous groups of athletes with SCI.[94]

CLINICAL CASE STUDY Sports and Recreation for Individuals with a Spinal Cord Injury

Patient History
Charlie Tomlinson is a 22-year-old man with T10 paraplegia, ASIA A diagnosis from a diving accident at age 16 years. He currently is a junior in college and is active with wheelchair sports and recreational activities.

Charlie lives with his family in a wheelchair accessible home and has two younger brothers who are 12 and 10 years of age. His primary interest is basketball, which he played before his injury. He has begun training for wheelchair racing. He enjoys winter and summer recreational activities, including skiing, softball, and kayaking.

Patient's Self-Assessment
Charlie wants to live an active life anchored by a range of sport activities. He is open to new activities and continually pushing his physical limits.

Clinical Assessment
Patient Appearance
- Height 6 feet 0 inches, weight 175 pounds, body mass index 23.7

Cognitive Assessment
- Alert, oriented × 3

Cardiopulmonary Assessment
- Blood pressure 116/64 mm Hg, heart rate at rest 76 beats/min, respiratory rate 13 breaths/min, effective (>360 L/min), vital capacity is within normal limits

Musculoskeletal and Neuromuscular Assessment
- Motor assessment reveals T10 ASIA A motor to the T10 level
- Deep tendon reflexes 3+ below the level of lesion

Integumentary and Sensory Assessment
- Skin is intact throughout, sensory intact to T10

Range of Motion Assessment
- Passive and active motion is within normal limits in both upper limbs.

- Straight leg raise is 105 degrees in both lower limbs and dorsiflexion is 8 degrees; all other motions in the lower limbs are within functional limits.

Mobility and ADL Assessment
- Independent with bed mobility
- Independent in transfers to all surfaces including wheelchair to floor
- Independent with pressure relief
- Independent in manual wheelchair maneuvering on all surfaces
- Independent in high-level wheelchair skills
- Independent in bowel and bladder care
- Independent in dressing
- Independent in driving

Evaluation of Clinical Assessment
Charlie Tomlinson is a 22-year-old man with T10 paraplegia, ASIA A diagnosis. He is active in wheelchair sports and is interested in pursuing wheelchair racing and other recreational activities.

Patient's Care Needs
1. Evaluation and prescription for an exercise arm crank test to assess the appropriate fitness levels
2. Strength testing for strength training prescription
3. Consultation for sports and recreation activities
4. Consultation for sports and recreation equipment
5. Education regarding fitness and wellness for safety and prevention of secondary complications after SCI

Diagnosis and Prognosis
Diagnosis is T10 paraplegia, ASIA A. Prognosis is excellent for improved strength training and exercise capacity for wheelchair sports and participation in recreational interests. In addition, prevention of secondary complications after SCI is good with adherence to the prescribed exercise program.

Preferred Practice Patterns*
Impaired Muscle Performance (4C), Impairments Nonprogressive Spinal Cord Disorders (5H), Primary Prevention/Risk Reduction for

Continued

CLINICAL CASE STUDY   Sports and Recreation for Individuals with a Spinal Cord Injury—cont'd

Cardiovascular/Pulmonary Disorders (6A), Primary Prevention/Risk Reduction for Integumentary Disorders (7A)

Team Goals
1. Team to complete an exercise arm crank test
2. Team to design and evaluate a wellness exercise fitness program for wheelchair sports
3. Team to educate Charlie regarding fitness and wellness for safety and prevention of secondary complications after SCI
4. Team to conduct a strength testing for improved upper body strengthening for sports-related activities
5. Team to consult about sports and recreation activities and equipment

Patient Goals
"I want to be able to be active and participate in any recreational activities I want to."

Care Plan
Treatment Plan & Rationale
- Completion of an exercise arm crank test for designing a wellness exercise fitness program for Charlie to enable primary prevention of secondary complications after SCI and for the development of an effective training program for wheelchair sports
- Completion of a strength training prescription after testing for maximal strength in key upper limb muscle groups for sports
- Practice with a variety of sports chairs and protective equipment for wheelchair sports
- Educate Charlie in sporting activity teams and mentors near his living environment and provide game rules for sporting activities of interest

Interventions
- Perform exercise and strength testing and exercise prescription.
- Educate patient on injury prevention for wheelchair and other sports activities.
- *Consultation with outpatient wellness and recreational therapy for wheelchair sports opportunities, appropriate equipment and protective gear

Documentation and Team Communication
- Team will document evaluation of strength and cardiorespiratory maximal tests.
- Team will meet to discuss options for wheelchairs that enable wheelchair sporting activities.
- Team will discuss patients knowledge of potential for injury, sporting equipment, and game rules.
- Team will discuss potential opportunities for experienced athletes to serve as resources for Charlie to pursue to make contacts as a new disabled athlete.

Follow-Up Assessment
- Reassessment of the exercise prescription every 4 weeks for 4 months
- Reassessment of any injuries related to sports as needed
- Follow-up to ensure engagement with a team or mentor to begin sporting lifestyle

Critical Thinking Exercises
Consider factors related to Charlie's desire for an active lifestyle that will influence his ability to pursue a complete range of sport and recreational activities. Especially consider the concepts of classification, training, and Charlie's ability to perform activities with or without special equipment. On the basis of the preceding case study summarization and outlined care plan, answer the following questions:
1. How would Charlie be classified for wheelchair sports? Describe the shortcomings of the classification system. What sport has moved from the classification system and how are the athletes classified?
2. Describe how you would instruct Charlie regarding wheelchair propulsion as he begins training for wheelchair racing.
3. What training errors must be avoided? What training considerations would be appropriate for wheelchair basketball and racing?
4. Regarding recreational skiing, softball, and kayaking, what equipment would be required?

*Guide to physical therapist practice, rev. ed. 2, Alexandria, VA, 2003, American Physical Therapy Association.

SUMMARY

There are numerous reasons for individuals with SCI to participate in sports, including maintaining fitness, social interaction, and improvement in self-esteem. When embarking on or expanding to a new sport, it is important to understanding appropriate training techniques necessary to prepare for the sporting event, including endurance, skill, and speed training along with the implementation of periodization. Strength training can incorporate free weights or machines, and the correct combination of sets and repetitions will focus the progression of the training regimen. There are numerous recreational and competitive sports in which individuals with SCI can participate. It is important for each athlete to understand the rules of classification, game rules, and the equipment needed for each sport. More competitive athletes may choose to engage in training for the Paralympics; representing their country requires extremely hard work, dedication, and continuous training but is extremely rewarding. Clinicians and researchers can support the athlete with knowledge of physiological and biomechanical training principles based on the evidence available. Physical or occupational therapists can help athletes apply research to their training regimens and often volunteer to classify athletes at athletic events. Encouraging patients to begin to explore athletic participation may provide them with an enjoyable form of life-long activity.

REFERENCES
1. Cook AM, Webster JG: *Therapeutic medical devices: application and design*, Englewood Cliffs, NJ, 1982, Prentice Hall.
2. Cooper RA: Contributions of selected anthropometric and metabolic parameters to 10K performance: preliminary study, *J Rehabil Res Dev* 29:29-34, 1992.
3. Wade J: A league of its own, *Rehab Manage* 6:44-51, 1993.
4. Cooper RA, Quatrano LA, Axelson PW et al: Research on physical activity and health among people with disabilities: a consensus statement, *J Rehabil Res Dev* 36:142-154, 1999.

5. Fletcher GF, Balady G, Blair SN et al: Statement on exercise: benefits and recommendations for physical activity programs for all Americans, *Circulation* 94:857-862, 1996.

6. Steadward R, Peterson C: *Paralympics: where heroes come*, Edmonton, Alberta, Canada, 1999, One Shot Publishing.

7. Fleck SJ: Periodized strength training: a critical review, *J Strength Cond Res* 13:82-89, 1999.

8. Harre D: *Principles of sports training: introduction to the theory and methods of training*, ed 1, Berlin, 1982, Sportverlag.

9. Pyne D: Designing an endurance training program. In *Proceedings of the National Coaching and Officiating Conference* (1996 Nov 30–Dec 3), Brisbane, 1996, Australian Coaching Council.

10. Bompa TO: *Periodization: theory and methodology of training*, ed 4, Champaign, IL, 1999, Human Kinetics.

11. Washburn RA, Figoni SF: High density lipoprotein cholesterol in individuals with spinal cord injury: the potential role of physical activity, *Spinal Cord* 37:685-695, 1999.

12. Chow J, Mindock L: Discus throwing performance and medical classification of wheelchair athletes, *Med Sci Sports Exerc* 31:1272-1279, 1999.

13. Seiler S, Institute for Sport, Agder College: Masters athlete physiology and performance (1998): http://home.hia.no/~stephens/. Accessed May 2004.

14. Norris SR, Smith DJ: Planning, periodization, and sequencing of training and competition: the rationale for a competently planned, optimally executed training and competition program, supported by a multidisciplinary team. In Kellmann M, editor: *Enhancing recovery: preventing underperformance in athletes*, Champaign, IL, 2002, Human Kinetics.

15. Abernathy PJ, Jurimae J: Cross-sectional and longitudinal uses of isoinertial, isometric, and isokinetic dynamometry, *Med Sci Sports Exerc* 28:1180-1187, 1996.

16. Garhammer J: Equipment for the development of athletic strength and power, *Natl Strength Cond Assoc J* 3:24-26, 1981.

17. Stone MH, Collins DC, Plisk S et al: Training principles: evaluation of modes and methods of resistance training, *Strength Cond* 22:65-76, 2000.

18. Richardson T: Program design: circuit training with exercise machines, *Natl Strength Cond Assoc J* 15:18-19, 1993.

19. Wathen D, Roll F: Training methods and modes. In Baechle T, editor: *Essentials of strength training and conditioning*, Champaign, IL, 1994, Human Kinetics.

20. Chestnut JL, Dockerty D: The effects of 4 and 10 repetition maximum weight-training protocols on neuromuscular adaptations in untrained men, *J Strength Cond Res* 13:353-359, 1999.

21. Moritani T, De Vries HA: Neural factors versus hypertrophy in the time course of muscle strength gain, *Am J Phys Med* 58:115-130, 1979.

22. Sale DG: Neural adaptation to resistance training, *Med Sci Sports Exerc* 20:S135-S145, 1988.

23. Sale DG, MacDougall JD, McComas AR: Effect of strength training upon motor neuron excitability in man, *Med Sci Sports Exerc* 15:57-62, 1983.

24. MacDougall JD, Ward GR, Sale DG et al: Biomechanical adaptation of human skeletal muscle to heavy resistance training and immobilization, *J Appl Physiol* 43:700-703, 1977.

25. Frontera WR, Meredith CN, O'Reilly KP et al: Strength conditioning in older men: skeletal muscle hypertrophy and improved function, *J Appl Physiol* 64:1038-1044, 1988.

26. Cooper RA: Wheelchair racing sports science: a review, *J Rehabil Res Dev* 27:295-312, 1990.

27. Harris G: *Wheelchair archery, USA, 2004, official rules:* www.wsusa.org/wsusa/Sports/archery.htm. Accessed May 19, 2004.

28. *Wheelchair track and field USA, 2004 competition rules for track and field and road racing:* www.wsusa.org/Sports/t-tfrules.doc. Accessed July 15, 2004.

29. Chow W, Kuenster AF, Lim YT: Kinematic analysis of javelin throw performed by wheelchair athletes of different functional class, *J Sports Sci Med* 2:36-46, 2003.

30. Cooper RA: Racing wheelchair crown compensation, *J Rehabil Res Dev* 26:25-32, 1989.

31. Cooper RA: Racing wheelchair rear wheel alignment, *J Rehabil Res Dev* 26:47-50, 1989.

32. Cooper RA: An international track wheelchair with a center of gravity directional controller, *J Rehabil Res Dev* 26:63-70, 1989.

33. Cooper RA: Contributions of selected anthropometric and metabolic parameters to 10K performance a preliminary study, *J Rehabil Res Dev* 29:29-34, 1992.

34. Cooper RA: Wheelchair racing sports science: a review, *J Rehabil Res Dev* 27:295-312, 1990.

35. Cooper RA, Baldini FD, Langbein WE et al: Prediction of pulmonary function in wheelchair users, *Paraplegia* 31:560-570, 1993.

36. Wang YT, Deutsch H, Morse M et al: Three-dimensional kinematics of wheelchair propulsion across racing speeds, *Adapt Phys Act Q* 12:78-89, 1995.

37. Morse M, Bleakney A: Marathon racing, *Sports'N Spokes* 29:5-6, 2002.

38. Strohkendl H: *The 50th anniversary of wheelchair basketball: a history,* New York, 1996, Waxmann.

39. Hedrick B, Byrnes D, Shaver L: *Wheelchair basketball,* Washington, DC, 1994, Paralyzed Veterans of America.

40. National Wheelchair Basketball Association: 2003-2004 *official rules and case book:* www.nwba.org. Accessed July 20, 2004.

41. Vanlandewijck YC, Daly DJ, Theisen DM: Field test evaluation of aerobic, anaerobic, and wheelchair basketball skill performances, *Int J Sports Med* 20:548-554, 1999.

42. Cooper RA: An arm-powered racing bicycle, *J Assist Tech* 1:71-74, 1989.

43. Janssen TWJ, Dallmeijer AJ, van der Woude LHV: Physical capacity and race performance of handcycle users, *J Rehabil Res Dev* 38:33-40, 2001.

44. *United States Fencing Association, 2004 official rules:* www.usfencing.org/. Accessed May 2004.

45. Love D: Reel adventure: underwater wonders, *Sports'N Spokes* 27:30-33, 2001.

46. Santos A: Football's the name, battery's the game! Here's how it's done legally, *Sports'N Spokes* 28:10-14, 2002.

47. Hopkins G: Bike on!, *Sports'N Spokes* 27:42-49, 2001.

48. Hens W: *2004 U.S. Wheelchair Weightlifting Federation (USWWF) official rules:* www.wsusa.org/Sports/weightlifting.htm. Accessed May 20, 2004.

49. Electric wheelchair soccer: www.efds.net. Accessed July 10, 2004.

50. Lapolla T: *2000 International rules for the sport of wheelchair rugby:* hattp://quadrugby.com/rules.htm. Accessed July 7, 2004.

51. Sail away, *Sports'N Spokes* 28:32, 2002.

52. International Foundation of Disabled Sailing: Racing rules of sailing 2001-2004: www.paralympic.org. Accessed June 6, 2004.

53. Boyd J: Underwater wonders, *Sports'N Spokes* 27:9-11, 2001.

54. International Paralympic Committee: *Official shooting rule book*(2002): www.paralympic.org. Accessed June 6, 2004.

55. Kurtz M: Difference makers, *Sports'N Spokes* 28:10-14, 2002.

56. Axelson P: It's all downhill, *Sports'N Spokes* 26:49-55, 2000.

57. Laskowski ER, Paul A: Snow ski injuries in the physically disabled, *Am J Sports Med* 20:553-560, 1992.

58. U.S. Sled Hockey Association (2004): www.sledhockey.org/. Accessed July 20, 2004.

59. National Wheelchair Softball Association: 2004 NWSA rules: www.wheelchairsoftball.com. Accessed July 20, 2004.

60. U.S. Wheelchair Swimming: 2001 Official rules: www.paralympic.org. Accessed June 10, 2004.

61. International Table Tennis Federation: 2000 ITTF rules: www.paralympic.org Accessed June 10, 2004.

62. International Tennis Federation: Wheelchair tennis handbook (2004): www.itfwheelchairtennis.com. Accessed June 10, 2004.

63. Michigan State University Disability Sports: http://edweb6.educ.msu.edu/kin866/menugovern.htm. Accessed July 27, 2004.

64. International Paralympic Committee: What is IPC?: www.paralympic.org. Accessed August 2, 2004.

65. U.S. Paralympics: www.usparalympics.org. Accessed July 27, 2004.

66. Paralymic Spirit 1996. Paralympic Spirit (S.E.A. Multimedia, CD-ROM for PC, 1996).

67. Malone LA, Gervais PL, Steadward RD: Shooting mechanics related to player classification and free throw success in wheelchair basketball, J Rehabil Res Dev 39:701-710, 2002.

68. Langbein WE, Maki KC: Predicting oxygen uptake during counter-clockwise arm crank ergometry in men with lower limb disabilities, Arch Phys Med Rehabil 76:642-646, 1995.

69. Langbein WE, Fehr LS, Edwards LC: A new wheelchair exercise test to assess anaerobic power and anaerobic work capacity of persons 55 years of age and older. In Langbein WE, Wyman DJ, editors: National veterans golden age games research monograph: health-related physical activity, Chicago, 1994, Hines VA Hospital.

70. Langbein WE, Maki KC, Edwards LC et al: Initial clinical evaluation of a wheelchair ergometer for diagnostic exercise testing: a technical note, J Rehabil Res Dev 31:317-325, 1994.

71. Van der Woude LHV, Bakker WH, Elkhuizen JW et al: Propulsion technique and anaerobic work capacity in elite wheelchair athletes, Am J Phys Med Rehabil 77:222-234, 1998.

72. Fullerton HD, Borckardt JJ, Alfano AP: Shoulder pain: a comparison of wheelchair athletes and nonathletic wheelchair users, Am College Sports Med 35:1958-1961, 2003.

73. Chow JW, Millikan TA, Carlton LG et al: Effect of resistance load on biomechanical characteristics of racing wheelchair propulsion over a roller system, J Biomech 33:601-608, 2000.

74. Morse M: Para-backhand pushing technique, Sport 'N Spokes 25:52-55, 1999.

75. Boninger ML, Baldwin M, Cooper RA et al: Manual wheelchair pushrim biomechanics and axle position, Arch Phys Med Rehabil 81:608-613, 2000.

76. Cooper RA: An exploratory study of racing wheelchair propulsion dynamics, Adapted Phys Activity Q 7:74-85, 1990.

77. Cooper RA: Contributions of selected anthropometric and metabolic parameters to 10K performance: preliminary study, J Rehabil Res Dev 29:29-34, 1992.

78. Glaser RM: Arm exercise training for wheelchair users, Med Sci Sports Exerc 21:S149-S157, 1989.

79. Glaser RM, Sawka MN, Brune MF et al: Physiological responses to maximal effort wheelchair and arm crank ergometry, J Appl Physiol 48:1060-1064, 1980.

80. Janssen TWJ, Dallmeijer AJ, van der Woude LHV: Physical capacity and race performance of handcycle users, J Rehabil Res Dev 38:33-40, 2001.

81. Rodgers MM, Gayle W, Figoni SF et al: Biomechanics of wheelchair propulsion during fatigue, Arch Phys Med Rehabil 75:85-93, 1994.

82. Hakkinen K, Pakarinen A, Kraemer WJ, et-al: Selective muscle hypertrophy, changes in EMG and force, and serum hormones during strength training in older women, J Appl Physiol 91,569–580, 2001.

83. Cooper RA, Bedi JF: Gross mechanical efficiency of trained wheelchair racers, Annu Int Conf IEEE Eng Med Biol Soc 12:2311-2312, 1990.

84. Abel T, Kröner M, Rojas Vega S et al: Energy expenditure in wheelchair racing and handbiking—a basis for prevention of cardiovascular diseases in those with disabilities, Eur J Cardiovas Prev Rehabil 10:371-376, 2003.

85. Boninger ML, Robertson RN, Wolff M et al: Upper limb nerve entrapments in elite wheelchair racers, Am J Phys Med Rehabil 75:170-176, 1996.

86. Curtis KA, McClanahan S, Hall KM et al: Health, vocational, and functional status in spinal cord injured athletes and nonathletes, Arch Phys Med Rehabil 67:862-865, 1986.

87. Whiteneck G: Learning from empirical investigations. In Menter R, Whiteneck G, editors: Perspectives on aging with spinal cord injury, New York, 1992, Demos Publications.

88. Cooper RA, Vosse A, Robertson RN et al: An interactive computer system for training wheelchair users, Biomed Eng App Basis Com 7:52-60, 1995.

89. Frontera W, Dawson D, Slovik D: Exercise in rehabilitation medicine, Champain, IL, 1999, Human Kinetics.

90. Alexander MJL: Aspects of performance in wheelchair marathon racing, J de l'ACSEPL 55:26-32, 1989.

91. Davis R, Ferrara M: The competitive wheelchair stroke, J Strength Cond Res 10:4-10, 1988.

92. O'Connor TJ, Robertson RN, Cooper RA: Three-dimensional kinematic analysis of racing wheelchair propulsion, Adapted Phys Activity Q 15:1-14, 1998.

93. Cooper RA, Boninger ML, Baldini FD et al: Wheelchair racing efficiency, Disabil Rehabil 25:207-212, 2003.

94. Brown DD, Knowlton RG, Hamill J et al: Physiological and biomechanical differences between wheelchair-dependent and able-bodied subjects during wheelchair ergometry, Eur J Appl Phys 60:179-182, 1990.

95. Patterson P, Draper S: Selected comparisons between experienced and non-experienced individuals during handrim wheelchair propulsion, Biomed Sci Instrum 33:477-481, 1997.

96. Vanlandewijck YC, Spaepen AJ, Lysens RJ: Wheelchair propulsion efficiency: movement pattern adaptations to speed changes, Med Sci Sports Exerc 26:1373-1381, 1994.

97. Vanlandewijck YC, Daly DJ: Wheelchair propulsion kinematics: movement pattern adaptations to speed changes in elite wheelchair rugby players, Proc Fifth Paralympic Cong 28:11-13, 2000.

98. Souza AL, Boninger ML, Koontz AM et al: Classification of stroke patterns in manual wheelchair propulsion, Proc 23rd Annu RESNA Conf Orlando, FL, 23:384-386, 2000.

99. Dallmeijer AJ, van der Woude LHV, Veeger HEJ et al: Effectiveness of force application in manual wheelchair propulsion in persons with spinal cord injuries, Am J Phys Med Rehabil 77:213-221, 1998.

SOLUTIONS TO CHAPTER 19 CLINICAL CASE STUDY

Sports and Recreation for Individuals with a Spinal Cord Injury

1. Charlie is in classification III (T6-10). The wheelchair sports classification system is based on a medical diagnosis but fails to account for functional performance capabilities of athletes with SCI in certain events using specialized sports equipment. Wheelchair basketball has led the formation of a functional classification system because the wheelchair acts as an equalizer during the game. The Paralympics classification system is based on a player's function on the court during competition specifically related to trunk movement and stability during actual basketball play. On the basis of their classification, players are assigned a point value. Teams are allowed a predetermined maximum number on the court and the sum of the point value of all players cannot exceed this predetermined number.

2. Efficiency with wheelchair propulsion is related to minimizing head motion, a lower trunk angle, a larger push angle, and higher peak elbow height during recovery. Charlie should receive visual instruction in which he can observe a demonstration of both efficient and inefficient techniques (see Figure 15-3, *B*). Experienced wheelchair racers increase the amplitude of their movements through greater shoulder and elbow extension angles at initial hand-to-rim contact and maximal time spent in propulsion versus recovery, and they have lower peak forces reached later in the propulsion cycle maintained for longer periods of time at elevated velocities. Wheelchair seating and position must be optimal to allow for the best trunk balance related to the level of injury.

3. Training errors that commonly occur include the following:
- Insufficient recovery time
- Demands imposed too quickly without sufficient time for adaptation (i.e., after an injury training load does not allow for appropriate recovery if it is increased too rapidly)
- Intensity of maximal and submaximal and volume of intensity is too high.
- Excessive attention and time spent in complex technical or mental aspects without enough down time
- Excessive number of competitions without recovery
- Training bias with insufficient balance
- Lack of trust in the coach

Every endeavor should be made to eliminate such errors in an effort to encourage participation and avoid athlete injury.

Training should implement five regimens into a periodization program: endurance, speed, skill, strength, and flexibility. Endurance and speed are necessary for both wheelchair basketball and racing. The length of a racing event should be considered and training should include approximately a 2K additional distance beyond the race to allow adequate preparation for changes in terrain and hills. In wheelchair basketball, the time of a game is known; however, interval training should be done for the sprints and directional changes required of the wheelchair during the game. Skill for basketball needs to be specific to the sport including plyometrics for catching. Throwing in multiple directions when the wheelchair is moving and one bounce coordination drills need continuous practice. The SAID principle, for strength training, describes the adaptation that occurs within muscle tissue when it is progressively stressed or overloaded. Age, sex, and type of event should be considered along with sufficient preseason training periods to determine the optimal strengthening

program. A comprehensive weight-training program can include exercises such as the bench press, overhead/military press, seated rows, lat-pulls, squats, and standing calf-raises. To prevent overtraining, at least 1 day should be spaced between each workout of this type, with athletes devoting off days to training regimens for skill, flexibility, endurance, or speed. Alternatively, Charlie can dedicate one day to an upper body workout, with the second day focused on the lower body. A more intense workout is required because only one half of the body is exercised per workout. The higher intensity occurs by use of heavier weights or by performing more sets or repetitions. The training program should include at least one off day to allow the body to recover from a more intense workout. Or, Charlie could opt for a push-pull workout, which divides the training program into three primary training days. The first day focuses on the chest and triceps area (the push day). The second day focuses on the back and biceps musculature (the pull day). The last day exercises the leg and shoulder musculature. This program permits very intense workouts because each body part has at least 3 days to recuperate. Yet even with three days of muscle recuperation, individuals should dedicate at least 1 day to other training regimens after the last day of the entire push-pull routine. Adequate prestretching and poststretching for the upper limbs should be required before wheelchair racing or basketball and for maintaining lower limb motion for optimal wheelchair positioning.

4. Charlie can choose between Alpine (i.e., downhill skiing), Nordic (i.e., cross-country skiing), and sit-skiing with monoski or bi-ski configurations. Assistive devices such as adaptive seating, backrests, cushions, tethering ropes, roll bars, and outriggers need to be evaluated for safety, support, and performance. Guides are recommended to assist new skiers down the slopes for direction and safety. Monoskis and bi-skis have become quite sophisticated and offer shock absorption systems, frames molded to body shape, and quick-release safety options. The outriggers that skiers use are an adapted version of a forearm crutch and a shortened ski. Outriggers provide extra balance and steering maneuverability that the typical ski pole does not.

Wheelchair softball is played in manual wheelchairs with footrests and uses a 16-inch slow pitch softball. Ten individuals play on each team and just as in rugby and basketball, players are classed on the basis of functional abilities and only a specified quantity can legally be active at one time. Playing fields have hard surfaces to allow for easier maneuverability of the wheelchairs, preserving the pace of the game. Charlie views softball as a recreational sport and his primary goal would be to find a team and follow the rules as outlined by Amateur Softball Association of America with some exceptions geared toward the wheelchair user.

Kayaking is a recreational sport in which Charlie could participate with a friend or by himself because his injury level is T10. Kayaks can be adapted to address balance needs for trunk stability by using outriggers. Because he is a beginner, Charlie may initially require or desire assistance, in which case tandem kayaks are available. A paddling partner or instructor seated in the stern of tandem kayaks can help with steering and paddling when necessary.

CHAPTER TWENTY

Wheelchair Transportation Safety

Gina Bertocci, PE, PhD

Fortunately, once your vehicle is perfectly suited to your injury, you will still be able to jump in your car and take off as quickly as you always did. But your stopping time is lengthened, so your tailgating days should be over! My EZ Lock system allows me to motor up the ramp into my van and engage the adapter under my wheelchair so I'm securely docked and ready to drive. I still finish my errands before 9 am.

Jeanine (C6-7 SCI)

In recognition of the importance for people with disabilities to function in society, in 1990 the U.S. Congress enacted the Americans with Disabilities Act (ADA) prohibiting discrimination against people with disabilities in employment practices, public accommodations, and telecommunication services.[1,2] Transportation services, by legislative definition, fall within the public accommodation category. Therefore public transportation service providers must accommodate individuals seated in wheelchairs who wish to travel. More recently, the 2001 New Freedom Initiative has cited integration of persons with disabilities into the workforce and the community as a priority, specifically noting transportation as a critical factor in meeting this priority.[3] In support of this initiative, the Director of Project Action reinforced the need for people with disabilities to use public transportation systems, indicating that one third of the 25 million transit-dependent people with disabilities report inadequate transportation as a significant barrier to successful integration into society. The National Institute for Disability and Rehabilitation Research (NIDRR) has further reported that 82% of wheelchair users indicate difficulty in using public transportation systems and nearly 39% report wheelchair access problems.[4]

The NIDRR Disability Statistics Report on Mobility Device Use in the United States further highlights the lack of integration of wheelchair users into society and the workplace, indicating that mobility device users are less likely to be employed than those not using mobility devices.[4] Roughly 25% of mobility device users are employed compared with approximately 75% in the nonmobility device-using population—a difference of 50%. This high rate of unemployment among wheeled mobility users further translates into lower economic status. Among all users of mobility devices including wheelchairs, walkers, canes, and crutches, roughly 21% live in poverty compared with 13% of the nonuser population. When comparing the working-age population, the report indicates that users of mobility devices are two and a half times more likely to live in poverty than are nonusers.[4]

Although there are no reliable statistics on the proportion of wheelchair users who remain seated in their wheelchairs when using private, public, and school transportation systems, it is likely that the proportion is high and that the numbers are increasing. Although many of these wheelchair users can transfer to a vehicle seat, in some transport situations they will choose to remain seated in their wheelchairs. For example, a wheelchair user may choose to transfer to a vehicle seat in his personal vehicle but will opt to ride seated in the wheelchair when using public transportation. Therefore devices capable of providing safe and independent wheelchair transport are likely to affect a significant portion of the 1.7 million wheelchair users.

BOX 20-1 | **Potential Benefits of Increased Safety and Independence in Motor Vehicle Transportation for Wheelchair Users**

- Improved integration into society
- Increased employment opportunities
- Increased educational attainment

With increased safety and independence in using motor vehicle transportation for all wheelchair users, the beneficial effects can be expected to include improved integration into society, increased employment, and increased educational attainment (Box 20-1). Access to safe public and private transportation services can be vital to providing wheelchair users access to work, education, and recreational environments—all essential to attaining equality of lifestyle in the United States.

A reasonable goal for wheelchair transportation is that all wheelchair users will be able to realize a level of safety equivalent to that afforded to passengers and drivers seated in federally regulated, original equipment manufacturer's (OEM) vehicle seats. To achieve this goal, wheelchairs must perform as a vehicle seat under all conditions and the wheelchair must be secured to the vehicle and the occupant restrained with a crashworthy occupant restraint. This systems approach, including a stable seating support surface, wheelchair securement, and occupant restraint, dictates that after-market adaptive devices that have not been federally regulated be used to provide safe wheelchair transport. Unfortunately, not all wheelchairs are designed to function as motor vehicle seats, placing wheelchair users at a higher risk of injury in a crash than their counterparts using OEM vehicle seats. Furthermore, as discussed later, some wheelchair securement systems can be cumbersome to use, often resulting in disuse or misuse. Vehicle-mounted occupant restraints are often unable to provide adequate protection across a wide range of occupant sizes because of poor belt fit. These compounded problems present unique challenges to providing safe travel for wheelchair-seated passengers and drivers (Box 20-2).

CRASH SAFETY ISSUES INFLUENCING WHEELCHAIR TRANSPORTATION

There is a paucity of data regarding injuries occurring during wheelchair transportation. The only published information has been from a study conducted by National Highway Traffic Safety Administration's (NHTSA) National Center for Statistics and Analysis.[5] This study examined the Consumer Product Safety Commission's National

Electronic Injury Surveillance System (NEISS) to identify cases of injury or death to wheelchair users involving vehicles that occurred during 1991-1995. During this period an estimated 7121 wheelchair users were injured in incidents involving motor vehicles, an average of 1500 persons each year, and 43 wheelchair users were fatally injured. In these events, improper or no securement was involved in 35% of incidents leading to injuries. Other classifications of events involved a nonmoving vehicle, collision between the wheelchair and motor vehicle (26%), lift malfunction (19%), transferring to or from a motor vehicle (15%), and falling off of a vehicle ramp (6%). Seventy-three percent (73%) involved wheelchair users who were 60 years of age or older. It is important to note that this study is limited in the following ways: (1) NEISS does not include medical facilities without emergency care, (2) NEISS obtains data from a sample of 91 of 6127 hospitals nationwide, and (3) NEISS is focused on injuries involving consumer products as opposed to motor vehicles. Such limitations may lead to underestimating the true level of injury occurring in association with wheelchair transportation. Additional studies that are focused on motor vehicle accidents involving wheelchair users are greatly needed. Information regarding failure modes of wheelchairs and wheelchair tiedowns and occupant restraint systems (WTORS) are necessary to assess the effectiveness of industry standards and can aid in updating these standards to ensure product effectiveness and safety.

The exposure of a wheelchair user seated in a vehicle during a crash is dependent on a number of factors, one of which is the size of the vehicle (Box 20-3). In large, fixed route public vehicles (i.e., greater than 30,000 pounds), maximum vehicle decelerations in frontal impacts are near 10 g, whereas in demand-type vehicles (<30,000 pounds), maximum vehicle frontal impact decelerations can be as high as 20 g.[6] These maximum deceleration values can be, and have been, used to define test conditions in wheelchair transportation standards and regulations.

Other factors that affect occupant exposure in a crash are the weight of the wheelchair and occupant. Wheelchairs and occupants with greater mass will experience or generate increased forces during an emergency driving maneuver or crash. During a frontal impact, the wheelchair securement system or tiedowns act to resist the forward motion of the wheelchair, whereas the forward motion of the occupant is countered by the lap and shoulder belts (Figure 20-1). In a rearward impact, the wheelchair tiedowns act to resist the rearward motion of the wheelchair, while the wheelchair seatback resists rearward motion of the occupant.

In smaller vehicles and where the occupant restraint loads pass through the securement system, loads on the securement system can be as much as 20 times (derived from 20 g) the combined mass of the occupant and wheelchair in a severe frontal impact (derived from Newton's law: Force = Mass × Acceleration). As an example, rear tiedown forces associated with a 20-g/30-miles per hour (mph) frontal impact of a 187-pound wheelchair with a 168-pound occupant restrained with a vehicle-anchored restraint system can be near 4700 pounds per rear tiedown.[7] In this given scenario, however, tiedown loads can vary greatly depending on the location of the wheelchair and occupant center of gravity, where rear tiedowns are secured to the wheelchair, whether the lap belt is anchored to the wheelchair or vehicle, the wheelchair seat angle, and other factors.[8] Because children typically have a lower mass, rear tiedown loads are substantially less than those associated with an adult wheelchair and occupant. For example, a 41-pound pediatric wheelchair with a seated 6-year-old occupant who weighs 55 pounds and is restrained with a vehicle-mounted restraint system will generate rear tiedown forces near 950 pounds in a 20 g/30 mph frontal impact.[8] Again, these loads can vary greatly, depending on the factors previously stated.

Regulations and standards have largely focused on frontal impact vehicle crashes because they are responsible for more than half of the serious injuries (67%) and fatalities (65%).[9] Regulations such as Federal Motor Vehicle Safety Standard (FMVSS) 208 Occupant Crash Protection[10] and FMVSS 222 School Bus Seating and Crash Protection[11] are based on these epidemiological findings associated with frontal impact. Therefore in an effort to protect wheelchair users during transport, the wheelchair must be oriented to maximize the effectiveness of occupant restraints. A forward orientation relative to the vehicle accomplishes this goal. Unfortunately, historically it has been common practice to transport wheelchair users in a sideways-facing orientation. Sideways-facing orientation prevents effective occupant restraint, allowing excessive occupant excursion in a crash and possible impingement of the torso with the armrest. Also, many wheelchair designs are not inherently strong when loaded laterally, leading in some cases to twisting of the wheelchair frame and an unstable support surface (Figure 20-2). Such a scenario would be associated with a high risk of injury.

Today users of wheelchairs desire to travel in a wide range of wheelchair types and sizes. In many cases these wheelchairs are not designed to function as a vehicle seat and may not be able to be effectively secured. For these reasons, when possible, wheelchair users should transfer to a vehicle seat and use the OEM occupant restraints that have been designed and tested to federal regulations. Unfortunately not all wheelchair users are willing or able to transfer to a vehicle seat, making it necessary to travel

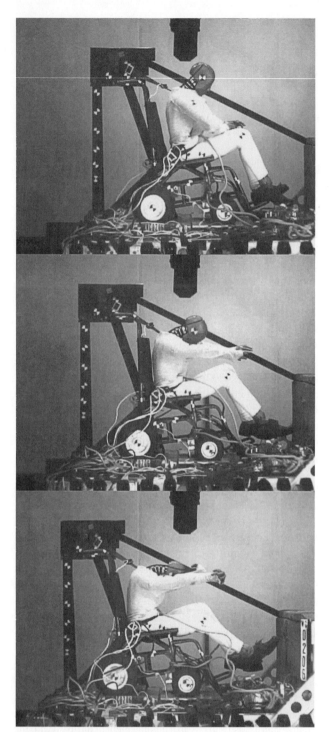

FIGURE 20-1 Wheelchair and anthropomorphic test device (ATD) response to 20 g/30 mph frontal impact sled test illustrating the nature of forces associated with such an event.

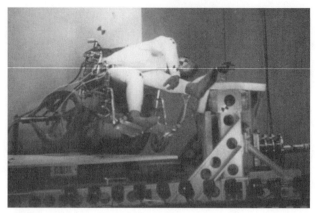

FIGURE 20-2 Consequences of sideways-facing wheelchair orientation in a frontal crash.

the forward motion of an occupant during emergency driving maneuvers and crashes. Restraints are designed to prevent occupant ejection from the vehicle and to prevent secondary collision with the vehicle interior (Clinical Note: Tips to Achieve Proper Fit and Position of Restraint Belt). Proper belt fit that positions belts over bony structures of the anatomy is of key importance. Such positioning will allow the crash forces to be distributed to body structures that are capable of carrying restraint loads while protecting soft tissues from injury. Soft tissues are unable to sustain high levels of loading without injury, and research has shown that such conditions can lead to serious injury. If the lap belt is allowed to slide onto the soft pelvic tissues, a phenomena known as submarining can occur, which can result in injury to internal organs or the spine.[12] Therefore a steep lap belt angle as viewed from the side is essential in preventing such injuries.[13] Additionally, the shoulder belt should be positioned so that it passes between the mid-point of the shoulder and neck as viewed from the front. Both the lap and shoulder belt must be in full contact with the body to be effective. It must be ensured that wheelchair components such as the armrests do not hold the belts away from the body.

CLINICAL NOTE	Tips to Achieve Proper Fit and Position of Restraint Belt

- Belt positioned over bony structures
- Steep lap belt angle (as viewed from the side)
- Shoulder belt angle (as viewed from the front) that positions belt at mid-point between neck and shoulder
- Belt loading distributed over largest area possible
- Belt in contact with occupant's pelvis and torso, not held away from occupant by wheelchair components (e.g., armrests)

Good belt fit also serves to distribute loading over the largest possible area, reducing localized stresses on the body. When properly positioned, restraints will prevent excessive occupant excursion. Some manufacturers of wheelchair occupant restraints have included webbing locks on their systems to prevent the shoulder belt from spooling out of the reel when activated, thereby limiting forward occupant excursion. This reduction in excursion is important to preventing impact with the vehicle interior.

seated in the wheelchair. Safe transport of a wheelchair user is dependent on the provision of (1) a structurally sound wheelchair that is capable of providing a stable seating support surface, (2) a wheelchair that is secured to the vehicle, and (3) an occupant who is effectively restrained in the wheelchair (Figure 20-3).

Occupant restraints are critical to protecting the occupant in a crash and have been responsible for injury reduction over the past 15 years. The intent of occupant restraints is to reverse or prevent

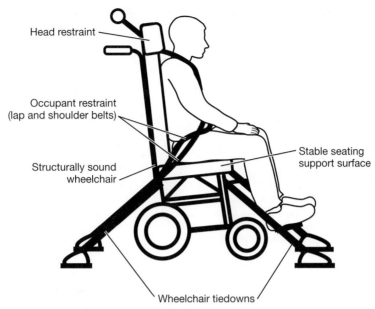

Head restraint

Occupant restraint
(lap and shoulder belts)

Structurally sound
wheelchair

Stable seating
support surface

Wheelchair tiedowns

FIGURE 20-3 Features that reduce wheelchair user injury risk in a crash.

WHEELCHAIR TRANSPORTATION TECHNOLOGIES

To safely transport an individual seated in their wheelchair, third-party add-on equipment is needed to secure the wheelchair and restrain the occupant. In other words, wheelchair transport equipment is not typically manufactured by the vehicle manufacturer but instead by another company specializing in these types of products.

In a wheelchair transportation scenario, the wheelchair is analogous to a vehicle seat and the securement system is analogous to the rigid anchoring of the seat to the vehicle floor. Over the past decades, wheelchair securement has evolved from rather primitive unsafe methods that have included bungee cords to methods that have been dynamically impact tested to verify their safety and crash performance. Despite their ability to secure a wheelchair under crash conditions, each of the securement systems has its advantages and disadvantages, which are discussed subsequently (Table 20-1).

Occupant restraint systems most often used in wheelchair transportation scenarios are similar to those found in personal vehicles and include both a lap and shoulder restraint. However, technological advances in occupant restraint designs, such as retractors and pre-tensioners, that can be found in recent model personal vehicles have not necessarily translated to the wheelchair transport environment. Because of poor muscle tone, some wheelchair users may require more that just a lap and shoulder belt, needing a four-point harness to provide postural stability and occupant protection during transport.

Wheelchair Securement Systems
Four-Point Tiedown Systems

The most common securement system in public transportation settings is the four-point tiedown system. This system consists of four webbing straps anchored to the vehicle floor and to the wheelchair. Two straps secure the front of the wheelchair and two straps secure the rear of the wheelchair. End fittings of the straps that attach to the wheelchair can be large hooks or loops of webbing that pass around the wheelchair and then reattach to the strap. Figure 20-4 shows an example of a four-point strap-type tiedown next to a secured wheelchair. Figure 20-5 shows four-point strap-type tiedown system securing a wheelchair and a three-point occupant restraint system restraining an occupant.

One advantage of four-point tiedowns is that they have been shown to be capable of passing a 20 g/30 mph frontal impact test, making them a safe securement option under crash conditions when used properly. This level of testing is the benchmark dynamic impact test required for compliance with the Society of Automotive Engineers (SAE) J2249 Wheelchair Tiedowns and Occupant Restraints for Use in Motor Vehicles Standard,[14] which is described in a subsequent section. Another advantage of strap-type tiedowns is that they are capable of interfacing with most wheelchairs that have exposed frames, requiring no special adapters.

Unfortunately, this commonly used securement system does have some disadvantages. First, tiedowns are cumbersome to use and do not allow wheelchair users to independently secure their wheelchair. An attendant or vehicle operator is, in most cases, required to secure the four straps to the wheelchair. In a public transport situation, this requires that the vehicle operator leave the driving station to secure the wheelchair. This is a time-consuming process that is not necessarily welcomed in fixed-route transit by either the wheelchair user or the other passengers. Also, wheelchair users may not be pleased with the intrusion that securing the tiedowns can involve. In personal transport settings the wheelchair user would be required to have another person secure him in the vehicle, requiring wheelchair users to be dependent on others. To enable wheelchair users to become fully engaged in society, independent transport should be a goal of all securement systems.

Another disadvantage of strap-type tiedowns is that it is often difficult to identify appropriate securement locations on wheelchairs that use shrouds or housings to encase their frames. This is often the case with power wheelchairs attempting to

TABLE 20-1 | Advantages and Disadvantages of Various Wheelchair Securement Systems

Securement System	Advantages	Disadvantages
Four-point tiedown	Safe under crash conditions when used properly Capable of interfacing with most wheelchairs that have exposed frames	Cumbersome/time consuming Wheelchair user must be dependent on others for securement Often difficult to identify appropriate securement locations on wheelchairs with shrouds or housings encasing their frames Misuse is common in public transportation settings Straps are subject to theft or being misplaced, leaving fewer than four straps for securement Straps often become damaged or soiled, which can lead to malfunctions in use
Docking systems	Typically automated, thus affording independence to users Reduced securement times Removes human judgment from securement, therefore ensuring that wheelchair is repeatedly secured appropriately	Not adopted for widespread use because of absence of universality in wheelchair adaptors Wheelchair adapter hardware can increase weight of wheelchair When mounted to the bottom of the wheelchair, adapters can decrease ground clearance When mounted to the rear of the chair, wheelchair adapters can increase overall length of the wheelchair More costly than four-point tiedown systems Requires maintenance of mechanical components
Other securement systems (e.g., clamping and rim pin systems)	None. It is strongly suggested that these securement systems be avoided to protect against unsafe transport	These systems have not been shown to be safe under vehicle crash conditions Some of these systems require that the wheelchair be oriented sideways in the vehicle, which is unsafe

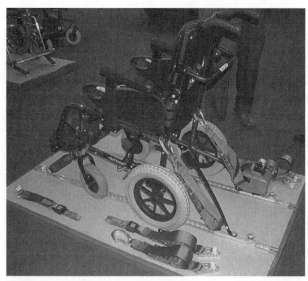

FIGURE 20-4 Wheelchair secured by a four-point strap-type tiedown system. (From Schneider LW, Manary MA: Wheeled mobility tiedown systems and occupant restraints for safety and crash protection. In Pellerito JA Jr, editor: *Driver rehabilitation and community mobility: principles and practice*, St Louis, 2006, Elsevier Mosby, Figure 17-5, p 364.)

provide a sleek appearance by covering the frame. As more wheelchairs begin to comply with the American National Standards Institute and Rehabilitation Engineering Society of North America (ANSI/RESNA) WC-19 Standard, which requires four accessible securement points to be included on wheelchairs, this problem will become less of an issue.[15]

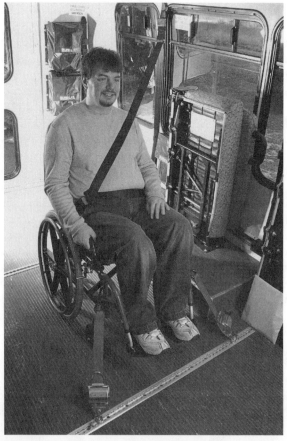

FIGURE 20-5 Wheelchair secured using four-point tiedowns and a three-point occupant restraint system. (Courtesy Sure-Lok, Bethlehem, PA.)

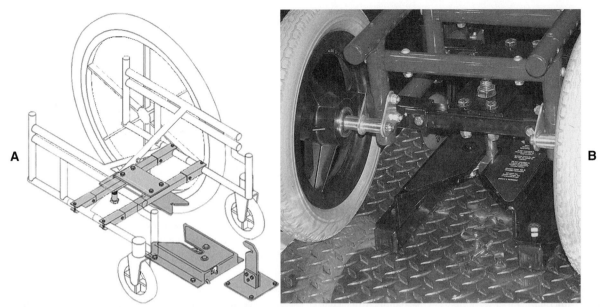

FIGURE 20-6 EZ Lock docking system for use in personal vehicles uses a vertical pin mounted to the underside of the wheelchair that engages the docking capture mechanism. **A,** Schematic of docking process, and **B,** rear view of wheelchair secured. (From Schneider LW, Manary MA: Wheeled mobility tiedown systems and occupant restraints for safety and crash protection. In Pellerito JA Jr, editor: *Driver rehabilitation and community mobility: principles and practice*, St Louis, 2006, Elsevier Mosby, Figure 17-8 A-B, p 365. Courtesy Constantine, Inc.)

It has also been documented that misuse of four-point tiedowns is common in public transport.[16] Despite the willingness of vehicle operators to secure wheelchairs, tight securement stations, compounded with a lack of identifiable securement points on wheelchairs and time constraints, tiedown straps can be difficult to engage under these conditions. A consequence of such a situation is using less than all four tiedown straps. Although four tiedowns, properly engaged, can provide suitable securement in a crash, the use of fewer than four tiedowns can seriously jeopardize safety during emergency driving maneuvers and in a crash.

Because tiedowns can lie loose about the vehicle floor, these straps are subject to theft and being misplaced, leaving fewer than four straps for securement. In addition, straps often become damaged and soiled lying loose about the floor. Such damage to tiedowns can lead to malfunctions in use.

Docking Systems

Another method of wheelchair securement is an automatic docking system. This type of securement relies on a special hardware adapter mounted on the wheelchair that engages with a capture system located in the vehicle. The docking system housing may be mounted on the vehicle floor or sidewall and may engage the wheelchair from the rear or bottom, depending on the system's design. Docking systems have been successfully demonstrated in personal vehicles for drivers but have not had widespread success in public transit. Docking systems used for wheelchair drivers typically engage by maneuvering the wheelchair forward toward the steering wheel, engaging a floor-mounted docking system.

A popular docking system, the EZ Lock system, that is used in personal vehicles engages an adapter positioned at the bottom of wheelchair (Figure 20-6, *A*). This wheelchair adapter presents a vertical pin protruding from the bottom of the wheelchair, which is captured by a docking system mounted on the vehicle floor when the wheelchair is driven forward into the docking station (Figure 20-6, *B*).

Newly available docking systems such as the Q'Straint QLK200 also are designed for securement of wheelchair drivers. This docking system also uses an adapter positioned beneath the wheelchair (Figure 20-7, *A*) that engages the docking system housing mounted on the floor of the vehicle (Figure 20-7, *B*). In this case the component that engages the low profile latching mechanism is a horizontally positioned metal tab.

A docking system developed by the Oregon State University uses two D-ring adaptors mounted to the rear of the wheelchair and has been used in public transit settings.[6] The D-rings extending from the rear of the frame (Figure 20-8, *A*) and spaced a distance equal to the frame width are captured by the docking system mounted in a vehicle (Figure 20-8, *B*). This docking system has been pilot tested in various demonstration projects throughout the United States.

Other types of docking systems exist on the market but all include an adapter that must be mounted on the wheelchair that will engage a capture mechanism mounted in the vehicle. Unfortunately, docking systems have not been adopted for widespread use because of the absence of universality in wheelchair adapters. Both the international and national standards processes are addressing this issue to promote docking system development and implementation.

There are a number of advantages to docking systems, but perhaps the most important is the independence that they afford wheelchair users. Docking systems are typically automated and do not require a vehicle operator or attendant to engage or disengage the wheelchair. This is a tremendous benefit to wheelchair users in all transportation settings and to public transit passengers and vehicle operators, who will realize reduced times associated with wheelchair boardings. Reduced securement times and reduced personnel involvement translate into cost savings

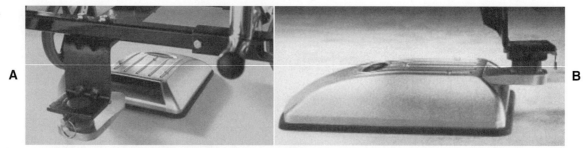

FIGURE 20-7 Q'Straint QLK200 docking system for use in personal vehicles uses (**A**) an adapter mounted to the underside of the wheelchair that (**B**) engages the docking capture mechanism. (Courtesy Q'Straint, Ft. Lauderdale, FL.)

for transit authorities. Docking systems also remove the human judgment from the securement process, ensuring that the wheelchair is repeatedly secured in a way that has been verified to be crashworthy through testing.

Docking systems do, however, have some disadvantages associated with them. First, docking systems require wheelchair adapter hardware that interfaces with the docking capture mechanism, which can increase wheelchair weight. Increased weight is more of a concern for manual wheelchair users propelling their wheelchairs than for those using power wheelchairs. In some cases, these wheelchair adapters may decrease wheelchair ground clearance when mounted to the bottom of the wheelchair or they may increase the overall length of the wheelchair when mounted at the rear. In addition, docking systems are a more costly securement option compared with four-point tiedowns, the most commonly used securement system in public transportation vehicles in the United States. Transit authorities may therefore be somewhat reluctant to replace their existing tiedown systems with docking systems. An additional cost consideration is the maintenance associated with docking systems that have a number of working mechanical components to accomplish their automation and securement. Certainly docking systems will have an increased maintenance cost compared with tiedown systems.

Other Securement Systems

Other types of wheelchair securement systems, such as clamping systems and rim pin systems, have also been used to secure wheelchairs to vehicles. However, these systems have not been shown to be safe under vehicle crash conditions. Some of these systems also require that the wheelchair be oriented sideways in the vehicle. It is strongly suggested that these securement systems be avoided to protect against unsafe transport.

Occupant Restraint Systems

In public transportation and private vehicle settings three-point occupant restraint systems are commonly provided for wheelchair users. This system is composed of a lap belt and shoulder belt that are manually positioned on the body. To ensure that an occupant restraint system is able to protect an occupant in a crash, it must meet the requirements of SAE J2249, which include dynamic testing.[14] Two different types of occupant restraint systems are available on the market for wheelchair users: an integrated restraint system and an independent

restraint system. Integrated restraints are anchored to the rear wheelchair tiedowns (Figure 20-9, *A*), whereas independent restraint systems are anchored directly to the vehicle floor (Figure 20-9, *B*).

Integrated restraints increase the force that the rear tiedowns experience in a frontal crash, carrying both the load on the wheelchair and occupant. Conversely, with independent restraint system designs, the load of the wheelchair and occupant are independently transmitted to the vehicle, reducing the load of the wheelchair tiedowns. Another important difference between these two restraint system designs concerns the resulting wheelchair and occupant kinematics in a frontal crash. It is possible with the independent restraint design for the wheelchair to load the back of the occupant because the forward motion of the wheelchair and occupant may be out of phase with each other. A large mass wheelchair may move further forward during frontal impact than the occupant, loading the torso of the occupant. This condition can lead to an increased risk of injury due to impingement of the occupant torso between the wheelchair and the occupant restraint belts.

There is much confusion in the field as to what constitutes a crashworthy occupant restraint system. In particular, postural belts are often erroneously assumed to be able to provide occupant protection in a crash. Often the presence of a postural lap belt is thought to satisfy the need for an occupant restraint, when in reality postural support belts are not crashworthy and are unable to protect occupants in a crash. In many cases postural support belts are anchored to the wheelchair with light-duty screws and grommets that would not be able to sustain crash level forces. In no instances must a postural belt be substituted for a crashworthy occupant restraint system.

Further complicating this issue of suitable lap restraints is the recent requirement of the ANSI WC-19 Standard that requires transit wheelchairs to be dynamically tested with an integrated, on-board lap belt.[15] Manufacturers must then offer their transit wheelchair with an integrated lap belt that has been certified as crashworthy. This lap belt will be distinguishable from a postural belt that has not been dynamically tested on the basis of its labeling certifying its compliance with ANSI WC-19. It is important that clinicians, transit providers, and consumers are aware of this difference between postural belts and crashworthy lap belts.

In some cases wheelchair users may require additional support to stabilize their torso during transport. Four- and five-point harnesses have been used in these situations to provide the occupant with additional postural support while still providing an adequate level of occupant protection.

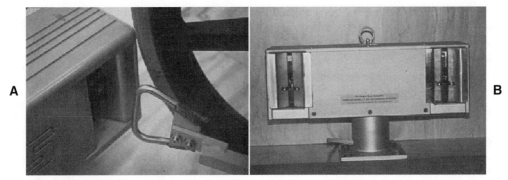

FIGURE 20-8 Oregon State University docking system for use in public vehicles. **A,** D-rings mounted on the rear of the wheelchair frame **B,** engage the docking system capture mechanism.

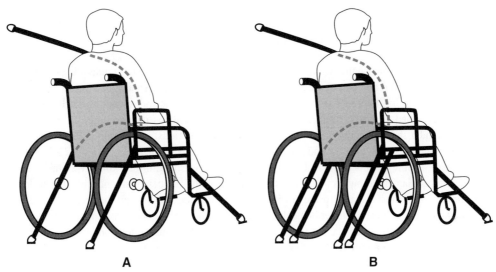

FIGURE 20-9 **A,** Integrated and **B,** independent three-point belt restraint and four-point strap-type tiedown system (Adapted from Society of Automotive Engineers: Recommended practice J2249 wheelchair tiedowns and occupant restraint systems for use in motor vehicles (surface vehicle recommended practice). In *SAE handbook,* Warrendale, PA, 1999, SAE.)

WHEELCHAIR TRANSPORTATION STANDARDS AND REGULATIONS
Regulations
Americans With Disabilities Act

In 1990 the U.S. Congress enacted the ADA, prohibiting discrimination against people with disabilities in employment practices, public accommodations, and telecommunications services.[1,2] By definition of this legislation, transportation services fall within the public accommodations category. The ADA has wide-reaching implications for transportation services because it requires both public and private transporters to accommodate people with disabilities who wish to travel in their wheelchairs. Virtually all modes of transportation, including buses, trains, and subways, are required to be accessible. ADA subpart B1192.23 addresses wheelchair accessibility in the vehicle, vehicle wheelchair lifts and ramps, and wheelchair securement devices.[1] The discussion in this chapter is limited to motor vehicles and only those items that relate to wheelchair safety in a moving vehicle (e.g., securement and occupant restraint).

The ADA states that at least two securement stations shall be provided on vehicles in excess of 22 feet in length and at least one securement station shall be provided on vehicles 22 feet in length

or less. In vehicles longer than 22 feet, at least one securement station shall secure the wheelchair in a forward-facing orientation; others can be either forward or rearward facing. In vehicles 22 feet long or less, the securement station may secure the wheelchair either forward or rearward facing. In those cases where wheelchairs will be oriented toward the rear of the vehicle, a padded barrier shall be provided at the rear of the wheelchair.

Securement systems complying with ADA must be capable of securing common wheelchairs and mobility aids. A common wheelchair is defined as a three- or four-wheeled device being no larger than 30 inches wide by 48 inches long and weighing no more than 600 pounds when occupied. Securement system performance is dependent on gross vehicle weight. In those vehicles weighing 30,000 pounds or more, securement systems must be capable of withstanding a forward longitudinal static load of 2000 pounds per leg or a minimum or 4000 pounds per wheelchair. On vehicles weighing up to 30,000 pounds, each leg of the securement device must withstand a 2500-pound forward static longitudinal load and a minimum of 5000 pounds per wheelchair. Additional securement system performance criteria include limiting the movement of the occupied wheelchair to no more than

2 inches in any direction under normal vehicle operating conditions. However, no test method is provided to evaluate whether the wheelchair meets this performance criteria.

The ADA also requires that a lap and shoulder belt be provided at each securement station. Occupant restraints are required to meet the applicable provisions of the FMVSS Code of Federal Regulation Title 49, Transportation Part 571 as a part of the ADA.[17]

Federal Motor Vehicle Safety Standard 222

FMVSS 222, School Bus Passenger Seating and Crash Protection, establishes occupant protection requirements for wheelchair users traveling on school buses.[18] This regulation focuses primarily on vehicle requirements. FMVSS 222 requires that each wheelchair station on a school bus have not less than four wheelchair securement anchorages, arranged in such a way that the wheelchair can be positioned in a forward-facing orientation. Wheelchair anchorage is defined as "the provision for transferring wheelchair securement or occupant restraint loads to the vehicle structure."[18] The wheelchair must be secured by a device that attaches to the wheelchair at two locations in the front and two in the rear. The securement device must be able to limit wheelchair movement, although limitations are not specified. Each of the vehicle anchorages must be able to withstand a statically applied load of 3033 pounds. Wheelchair stations must also provide a lap and shoulder belt along with an anchorage for the shoulder belt and not less than two floor anchorages for the lap and shoulder belt combination. Each lap belt anchorage point must also be capable of withstanding a 3033-pound static load, and the shoulder belt vehicle anchorage point must withstand a 1516-pound static load.

One of the major shortcomings of both the ADA and FMVSS 222 is the use of statically applied loads to evaluate securement system and occupant restraint performance. Such loading conditions do not replicate the dynamic environment that these systems would be subjected to in a crash. Therefore, the true crash performance of securement and occupant restraint systems complying with either the ADA or FMVSS 222 remain unknown. In contrast, voluntary industry wheelchair transportation standards have chosen a more applicable approach, requiring that systems be subjected to dynamic testing, better simulating a real-world crash event.

Wheelchair Transportation Standards

Wheelchair transportation standards development has been divided into two primary areas: the first area is devoted to wheelchair securement and occupant restraint, and the second focuses on the wheelchair as a motor vehicle seat (Box 20-4). These standards are voluntary industry standards and currently have not been legislated. Therefore manufacturer compliance with standards is largely dependent on consumer demand for transport-safe products.

Society of Automotive Engineers Recommended Practice J2249: Wheelchair Tiedowns and Occupant Restraint Systems for Use in Motor Vehicles

Society of Automotive Engineers Recommended Practice J2249 Wheelchair Tiedowns and Occupant Restraint Systems for Use in Motor Vehicles was adopted in 1996 and revised in 1999.[14]

BOX 20-4	Primary Goals of Wheelchair Transportation Standards

- SAE RP J2249: Provides design requirements, test methods and labeling requirements for wheelchair tiedown and occupant restraint systems; WTORS must be dynamically tested
- ANSI/RESNA WC-19: Provides design requirements, test methods, and labeling requirements for wheelchairs intended to function as a motor vehicle seat; wheelchairs must be dynamically tested
- ANSI/RESNA WC-20: Currently under development with the goal of providing methods to evaluate wheelchair seating system crashworthiness independent of the frame to which it may be coupled

---

The primary goal of this standard is to evaluate the performance of devices or systems designed to secure a forward-facing wheelchair in a vehicle and restrain a wheelchair-seated occupant. This standard contains design requirements, labeling requirements, user instructions, installation instructions, and testing requirements for WTORS. The scope of J2249 addresses WTORS designed for frontal impact that are suitable for use in all vehicles (i.e., public and personal) and with all wheelchair types. WTORS must include both lap and shoulder belts as a part of their system. Securement of the wheelchair may be attained through a variety of methods including four-point strap-type tiedowns or docking systems.

Perhaps the hallmark of SAE J2249 is the requirement that WTORS must be dynamically tested. Test procedures specify that a 20 g/30 mph frontal impact sled test must be used to evaluate WTORS securing a surrogate wheelchair and restraining a 50th percentile male anthropomorphic test device (ATD). The surrogate wheelchair is a reusable and repeatable 187-pound wheelchair (Figure 20-10). The 50th percentile male ATD has a mass of 168 pounds and represents an average-sized male. Both the surrogate wheelchair and the ATD load the WTORS in a repeatable fashion to evaluate their dynamic strength (see Figure 20-1). Compliance with the standard requires that wheelchair and occupant excursions are within established limits during the dynamic test and that there is no sign of WTORS failure after the test.

The standard also requires that WTORS be subjected to a test for partial engagement of tiedowns to prevent erroneously perceived engagement and also a test for webbing slippage through adjustment devices. SAE J2249 design requirements stipulate front and rear tiedown angles (Figure 20-11), lap belt angles (Figure 20-12), and shoulder belt anchorage zones (Figures 20-13).

A number of WTORS on the market today comply with SAE J2249, most of which are four-point tiedown systems. These WTORS are suitable for use in personal vehicles and public vehicles because they have been tested at a severe crash pulse. Future versions of the standard will likely address the performance of WTORS under rear- and side-impact conditions.

American National Standards Institute and Rehabilitation Engineering Society of North America WC-19: Wheelchairs Used as Seats in Motor Vehicles

The ANSI/RESNA WC-19 Standard: Wheelchairs Used as Seats in Motor Vehicles (Vol, 4/Section 19) was adopted in 2000.[15] The primary goal of this standard is the provision of wheelchairs that are crashworthy and suitable to function as a motor vehicle seat, providing a stable support surface for the occupant. This standard addresses both adult and pediatric wheelchairs used in a forward-facing orientation in both public and personal vehicles. ANSI WC-19 provides design requirements, labeling requirements, user instructions, and test requirements for wheelchairs used as forward facing motor vehicle seats or transit wheelchairs.

ANSI WC-19 requires that wheelchairs with an appropriately sized ATD to be dynamically tested to a 20 g/30 mph frontal impact crash pulse, the same pulse used to evaluate WTORS in SAE J2249. When a wheelchair is evaluated, it is secured to the sled with a surrogate WTORS that provides repeatability in testing. The surrogate WTORS also includes lap and shoulder belts for occupant restraint. To achieve a successful dynamic test, ATD and wheelchair excursion must be within specified limits and the wheelchair must not show any visible evidence of failure. ATD excursion measures include forward and rearward head excursion, as well as forward knee excursion. Seat integrity is assessed through a comparison of the ATDs pretest to posttest H-point (hip) vertical displacement, with a limit of no more than a 20% difference.

The inclusion of four securement points on all transit wheelchairs is a primary design requirement of WC-19. This requirement was instituted in an effort to improve compatibility between wheelchairs and four-point tiedown systems. As stated earlier, many wheelchairs do not provide easy access to potential securement points on the wheelchair frame, leading to poor securement techniques or great deliberation on the part of the vehicle operator in deciding on an appropriate securement location. With fixed securement points on the wheelchair, crash performance of the wheelchair will have been evaluated with specific securement point locations that can be repeatedly used during transport, removing the guesswork from selecting securement points. ANSI WC-19 requires that securement points have a specified geometry that is capable of engaging hook-type and strap-type end fittings of tiedowns, and a WC-19 securement point must be labeled with a hook icon to identify its location on the wheelchair (Figure 20-14).

ANSI WC-19 also requires that transit wheelchairs be equipped with integrated lap belts. The wheelchair must be tested with an

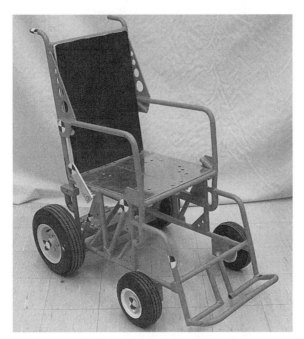

FIGURE 20-10 SAE J2249 surrogate wheelchair used for dynamically testing WTORS. (From Schneider LW, Manary MA: Wheeled mobility tiedown systems and occupant restraints for safety and crash protection. In Pellerito JA Jr, editor: *Driver rehabilitation and community mobility: principles and practice*, St Louis, 2006, Elsevier Mosby, Figure 17-6 A, p 364.)

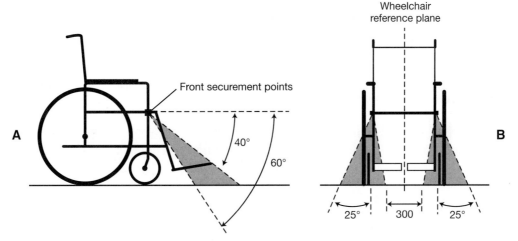

FIGURE 20-11 SAE J2249 preferred angles of front and rear tiedown straps. Front tiedowns should be angled out for lateral stability when possible. (Adapted from Society of Automotive Engineers: Recommended practice J2249 wheelchair tiedowns and occupant restraint systems for use in motor vehicles (surface vehicle recommended practice). In *SAE handbook,* Warrendale, PA, 1999, SAE.)

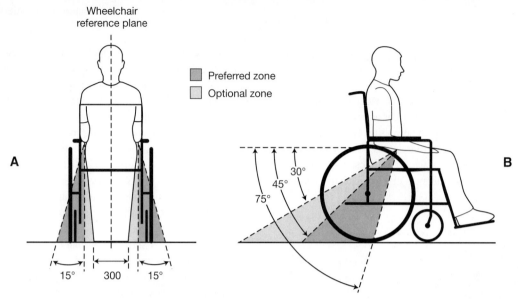

FIGURE 20-12 SAE J2249 preferred lap belt angles (Adapted from Society of Automotive Engineers: Recommended practice J2249 wheelchair tiedowns and occupant restraint systems for use in motor vehicles (surface vehicle recommended practice). In *SAE handbook,* Warrendale, PA, 1999, SAE.)

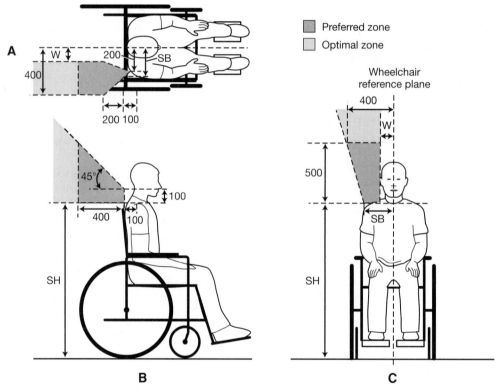

FIGURE 20-13 SAE J2249 preferred and optional zones for upper vehicle anchor point of shoulder belt. (Adapted from Society of Automotive Engineers: Recommended practice J2249 wheelchair tiedowns and occupant restraint systems for use in motor vehicles (surface vehicle recommended practice). In *SAE handbook,* Warrendale, PA, 1999, SAE.)

Typical Values of Shoulder Height, Half Shoulder Breadth, Half Neck Breadth, and Seat Height for Different-Sized Occupants Used to Establish Shoulder Belt Anchorage Location

Occupant Size	Shoulder Height (SH)	Half Shoulder Breadth (SB)	Half Neck Breadth (W)	Seat Height
Six-year-old child	775	130	50	380
Small female	1000	175	75	450
Mid-size male	1100	200	75	500
Large male	1200	210	75	550

All dimensions in millimeters.
From Society of Automotive Engineers: Recommended practice J2249 wheelchair tiedowns and occupant restraint systems for use in motor vehicles (surface vehicle recommended practice). In *SAE handbook,* Warrendale, PA, 1999, SAE.

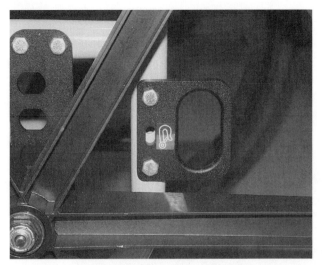

FIGURE 20-14 Close-up of ANSI WC-19 wheelchair securement point. (From Schneider LW, Manary MA: Wheeled mobility tiedown systems and occupant restraints for safety and crash protection. In Pellerito JA Jr, editor: *Driver rehabilitation and community mobility: principles and practice*, St Louis, 2006, Elsevier Mosby, Figure 17-11 B, p 368.)

on-board lap belt that must be made available to the consumer. The lap belt must be equipped with a standardized pin bushing that can interface with a vehicle-mounted shoulder belt. The integrated lap belt requirement is intended to improve lap belt fit and to avoid poor belt fit and reduce wheelchair interference that might be present with vehicle-mounted restraint systems. Recommended integrated lap belt angles are specified in ANSI WC-19 and are the same as those specified in SAE J2249 (see Figure 20-12).

ANSI WC-19 also includes a test to evaluate the lateral stability of a transit wheelchair. The purpose of the test is to promote transit wheelchair designs that provide a stable seating support surface and comfortable ride for occupants during normal and emergency driving maneuvers. The test procedure, which simulates an emergency vehicle turn, mounts a wheelchair with a restrained ATD on a tilt table platform that is raised to 45 degrees. The lateral displacement of a specific point on the wheelchair relative to the platform is measured and is to be reported in presale literature.

Manufacturers are free to locate wheelchair securement points within ANSI WC-19 prescribed front and rear zones. However, securement points must be easily accessible from the side of the wheelchair, and the tiedown path from the vehicle floor anchor to the wheelchair securement point must be free from any interference or sharp edges.

Despite the requirement for an integrated lap belt, wheelchair users may still need to use vehicle-mounted occupant restraints in some vehicles (in those cases where a separate shoulder belt is not available to interface with the integrated lap belt pin bushing); therefore ANSI WC-19 contains a test to evaluate the wheelchair's accommodation of vehicle-mounted occupant restraints. The test procedure assesses belt fit on the ATD, belt proximity to sharp edges, and whether the belt has a clear path without interference from the wheelchair. Results are assigned a categorical rating of poor, good, or excellent, which must be disclosed in presale literature.

American National Standards Institute and Rehabilitation Engineering Society of North America WC-20: Seating Devices for Use in Motor Vehicles

Despite an effort with ANSI WC-19 to evaluate wheelchair crashworthiness, the addition of often used after-market or optional wheelchair seating systems will invalidate previous ANSI WC-19 wheelchair testing and leave questions regarding how the combined wheelchair frame and seating systems will perform in a crash. Consequently, wheelchairs using after-market seating systems may not be impact tested to evaluate their ability to withstand crash-level forces. In addition, replacement seating systems provided in the field, which differ from those provided with an ANSI WC-19–approved wheelchair, will invalidate compliance and will not have been tested in combination with the ANSI WC-19 wheelchair frame. Therefore methods to evaluate wheelchair seating system crashworthiness, independent of the numerous wheelchair frames that it may be coupled with in the field, are needed.

Toward that end, ANSI/RESNA has organized efforts to address after-market transit wheelchair seating. The ANSI/RESNA Seating Devices for Use in Motor Vehicles Standard (Vol. 4/Section 20) is currently under development. This standard includes a 20 g/30 mph frontal impact sled test to evaluate commercial seating systems mounted on a surrogate wheelchair base (SWCB). The SWCB is a reusable wheelchair base that allows commercial seating systems to be mounted on its frame for testing purposes (Figure 20-15, *A*). The SWCB is able to accommodate a range of seating sizes from pediatric to adult, as well as a wide range of seating system hardware. It also is equipped with adjustable seat back canes and adjustable caster mountings to alter wheel or frame stiffness. The SWCB has been validated against commercial wheelchairs and their seating systems to ensure that similar loading is imparted to seating systems mounted on the SWCB (Figure 20-15, *B*). The standard will also include a test for rating a seating system's accommodation of vehicle-mounted occupant restraints.

BRIEF SYNOPSIS OF WHEELCHAIR TRANSPORTATION SAFETY RESEARCH

Early wheelchair transportation research primarily focused on efforts needed to advance standards development. This early research worked toward the development of a repeatable frontal impact test using a reusable surrogate wheelchair.[19] As a part of the standards effort, a computer simulation model was used to investigate the effects of wheelchair tiedown system characteristics, crash pulse corridor, and seated posture on tiedown and belt loading, wheelchair excursions, and occupant crash response.[20] Studies have also investigated the injury risk associated with using a wheelchair as a motor vehicle seat, examining the effects of crash pulse,[20] securement point location,[20,21] restraint configuration,[22,23] and seated posture.[20]

Supporting the fact that wheelchairs are often not designed to sustain crash-level forces, component testing studies have shown that casters, seat attachment hardware, and seat support surfaces often fail at loads similar to those imposed in a frontal impact crash.[24-27] Unfortunately, design criteria to guide manufacturers in the development of transit wheelchairs and wheelchair seating systems are relatively scarce. Information related to

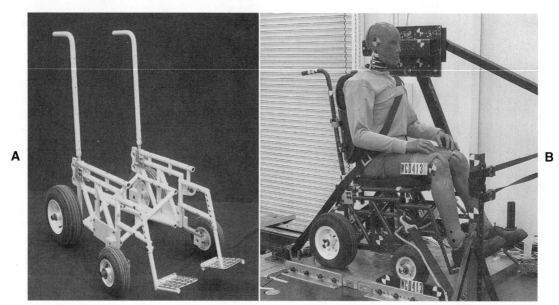

FIGURE 20-15 **A,** ANSI WC-20 SWCB on which wheelchair seating systems are installed for frontal dynamic testing of systems independent of a specific wheelchair frame. **B,** SWCB with seating system and mid-size male ATD test setup on University of Michigan Transportation Research Institute sled. (From Schneider LW, Manary MA: Wheeled mobility tiedown systems and occupant restraints for safety and crash protection. In Pellerito JA Jr, editor: *Driver rehabilitation and community mobility: principles and practice*, St Louis, 2006, Elsevier Mosby, Figure 17-14 A-B, p 370.)

transit wheelchair design criteria that exist in the literature has largely been derived from computer simulation of frontal impact events.[7,21-23] Recent efforts have also included an investigation of pediatric wheelchair and frontal seating impact loading by using a combination of sled testing and computer simulation.[8] This work has shown that numerous factors (e.g., rear wheelchair securement height relative to the wheelchair center of gravity, seat stiffness, seat angle) can influence loads that wheelchairs and seating systems are exposed to in a crash. Findings suggest that manufacturer design decisions can greatly affect the crashworthiness of wheelchairs and their seating. Although the performance of all wheelchair load-carrying components is important to occupant crash protection, seat design and integrity are of particular concern because vehicle seat characteristics and failure have been linked directly to injury risk in motor vehicle crashes.[12,28-34] Frontal impact sled tests (20 g/30 mph) of commercial wheelchairs have shown seating system failures to be relatively common.[35] Seat attachment hardware, seat support surfaces, and seat backs on rebound are among the most common components to fail under frontal impact conditions. Recently seat back performance under rear impact conditions has also been investigated by use of an instrumented seat back that assessed seat back loading and deflection during rear impact sled tests.[36]

Previous research that attempted to elucidate wheelchair seat loading under crash conditions consisted of both computer simulation studies and limited sled testing. Computer simulation studies have shown that frontal impact seat forces are dependent on crash pulse, rear securement point location, seat characteristics, and occupant restraint configuration.[7,20-23] A limited series of frontal impact sled tests

conducted by Gu and Roy[23] with disc-type load cells incorporated into the surrogate wheelchair and using a Hybrid III 50th percentile male test dummy measured seat loads. Shaw also estimated seat loading in frontal impact sled testing using pressure-sensitive film placed on the seat and load cells located beneath the front wheels of commercial manual wheelchairs with various types of seating systems (e.g., sling, rigid foam mounted on plywood).[37] In these tests Shaw estimated vertical seat loads and found that higher loads were associated with the more rigid seating systems. Four frontal impact tests conducted by Bertocci and Manary[38] used the SAE J2249 surrogate wheelchair and evaluated seat loads using disc-type load cells incorporated into the wheelchair seat and also evaluated the effects of rear securement point location.

Although this research provides an approximation of wheelchair seat loading under 20 g frontal impact conditions, limitations exist. Experimental measurement techniques used in sled tests conducted by Shaw were limited because seat loads were estimated from measurements recorded at only the front wheels and did not account for that portion of the seat load that may be distributed over the rear wheels. Gu and Roy's[23] testing used measurement techniques directly assessing seat loads, but unfortunately only one sled test was conducted at the 21 g/30 mph level; all others were below this crash severity. Recent frontal impact tests conducted by Bertocci and Manary are also somewhat limited and can be used only as a guide because seat loads were assessed using the SAE surrogate wheelchair, which is more rigid than a commercial wheelchair.[38]

Although such research represents a preliminary effort toward development of transport-safe wheelchairs and wheelchair seating, additional efforts are needed to advance safe wheelchair transportation. Testing and computer simulations to date have mostly been conducted with a 50th percentile male test dummy; only one study has been conducted to evaluate seating loads associated with 6-year-old child-sized ATD.[8] Furthermore, studies have evaluated seat loading primarily in frontal impact conditions; little effort has been undertaken to study seat loading in rear and side impact, which are likely to impose very different loading conditions. Wheelchair seat backs are subjected to unique loading conditions in rear impact crashes because they serve to resist occupant motion, yet only one preliminary study has been conducted to quantify seat back or wheelchair loading in rear impact. More detailed investigational studies, such as those conducted in the automotive industry, are also needed to evaluate the effects of wheelchair seating design on injury risk. Clearly additional guidance is needed to provide wheelchair manufacturers with guidance related to seating system design for transport-safe wheelchairs.

Securement technology research has been fairly limited. Despite reported problems, four-point strap-type tiedown systems are still the most commonly used wheelchair securement system in public transportation. These problems as they relate to the transporter were highlighted by Hardin et al[16] in a survey of 270 paratransit and transit agencies located primarily in Florida. The identified issues included an excessive amount of time required to secure a mobility device and difficulty in securing mobility devices, particularly three- and four-wheeled scooters. The report also suggests that the intent of the ADA will not be fulfilled until these deficiencies have been resolved. Transporter-reported problems in conjunction with wheelchair user–reported problems highlight the need for alternative solutions in securement. Docking systems offer a promising automated solution that would allow wheelchair users to independently secure their wheelchairs and would remove the human error associated with using tiedowns. However, docking systems have not been very successful in public transport because of the lack of a standardized approach to interfacing the wheelchair and docking system. A universal docking interface adapter geometry has been proposed and is moving toward standardization.[39,40] This universal adapter, which would be mounted on the rear of a wheelchair, resembles an upside-down U-shaped bar that would engage the vehicle mounted docking system. It is believed that this approach could promote the development and commercialization of docking systems through the standardization of a universal docking interface. Ultimately this could provide wheelchair users the freedom to travel independently without having to rely on attendants or vehicle operators to secure wheelchairs.

CLINICAL CASE STUDY | Wheelchair Transportation Safety

Client History

Bruce Benson is a 60-year-old man with a C5 tetraplegia, ASIA A diagnosis. He sustained his injury 4 months ago in a motor vehicle accident. He has completed both his acute inpatient and rehabilitation care. Bruce is orthopedically and medically stable.

Bruce is a salesman for a large manufacturing firm. He plans to return to his job, which includes office work and sales presentations. He will purchase a van for transportation and use it for travel between home and the office but rely on public transportation between the office and other business locations. Bruce uses a power reclining wheelchair and has a manual wheelchair for backup use. He lives with his wife, age 48 years, and their two children. His wife works as a social worker; their older son is a junior in college and their daughter is a senior in high school.

Client's Self-Assessment

Bruce plans to return to work as soon as he has gained his certification to drive a van using hand controls. Before his injury, he was instrumental in helping establish his city's fully accessible public transit system that allows wheelchair users to board and ride all buses and travel safely. All buses are equipped to board wheelchair riders using a lift at the front of the bus, and designated spaces are provided for forward-facing securement of the rider in his wheelchair. An on-call van service is available as well.

Clinical Assessment
Client Characteristics
• Height 5 feet 11 inches, weight 205 pounds, body mass index 28.6

Cognitive Assessment
• Alert, oriented × 3

Cardiopulmonary Assessment
• Blood pressure 125/80 mm Hg, heart rate at rest 72 beats/min, respiratory rate 14 breaths/min, cough flows are ineffective (<360 L/min), vital capacity is reduced (between 1.5 and 2.5 L)

Musculoskeletal and Neuromuscular Assessment
• Motor assessment reveals C5 ASIA A
• Deep tendon reflexes 3+ below the level of lesion

Integumentary and Sensory Assessment
• Skin is intact throughout, sensory intact to C5.

Range of Motion Assessment
• Passive and active motion is within normal limits in both upper limbs.
• Straight leg raise is 90 degrees in both lower limbs and dorsiflexion is 0 degrees; all other motions in the lower limbs are within functional limits.

Mobility and ADL Assessment
• Dependent with bed mobility
• Moderate assistance required for transfer board transfers between level surfaces and maximal assistance for uneven transfers
• Independent with pressure relief

CLINICAL CASE STUDY Wheelchair Transportation Safety—cont'd

- Independent with power wheelchair mobility
- Independent maneuvering manual wheelchair with splints and gloves for short distances only
- Dependent in bowel and bladder care
- Minimal to moderate assistance required for upper body dressing
- Dependent in lower body dressing
- Dependent in auto driving

Evaluation of Clinical Assessment

Bruce Benson is a 60-year-old man with a C5 tetraplegia, ASIA A diagnosis from a motor vehicle accident 4 months ago. He is orthopedically and medically stable, has completed rehabilitation care. Bruce is currently using an ANSI WC19 compliant wheelchair and is in the process of selecting a van for transportation.

Client's Care Needs

1. Consultation for appropriate adapted van—equipped with wheelchair securement system, occupant restraints, and wheelchair lift/ramp
2. Consultation with instructor of disabled drivers training program
3. Instruction regarding transportation safety and the proper use of occupant restraints and wheelchair securement system installed in vehicle
4. Instruction regarding appropriate and safe use of wheelchair lift or ramp installed in vehicle

NOTE: Client already uses an ANSI WC19–compliant wheelchair.

Diagnosis and Prognosis

Diagnosis of C5 tetraplegia, ASIA A. Prognosis for full independence for transportation with an adequately adapted van with necessary safety features. Independent with certain types of public transportation

Preferred Practice Patterns*

Impaired Muscle Performance (4C), Impairments Nonprogressive Spinal Cord Disorders (5H), Primary Prevention/Risk Reduction for Cardiovascular/Pulmonary Disorders (6A), Primary Prevention/Risk Reduction for Integumentary Disorders (7A)

Team Goals

1. Team to ensure client's independence in use of the wheelchair mechanical lift or ramp to enter/exit the van
2. Team to instruct for independence and safety in the use of occupant restraints and wheelchair securement system
3. Team to teach patient to instruct others regarding proper use of wheelchair lift or ramp, as well as occupant restraints and wheelchair securement system
4. Team to schedule community travel to ensure independent access and safe use of public transportation system, including lift/ramp, occupant restraint system, and securement system use

Client Goals

"I want to be able to get where I need to go."

Care Plan
Treatment Plan and Rationale

- Evaluate optimal vehicle adaptations for van driving, access to vehicle, wheelchair securement, and occupant restraint.
- Schedule consultation as needed for van purchase.
- Discuss time line for the written and behind-the-wheel tests.
- Review travel safety instructions when functioning as a driver and as a passenger.
- Review proper use of wheelchair securement system, occupant restraint system, and lift/ramp.

Interventions

- Evaluate optimal vehicle adaptations for van driving with relevant auto vendors.
- Evaluate options for vehicle assess (e.g., lift or ramp).
- Evaluate options for wheelchair securement and occupant restraint with van modifier.
- Complete consultation for van purchase in conjunction with caseworker to determine insurance support.
- Prepare client for and schedule the written and behind-the-wheel driver's tests.
- Review travel safety instructions with patient and family when functioning as a driver and as a passenger. This must include proper use of the wheelchair securement system, occupant restraint system, and lift/ramp.

Documentation and Team Communication

- Weekly progress notes with team meetings as needed
- Discuss and document decisions about choice of van and vehicle adaptations.
- Record results of driver's tests.
- Document and discuss knowledge of instructional content on vehicle safety measures and proper use of wheelchair securement system, lift/ramp, and occupant restraint system.

Follow-Up Assessment

- Contact client 1 month after adaptable van purchase to discuss questions regarding use of transportation safety equipment in van and during use of public transportation

Critical Thinking Exercises

Consider factors, especially lifestyle and type of wheelchair, that may influence Bruce's education regarding independent and safe transportation whether driving his accessible van or using public transportation. These questions are posed as coming from the client to the rehabilitation caregiver to obtain information and advice.

1. What wheelchair orientation relative to the front of the vehicle is safest during transport? Why?
2. What wheelchair securement system should be used when I am seated in my wheelchair?
3. What do you advise regarding the use of occupant restraint systems; must both the lap and shoulder belts be used at all times during transport?

*Guide to physical therapist practice, rev. ed. 2, Alexandria, VA, 2003, American Physical Therapy Association.

SUMMARY

Safe transportation is essential to providing wheelchair users access to work, school, and recreation. Wheelchair-seated travelers must have a level of safety equivalent to those traveling seated in motor vehicle seats. Meeting this goal depends on proper wheelchair securement, appropriate occupant restraints, and a wheelchair that is able to withstand crash-level forces.

Voluntary industry standards addressing the design, testing, and labeling of wheelchair tiedowns, occupant restraints, and wheelchairs exist to aid manufacturers in the development of these products for frontal impact conditions. Commonly used wheelchair securement technologies include both four-point strap-type tiedowns and docking systems. Some wheelchair models are now commercially available that have a proven ability to withstand frontal impact crashes. Occupant restraint systems for use in wheelchair transportation include both vehicle-anchored restraints and wheelchair-anchored restraints.

Challenges remain in the provision of safe wheelchair transportation and include the proper and effective usage of securement systems, achieving proper belt fit in occupant restraint usage, and increasing the numbers and types of transport-safe wheelchairs available. Research to advance safety in the wheelchair transportation field has included, but is not limited to, evaluation of test methods for the development of industry standards, development of design guidelines for wheelchairs and securement systems, identification of wheelchair failure modes under crash conditions, identification of problems with the use of securement systems in transportation settings, and development of methods to advance the use of docking system technologies to allow for wheelchair user independence in the securement process. Much work in the area of effective legislation, standards development, and research remains to be done to ensure the safe transport of those traveling seated in their wheelchairs in motor vehicles.

REFERENCES

1. Americans with Disabilities: *Act of 1990 (PL 101-336, 26 July 1990), 104 United States Statutes at Large*, Washington, DC, 1990, Government Printing Office, pp 327-378.

2. Architectural and Transportation Barriers Compliance Board: *Americans with Disabilities Act (ADA) accessibility guidelines for transportation vehicles*, 36 Code of Federal Regulations Part 1192, Federal Register 56 (173), 1991.

3. *Fulfilling America's promise to Americans with disabilities: new freedom initiative, 2001*: http://www.whitehouse.gov/news/freedominitiative/freedominitiative.html Accessed July 20, 2006.

4. Kaye H, Kang T, LaPlante M: *Disability statistics report—mobility device use in the United States*, Washington, DC, 2000, U.S. Department of Education, National Institute of Disability and Rehabilitation Research.

5. National Highway Traffic Safety Administration: *National Center for Statistics and Analysis, wheelchair users' injuries and deaths associated with motor vehicle related incidents: research note*, Washington, DC, 1997, NHTSA.

6. Hunter-Zaworski K: The mechanics of mobility aid securement/restraint on public transportation vehicles, *Transportation Res Record* 1378:45-51, 1993.

7. Bertocci GE, Szobota S, Ha D et al: Development of frontal impact crashworthy wheelchair seating design criteria using computer simulation, *J Rehabil Res Dev* 37:565-572, 2000.

8. Ha D, Bertocci G, Jategaonkar R: Development and validation of a frontal impact 6 yr old wheelchair seated occupant computer model, *Assist Technol* Vol. 19.4, 2007.

9. National Highway Transportation Safety Administration: *2005 Traffic facts overview*, Washington, DC, 2005, NHTSA.

10. Code of Federal Regulations, Title 49, Transportation, Part 571.208, *Occupant crash protection*, Washington, DC, 2003, National Archives and Records Service, Office of the Federal Registrar.

11. Code of Federal Regulations, Title 49, Transportation, Part 571.222, *School bus seating and crashworthiness*, Washington, DC, 1998, National Archives and Records Service, Office of the Federal Registrar.

12. Viano D: *Influence of seat back angle on occupant dynamics in simulated rear-end impacts, SAE paper No. 922521*, Warrendale, PA, 1992, SAE.

13. Viano D, Arapelly S: *Assessing the safety performance of occupant restraint systems, SAE paper No. 902328*, Warrendale, PA, 1990, SAE.

14. Society of Automotive Engineers: *Recommended practice J2249 wheelchair tiedowns and occupant restraint systems for use in motor vehicles (surface vehicle recommended practice), SAE handbook*, Warrendale, PA, 1999, SAE.

15. American National Standards Institute/Rehabilitation Engineering Society of North America, Subcommittee on Wheelchairs and Transportation: Wheelchairs used as seats in motor vehicles, *ANSI/RESNA Vol 1; Section 19*, 2000.

16. Hardin J, Foreman C, Callejas L: *Synthesis of securement device options and strategies, technical report No. 416-07*, Tampa, FL, 2002, National Center for Transit Research.

17. Code of Federal Regulations, Title 49, Transportation, Part 571.209, *Seat belt assemblies*, Washington, DC, 1999, National Archives and Records Service, Office of the Federal Registrar.

18. Department of Transportation: *Federal motor vehicle safety standards (FMVSS), part 571: 222, school bus passenger seating and crash protection (standard)*, Washington, DC, 1977, Department of Transportation.

19. Shaw G, Lapidot A, Scavinsky M et al: *Interlaboratory study of proposed compliance test protocol for wheelchair tiedowns and occupant restraint systems, SAE paper No. 94229*, Warrendale, PA, 1994, SAE.

20. Kang W, Pilkey W: Crash simulations of wheelchair occupant systems in transport, *J Rehabil Res Dev* 35:73-84, 1998.

21. Bertocci GE, Hobson DA, Digges K: Development of transportable wheelchair design criteria using computer crash simulation, *IEEE Trans Rehabil Eng* 4:171-181, 1996.

22. Bertocci GE, Digges K, Hobson DA: Shoulder belt anchor location influences on wheelchair occupant crash protection, *J Rehabil Res Dev* 33:279-289, 1996.

23. Gu J, Roy P: *Optimization of the wheelchair tiedown and occupant restraint system*. Presented at the 15th International Technical Conference on Enhanced Safety of Vehicles, Melbourne, Australia, 1996.

24. Bertocci GE, Esteireiro J, Cooper RA et al: Testing and evaluation of wheelchair caster assemblies subjected to dynamic crash loading, *J Rehabil Res Dev* 36:32-41, 1999.

25. Bertocci GE, Ha D, Deemer E et al: Evaluation of wheelchair seating crashworthiness: drop hook type attachment hardware, *Arch Phys Med Rehabil* 82:534-540, 2001.

26. Bertocci GE, Ha D, van Roosmalen L et al: Evaluation of wheelchair drop seat crashworthiness, *Med Eng Phys* 23:249-257, 2001.

27. Ha D, Bertocci GE, Deemer E et al: Evaluation of wheelchair seating system crashworthiness: combination wheelchair seat back surfaces and attachment hardware, *J Rehabil Res Dev* 37:555-563, 2000.

28. Warner C, Stother C, James M et al: *Occupant protection in rear end collisions II: the role of seat back deformation in injury reduction, SAE paper No. 912914*, Warrendale, PA, 1991, SAE.

29. Strother C, James M: *Evaluation of seat back strength and seat belt effectiveness in rear impact, SAE paper No. 872214*, Warrendale, PA, 1997, SAE.

30. Saczalski KJ, Syson SR, Hille RA et al: *Field accident evaluations and experimental study of seat back performance relative to rear-impact occupant protection, SAE paper No. 930346*, Warrendale, PA, 1993, SAE.

31. National Highway Traffic Safety Administration: *Preliminary assessment of NASS CDS data related to rearward seat collapse and occupant injury*, Washington, DC, 1997, U.S. Department of Transportation.

32. Blaisdell DM, Levitt AE, Varat MS: *Automotive seat design concepts for occupant protection, SAE paper No. 930340*, Warrendale, PA, 1993, SAE.

33. Adomeit D: *Seat design—a significant factor for safety belt effectiveness*, SAE paper No. 791004, Warrendale, PA, 1979, SAE.

34. Aibe T, Watanabe K, Okamoto T et al: *Influence of occupant seating posture and size on head and chest injuries in frontal collision*, SAE paper No. 826032, Warrendale, PA, 1982, SAE.

35. Manary M, Woodruff L, Bertocci G et al: *Patterns of wheelchair response and seating-system failures in frontal-impact sled tests*, Presented at the Atlanta, GA, 2003, RESNA Conference.

36. Manary M, Schneider L: *Wheelchair seatback loads and deflection in rear impacts*, Presented at the Orlando, FL, 2004, RESNA Conference.

37. American National Standards Institute/Rehabilitation Engineering Society of North America: Seating insert evaluation sled tests, Charlottesville, VA, 1996, University of VA Auto Safety Lab.

38. Bertocci GE, Manary M, Ha D: Wheelchairs used as seats in motor vehicles: seat loading in frontal impact testing, *Med Eng Phys* 23: 679-685, 2001.

39. Hobson DA: Wheelchair transport safety—evolving options, *J Rehabil Res Dev* 37, vii-xv, 2000.

40. International Standards Organization: *10542–3 Technical systems and aids for disabled or handicapped persons, wheelchair tiedown and occupant-restraint systems-part 3: docking type tiedown systems (standard)*, Geneva, 2005, International Standards Organization.

SOLUTIONS TO CHAPTER 20 CLINICAL CASE STUDY

Wheelchair Transportation Safety

1. Research based on motor vehicle accidents and associated injury outcome indicates that more than half of all serious injuries and fatalities occur during frontal impact collisions. Accordingly, a forward-facing wheelchair orientation is key to maximize the effectiveness of the occupant restraint system.

It would be ideal for an individual to transfer into the original equipment manufacturer's vehicle seat and use occupant restraints that have been designed and tested to meet federal regulations. Unfortunately, transfer to a vehicle seat is likely not feasible at a C5 level of injury. Safe transport therefore should include (1) a structurally sound wheelchair that is capable of providing a stable seating support surface (preferably compliant with ANSI WC19), (2) a securement system to secure the wheelchair to the vehicle, and (3) an occupant restraint system that includes both a lap and shoulder belt.

Proper belt fit positioned over bony structures versus soft tissue is important. Good belt fit serves to distribute restraining loads over the largest possible area. Some manufacturers of wheelchair occupant restraints have included webbing locks on their systems to prevent the shoulder belt from spooling out of the reel when activated, thereby limiting forward occupant excursion. This reduction in excursion can be important in preventing impact with the vehicle interior.

2. It is essential that a wheelchair be secured during transportation as even an abrupt turn can lead to wheelchair tipping and thus risk of injury to the occupant. A four-point tiedown system is the most commonly found wheelchair securement system used in public transportation. When properly used, this securement system is capable of withstanding a 30 mph/20 g frontal crash. For the securement system to be effective, it is important that all four tiedowns— two in the front and two in rear of the wheelchair—be used. An automatic docking system could provide Bruce with independent securement of his wheelchair in a private vehicle. However, use of a docking system would require that an adapter be attached to the wheelchair for interface with the docking system.

3. In addition to a wheelchair securement system, an occupant restraint system must also be provided in the vehicle. The occupant restraint system should be composed of a lap belt and shoulder belt that can be positioned properly on the body to provide effective crash protection. When properly positioned, belt restraints will prevent excessive occupant forward excursion, and thus secondary impact with the vehicle interior. A lap and shoulder belt should be used at all times during transportation to optimize occupant protection. Furthermore, the occupant restraint system must meet SAE J2249 requirements, which includes dynamic testing. It is important to note that positioning or postural belts are not crashworthy and have not typically been designed to provide occupant protection in a crash. The ANSI/RESNA WC-19 Wheelchairs Used as Seats in Motor Vehicles Standard was adopted in 2000 to ensure that a wheelchair is crashworthy and suitable to function as a motor vehicle seat, providing a stable support surface for the occupant. One requirement of this standard is that the wheelchair be dynamically tested with an integrated lap belt that is suitable for crash purposes. This requirement is intended to improve lap belt fit and reduce wheelchair interference that might be present with vehicle-mounted restraint systems. ANSI WC-19 also requires that the lap belt be equipped with a standardized pin bushing that interfaces with a vehicle-mounted shoulder belt. Although an integrated lap belt is recommended for use during transport, users may still require the use of vehicle-mounted occupant restraints in some cases. ANSI WC-19 therefore contains a test to evaluate the wheelchair's accommodation of vehicle-mounted occupant restraints. The results are assigned a categorical rating of poor, good, or excellent, which must be disclosed in presale literature.

CHAPTER TWENTY-ONE

Transportation, Driving, and Community Access

Katharine Hunter-Zaworski, PE, PhD, and Richard Nead, CDRS

I've visited over 38 countries researching and promoting accessibility based on ability. The everyday challenges that I faced during my early travel have been blunted somewhat as the world became friendlier for people traveling in wheelchairs. [But I remember my first trip] to the famous Colosseum in 1999. It was not an accessible tourist attraction and I was limited to moving around in a small section of the ground level tier. As I watched my wife Pat follow a guided tour, I felt a deep sadness overcome me. I was thrilled that she was able to have that whole experience but I wanted to have it as well. For the first time, I really felt as if I was missing out on something because I am confined to a wheelchair. I wanted to climb those stairs and hear more about the gladiators fighting and all the other fascinating stories surrounding this work of art.

Scott (T8 SCI)

Accessible transportation is essential for an independent lifestyle, especially for people with temporary or permanent impairments. Transportation, whether by public or private vehicle, allows individuals and groups to travel from one point of the community to another. These journeys are referred to here as trip chains, composed of incremental segments or links. Each of the links must be accessible for the total trip to be considered accessible. There are many places where the links can break and make the total trip inaccessible or impossible. As each link is discussed, the new language of accessible transportation is introduced, and definitions include context or application. In addition to trip chain, the specific terminology includes trip purpose, trip payment options, transportation mode choices, family of services, community access, land use, transportation challenges, travel training, transportation amenities, and virtual transportation.

In the United States, most trips are made by single-occupancy private automobiles, including trips made by people with spinal cord injury (SCI). Although the focus of this chapter is on accessible community public transportation for people using wheelchairs and community access, it also addresses private vehicle adaptation, driver education, and licensing.

This chapter is written from the perspective of professionals who have worked both inside and outside the health care field. The authors bring experience in clinical rehabilitation, barrier-free transit design,[1,2] the National Center for Accessible Transportation, and hands-on expertise in developing and collaborating with transportation planners and policy makers throughout the Pacific Northwest, where transit systems for urban, suburban, and rural communities are among the most innovative and progressive in accommodating people with disabilities. They believe that mobility is a basic need and requirement for healthy living. Without the ability to get around independently, people become excluded from community life and are unable to avail themselves of opportunities to enrich their lives.

UNDERSTANDING ACCESSIBLE TRANSPORTATION

It is important that rehabilitation professionals, practitioners, and people with SCI understand the world of transportation, specifically the world of accessible transportation. Accessibility is defined as both "a measure of the ability or ease of all people to travel among various origins and destinations" and for people

with disabilities as "the extent to which facilities are free of barriers and usable by persons with disabilities including wheelchair users."[3] Although the needs of people with SCI are most germane to this discussion, in terms of accessible transportation, the diversity of people with disabilities must be considered.

It is assumed that the majority of the people with SCI are users of wheeled mobility aids. Therefore it is very important that the rehabilitation team consider the transportation needs of their clients when prescribing those mobility aids. For example, a person who drives while seated in his mobility aid must have a wheelchair that is robust and can withstand the forces encountered in a private vehicle (see Chapter 20). On the other hand, if a person transfers from his mobility aid to drive a vehicle, then the wheelchair must be light enough to permit the user to safely and conveniently stow it away during transit. For clients who use public transportation, where it is assumed they will remain in the wheelchair during transport, the mobility aid must be strong enough to be safely secured. In addition, it is important to consider the overall size of the mobility aid in relation to the transportation vehicle.

All aspects of the accessible trip chain are examined (Figure 21-1). There are certain topics, however, that are not discussed, such as the Americans with Disabilities Act (ADA) and its corresponding regulations, except to say that the ADA mandates that public transportation services not discriminate against people with disabilities in the provision of their services and that they comply with the requirements of accessibility in newly purchased vehicles.[4] This is a purposeful omission because the ADA and the related regulations set minimum standards for accessibility and do not provide universal access for all people. For additional regulations concerning the ADA, the reader is referred to the resources located at the U.S. Access Board.[5,5a]

There are many communities in the United States that go above and far beyond the legal regulations of the ADA and provide a high level of accessible public or community transportation. It is also interesting to note that many of the communities that are the most accessible for people who use wheelchairs began providing accessible transportation long before there was an ADA. In addition, these communities also have more accessible infrastructure.

Any discussion of accessible community transportation needs to embrace the concept of universal design. Universal design

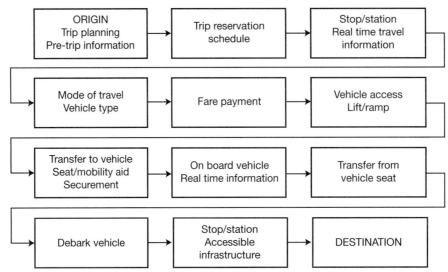

FIGURE 21-1 Links on a trip chain.

implies use by all people rather than targeted design for one or two user groups (see Chapter 14). For example, a curb cut is beneficial for people who use wheeled mobility aids (e.g., the full range of wheelchairs, scooters, and walkers) and for parents with strollers and travelers with wheeled luggage (Figure 21-2, A). A close-up reveals that gradual grading and a space or cut wide enough to accommodate several walkers or a large power wheelchair are optimal (Figure 21-2, B). It should be noted that some curb cuts that are not well designed or maintained may be hazardous to people with visual impairments, who may not delineate the edge of the curb cut and the start of a crosswalk. Universal design benefits all age and ability groups by ensuring that the activities of daily living are easy to accomplish rather than being encumbered with challenges.

Total Trip

When considering the total trip, the trip chain, level of service, and user expectations must be taken into account. Every trip has a start and end point, or to be more technical, an origin and a destination.[6] In terms of community or public transportation, an origin and destination can be categorized into four major types:

- Door to door
- Curb to curb
- Stop to stop
- Point to point

Many social service agencies provide transportation services from the door of a personal residence to the door at the destination. In reality this often extends into a building and is better defined as door through door.

Trip Chain

Almost all public transit agencies with regular fixed-route schedules also provide a curb-to-curb service designed to serve people with disabilities unable to use regular transit service because of the nature of their conditions. The reason for this differentiation has to do with operational and insurance policies that are linked to minimum federal standards or requirements. In reality, many individual operators who provide curb-to-curb service will

escort a passenger to the door and those who provide door-to-door service may provide door-through-door service. It is important, however, to understand that when public transit crosses the threshold into a residence, business, or other facility, it represents a level of service that public agencies are not prepared to provide.

Trip Origin: Accessible Housing Component

When a trip's origin and destination are discussed in the terms of the trip chain, both are generally buildings. It is difficult to control access to buildings in the community, although most public or government buildings and all new construction should be accessible as a result of the ADA. One of the challenges for most people with disabilities, however, is finding accessible housing in the first place and then linking that housing with an accessible transportation system. In many cities with well-developed public transportation systems, the price of real estate near stops and stations is proportional to the distance from the transit stop or station.

For many individuals with mobility impairments, housing options are limited both in terms of physical access and affordability. Accessible and affordable housing is even more of a problem for individuals who need temporary or short-term housing as a result of an outpatient therapy program or education and training assignment. For most people who have SCI, life has been changed forever and occasionally these individuals must relocate completely. This relocation can be even more challenging if it also involves a move from a rural to an urban environment. It is important that transportation, and public transportation in particular, be a consideration in the housing decision for people with SCI.

Level of Service

Level of service describes the amount of transit service that is provided in a community or the quality of a certain aspect of transportation performance that is being measured. In general, transportation performance measures range from level of service grade A, that is, uncongested or excellent to level of service grade F, that is, very congested or unacceptable. In the context of this discussion, level of service refers to the amount of transit service that is provided, and it is not a performance measure.

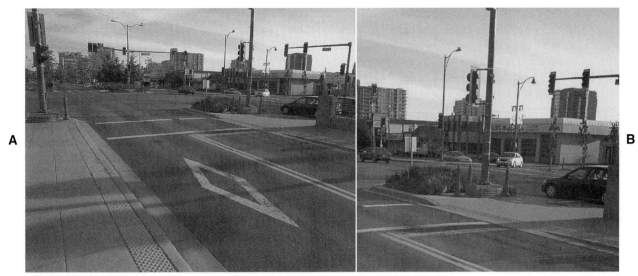

FIGURE 21-2 **A,** Overview of intersection showing wide sidewalks for wheelchair access and curb cuts at cross walks. **B,** Close up of curb cuts.

User Expectations

User expectations for transportation services vary as a function of location. There are many differences related to function of transportation depending on its location in urban, rural, or suburban areas. In general, people residing in rural or less densely populated areas have fewer public transportation options. There are also huge variations between the services available among the 50 states. Some states promote and support accessible public transportation and others are less supportive. Individuals residing in large urban areas that have strong public transit will usually have more flexibility for accessible transportation services, whereas people in rural environments will have very limited access to any form of public transportation and may only have access to private transportation provided by family members, neighbors, or friends.

Trip Purpose

There are various categories of trip purposes: medical and therapy, education or training, work, shopping, family, and recreation. There is often a very strong correlation between the trip purpose, the funding source for the trip or trip payment, and the method or mode that is used to provide that trip for a person with disabilities. Specialized transit services that are provided as a result of a request for a service that requires a relatively high level of assistance are discussed subsequently but may include paratransit, demand responsive, specialized services, dial-a-ride, or flexible schedule services.

Individuals with SCI who do not drive and are not on a public transportation route may need to use specialized transportation services. One of the major drawbacks to these types of service is the return trip, particularly if a medical appointment is delayed. Travelers who use specialized services often have to wait for a return trip for appointments that have an uncertain completion time. This can be a source of frustration when long delays occur because of delayed medical appointments.

Funding methods for the trip may determine how the trip is taken. This may change in the future as the federal agencies that have responsibility for transportation better coordinate transportation services. Currently, there are more than 62 federal agencies that fund transportation services. The Department of Transportation, with its partners at the Departments of Health and Human Services, Labor, and Education, has renewed interest in coordination of public transportation services. Many trips for medical, education, and training are not determined by the user's functional capabilities but rather by the source of funds and local service providers. For example, a client may use paratransit service for a medical or therapy trip but have to use accessible fixed route service, if it is available, when shopping or for recreational trips.

TRANSPORTATION MODE CHOICES
Demand-Responsive Transportation Modes

Demand-responsive services are defined as "a passenger car, van, or bus with fewer than 25 seats operating in response to call from a passenger or his agents to the transit operator, who then dispatches a vehicle to pick up the passenger and transport him to his destinations."[3] A clients with disabilities operation provides vehicles to respond to special need requests and may service several passengers at the same time who are going to separate destinations. They may also contract on a temporary basis to cover a fixed-route or schedule.[3]

In urban environments, demand-responsive service is a parallel service that is often provided by transit operators or contractors and only to people who meet set eligibility requirements as defined by the ADA or the local operator. Often in rural and suburban communities demand-responsive service is the only service that is available for clients with disabilities and it may or may not serve everyone. Such specialized services are generally much more expensive on a per passenger mile basis than are fixed-route transportation services.

Transportation agencies officially will not prioritize trips according to trip purpose, but in reality, where demand for specialized transportation services exceeds the supply, many of these trips are prioritized. In almost all circumstances medical trips are given the highest priority and trips for socialization are given a lower priority. As discussed previously, there is often a strong correlation among the trip purpose, funding source for the trip or trip payment, and method or mode that is used to provide that trip for a person with disabilities.

In most cases, trips that are made on a regular schedule are called subscription trips. These can include trips to school, work, or regular medical or therapy appointments. When an individual uses demand-responsive transportation, these trips often are set up with only one phone call and continue on a regular schedule until they are canceled. These trips are convenient for the rider and also allow the operator to create a regular base of operations. Other trips that are more random without a regular pattern are general paratransit. These trips may be booked the same day, but for many agencies these trips must be scheduled at least 24 hours in advance, and same-day requests are likely to be handled on a space-available basis.

Fixed-Route Transportation Modes

Transportation service that is provided on a daily basis with a fixed schedule and follows a defined route along which vehicles stop to pick up and deliver passengers is known as a fixed-route transportation mode.[3] Each fixed-route trip runs between the same origin and destination.

Fixed-route service also may include variations such as route deviation service, where the vehicles deviate from the fixed route on a discretionary basis to serve a special need. Many regular transit agencies provide mid-day route deviation service to transport seniors to meal sites.

FAMILY OF TRANSPORTATION SERVICES

A large range exists within the family of transportation services from accessible taxis to commuter rail service. Thus it is important to present and discuss the most common types of transit modes and the service characteristics of each. Note that not all these modes are available in all parts of the United States, and some of these modes are new.

Within the family of services there is also a range of requirements for independent travel. An individual's personal level of independence can change as a result of weather, terrain, and time of day; therefore, a choice of transportation options is very important. It can be noted that travel by fixed-route transit requires access to the bus stops, and for many communities this is a major problem. For many people with disabilities, however, paratransit transportation is viewed as a separate, segregated service, whereas fixed-route service is more inclusive and promotes normalization.

The promotion of independence is the goal for the rehabilitation team as well as public transportation providers. In a successful rehabilitation process, there is a large transition from dependence to independence. This is reflected in the need for people to start with transportation that may include the use of a stretcher chair and nonemergency medical transportation to independent travel on fixed-route transit

systems or driving their own vehicles. For many individuals these transitions may take months or even years to accomplish. Since the passage of the ADA, many transit operators require that users qualify or be eligible for demand-responsive service. Unfortunately, many of these operators do not consider that eligibility can change as a function of weather, trip origin, or destination. Many transit agencies have embarked on passenger assistance and training programs that help users of demand-responsive service transition to accessible fixed-route service.

Demand-Responsive Transportation Services

The modes of transportation provided by demand-responsive operations range from nonemergency medical transportation in cabulances up to 20 to 25 passenger vans. Cabulances may be special-purpose vehicles that are used for nonemergency medical transport or an ambulance that is not being used for emergency medical transport. These vehicles can accommodate stretchers and chairs and generally only one or two passengers at a time. The cost per ride for this form of transport is the most expensive form of demand-responsive service.

Accessible taxis are an important member of the demand-responsive family of services. New taxis are being made to accommodate wheelchairs and other mobility aids and are often available for after-hours and weekend transportation (Figure 21-3). In general, accessible taxis are special-purpose vehicles or adapted vans operated by regular taxi operators under contract to transit companies to provide special transportation services. Both cabulances and accessible taxis have limited capacity that make the cost per ride of each service higher than for other higher capacity modes.

Although individuals who want to use ADA paratransit services must go through an eligibility process, service has increased and improved substantially since its implementation in 1991 (Figure 21-4).[7] Perhaps the biggest difficulty to ensuring its demand-response promise is that, as service improves, more people want to use it.[8]

Demand-responsive service is provided by use of vans, shuttle buses, and small buses that are equipped with lifts or ramps. In some communities, passenger cars are also part of the fleet of vehicles and require that mobility aid users transfer to a regular seat. It should be noted that all these vehicles are generally lighter than 20,000 pounds gross vehicle weight and their performance characteristics are very different from those of the vehicles used in fixed-route transit operations. The lighter weight of these vehicles together with the transmission and braking systems require that all mobility aids must be properly secured with an approved wheelchair securement system and that all passengers should be provided with approved passenger restraint systems (see Chapter 20).[9,10]

Fixed-Route Transportation Services

Accessible fixed-route services are generally considered curb to curb. For the total trip chain to be accessible, the civil infrastructure that includes walkways and sidewalks that connect to the trip origin and destination must also be accessible. There is a hierarchy of infrastructure that is associated with these services, which

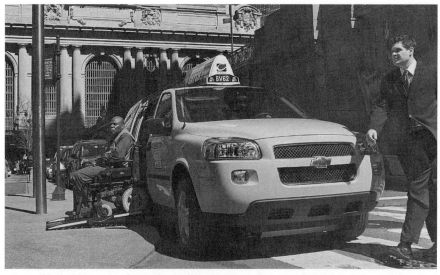

FIGURE 21-3 Accessible taxi (Courtesy of United Spinal Association, Jackson Heights, NY, and photographer, Emile Wamsteker.)

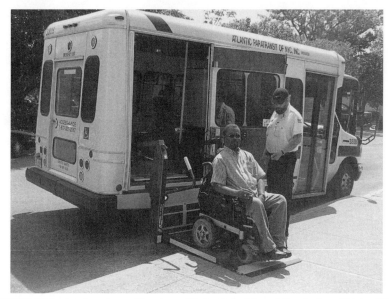

FIGURE 21-4 Paratransit van. (Courtesy of United Spinal Association, Jackson Heights, NY.)

ranges from an unimproved bus stop to a multimodal passenger terminal. Infrastructure, stops, and terminals are discussed later.

Note that within each transportation mode there are subsets of vehicle types. For example, fixed-route bus transit service may include 30-, 35-, 40-, or 45-foot low- or high-floor transit buses, double-decker buses, and articulated transit buses. The main difference between a low-floor and high-floor bus is that an accessible high-floor bus has a lift at the front or rear door (Figure 21-5, *A*) and a low-floor bus has a ramp (Figure 21-5, *B* and *C*). Many transit agencies are only purchasing low-floor vehicles because these are more popular with older passengers. Low-floor transit vehicles, however, may not be used in areas that do not have sidewalks because the slope on the ramp is much too steep to be accessible for people who use wheeled mobility aids.[11]

Articulated buses are typically 60 feet long and articulate or rotate in the center (Figure 21-6, *A*). The wheelchair securement area is usually in the front portion of the vehicle,

where the ride quality is better as well. Most new articulated buses are low-floor models with ramps located at the front door. Traditional buses may have front or back door ramps or lifts (Figure 21-6, *B*).

There also are new designs for transit buses that will be coming on line as cities develop bus rapid-transit (BRT) systems. This service usually includes operational amenities that are found on rail transit modes. One of the key distinguishing features of BRT is off-vehicle fare collection, which works well in urban rail services (Figure 21-7, *A* to *C*). By removing fare collection from the vehicle, all the vehicle doors can be used to load and unload passengers. This single feature can affect the design and operation of the vehicles and related infrastructure. BRT is a useful form of bus transit in transit corridors that require high-volume bus service but do not have the population density to support investment in light rail infrastructure. In many cities, BRT is regarded as a bridging technology that will

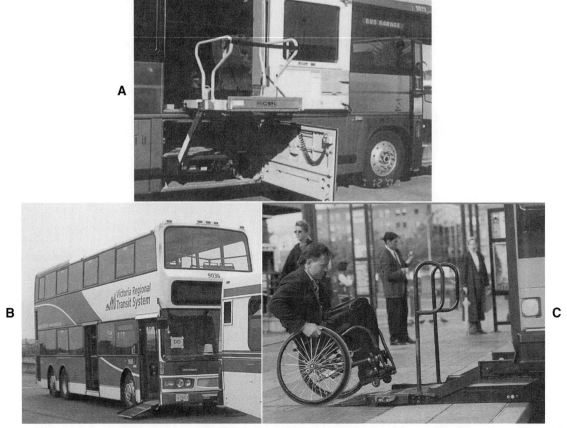

FIGURE 21-5 BRT vehicle that has doors thar open on both side if the vehicle. **A,** High floor bus lift accessing an over the road bus. **B,** Low-floor bus ramp. **C,** Low-floor lift with person in wheelchair boarding bus. (**A** and **B,** Courtesy National Center for Accessible Transportation, Corvallis, OR. **C,** From Pellerito JM Jr: *Driver rehabilitation and community mobility: principles and practice,* St Louis, 2006, Elsevier Mosby, p 309.*)*

be replaced in the long term (i.e., 20 to 50 years) with higher-capacity light rail technologies.

Urban Rail Technologies

Urban rail technologies range from modern street cars and light rail systems to heavy rail subways and commuter rail systems. The extent of usefulness of rail technology is related to population and land use density, urban form, and the overall maturity of the urban area. A street car is a single unit vehicle, whereas light rail systems usually consist of two vehicles or a married pair that are linked together as multivehicle trains. In general, as the rail systems get heavier there are more cars in the train.

Many of the older or legacy systems were constructed long before there was any consideration about access by people who use wheeled mobility devices. All newly constructed urban rail systems are designed to be fully accessible, and the new vehicles or rolling stock are also designed and constructed to permit full access by people who use wheelchairs. The operating characteristics of rail transit in general do not necessarily require the use of mobility aid securement systems. Street cars and light rail vehicles, however, operate on the streets and should be equipped with securement equipment. Light rail and heavy rail systems that operate exclusively on isolated guideways do not require mobility aid securement devices.

This is because of the mass of the vehicle, the right of way, and the train's operating characteristics.

Intercity Public Transportation Services

Intercity public transportation is usually provided by commuter rail, Amtrak, over-the-road buses (OTRB), passenger ferry systems, and air travel. Intercity public transportation is now supposed to be fully accessible, and commuter rail station access in Vancouver, British Columbia, provides a good example (Figure 21-8, *A* and *B*). The reality, however, is that in many parts of the United States it is very challenging to travel from one urban area to another by accessible surface transportation.

Amtrak

Amtrak is a national company, but there are significant regional differences in the age, design, and level of accessibility of the equipment. All of Amtrak's passenger rolling stock is accessible. There are, however, differences in the vehicles depending on the region. From Chicago west, Amtrak operates bilevel and single-level vehicles that are equipped with on-board ramps. In the Northeast corridor, most of the platforms are high level and there are bridging ramps. In the east and south wayside lifts that are station based are used to access the trains from low platforms (Figure 21-9).

One of the disadvantages of the bilevel trains is that only the first level is accessible. On the new Acela and Cascadia high-speed

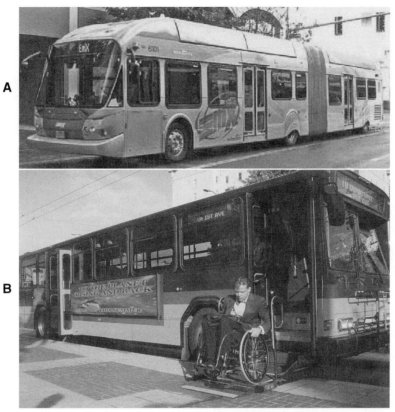

FIGURE 21-6 Fixed route transit. **A,** Articulated bus rapid transit vehicle. **B,** Low-floor vehicle with person in wheelchair disembarking. (**A,** Courtesy National Center for Accessible Transportation, Corvallis, OR. **B,** From Pellerito JM Jr: *Driver rehabilitation and community mobility: principles and practice*, St. Louis, 2006, Elsevier Mosby, p. 519.)

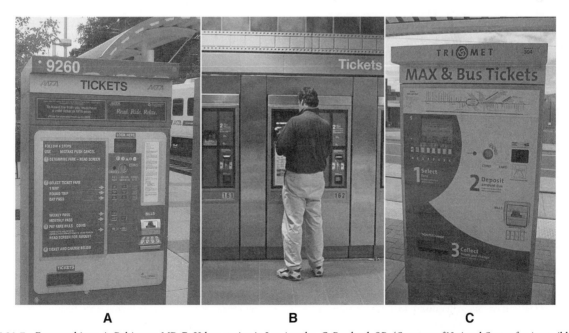

FIGURE 21-7 Fare machines. **A,** Baltimore, MD. **B,** Urban station in Los Angeles. **C,** Portland, OR. (Courtesy of National Center for Accessible Transportation, Corvallis, OR.)

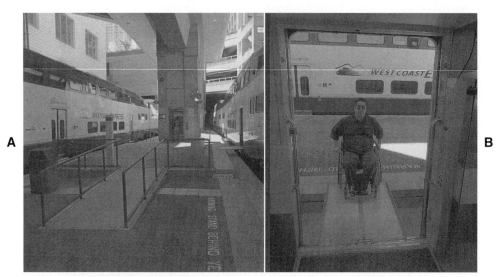

FIGURE 21-8 Intercity rail transit. **A,** Access ramps at Vancouver, BC, station. **B,** Individual in wheelchair coming on board train. (Courtesy of National Center for Accessible Transportation, Corvallis, OR.)

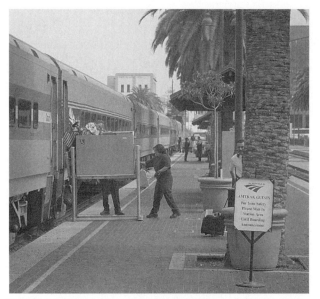

FIGURE 21-9 Wheelchair lift at Amtrak station in San Diego. (Courtesy of National Center for Accessible Transportation, Corvallis, OR.)

rail service that runs on the east and west coasts, respectively, the new trains are very accessible for people who use wheeled mobility aids. Amtrak maintains a special Web site for travelers with disabilities and special needs (www.Amtrak.com/plan/accessibility.html).

Over-the-Road Buses

Since 1998, OTRB have been required to be accessible. Federal regulations, however, only require access to the vehicle and specify mobility aid securement and passenger restraint. The on-board restrooms do not have to be accessible as long as the bus stops every hour because it is assumed that the restrooms at the regular bus stops meet the ADA requirements for accessibility. OTRB operators must provide accessible service when requests are made 48 hours in advance of the need.[12]

Passenger Ferry Service

In cities such as San Francisco, Seattle, New York, Boston, and Vancouver, British Columbia, passenger ferry service is an integral part of the public transportation system. There are many physical challenges to providing accessible passenger ferry service in areas where there are tidal effects. In Vancouver, the SeaBus has been accessible from the beginning. The actual ferries are completely barrier free (Figure 21-10, *A*), and the docks are accessed by elevators and long ramps. The ramp is designed so that even in extreme tidal events it is still accessible. In addition, ingress and egress paths have been designed for maximum universal mobility (Figure 21-10, *B*).

Other cities have made progress in retrofitting existing infrastructure to improve access to passenger ferry service. New retrofits are also addressing many problematic on-board circulation barriers to provide accessible access to restrooms as well as all areas of the ship.[13]

Air Travel

In the United States, air travel is among the most important intercity travel services, especially for trips that are over 500 miles. Aircraft can be categorized according to size: wide-body aircraft have two aisles; narrow-body aircraft have a single aisle and, in general, have more than 100 seats; and regional aircraft usually have fewer than 100 seats. Wide-body aircraft are more accessible than the narrow-body aircraft, which are considerably more accessible than regional aircraft.

The aviation industry is currently struggling for economic survival, and as a result more and more trip segments are provided by smaller regional aircraft that are much more energy efficient to operate. Narrow aisle chairs are designed to move along the aisle easily between rows of seats (Figure 21-11, *A*) and are sometimes used to board individuals with SCI on smaller aircraft (Figure 21-11, *B*). Many challenges related to air travel for people with SCI include the following:

- Transfer to aisle chair for boarding aircraft
- Use of on-board aisle chairs for access to lavatory
- Care and stowage of personal wheelchairs

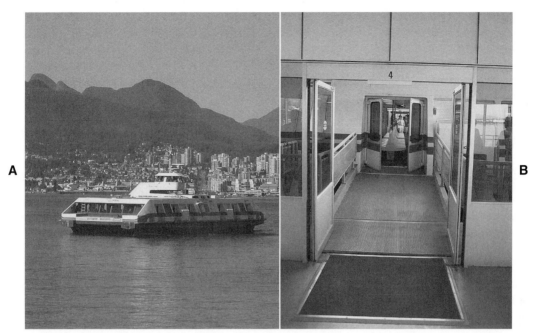

FIGURE 21-10   SeaBus in Vancouver, BC. **A,** A fully accessible ferry pulls into the harbor. **B,** Carefully designed universal exit ramps to accommodate walkers, strollers, and wheelchairs. (Courtesy National Center for Accessible Transportation, Corvallis, OR.)

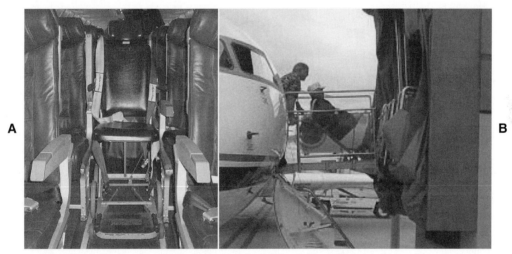

FIGURE 21-11   Air travel can be challenging for individuals who use wheelchairs. **A,** The aisle chair is designed to move between seats in the narrow aisles. **B,** Individual being wheeled from the plane on an aisle chair and up ramp into the terminal. (Courtesy National Center for Accessible Transportation, Corvallis, OR.)

Airline Web sites include detailed information for travelers with disabilities, but airlines also like to talk directly with customers with special needs to make sure that their requests for assistance are arranged appropriately (Client's Perspective: Successful Air Travel With Spinal Cord Injury). Travelers with disabilities should call 24 to 48 hours ahead of travel to confirm arrangements for special service requests. This does not guarantee that the trip will go seamlessly because difficulties can always arise at transfer points. Seasoned travelers with disabilities will often try to arrange nonstop flights, to help simplify travel arrangements and reduce the amount of special handling of their wheelchairs. Some rehabilitation facilities work directly with airports and airlines to arrange for air travel training sessions for their clients to practice accessing the airport

and aircraft. At Hartsfield International Airport in Atlanta, the airlines and airport, in cooperation with local rehabilitation centers, coordinate a travel training program for rehabilitation clients on a regular basis. This program has been so successful that it has been implemented at other large airports. Such training sessions help to build traveler confidence and provide excellent opportunities for airport and airlines staff to get to know the special needs of the traveler without the time pressure of an actual air travel schedule.

Personal Vehicles

The goal of rehabilitation is to maximize independence, which often includes preparing the client to drive an adapted personal vehicle. Accessible personal transportation can be the key to community access, especially when community-based public transportation is not available. Adapted vehicles are as personalized as mobility aids. If a person with SCI is going to transfer to drive a car, then it is necessary that he can both access the vehicle and store the mobility aid independently. Manual wheelchair users who drive their own vehicles transfer to the vehicle seat and, therefore, enter and leave the vehicle on the driver's or left side (Figure 21-12, *A*). Similarly, if a person is going to drive a van from his mobility aid, then it is important that the wheelchair can be secured and can also withstand the dynamic forces that the vehicle and driving impose on it. Many power mobility aid users who drive their own vehicles drive from their wheelchair and enter and leave their vehicles by a ramp or lift on the passenger or right side (Figure 21-12, *B*).

There are similar arguments for individuals who use public transportation, and chief among them is that the mobility aid be maneuverable enough to access the transportation vehicle and strong enough to be secured on the transit vehicle. It is also important to note that there should not be any differentiation in auto insurance related to the use of hand controls; however, prior accident and claims history could affect insurance rates. It is important for the rehabilitation team to consider the client's transportation options when

prescribing mobility devices (Clinical Note: Considerations to Ensure a Wheelchair Appropriate to Client's Modes of Transportation).

Location, size, and availability of accessible parking are essential elements related to driving adapted vehicles (Figure 21-13). It is important that there are a variety of accessible parking spaces that accommodate adapted vans and personal automobiles. The inventory of accessible parking spaces should always include accessible spaces that allow people who use wheelchairs to safely access their vehicles from either side. It is also important that parking regulations are enforced to ensure that only authorized users use accessible parking spaces. In addition, individuals with SCI who drive need to think ahead about vehicle maintenance and road-side emergency plans (Client's Perspective: Vehicle Breakdowns).

DRIVER REHABILITATION EVALUATION PROCESS

Independent access to the community is the direct goal for those involved in a driver rehabilitation program (DRP). Advancements in technology have made it possible for more people with SCI to cross the threshold to independence through mobility by allowing many who were once considered nondriving candidates to drive their own vehicles. A person can access a DRP through the referral by a physician on his rehabilitation team. Programs developed for clients with SCI consist of one of four evaluation categories:

- Nondriver transport consultation by using a van
- Van transport evaluation with vehicle modification to include future driving

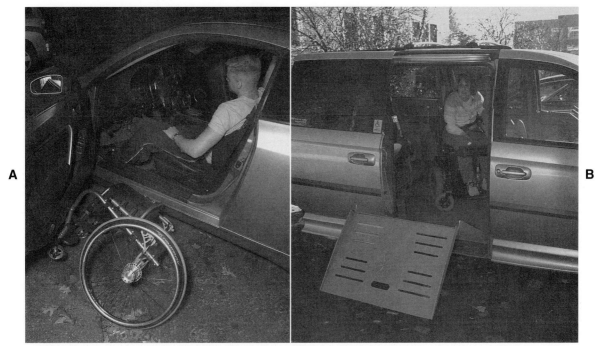

FIGURE 21-12 Personal vehicles. **A,** Man has transferred into his car seat and gets ready to break down and load rigid frame wheelchair across his lap; the car's hand controls give its interior the feel of a cockpit. **B,** Woman with C6 SCI raises ramp after entering her modified van and begins to turn her power wheelchair so that it is in position to be secured with her EZ-lock system.

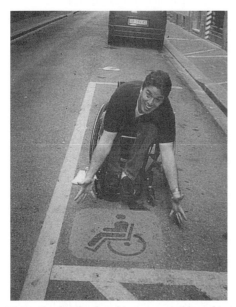

FIGURE 21-13 Eureka! I've found it—an accessible parking space on a street in Europe.

- Van transport evaluation for full driving considerations
- Sedan transport evaluation for full driving considerations

Each of these evaluations can be broken down into several categories for individualized assessment to customize the assessment for each client as it pertains to the overall objective. The capacity to independently access the community for social, vocational, and family-oriented activities is a privilege many take for granted. It is second nature for a majority of people to jump in their cars and drive to these functions. Medical compromise

such as SCI often hinders the ability to participate in community events. SCI and its subsequent level of disability alter current driving status in both access and licensure issues.

Most comprehensive rehabilitation facilities include a DRP as a part of the team treatment approach. At varying intervals of the rehabilitation process, consultation with a driver rehabilitation specialist (DRS) familiar with SCI can help clarify transportation issues as they arise. In all instances, it is imperative that a comprehensive driver evaluation series be administered and adhered to. A DRS certified through the Association of Driver Rehabilitation Specialists is best qualified to work with the medical team and mobility equipment dealer toward a satisfactory outcome: enabling the person with SCI renewed access to the community via his own vehicle. Table 21-1 is an abbreviated overview of a DRP for each of the four vehicle evaluations.

Evaluation
Basic Interview
The DRS uses this interview to gather personal information from the client such as name, address, telephone number, and driver's license number and status as applicable. SCI level and type are discussed in relation to driving being a viable option for the candidate. Medications also are addressed to assess whether they will affect the individual's capacity to operate a motor vehicle in any adverse way. In addition, spasm and seizure information may have licensing implications in some states. In New Jersey, for example, several scenarios exist. In most instances, an individual must be free from recurrent seizures for 1 year to be considered a driving candidate from a legal standpoint. A singular seizure at the time of trauma or a medication-induced seizure, however, may be waived through the Division

TABLE 21-1 | Base Evaluation for Each Driver's Training Category

	Nondriver Consultation Using a Van	Van: Transport Evaluation With Vehicle Modification	Van: Full Driving Considerations	Sedan: Full Driving Considerations
Basic interview	X	X	X	X
Clinical assessment		D	X	X
Seating assessment	X	X	X	X
Static behind the wheel		D	X	X
Dynamic behind the wheel			X	X
Training categories			X	X
Licensure			X	X
Equipment prescription	X	X	X	X
Transportation alternatives	X	X		
Follow-up services	O	X	X	X
Intervention alternatives	X	X	X	X

X, All instances; O, client option; D, determined by case.

of Motor Vehicles Medical Fitness Unit. The attending physician can facilitate this by verifying, in writing, that the client had been seizure free since the event. Specific requirements for each state should be explored.

Clinical Assessment

Clinical assessment has been shown to predict crash-related risk and possible failure during community on-road evaluations.[14] After it is determined the client is a potential driving candidate, a member of the DRP team provides a thorough assessment by using a series of standardized tests that document visual skills, reaction time, and physical responses. Visual assessment normally includes testing for acuity, depth perception, useful field of view, color perception, and other occulomotor skills. Some states use visual acuity as the only requirement for licensure whereas many others include a field of view requirement as well. The client's physical status, such as muscle strength, active range of motion (AROM), spasticity, trunk balance, and transfer skills are assessed. Reaction time is tested using the client's most reliable extremity. Results of this assessment help to determine which extremity is most appropriate for operating primary control systems that include acceleration, braking, and steering.

In most instances, where head injury is not indicated, a cognitive and perceptual evaluation may be minimized or eliminated altogether. In instances where cognitive and perceptual deficits are indicated, such as seen with a dual diagnosis of SCI and traumatic brain injury, a more in-depth assessment is administered. Areas of assessment may include processing speed, memory, concentration, attention to detail, judgment, problem solving, and decision making. On completion of the clinical assessment, the client's prognosis is determined and his motivation level is discussed. The DRP member then makes recommendations regarding driving and the client's long-term goals.

Seating Assessment

Seating choices coincide with the client's clinical assessment and long-term driving goals. The primary DPR goal is to ensure that the mobility device will interface with the proposed driving scenario. Manual wheelchair considerations that may need to be addressed include frame type, seating systems, weight of original chair, weight of chair with tiedown hardware, and the client's ability to propel, fold, disassemble, and load the chair into a sedan.

When a scooter is being considered, it is important to assess the client's ability to transfer from the scooter to the driver's seat, the ability to secure the scooter for safe transit before transfer, the ability to break down the scooter, the ability to operate an assistive loading device, and the ability to ambulate to the driver's station.

Seating system and positioning for a power wheelchair includes lateral supports, chest straps, chest harnessing, securement lock functions, and clearances of footrests and battery supports. In all instances, the client's height when seated in his mobility device and the width of the chair will affect his ability to enter and egress from a vehicle without modifications to existing clearances.

Program Stages

Static Behind-the-Wheel Assessment

After reviewing the results of the previous assessments, the DRS and client make their first contact with an actual vehicle. Whether the client is transferring to a sedan or driving from a wheelchair, entry and egress issues are always addressed first. Independence in this function is essential, or other avenues must be pursued to facilitate this independence. Positioning in the driver's station, appropriate interface with the intended controls, and preparation to drive follows. At this point steering options are explored, starting from simple (i.e., power steering) to more complex (i.e., digital or unilever) systems until an appropriate interface is achieved (Figure 21-14). The same is completed for accelerator and braking. On completion of the primary control interface decision, secondary controls such as headlamps, wipers, horn, and dimmer switch are evaluated for independent activation.[15] These trials will result in an idea of what may or may not need to be controlled by a remote unit in the client's vehicle of choice.

Driving Simulation

Computer technology has dramatically improved and made simulated learning equipment interfaces realistic and interactive. These simulators can now alter the environment in response to the driver's evaluation such as turning, acceleration, and braking (Figure 21-15, *A*). Such an interactive approach offers a unique opportunity for a driver's evaluation to take place along any point in the continuum of the rehabilitation process (Figure 21-15, *B*). Driving simulators offer less expensive and restricted ways to practice before venturing into the community environment. This is particularly useful in clients with SCI where hand controls require new learning skills. Use of simulators also causes less stress, allowing clients low-risk practice while they build confidence in preparation for driving on the road.

Although driving simulators do not replace traditional methods of evaluation, including dynamic behind-the-wheel driving, they can provide a risk-free opportunity for a client to demonstrate his abilities. The results provide clinicians with objective information on which to base appropriate instruction including

on-road driving. When a client is unable to perform well with the simulator, the client is more likely to understand that he is not yet ready for the open road.[16] Still, a driving simulator is only one part of a comprehensive driver rehabilitation program because more research is needed to demonstrate its validity in predicting on-road performance.

Dynamic Behind-the-Wheel Assessment

After decisions about the appropriate interfaces with primary controls, wheelchair securement, and occupant restraint have been made (see Chapter 20), the element of motion is added. When dynamics are introduced to the formula, it is not uncommon to fine tune the initial setup. Often systems that looked appropriate statically will not produce the desired results at higher speeds. A client who is properly interfaced with primary and secondary systems must be capable of operating any one function at any given time in all traffic densities and scenarios. This can only be fully addressed during dynamic driver training.

Training Strategies

The training process fully focuses on the client's trunk stability and endurance as well as operation of systems and unit control. In addition, the tasks of basic driving skills through comprehensive defensive driving patterns must also be addressed and emphasized. On-road driving begins in low-impact settings such as parking lots and progresses through city and expressway situations.[17] Some training is conducted in facility vehicles with follow-up training conducted in the client's newly adapted vehicle. Activities include visiting drive-through windows, toll booths, and service stations for fuel fill-ups and may present interesting challenges for some drivers with SCI.

Licensing

In a majority of states, a driver must possess a classified license to drive a vehicle adapted or modified to meet a medical need. For example, to gain medical clearance in the state of New Jersey, a

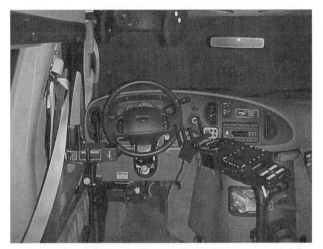

FIGURE 21-14 Full console. (From Pellerito JM Jr: *Driver rehabilitation and community mobility: principles and practice*, St. Louis, 2006, Elsevier Mosby, Fig. 11-10, p. 250.).

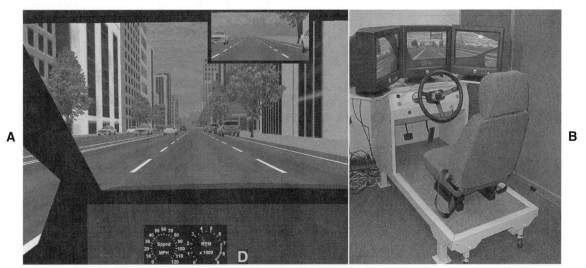

FIGURE 21-15 Driving simulation. **A,** STISIM Drive computerized graphic imagery. **B,** STISIM three-monitor system. (From Pellerito JM Jr: *Driver rehabilitation and community mobility: principles and practice*, St. Louis, 2006, Elsevier Mosby, Figs. 10-2 and 10-3, p. 224, 229. Courtesy Systems Technology, Hawthorne, CA.)

driver must present himself to the licensing authorities and pass both vision and road test requirements. After passing these examinations, he is classified with a number 5 code with an attached endorsement. This endorsement indicates the type of equipment he is classified to operate. Failure to obtain the proper classified license can result in loss of driving privileges and loss of insurance coverage and incurs a safety risk to the driver and others in the community.

Handicap parking privileges may be obtained through application in collaboration with the client's physician to the state Division of Motor Vehicles (Box 21-1).

Equipment Prescription

When the client has completed training and licensure requirements, the DRS will develop a final prescription for vehicle modification and adaptive driving controls that best fit the client's needs. This prescription becomes the basis on which the final product will be built, and the vendor charged with building the vehicle must strictly adhere to its specifications. The prescription eliminates the requirement for the client to pay sales tax on the modifications and adaptations applied to the base vehicle.

The DRS also continuously explores base vehicle options with the client. When the purchase of the base vehicle is considered, there are certain standard and optional features that may be required. Specifications will vary from client to client and similar diagnoses can produce very different requirements. Before purchasing a base vehicle, it is essential that a person with SCI consult with a DRS to prevent costly mistakes.

Transportation Alternatives

In instances in which an individual is not considered to be a driving candidate, alternative means of transportation will be explored. When caregivers will be present, a vehicle can be modified or adapted for transportation use only, but this can be costly. In situations where an individual may be independent by using mobility assistive technology, mass transit may be used. Services such as Red Cross, Access Link, County Paratransit, and others also can be used to access the community.

Follow-Up Services

Follow-up services are initially conducted at the adapted van vendor's place of business. It normally includes initial fittings in the client's vehicle of choice, subsequent fittings before van completion, and a final fitting at completion. During these phases of construction, vehicle checks for adherence to prescription can be conducted. After completion of the vehicle, a final check is conducted with the client and is conducted much like a static and dynamic behind-the-wheel sequence. If needed, subsequent training with the client's new vehicle is conducted as well.

Intervention Alternatives

At any time during the program stages, a client may be referred to alternative rehabilitation services. Normally this occurs when a problem arises in the projected driving pathway that can be corrected through another rehabilitation intervention (Clinical Note: Intervention Alternatives That May Occur During Driver Retraining Program). In all cases, these referrals are suggestions, and the client's medical team must deem them appropriate before they can be carried out.

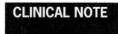

CLINICAL NOTE **Intervention Alternatives That May Occur During Driver Retraining Program**

- Referral to occupational therapy for transfer training, wheelchair management, and loading techniques
- Referral to physical and occupational therapy to work on muscle strength, AROM, and trunk balance
- Referral to wheelchair seating clinic to solve deficiencies in the mobility assistive device
- Referral to vision clinic to determine whether observed driving pattern inconsistencies are visually oriented

Driving Considerations Related to Level of Spinal Cord Injury

Individuals with SCI have differing capabilities within similar injury levels. The following descriptions are based on the American Spinal Injury Association (ASIA) scale of complete SCI for cervical-level injuries.

Above C4 to C5

A client with an injury about C4 to C5 will, in most cases, not be a viable driving candidate. He will require a van transporter evaluation in helping secure an appropriate vehicle to meet client, family, and caregiver needs. Consideration will be given to the client's location in the vehicle to maximize his ability to participate in events during the ride. Entry and egress clearances, as well as wheelchair securement and occupant restraints, are important issues.

C4 to C5

An individual with a C4 to C5 level of injury will likely drive a minivan or a full-size van from a power wheelchair. Trunk stability will be a major issue with seating systems; chest straps and lateral supports will likely be used as well. Entry and egress issues will likely involve floor cuts that will bring the client's eye line to the level suitable for appropriate driving. Primary control operation will be on the high-tech side, including power-assisted controls for acceleration, braking, and steering. Steering modifications may include removal of the steering column and the use of a steering interface on a horizontal rather than a vertical plane. New high-tech digital steering systems can be supplied, allowing for the original column, wheel, and air bag to remain intact. All secondary controls for headlamps, horn, heater, and air conditioner will probably require remote locations. Consoles consisting of membrane-activated switches, auditory signals, or voice activation can be strategically located, allowing for ease in activation. Vehicle modification and driving adaptation costs can range from $50,000 to $80,000.

C6

A client with a C6 injury will usually drive a minvan or a full-size van from a power wheelchair; however, he may drive from a manual wheelchair or, in rare instances, a transfer seat. The majority of clients will require high-tech interventions in the form of reduced effort for primary control operation. System reductions are completed by qualified mobility equipment dealers. Mobility equipment dealers associated with National Mobility Equipment Dealers Association are rated for their qualifications to perform modification and adaptation tasks and should be given primary consideration for the work. A client with this injury level may be capable of operating a mechanical hand control for acceleration and braking with system reduction (Figure 21-16). Costs for mechanical controls range from $500 to $800 versus a power-assisted control from $8500. Some original equipment secondary controls may be accessible to the client, lessening the complexity of required remote controls.

C7

More individuals with C7 lesions will be seen in vans rather than in sedans. A sedan becomes a viable option for a person who can load his manual wheelchair independently or with the use of a power-assistive device. To use a car top wheelchair carrier (see Figure 8-30), a client's chair must have a foldable frame and easily removed seating systems. In many instances, legrests must also be removable to store a chair in a car top container. These storage containers are electrically controlled, requiring the client to have the capacity to assemble and disassemble the chair and assist with its folding and unfolding.

In most instances, standard power steering and braking resistances will be suitable with use of mechanical hand controls. For steering purposes, a person with limited hand function may benefit form a spinner knob or V-grip device (Figure 21-17, A and B).

Many clients using a van will more than likely access the driver's station by using a six-way power transfer seat rather than driving from a wheelchair. This seat base will move front to back and up and down and rotate 90 degrees to assist the individual's independent transfers (Figure 21-18).

C8 and Below

A client with a C8 and below injury should easily access a sedan by using standard resistances in primary control functions. The client's trunk stability is less of an issue but still must be evaluated. Wheelchair management issues are still

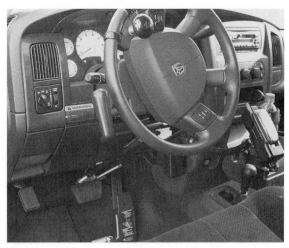

FIGURE 21-16 Hand controls. (From Pellerito JM Jr: *Driver rehabilitation and community mobility: principles and practice*, St. Louis, 2006, Elsevier Mosby, Fig. 11-7, p 246.)

present; however, use of power assistive devices and manual loading become less cumbersome (see Figures 21-12, *A*, and 8-29, *A* and *B*).

BARRIERS TO TRANSPORTATION AND COMMUNITY ACCESS

Regardless of whether an individual is able to access his community by driving a vehicle, there may be other barriers to transportation and community access. Every community has its own personality and unique characteristics, which influence accessibility to transportation and the community. These are referred to as soft barriers, such as local politics and attitudes, and hard barriers, including climate and topography.

It is much harder to make a community on a hillside accessible, and it is impossible to change the weather! At the same time there are communities built on steep hills that have made accessibility a priority. An example of this is downtown Seattle, Washington. Other communities embrace and welcome people with disabilities—two examples of which are Berkeley, California, and Eugene, Oregon.

Among the most limiting factors for people who use mobility aids and are public transportation dependent are the service hours and the service area. There are almost no transit systems that operate 24/7, so the question then becomes: what are the other options? Many smaller communities have limited available transit and no alternative or accessible taxi service. For communities that do have accessible taxi service, operators often charge extra drop fees for people who use mobility aids or have service restrictions that make taxi service outrageously expensive.

In addition, wheeled mobility aids are constantly changing and many new devices are not transportable either because they cannot be secured or because they are too large to fit on a vehicle lift or ramp. For individuals on fixed incomes, the cost of transportation is another barrier to community access. Some of trips for medical appointments, therapy treatment, and education may be paid for by insurance or

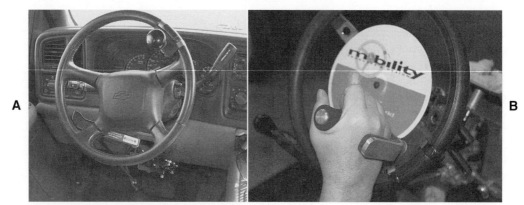

FIGURE 21-17 Steering aids. **A,** Spinner knob. **B,** V-grip device. (From Pellerito JM Jr: *Driver rehabilitation and community mobility: principles and practice*, St. Louis, 2006, Elsevier Mosby, Figs. 11-1 & 11-2, p. 243.)

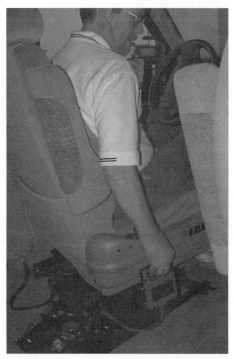

FIGURE 21-18 Six-way power transfer seat. (From Pellerito JM Jr: *Driver rehabilitation and community mobility: principles and practice*, St. Louis, 2006, Elsevier Mosby, Fig. 11-9, p. 248.)

other sources, but trips that improve the quality of life such as family visits and recreation are not covered and may be too expensive.

Full access to transportation and the community means that every link on the trip chain must be accessible and affordable. This includes the civic infrastructure, public buildings, parking, and bus stops and all the walkways and sidewalks that link the community together. The removal of the hard barriers can be accomplished by a community's commitment to and enforcement of a universal and barrier-free design.

Soft barriers—attitudinal and political barriers—are often more difficult to overcome. A young man who sustained a T4 spinal cord injury 5 years ago was recently interviewed about accessible transportation and community access. His

first comment was, "I don't use public transportation because I don't like the way people look at me." During his early rehabilitation process, he used a cabulance and then tried a dial-a-ride service. He did not like the dial-a-ride service because most of the other passengers were older adults and he really wanted to be independent. For a very short time he used fixed-route public transportation. Now he drives his own vehicle. This young man felt undignified traveling on public transportation and he did not like being stared at by other passengers, which only reinforced his self-consciousness. He is very typical of people with an SCI who transition from dependence to fully independent transportation.

ACCESSIBLE COMMUNITY INFRASTRUCTURE
Bus Stops

Basic accessible community infrastructure includes rights of way such as sidewalks, walkways, and curb cuts. For the total trip to be fully accessible, the path of travel to and from the vehicles must be free of obstacles. This includes bus stops, stations, terminals, and parking lots.[18,19] An accessible bus stop does not just include the stopping area but also the access right of way to and from the bus stop (Figure 21-19, *A*). A bus stop is accessible if a transit vehicle's ramp or lift can be safely deployed and accessed safely by people using wheeled mobility aids. In technical terms, an accessible bus stop also includes the pavement infrastructure or pad where the bus stops. The pavement in this area needs to be reinforced to accommodate the resting weight of the bus. A continuously accessible path also needs to be available to and from the bus stop (Figure 21-19, *B*). In addition, bus route and schedule information must be accessible for people standing as well as those seated in wheelchairs (Figure 21-19, *C*).[20]

In areas where there are no paved sidewalks, a high-floor bus is often more accessible and safer for people who use wheeled mobility aids. The ramp on low-floor buses is designed to bridge the area between the top of the sidewalk and not the street level. The location of the bus stop is also important. A good rule of thumb is to locate a bus stop where traffic conflicts are minimized. This means locating a bus stop on the same side of the street as the trip destination, or locating bus stops in a way that minimizes the number of streets a person must cross in transferring from one bus to another.

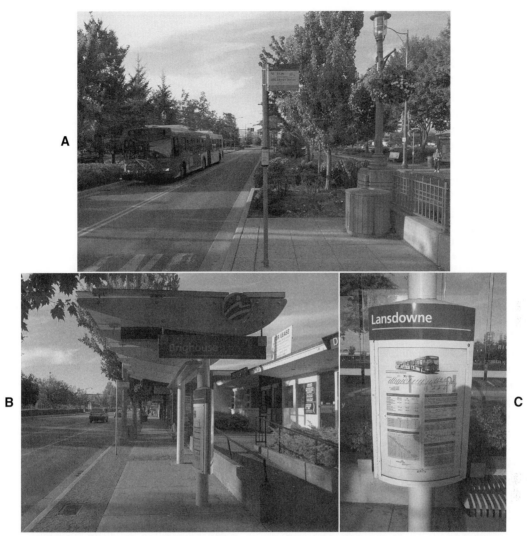

FIGURE 21-19 Community Transit Center in Vancouver, British, Columbia. **A,** Specially designed areas for buses to pick up passengers with wide sidewalks, clearly marked cross walks, and curb cuts designed to accommodate manual and power wheelchairs. **B,** Transit station with ramp access, kiosks, and universally designed friendly route information at eye level for people who are standing but easy to read from a seated position as well. **C,** Close-up of route information sign. (Courtesy National Center for Accessible Transportation, Corvallis, OR.)

As new intersections are designed and new traffic signals are introduced, all these intersections should be equipped with accessible pedestrian technologies.[21] In general, an accessible pedestrian signal refers to the technologies associated with the pedestrian button and walk signal indicators. These technologies are designed to make it easier for people with visual impairments to navigate the right of way.[22,23] There are new standards for the design and construction of the pedestrian right of way to make the infrastructure accessible to users of wheeled mobility aids.[24]

Passenger Drop-Off Areas

It is important that transit facilities are equipped with passenger drop-off areas, sometimes called "Kiss and Ride," to permit the safe transfer of people who use wheeled mobility aids. The drop-off area should be as close to the facility entrances and elevators as possible and the path from the drop-off site to the terminal should also be fully accessible. Park-and-ride facilities also should provide a mix of van-accessible and car-accessible parking spaces. All parking spaces should permit safe access and egress to and from the vehicle. Parallel parking should be avoided because the driver who accesses the vehicle from the driver's side (i.e., left side of the vehicle) would have to transfer into and out of a mobility aid in traffic. The path from the accessible parking spaces should minimize conflicts with moving traffic and should also be located as close as possible to the terminal facility.

Transit Amenities: Kiosks, Smart Cards, Automatic Teller Machines

In the electronic age, more and more transit agencies are using fare machines (see Figure 21-7), electronic information kiosks, automatic teller or transaction machines, and vending machines. As new technologies emerge, it is important that all these devices are installed for use by people who use wheelchairs or have visual impairments. Each of these devices should be universally accessible. In transit facilities that use turnstiles as part of the ticketing process, it is important that there are sufficient numbers of accessible turnstiles for people who use wheeled mobility aids, luggage carts, and mothers with strollers.[25]

A key element in any transit trip is fare payment, and many large transit agencies are developing electronic fare payment systems. Electronic fare payment has been shown to reduce costs and improve efficiency. Electronic fare payment includes a variety of media, such as Smart Cards, magnetic strips, or contactless cards. Most of these are generally prepaid fare media and transit passes. One of the challenges has been the development of accessible fare machine technology. These machines are still evolving at the same time that sophisticated Smart Cards are also evolving. In the future, transit riders will not put cash in a fare box. In addition, after fare boxes are removed from transit vehicles, there will be more options for access onto and off of transit vehicles. Currently, the fare box location and design on many vehicles limits the size of wheelchair that can access the vehicle.

In the past, the location of accessible public telephones was an important consideration in the design of transit facilities, but with the proliferation of cell phones fewer public pay phones are now available. The design and placement of emergency phones is, however, still an important consideration.

Many transit systems are installing real-time passenger information systems at bus stops, stations, and on board vehicles. This information can be particularly useful for people with wheelchairs. If passengers know about delays, they can seek safe places to wait. This helps to minimize exposure to inclement weather and decrease general vulnerability. It is important that these devices are placed in the unobstructed line of sight of people who use wheelchairs.

Accessible Buildings

After the passage of the ADA in 1990, many public agencies were concerned with providing access to public buildings. The challenges of the second decade include internal building circulation, accessible restrooms, and accessible paths and routes through buildings. After September 11, 2001, emergency building evacuation has become a huge challenge. New safety procedures need to be developed and instituted that ensure that all people can be safely evacuated in a timely manner. This is a new challenge for designers and operators of buildings. Previously, areas of safe refuge were designated as places for people with mobility impairments to go to and wait for emergency personnel for evacuation. For many people this is not an acceptable solution. Many buildings are now being equipped with emergency evacuation chairs that can quickly move people down stairs.

For privately owned and operated facilities, there are still enormous barriers. Building proprietors need to be educated to understand that universal access is simply good business. Stores that are accessible to people who use wheeled mobility aids are easier for everyone and make shopping a much more enjoyable experience for all. Most medical facilities are accessible; however, many hospital emergency departments and immediate-care facilities are not equipped to handle patients who use wheelchairs—few have examining tables that can be raised or lowered to accommodate easy transfers to and from wheelchairs.

Offices, schools, restaurants, and recreational facilities are still not fully accessible to people who use wheelchairs, which limits full integration and community access. In communities where these facilities are accessible, there are more opportunities for full integration into community activities by all people (Client's Perspective: Accessibility in the Community). Accessible community centers and gymnasiums provide opportunities for adaptive recreation programs that benefit people of all ages.[26,27]

THE CLIENT'S PERSPECTIVE | Accessibility in the Community

I appreciate living life as a person with SCI under the ADA for a variety of reasons. First, I have lived with a C5 to C6 SCI since 1981, which was before the ADA was enacted. Living life 2 feet closer to the ground was more difficult then because curb cuts, handicapped parking, and ramps into buildings were not easy to find before 1990. Passage of the ADA replaced and put teeth behind accessibility laws that were already on the books but had not been universally enforced.

The ADA is designed to prohibit discrimination of any kind against people with disabilities. For example, companies can no longer legally deny workers with disabilities job opportunities. New construction must be totally ADA compliant. And services readily available to the nondisabled community must be offered to the disabled community as well.

I am in charge of ADA enforcement at one of the major sports and entertainment complexes in the country—Meadowlands SportsComplex, which encompasses Giants Stadium and the Continental Airlines Arena. I protect and enforce the rights of those who fall under the guidelines of the ADA and I truly enjoy my job and all the challenges associated with it.

As much as the ADA has helped people with a disability lead more productive and active lives, there are problems with abuse. Far too many companies and businesses claim they do not fall under the auspices of the ADA to make their environments more accessible. The avalanche of people who get and misuse handicapped parking privileges make finding accessible parking even harder than in the days before ADA.

Could enforcement of the ADA be better? Yes. But, for the majority of people who live with a disability, life without the ADA would be far more difficult.

Michael Smith

TRAVEL TRAINING

The goal of travel training is to develop mobility and navigation skills that maximize independence and freedom and move individuals to the most independent mode of travel. It should be realized that this mode is influenced by and may change as a function of weather, health, and trip origin and destination. Travel training is a formal program that is usually instituted by a transit agency in partnership with advocacy groups to develop training programs that meet the individual needs of travelers with special needs. Many rehabilitation facilities have formal programs where a transit vehicle is taken to the rehabilitation facility and people practice getting on, moving around in, and getting off transit vehicles. This provides a training opportunity for people to learn how to access and egress a vehicle without affecting the schedule of a vehicle in regular service. It also provides rehabilitation professionals with an opportunity to evaluate their client's capabilities for independent travel. It is recommended that rehabilitation professionals who are responsible for the prescription of mobility devices also be involved with travel training to ensure that appropriate mobility aids are prescribed.

Many transit agencies also have travel buddy programs for new travelers. A travel buddy is a person who provides an extra level of support for people with disabilities while they develop independent travel skills. At large transit facilities, travel hosts may also provide special assistance during transfers. Many times the travel host and travel buddy are people who also have disabilities and, therefore, have first hand knowledge of many of the challenges involved in independent travel.

VIRTUAL TRANSPORTATION

The integration of computers into personal lifestyles has created many opportunities for people with disabilities. Indeed, for many people with disabilities, the computer has become their connection to the world, for others it provides an opportunity to learn and work from home, and yet others can remain in their home and community but still be linked to the world around them.[28]

Trip Planning

Most transit systems in the United States already have on-line trip planning information or will have in the near future. This enables a traveler to know all about the trip before he leaves home (Client's Perspective: Travel Planning). Some of the systems provide detailed maps that not only include transit information but also information on local attractions near the trip origin and destination as well as about fares and transfers. Systems that provide real-time information also provide updates on service changes resulting from local incidents. Many on-line trip planning systems permit the traveler

to look at all the travel options and select the best combination of schedule, vehicle, and fare for his particular needs.

Telecommuting and In-home Services

Telecommuting is changing how many individuals live and work. Telecommuting reduces the need for travel and allows many people with disabilities to work directly from home. This eliminates the need for a daily commute to the office and provides a new level of flexibility in lifestyle.

Distance education, e-campuses, and on-line learning bring the world of education and training resources into the home. It is possible for an individual to complete a college degree at home. Others find that the Internet brings the world directly to them. Many people use on-line shopping for essentials such as groceries and medicines. On-line shopping is a vital link to living independently. The other side of the picture is that remaining at home all the time can increase an individual's isolation. So, as in all things, it is a question of balance.

ADVOCACY: WHOSE RESPONSIBILITY IS IT?
Users

Users of accessible transportation services have a responsibility to ensure that all aspects of the trip chain are accessible, by having and communicating reasonable expectations for service delivery. Users of public transportation resources have opportunities to be their own advocates (Box 21-2). The biggest impact that users can make is through their use of public transportation resources and encouragement of providers to find ways to make service improvements.

Providers

The community at large and transportation providers in particular are responsible for providing public transportation and community access that is barrier free. In addition, providers share a responsibility to ensure that the infrastructure, vehicles, and equipment are clean and well maintained. The total trip chain must also be accessible and travelers must feel safe and secure and be able to travel with dignity.

Rehabilitation Team

The rehabilitation team has responsibility to ensure the correct prescription of wheeled mobility aids to maximize user independence. Community access and accessible transportation are essential for quality of life; therefore wheelchairs that promote independence and take all aspects of the user's lifestyle into account should be prescribed to maximize these opportunities. Transportation is a key to all aspects of independent living and transportable mobility aids are essential for safe and dignified travel.

THE CLIENT'S PERSPECTIVE | Travel Planning

When you are getting ready to take a trip, call the Chamber of Commerce in your destination city to find out what accessible transportation is available. Many large cities now offer a variety of accessible transportation options, and some car rental agencies have wheelchair-accessible vehicles available. Also check the Internet to find listings for wheelchair-accessible van rentals.

Another helpful resource is the National Spinal Cord Injury Association Web site (www.spinalcord.org), which lists different transportation options throughout the country and the United Kingdom and provides links to accessible overseas travel.

Always contact your hotel in advance to make sure their shuttle service is accessible and reconfirm all arrangements before your arrival. When traveling by air, contact the airline carrier directly to find out what their requirements and restrictions are and to inform them of any accommodations YOU may require. Get to the airport early because you will board first. If you use a manual wheelchair, have it gate-checked and placed onboard with you. Power chair users need to check with the airlines about how their chairs will be stored. Pack all removable wheelchair parts in a duffle bag that you bring with you and store them in the overhead storage compartment so they are not lost or broken. Pack your medications, a change of clothes, and any other necessary supplies in your carry-on luggage, not in checked baggage.

Train and bus services also have Web sites that list information important to people with SCI.

Scott Chesney

BOX 21-2 | **Being Your Own Advocate**

- Participate on citizen advisory boards.
- Provide instruction to those who give you assistance.
- Provide constructive comments for continuous community improvement.

CLINICAL CASE STUDY | Transportation and Accessibility Case 1

Patient History

William "Bill" Mead is a 63-year-old man with a C5 tetraplegia, ASIA A diagnosis. He is 30 weeks post injury. He has completed rehabilitation and is medically stable. His home renovations have just been finished and he is researching transportation options for his return to work and for leisure.

Bill is a financial advisor for a large company. He intends to return to work, which includes both office time and client visits. Currently he is working part time from home. He uses a power tilt-in-space wheelchair and has a manual wheelchair for backup. He and his wife Sarah, age 60 years, live 30 minutes from his office. Sarah is an office assistant in a dental office. She is in excellent health and is currently Bill's primary caretaker with assistance from their two sons who live about 20 minutes away. Bill also has assistance from an attendant, who provides him with personal care 3 hours of morning help 6 days a week and 3 hours two nights a week. He and Sarah have been looking at adapted vehicles to accommodate their transportation needs and will explore his ability to drive this vehicle.

Patient's Self-Assessment

Bill has always been a go-getter and is determined to resume his lifestyle as soon as possible.

Clinical Assessment
Patient Appearance

- Height 6 feet, weight 200 pounds, body mass index 27.1

Cognitive Assessment

- Alert, oriented × 3

Cardiopulmonary Assessment

- Blood pressure 110/62 mm Hg, heart rate at rest 72 beats/min, respiratory rate 14 breaths/min, cough flows are ineffective (<360 L/min), vital capacity is reduced (between 1.5 and 2.5 L)

Musculoskeletal and Neuromuscular Assessment

- Motor assessment reveals C5 ASIA A.
- Motor and sensory are intact to C5.
- Upper limb 4/5 for biceps, trapezius, and deltoids; 3/5 for wrist extensors; 0/5 for remaining upper limb muscles; lower limb key muscle grades are 0/5
- Deep tendon reflexes 3+ below the level of lesion

Integumentary and Sensory Assessment

- Skin is intact throughout, sensory intact to T4 (sensory zone of partial preservation from C6 to T4)

Range of Motion Assessment

- Passive and active motion is within normal limits in both upper limbs.
- Straight leg raise is 88 degrees in both lower limbs and dorsiflexion is 0 degrees; all other motions in the lower limbs are within functional limits.

Mobility and ADL Assessment

- Dependent with bed mobility
- Requires moderate to maximal assistance for transfer board transfers from wheelchair to bed
- Dependent in shower chair transfers
- Independent with pressure relief
- Independent in power wheelchair maneuvering on all surfaces and manual wheelchair propulsion with bilateral wrist splints and wheelchair lugs for 100 feet
- Dependent in bowel and bladder care and bathing

- Requires moderate assistance for upper body dressing and is dependent in lower body dressing

Evaluation of Clinical Assessment

William "Bill" Mead is a 63-year-old man with a C5 tetraplegia, ASIA A diagnosis. He is 30 weeks post injury. He has strong family support and is seeking consultation for transportation needs.

Patient's Care Needs

1. Consultation for transportation needs
2. Consultation for driver's training evaluation

Diagnosis and Prognosis

Diagnosis of C5 complete tetraplegia, ASIA A, with a sensory zone of partial preservation from C6 to T4. Prognosis is for return to work and leisure activities with appropriate transportation.

Preferred Practice Patterns*

Impaired Muscle Performance (4C), Impairments Nonprogressive Spinal Cord Disorders (5H), Primary Prevention/Risk Reduction for Cardiovascular/Pulmonary Disorders (6A), Primary Prevention/Risk Reduction for Integumentary Disorders (7A)

Team Goals

1. Team to advise regarding appropriate vans for transportation to and from work and within the community that will be driven by a family member or attendant.
2. Team will evaluate the client's ability to drive an adapted van.
3. Team to advise regarding public transportation options for work or leisure.

Patient Goals

"I want to be able to get where I need to with the least hassle."

Care Plan
Treatment Plan and Rationale

- Provide options for van adaptations.
- Examine independent driving capacity with an adapted vehicle,
- Evaluate the trip from home to work and leisure for optimal route with fewest barriers to public transportation.

Interventions

- Occupational therapist or driver's training specialist provides options for van adaptations as a passenger and a driver.
- Driver's training specialist evaluates the client's potential for independent driving of an adapted vehicle.
- Occupational therapist completes a home and community evaluation to select optimal route for work and leisure by public transportation.
- Education regarding transportation resources for traveling with a disability

Documentation and Team Communication

- Team will consult with vendors for vans and case managers for insurance support for van purchase.
- Team will consult with vendors, occupational therapists, and driver's training specialist to determine optimal van adaptations to function as a driver or a passenger.
- Team will consult with driver's training specialist to determine client's potential for independent driving.
- Team will consult with occupational therapist to discuss barriers in public transportation for necessary trips to work.
- Team will prepare consultation report and transportation resource guide.

CLINICAL CASE STUDY — Transportation and Accessibility Case 1—cont'd

Follow-Up Assessment
- Reassessment at van delivery
- Follow-up for behind-the-wheel training, if appropriate, with new van
- Reassessment per patient request for transportation resources

Critical Thinking Exercises
Consider factors related to lifestyle and work that will influence Bill's mobility and transportation needs as well as his ability to meet the complex demands of often being out of the office with clients.

1. What type of vehicle would you recommend to enable Bill and his wife to plan social events?
2. What are considerations for the trip chain when he is visiting clients? How much time should he allot when meeting a client 45 minutes from his home?
3. What advice would you offer Bill when he is planning a vacation by train and in a city with bus service?
4. When visiting a client, what information should Bill gather from the client to prepare for adequate trip planning?

*Guide to physical therapist practice, rev. ed. 2, Alexandria, VA, 2003, American Physical Therapy Association.

CLINICAL CASE STUDY — Transportation and Accessibility Case 2

Patient History
Peter Kapps is a 27-year-old man with T12 paraplegia, ASIA A diagnosis. He was injured in a motor vehicle accident. He is now 24 weeks post injury and has completed both inpatient and outpatient rehabilitation. Peter is planning on returning to work in September for the start of school.

Peter is the athletic director at a high school. He has a manual wheelchair and intends to purchase a racing wheelchair. The high school is making accommodations so that his office and a bathroom nearby will be fully accessible. There is an elevator in the building. Peter's wife works at the same high school as a guidance counselor. They have a 2-year-old daughter and own a ranch home that is being renovated to improve wheelchair accessibility.

Patient's Self-Assessment
Peter is intent on regaining his mobility and looking forward to the active pace of working with high school students and wheelchair athletics.

Clinical Assessment
Patient Appearance
- Height 5 feet 9 inches, weight 140 pounds, body mass index 20.7

Cognitive Assessment
- Alert, oriented × 3

Cardiopulmonary Assessment
- Blood pressure 120/76 mm Hg, heart rate at rest 72 beats/min, respiratory rate 12 breaths/min, vital capacity is within normal limits

Musculoskeletal and Neuromuscular Assessment
- Motor assessment reveals T12 paraplegia, ASIA A
- Motor and sensory are intact to T12
- Deep tendon reflexes are 2+ in the upper limbs and 0 in the lower limbs.

Integumentary and Sensory Assessment
- Skin is intact throughout, sensory intact to T12.

Range of Motion Assessment
- Passive and active motion is within normal limits in both upper limbs.
- Straight leg raise is 100 degrees in both lower limbs and dorsiflexion is 5 degrees; all other motions in the lower limbs are within functional limits.

Mobility and ADL Assessment
- Independent with bed mobility
- Independent in transfers to all surfaces including floor
- Independent with pressure relief
- Independent in manual wheelchair maneuvering on all surfaces
- Independent in high-level wheelchair skills
- Independent in bowel and bladder care
- Independent in dressing
- Independent in driving

Evaluation of Clinical Assessment
Peter Kapps is a 27-year-old man with T12 paraplegia, ASIA A diagnosis. He is seeking consultation for his transportation needs for both work and leisure.

Patient's Care Needs
1. Consultation for driver's training evaluation
2. Consultation for driving vehicle with adaptations and wheelchair transport mechanism

Diagnosis and Prognosis
Diagnosis of T12 paraplegia, ASIA A. Prognosis excellent for return to work and leisure activities with appropriate transportation

Preferred Practice Patterns*
Impaired Muscle Performance (4C), Impairments Nonprogressive Spinal Cord Disorders (5H), Primary Prevention/Risk Reduction for Cardiovascular/Pulmonary Disorders (6A), Primary Prevention/Risk Reduction for Integumentary Disorders (7A)

Team Goals
1. Team to advise about driver's training evaluation
2. Team to advise about appropriate vehicle for transportation to and from work and within the community
3. Team to advise regarding the accessibility of public transportation for work or leisure

Patient Goals
"I want to be able to go anywhere."

Care Plan
Treatment Plan and Rationale
- Refer to a driver's training specialist for a driver's training evaluation.
- Provide recommendations to the occupational therapist and family for vehicle options.

Continued

CLINICAL CASE STUDY Transportation and Accessibility Case 2—cont'd

- Provide options for vehicle driving adaptations and wheelchair transport.
- Conduct a community trip evaluation to determine possible barriers to travel to work and leisure activities.

Interventions
- Evaluate ability to drive independently.
- Discuss vehicle options with client and family and suggest contact with insurance company or case worker for reimbursement questions.
- Provide information about options for vehicle adaptations for independent driving and options for wheelchair transport.
- Provide resources for independent travel for persons with disabilities.

Documentation and Team Communication
- Team will document independent driving ability.
- Team will document vehicle and adaptation selection.

- Team will report ability to transport wheelchair for travel needs.
- Team will provide consultation report and transportation resource guide.

Follow-Up Assessment
- Reassessment per patient request and on delivery of adapted vehicle

Critical Thinking Exercises
Consider factors related to lifestyle and work that will influence Peter's mobility and transportation needs and his ability to maintain his stamina in the fast-paced environment of a high school and the sports arena.
1. What type of vehicle would you recommend for Peter and his wife so that they can commute to school together?
2. What are considerations for the trip chain when going to and from work? How much time should Peter allot each way for a typical commute of 15 minutes?
3. What advice would you give this client when he plans a vacation by air with a car rental?

*Guide to physical therapist practice, rev. ed. 2, Alexandria, VA, 2003, American Physical Therapy Association.

SUMMARY

We have traveled through the trip chain and explored terminology related to accessible transportation and community access. This chapter has provided an overview of a number of challenges associated with accessible transportation. The discussion has also embraced a number of topics not usually considered in discussions of accessible transportation. A key issue is the need for the rehabilitation team to consider transportation and community access when prescribing mobility aids. Components of a trip, transportation modes, and services are discussed. A drivers training rehabilitation program is detailed including evaluation criteria for specific injury levels. Barriers to transportation and community access are outlined, emphasizing the need for advocacy to eliminate these barriers. The chapter discusses the importance of responsibility by all parties to ensure that community infrastructure and transportation are accessible. Community infrastructure including bus and train stops and transit amenities are presented as well as other modes of transportation such as passenger ferry services and air travel. It is important that all links on a trip chain are accessible so that travel is safe, seamless, and dignified.

REFERENCES

1. Hunter-Zaworski KM: *Barriers and safety risks for transportation disadvantaged air travelers,* Transportation Research Record 1098, Washington, DC, 1986, Transportation Research Board.
2. Hunter-Zaworski KM: A synopsis of accessibility features of Skytrain-Vancouver's rapid transit system, *ITE J* 59:23-27, 1989.
3. Paul Ryus: *Transit capacity and quality of service manual,* ed 2,TCRP Report #100,Washington, DC, 2003, National Academies.
4. Blackwell TL, Krause JS, Winkler T, Stiens SA: *Spinal cord injury desk reference: guidelines for life care planning and case management,* New York, 2001, Demos Medical Publishing.
5. US Access Board: ADA access guidelines for transportation vehicles (ADAAG) (as amended through 1998).
5a. US Access Board; revised draft. *Guidlines for public rights of way,* November 23, 2005.
6. Hunter-Zaworski KM: A study of human factors of elderly and handicapped passengers in public transportation safety. In Norrbom CE, Stahl A, editors: *Mobility and transport for elderly and disabled persons,* Reading, UK, 1991, Gordon and Breach Science Publishers.
7. Moakley T: Paratransit: love it or leave it? *Action Online* (United Spinal Association) July: 18-19, 2007.
8. Weisman JJ: Mass transit access: we were there, *Action Online* (United Spinal Association) July, 12-13, 2007.
9. Hunter-Zaworski KM: *The mechanics of mobility aid securement/ restraint on public transportation vehicles,* Transportation Research Record 1378, Washington, DC, 1993, Transportation Research Board.
10. Hunter-Zaworski KM, Zaworski JR: *Progress in wheelchair securement: 10 years since the American with Disabilities Act,* Transportation Research Record 1779, Washington, DC, 2002, Transportation Research Board.
11. Hunter-Zaworski KM, Zaworski JR: *Auto engaging mobility aid securement systems and low floor buses,* Transportation Research Record 1671, Washington, DC, 1999, Transportation Research Board.
12. Federal Register: *ADA accessibility guidelines for transportation vehicles: over the road buses,* 36 CFR 1192, September 28 , 1998 .
13. U.S. Access Board: *Revised draft guidelines for passenger vessels and supplementary materials,* July 2006.
14. Korner-Bitensky N, Sofer S, Kaiser F: Assessing the ability to drive following an acute neurological even: are we on the right road ?*Can J Occup Ther* 61:141-148, 1994.
15. Jones DG: Assistive devices for driving. In Goldberg B, Hsu JR, editors: *Atlas of orthosis and assistive devices, ed 3,* St. Louis, 1997, Mosby–Yearbook.
16. Pellerito JM Jr: *Driver rehabilitation and community mobility: principles and practice,* St. Louis, 2006, Elsevier Mosby.
17. Nead RW: Behind the wheel driver training, In Bain BK, Leger D, editors: *Assistive technology: an interdisciplinary approach,* New York, 1997, Churchill Livingston.
18. Dawson D: Designing accessible facilities in the public right of way, *ITE* 74:46-48, 2004.
19. Windley S: Toward accessible public rights of way, *ITE* 74:42-45, 2004.

20. Hunter-Zaworski KM, Kloos W, Donaker A: *Bus priority at traffic signals in Portland: the Powell Boulevard Pilot Project,* Transportation Research Board Record 1503, Washington, DC, 1998, Transportation Research Board Record.

21. Ashmead DH, Wall R, Bentzen BL et al: Which crosswalk? Effects of accessible pedestrian signal characteristics, *ITE J* 74:26-32, 2004.

22. Bentzen BL, Barlow JM, Franck L: Speech messages for accessible pedestrian signals, *ITE J* 74:20-25, 2004.

23. Hunter-Zaworski KM: *Improving bus accessibility systems for persons with sensory disabilities,* Transportation Research Record 1671, Washington, DC, 1999, Transportation Research Board.

24. Accessible Pedestrian Intersections: http://www.walkinginfo. org/aps; Detectable warnings: http://www.access-board.gov/ publications/DW%20Synthesis/report.htm; Update on detectable warning systems: http://www.access-board.gov/adaag/dws/ update.htm.

25. National Academy of Sciences/Transportation Research Board: Transit cooperative research program: *Synthesis project panels* 1988-2003.

26. Federal Register: *ADA accessibility guidelines for buildings and facilities: recreation facilities,* 36 CFR 1191, September 3, 2002.

27. Federal Register: *ADA and ABA accessibility guidelines for buildings and facilities,* 36 CFR 1191, July 23 , 2004.

28. Hunter-Zaworski KM: *The next frontier in accessible traveler information systems: world wide web-based information systems,* Transportation Research Record 1671, Washington, DC, 1999, Transportation Research Board.

SOLUTIONS TO CHAPTER 21 CLINICAL CASE STUDY

Transportation and Accessibility Case 1

1. Bill will require a van with a side lift and a lock down for the power wheelchair. His wife Sarah could be driving the vehicle so she should be comfortable and confident with all aspects of managing the vehicle and the controls for the lift and lock down. If Bill later meets the requirements for independent driving, then he will drive himself with the same for entry and egress and securement of his wheelchair.

2. Bill will benefit from a subscription service that is willing to meet his expectations for door-through-door service and on a relatively infrequent schedule with varying distances and locations. Accessible taxis may be one possibility because of the flexibility with service times; however, this may be an expensive transportation alternative. A private driver may be another alternative, with the van that they plan to purchase. The cost of a driver versus accessible taxis should be compared. If possible, Bill can drive himself after driver evaluation and completing a driver rehabilitation program. Daily time calculations need to consider Bill's maximum activities of daily living (ADL) preparation time, plus time to enter and exit the vehicle, travel distance with traffic considerations, and building access time. Thus, if Bill's morning ADL requires 1.5 hours, 10 minutes for vehicle entrance and exit, 45 minutes on the road, and 10 minutes to access the building, the total trip time will over 2½ hours to reach his first appointment with a return time of approximately an hour.

3. Vacation planning by train and city bus service will take a significant amount of preparation considering the accessibility needs with a power wheelchair. Full access to transportation and the community means that every link on the trip chain must be accessible and affordable, which is the goal of the preparation. Accessible fixed-route service must consider not only the train and bus entrance and exit accessibility but also walkways and sidewalks that connect to the trip origin and destination. This client may have difficulty with low-floor vehicles because the ramp may be too steep. Ideally, BRT system availability should be considered in the planning because it will most likely enhance access.

When train travel is considered, the region for the vacation should be chosen carefully. All of Amtrak's passenger rolling stock is accessible; however, in the region east of Chicago and south of Washington, DC, station lifts are required to access the train. In the west, all trains are equipped with on-board lifts. Again, coordination between train and bus transportation must be planned, noting regional differences with door-to-door accessibility. The use of on-line trip planning is advisable.

4. When client visits are set up, preparation must include determination of the site's accessibility. The building access, availability of accessible parking, walkways and sidewalks, and the bathroom must be taken into consideration. Using a template of questions to plan ahead will help ensure the ease of the entire trip chain and provide for accurate timing.

SOLUTIONS TO CHAPTER 21 CLINICAL CASE STUDY

Transportation and Accessibility Case 2

1. Peter could potentially use a vehicle that allows for mobility and store his manual wheelchair in a car. When selecting the car, however, consideration also should be given to placement of his daughter's car seat and room for groceries and other items that are needed on a regular basis. Transfers should be practiced to and from the driver and passenger sides of the vehicle and Peter's wheelchair to plan for optimal safety regarding the transfer-related height of the seats and to maximize independence. If the couple's schedules do not correspond, two vehicles may be required. Should Peter purchase a racing wheelchair, storage of this chair may also be a consideration in vehicle selection.

2. The total trip chain for Peter must consider morning ADL preparation, child care, access in and out of the vehicle, and entrance time from the parking lot to his office in the school. If morning preparations take 1 hour, car entrance with the manual wheelchair and getting his daughter into her car seat 15 minutes, drop off at child care time 15 minutes, 15-minute drive time, car and wheelchair exit 10 minutes, and finally parking lot to the office 15 minutes, the total morning transportation time will be 2 hours and 10 minutes.

3. Air travel and car rental for a vacation requires a significant amount of preparation time. This family will need to consider accessibility with the manual wheelchair and adequate accommodation from the airlines in addition to plans for their daughter and her car seat for both air travel and car rental. A wide-body aircraft and nonstop flight would be desirable, so calling the airline in advance is appropriate to ensure ease of access for both Peter and his daughter. Air travel preparation includes transfer to the aisle chair for boarding the aircraft, the use of the on-board chair to access the lavatory, and storage of the Peter's wheelchair.

When selecting the rental car, Peter and his wife will need to decide whether both of them will be driving. Peter will need to be comfortable accessing the vehicle, and if he will be sharing the driving, hand controls for accelerating and braking will be required. Therefore the cost of the rental may increase and a rental agency that provides hand controls must be found. On-line trip planning may help with information gathering and planning.

CHAPTER TWENTY-TWO

Functional and Psychosocial Aspects of Aging with Spinal Cord Injury

Bryan Kemp, PhD, and Lilli Thompson, PT

When I got hurt 26 years ago, they told my family I wasn't going to make it. Back then they didn't have much to offer. Turns out I was one of the ones that hung around to see what the future would hold. I've learned you can't be bitter and you have to keep busy or you'll go downhill. I can do everything everyone else does, except kick a football. I've found that things have gotten better over the years because I keep working on it. I get over my fears, take chances, do things for myself, and think positive. I still have lots of plans for the next 20 years...and I think I'm going to make it. I've been blessed.

Booker (age 65, C6 SCI)

Individuals with a spinal cord injury (SCI) are living longer than ever before.[1] Over the last 50 years, life expectancy has increased to about 85% of normal compared with the nondisabled population and, consequently, close to 40% of all people with SCI are now over the age of 45 years.[2] This is a dramatic change from the 1940s, when life expectancy after onset was usually measured in months instead of decades. Today, most people with SCI can expect to live into their 60s, 70s, and beyond. The nature and quality of these added years, however, are what is at question.

The topic and the importance of aging with SCI are new. It is only during the last several years that investigators have begun to delineate the changes that occur in people with SCI as they age. What has emerged is a complex set of medical, functional, psychological, and social issues that were unknown until recently. Previous chapters focused on health, function, and psychosocial issues in the more acute phases of SCI. This chapter focuses on the functional issues and psychological considerations that emerge as individuals live long term and age with SCI.

It is apparent from the findings to date that individuals with SCI do not age in a typical manner. Instead of enjoying good health and functioning easily until late in life, a large proportion of people with SCI have significant health and functional problems, often beginning in their 40s or 50s or as early as 15 to 20 years after onset of injury (Box 22-1). These changes can affect daily life, including employment, leisure, and family life. Quite naturally, these changes can also affect psychological health. The very quality of life (QOL) developed over years of working out accommodations to the SCI and developing a satisfying lifestyle can be eroded or severely threatened by the loss of hard-won abilities and independence. This chapter is based on scientific research to guide practical and efficient clinical practice and includes changes in function, symptoms associated with functional loss, QOL, life satisfaction, psychological distress, and the role of social support and family.

INTERACTION OF PSYCHOSOCIAL FACTORS, HEALTH STATUS, AND FUNCTIONING IN SPINAL CORD INJURY
Biopsychosocial Perspective
SCI is both a neurological catastrophe and a life-changing event that affects an individual biologically, functionally, and psychosocially. It is impossible to consider one area without considering

---

> **BOX 22-1 | Aging with Spinal Cord Injury**
>
> - Individuals are living longer with SCI than ever before.
> - New medical and functional problems occur 15 to 20 years after onset.
> - Medical and functional problems can affect quality of life for people with SCI.

the others, for these parts are intimately related. Ultimately, the best measure of successful outcome will depend on how well a person can function in life after SCI. The way he functions on a daily basis and his ability to work and to be independent, however, cannot be considered as being simply the result of physical attributes such as strength, endurance, and health. Psychological factors have a major impact on functioning as well. Motivation, personality traits, and depression affect functioning too. Likewise, social factors such as social support, community accessibility, and public attitudes also influence functioning. It logically follows, then, that age-related problems with functioning can be due to any of a number of biological, psychological, or social issues. It is the rehabilitation professional's role and responsibility to help discover barriers to function and address them. It can even be argued that the medical, psychological, and social professionals on the rehabilitation team work primarily to remove barriers to improving functioning, whereas the rehabilitation therapists (physical therapist, occupational therapist, speech therapist, vocational therapist, and recreation therapist) primarily promote functioning.

In essence, the biopsychosocial principle states that there is an inherent link among biological, psychological, and social variables in terms of how they affect function. This principle is simply a shorthand way of describing the important influence each of these spheres has on each other and on function (Figure 22-1).

The importance of this principle to understanding aging with SCI is critical. Individuals with SCI age prematurely in some aspects. They develop medical illnesses earlier than their nondisabled counterparts, their physiological reserves are lower than those of people without disabilities, their tolerance for added stress is lower, and life changes often increase more quickly with age. Biological, psychological, social, and functional spheres become increasingly interdependent with aging. The net result is that the average 50-year-old person with SCI often has medical, functional, and social needs akin to those of a 70-year-old person without a prior disability. And like any older adult, someone aging with SCI can easily go from a state of good health and function to poor health and function if any of a variety of medical, psychological, or social problems develop. The interrelationships can have a positive effect as well. If health status is improved, essential resources are acquired, or mental health conditions treated, an individual's function, health, and psychosocial status may all benefit.

Functional Changes While Aging

Functional demands range along a continuum, and aging changes can affect any point on this continuum. The basic life maintenance activities such as mobility, self-care, and communication are at one end of the continuum. The other end includes abilities that contribute to productive participation in society such as being able to work and participate in family, social, leisure, and recreational activities. In early rehabilitation the emphasis is on regaining abilities with the basics of life maintenance functions and establishing resources to reintegrate into life roles (Figure 22-2). Once achieved, most individuals do not expect to need future therapy services for these fundamental activities of mobility and self-care, yet changes with age can affect both basic and complex functions.

After the early rehabilitation phases of adjustment and skill acquisition, many individuals successfully reintegrate into life roles and lead full, meaningful, and productive lives despite significant

SCI impairment. From a functional perspective the next phase is a plateau. The fundamental levels of function are essentially maintained over a period of time. A means to successfully manage the functional demands of life with a physical impairment is established. Unless new or continuing health conditions arise that require specialty care, many people have very little contact with rehabilitation specialists beyond routine checkups and equipment updating. The primary health care need is to attend to regular health maintenance issues. In essence, life carries on and the important life events tend to involve changes in family, friendships, vocation, and recreation or leisure activities. A decline in functional abilities marks the latter phase of functioning. The functional decline may be gradual or marked and represents the combined effect of the physiological processes of aging overlapping with the impairment of SCI. Contact with specialists in rehabilitative services or other health care specialties is often necessary and highly recommended to adequately address the physical, functional, and psychosocial needs that arise during this phase of change.

The World health Organization's *International Classification of Functioning, Disability, and Health,* known as ICF (see Figure 5-2), provides a framework to understand the points of impact that primary impairment of SCI and aging changes have on the body systems, performance, and functioning.[3,4] The health condition represents the disorder, disease, or pathology (injury). The primary condition is the SCI and other health conditions that may exist as secondary or comorbid conditions (e.g., diabetes, cardiovascular disease [CVD], depression). Health conditions can have an impact on body functions and structures, activity, and participation. Loss of structure or function at the organ system level may impair the body (e.g., increased spasticity, muscle weakness, pain, contractures). Activity, similar to functional limitations, occurs at the level of the individual and represents the ability to perform activities considered normal for humans (e.g., moving, walking, eating, dressing, bathing, toileting). Participation reflects the ability to engage in societal-level roles such as family and home responsibilities, working, and leisure or social activities. Contextual factors consider the impact of the environmental and personal characteristics on the organ system, the person, and societal levels. Environmental and personal factors might include the resources, health behaviors, motivation, and attitudes (either personal or community) that influence disablement. Age-related health, function, and psychosocial changes can have an effect at any point within the model.

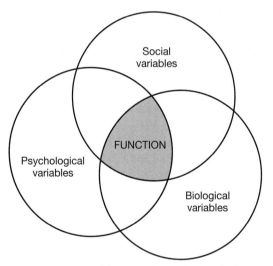

FIGURE 22-1 Diagram of the biopsychosocial principle illustrates the interrelationship of psychological, social, and emotional variables.

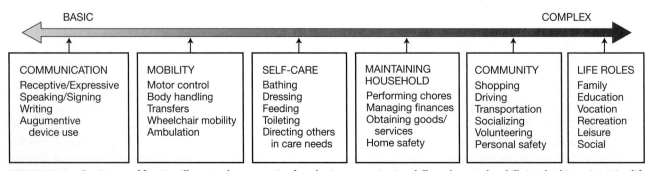

FIGURE 22-2 Continuum of function illustrates the progression from basic communication skills to the complex skills involved in maintaining life roles.

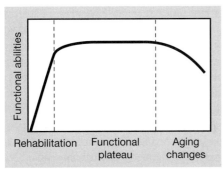

FIGURE 22-3 Diagram of the functional plateau illustrates the relatively stable period between rehabilitation and aging.

The fear of functional loss with aging may lurk in the background thoughts of some, or it may be openly expressed as a concern by others. In any case, it is not a surprise that anxiety and distress result when the well-maintained plateau of function takes a downward turn and once routine activities begin to feel more difficult or impossible to perform. These feelings seem legitimate when considering the relatively young ages of those experiencing changes and that these changes are comparable to the late-life changes of older adults from the general population.

Research on aging in the general population and geriatrics provides the benchmark to understand the differences in the aging process for people with SCI. Capacity and function are affected by age-related changes in organ systems regardless of whether an individual is living with a preexisting impairment. Functional capacity of the neuromuscular, musculoskeletal, and cardiopulmonary systems decline with advancing age in the general population.[5,6] Organ system changes usually do not affect function until late life for people without preexisting impairments. The same is not true for individuals with SCI where the physiological reserves are lower. A relatively minor decline in a major organ system can result in considerable functional consequences for someone with lower reserve capacity. In people with SCI, the overlapping effects of the primary impairment and the age-associated system changes result in functional problems developing in younger age groups. For example, bone loss or osteopenia can lead to osteoporosis and increased fracture risks with advancing age in the general population. The osteoporosis resulting from paralysis and mobility impairment in individuals with SCI compounds the fracture risk at a much younger age. In older adults, skeletal muscle fiber loss or sarcopenia can lead to decreased force production in muscles. Even slight losses in muscle strength in people with SCI can significantly affect functional abilities.

Thinning of the epidermis and decreased lean body mass results in increased skin fragility with advancing age. For someone with long-standing SCI, a decrease in skin resilience increases the risk for pressure ulcers even when they were never a problem in the past. Declines in physical activity tolerance can result from decreased cardiopulmonary function in older adults. Individuals with SCI have disproportionately higher rates of CVD, pulmonary dysfunction, and metabolic disorders and a high mortality rate from cardiovascular disease and pneumonia compared with nondisabled populations.[7-11] Declines in any of these systems with age can have significant health and functional consequences (Figure 22-3).

Another concern is the greater susceptibility to specific musculoskeletal pathological conditions that can directly affect function. People with SCI are at risk for acute and chronic overuse injuries from the increased and abnormal functional demands on muscles and joints of the upper extremities and spine. The margin to absorb additional conditions in the musculoskeletal system is very limited and can create dramatic change in functional abilities (Clinical Note: Spinal Cord Injury as Primary Impairment).

CLINICAL NOTE Spinal Cord Injury as Primary Impairment

- SCI increases susceptibility to certain health and musculoskeletal conditions.
- SCI reduces the capacity to absorb the steady age-related declines over time.

Do recognizable symptoms precede changes in function, and if so, are interventions effective to prevent the progression into full loss of function? What are the appropriate goals when someone with SCI has a decline in functional abilities? Can the changes be reversed or are accommodations to the changes the most effective strategy? These are all-important questions for clinicians, researchers, and consumers to consider.

Studies of specific physical symptoms commonly reported by individuals living long term with an SCI include high rates of new muscle and joint pain, generalized fatigue, and loss of muscle strength. Indications from preliminary studies have identified a relationship between the development of new pain, problems with fatigue, and new muscle weakness and a subsequent loss of functional abilities in people with long-term SCI.[12] No one single health or physical condition can explain the development of these problems. It is likely a combination of overlapping physical, physiological, and psychological factors that contribute to the symptoms and loss of function. Investigations of interventions to address these symptoms have to look specifically at the underlying etiology and the functional activities at risk. Whether the functional decline can be completely reversed is highly dependent on the etiology. Nevertheless, prudent thinking suggests the need to plan for progressive functional changes with a goal of preserving valued activities by modifying performance.

Pain

Pain is a frequent problem for people with SCI. Reports range from 34% to 94% prevalence rates.[13] Extensive literature exists on pain prevalence, classification of pain types, and options for treatment in persons with SCI.[14-18] The pertinent issue in the study of aging with SCI and pain are when pain becomes a new problem, for instance, when chronic pain is exacerbated or new pain develops from a new source and creates the potential for additional disability or functional decline. Chronic neuropathic pain developed just after injury and experienced at or below the injury level has prevalence rates as high as 94% in some SCI populations. This type of pain results from the original lesion and the residual damage to neurological structures and surviving tissue.[15] Individuals with SCI often are involved in life-long management of neuropathic pain. In contrast to the continuous neuropathic pain, new pain above the level of the SCI is frequently musculoskeletal or neuromuscular in nature. This type of pain is what usually creates new problems for people aging with SCI, although it is highly recommended that any new pain condition undergo a thorough evaluation to rule out a new central condition such as a syringomyelia.

Musculoskeletal impairments are the most common cause of functional loss in the general population.[19] Similarly, new musculoskeletal problems are frequently reported in individuals aging with SCI and can have a dramatic impact on function.[20-22] Abnormal biomechanical demands on specific muscles and joints create stresses on the musculoskeletal system. For example, the shoulder joint was anatomically designed for multidimensional mobility to perform prehensile functions rather than for weight bearing and stability of the body. Yet many people with SCI rely heavily on the upper extremities for weight bearing with transfers, propping, wheeling, and walking with assistive devices. Upper limb pain is one of the most common problems in the long-term SCI population and the incidence and severity increases with longer duration of SCI.[23-29]

Sie et al[27] determined the prevalence of upper limb pain in a group of 239 individuals with SCI who were an average of 37 years of age and 12 years after injury.[27] Fifty-five percent of those with tetraplegia had upper limb pain and 46% had shoulder pain specifically. Sixty-four percent of the group with paraplegia had upper limb pain and the most common symptoms were associated with carpal tunnel syndrome (CTS) of the wrists, followed by shoulder pain. Cervical pain and back pain are also common in people with SCI. Abnormal stresses on the spine result from functioning in a seated position. Long-term and repetitive suboccipital extension is often necessary for the seated individual to converse with a person standing beside their wheelchair. Frequent and more extensive cervical rotation is often required to look over the shoulder if the trunk is stabilized in a chair. In the thoracic and lumbar spine weak or paralyzed trunk musculature, poor postural support, and the sequela of spine stabilization methods after the initial SCI compound the stresses on the spine.

New or exacerbated pain conditions can have an additional disabling effect on people with preexisting mobility impairments. A seemingly minor musculoskeletal problem can cause a marked decrease in mobility and loss of functional independence with critical abilities. The Rehabilitation Research and Training Center (RRTC) on Aging with a Disability in Downey, CA, investigated the impact of pain on function in people with SCI.[30] Pain primarily interfered with abilities to perform self-care, home responsibilities, and family activities in the population with SCI. Pain had a two to four times greater impact on basic functional tasks compared with a nondisabled control group. The nondisabled group identified recreation as the activity most disrupted by pain, in contrast to the basic self-care and life support activities reported by people with a preexisting impairment.

Management and treatment of pain is a complex process in any population and the complexity is magnified in individuals with SCI. As in any case, the specific etiology of the pain should be identified to appropriately direct treatment. Circumstances exist where the underlying etiology remains elusive and treatment is directed at pain management. Therapy-based treatments for musculoskeletal pain include use of manual therapy techniques,

therapeutic modalities, therapeutic exercises, pacing strategies, biofeedback, relaxation techniques, and the addition of assistive or adaptive equipment. To avoid continual reinjury, education and functional retraining to modify activities is an important component of treatment in the SCI population. Appropriate pharmacological treatment can enhance therapy-based outcomes.

Challenges arise when pain is acute, severe, and easily aggravated by essential functional activities. Providing pain relief measures while preserving range of motion and strength is the focus. Active rest of the body part is important when a person has highly irritable levels of pain. Resting a body part without completely obstructing function is sometimes impossible if the painful part is critical to essential life functions. For example, an acute biceps tendon tear in an individual with C7 tetraplegia who pushes a manual wheelchair, transfers independently, and works full time is difficult to manage in the traditional mode. Use of the upper limb for functional tasks must continue to a certain extent while the acute injury is resolving. Arranging the environment to minimize use of the affected limb is essential during healing phases. Leading with the painful shoulder during transfers, adjusting the surface heights to level the transfers, or using a transfer board versus a depression technique can preserve the function and may protect the painful upper limb. When the pain is relieved with rest; responds to therapeutic techniques; occurs only with specific movements, postures, or activities; or is rated as low to mid range for severity, then a slow progression back to modified daily activities is recommended. Guarding against exacerbation of the painful condition and avoiding the specific movements or postures that aggravate the problem is important.

The use of a sports medicine philosophy is helpful. With high-caliber athletes the goals are to treat acute conditions quickly and effectively and return athletes to the sport while preventing future reinjury. Professional athletes' very livelihood depends on the ability to play the game just as a person with SCI depends on functional abilities for his functional livelihood. Therefore when someone with SCI has a musculoskeletal problem, immediate, effective, comprehensive, and professional treatment is advised to address the issue and to prevent potential progression into a chronic condition.

Pain caused by overuse or atypical use of the musculoskeletal system may respond to changes in performance techniques to specifically protect painful structures. The demands on the shoulder muscles for functional activities have been investigated and provide a basis for development of clinical interventions for shoulder dysfunction. Perry et al[31] identified the timing and intensity of the shoulder muscles during lateral transfers. The thoracicohumeral muscles were identified as playing a protective role in preventing impingement of the glenohumeral joint during lateral transfers, and a difference in the demands on muscle groups was identified between the leading and trailing limbs. In addition, Mulroy et al[32] described the critical role of the rotator cuff muscles in wheelchair propulsion and the high risk for muscle fatigue during prolonged wheelchair propulsion.

Shoulder pain has been attributed to the increased weight-bearing demand for mobility, muscle imbalances in the shoulder girdle, poor postural alignment from trunk paralysis, and the need to function from a seated position. Rotator cuff tendonitis, subacromial bursitis, degenerative joint disease, rotator cuff tears and adhesive capsulitis, biceps tendonitis and tears, myofascial pain syndrome, and fractures or dislocations have been identified as potential conditions resulting in shoulder pain. The subacromial region is especially vulnerable to impingement in people with SCI, given the functional demands on the shoulder joint. A relative weakness of the shoulder rotator cuff muscles and adductors compared with the strength of the deltoid muscles increases the risk of subacromial impingement. A common mechanism of impingement occurs during upper limb weight bearing. Without adequate stability, the humeral head is driven upward into the acromion process and coracoacromial arch; another mechanism occurs when the greater tuberosity impinges on this space during abduction of the arm.

Curtis et al[18] proposed a shoulder muscle strengthening and stretching intervention to decrease the shoulder pain experienced during functional activities. The program was based on the premise that anterior shoulder muscle tightness, relative weakness of posterior muscles, and repeated subacromial impingement contributes to shoulder pain. Valuable information to guide clinical interventions has been provided by research investigating the role of the rotator cuff muscles during specific activities.[31,33, 34] In addition, the effect of muscle strength imbalances on performance[23] and the sources of pain in people with specific impairments have been studied.[25,27,35] This research provided clinicians with a better understanding about how interventions and modified activities can be applied to changes in wheelchairs and walking ergonomics, changes in wheeling and transferring biomechanics, and performance of specific exercises to strengthen and stretch key muscles and joint structures.

Fatigue

Fatigue may refer to a variety of symptoms. There are several types of fatigue: central, peripheral, and mental. Central fatigue is a generalized lack of energy, feeling exhausted or tired. When this exhaustion is beyond reasonable or expected on the basis of the activity level, it is abnormal. Peripheral fatigue refers to muscle weakness (the decreased ability to generate force) or lack of muscle endurance (an inability to generate repetitive force). Mental fatigue describes an inability to focus, concentrate, or maintain alertness because of feeling tired or sleepy.

Individuals aging with SCI have reported each of these forms of fatigue. Mental fatigue may be related to medication side effects, mental health issues, or sleep disruptions that go along with having an SCI. Peripheral fatigue is often a neurological or musculoskeletal-based issue and relates to a change in muscle performance. Central fatigue is probably the most complex and difficult to explain. Although the presence of central fatigue is a common symptom of people with long-term physical impairments, including SCI, it is not always fully investigated or addressed.[36,37] Adding to the difficulties are the multiple factors that may contribute to fatigue, such as underlying medical conditions, side effects of medications, poor diet, inadequate rest, depression, stress, and overwork of the body.

Two primary factors contribute to fatigue in individuals with SCI. First, excess fatigue may result from the high level of physical demands required to perform daily activities with a movement impairment and a portion of volitional muscle paralysis. Janssen

et al[38] reported excessive and prolonged cardiovascular demands in individuals with tetraplegia when performing routine activities such as lifting objects, pushing a wheelchair outdoors, ascending ramps and curbs, showering, and getting into and out of a car. The cardiovascular response far exceeded the demand for the nondisabled population performing comparable activities. The second issue contributing to fatigue may relate to the increased susceptibility to secondary medical and psychological conditions compared with a nondisabled population. High rates of fatigue may be a symptom of underlying health conditions or reflect the side effects of medications used to manage secondary conditions in people with long-term SCI. Medical problems such as anemia, thyroid dysfunction, diabetes, urinary tract infections, kidney dysfunction, depression, sleep apnea, and respiratory or heart disease can all cause fatigue.

Medications common to the SCI population such as muscle relaxants, pain medications, antidepressants, and sedatives have fatigue as a side effect. Aging changes in metabolic and kidney function create another medication issue to be aware of. The clearance rates of some medications slow with advancing age, and the interactive effect of residual muscle paralysis may magnify this problem in people with SCI. Medication in the system can build up over time. This is a problem when the dosages are not adjusted to account for the aging effect. As a result, side effects such as fatigue can become more pronounced. A routine review of medication and dosage is highly recommended.

Fatigue can be an extremely debilitating condition. Investigations of the effect of fatigue on individuals aging with SCI are just emerging. Fatigue has been studied more extensively in people with other disabling impairments such as postpolio syndrome or multiple sclerosis. A continuing investigation by the RRTC on aging with a disability has found comparable fatigue levels and impact in people with postpolio syndrome, cerebral palsy, rheumatoid arthritis, and SCI.[30] These findings provide a glimpse of the significant effect fatigue has on daily function. People describe giving up activities such as recreation, social outings, or any activity considered extraneous in an attempt to preserve work, self-care, and chores. Many individuals struggle to continue working despite extreme problems with fatigue because the loss of employment would have significant personal and financial consequences. McNeal et al[39] investigated the work problems reported in people aging with SCI and found that 41% of the workers reported fatigue or pain as the primary physical problem. Progression of fatigue can result in early retirement, or in the case of younger workers, the decision to just give up work completely. Fatigue can eventually interfere with the ability to manage self-care and home responsibilities. Some individuals essentially shorten the active hours in the day by limiting the amount of time they are up and engaging in activities. By staying in bed later or lying down earlier in the afternoon or evening to rest the body, the day begins to shrink to only a few productive hours.

The cause of fatigue has to be thoroughly investigated to determine appropriate interventions for treatment. New generalized fatigue that interferes with daily function has to be considered abnormal. Health care providers should routinely ask about changes in energy levels and encourage discussion about the problem if it exists. Thorough evaluation and assessment may identify the source of the new symptoms and rule in or out fatigue causing medical conditions. This information allows clients and health care providers to make informed decisions about the best course of treatment and management. Direct management of fatigue involves reducing the fatigue and minimizing the impact on function.

Use of pacing techniques and lifestyle changes are recommended to conserve energy. Prioritizing activities and energy use helps identify the activities that are of value, bring meaning, and enhance the QOL of the individual. These types of activities should be considered a priority to preserve, at least in some form. Extraneous tasks or those of lesser value to the individual may be modified, completely stopped, or given over to others. Energy for the most meaningful activities can be preserved by using assistance for high-energy demand tasks or by improving the efficiency of task performance. For instance, if assistance (either from equipment or another person) helps make bathing and dressing more efficient, energy to participate in personally important community or social activities may be preserved. Another consideration is using powered mobility either for part-time or full-time mobility. A change in the equipment used for primary mobility can be very difficult for some to consider because many view it as a symbol of increased disability. In reality, the device may decrease the disability created by fatigue or pain and enhance functional mobility. This actually results in a decrease in the disability. In hindsight, people have wondered why they delayed or resisted accepting new functionally enhancing technology once they become accustomed to its use.

Adopting the perspectives necessary to manage fatigue and pain sometimes requires a dramatic shift in philosophy. Changing the way one approaches life to conserve energy is not always easy. People need assistance, encouragement, and strategies that work specifically for them. Professional, peer, and family support can assist people who are making these changes. Successful fatigue management is a continuous learning process that requires practice and patience. Making multiple small changes in energy use throughout the day may achieve a relatively larger impact on overall energy and is often more successful than giving up a major meaningful activity completely. For example, if mobility efficiency is improved, assistance is obtained with chores, and rest breaks are taken regularly, sufficient energy may be conserved to continue other more valued activities.

Understanding the relationship between fatigue and known medical, psychological, and physical causes will help direct treatment. Fatigue may be the consequence of age-related losses in physical capacity, declines in muscle function, or cardiopulmonary dysfunction. If fatigue is a result of physical demands that exceed a declining capacity, then interventions must focus on reducing the physical strain of daily function and increasing the individual's physical capacity. Interventions to increase capacity and prevent deconditioning will provide a greater margin of reserve in individuals as they age. If the primary culprit of declines in energy level is new medical, psychological, or physiological conditions, then treatment is directed at those conditions.

Weakness

Objective confirmation of new muscle weakness in individuals with SCI is often problematic. To document a change it is necessary to have access to an objective baseline measure that can confirm a change in force production in a muscle group. Manual muscle testing (MMT) is the common clinical measure of strength (force production) used in rehabilitation settings and it is often not sensitive or objective enough to detect small-magnitude force changes among different testing therapists. Another common factor in the SCI population is that prior records of muscle strength were likely acquired during acute rehabilitation when muscle strength is in a state of change as a result of new functional demands and the neurological recovery processes. Dynamometry or isokinetic testing can provide a more objective measure, but the latter issue is still relevant. Therefore loss of strength in key muscle groups may not be recognized by clinicians until the patient identifies the problem. At this point, strength declines have probably crossed below a critical functional threshold and are now affecting a functional activity. Changes in hand function, changes in transfer abilities, difficulty lifting objects, or wheeling the chair are common problems associated with upper limb weakness. New difficulty or inability to stand from a chair, walk a customary distance, climb stairs or inclines, or frequent falls coincide with lower limb weakness. Depending on the original muscle capacity, significant changes in strength may have occurred before the decline is recognized by the change in functional activity, or only a small change occurred in a key muscle (or muscle group) with marginal capacity.

Self-reports of feeling weaker are reported in studies of aging changes in people with SCI.[40-42] Various etiologies may explain new weakness, including new neurological abnormalities, metabolic dysfunction, or deconditioning. In a sample of 150 people with an average of 13 years' duration of SCI, 11% attributed functional declines to loss of muscle strength. Bursell et al[43] investigated the etiology of self-reported weakness in a group of individuals with long-standing SCI and found a high percentage with new neurological abnormalities. The group consisted of 502 participants with an average age of 51 years and duration of injury of 16 years. Nineteen percent reported new weakness or sensory loss. Clinical examination, electrodiagnostic testing, and neuroimaging confirmed neurological abnormalities of a central or peripheral nature in 14% of those with new weakness. Common central conditions included posttraumatic syringomyelia and myeloradiculopathy. Peripheral etiologies resulted primarily from ulnar nerve entrapment and carpal tunnel–type syndrome. These findings confirm the need to fully investigate the subjective reports concerning new weakness. It also indicates that individuals appear reliable in recognizing the new weakness and that clinicians should attend to reports of strength changes in their patients.

Sarcopenia, joint or muscle pain, and deconditioning are other conditions that contribute to declines in muscle performance. Sarcopenia or the loss of muscle mass with age contributes to declines of contractile strength in older adults. The negative effects of disuse and age-associated weakness are responsive to exercise interventions when appropriately applied. Fiatarone et al[44] demonstrated an improvement in functional performance and muscle strength after exercise programs in elderly nursing home residents. Muscles weakened by deconditioning in people with SCI are generally responsive to the same types of strengthening principles applied to the able-bodied populations, although special consideration is necessary for muscle groups affected by peripheral or nerve root injury or those susceptible to overuse syndromes when determining how to appropriately use muscle strengthening techniques. Weakness associated with musculoskeletal pain can be treated with a progressive increase in muscle activity once the musculoskeletal condition is addressed.

Bracing to support joints and protect weakened muscles may be indicated to preserve functional use of extremities resulting from new weakness with aging. The same principles of bracing and splinting applied in early rehabilitation processes are relevant to those with new weakness later in life. Wrist-hand orthosis can maintain certain hand functions at risk because of weakness. Positional splinting can prevent loss of function from joint contractures or muscle shortening. Custom-designed bracing is usually necessary to meet the unique needs of people with an SCI. Off-the-shelf models generally do not address the specific needs of this population. Generic orthoses may fit poorly and create skin ulcers in insensate skin. The variability of hand size and shape and the movement precision required for hand function usually dictate the need for customized hand orthosis. Problems with edema, spasticity, and lack of skin sensation generally indicate a need for customized lower limb orthotics.

Rehabilitation Issues

The functional changes with age are important issues for clinicians to be aware of in any setting. Those who provide services to individuals with SCI specifically, whether in early rehabilitation or throughout the life span, have a particular need to understand the potential for declines in function. Clinicians in other settings, such as outpatient clinics or acute-care hospitals, also have contact with individuals living with SCI and can play a critical role in addressing these changes. The rehabilitation teams providing initial rehabilitation services are in a strategic position to influence future function. There are both broad and specific recommendations for early rehabilitation to help shape activity performance and lifestyles to prevent or attend to problems.

First, clinicians have to maintain a long-term life perspective when guiding decisions. Some patients may not be able to picture themselves living a long full life with paralysis but their team members can. This view is an important one because it influences health behaviors and life goals (Clinical Note: Rehabilitation Considerations). When patients see the team considering and discussing the effect of early rehabilitation decisions on later life function, they understand the importance of adopting similar habits. Clinicians should teach patients to anticipate, recognize, and manage changes in health and function. Patients should learn movement skills that protect the musculoskeletal system and that are biomechanically sound and efficient. Health promotion and health maintenance practices should be discussed, such as maintaining a healthy diet and weight, smoking cessation, and identifying a means and method to exercise safely. The philosophy of pushing the body 110% in every facet of life should be tempered to consider the long-term effects. Striving to maximize capacity is appropriate, but overusing the body on a constant basis will have negative consequences. Patients should be encouraged to educate themselves about health and functional issues so that they can make appropriate decisions throughout their lifetimes and

effectively advocate for necessary services. Last, patients should be encouraged to attend to health maintenance issues and reconnect with specialty rehabilitative services if symptoms associated with functional changes arise.

CLINICAL NOTE   **Rehabilitation Considerations**

- Educate patients regarding long-term life perspective.
- Promote health maintenance and disease prevention practices.
- Encourage efficient and biomechanically sound movement.
- Teach the skills to recognize and address functional changes.
- Encourage clients to educate and advocate for themselves.
- Identify the role rehabilitation specialists can play in late life issues.
- Encourage each individual to "Live well, long, and healthy lives!"

Relationships of Life Satisfaction to Health and Function While Aging

One of the more important ways that psychological variables influence successful aging, with or without SCI, is through life satisfaction. There is ample evidence to support the idea that in the general aging population there is an association between life satisfaction, health, and functioning and that this is a two-way relationship. Birren et al[45] have shown that good health and functioning leads to higher life satisfaction and higher life satisfaction leads to better health and function. Without an adequate degree of life satisfaction, life can become dull and drab. As people with SCI age, and as health and function are challenged, it follows that there could be problems maintaining life satisfaction.

Several research studies have examined life satisfaction among individuals living with and aging with SCI. Most research has used multi-item scales to assess life satisfaction. That is, life is divided into several areas, such as family, income, recreation, and friendships, and each part is rated, typically on a 4-point scale. Fuhrer et al[46] used an 11-item scale, and Post et al[47] used a similar method. Such approaches can also be used in clinical practice. An 11-item life satisfaction scale (usually with 4-point answers of very satisfied, mostly satisfied, somewhat satisfied, and generally dissatisfied) can be easily given to patients and it will provide valuable information about overall life and areas that could be improved.

Crewe[48] conducted a study by questionnaire and interviews of 128 people with SCI and 66 of their significant others (parent or spouse). She also compared her results with those of Flanagan, who had conducted national surveys of QOL among nondisabled individuals of various ages during the previous decade. In the 30-year-old age group, people with SCI were significantly less satisfied than individuals who were not disabled in the areas of employment, finances, sexual adjustment, and health. Other studies have also shown that people with SCI are generally less satisfied with several areas of life compared with nondisabled individuals and also have lower life satisfaction than those with other forms of impairment.[46,49]

An important question is how much does health and function relate to life satisfaction? What kind of health problems? What kind of function? If the seriousness of the SCI itself is considered, it is clear from available evidence that the level of impairment does not relate to life satisfaction to any appreciable degree in people living long term with SCI. This may run counter to intuition, but several studies show this to be true. Fuhrer[50] reviewed 19 different studies and found little evidence of a relationship between level of SCI injury and life satisfaction. Similar results have been reported by others.[41,46,47,51] The clinical significance of these results is that level of injury has little bearing on life satisfaction and therefore other things are more important. Individuals with tetraplegia can be just as satisfied with life as people with paraplegia. Any differences in life satisfaction are thus due to factors other than the level of injury. One such factor is the presence of secondary health conditions. Individuals with SCI are prone to secondary conditions such as respiratory infections, pressure ulcers, CVD, diabetes, pain, spasms, edema, and urinary tract infections. These problems do affect life satisfaction. The higher the number of secondary health problems, the lower life satisfaction becomes.[47,52] Thus managing these health problems and staying healthy are more important than the level of SCI itself in determining life satisfaction.

In a similar way, not all function relates equally to life satisfaction. Functioning can be described as activities of daily living (ADLs), instrumental activities of daily living (IADLs), and social functioning. It is primarily the latter that has shown strong relationships to life satisfaction. In his review of 19 studies, Fuhrer[50] looked at how life satisfaction correlated with measures of ADL, IADL, and social functioning. Social functioning was the only kind that was significantly related to life satisfaction. Thus employment, family participation, recreation, and community integration are the best correlates of life satisfaction.

What about when individuals with SCI grow older? How is life satisfaction affected? As could be predicted from the previous discussion, as long as health stays good and social functioning remains fairly stable, life satisfaction should stay high. As a matter of fact, the longer a person lives with an SCI, the higher life satisfaction becomes. That is, there is a positive correlation between duration of SCI and life satisfaction. Apparently, as more time goes by, people develop more satisfying lives. Moreover, the key element is duration of SCI because there is practically no correlation between age, per se, and life satisfaction.[47,49,53] The reason that duration of injury is related to life satisfaction while age is not probably relates to the fact that an SCI can have its onset at any age. In fact, about 25% of people are older at the time of onset and they naturally have relatively short durations compared with people with an early-life onset. Moreover, the chance of development of health or functional problems goes up with age, so the risk of lower life satisfaction goes up. Gerhart et al[40] studied individuals with SCI in England who were at least 20 years post onset and at least 50 years of age. They found that as duration of injury increased, life satisfaction also increased—a finding common to other studies. Gerhart et al[40] then compared life satisfaction between people who had changed function and those who had not and found that individuals who changed reported lower life satisfaction.

Relationships of Social Support to Health and Function

Another example of the biopsychosocial principle is when a psychosocial factor is important for buffering the effects of stress and poor health. Such a factor that helps to deal with adversity is the role of social support. Two aspects of social support are generally described, the practical and the emotional, but it is the latter that is of primary importance here. By emotional support is meant communications that signify that a person is valued, understood, and appreciated by others. The others can be friends, family, spouse, or children. Although elaborate instruments have been developed to assess social support, assessment can be quite straightforward and is very predictive of how well a person will do in rehabilitation and over the long term. Having people rate how much they feel supported by family and friends using this definition and asking if they have at least one very close confidant (someone they can confide in) is sufficient for clinical purposes.

In 1971, Kemp and Vash[54] measured productivity (both employment and other activities) among individuals with either paraplegia or tetraplegia who were at least 5 years post onset. The results indicated that with adequate social support, people with tetraplegia were just as productive as individuals with paraplegia. Without good social support, however, people with tetraplegia were much less productive than persons with paraplegia. In other words, there was a statistical interaction between degree of disability and social support. This interaction illustrates the buffering effect of social support: as more stress occurs, support shows a larger role. Overall, life with tetraplegia is more stressful than life with paraplegia, but good social support buffers this added stress.

Aging brings with it, in both those with and without disability, an increased risk for stressful life events. Health problems, loss of friends, decreased function, relocation of children, death of spouse, and so forth all increase with age. Thus it is even more important for individuals with SCI to have developed good social support relationships as they age. McColl and Rosenthal[41] studied the resource needs of men aging with SCI. Their sample consisted of 70 men who had an SCI for at least 15 years. Half their sample was over age 50 years and half was under 50 years old. Successful aging was measured by life satisfaction and adjustment to disability scales and by a measure of depression. A social support scale measured three aspects of support: informational, instrumental, and emotional. Function was measured by the Functional Independence Measure (FIM) (see Figure 6-13). All three aspects of social support predicted life satisfaction, adjustment, and the absence of depression. These authors, like others, concluded that objective indicators of severity of impairment and ADL or IADL performance are weakly related to life satisfaction, but social support is strongly related.

For the practicing therapist or allied health professional, the message is clear. Assessment of social support is an important part of any clinical evaluation. Social support buffers against health problems and is strongly related to life satisfaction.[55] Although social support does not necessarily diminish with age, its importance may actually increase with the age of the person with SCI because health problems and functional losses increase with age. Level of injury, age, and duration of SCI do not appear to be strongly related to developing or maintaining social support. What is probably more important to garnering support is the personality of the person with SCI. The capacity to be optimistic, somewhat extroverted, open to sharing experience, self-responsible, and interested in others' well-being will set the stage for developing good social support relationships.

Relationships of Psychological Distress to Health and Functioning

Of all the psychological variables of importance for their direct impact on health and daily function, none is more important for the therapist and allied health professional to understand than distress. And the most important form of distress relevant to SCI and other impairments is depression. The diagnosis and management of depression is discussed in a following section. For now, it is sufficient to realize that either a moderate or a severe level of depression in a person with SCI causes excess disability, poor health, and lower life satisfaction.

Depression is the number one mental health problem among individuals with disability (Clinical Note: Depression in Patients with Spinal Cord Injury). Unfortunately, depression often goes unrecognized and is poorly assessed and greatly undertreated in rehabilitation and community settings alike. Depression is often overlooked as a separate disorder because the symptoms of it may seem to be normal or even expected in a person with SCI. Certainly, discouragement, frustration, poor sleep, lack of optimism, poor endurance, troubled interpersonal relations, and health concerns do occur in people who have a disability. However, depressed affect that goes beyond discouragement and irritability, including early morning awakening, hopelessness, poor learning capacity, excess fatigue, lack of pleasure, and thoughts of suicide, are not normal and unless these symptoms are actually assessed, it is easy to confuse normal adjustment difficulties with these abnormal responses.

> **CLINICAL NOTE** **Depression in Patients with Spinal Cord Injury**
>
> - Depression greatly affects health and functioning.
> - Depression is the major mental health problem affecting individuals living with and aging with SCI.
> - Clients with SCI need ongoing screening or assessment for depression along with life satisfaction and social support.

Evidence suggests that current age is not related to depression within SCI samples.[41,46,49] However, this relationship needs further explanation. First, age may actually be related to depression, but we simply lack the longitudinal data to know. That is, depression and health problems are highly associated, and as people with SCI age, their health problems increase.[11] Older adults with depression who have health problems have shorter life expectancies than do those who are not depressed.[56] Therefore it is quite possible, and even likely, that people with SCI who are depressed are less likely to live into late life and this in turn obscures the relationship between depression and age. Second, there is a relationship between age at onset and depression. The older an individual is at the age of onset (particularly over the age of 50 years), the greater the likelihood of depression.[57]

The reported prevalence of depression in people with SCI who are at least 1 year post onset varies between 25% and 40%, depending on the study's sample characteristics, the measure used, and how the data were analyzed. McColl and Rosenthal[41] found a 40% rate of depression with the Centers for Epidemiological Studies (CES-D) measure. Fuhrer et al[46] found higher average scores in people with SCI compared with nondisabled samples.

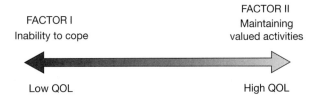

FACTOR I
Inability to cope

FACTOR II
Maintaining valued activities

Low QOL   High QOL

FIGURE 22-4 A quality of life continuum illustrates the divergences between an inability to cope with low quality of life and the ability to maintain valued activities associated with high quality of life.

Kemp and Krause[49] found a 42% prevalence rate. Although Decker and Schulz[58] did not find higher mean scores on the CES-D, they did not compute the percent of people falling above cut off scores for depression. The Consortium for Spinal Cord Medicine Clinical Practice Guidelines indicates a prevalence rate across studies of 30% to 35%.[59]

Whichever prevalence rate is selected, two points are important. First, these rates are two to three times higher than in the nondisabled population. Second, depression itself is a disabling condition. In the presence of SCI, depression can cause an increase in health problems, disability, and withdrawal from community activities.[49]

Fortunately, depression is a very treatable disorder with today's improved antidepressant medicines and focused psychotherapy. Kemp et al[60] have been treating depression with success. In one study treating depression in individuals with SCI, a group of 27 with major depression were compared with an untreated group over a 1-year period. Most of the people who were treated (with medicine and psychotherapy) decreased their levels of depression by an average of 57%, increased their community activities over 100%, and increased their life satisfaction from an average somewhat satisfied score to a mostly satisfied average score.

MAINTAINING QUALITY OF LIFE WHILE LIVING WITH SPINAL CORD INJURY

There is an obvious link between life satisfaction and depression. Together, they can be seen to anchor the opposite ends of a QOL continuum (Figure 22-4). People who experience high QOL are happy with most aspects of their lives, they are energetic and optimistic; life is good and it's difficult to imagine how it could get much better. At the other end of the continuum, we find distress, despair, and depression. At the low end, it's hard to imagine how life could get much worse. The value and meaning of life are often missing and the option of not living may look better than living with such despair. In the middle of the QOL scale is a life that is neither happy nor unhappy, a getting by attitude, life is so-so. The issue of what relates to QOL among individuals living with SCI is the topic in a following section.

Objective Versus Subjective Measures of Quality of Life

QOL has been measured two different ways in research. First, the objective approach measures observable indices such as employment status, income, home ownership, number of medical problems, and marital status. Second is the subjective method, which measures the respondent's own views of his QOL without regard to objective indices. Both QOL measurement approaches have been reviewed by Fuhrer,[50] Gill and Feinstein,[61] and Dijkers.[53] Subjective approaches are favored here. The basic arguments in favor of a subjective QOL approach are as follows:

- Self-appraisal is correct for the person himself because he is the best judge of his own life
- Subjective appraisals often are based on things that are not obvious, such as the quality of a person's primary relationship
- Assessment of subjective QOL allows researchers to focus on what correlates with high and low QOL, whether there are other subjective factors or objective factors

Two-Factor Theory of Quality of Life over the Life Span

A review of the literature on the topic of QOL in SCI indicates that the correlates of low QOL are quite different than the correlates of high QOL. Low QOL has been found to be correlated with a poor attitude toward disability, low interpersonal support, multiple losses, poor coping ability, diminished health, poor daily functioning, and less adaptive personality traits.[59,62,63] High QOL, however, seems not to be just the reverse of these. High QOL correlates with a variety of other things, including positive engagement in social and community activities, a sense of purpose in life, rewarding social interactions, the productive use of time, and the presence of some pleasurable activities.[47,50,52,53,64] These findings suggest a two-factor theory of QOL. In a two-factor theory that tries to account for phenomena at opposite ends of a continuum, one factor often explains one end of the continuum whereas a different factor altogether accounts for the opposite end of the continuum. In the case of QOL as it relates to individuals with SCI, the same can be said. One factor, which consists of several variables, can be used to account why those with SCI become distressed and depressed (low QOL) but a separate factor accounts for positive QOL. The factor that seems to best account for distress and depression is the inability to cope. Coping itself is a complex phenomenon that is described later, but the inability to cope implies that the person is not capable of dealing with the multitude of changes and losses brought about by the SCI initially or subsequently as he ages.

The second factor, which accounts for high QOL, might be summarized as "maintaining valued activities." To have high life satisfaction, not only must a person be able to cope with losses, changes, and new challenges but also must find a way to develop and maintain valued activities and experiences. This is probably why research shows that the ability to perform basic ADLs is unrelated to life satisfaction (these are just activities everyone has to do) but social relationships are related to life satisfaction (because they provide meaningful activity).

The kinds of activities that provide valued and meaningful experience change over the life span. In early life, up to about age 18 years, the principal important activities are pleasure seeking. Activities that provide fun, excitement, adventure, and sensation are valued. From roughly age 18 to age 60 years, important activities revolve around success and achievement. People strive to become someone, to make a good living, to accomplish their goals, to have a career, or to raise a family. In

later life, certainly by about age 60 years, a principal task is to find meaning and purpose through activities. This may involve new roles such as becoming a grandparent or through travel or spiritual growth. At this stage of life, it's not that pleasure and success are unimportant but rather that other aspects of life begin to take on greater importance. Thus, what is important for maintaining valued experiences evolves across the life span. If therapists want to know what contributes to a person's QOL, asking the person to describe the presence and absence of these kinds of activities is helpful.

RECOGNIZING AND SCREENING FOR DEPRESSION IN INDIVIDUALS LIVING WITH SPINAL CORD INJURY
Importance of Depression

It is vital that therapists and other clinicians be able to recognize, and when appropriate, refer individuals with SCI who are suspected of being depressed (Clinical Note: Prevalence of Depressive Disorders in Individuals with Spinal Cord Injury). Depression represents an abnormal response, usually to losses or multiple losses, that becomes a full-fledged biopsychosocial disorder when it reaches full proportions. Depression is the most common and the most serious secondary condition of a psychiatric nature among individuals with SCI, affecting 30% to 40% of clients with SCI. The 1998 clinical practice guidelines for primary care physicians, *Depression Following Spinal Cord Injury*, cites many studies showing the impact of depression.[59] In another study, conducted at Shepherd Rehabilitation Center in Atlanta, Krause studied 1300 people with SCI by use of a variety of health, life satisfaction, and daily functioning measures and found that depression was highly correlated with every one of them.[57]

CLINICAL NOTE | **Prevalence of Depressive Disorders in Individuals with Spinal Cord Injury**

- Thirty to forty percent of patients with SCI have depression severe enough that it interferes with daily function.
- Clinicians need to be aware of this common problem.
- Clinicians need to recognize and properly refer clients with this disorder.

Recognizing depression in a person living with and aging with SCI is difficult, not only because symptoms of each condition overlap, but because clinicians and individuals with SCI are hesitant to explore and probe the kinds of thoughts and feelings that would reveal a depressive disorder. After all, is anyone really comfortable discussing thoughts of death, gloomy feelings, or how unsuccessful they feel? Nevertheless, a clinician always needs to be ready to entertain the existence of depression, particularly if the client:

- Functions at less than expected levels given his injury and disability
- Reports with vague descriptions of pain, fatigue, poor sleep, or digestive problems
- Has health problems that appear to relate to poor self-care
- Causes other people to report that he is harder to get along with or is moody

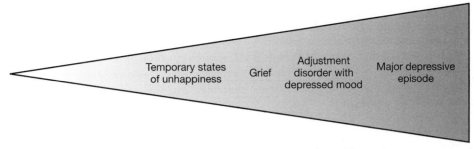

FIGURE 22-5 A spectrum of depressive disorders common in SCI illustrates the range of mood from unhappiness to major depressive episode.

Understanding Depressive Disorders

The term depression actually applies to a variety of disorders, all of which are characterized by a change in mood as the principal feature. So, to be accurate, there is a family of depressive disorders. The individual disorders have different diagnostic terms depending on the severity of the disorder. Together, depressive disorders can be thought of as existing on a continuum or spectrum, from less severe to very severe. Some different diagnostic terms applied to these depressive disorders are dysphoria, adjustment disorder with a depressed mood, or major depressive episode. The spectrum concept and some of the depressive disorders making up this spectrum is illustrated in Figure 22-5. Usually less severe disorders resolve with time, understanding, and support from others. Moderately severe disorders usually require psychotherapy of several months' duration. Severe major depressive disorders usually respond best to psychotherapy and antidepressant medication. So how do you determine whether a person has a depressive disorder and how severe it is? This is determined by three parameters.

The most important thing to consider is the number and kind of symptoms the person has. To qualify for a depressive disorder, at least of a moderate degree, the person must have a change in mood that is not typical of him. The mood change can be sadness but it can just as easily be irritability, anger, indifference, or apathy. This mood change should have existed for 3 to 6 weeks. The person also has to have some additional symptoms in the following domains:

- Cognitive change: decreased memory or concentration, hopeless thoughts, self-blame, irrational beliefs
- Behavioral change: self-neglect, poor work performance, poor interpersonal relations, few pleasurable activities
- Physiological change: fatigue, poor sleep, lack of sexual ability, poor appetite, pain

Importantly, these symptoms cannot be the result of other causes such as a medical condition (e.g., hypothyroidism), a neurological deficit (e.g., dementia), or a different psychiatric disorder (e.g., schizophrenia).

Everything else considered, fewer symptoms (i.e., some mood change plus three to four others) imply a moderate level of depression, such as an adjustment disorder with a depressed mood, whereas a profound mood change plus six to eight other symptoms implies a major depressive disorder. In addition to symptoms, two other factors need to be considered. First is the effect of these symptoms on daily function. A greater effect on daily functioning implies a more severe depressive disorder. In fact, it is sometimes hard to elicit symptoms from a severely depressed individual, so a greater emphasis has to be placed on function. For someone with SCI, altered functioning is probably a bigger tip-off to the presence of depression than in nondisabled individuals. Second, in helping to determine the severity of depression, it is important to know how readily the symptoms are changed by providing the relatively simple elements of support, understanding, counseling, and time. Symptoms that are relieved with these relatively simpler techniques imply a less serious disorder. Symptoms that do not respond to these methods, however, suggest that a more severe disorder is present. Thus it is important to ask each client about his symptoms, about how long the symptoms have been going on, whether the symptoms are atypical (he will tell you), what changes in daily or social functioning have occurred, and whether anything makes it better.

Several screening instruments for depression are available in the literature, such as the Beck Depression Inventory[65] and the Geriatric Depression Scale.[66] Another scale, the Older Adult Health and Mood Questionnaire, was developed specifically for adults who have a disability (Box 22-2).[67] It has proven valuable with adults at any age who have a disability, not just older adults. It contains two kinds of items: those that reflect a change in mood (all the odd-numbered items) and those that reflect cognitive, behavioral, or physiological symptoms (all the even-numbered items). The critical answer for each question is true, and the total number of true answers provides a reliable indication of possible depression. Scores from 0 to 5 are considered normal or mild depression, and scores from 6 to 10 suggest some form of moderate depressive disorder (such as an adjustment disorder with a depressed mood). Scores above 11 indicate the strong likelihood of a severe depressive disorder. In moderate and severe cases, the clinician should make sure that both odd and even items are endorsed. A pattern of endorsement of only even-numbered items, particularly if they pertain to behavioral and physiological items, would suggest that this is not a depressive disorder but is the manifestation of the effects of the disability or related health problems.

Causes of Depression in Spinal Cord Injury

Moderate depressive disorders primarily have psychological factors as their cause, particularly the person's difficulty coping with losses and changes. Severe forms of depression have both psychological and neurological causes that impair basic processes of adaptive and integrative behavior. Psychologically, the mechanisms involved in coping with adverse life events seem to break down in individuals who become depressed. Coping itself is a complex process involving interpersonal, attitudinal, and

BOX 22-2 | The Older Adult Health and Mood Questionnaire

1. My daily life is not interesting ....T or F
2. It is hard for me to get started on my daily chores and activities .... T or F
3. I have been more unhappy than usual for at least a month..T or F
4. I have been sleeping poorly for at least the last month ....T or F
5. I gain little pleasure from anything ....T or F
6. I feel listless, tired, or fatigued a lot of the time ....T or F
7. I have felt sad, down in the dumps, or blue much of the time during the last month ....T or F
8. My memory or thinking is not as good as usual ....T or F
9. I have been more easily irritated or frustrated lately ....T or F
10. I feel worse in the morning than in the afternoon ....T or F
11. I have cried or felt like crying more than twice during the last month .... T or F
12. I am definitely slowed down compared with my usual way of feeling .... T or F
13. The things that used to make me happy don't do so anymore .... T or F
14. My appetite or digestion of food is worse than usual ....T or F
15. I frequently feel like I don't care about anything anymore .... T or F
16. Life is really not worth living most of the time ....T or F
17. My outlook is more gloomy than usual ....T or F
18. I have stopped several of my usual activities ....T or F
19. I cry or feel saddened more easily than a few months ago ....T or F
20. I feel pretty hopeless about improving my life ....T or F
21. I seem to have lost the ability to have any fun ....T or F
22. I have regrets about the past that I think about often .... T or F

From Kemp BJ, Adams BA: The Older Adult Health and Mood Questionnaire: a measure of geriatric depressive disorder, *J Geriatr Psychiatry Neurol* 8:162-167, 1995.

personality factors. Recent research and theoretical developments by Lazarus and Folkman[68] and others have resulted in a multifactorial model of coping (Figure 22-6). This model not only has been helpful in directing research, but it is clinically useful because it helps to illustrate how people cope and, when coping breaks down, what aspects might be involved.

The stress-coping model, as it is called, starts with the adverse life events people are faced with and ends with the quality of their coping, whether good, poor, or in between. Depression would be an example of a poor coping outcome. Between the adverse events and the coping outcomes are four key variables. These are termed (1) appraisal—the meaning and interpretation people give to the events and changes in their lives, (2) their coping methods—what they actually try to do to deal with the stressful live events, (3) the amount of social support people receive, and (4) the person's underlying personality. The model proposes that when any part of the coping process breaks down or is faulty (too many adverse life events, irrationally negative interpretations of them, little social support, maladaptive personality traits, or poor coping methods), then coping will be difficult and the outcome will be poor. If the components of coping are positive, then the result will be as good as possible.

Undeniably, someone living long term with an SCI faces many adverse life events. Health, functional, economic, social, environmental, and personal problems happen frequently. Additionally, some people may never have learned how to cope with such adversity or may have questionable support or a poor outlook. This would predict a poor outcome. On the other hand, another person with exactly the same injury may maintain a realistic outlook, have good support and coping resources, and will have a reasonably adequate outcome. In every case of major or moderate depression, at least one of these four components will be significantly abnormal. Psychotherapy that is based on this model tries to correct and improve these components.

Major depression also involves alterations in biology and psychological coping. Among other things, profound changes in brain neurotransmitters—the chemical substances responsible for transmitting messages between cells—occur in major depression. Different neurotransmitters are involved in different kinds of systems: motor, sensory, cognitive, or affective. The two main neurotransmitters that are deficient in depression are serotonin and norepinephrine; in depression too little of these chemicals gets across the synapse. Antidepressant medications help to make these neurotransmitters more available postsynaptically. Medicines commonly given for depression include Paxil (paroxetine), Zoloft (sertraline), Prozac (fluoxetine), and Celexa (citalopram). After a person takes a medicine for a sufficient time, enough neurochemical changes occur to ease the depression, improve behavior and outlook, and allow the individual to be able to profit from psychotherapy. Without these medicines, progress in recovery from psychotherapy is often much slower. Most people continue to take a medicine for about one year, after which the drug is slowly reduced.

Age Differences Related to Development of Depression

Most research concerning aging and depression in individuals with SCI has looked at three issues: current age, duration of SCI, and age at onset. Neither of the first two variables is strongly related to the prevalence of depression. The latter variable, however, is moderately related, with later age onsets having a higher prevalence.[57]

Although the prevalence of depression is not highly age related, there are still age differences in the display of depression. In older nondisabled adults, for example, depression is more likely to be displayed as irritability than it is in younger people. Another age difference may involve the number and rate of adverse life events younger and older adults with SCI have to cope with. Health and functional problems increase with age in SCI. Individuals can usually cope with about one major life event every 6 months. At a higher rate than that, coping resources are greatly taxed.

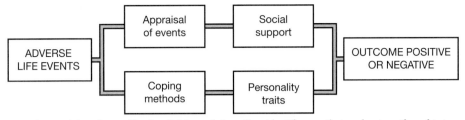

FIGURE 22-6 A stress-coping model can be used by the clinician to help a client identify areas that can be strengthened to improve coping skills and others that may be the cause when coping breaks down.

IMPACT OF AGE CHANGES ON THE FAMILY
Understanding the Family: Individuals and the Group

As individuals with SCI age, health and functional problems often increase. This change not only has an impact on the individual with the SCI but can affect the family as well. Families are the biggest source of support for all people with disabling conditions. In the case of SCI, when assistance is required, families provide more than 70% of it. The remaining help is provided by paid attendants or friends. Family assistance may come from spouse, parents, siblings, or children. The better a family is able to meet the needs of the person with SCI at the same time that it meets its own needs, the better the health, functioning, and quality of life will be for the individual with SCI.

SCI can be stressful for both the individual who has it and for the family. Rates of divorce among those who were married at the time of injury are higher among people with SCI than among people who are not disabled,[69] and a smaller percentage of single people with SCI marry after onset compared with those who are not disabled.[70] In addition, measured depression is higher among spouses of people with SCI 1 year after onset than it is among those without SCI,[71] and stress in spousal caregivers of people with SCI is higher than in spouses who are not providing additional assistance for someone with a disability.[72]

Families are difficult to assess because they are made up of individuals, but these individuals also constitute a group. Therefore, it is essential in understanding families to understand both the individuals who make it up as well as the group dynamics that describe how the family functions. Among the first things that should be done in assessing families is to identify who is in the family, the quality of their relations with each other, and who is/are the principal sources of support. Who constitutes the family differs by the age at onset of the SCI. Below the age of 25 years, the family is usually the nuclear family, meaning that the person with SCI is not married and the principal relationships are to parents and siblings. After age 25 years, at least half of people with SCI are married. Their principal relationships are to their spouses and children and secondarily to their parents and siblings. When SCI occurs to a married person, the spouse becomes the principal source of family assistance if any is needed. As individuals age with SCI, many experience functional changes and the need for more assistance. Research by Gerhart et al[21] and Thompson et al[73] shows that about 25% of those aging with SCI undergo functional changes that will require increased assistance, particularly with chores, toileting, bathing, and

transfers. Thompson et al[73] further assessed who helped these individuals with increased assistance and found that much the same pattern emerged as is reported for assistance before age-related changes: spouses and older children for married people, and parents, siblings, or adult children for single or divorced individuals. A genogram can be a useful tool for both describing the individuals in a family and their interactions and availability to give assistance as needed.

Identifying Family Members: The Genogram

The genogram is a diagramming tool developed in genetic research and family medicine to help capture, on paper, all the persons in a family. A simplified sample is presented in Figure 22-7. In this figure, squares represent males and circles represent females. Solid lines indicate a marital or offspring bond. A solid line with a crossed line through it represents a separated relationship (e.g., divorce) and a solid line with zigzag cross lines through it represents a conflicted relationship. Deaths are indicated by crossing out the square or circle. Offspring are indicated in their birth order from left to right. The identified patient or person with SCI is indicated by an arrow. The primary care provider can be indicated by a symbol, such as a star. The names, ages, locations, and major health problems of each individual are indicated in or beside each square or circle. The genogram usually starts with the parents or grandparents.

This diagram shows that Bob, who has SCI, lives in Long Beach with his wife, Anne, and their two sons, Fred, age 10 years, and John, age 16 years. Bob is 46 years old and has had his SCI since 1980. Anne is his wife and his principal assistance, but she has rheumatoid arthritis. Bob's dad is alive, but has Alzheimer's disease; Bob's mother is deceased from cancer. Bob has two sisters but they live in different states. Bob was married once before, to Linda, and they had a child, Becky, who is 23 years old and is married to Tim.

This family is at high risk of considerable stress. Bob and Anne both have disabilities, Bob's father has Alzheimer's disease, and Bob and Anne's two children are still in school. This family system may hold together as long as additional stress does not occur. However, that is unlikely. Bob has a high-level injury. Bob's father will get worse, Anne's arthritis may flare and Bob may develop new problems as he ages. Bob's dad will probably need support from Bob or Anne because the other siblings are out of the state. The main point is that a genogram ensures that a picture of the family is captured, its strengths

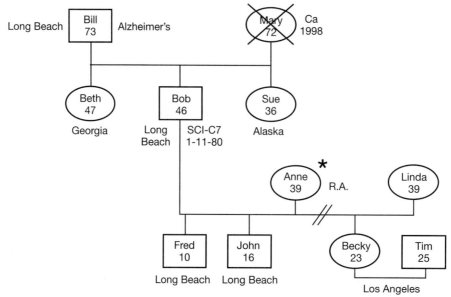

FIGURE 22-7 A genogram of the family unit ensures that a picture of the family is captured, revealing its strengths and vulnerabilities. This allows assessments to be made of at-risk members and a plan implemented to follow or assist them.

and vulnerabilities can be revealed, assessments can be made of at-risk members, and a plan to follow or assist them can be implemented.

Family Dynamics

From a functional point of view, it is necessary to understand how a family operates as a unit. When the focus is on the family unit, it is important to consider how well the family functions along certain lines. Four such parameters are:

- Communication—how fully people communicate with each other
- Cohesion—how well people work together
- Support—how much people support each other, not just the person with SCI
- Adaptability—how adaptable the family is to changing demands

Experience shows that family members can make reliable judgments of these parameters.[24] Further, these dynamics relate to important outcomes, such as how individuals cope with aging-related changes.

It is unknown what percent of families that include an individual with an SCI perform very well, moderately well, or poorly in terms of incorporating the needs of that member who is aging with SCI into family life with minimal stress. Some of the important predictors of family adaptability include the stress levels and health status of each of the family members, its history of working together, and any conflicts between individual members of the family.

Helping Families to Cope with the Problems of Aging

Depending on the stress level of individual members and the functioning of the family unit, different kinds of interventions can be developed to assist them. At least three different levels of assistance can be defined.

1. Education: All families should be taught about age-related changes in SCI. Medical, functional, vocational, and psychosocial changes that occur to individuals aging with SCI and what to do about them need to be presented to every family. In addition, families need to learn about community resources, assistive technology, and recognizing and managing stress.

2. Counseling: Some percentage of families need counseling to help them develop better coping skills; to express and understand common but difficult emotions such as resentment, frustration, and guilt; and how better to support each other. Families needing counseling are more or less normal but are showing signs of stress.

3. Therapy: A small percentage of families (10% to 15%) are dysfunctional enough that the care and well-being of everyone in the family, including the person with SCI, is affected. In these families, one or more members has a definable disorder or else the family's functioning on those four parameters is so poor that they cannot provide each other with basic needs of family life. These families may display what Holicky[74] described as burden, role fatigue, conflict, or hostility.

CLINICAL CASE STUDY Aging and Spinal Cord Injury

Patient History

Samuel Gross is a 71-year-old man with a C6 tetraplegia American Spinal Injury Association (ASIA) A diagnosis. He sustained his SCI 31 years ago as the result of a motor vehicle accident. Sam is a retired financial consultant. He and his wife have two grown children. Their daughter, age 36 years, has two young children, ages 2 and 4 years, and his son, age 34 years, also has two children, ages 5 months and 3 years. His children live nearby, but his son has just been transferred out of state, 300 miles away.

Sam's wife is 62 years old and works as an elementary school teacher. Sam has recently had right shoulder tendonitis and is currently not able to propel his wheelchair or drive his van. He has also developed a small left ischial pressure ulcer, which is healing. He has started a course of physical therapy for his shoulder.

Patient' Self-Assessment

Sam feels he has been lucky since his injury at age 40 years. His career was not altered significantly and he continued to be able to provide for his family, including sending both children through college. Since his injury, Sam has had an aide who comes 2 hours every morning to help him with bathing, bowel and bladder care, and dressing. His health has been good and he only has had some minor issues including a couple of urinary tract infections, one sacral pressure ulcer that required one week of hospitalization, and a couple of bouts of pneumonia. He has some growing concerns, however, brought into focus by his shoulder pain and is considering switching to a power wheelchair. He is also sad that his son will be moving. He has enjoyed having his grandchildren nearby and being able to see them two to three times a week. Sam is fortunate to be an avid reader and enjoys using his computer.

Clinical Assessment
Patient Appearance

- Height 5 feet 10 inches, weight 180 pounds, body mass index 25.8

Cognitive Assessment

- Alert, oriented × 3

Cardiopulmonary Assessment

- Blood pressure 128/80 mm Hg, heart rate at rest 76 beats/min, respiratory rate 12 breaths/min, cough flows are ineffective (<360 L/min), vital capacity is reduced (between 1.5 and 2.5 L)

Musculoskeletal and Neuromuscular Assessment

- Motor assessment reveals C6 ASIA A, sensory C6
- Deep tendon reflexes 3+ below the level of lesion

Integumentary and Sensory Assessment

- Left ischial pressure ulcer, 3 × 4 × 2 cm, sensory intact to C6

Range of Motion Assessment

- Passive and active motion is within normal limits in the left upper limb; the right shoulder is limited as follows:

	Active range of motion (degrees)	Passive range of motion (degrees)
Flexion	110	115
Abduction	90	95
Internal rotation	50	55
External rotation	30	38

- Straight leg raise is 80 degrees in both lower limbs and dorsiflexion is 0 degrees; all other motions in the lower limbs are within functional limits.

Mobility and ADL Assessment

- Sam requires minimal to moderate assistance with bed mobility and transfers to all surfaces.
- Sam is independent with pressure relief.
- Sam is currently dependent in manual wheelchair maneuvering on all surfaces.
- Sam is dependent in all self-care ADLs.
- Sam is currently unable to drive.

Evaluation of Clinical Assessment

Samuel Gross is a 71-year-old man with a C6 tetraplegia ASIA A diagnosis. He sustained his SCI 31 years ago from an MVA. He began attending outpatient physical therapy 1 week ago for shoulder pain and decreased functional ability.

Patient's Care Needs

1. Interventions for physical therapy to restore pain-free right shoulder and return it to prior level of function
2. Assess need for seating clinic referral
3. Education regarding prevention of worsening of wound
4. Evaluation for psychology services

Diagnosis and Prognosis

Diagnosis is C6 complete tetraplegia, ASIA A with a prognosis of full recovery of right shoulder to prior level of pain-free function.

Preferred Practice Patterns*

Impaired Muscle Performance (4C), Joint Mobility, Motor Function, Muscle Performance, and Range of Motion Associated With Localized Inflammation (4E), Joint Mobility, Motor Function, Muscle Performance, and Range of Motion Associated With Fracture (4G), Primary Prevention/Risk Reduction for Cardiovascular/Pulmonary Disorders (6A), Impaired Integumentary Integrity Associated with Superficial Skin Involvement (7 B)

Team Goals

1. Team to improve patient's right shoulder pain-free range of motion and strength
2. Team to educate patient on prevention of future pressure ulcers and current wound care
3. Patient to improve cardiopulmonary capacity

Patient Goals

"I want to be able to control my own wheelchair again, even if it is a power chair, and drive again without any shoulder pain."

Care Plan
Treatment Plan and Rationale

- Initiate physical therapy interventions for the reduction of pain in client's right shoulder and restoration of function to prior level.
- Educate patient about prevention strategies for pressure relief to avoid future pressure ulcers.
- Initiate cardiopulmonary fitness training to improve aerobic capacity for functional activities and prevention of future pneumonias.
- Schedule patient for psychology evaluation.

Interventions

- Outpatient physical therapy therapeutic exercise, neuromuscular re-education, functional activities training, and modalities for reduction of pain, aerobic exercises, and wound prevention education

Continued

CLINICAL CASE STUDY Aging and Spinal Cord Injury—cont'd

Documentation and Team Communication
- Team consultation for adjustment to life changes and probable wheelchair clinic consultation

Follow-Up Assessment
- Biweekly team conferences for timely attainment of goals
- Reassessment for consultation with other services

Critical Thinking Exercises
Consider factors that will influence patient education, physical therapy, and team care decisions unique to Sam's SCI associated with his aging and his concerns about his son's family move when answering the following questions:

1. Describe from a biopsychosocial perspective the issues in this clinical case.
2. What age-related changes would Sam be at higher risk for? What must be considered that could further affect Sam's function?
3. List three suggestions that could be implemented to manage Sam's pain.
4. What would you expect regarding Sam's life satisfaction? What issues related to social support are affecting Sam's health status?
5. List signs and symptoms of depression that you, as the clinician, should be aware of when observing Sam.

*Guide to physical therapist practice, rev. ed. 2, Alexandria, VA, 2003, American Physical Therapy Association.

SUMMARY

Aging with SCI is often accompanied by health and functional changes. These additional challenges, in turn, can affect psychological outcomes such as quality of life. In addition, several psychosocial variables affect how well individuals with SCI will age and function. Among these are social support, coping ability, depression, and the role of the family. Increasing age of both the individual with SCI and his family adds to the importance of these factors. It is important for the clinician to be able to identify and assess these factors and to make referrals when appropriate.

REFERENCES

1. National Spinal Cord Injury Statistical Center: *Spinal cord injury: facts and figures at a glance,* Birmingham, 1995, University of Alabama.
2. Berkowitz M: *The economic consequences of traumatic SCI,* New York, 1993, Demos.
3. Jette AM: Special issue: physical disability, *Phys Ther* 74:379-503, 1994.
4. World Health Organization: *International classification of functioning, disability and health (ICF):* www3.who.int/icf/. Accessed November 15, 2006.
5. Baumgartner RN: Body composition in healthy aging, *Ann N Y Acad Sci* 904:437-448, 2000.
6. Hughes VA, Frontera WR, Wood M et al: Longitudinal muscle strength changes in older adults: influence of muscle mass, physical activity and health, *J Gerontol Biol Sci* 56A:B209-B217, 2001.
7. Bauman WA, Spungen AM: Body composition in aging: adverse changes in able-bodied persons and in those with spinal cord injury, *Top Spinal Cord Inj Rehabil* 6:22-26, 2001.
8. Linn WS, Adkins RH, Gong H et al: Pulmonary function in chronic spinal cord injury: a cross-sectional survey of 222 Southern California adult outpatients, *Arch Phys Med Rehabil* 81:757-763, 2000.
9. Bauman WA, Spungen AM, Adkins RH et al: Metabolic and endocrine changes in persons aging with spinal cord injury, *Assist Technol* 11:88-96, 1999.
10. Ragnarsson KT: The cardiovascular system. In Whiteneck GG, editor: *Aging with spinal cord injury,* New York, 1993, Demos.
11. Whiteneck G, Charlifue MA, Frankel HL et al: Mortality, morbidity, and psychosocial outcomes of persons spinal cord injured more than 20 years age, *Paraplegia* 30:617-630, 1992.
12. Thompson L, Yakura J: Aging related functional changes in person with spinal cord injury, *Top Spinal Cord Inj Rehabil* 6:69-82, 2001.
13. Siddall PJ, Taylor DA, Cousins MJ: Classification of pain following spinal cord injury, *Spinal Cord* 35:69-75, 1997.
14. Bryce TN, Ragnarsson KT: Epidemiology and classification of pain after spinal cord injury, *Top Spinal Cord Inj Rehabil* 7:1-17, 2001.
15. Yezierski RP: Identification of therapeutic targets and the development of novel treatments for spinal cord injury pain, *Top Spinal Cord Inj Rehabil* 7:93-105, 2001.
16. Rintala D, Loubser P, Castro J et al: Chronic pain in a community-based sample of men with spinal cord injury: prevalence, severity and relationship with impairment, disability, handicap and subjective well-being, *Arch Phys Med Rehabil* 79:604-614, 1998.
17. Yezierski RP: Pain following spinal cord injury: the clinical problem and experimental studies, *Pain* 68:185-194, 1996.
18. Curtis KA, Tyner TM, Zachary L et al: Effect of a standard exercise protocol on shoulder pain in long-term wheelchair users, *Spinal Cord* 37:421-429, 1999.
19. U.S. Department of Health and Human Services, Public Health Service: *Evaluation of the musculoskeletal diseases program,* Rockville, MD, 1984, NIH Publication. pp 84–109.
20. Halstead LS, Rossi CD: New problems in old polio patients: results of a survey of 539 polio survivor, *Orthopedics* 8:845-850, 1985.
21. Gerhart KA, Bergstrom E, Charlifue MA et al: Long-term spinal cord injury: functional changes over time, *Arch Phys Med Rehabil* 74:1030-1034, 1993.
22. Murphy KP, Molnar GE, Lankasky K: Medical and functional status of adults with cerebral palsy, *Dev Med Child Neurol* 37:1075-1084, 1995.
23. Burnham RS, May L, Nelson E et al: Shoulder pain in wheelchair athletes: the role of muscle imbalance, *Am J Sports Med* 21:238-242, 1993.
24. Campbell ML: *Aging with disability: post-polio, rheumatoid arthritis, and stroke,* Downey, CA, 1996, Rehabilitation Research and Training Center on Aging with Disability, Rancho Los Amigos Medical Center.
25. Curtis KA, Drysdale GA, Lanza D et al: Shoulder pain in wheelchair users with tetraplegia and paraplegia, *Arch Phys Med Rehabil* 80:453-457, 1999.
26. Pentland WE, Twomey LT: Upper limb function in persons with long term paraplegia and implications for independence, *Paraplegia* 32:219-224, 1994.
27. Sie IH, Waters RL, Adkins RH et al: Upper limb pain in the post-rehabilitation spinal cord injured patient, *Arch Phys Med Rehabil* 73:44-48, 1992.

28. Subbarao J, Kopfstein J, Turpin R: Prevalence and impact of wrist and shoulder pain in patients with spinal cord injury, *J Spinal Cord Med* 18:9-13, 1995.

29. Gellman H, Sie I, Waters RL: Late complications of the weight-bearing upper limb in paraplegic patient, *Clin Orthop* 233:132-135, 1998.

30. Rehabilitation Research and Training Center on Aging with a Disability: *Natural course study of aging with a disability*, Downey, CA, 2001 unpublished RRTC report.

31. Perry J, Gronley JK, Newsam CJ et al: Electromyographic analysis of the shoulder muscles during depression transfers in subjects with low-level paraplegia, *Arch Phys Med Rehabil* 77:350-355, 1996.

32. Mulroy SJ, Gronley JK, Newsam CJ et al: Electromyographic activity of shoulder muscles during wheelchair propulsion by paraplegic persons, *Arch Phys Med Rehabil* 77:187-193, 1996.

33. Newsam CJ, Rao SS, Mulroy SJ et al: Three dimensional upper limb motion during manual wheelchair propulsion in men with different levels of spinal cord injury, *Gait Posture* 10:223-232, 1999.

34. Gronley JK, Newsam CJ, Mulroy SJ et al: Electromyographic and kinematic analysis of the shoulder during four activities of daily living in men with C6 tetraplegia, *J Rehabil Res Dev* 37:423-432, 2000.

35. Waters RL, Sie IH: Upper limb changes with SCI contrasted to common aging in the musculoskeletal system, *Top Spinal Cord Inj Rehabil* 6:63-70, 2001.

36. Price RK, North CS, Wessely S et al: Estimating the prevalence of chronic fatigue syndrome and associated symptoms in the community, *Public Health Rep* 107:514-522, 1992.

37. Walker EA, Katon WJ, Jenelka RP: Psychiatric disorders and medical care utilization among people in the general population who report fatigue, *J Gen Intern Med* 8:436-440, 1993.

38. Janssen TWJ, Van Oers CAJM, Van der Woude LHV et al: Physical strain in daily life of wheelchair users with spinal cord injuries, *Med Sci Sports Exerc* 26:661-670, 1994.

39. McNeal DR, Somerville BS, Wilson DJ: Work problems and accommodations reported by persons who are post polio or have a spinal cord injury, *Assist Technol* 11:137-157, 1999.

40. Gerhart KA, Koziol-McLain J, Lowenstein SR et al: Quality of life following spinal cord injury: knowledge and attitudes of emergency care providers, *Ann Emerg Med* 23:807-812, 1994.

41. McColl MA, Rosenthal C: A model of resource needs of aging spinal cord injured men, *Paraplegia* 32:261-270, 1994.

42. Thompson L: Functional changes in persons aging with spinal cord injury, *Assist Technol* 11:123-129, 1999.

43. Bursell JP, Little JW, Stiens SA: Electrodiagnosis in spinal cord injured persons with new weakness or sensory loss: central and peripheral etiologies, *Arch Phys Med Rehabil* 80:904-909, 1999.

44. Fiatarone MA, O'Neill EF, Ryan ND et al: Exercise training and nutritional supplementation for physical frailty in very elderly people, *N Engl J Med* 330:1769-1775, 1994.

45. Birren JE, Sloane RB, Cohen GD: *Handbook of mental health and aging*, New York, 1992, Academic Press.

46. Fuhrer MJ, Rintala DH, Hart KA et al: Relationship of life satisfaction to impairment, disability, and handicap among persons with spinal cord injury living in the community, *Arch Phys Med Rehabil* 73:552-557, 1992.

47. Post MWM, de Witte LP, van Asbeck FWA et al: Predictors of health status and life satisfaction in spinal cord injury, *Arch Phys Med Rehabil* 79:395-401, 1998.

48. Crewe N: Quality of life: the ultimate goal in rehabilitation, *Minn Med* 163:586-589, 1980.

49. Kemp BJ, Krause JS: Depression and life satisfaction among people ageing with post-polio and spinal cord injury, *Disabil Rehabil* 21:241-249, 1999.

50. Fuhrer MJ: The subjective well-being of people with spinal cord injury: relationships to impairment, disability, and handicap, *Top Spinal Cord Inj Rehabil* 1:56-71, 1996.

51. Cushman LA, Hassett J: Spinal cord injury: 10 and 15 years after, *Paraplegia* 30:690-696, 1992.

52. Krause JS: Adjustment after spinal cord injury: a 9-year longitudinal study, *Arch Phys Med Rehabil* 78:651-657, 1997.

53. Dijkers M: Quality of life after spinal cord injury: a meta-analysis of the effects of disablement components, *Spinal Cord* 35:829-840, 1997.

54. Kemp BJ, Vash CL: Productivity after injury in a sample of spinal cord injured persons: a pilot study, *J Chronic Dis* 24:259-275, 1971.

55. Cobb S: Social support as a moderator of life stress, *Psychosom Med* 38:300-314, 1976.

56. Murphy E, Smith R, Lindesay J et al: Increased mortality rates in late-life depression, *Br J Psychiatry* 152:347-353, 1988.

57. Krause JS, Kemp BJ, Coker JL: Depression after spinal cord injury: relation to gender, ethnicity, aging, and socioeconomic indicators, *Arch Phys Med Rehabil* 81:1099-1109, 2000.

58. Decker SD, Schulz R: Correlates of life satisfaction and depression in middle-aged and elderly spinal cord-injured persons, *Am J Occup Ther* 39:740-745, 1985.

59. Consortium for Spinal Cord Medicine: *Depression following spinal cord injury: a clinical practice guideline for primary care physicians*, Washington, DC, 1998, Paralyzed Veterans of America.

60. Kemp BJ, Kahan JS, Krause JS et al: Treatment of major depression among persons with spinal cord injury: changes in depressive symptoms, life satisfaction and community activities over six months, *J Spinal Cord Med* 27:35-41, 2004.

61. Gill TM, Feinstein AR: A critical appraisal of the quality of life measurements, *JAMA* 272:619-626, 1994.

62. Elliott TR, Frank RG: Depression following spinal cord injury, *Arch Phys Med Rehabil* 77:816-823, 1996.

63. Cairns D, Baker J: Adjustment to spinal cord injury: a review of coping styles contributing to the process, *J Rehabil* 59:30-33, 1993.

64. Hansen NS, Forchheimer M, Tate DG et al: Relationships among community reintegration, coping strategies, and life satisfaction in a sample of persons with spinal cord injury, *Top Spinal Cord Inj Rehabil* 4:56-72, 1998.

65. Beck AT, Beck RW: Screening depressed patients in family practice: a rapid technique, *Postgrad Med* 52:81-85, 1972.

66. Yesavage JA, Brink TL, Rose TL et al: Development and validation of a geriatric depression screening scale: a preliminary report, *J Psychiatr Res* 17:37-49, 1983.

67. Kemp BJ, Adams BA: The Older Adult Health and Mood Questionnaire: a measure of geriatric depressive disorder, *J Geriatr Psychiatry Neurol* 8:162-167, 1995.

68. Lazarus RS, Folkman S: *Stress appraisal and coping*, New York, 1984, Springer Verlag.

69. DeVivo MJ, Fine PR: Spinal cord injury: its short-term impact on martial status, *Arch Phys Med Rehabil* 66:501-504, 1985.

70. DeVivo MJ, Richards JS: Marriage rates among person with spinal cord injury, *Rehabil Psychol* 41:321-339, 1996.

71. Richards JS: Psychological adjustment to spinal cord injury during first postdischarge year, *Arch Phys Med Rehabil* 67:362-365, 1986.

72. Weitzenkamp BA, Gerhart KA, Charlifue SW et al: Spouses of spinal cord injury survivors: the added impact of caregiving, *Arch Phys Med Rehabil* 78:822-827, 1997.

73. Thompson ML, Kemp BJ, Adkins RH: Functional changes in persons aging with spinal cord injury, *J Spinal Cord Med* 2:55, 1999.

74. Holicky R: Caring for the caregivers: the hidden victims of illness and disability, *Rehabil Nurs* 21:247-252, 1996.

SOLUTIONS TO CHAPTER 22 CLINICAL CASE STUDY

Aging and Spinal Cord Injury

1. Sam's health status and functional ability has changed recently after 31 years of coping with his SCI. His independence has been drastically altered with ADLs, IADLs, wheelchair propulsion, and driving as a result of tendonitis in his right shoulder. He has most likely become dependent on his wife and other family members for assistance with activities he previously was independent performing. Fear related to loss of function may be present with this client. In addition, Sam is at risk for continuing decline in his health status because of increased time in bed to allow the healing of his ischial pressure ulcer and decreased activity levels from not propelling his wheelchair. Fortunately he is undergoing physical therapy; however, special attention needs to be given to other potential problems related to aging.

Psychological factors need to be assessed as well, such as motivation, his personality traits, and signs of depression that may affect Sam's overall health status and quality of life. Although he appears to have a strong social support system, which is the most important element of overall life satisfaction, a shift is about to take place because his son has been transferred and will be moving a significant distance away. The move's impact on the family and Sam's social support structure may be more important than his shoulder pain. It is critical that the clinician understand the social support structure of the client. A genogram may be used to assist clinician and client in understanding the social support relationships.

2. Age-related issues include osteopenia (osteoporosis with increased fracture risk) and sarcopenia (loss of muscle skeletal muscle fiber) that affect both strength and endurance. Sam is experiencing decreased skin resilience and is further functionally limited as a result of bed rest to facilitate skin healing. Pulmonary dysfunction would place him at higher risk for infections such as pneumonia. CVD is more prevalent in individuals with SCI and he may currently be at greater risk because of his decreased function. Finally Sam may also be at risk for metabolic disorders.

3. To decrease the probability of increased pain in Sam's right shoulder and to provide for proper shoulder rest, ADL and IADL activities that cause impingement or need to be performed in a position that aggravates Sam's symptoms should be performed with caregiver assistance. Transfers may need to be performed dependently to provide adequate rest of the shoulder injury or Sam's right shoulder should be the leading limb with a transfer board transfer. An electric wheelchair is a feasible solution for transportation and may allow Sam to drive if driving does not aggravate his shoulder. He must still perform strengthening activities within pain-free limits and range of motion of his shoulder must be preserved. As Sam heals, a shoulder strengthening and stretching program needs to be designed and taught to enable him to prevent future reinjury.

4. Sam has been adjusting to and coping with his injury for 31 years. Because there is a positive correlation between duration of SCI and life satisfaction, it is expected that Sam will have higher life satisfaction than a newly injured individual of the same age. His son's transfer and move present an added stress for Sam. Assessment of social support and the changes that may occur related to his son's relocation should be monitored. The emotional support provided by his current relationship with his son and the family unit may change and Sam may be at risk for requiring social support and suggestions for additional methods of coping.

5. Depression is the number one mental health problem among individuals with disability. Therefore this particular time in Sam's life must be observed closely by health care professionals because he may be at greater risk for depression with the functional and social changes he is experiencing. His clinician needs to be a keen communicator, use strong listening skills, observe Sam's behavior carefully, check in with family members, and use tools such as QOL measures to monitor for signs of depression to make sure such signs do not go unrecognized. Strategies for detecting depression include the following:

- Patient's function is less than expected given his level of injury.
- Patient reports vague descriptions of pain, fatigue, poor sleep habits, or digestive problems.
- Patient develops health problems that appear to relate to poorly looking after himself.
- Caregivers or others report that the client is harder to get along with or is moody (in Sam's case increased irritability may well be noted).

The number and kinds of symptoms noted using such detection hints should assist in identifying possible depression and its severity. Although function and decline of function are key elements in determining signs and symptoms of depression, Sam already has a change in function as a result of his shoulder impairments and skin problems. Using a screening scale would be a helpful method to establish a baseline and detect increased change. In addition, the stress-coping model could be applied to this case to facilitate interventions that may be most helpful in assisting Sam (such as his appraisal of his son's transfer). Family considerations and changes with his son's transfer may be particularly important in this case.

CHAPTER TWENTY-THREE

Quality of Life After Spinal Cord Injury

Claire Z. Kalpakjian, PhD, MS, Martin Forchheimer, MPP, and Denise G. Tate, PhD

The best way to describe the journey back to a full and rewarding life by an individual with an SCI is to imagine the mixed emotions that we all feel on the first day of school, a first date, a first day at a new job, or pretty much any new experience. While there is always overwhelming excitement associated with taking the next step in life, recognizing the accomplishments that have brought us up to this very moment, there are also feelings of fear and uncertainty because we face a whole new world. We have concerns about whether or not we are prepared to meet the challenges ahead. So too the individual with an SCI sees life from a whole new perspective, not just physically, but emotionally, mentally, and spiritually as well. We need guidance to prepare for these life-altering experiences, but ultimately it is only through trial and error that we can establish the most beneficial and effective daily routine and set the standard for our quality of life. Our attitude is the key component to the equation of reintegration into life…and that is a choice.

Scott T-8 SCI

CHALLENGE OF DEFINING QUALITY OF LIFE

It is widely recognized that defining and conceptualizing quality of life (QOL) is a challenging and difficult endeavor. For example, in a 1997 review of QOL literature, Cummins[3] found 27 different published definitions. Arguably, there is no singular, best definition. This is due in part to the large number of disciplines in which QOL research has been conducted, all of which have informed and enriched its general framework. Taillefer et al[2] argue that for its own survival as a scientific concept, definitions of QOL should not vary from research to research but be able to stand alone. It otherwise risks being reduced to an unspecified, yet ubiquitous, variable that must be included in any clinical study, regardless of its definition.

In the United States, the term *quality of life* was first introduced in the 1950s as a political slogan and was considered only with respect to entire populations. Attempts to address QOL at the societal level were initiated by President Eisenhower's Commission on National Goals.[3] Later, in the 1970s the concept began to be used in reference to the individual.[4] Some of the earliest work in QOL was conducted in the fields of economics,[5] oncology,[6] and gerontology[7] and focused on physical status, symptoms, and functional well-being. This orientation was narrow in focus, concerned exclusively with physical health, and as such conformed with the biomedical model.[8] This orientation had a wholly deficit basis and excluded any subjective elements.

Subsequent conceptualizations broadened this approach, adding mental health into the mix. One primary modification was that QOL became viewed as a subjective experience.[9] A second was that QOL was generally seen as being dynamic, responsive to changes in a person's situation over time.[10] A third was that QOL could be viewed as having both positive and negative aspects.[11] Finally, common to many contemporary conceptualizations, QOL was described as multidimensional and that comprehensive appraisal requires taking into account environmental factors such as social well-being.[12] Although no uniform definition of QOL is acceptable, most discern QOL as a temporal experience of relative satisfaction with life that can only be appraised by the individual.

Multidimensional Versus Global Conceptualizations

As previously noted, it is common to conceptualize QOL in a multidimensional fashion. The number of dimensions of which QOL is purported to be composed varies across research, although physical, emotional, and social dimensions are common to most schema. In contrast to this is a global school of thought that holds that QOL is intrinsically a functional configuration of properties (i.e., gestalt). In such, people assess their QOL by global self-appraisal and any attempt to disaggregate it is untenable. Although this approach does not discount the importance of physical, social, material, and other forms of quality of well-being, it holds that they do not equate to QOL alone or in conjunction. Those that adhere to the multidimensional school of thought have argued that global QOL is essentially a proxy for current emotional status.[13]

Objective Versus Subjective Debate

There has long been debate over the very nature of QOL—definitions aside—and whether it is, at its core, objective or subjective. Early investigations of QOL, particularly in the field of economics, were primarily objective, predicated on the notion that resources, financial and otherwise, determined QOL. Objective indicators can be defined as the sum total of an individual's scores on characteristics that can be objectively determined, such as income or meals per day. This approach encompasses an individual's actual status, behaviors, and possessions that are considered to be central to QOL and preconditions of life quality.

Later, the subjectivity of QOL began to emerge and today dominates its overarching conceptualization. Subjective definitions of QOL include well-being, life satisfaction, morale, and happiness.[14] Diener et al[15] describe three components of subjective well-being (the term typically used when referring to subjective QOL): positive affect, negative affect, and life satisfaction. The two former refer to emotional aspects of QOL whereas the latter encompasses cognitive-judgmental aspects of QOL.

There is a third general approach to QOL from the field of economics, termed quality-adjusted life years. This is based on the principle that benefit can be measured in terms of effect on life expectancy adjusted for QOL. This approach has been used

BOX 23-1 | Quality of Life Indices

Objective: Measurable Information
- Physical or health status
- Financial status
- Resources for ease of ADL

Subjective: Self-Rated Markers
- Well-being
- Life satisfaction
- Morale
- Happiness

BOX 23-2 | Components of Response Shift

- Recalibration—change in internal measures of independence and life events: transporting in a wheelchair independently compared with walking or connecting with loved ones by Internet instead of driving to visit
- Reprioritization—determining the importance of independence in different tasks: designing the landscape of the yard compared with performing it or working from home 2 days a week to allow for more self-care time instead of 5 days in the office
- Reconceptualization—viewing the meaning of independence within a construct: eating a meal independently with adaptive equipment and set-up help compared with not needing adaptive equipment and help or having your grandchild climb up the wheelchair into your lap instead of picking the child up

to provide rationales for allocation of health care resources, increasingly challenging with burgeoning health care costs. It may also be used as justification for treatment selection between individuals, favoring those who have the potential to gain the most (Box 23-1).

Health-Related Quality of Life

Health-related QOL (HRQOL) is a specified approach to defining QOL by use of either subjective or objective components. The term is used in medical and allied health literature to refer to those components of overall QOL that are directly affected by health, disease, disorder, and injury.[14] HRQOL components can include signs, symptoms, treatment side effects, and physical, cognitive, emotional, and social functioning. They can be disease or disability specific or more generic to include outcomes related to a broader category, such as spinal cord injury (SCI).

During the progression of physical disability, HRQOL components can interact with non-health-related QOL dimensions in a number of situations, as shown later in a review of factors associated with QOL after SCI. Non-health-related QOL dimensions may affect an individual's capacity to cope with disability and respond to interventions.[14] In addition, disease and disability can affect the capacity to enjoy dimensions of life other than those directly limited by the disease or disabling condition.[16]

Although HRQOL focuses on QOL as it relates to health, health is often conceptualized in exceptionally broad and subjective terms, as can be seen by this 1984 definition: "HRQOL are those attributes valued by people, including their resultant comfort or sense of well-being; the extent to which they are able to maintain reasonable physical, emotional and intellectual function; and the degree to which they retain their ability to participate in valued activities with the family, in the workplace and in the community."[17] Moreover, unlike measures of life satisfaction that are most commonly used with healthy populations and whether it is called HRQOL or QOL, research on QOL has been primarily conducted with ill or disabled populations.[18] If HRQOL is used to denote that construct appraised by certain biomedically oriented assessment instruments such as the Sickness Impact Profile,[19] then the distinction between HRQOL and QOL is a gross one. Other HRQOL instruments, such as the Patient Generated Index measures, blur the distinction, however, closely adhering to what is intended by good measures of QOL.

Response Shift in Quality of Life

More recently, the concept of response shift has been identified as key to measuring QOL in relation to changes in health status. Response shift refers to a change in the evaluation of QOL as a result of changes in internal standards, values, and conceptualizations.[10] This way of understanding changes in QOL is particularly pertinent to people who have SCI because it is frequently precipitated by sudden significant changes in health condition or physical functioning. These changes leading to alteration in assessment of QOL are also referred to as recalibration, reprioritization, and reconceptualization (Box 23-2).

After SCI, individuals experience considerable changes in their health, the ability to complete activities of daily living, personal relationships, social environment, and community integration. It is precisely because of these drastic changes that response shift so frequently occurs among people with SCI. Loss of independence to some degree is nearly a universal experience after SCI and recalibration, reprioritization, and reconceptualization of response shift can be illustrated by adjusting to this loss of independence. Recalibration is to change internal standards of measurement: what is the frame of reference for determining amount of independence? Reconceptualization is a redefinition of the target construct: what does it mean to be independent? Finally, reevaluation is to determine how important the target construct is: how important is independence in the larger context of life? Thus, response shift is the change in meaning of an individual's self-evaluation of a target construct, in this example independence, resulting from the combination of these three things.

The underlying process of response shift is iterative and dynamic in nature.[10] Life after SCI is similarly dynamic. For example, changes related to aging with a physical disability and the attendant shifts in functional independence can all serve to restart the process of response shift over again.

Conceptualization of Quality of Life in Spinal Cord Injury

Several studies have examined how people with SCI themselves conceptualize QOL by using a qualitative method of inquiry. Qualitative methods are closely aligned with the subjective perspective of QOL, allowing participants' "voices to be heard" and providing researchers with an opportunity to uncover aspects of QOL that might fail to be observed by use of more common quantitative methods.[20]

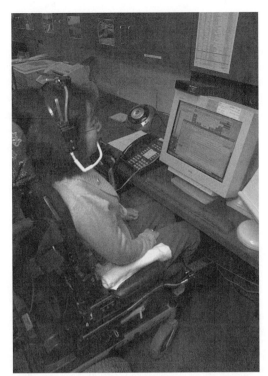

FIGURE 23-1 The ability to work regardless of level of SCI provides an individual with social contacts, exposure to a broad environment, mental acuity, feelings of self-worth, facility to use a wide variety of skills, and the opportunity to earn income. This woman with tetraplegia uses a specialized head set to interact with her computer.

TABLE 23-1	Subjective Aspects of Quality of Life	
Personal Expectations	Personal Evaluations	Personal Achievements
Aspirations	Coping	Accomplishments
Desires	Enjoyment and happiness	Career
Goals	Health	Education
Needs	Perceived good life	Possessions
Standards	Satisfaction	Recognition
Values	Well-being	Relationships

Data from Dijkers M: Quality of life after spinal cord injury: a metaanalysis of the effects of disablement components, *Spinal Cord* 35:829-840, 1997; Dijkers M: Measuring quality of life: methodological issues, *Am J Phys Med Rehabil* 78:286-300, 1991; Dijkers M: Correlates of life satisfaction among persons with spinal cord injury, *Arch Phys Med Rehabil* 80:867-876, 1999;

Boswell et al[21] examined definitions of QOL among 12 individuals with SCI by using moderated small focus groups. Participants characterized QOL as inherently subjective, meaning different things to different people. It was also considered to be developmental in nature and influenced by how closely life goals were met. Attitude toward life was recognized as one of the most significant influences on QOL. Opportunities to work (Figure 23-1) and level of resources were two of the other key domains influencing QOL after SCI, the latter in part serving as a foundation for a positive attitude.

Duggan and Dijkers[20] used individual interviews to examine QOL in a sample of 40 community-dwelling individuals with SCI. Participants were asked to define QOL, which most had difficulty doing. Many perceived QOL as something dynamic, subjective, and "elastic" and as something generated out of their personal experiences. When asked to assess their QOL, some people used an internal benchmark, for example, comparing their lives before injury, immediately after injury, or at some point in the future. Others used external references, for example, comparing their lives to what they imagined others' lives were like. Indeed, subjective aspects of QOL often include personal expectations, personal evaluations, and personal achievements (Table 23-1).

Shifting Priorities After Spinal Cord Injury

As the process of recalibration and accommodation after disability begins, with concomitant changes in health and functional capacity, individuals with SCI also begin to experience changes in values and the meaning of life events. Some researchers speculate that unattainable goals may be devalued and those things that are achievable become more highly valued in an effort to enhance QOL.[22,23] In the study by Boswell et al,[21] participants described how their perspective of QOL changed by reassessing their priorities after injury, with cognitive abilities assuming greater importance in their lives. Weitzenkamp et al[24] found that, among men who were many years after injury, the criteria they used to assess their QOL changed over time and differed from those of a nondisabled comparison group. For those with SCI, family relationships, quiet leisure activity, and creative expression were more likely rated as important or very important. In addition, priority rankings were related to what the individuals with SCI had actually attained or achieved. For example, those working tended to rate work as a higher priority than did those who did not.

Similar findings were noted in a recent study by Tate et al[25] of women with SCI whose coping mechanisms were investigated in relation to their effect on overall QOL. Coping refers to the thoughts and behaviors that an individual person uses to regulate distress and to maintain positive well-being. The coping processes that are necessary for response shift involve realistic appraisal of changing circumstances. This perspective was found in women with SCI who demonstrated successful coping and adaptation also exhibiting realistic appraisal of their circumstances, whereas avoidance coping was observed in those who were categorized as poor copers. Women who coped well with their SCI in spite of a lack of resources and support seemed to be able to make meaning in the face of adversity. For them, response shift appeared to work very effectively and practicing the art of living involved finding personal meaning and still beholding the goodness in life, even when the circumstances surrounding them were horrific (involving personal abuse and violence).

One final caveat is important when considering these conceptualizations of QOL by people with SCI. Although there is little doubt that priorities shift after injury and over the course of disability, it is important to recognize that those core domains of QOL valued by people with SCI are shared across populations. It is perhaps more accurate to say that people with SCI highly value those domains of human contact and connection, as does the population at large, but with a greater emphasis on resources and independence, making their lives easier and healthier (Box 23-3).

BOX 23-3 | **Factors Influencing Quality of Life in Individuals with SCI Tetraplegia**

- Social and family networks, particularly marriage after injury is associated with greater QOL; freqency of social contact, irrespective of the reason, enhances QOL.
- Attitude and outlook have direct influence on QOL.
- Functional losses have an impact on QOL in part through restricting social functioning.
- Bowel and bladder function have an indirect effect on QOL through thier impact on social functioning; that is, the pontential for embarrassment by bowel accidents or urinary leakage has been associated with limited social connectivity.
- Community participation and employment have direct and indirect effects on QOL through increased opportunities for social connection and meaningful and productive activity.

Outside Looking In: Outsiders' Perspectives

Discrepancies between self-ratings of QOL and the views of outsiders estimating QOL after SCI have implications not only for measurement but also for family dynamics, social relationships, and even decisions to end life after high-level SCI. Hammell[26] keenly observes that health care professionals consider themselves to have "knowledge" whereas patients have "beliefs" that can affect the clinician's approach to understanding subjective QOL after SCI. This bias about what life is like after SCI and its quality can affect treatment given during emergency care and expectations of patients during acute rehabilitation, both of which can have serious consequences on the individual receiving care. Examining the congruence, or lack thereof, between self-ratings of QOL by those with SCI and what their families, health care providers, or nondisabled peers believe is their QOL gives a unique insight into the subjectivity of QOL after SCI.

Gerhart et al[27] conducted a study of emergency care providers (e.g., nurses, emergency medical technicians, and physicians) and their attitudes toward QOL after SCI. This comparison highlighted substantial discrepancies between how satisfied people with SCI were with their lives and how emergency care providers imagined their QOL would be after a tetraplegic SCI. For example, although 92% of the group with SCI was glad to be alive, only 18% of the emergency care provider group imagined they would be glad to be alive after such an injury. Although 86% of the group with SCI reported their QOL as average to above average, only 19% of the emergency care providers imagined their QOL would be as high. In general, those who had the bleakest outlook on life after SCI were least likely to favor aggressive intervention after injury, which can have serious implications for patients.

Emergency care providers also imagined that individuals with tetraplegia were less active than they actually were. Finally, their estimates of being sexually active with tetraplegia (10%) were far below the actual report of those people (66% not using respirators and 25% using respirators). The investigators of this study argue that such discrepancies between what emergency care providers imagine life is like after a tetraplegic SCI and the reality of life for many people with tetraplegia have serious implications for delivery of care and for how these attitudes can negatively affect families and patients because they are often the first medical personnel to interact with them.

Patterson et al[28] addressed the question of discontinuing life support early in the care of patients with high-level tetraplegia and the special problems that arise in making such decisions. Negative biases about QOL after SCI held by medical personnel can increase the possibility of a too-hasty decision resulting in the premature death of someone who would have lived a happy and productive life (Clinical Note: Quality of Life Perspectives and Impact on Care). They argue that until the patient is able to fully appreciate what life may be like after a full course of rehabilitation, decisions about life support should be delayed.

CLINICAL NOTE **Quality of Life Perspectives and Impact on Care**

- Although priorities after injury change, between 80% and 90% of people with SCI perceive their QOL as average or above average.
- Fewer than 20% of emergency care providers surveyed imagined that their QOL after tetraplegia would be high.
- Outsiders' bias about QOL of individuals with SCI may adversely affect family dynamics, social relationships, quality of care, and end-of-life decisions for those with high-level SCI.
- Determination of QOL must be determined by each individual with SCI.

Comparisons with Population Norms

As described previously, there is a prevailing assumption that SCI will necessarily reduce QOL, and comparisons with nondisabled samples have borne this out to some degree,[29] but this is not a universal finding nor are differences typically large (Figure 23-2). In 1978, in perhaps the most widely cited survey of QOL after SCI, Brickman et al[30] compared people who had sustained SCI with lottery winners and tracked their relative QOL over time. To the surprise of many, over time, individuals with SCI fared no worse or better than lottery winners in their QOL. In a meta-analysis, Dijkers[29] found that, although QOL was lower in SCI than the population in general, differences tended to be small. Despite this and subsequent evidence that SCI does not necessarily devastate QOL (and that over time QOL does improve), pessimistic expectations remain firmly entrenched.

Schulz and Decker[31] interviewed 100 middle-aged and older adults with SCI who were an average of 20 years post injury and found that QOL along with emotional well-being was only slightly below population means. Westgren and Levi[32] compared a group of Swedish adults with SCI to a nondisabled community sample and found that QOL was significantly lower for those with SCI. Kreuter et al[33] compared Swedish SCI, traumatic brain injury (TBI), and community samples and found that people with SCI reported lower QOL than the community sample, whereas those with TBI were similar to the community sample. Post et al,[34] using a Dutch sample, also found that people with SCI reported lower QOL than did a nondisabled community sample, except in the area of family life. Nevertheless, their overall QOL ratings were still good to high.

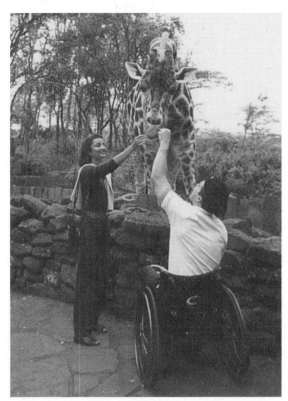

FIGURE 23-2 This couple enjoys community activities and attractions. They both consider the additional challenges to activities of daily life and mobility that are associated with paraplegia to be part of their normal routine; more time may be needed in their schedule but that does not deter an active lifestyle.

MEASUREMENT OF QUALITY OF LIFE

Understanding of the fundamental conceptual issues of QOL has often taken a back seat to development and use of assessment instruments.[35] The effects of this are clearly unfortunate because, regardless of whether many of these instruments seemingly have sound psychometrics, their findings can lead to misinference. Most of the issues of measurement follow from those of definition: because there is no singular definition of QOL, there is no correct way to measure it. Appropriateness is in part a function of whether the approach to measurement is congruent with the conceptualization of QOL adopted. Several fundamental issues in QOL measurement have been raised over time in addition to overarching considerations, which are reviewed.

Generic Versus Condition-Specific Assessment

Among the most basic issues of QOL assessment are the following: what should be assessed? what should be the scope of assessment? Because QOL is a universal issue, it follows that the fundamental issues for assessment should be common across the entire population regardless of disability status or otherwise. The term QOL has a meaning. It is debatable whether this is also true of the term "SCI QOL," which is arguably all that can be assessed by SCI-specific measures. In addition, use of well-written generic measures minimizes the degree to which instruments will be differentially interpreted by subpopulations.

Finally, although generic measures allow for the development of group norms or benchmarks, highlighting issues common among certain subpopulations, these can be defined by attributes other than health condition (e.g., economic status and urbanicity).

Although generic measurement of QOL captures the broadest possible spectrum of domains in a consistent manner, reliance on this approach to assessment forgoes a level of precision that can only be obtained through condition-specific appraisal or qualitative approaches, which are fundamentally still less generic. The global issues of QOL, such as emotional and physical well-being, are experienced by everyone, but arguably there are certain factors that tend to be uniquely salient to people with certain conditions. For example, although restrictions in ability to complete activities of daily living can be of great importance for the understanding of QOL for some subpopulations (e.g., SCI) it is not for others (e.g., nondisabled individuals), and moreover, its assessment cannot be appropriately determined with one-size-fits-all questions that can be incorporated in a universal QOL assessment tool. In addition, one of the values of QOL assessment is to evaluate the effects of a course of treatment, and it is unclear whether global evaluation is sufficiently sensitive for this purpose (Clinical Note: Generic Measurement Tools for Quality of Life).

CLINICAL NOTE **Generic Measurement Tools for Quality of Life**

- Allow development of group norms or benchmarks
- Capture broadest spectrum of domains consistently
- Deficient in precision; not qualitative
- Lack sensitivity to evaluate treatment course
- Base choice of generic versus individualized assessment on content interest

---

Some have argued for the use of condition-specific measurement as an adjunct to generic appraisal.[36] Condition-specific QOL instruments are most commonly associated with oncology, and include the Functional Living Index–Cancer[37] and the Cancer Rehabilitation Evaluation System–Short Form.[38] Two condition-specific instruments have been used with SCI: the Life Situation Questionnaire–Revised[39] and the Spinal Cord Injury Quality of Life-23.[40] Whether it is appropriate to measure QOL using condition-specific instruments is largely a function of the specific purpose of the investigation.

Individualization

Most QOL measurement is based on a process whereby researchers develop sets of domains, items to embody these, and means of aggregating these into a global score or a set of indices. There are various ways in which this process may be accomplished. The domains generally reflect the conceptualization of QOL held by the authors of the measure. The choice of items may be derived from their personal judgment or that of some panel of experts, or it may be based on prior research conducted to determine the most salient items, such as qualitative interviews. Similarly, weighting may be based on these same techniques, psychometric procedures such as factor analysis, or some combination thereof. Regardless of how these instruments are developed, what they share in common is that they lack individualization; all respondents answer the same questions regardless of their situations and values. The Short Form-36 (SF-36)[41] which is the most commonly used QOL instrument, is an example of a standardized measure of QOL.

At the other end of the spectrum are individualized measurement approaches in which respondents are responsible for generating the domains pertinent to their own QOL and the relative importance or weights for each. These methods are less common in large-scale studies. As a group, these are referred to as patient-generated outcome measures. To the degree that these individualized measures of QOL incorporate information about meaning and value, they provide much more information than do standardized instruments, which assume domain importance a priori. Standardized instruments may wholly omit domains of importance to some individual's QOL while attending to areas that they may not value highly.[35] Finally, individualized instruments are more receptive to respondents' experience of response shift.

Conversely, although the information provided by individualized measures of QOL may have greater depth, they have less breadth; respondents do not provide information on as wide an expanse of topics as they do on some standardized instruments. Standardized instruments follow from conceptual frameworks, collecting information about domains deemed pertinent on the basis of prior work. Although the domains covered are not selected by the respondents, the rationale underlying their selection is deemed to have universal importance. In using individualized measures of QOL, researchers may forgo the ability to address questions about established constructs of interest. The validity of any instrument is limited by the burden that it places on respondents, and some of the established individualized measures of QOL are inappropriate for some subpopulations because of the requisite cognitive processing that their use entails. As with the preferability of generic and condition-specific measures of QOL, there is no simple answer to the question of which is better, individualized or standardized measures of QOL; this depends on the purpose and context of the assessment.

Psychometrics

Fundamental issues with measurement of QOL are those of assessment of reliability and validity. The issue is not that QOL instruments have not been rigorously evaluated, but rather that the traditional means of conceptualizing and assessing psychometric properties are not appropriate when applied to QOL. This is a function of appraisal and response shift, which are integral to QOL.[42] Standard psychometric analysis is based on the assumption that individual differences in scale usage reflect measurement error. In contrast and as discussed previously in the section on response shift, assessment of QOL involves a combination of standards of measurement, values, and meaning, all of which intrinsically differ across people and within people over time. Standard psychometric analysis is based on the concept that there is an underlying correct score that is unrelated to the attributes of an instrument's respondent. This is not true

for QOL, which cannot be disentangled from the person doing the appraising. Item response theory, which has advantages over standard psychometric procedures in many ways, shares its limitations when it comes to QOL because it also assumes an invariant underlying construct.

Given that different people apply different standards, values, and meanings in responding to questions about QOL, it is questionable whether interrater reliability is even a meaningful construct. Similarly, in light of the dynamics of response shift, it is hard to interpret test-retest reliability. Although response shift tends toward maintenance of homeostasis, elevating observed reliability,[10] countervailing forces can result in appropriately low levels. Construct validity is also difficult to assess with QOL. Construct validity is said to exist when scores on one instrument correlate highly with another assessing a similar construct, lowly with measures of dissimilar ones and when they discriminate between people with dissimilar statuses. Considering the dynamics of the appraisal process it is not readily apparent when it is appropriate to expect measures to have high or low correlations. QOL, as discussed previously, is an amorphous construct. Although physical and emotional well-being, pain, sexual satisfaction, and many other constructs can all be readily defined distinctly, they can all also be experienced as QOL. It is not uncommon for high correlation to be observed among the scale scores for multidimensional QOL instruments. Whether this indicates relationships among these dimensions, response set issues, appraisal, or low construct validity is not transparent.

Although the nature of these problems is clear, their solutions are not; it is also unclear how substantial the resulting problems are. One step in this process of resolving these problems may involve assessment of "internal construct validity," or the degree to which the questions on an instrument elicit the desired process of appraisal from respondents.[42] This would entail a process of qualitative interviewing. Knowledge of the appraisal parameters could be used to gain a sense of the impact of response shift. It could also be used in the selection of variables for new QOL instruments. This argues in favor of some of the individualized measures of QOL because, in completing several of these, respondents provide information that directly addresses the appraisal process. During recent years, major efforts have also been made to formally measure the components of response shift.[43]

Measures of Quality of Life

Specific instruments assessing QOL vary from generic to condition specific. Accompanying the rising interest in QOL in the last several decades, some might argue that there are as many instruments as there are definitions of QOL, restricting the maturation of this field of inquiry.[26,44] There are more than two dozen QOL instruments; a select few are briefly described to illustrate these issues of QOL measurement.

Generic Instruments

The SF-36[41] and SF-12[45] are the two most widely used measures of HRQOL. For example, a recent Medline search found more than 4000 studies using the SF-12 or SF-36, 29 of them among people with SCI, including two studies that validated the SF-36 as being appropriate for use with this population.[46,47] The SF-12 was used by the Model SCI Care Systems between 1995 and 2000. Norms have been established for 13 chronic illnesses and for subgroups of the U.S. general population, but no SCI norms have been established to date. The SF-36 has eight scale scores and physical and mental summary scales. The SF-12 contains only the two summary scales.

The WHOQOL-BREF[48] is a 26-item standardized measure based on the World Health Organization's work on QOL. The instrument has four scales: physical health, psychological status, social relationships, and environment. A recent study of the attributes of WHOQOL-BREF when used with people with SCI concluded that it was suitable.[49]

Global Measures

Although the Satisfaction with Life Scale (SWLS),[15] was developed for use in the general population, it has been used far more than any other global measure in SCI research. It defines life satisfaction as the global assessment of QOL on the basis of each individual's uniquely selected criteria, which are appraised by a cognitive judgmental process.[50] Because life satisfaction is experienced globally, the SWLS approach to appraisal is to query respondents about their overall life experiences rather than about the various facets of life. The instrument has five questions; scores can range from 5 to 35.

Individualized Measures

The Schedule for the Evaluation of Individual Quality of Life—Direct Weighting (SEIQoL-DW)[51] is one of the few individualized instruments in common usage in which respondents determine the pertinent domains for assessment; research has been specifically conducted using it with individuals with SCI.[52] Although some have argued that the global instruments, such as the SWLS, are also implicitly individualized because there are no domains; and thus the terms of appraisal are not pre-established,[35] this group is generally considered restricted to domain-based instruments. The SEIQoL is based on the idea that QOL is "the extent to which our hopes and ambitions are matched by experience."[53] As such, QOL cannot be appraised without weighting in terms of self-appraised importance; doing well in a domain that is important to a person has a greater impact on QOL than does doing equally well in one of less import. The SEIQoL-DW asks respondents to nominate the five areas of life that are most important to their experience of QOL; their status in each of these life areas, from as good as possible to as bad as possible; and the relative importance of each. Scores are based on an integration of importance and status assessments. The SEIQoL-DW has advantages over many other individualized measures in being easier to administer and complete and in that respondents are required to list the relative importance of the five areas; it is less prone to problems of response set than are many measures. Moreover, the information about what areas are nominated can serve as a starting point for assessing response shift.

Spinal Cord Injury–Specific Instruments

The Life Situation Questionnaire—Revised (LSQ-R)[39] was developed on the basis of the idea that even measures of QOL designed for people with physical disabilities in general cannot sufficiently address the dynamics of all issues pertinent to SCI. The LSQ-R contains 43 items and seven scales that were constructed by use of factor analysis: Engagement, Negative Affect, Health Problems, Finances, Career Opportunities, Living Circumstance, and Interpersonal Relations. The LSQ-R's scales have high levels of reliability and validity as assessed across a large sample of people with SCI and across subsamples on the basis of sex, race, and geographical region.

The goal of the Spinal Cord Injury Quality of Life-23[40] was to combine four standardized, established measures of general QOL with two SCI-specific ones and through statistical techniques reduce these measures to arrive at a tool that would comprehensively appraise the QOL experience among people with SCI. Across the initial instruments there were 22 scales and 205 items. The final instrument contains three scales: mental health (e.g., absence of depression), physical and psychological dysfunction (e.g., limitations in mobility and social activity), and SCI-specific problems (e.g., loss of independence) (Clinical Note: Spinal Cord Injury–Specific Quality-of-Life Measurements and Analysis).

CLINICAL NOTE — **Spinal Cord Injury–Specific Quality-of-Life Measurements and Analysis**

- Set specific domains for QOL in people with SCI
- Include organic dynamics of response shift, coping, and values that may influence construct
- Integrate documented importance and status of assessments
- Combine comprehensive scales including mental health, physical and psychological dysfunction, and SCI-specific problems

---

FACTORS AFFECTING QUALITY OF LIFE AFTER SPINAL CORD INJURY

One of the greatest challenges to understanding the factors that affect QOL after SCI, or QOL in general, is the complexity and interrelationships of these factors.[44] These interrelationships create indirect associations with QOL, further muddying the waters in attempts to clarify what can directly diminish or improve QOL. Rather than an exhaustive review, the following section serves as a general overview and introduction to the empirical and extant literature on QOL after SCI, highlighting the key issues for more in-depth examination.

Demographic and Injury Factors

Demographic and injury factors reflect those characteristics that are largely immutable. Although injury factors in particular are assumed to exert strong influence over QOL, the empirical literature is decidedly equivocal. It could be argued that the belief that such immutable factors serve to necessarily diminish QOL can lead to unfounded pessimism that has the potential to adversely affect not only people with SCI and their expectations for their lives after injury, but also care providers, whose attitudes can have a substantial impact on the people they treat. Despite evidence to the contrary, associations between QOL and injury factors are neither simple nor direct nor do they necessarily prescribe an individual to a life devoid of quality dependent solely on level of injury.

Demographics

In general, weak associations have been found between QOL and demographic factors. In a meta-analysis of 22 QOL and SCI studies, Dijkers[54] found that women tended to rate QOL slightly higher than men and that white non-Hispanics had better QOL than African Americans and Hispanics. Putze et al[55] also found that being male was associated with lower QOL.

The relationship of age and QOL has been equivocal. In Dijkers' meta-analysis, the lowest and highest age groups had the highest QOL.[54] McColl et al[56] found that age was directly and indirectly (by health problems and fatigue) related to QOL in chronic SCI. Ville and Ravaud,[44] in a large study of 1668 individuals with tetraplegia in France (the Tetrafigap Survey) found no main effects of age on QOL, largely because of its association with many other variables. They also found that education had no main effect on QOL because of its association with professional situation and financial resources, both of which did have a main effect on QOL. On the contrary, lower education also was found to be associated with poor QOL in Dijkers' meta-analysis.[29]

Level and Severity of Injury

Injury factors such as level and severity are often those characteristics first considered to diminish QOL after SCI given their dramatic impact on nearly all aspects of life. A long-standing presupposition has been that the level of injury itself serves to reduce QOL in a direct manner; however, the literature is equivocal on this point and often suggests that level of injury indirectly affects QOL through its effect on functioning.[57]

McColl et al[56] found that level of injury indirectly affected QOL via the perception of accelerated aging and disability-related problems, such as dependence, accessibility, and transportation among individuals with long-term SCI (20 years or more). No direct relationship between injury level and QOL was found. Similarly, Westgren and Levi[32] and Kreuter et al[33] found no direct relationship between level of injury and health-related QOL in Swedish samples. Manns and Chad[58] did not find significant differences among those with tetraplegia and paraplegia in terms of QOL when studying the effects of fitness and physical activity on QOL in a Canadian sample.

With a qualitative, ethnographic approach (i.e., understanding an experience from the insider's point of view), Manns and Chad[59] found that nine domains of life considered important for QOL were similar between those with paraplegia and tetraplegia; however, physical function and independence and physical well-being appeared to affect the QOL of those with tetraplegia to a greater extent (Box 23-3).

Use of Ventilator and High-Level Spinal Cord Injury

As previously discussed, there is an entrenched assumption that high-level SCI, and use of a ventilator in particular, necessarily diminish QOL to the extent that continuation of life itself may be called into question.[28] Empirical investigations of QOL, however, with a focus on high-level SCI have been sparse. Hammell[26] asserts that this gap in understanding has serious implications for informed consent and medical treatment given the pervasive belief in Western culture that life would not be worth living with high-level SCI. Despite these long-held assumptions, research points to very different conclusions.

Hall et al[60] compared 82 individuals with high-level tetraplegia (C1 to C4), 16 of whom were ventilator-assisted and 66 of whom were ventilator-independent, in terms of their respective QOL. Both groups rated their QOL high, with those who needed ventilator assistance similar to those who were ventilator independent. Bach and Tilton[61] also compared people with complete tetraplegia by ventilator use and respiratory independence and found no differences between ratings of QOL. Warschausky et al[62] examined differences in QOL in individuals with high tetraplegia using ventilators, not using ventilators, and people using ventilators because of other disabling conditions. No differences in QOL, conceptualized by HRQOL, global cognitive appraisal, and individualized-judgmental, were found between groups.

Functional Status

Functional status typically refers to the ability to physically perform activities such as self-care, being mobile, and independence at home or in the community. In rehabilitation, there has long been an emphasis on the impact of functional status on QOL. Ville et al[44] argue that most QOL scales are dominated by items related to functional status reflecting the a priori assumption that functional independence is directly linked to QOL. They suggest, however, that it may be more accurate to say that it is the impact of functional status by limitations on social activity that reduce QOL, adding another layer of complexity to the link between SCI and QOL. In addition, the perception of handicap or the degree to which the impairment limits participation also has been found to be associated with QOL.[63]

Dijkers[29] found a weak and generally nonsignificant relationship between impairment (i.e., level of injury) and QOL; disability (or the impact of injury on functioning) tended to have a stronger relationship to QOL, but this was not consistently found. When the relationship was found, disability was most robustly and consistently associated with QOL in a negative direction so that higher QOL was associated with less disability.[29]

In the Tetrafigap Survey, Ville and Ravaud[44] found a complex relationship between impairments resulting from SCI and QOL. They found that functional independence in general was linked to QOL only when it related to situations in which the dependence created embarrassment from sociocultural taboos. The greater the level was of perceived disability, then the lower the QOL. Similarly, the evolution of independence after rehabilitation was associated with higher QOL.[44]

The Tetrafigap Survey also highlighted another layer of complexity in the association between functional status and QOL by examining the effect of functional losses on restricting social activity, cautioning that the effects of functional losses should not be viewed simply as an inability to do but must also take into account the social meaning of such activities (and losses) and the way in which assistance from others will affect day-to-day social interactions.[44] In general, their analysis with sociological and clinical variables indicated that declines in functional status attenuate the association between sociological variables and QOL, particularly those that restrict mobility, travel, and outings.

In examining how perceived causes of change in function impacted QOL, Price et al[64] found that factors perceived to threaten function such as pain and loss of strength were also those factors that negatively affected QOL, although in a smaller proportion of participants. The investigators argued that by being more easily identifiable, physical threats to function and QOL were the most robust in this study. Manns and Chad[58] examined the relationship among physical activity, fitness, and handicap and QOL and found no relationship between the latter and physical activity and fitness.

Time After Injury

As discussed in regard to response shift, QOL rating and the relative importance of life domains may shift over time. Examining the relative stability (or instability) of QOL after injury during early phases of rehabilitation and over the long term gives insight into the process of adjustment and accommodation and the dynamics of response shift in the context of SCI. In general, a positive relationship has been found between time since injury and QOL.[32,65] Research also has found that QOL remains relatively stable after the first years after injury. Nevertheless, limitations in measurement should always be considered when examining stability over time.

Crewe and Krause[66] conducted one of the first longitudinal studies examining long-term psychological adjustment in individuals with SCI. Individuals involved in a longitudinal study beginning in 1975 and were at least 2 years after injury when joining the study completed a series of interviews. Only satisfaction with employment increased over an 11-year period; other domains of QOL were relatively stable over time. Examining the stability of QOL in from acute and postacute (6 months) stages, Kennedy and Rogers[67] also found that ratings of QOL were generally stable. On the contrary, Lucke et al[68] found that QOL declined 3 and 6 months after injury.

Dijkers[54] similarly found a positive relationship between years living with SCI and QOL. In contrast, Post et al[34] found no specific relationship between time since injury and QOL. McColl et al[56] found that individuals who believed they were aging more quickly than others had a lower QOL than those who did not believe they were aging more quickly.

Some studies have found age at time of injury also contributes to QOL. Kannisto et al[69] in Finland compared three subgroups of SCI (in those who sustained SCI as a child, newly injured, and chronic SCI) on indices of health-related QOL. Results indicated that those who were injured as children had significantly higher health-related QOL than the other two groups. The Tetrafigap Survey also found younger age at injury associated with better QOL after controlling for sex and current age.[44]

Cause of Injury

Few studies have examined the impact of mechanism of injury on QOL and those that have found few differences. With use of a case-controlled design with a U.S. sample of individuals matched on age, education, sex, race, marital status, occupational status, injury duration, and impairment level, Putzke et al[70] examined the effects of SCI caused by gunshot versus other mechanisms of injury (e.g., vehicular). They found no meaningful differences between the two groups on QOL measures but noted that those at a higher risk of sustaining a gunshot injury also may be exposed to other factors (e.g., socioeconomic circumstances) that can have a

negative impact on QOL. Post et al[71] similarly did not find cause of injury (e.g., traffic accident, sports injury, occupational injury) to be significantly related to life satisfaction in their Dutch sample. In another study, however, Putzke et al[55] did find that violent injury was associated with poorer QOL.

Secondary Conditions

Secondary conditions are a fact of life for people with SCI with an impact on overall health that ranges from nuisance to life threatening. Outpacing renal failure, respiratory complications are now the leading cause of death after SCI.[72] And although life expectancies have continued to increase with advances in emergency and rehabilitative care, the specter of health complications looms ever present.

Health problems associated with SCI (in aggregate) have been found to be directly related to diminished QOL; fatigue also has been indirectly related to QOL by health problems.[56] Dijkers[54] found weak, but significant associations between number of hospitalizations in the prior year and pressure ulcers and QOL. Westgren and Levi[32] also found neurogenic pain, spasticity, and neurogenic bladder and bowel problems were associated with lower health-related QOL in a Swedish sample.

One of the more common problems after SCI is pain[73] and its relationship to QOL has been examined in several studies. Putzke et al,[74] in two interrelated studies involving 270 individuals in a case-controlled, repeated-measures design, found a significant relationship between pain interference and diminished QOL that was mediated by a change in pain interference from year 1 to year 2. For those individuals whose pain interference worsened from year 1 to year 2, QOL accordingly declined; the converse also was true in that QOL increased as pain improved from year 1 to year 2. For individuals whose pain did not change during this time, there was also no significant change in QOL ratings.

In addition to a negative association of pain and QOL, the Tetrafigap Survey[44] also found that, although pressure sores and contractures were indirectly linked to QOL, urinary leakage was directly associated with diminished QOL. It was presumed that this direct link was due to the embarrassing social connotation of incontinence and its impact on social relations. Hicken et al[75] examined the impact of requiring assistance for bladder and bowel management on QOL and HRQOL with a case-controlled design at 1-year follow up. Those who were dependent on assistance had significantly lower QOL than those who were independent in these functions. Creating and maintaining new social relationships was negatively affected by requiring assistance. The relationship between dependence for bladder and bowel management may be tied to fear and embarrassment over accidents, increased time demands for managing these functions, and the frustration, discomfort and increased health problems. Branagan et al[76] similarly found that the use of colostomy in bowel management improved QOL in their sample. Reitz et al[77] also found a positive association between good bladder management and higher QOL.

Psychosocial and Interpersonal Factors

Broadly, psychosocial factors capture the psychological and social context in which the individual functions. Within the psychosocial framework are intrapersonal and interpersonal dynamics influencing QOL. Intrapersonal factors reflect intrinsic characteristics of the individual that can be fluid and influenced by intervention, such as emotional well-being, attitude, and outlook; these elements are in contrast to personal characteristics, such as demographics, which are immutable. Interpersonal factors reflect those dynamics between individuals or groups, such as family, friends, and the larger social community in which an individual resides.

Emotional Well-Being and Attitude

Emotional well-being has been used interchangeably with QOL and the directionality of this relationship is not always clear. For example, in a large Finnish study (nondisabled respondents) global QOL judgments were found to be based largely on current emotional state.[13] Emotional state mediated the relationship between other predictors of QOL and global QOL ratings. Pointing to the difficulty in understanding the directionality of this relationship, two explanations are offered: (1) mood increases access to information about an individual's life—a bad mood increases access to negative quality of life information or (2) people use mood as the information on which to base their judgment of QOL.

Attitude and outlook also can play a role in QOL after SCI. In the study of Boswell et al,[21] attitude toward life was considered to be one of the most important influences on QOL after SCI. Boschen[78] found a modest but significant relationship between locus of control and self-concept and QOL, suggesting that those individuals who are more confident and self-assured will enjoy greater QOL after SCI. Brown et al[79] investigated the relationship between attributions for responsibility for injury and HRQOL as a long-term outcome and found no significant relationship between the two.

Perceived control has been shown to play a role in QOL after SCI as well. For example, Schulz and Decker[31] found a strong relationship between emotional well being and QOL and perceived control as did Boschen.[78] May and Warren,[80] however, did not find the expected relationship between locus of control and QOL, although the reason for this lack of association was not clear. In their study, QOL was associated with self-esteem.

THE CLIENT'S PERSPECTIVE   Striving for My Best Life

I hope always to continue evolving and experiencing new challenges. A few years ago I developed a list of things I have learned since my disability, and I'd like to share them, David Letterman style:

11. We need to laugh at ourselves, have FUN, and try to stay light about life. My life since my injury has been one ironic and ridiculous experience after another and laughing has made it all quite bearable. My silver lining is good parking, great concert or theater tickets, and experiencing the generosity of others on a daily basis.

10. It is important and even necessary to challenge ourselves and take risks. We need to go outside our comfort zone so that we understand more about who we are. My skiing friends call this the "YIKES ZONE" because it can be pretty sketchy, but it's where our skills, knowledge, and ability are tested, and it offers the greatest pay-off. Don't be afraid to go there.

9. Appreciate each moment for it will be gone in a second. The past has happened, it's over, and you can't change it. The future is unknown. Being present in each moment is our only reality.

8. We must approach ourselves as WHOLE people. Our body is merely a temporary container that houses who we REALLY are—our mind and spirit. It's important to take good care of our physical selves, but not at the expense of neglecting our mind and spirit because independence lies within our mind and any cure lies within our spirit.

7. Our whole is greater than the sum of our parts. We are called to be uniquely our own so that we can discover what is special inside us, improve on it, and give it away so that the greater whole can benefit.

6. We won't learn anything about our true selves without failing. Every negative experience is an opportunity to learn and gain more knowledge about ourselves.

5. We shouldn't limit ourselves and decide what we can and cannot do until we give it a try. A good friend who is a fellow adaptive ski instructor always says: "Never say 'can't' without adding a 'yet' at the end of the sentence." I NEVER want to look back on my life and think I wish I would've...

4. Confidence and self-esteem will get us everywhere and attitude is everything. It is totally and completely freeing to understand that we have a choice about how we handle everything that comes our way. We don't necessarily have a say in what happens to us, but we sure can choose how we will deal with it.

3. It's not what we HAVE; it's what we DO with what we have that matters.

2. We won't get very far in life without each other. The love and support we give and receive from our peers, friends, and family are our greatest assets.

1. WALKING IS OVERRATED.

Sarah Everhart Skeels

Social and Family Networks

The frequency with which individuals get out of their home environment and are socially active has been shown repeatedly to enhance QOL. In the Tetrafigap Survey, the frequency, not the reason for it, of going out of the home was positively related to QOL. Nor did it matter whether invitations to socialize were offered or received—it was simply seeing other people that enhanced QOL for that study's participants.[44] The Tetrafigap Survey also found that having or not having children was associated with QOL dependent on whether children were born before or after the injury. On average, those with at least one child born after injury had the highest QOL relative to those with no children and those born before injury, respectively. Benony et al,[81] in comparing individuals with SCI with nondisabled controls, found that social support was higher for the SCI participants and was generally satisfactory and associated with better QOL. Schulz and Decker[31] found a positive relationship between QOL and social support, the amount of social contact, and satisfaction with the quality of social contacts.

Marriage

Marriage has been shown to be a powerful ally in maintaining a high degree of QOL in both SCI and nondisabled populations (Figure 23-3). In a meta-analysis, Dijkers[29] found married

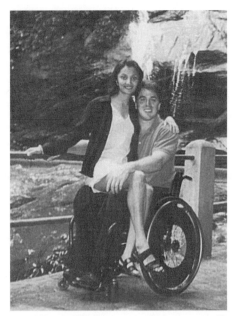

FIGURE 23-3   SCI certainly does not preclude romance. The love evidenced by this couple listening to the waterfall behind them is an important reminder of the daily fun, support, and appreciation couples can bring to marriage.

BOX 23-4 | *Healthy People 2010* **Disability and Secondary Conditions Objective**

- Reduce the proportion of adults with disabilities who report feelings such as sadness, unhappiness, or depression that prevent them from being active
- Increase the proportion of adults with disabilities who participate in social activities
- Increase the proportion of adults with disabilities reporting sufficient emotional support
- Increase the proportion of adults with disabilities reporting satisfaction with life
- Reduce the number of people with disabilities in congregate care facilities, consistent with permanency planning principles
- Eliminate disparities in employment rates between working-aged adults with and without disabilities
- Increase the proportion of health and wellness treatment programs and facilities that provide full access for people with disabilities
- Reduce the proportion of people with disabilities who report not having the assistive devices and technology that they need
- Reduce the proportion of people with disabilities reporting environmental barriers to participation in home, school, or community activities

Adapted from U.S. Department of Health and Human Services: *Healthy people 2010: understanding and improving health,* ed 2, Washington, 2000, U.S. Government Printing Office.

---

individuals reported the highest QOL and separated individuals the lowest. Looking at marital status 1 year after injury, Putzke et al,[82] using a case-controlled design, found that individuals who were single reported a lower level of life satisfaction than did their married counterparts; the former also had lower levels of self-reported social integration and economic self-sufficiency. Similarly, Kreuter et al[33] found that those with SCI or TBI who were married reported better QOL than their single counterparts. McColl et al[83] also found that marriage was a significant predictor of QOL over time and was particularly important as an individual aged. The loss of a spouse, who is often the central social support mechanism, was a significant factor associated with depressed mood.

The Tetrafigap Survey[44] found an interesting association between marriage and subjective well-being that was explained by the timing of marriage relative to the onset of injury. For couples who were married before injury, subjective well-being was the lowest, whereas those who married after injury reported the highest subjective well-being relative to those who lived alone (before and after the injury) and those whose partner was deceased. The investigators propose that a marriage partner becomes a source of social support only if he or she joins the person with SCI freely and being fully aware of the situation. Conversely, the partner present before injury does not freely choose their situation, but rather is forced to face the burden imposed by the injury.

Sexuality

SCI can dramatically affect the ability to engage in and enjoy sexual expression, affecting satisfaction with partnerships and sexuality and QOL as a whole. Although sexual functioning in men after SCI has typically received the majority of attention in the extant literature, both men and women have expressed dissatisfaction with their sexuality after injury.

Benony et al[81] found that sexuality was a source of dissatisfaction regardless of marital status. Hultling et al[84] examined the effects of oral sildenafil citrate (Viagra) on quality of life for men with erectile dysfunction from SCI. Examining various dimensions of QOL, including those specific to overall satisfaction with sex life and sexual relationship with parting, men using sildenafil versus placebo reported significantly greater satisfaction with their sex lives, being less bothered by the impact of erectile problems, and improvements in overall emotional well-being and depression. Reitz et al[77] found that sexual satisfaction was associated with relationship to partner, the ability to move, and mental well-being.

Community and Environmental Factors

Community and environmental factors may restrict a person's ability to expand outward from interpersonal relationships and social networks and thereby affect the QOL after SCI. In particular, an individual's ability to access the community and increase social interaction has been shown to be a key factor in enhancing QOL. Unfortunately, the many architectural barriers in the environment that people with SCI face when trying to access their communities further entrench and subsequently increase the negative pressure those barriers have on restricting participation in work, community life, and social interaction. Although the objectives outlined by the U.S. Department of Health and Human Services *Healthy People 2010* disability and secondary conditions[85] concentrate on a range of QOL issues, approximately half focus on community and environmental access (Box 23-4).

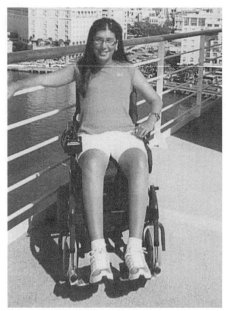

FIGURE 23-4 When an individual with SCI learns skills that foster independence and accepts the challenges of navigating her community, the payback comes in the form of warm sunshine, meeting new people, and the glow of self-sufficiency.

Community Participation

The positive relationship between QOL and community participation has been consistently found in the research, emphasizing the importance of access to community after SCI not only by reduction of architectural barriers but also social barriers (Figure 23-4). For individuals who were 1 to 2 years post injury, Richards et al[86] found that access to the community improved over time, making a significant contribution to QOL. The Tetrafigap Survey also found that participating in any activity (except television watching), be it paid or unpaid work, outdoor leisure, or simply leaving home, was linked to better QOL.[44]

Residence

In his meta-analysis, Dijkers[29] found that those who resided in nursing homes or had long-stay hospitalization had the lowest QOL. Similarly, in a matched sample of those with SCI living in nursing homes and those living in the community it was found that QOL was rated lower by the nursing home sample.[87] Interestingly, there were no differences on a measure of social functioning. When examined more closely, social contacts were found to vary between groups. Those individuals residing in nursing homes had more contact with strangers, roommates, and friends while those residing in the community had more contact with immediate family members and relatives.

Employment and Professional Activity

In general, employment has been found to be positively associated with QOL and given what is known about social connection and QOL, this is not surprising. In fact, for many regardless of disability, work is the primary way in which people make social connections. Dijkers[29] found that individuals who were employed competitively enjoyed the highest QOL; students and homemakers reported higher QOL than those who were retired or unemployed. Unemployment's negative association with QOL has been found elsewhere.[55] Interestingly, Benony et al[81] found that individuals with SCI, in comparison with a nondisabled sample, did not value career as highly, which may reflect the findings of Weitzenkamp et al[24] about activities that cannot be pursued as easily after SCI becoming less valued.

CLINICAL CASE STUDY Quality of Life

Patient History

Jared Brown is an 18-year-old man with a diagnosis of C5 tetraplegia, American Spinal Injury Association (ASIA) A resulting from a motor vehicle accident. He was a passenger in a car driven by a man who had been drinking heavily. The driver did not survive the accident.

Jared underwent an anterior fusion procedure from C4 through C6 and was in halo traction for 12 weeks. His acute-care stay was uncomplicated and he was discharged to a subacute facility 3 weeks after his injury. Jared was admitted to an acute rehabilitation program 3 days ago after the halo orthosis was removed.

Jared lives with his mother and 13-year-old sister in a two-family walk-up building. His mother currently receives unemployment and food stamps for the family. His parents are divorced; his father's location is unknown. Jared is a high school senior and he was working part time at a local convenience store. He has been an average student with a low-C grade average.

Patient's Self-Assessment

Jared was hoping to go to community college next year. Now he is confused, angry, and unable to focus on the future.

Clinical Assessment
Patient Appearance
- Height 5 feet 11.5 inches, weight 150 pounds, body mass index 20.6

Cognitive Assessment
- Alert, oriented × 3

Cardiopulmonary Assessment
- Blood pressure 110/62 mm Hg, heart rate at rest 68 beats/min, respiratory rate 16 breaths/min, cough flows are ineffective (< 360 L/min), vital capacity is reduced (between 1.5 and 2.5 L)

Musculoskeletal and Neuromuscular Assessment
- Motor assessment reveals C5 ASIA A
- Deep tendon reflexes 3+ below the level of lesion

Integumentary and Sensory Assessment
- Skin is intact throughout, sensory intact to C5.

CLINICAL CASE STUDY Quality of Life—cont'd

Range of Motion Assessment
- Passive and active range of motion is within normal limits in both upper limbs.
- Straight leg raise is 95 degrees in both lower limbs and dorsiflexion is 2 degrees bilaterally; all other motions in the lower limbs are within functional limits.

Mobility and ADL Assessment
- Dependent with bed mobility
- Dependent in transfers to all surfaces
- Dependent with pressure relief
- Dependent in manual wheelchair maneuvering on all surfaces
- Dependent in bowel and bladder care
- Dependent in upper body dressing and in lower body dressing
- Currently unable to drive

Evaluation of Clinical Assessment
Jared Brown is an 18-year-old man with a C5 tetraplegia, ASIA A diagnosis resulting from a motor vehicle accident. He was injured 12 weeks ago. He has been in an acute rehabilitation hospital for 3 days and the team is completing its evaluation.

Patient's Care Needs
1. Team evaluation and treatment to maximize functional outcomes
2. Consultation for necessary social, vocational, psychological, and additional skilled professional services as indicated
3. Education regarding his diagnosis, fitness and wellness for safety, and prevention of secondary complications after SCI

Diagnosis and Prognosis
Diagnosis is C5 complete tetraplegia, ASIA A, with a prognosis of total assist to some assist with equipment setup for activities of daily living (ADL) and independence with power wheelchair mobility. Jared has innervation to biceps and most shoulder muscles and should be able to perform some ADLs with help for setup (e.g., dressing upper body). Muscle transfer may be considered in the future to enable more function through elbow extension.

Preferred Practice Patterns*
Impaired Muscle Performance (4C), Impairments Nonprogressive Spinal Cord Disorders (5H), Primary Prevention/Risk Reduction for Cardiovascular/Pulmonary Disorders (6A), Primary Prevention/Risk Reduction for Integumentary Disorders (7A)

Team Goals
1. Team to evaluate and establish functional goals for discharge
2. Team to evaluate home for accessibility needs
3. Team to evaluate for wheelchair seating and propulsion
4. Team to devise education plan for Jared and his family focused on care and assistance needs
5. Team to advise on possibilities for future muscle transfers to increase upper limb function depending on recovery of strength
6. Team to structure a plan for Jared's education regarding prevention of secondary complications after SCI (e.g., pressure ulcer prevention, pulmonary hygiene, fitness and wellness goals)

Patient Goals
"I want to walk."

Care Plan
Treatment Plan and Rationale
- Complete a pulmonary assessment specific for peak cough flows, vital capacity, and oxygen saturation during functional wheelchair tasks.
- Initiate a patient and caregiver educational plan for pulmonary and skin management, bowel and bladder management, and range of motion maintenance.
- Schedule a wheelchair seating evaluation considering assistive technology device needs on the wheelchair for electronic ADLs.
- Schedule a home evaluation to determine assistive technology needs to enhance independence in management of home environment, accessibility, and needs for additional home modifications and a specialized pressure relief bed.
- Recommend psychological and vocational evaluations.

Interventions
- Skilled multidiscipline services to optimize patient outcomes and available resources
- Seating clinic evaluation for prescription of wheelchair
- Needs assessment for assistive device and home modification
- Education across disciplines on skin care, pulmonary hygiene, bowel and bladder management
- Psychological and vocational evaluations

Documentation and Team Communication
- Team will document evaluations and schedule team meeting.
- Team will discuss and document short- and long-term goals and communicate these to the patient and family, including educational plan, functional mobility, home modifications, assistive technology, and durable medical equipment.
- Team will document wheelchair prescription and communicate assistive technology goals for electronic ADLs on wheelchair and at home.
- Team will communicate and document patient's adjustment to SCI.

Follow-Up Assessment
- Reassessment of team goals every 2 weeks
- Reassessment for consultation with other services

Critical Thinking Exercises
Consider factors that will influence patient education, therapy, and team care decisions unique to Jared's spinal cord injuries when answering the following questions:
1. Considering Jared's age and socioeconomic status, what critical factors might the acute rehabilitation team prioritize to ensure an ultimately positive impact on the response shift and future QOL of this individual?
2. What factors could positively affect Jared's social interactions and therefore have a positive impact on his QOL?
3. What intrapersonal factors would be most beneficial to Jared's positive QOL?

---

*Guide to physical therapist practice, rev. ed. 2, Alexandria, VA, 2003, American Physical Therapy Association.

SUMMARY
Expectations about what life will be like after SCI and the quality of that life may be, in many ways, among the most critical aspects of well-being and good health in people with SCI. Perhaps one of the most important findings in the empirical literature is that, although QOL after SCI is often rated lower in comparison with a nondisabled population, these differences are not large enough to warrant unquestioned pessimism about the QOL that can be achieved after SCI. In fact, many people with SCI enjoy a high QOL in clear contrast to the expectations of others. Examining

expectations of what their own QOL would be like after such an injury, it is clear that people without SCI expect that they would find little in their lives with which to be satisfied and this erroneous expectation can have far-reaching implications. These assumptions can compromise the dynamic between patient and health provider, compromise what treatment is offered, and even call into question whether life should be continued. For families and friends, these assumptions can compromise relationships and communication in particular.

There is no single factor that has been shown to absolutely improve or diminish QOL in the context of SCI or in any other context for that matter. In fact, the empirical evidence shows that there is an intricate web of factors that weave together to influence QOL. Similarly, response shift and the re-evaluation of priorities, goals, and values provide an important insight into the adjustment process and help to lay the foundation for future treatment approaches aimed at improving QOL after SCI and other disabling injuries.

Although researchers will continue to struggle with the Gordian knot that is the definition and measurement of QOL, many people with SCI will go on to live productive and active lives, with meaningful re-evaluation of what they value in their lives. They will defy the entrenched pessimism that their injuries will necessarily diminish their QOL and many will consider their lives to be more meaningful and rich after injury than they had before because of the opportunity to re-examine what they value most.

REFERENCES

1. Cummins R: Assessing quality of life. In Brown R, editor: *Quality of life for people with disabilities: models, research and practice*, Cheltenham, 1997, Stanley Thornes.
2. Taillefer MC, Dupuis G, Roberge MA et al: Health-related quality of life models: systematic review of the literature, *Soc Indicators Res* 64:293-323, 2003.
3. Weisgerber R: *Quality of life for persons with disabilities: skill development and transitions across life stages*, Gaithersburg, MD, 1991, Aspen.
4. Wolfensberger W: Let's hang up "quality of life" as a hopeless term. In Goode D, editor: *Quality of life for persons with a disability: international perspectives and issues*, Cambridge, MA, 1994, Brookline Books.
5. Galbraith JK: Economics and quality of life, *Science* 145:117-123, 1964.
6. Holmes HA, Holmes FF: After ten years, what are the handicaps and life styles of children treated for cancer? An examination of the present status of 124 such survivors, *Clin Pediatr (Phila)* 14:819-823, 1975.
7. McKinsey ME: Applying research and training to improve life for the aged, *Geriatrics* 30:80-84, 1975.
8. Fuhrer M: Subjectifying quality of life as a medical rehabilitation outcome, *Disabil Rehabil* 22:481-489, 2000.
9. Fuhrer MJ: Subjective well-being—implications for medical rehabilitation outcomes and models of disablement, *Am J Phys Med Rehabil* 73:358-364, 1994.
10. Sprangers MAG, Schwartz CE: Integrating response shift into health-related quality of life research: a theoretical model, *Soc Sci Med* 48:1507-1515, 1999.
11. Huppert FA, Whittington JE: Evidence for the independence of positive and negative well-being: implications for quality of life assessment, *Br J Health Psychol* 8:107-122, 2003.
12. Cella D, Tulsky D, Gray G et al: Functional assessment of cancer therapy scale: development and validation of the general measure, *J Clin Oncol* 11:570-579, 1993.
13. Heinonen H, Aro AR, Aalto A-M et al: Is the evaluation of the global quality of life determined by emotional status?, *Qual Life Res* 13:1347-1356, 2004.
14. Tate D, Dijkers M, Johnson-Green L: Outcome measures in quality of life, *Top Stroke Rehabil* 2:1-17, 1996.
15. Diener E, Emmons R, Larsen J et al: The satisfaction with life scale, *J Pers Assess* 49:71-75, 1985.
16. National Institutes of Health: *Quality of life assessment: practice, problems, and promise: proceedings of a workshop*, Bethesda, MD, 1990, The Institutes.
17. Wenger NK, Mattson ME, Furberg CD et al: Assessment of quality of life in clinical-trials of cardiovascular therapies, *Am J Cardiol* 54:908-913, 1984.
18. Hyland ME, Sodergren SC: Development of a new type of global quality of life scale, and comparison of performance and preference for 12 global scales, *Qual Life Res* 5:469-480, 1996.
19. Gilson BS, Gilson JS, Bergner M et al: The sickness impact profile: development of an outcome measure of health care, *Am J Public Health* 65:1304-1310, 1975.
20. Duggan C, Dijkers M: Quality of life after spinal cord injury: a qualitative study, *Rehabil Psychol* 46:3-27, 2001.
21. Boswell BB, Dawson M, Heininger E: Quality of life as defined by adults with spinal cord injuries, *J Rehabil* 64:27-32, 1998.
22. Myers D, Diener E: The pursuit of happiness, *Sci Am* 274:70-72, 1996.
23. Heckhausen J, Schultz R: A life-span theory of control, *Psychol Rev* 102:284-304, 1995.
24. Weitzenkamp DA, Gerhart KA, Charlifue SW et al: Ranking the criteria for assessing quality of life after disability: evidence for priority shifting among long-term spinal cord injury survivors, *Br J Health Psychol* 5:57-69, 2000.
25. Tate D, Duggan C, Roller S et al: Stress and coping over the life course: a perspective on women with spinal cord injury. Final report. Ann Arbor, MI, 2005, University of Michigan Health System, Department of Physical Medicine and Rehabilitation.
26. Hammell KW: Exploring quality of life following high spinal cord injury: a review and critique, *Spinal Cord* 42:491-502, 2004.
27. Gerhart KA, Koziolmclain J, Lowenstein SR et al: Quality-of-life following spinal-cord injury—knowledge and attitudes of emergency care providers, *Ann Emerg Med* 23:807-812, 1994.
28. Patterson DR, Miller-Perrin C, McCormick TR et al: When life support is questioned early in the care of patients with cervical-level quadriplegia, *N Engl J Med* 328:506-509, 1993.
29. Dijkers M: Quality of life after spinal cord injury: a metaanalysis of the effects of disablement components, *Spinal Cord* 35:829-840, 1997.
30. Brickman P, Coates D, Janoff-Bulman R: Lottery winners and accident victims: is happiness relative?, *J Pers Soc Psychol* 36:917-927, 1978.
31. Schulz R, Decker S: Long-term adjustment to physical disability: the role of social support, perceived control and self-blame, *J Pers Soc Psychol* 48:1162-1172, 1985.
32. Westgren N, Levi R: Quality of life and traumatic spinal cord injury, *Arch Phys Med Rehabil* 79:1433-1439, 1998.
33. Kreuter M, Sullivan M, Dahllof AG et al: Partner relationships, functioning, mood and global quality of life in persons with spinal cord injury and traumatic brain injury, *Spinal Cord* 36:252-261, 1998.
34. Post M, Van Dijk A, Van Asbeck F et al: Life satisfaction of persons with spinal cord injury compared to a population group, *Scand J Rehabil Med* 30:23-30, 1998.

35. Dijkers MP: Individualization in quality of life measurement: instruments and approaches, *Arch Phys Med Rehabil* 84:S3-S14, 2003.

36. Cella D, Nowinski CJ: Measuring quality of life in chronic illness: the functional assessment of chronic illness therapy measurement system, *Arch Phys Med Rehabil* 83:S10-S17, 2002.

37. Schipper H, Clinch J, McMurray A et al: Measuring the quality of life of cancer patients: the Functional Living Index-Cancer: development and validation, *J Clin Oncol* 2:472-483, 1984.

38. Schag CAC, Ganz PA, Heinrich RL: Cancer Rehabilitation Evaluation System–Short Form (CARES-SF): a cancer specific rehabilitation and quality-of-life instrument, *Cancer* 68:1406-1413, 1991.

39. Krause JS: Dimensions of subjective well-being after spinal cord injury: an empirical analysis by gender and race/ethnicity, *Arch Phys Med Rehabil* 79:900-909, 1998.

40. Lundqvist C, Siosteen A, Sullivan L et al: Spinal cord injuries: a shortened measure of function and mood, *Spinal Cord* 35:17-21, 1997.

41. Ware J SK, Kosinski M, Gandek B: *SF-36 health survey: manual and interpretation guide*, Boston, 1993, Heath Institute, New England Medical Center.

42. Schwartz CE, Rapkin BD: Reconsidering the psychometrics of quality of life assessment in light of response shift and appraisal, *Health Qual Life Outcomes* 2:2-16, 2004.

43. Schwartz CE, Sprangers MA: Methodological approaches for assessing response shift in longitudinal health-related quality-of-life research, *Soc Sci Med* 48:1531-1548, 1999.

44. Ville I, Ravaud JF: Subjective well-being and severe motor impairments: the Tetrafigap survey on the long-term outcome of tetraplegic spinal cord injured persons, *Soc Sci Med* 52:369-384, 2001.

45. Ware JE Jr, Kosinski M, Keller SD: A 12-item short-form health survey: construction of scales and preliminary tests of reliability and validity, *Medical Care* 34:220-233, 1996.

46. Forchheimer M, McAweeney M, Tate DG: Use of the SF-36 among persons with spinal cord injury, *Am J Phys Med Rehabil* 83:390-395, 2004.

47. Andresen EM, Fouts BS, Romeis JC et al: Performance of health-related quality-of-life instruments in a spinal cord injured population, *Arch Phys Med Rehabil* 80:877-884, 1999.

48. WHOQOL Group: Development of the World Health Organization WHOQOL-BREF quality of life assessment, *Psychol Med* 28:551-558, 1998.

49. Jang Y, Hsieh CL, Wang YH et al: A validity study of the WHOQOL-BREF assessment in persons with traumatic spinal cord injury, *Arch Phys Med Rehabil* 85:1890-1895, 2004.

50. Shin DC, Johnson DM: Avowed happiness as an overall assessment of the quality of life, *Soc Indicators Res* 5:475-492, 1978.

51. Hickey AM, Bury G, O'Boyle CA et al: A new short form individual quality of life measure (SEIQoL-DW): application in a cohort of individuals with HIV/AIDS, *BMJ* 313:29-33, 1996.

52. Warschausky S, Dixon P, Forchheimer M et al: Quality of life in persons with long-term mechanical ventilation or tetraplegic SCI without LTMV, *J Spinal Cord Med* 27:S93-S97, 2004.

53. Ruta DA, Garratt AM, Leng M et al: A new approach to the measurement of quality of life: the Patient-Generated Index, *Med Care* 32:1109-1126, 1994.

54. Dijkers M: Correlates of life satisfaction among persons with spinal cord injury, *Arch Phys Med Rehabil* 80:867-876, 1999.

55. Putzke JD, Richards JS, Hicken BL et al: Predictors of life satisfaction: a spinal cord injury cohort study, *Arch Phys Med Rehabil* 83:555-561, 2002.

56. McColl MA, Arnold R, Charlifue S et al: Aging, spinal cord injury, and quality of life: structural relationships, *Arch Phys Med Rehabil* 84:1137-1144, 2003.

57. Dijkers M: Measuring quality of life: methodological issues, *Am J Phys Med Rehabil* 78:286-300, 1999.

58. Manns PJ, Chad KE: Determining the relation between quality of life, handicap, fitness, and physical activity for persons with spinal cord injury, *Arch Phys Med Rehabil* 80:1566-1571, 1999.

59. Manns PJ, Chad KE: Components of quality of life for persons with a quadriplegic and paraplegic spinal cord injury, *Qual Health Res* 11:795-811, 2001.

60. Hall K, Knudsen S, Wright J et al: Follow-up study of individuals with high tetraplegia (C1-C4) 14 to 24 years postinjury, *Arch Phys Med Rehabil* 80:1507-1513, 1999.

61. Bach JR, Tilton MC: Life satisfaction and well-being measures in ventilator assisted individuals with traumatic tetraplegia, *Arch Phys Med Rehabil* 75:626-632, 1994.

62. Warschausky S, Dixon P, Forchheimer M et al: Quality of life in persons with long-term mechanical ventilation or tetrapelgic SCI without long-term mechanical ventilation, *Top Spinal Cord Inj Rehabil* 10:94-101, 2005.

63. Hansen NS, Forchheimer M, Tate DG et al: Relationships among community reintegration, coping strategies, and life satisfaction in a sample of persons with spinal cord injury, *Top Spinal Cord Inj Rehabil* 1998; 4:56-72, 1998.

64. Price GL, Kendall M, Amsters DI et al: Perceived causes of change in function and quality of life for people with long duration spinal cord injury, *Clin Rehabil* 18:164-171, 2004.

65. Richards J, Bombadier C, Tate D et al: Access to the environment and life satisfaction after spinal cord injury, *Arch Phys Med Rehabil* 80:1501-1506, 1999.

66. Crewe N, Krause J: An eleven-year follow-up of adjustment to spinal cord injury, *Rehabil Psychol* 35:205-210, 1990.

67. Kennedy P, Rogers B: Reported quality of life of people with spinal cord injuries: a longitudinal analysis of the first 6 months postdischarge, *Spinal Cord* 38:498-503, 2000.

68. Lucke KT, Coccia H, Goode JS et al: Quality of life in spinal cord injured individuals and their caregivers during the initial 6 months following rehabilitation, *Qual Life Res* 13:97-110, 2004.

69. Kannisto M, Merikanto J, Alaranta H et al: Comparison of health-related quality of life in three subgroups of spinal cord injury patients, *Spinal Cord* 36:193-199, 1998.

70. Putzke J, Richards J, DeVivo M: Quality of life after spinal cord injury caused by gunshot, *Arch Phys Med Rehabil* 82:949-954, 2001.

71. Post M, Witte L, Van Asbeck F et al: Predictors of health status and life satisfaction in spinal cord injury, *Arch Phys Med Rehabil* 79:395-401, 1998.

72. DeVivo MJ, Krause JS, Lammertse DP: Recent trends in mortality and causes of death among persons with spinal cord injury, *Arch Phys Med Rehabil* 80:1411-1419, 1999.

73. Widerstrom-Noga EG, Turk DC: Exacerbation of chronic pain following spinal cord injury, *J Neurotrauma* 21:1384-1395, 2004.

74. Putzke JD, Richards JS, Hicken BL et al: Interference due to pain following spinal cord injury: important predictors and impact on quality of life, *Pain* 100:231-242, 2002.

75. Hicken BL, Putzke JD, Richards JS: Bladder management and quality of life after spinal cord injury, *Am J Phys Med Rehabil* 80:916-922, 2001.

76. Branagan G, Tromans A, Finnis D: Effect of stoma formation on bowel care and quality of life in patients with spinal cord injury, *Spinal Cord* 41:680-683, 2003.

77. Reitz A, Tobe V, Knapp PA et al: Impact of spinal cord injury on sexual health and quality of life, *Int J Impotence Res* 16:167-174, 2004.

78. Boschen KA: Correlates of life satisfaction, residential satisfaction, and locus of control among adults with spinal cord injuries, *Rehabil Counsel Bull* 39:230-243, 1996.

79. Brown K, Bell M, Maynard C et al: Attribution of responsibility for injury and long-term outcome of patients with paralytic spinal cord trauma, *Spinal Cord* 37:653-657, 1999.

80. May LA, Warren S: Measuring quality of life of persons with spinal cord injury: external and structural validity, *Spinal Cord* 40:341-350, 2002.

81. Benony H, Daloz L, Bungener C et al: Emotional factors and subjective quality of life in subjects with spinal cord injuries, *Am J Phys Med Rehabil* 81:437-445, 2002.

82. Putzke J, Elliott T, Richards J: Marital status and adjustment 1 year post spinal cord injury, *J Clin Psychol Med Set* 8:101-107, 2001.

83. McColl M, Stirling P, Walker J et al: Expectations of independence and life satisfaction among ageing spinal cord injured adults, *Disabil Rehabil* 21:231-240, 1999.

84. Hultling C, Giuliano F, Quirk F et al: Quality of life in patients with spinal cord injury receiving VIAGRA® (sildenafil citrate) for the treatment of erectile dysfunction, *Spinal Cord* 38:363-370m, 2000.

85. U.S. Department of Health and Human Services: *Healthy people 2010: understanding and improving health,* ed 2, Washington, 2000, U.S. Government Printing Office.

86. Richards JS, Bombardier CH, Tate D et al: Access to the environment and life satisfaction after spinal cord injury, *Arch Phys Med Rehabil* 80:1501-1506, 1999.

87. Putzke J, Richards J: Nursing home residence: quality of life among individuals with spinal cord injury, *Am J Phys Med Rehabil* 80:404-409, 2001.

SOLUTIONS TO CHAPTER 23 CLINICAL CASE STUDY

Quality of Life

1. The concept of response shift is considered key to measuring QOL in relation to changes in health status and it encompasses three fundamental components: recalibration, reprioritization, and reconceptualization. Recalibration helps to shift an individual's view of self so that he may establish a new frame of reference for independence. Team focus on the acquisition of financial resources in this case will be crucial to obtain the high-technology equipment that will be necessary to ensure Jared's greatest functional independence. Reprioritization of goals will need to take place and Jared's age could work in a positive or negative way. Appropriate career guidance is important to constructively point out encouraging directions and opportunities that could enhance his QOL. Reconceptualization with team and peer support may help Jared define what it means to be independent.

Jared has a high-level injury; team members will need to use effective and assertive communication techniques to make sure his needs are met both at home and in the community. The team must consider education the top priority for this individual. Higher levels of education are associated with a higher perception of QOL as well as with better work opportunities that include higher income and good benefits. Completion of his high school education and admission to college are the first steps toward a realistic job and potential career advancement that are critical for optimal outcomes. Opportunities to work and level of resources have been identified as key factors influencing QOL after SCI.

Establishment of a reliable bowel and bladder routine is another high priority that is valuable for planning related to education and social interactions to ensure avoidance of potential social embarrassment.

2. Social interactions are potentially important to a positive impact on QOL in Jared's case. He will need to be mobile to travel to and engage in social activities. Therefore, the team needs to prioritize opportunities for mobility and transportation for social interaction, which are assessed as significant to QOL by most individuals with SCI. As previously noted, reliable bowel and bladder routine will facilitate social engagement by reducing the potential for embarrassment.

Team help finding accessible housing that considers Jared's level of care needs will be another important step in this clinical case. Team help to optimize financial assistance must be completed early in the rehabilitation phase so that this low-income family can find resources that will play a pivotal role in maximizing Jared's independence.

3. Attitude toward life is recognized to significantly influence quality of life. Opportunities to work and level of resources are two of the main domains influencing QOL after SCI, the latter in part serving as a foundation for a positive attitude. Other influences on QOL include the ability to regulate distress with behaviors that help to maintain a positive emotional well-being and prevention of health complications because health decline may indirectly affect Jared's QOL. Jared's high level of injury will cause acceleration in deconditioning processes; therefore, fitness regimens also should be established.

Counseling about sexuality must begin early because it has been documented as an area of dissatisfaction after SCI. Because Jared is young, this will be an important area for the team to address as well as where resources may be available after his formal rehabilitation has ended. Jared will need guidance to redirect his understanding of what encompasses sexuality while he learns about his own sexuality.

Index

Page numbers followed by f indicate figures; t, tables; b, boxes.

TRY IT NOW!

Improve your understanding of treatment techniques with the companion DVD!

The enclosed DVD captures key therapeutic interventions designed to help you understand, practice, teach, and study highly specific movements.

Video segments clearly demonstrate specific therapeutic interventions, featuring footage of:

- Basic and advanced **position changes**

- **Transfers to multiple surfaces,** including floor and car transfers

- **Ambulation training** for complete and incomplete injuries

- High-level **wheelchair activities**

- **Electronic aids** to daily living

- **And much more!**

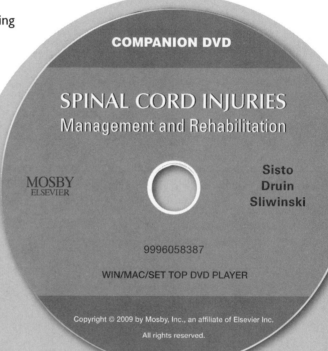

As an added bonus, the DVD includes interviews with six patients who have spinal cord injuries, including tetraplegia, paraplegia, and quadriplegia, discussing how their injuries affect their daily lives.

Simply insert the DVD into your computer or DVD player to get started now!

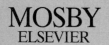

MOSBY
ELSEVIER